Orthopaedic Knowledge Update 3

Home Study Syllabus

American Academy of Orthopaedic Surgeons

Acknowledgments

Orthopaedic Knowledge Update 3
Home Study Syllabus

Published by the
American Academy of Orthopaedic Surgeons
222 South Prospect Avenue
Park Ridge, Illinois 60068
January 1990

The material presented in this *Orthopaedic Knowledge Update 3: Home Study Syllabus* has been made available by the American Academy of Orthopaedic Surgeons for educational purposes only. This material is not intended to represent the only, or necessarily the best, methods or procedures for the medical situations discussed, but rather is intended to present an approach, a view, statement, or opinion of the author(s) or producer(s), which may be helpful to others who face similar situations.

First Edition
Copyright 1990 by the
American Academy of Orthopaedic Surgeons

Library of Congress Cataloging in Publication Data
88-645327
ISBN 0-89203-035-6

American Academy of Orthopaedic Surgeons
Thomas C. Nelson, Executive Director
Fred V. Featherstone, MD, Deputy Executive Director
Mark W. Wieting, Director, Communications and Publications
Marilyn L. Fox, PhD, Assistant Director, Publications
Wendy O. Schmidt, Senior Editor

Ad Hoc Committee on Home Study
Robert Poss, MD, Chairman
Robert W. Bucholz, MD
Dale M. Daniel, MD
John W. Frymoyer, MD
Richard H. Gelberman, MD
Victor M. Goldberg, MD
Robert N. Hensinger, MD
James H. Herndon, MD
Stephen J. Lipson, MD
Bernard F. Morrey, MD
Paul M. Pellicci, MD
Robert W. Winquist, MD

AAOS Board of Directors, 1989
Newton C. McCollough III, MD, President
John B. McGinty, MD, First Vice-President
Augusto Sarmiento, MD, Second Vice-President
Robert N. Hensinger, MD, Secretary
Robert H. Haralson, MD, Treasurer
Reginald R. Cooper, MD
Thomas B. Dameron, Jr., MD
Kenneth E. DeHaven, MD
Letha Y. Hunter-Griffin, MD
Joseph M. Lane, MD
Thomas C. Nelson (ex officio)
J. Elmer Nix, MD
James F. Richards, Jr., MD
Bernard A. Rineberg, MD
William J. Robb, MD
Dempsey S. Springfield, MD
Roby C. Thompson, Jr., MD

Computer Consultants
B. Kaye Boles, PhD
Joseph A. Buckwalter, MD
Henry R. Cowell, MD
Gregory Crane, PhD
David W. Hennage, PhD
Mark J. Koris, MD
Jeffey D. Reuben, MD, PhD
Mark W. Wieting

Consultants
Marc A. Asher, MD
Robert H. Fitzgerald, Jr., MD

Reviewers
Clifford Colwell, MD; Mark Gebhardt, MD; Julie Glowacki, PhD; Harold Kitaoka, MD; Jennifer Kriegler, MD; James Maguire, MD; John Makley, MD; Mini Pathria, MD; Hamlet A. Peterson, MD; Robert Recker, MD; James Redford, MD; Donald T. Reilly, MD; Cynthia Rutherford, MD; Fred Shapiro, MD; Dempsey S. Springfield, MD; William H. Thomas, MD; George Thompson, MD; Thomas S. Thornhill, MD; Lawrence V. Tkach, MD; Andrew Weiland, MD; John H. Wilber, MD; Kaye E. Wilkins, MD

Contents

Lower Extremity

Contributors

Bone Grafts	Gary E. Friedlaender, MD *New Haven, Connecticut*
Soft-Tissue Implants	Freddie H. Fu, MD Vincent J. Silvaggio, MD *Pittsburgh, Pennsylvania*
Prostheses: Implant Materials and Methods of Fixation	Myron Spector, PhD *Boston, Massachusetts*
Microsurgery	Thomas M. Brushart, MD *Lutherville, Maryland*
Pain	F. Michael Ferrante, MD *Boston, Massachusetts*
Spinal Cord Monitoring	Clyde L. Nash, Jr., MD *Cleveland, Ohio*
Anesthesia for Orthopaedic Surgery	Mercedes Concepcion, MD *Boston, Massachusetts*
Congenital Abnormalities	Michael J. Goldberg, MD *Boston, Massachusetts*
Gait and Neuromuscular Disorders	Sheldon Simon, MD *Columbus, Ohio*
Rehabilitation: Amputation, Prosthetics, and Orthotics	Robert Waters, MD Richard Chambers, MD *Downey, California*

Upper Extremity Task Force

Section Editor	James H. Herndon, MD *Pittsburgh, Pennsylvania*
Upper Extremity: Pediatric Reconstruction	L. Andrew Koman, MD *Winston-Salem, North Carolina*
Throwing Injuries in the Athlete	Frank W. Jobe, MD Ronald E. Glousman, MD *Inglewood, California*
Shoulder: Trauma and Related Instability	Brian J. Galinat, MD *Wilmington, Delaware* Russell F. Warren, MD *New York, New York*
Shoulder: Reconstruction	Louis U. Bigliani, MD Evan L. Flatow, MD *New York, New York* Edward V. Craig, MD *Minneapolis, Minnesota*
Elbow and Forearm: Trauma	William P. Cooney III, MD *Rochester, Minnesota*
Elbow and Forearm: Reconstruction	Bernard F. Morrey, MD *Rochester, Minnesota*
Wrist and Hand: Trauma	William Bowers, MD *Richmond, Virginia* Peter C. Amadio, MD *Rochester, Minnesota*
Wrist and Hand: Reconstruction	James H. Herndon, MD *Pittsburgh, Pennsylvania*

Spine Task Force

Section Editor	Stephen J. Lipson, MD *Boston, Massachusetts*
Cervical Spine: Pediatric and Reconstructive Aspects	Charles R. Clark, MD *Iowa City, Iowa*
Cervical Spine and Cord: Trauma	Alan M. Levine, MD *Baltimore, Maryland*
Thoracolumbar Spine: Pediatric Aspects	John B. Emans, MD *Boston, Massachusetts*

Thoracolumbar Spine: Trauma — Steven R. Garfin, MD
San Diego, California

Thoracolumbar Spine: Reconstruction — Michael J. Murphy, MD
New Haven, Connecticut

Lumbar Spine — Neil Kahanovitz, MD
New York, New York

Lower Extremity Task Force

Section Editors — Dale M. Daniel, MD
San Diego, California
Paul M. Pellicci, MD
New York, New York
Robert A. Winquist, MD
Seattle, Washington

Pelvis, Hip, and Femur: Pediatric Aspects — Stephen W. Burke, MD
New York, New York

Pelvis and Acetabulum: Trauma — Joel M. Matta, MD
Los Angeles, California
Timothy Bray, MD
Reno, Nevada

Hip: Trauma — Joseph D. Zuckerman, MD
New York, New York

Femur: Trauma — Kenneth D. Johnson, MD
Nashville, Tennessee

Pelvis, Hip, and Femur: Reconstruction — Paul M. Pellicci, MD
New York, New York

Knee and Leg: Pediatric Aspects — Dennis R. Wenger, MD
San Diego, California

Knee and Leg: Soft-Tissue Trauma — Dale M. Daniel, MD
San Diego, California
Robert A. Teitge, MD
Warren, Michigan
William A. Grana, MD
Oklahoma City, Oklahoma
David M. Brody, MD
Norwalk, Connecticut

Knee and Leg: Bone Trauma — Fred Behrens, MD
Cleveland, Ohio

Knee and Leg: Reconstruction — James A. Rand, MD
Rochester, Minnesota

Ankle and Foot: Pediatric Aspects — James R. Kasser, MD
Boston, Massachusetts

Ankle and Foot: Trauma — Bruce J. Sangeorzan, MD
Sigvard T. Hansen, Jr., MD
Seattle, Washington

Ankle and Foot: Reconstruction — Andrea Cracchiolo III, MD
Los Angeles, California

Preface

Ten years ago, the American Academy of Orthopaedic Surgeons perceived a need for an educational medium that would help orthopaedic surgeons remain current in an ever-expanding field. The central product of this effort was a home study syllabus, the purpose of which was stated in the foreword to *OKU I*: to be "useful in daily practice as a narrative to be read, a reference to be consulted, and a guide providing direction to more detailed information." That the Academy's perception of this need was correct was evidenced by the resounding successes of *OKU I* and *OKU 2*.

Orthopaedic Knowledge Update 3 strongly adheres to the original intent and organization of its predecessors. However, it represents an evolution in style and content that attempts to meet the rapidly changing nature of our field. *OKU 3* is the last of three volumes reviewing and synthesizing the orthopaedic literature of the 1980s, and, therefore, it summarizes to some extent the progress made in this decade, and focuses the reader's attention on some of the important unresolved questions to be answered as we begin the next. To that end, each chapter in the General Knowledge Section concludes with a brief discussion of the trends in each field. In the anatomic sections (the Upper Extremity, the Spine and the Lower Extremity), each chapter includes a discussion of current controversies so that the reader can assess the arguments for and against different opinions regarding these unresolved questions.

A particularly difficult task for those involved in producing this syllabus was striking a proper balance between recent basic and clinical information (the update) and background material sufficient to provide an appropriate perspective, while at the same time keeping the volume small enough so that it would continue to be a portable and "friendly" reference. We have chosen to resolve this dilemma in the following way: Subjects new to this volume (such as child abuse, anesthesia in orthopaedics, pain, throwing injuries, and blood and blood components), are presented in a broad perspective. However, for previously presented subjects being updated, the reader is referred to the previous volumes for background material.

OKU 3 is based on the literature published between April 1985 and Dec 31, 1988, although some important articles published before 1985 are cited. When possible, 1989 publications have also been included. Each chapter contains an annotated bibliography and a list of "Keywords" to help the reader explore any subject of interest in greater depth. Like the previous edition, *OKU 3* will serve as a resource for the orthopaedic self-assessment examinations that will appear later in 1990.

The *OKU 3* home study syllabus is supplemented by a set of audio cassettes, and a new learning medium: a home computer CD-ROM (compact disk, read only memory) disk that will contain the contents of *OKU I*, *OKU 2*, and *OKU 3*, along with the full texts of as many of the references cited in these volumes as possible. This pilot project in the use of home computers for learner-centered education attempts to bring currently available electronic media into home education. It provides the user with a mechanism by which to study the past ten years of progress on any subject addressed in the *OKU* series. The choice of CD-ROM as the medium for home computer education in 1990 was based on its growing popularity and acceptance, and the reasonable cost of the hardware and software required for home use. As emerging interactive video technologies mature, they may augment and/or supplant CD-ROM in the future.

The authors, section editors, and the Board of Editors have made every effort to provide an update that is as objective as possible. Each manuscript has been reviewed by at least two, and often by three, reviewers. Each manuscript was initially reviewed by a section editor in conjunction with the members of his task force. In that way, experts in a particular field criticized and revised each manuscript. The revised manuscripts were then rereviewed by the Board of Editors and, when appropriate, sent to external reviewers as well. The information presented, therefore, represents the best efforts of the contributors to this volume to assess the current literature objectively and fairly.

A project of this magnitude depends for its success on the contributions of many people. I am indebted to the dedicated effort of the authors, section editors, and the Board of Editors. These are not unbusy individuals; yet, they found time in their already overcommitted schedules to contribute to the success of this project. Because this is the first *OKU* volume to be produced in its entirety by the Academy, special admiration and thanks are extended to the Academy staff: Thomas C. Nelson, Fred V. Featherstone, MD, Mark W. Wieting, Marilyn L. Fox, PhD, Wendy O. Schmidt, and Geraldine H. Dubberke. In particular, Wendy Schmidt deserves recognition for her overall management of the editorial process and superb editing. Mark Wieting served as director of the project and coordinated the efforts of the Academy staff involved in the project. David Hennage, PhD, deserves great credit for guiding the CD-ROM project.

I wish to pay special tribute to my predecessors, Marc A. Asher, MD, and Robert H. Fitzgerald, Jr., MD. They brought an idea of great promise to fruition, and it is on that solid foundation that *OKU 3* was built. All who have been associated with this effort are pleased and privileged to present to the fellows of the American Academy of Orthopaedic Surgeons and to our orthopaedic colleagues throughout the world the third volume of *Orthopaedic Knowledge Update*.

Robert Poss, MD
Editor

I
General Knowledge

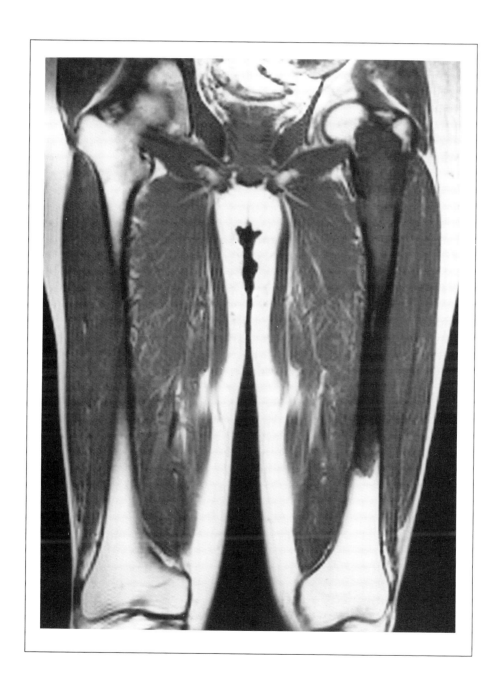

1

Imaging of the Musculoskeletal System

In the past few years dramatic changes have occurred in the field of diagnostic imaging. In large part, these changes have been related to the introduction and refinement of techniques, such as computed tomography (CT), magnetic resonance imaging (MRI), and single-photon emission computed tomography (SPECT), that rely on computer analysis of imaging data. Many investigations have confirmed that such methods can be effectively applied to the analysis of musculoskeletal disorders, although the precise methods continue to undergo modification and the advantages of one technique over another in many clinical situations have not been clearly defined. The newer imaging methods provide a unique challenge to the orthopaedic surgeon; the cross-sectional displays require of the observer a thorough comprehension of anatomic relationships and, in the case of MRI, knowledge of the biochemical composition and environment of normal and abnormal tissues so that the images are interpreted properly.

Imaging Techniques

Magnetic Resonance Imaging

The advantages of MRI over other methods are numerous and include, foremost, its reliance on the principles of magnetism rather than on the use of ionizing radiation. MRI shares with CT an ability to provide sectional images of the human body and does so with greater contrast resolution and equal or greater spatial resolution. Like nuclear medicine, it can provide physiologic data and does so without the need for radiation-emitting pharmaceutical agents. Like ultrasonography, MRI allows analysis of the internal composition of tissues. Like angiography, it can provide information about the anatomy of blood vessels, and, like arthrography, about intra-articular and periarticular structures such as cartilage and ligaments but without the need for iodinated contrast material. MRI can delineate the spinal cord (as well as the brain) without the injection of contrast agents and provide detail far superior to that of myelography. In short, MRI is capable of generating high-quality sectional representations of the human body from any angle or perspective, providing both anatomic and physiologic data without the use of ionizing radiation.

The examiner must ensure that the technical parameters chosen are the ones best suited to answer the clinical questions being posed. Before imaging, decisions must be made regarding the selection of the appropriate coil, the proper slice thickness, the slice spacing, the plane of section, the optimal pulse sequence, and the number of signal excitations. Although MRI of the musculoskeletal system has traditionally employed the spin-echo technique, interest in rapid or fast-scan imaging has evolved in an attempt to reduce examination time and, thereby, lower the cost of the procedure. Gradient-echo imaging, which includes such techniques as fast low-angle shot (FLASH), free-induction steady-state precession (FISP), and gradient-recalled acquisition steady-state (GRASS), employs a shorter flip angle that results in more rapid recovery of magnetization. Although gradient-echo techniques allow faster acquisition of imaging data, other advantages and possible disadvantages of these methods are not yet clear and will become apparent only through careful comparison with conventional spin-echo sequences. Preliminary data indicate that certain fast-scanning techniques, as well as methods that utilize chemical shift imaging (such as the chemical shift selective [CHESS] sequence), may demonstrate disorders of hyaline cartilage more effectively by providing better contrast resolution between the low-signal intensity of cortical bone, synovial tissue, and ligaments and the high-signal intensity of hyaline cartilage. An additional technique, the short T_1 inversion recovery (STIR) pulse sequence, has been found to facilitate the detection and localization of malignancy.

A variety of surface coils have been developed to improve the ratio of signal to noise during MRI. These coils are positioned as close to the region of interest as possible and, ideally, have a size and configuration that complement the anatomy of the area to be examined. For large parts, such as the pelvis, a body coil is usually employed; for smaller parts, such as the knee, shoulder, wrist, temporomandibular joint, and spine, smaller coils are appropriate. In some instances, specially designed surface coils allow simultaneous acquisition of imaging data from the right and left sides of the body, allowing the examination to be performed in less time.

The development of contrast media for MRI has received a great deal of attention. To date, the major focus of investigation has been to identify compounds that have an extracellular fluid distribution and possess paramagnetic properties that can augment the magnetic resonance images. Gadolinium diethylenetriaminepentaacetic acid (gadolinium-DTPA) has been the compound most often studied. Evidence to date indicates that gadolinium-DTPA effectively enhances defects in the blood-brain barrier, renal excretory capacity, inflammatory lesions, and certain tumors. This paramagnetic contrast medium has a strong effect on the T_1 relaxation time of protein; because of these properties, gadolinium-DTPA enhances edematous structures in the T_1-weighted images. Orthopaedic applications of magnetic resonance images enhanced by gadolinium-DTPA include, principally, the differentiation of recurrent disk herniation and scar formation in patients with new or continuous clinical manifestations after spinal surgery. However, this technique also shows promise in the further delineation of soft-tissue tumors and synovial inflammatory processes.

To enhance the efficacy of MRI in evaluating intra-articular soft-tissue structures, an MRI arthrographic technique has been described in which saline is injected into the joint before the MRI is done. Because fluid appears bright on T_2-weighted images, the definition of ligaments or cartilage is improved and small chondral defects become visible. This method, which employs an iatrogenic effusion, is not indicated in patients who have joint effusions (Fig. 1) and, in all cases, adds a degree of "invasiveness" to the examination. The precise role of magnetic resonance arthrography remains to be clarified.

As in other imaging methods, certain artifacts in MRI limit the usefulness of the examination in some patients. Although MRI presents potential hazards in individuals with cardiac pacemakers, electrical implants, prosthetic cardiac valves, and aneurysm clips because of induced currents in the lead wires (in the case of pacemakers) or significant torque and longitudinal force (in the case of surgical clips), MRI can be successfully performed on most such patients and image quality may be better than that obtained by CT.

Chemical-shift-misrepresentation artifacts have been described in relation to soft-tissue interfaces where fat and tissues with a high water content are closely apposed. These artifacts can lead to erroneous estimates of the thickness of cortical bone in the appendicular or axial skeleton. Modifications in the MRI technique generally overcome these problems.

Although the image provided by MRI is anatomically similar to that produced by CT, the appearance of flowing blood or cerebrospinal fluid on MRI has no correlate in CT. Indeed, flowing blood can appear bright or dark, depending on the velocity and the specific MRI technique. Although slowly flowing blood (as in the veins) generally appears bright and rapidly flowing blood (as in the arteries) generally appears dark, careful analysis of flow phenomena in MRI underscores the complexity and variability of the signal characteristics of the fluid, making it difficult to diagnose aneurysms, thrombi, and other vascular disorders.

MRI spectroscopy remains an experimental technique with the potential of noninvasively measuring important metabolites in living tissue. This method allows analysis of high-energy phosphates, lactate, and pH and, thus, laboratory detection of metabolic changes produced by tissue anoxia or ischemia. Although clinical evaluation of MRI spectroscopy has been restricted by the lack of suitable instrumentation and the inability to obtain MRI spectra from selected regions of the body, these difficulties have now been largely overcome. This should lead to increased use of this method as a clinical and research tool in the years ahead.

Computed Tomography

CT remains the most widely available cross-sectional imaging method and its musculoskeletal applications have been detailed in hundreds of scientific articles. Its spatial resolution is similar to that of MRI but inferior to that provided by routine radiography. Conversely, its contrast resolution is far superior to that of conventional radiography, but inferior to that of MRI. Many studies comparing the benefits of CT and MRI in the evaluation of musculoskeletal disorders have generally indicated the superiority of MRI; however, CT remains the better method for defining abnormalities of cortical bone and detecting calcification or ossification.

Unlike MRI, which allows acquisition of image data in any plane, initial image acquisition in CT is guided by the geometry of the human body. For structures in the axial skeleton and for some in the appendicular skeleton, CT scans normally are acquired in the transverse or transaxial plane. CT examinations of small, peripherally located parts, such as the hand, wrist, or foot, however, allow a choice with regard to positioning of the area to be examined; therefore, direct coronal or sagittal planes, or both, may be used in such instances.

It should be recognized that a "stack" of consecutive slices acquired by CT provides complete information about a three-dimensional volume. Therefore, when such a set of contiguous axial scans is acquired, it is still possible to produce an image by reconstruction or rearrangement of the data in essentially any desired plane (Fig. 2). Indeed, in some instances, a curved plane can be selected when it is believed it will enhance the diagnostic information. It is these techniques that have led to the popularity of multiplanar reformatted images for the analysis of certain structures, such as the spine. Fundamental to the concept of reformatted CT images is the realization that the method does not provide new data but, in reality, demonstrates the same data (with some loss of spatial resolution) in a different manner.

A natural extension of data reconstruction has been the development of three-dimensional imaging techniques that have been applied primarily to CT but can also be used for MRI. The quality and accuracy of three-dimensional images are improved when thin adjacent slices are available. One popular method used to generate three-dimensional images employs surface displays. That is, the edge or surface of the desired structures is viewed as though all remaining tissue were removed. The end result is a contour for each CT section that outlines the bone (or the soft tissues). The contours are stacked according to the sepa-

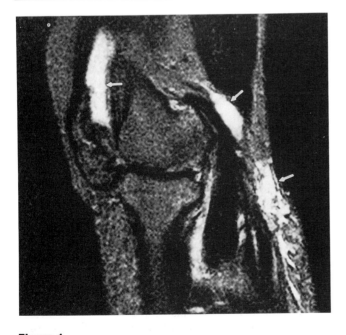

Figure 1

Magnetic resonance imaging. Identification of fluid. Patient with ruptured popliteal cyst. A sagittal T_2-weighted image of the knee reveals bright fluid (arrows) in the joint and synovial cyst, with extravasation of fluid into the posterior soft tissues.

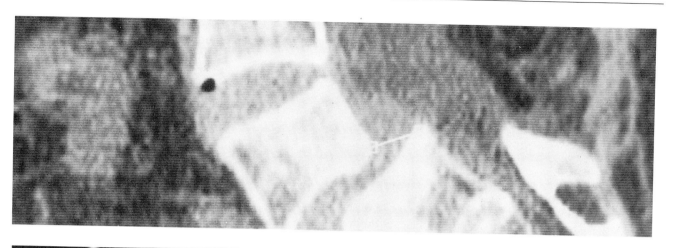

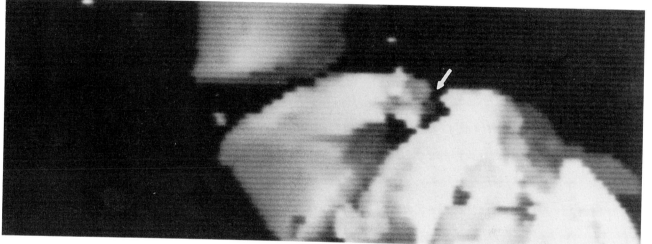

Figure 2

Computed tomography. Two- and three-dimensional image reformation in spondylolisthesis. Sagittal **(top)** and three-dimensional **(bottom)** representations of transaxial CT data reveal the extent of spondylolisthesis at the L5-S1 level and spondylolysis (arrow). Note the diskal vacuum phenomenon **(top).**

ation between slices, and a "three-dimensional" image is then displayed on a two-dimensional screen, using a light source in which objects close to the viewer appear brighter and those farther away appear darker. A second popular method is volumetric rendering in which all the information, not just the surface boundaries, is used in the generation of the three-dimensional display. In either case, the resultant images can be rotated in any axis, sectioned in any plane, or presented in a movie format. Currently, three-dimensional CT imaging methods are employed most widely in evaluation of traumatic disorders of anatomically complex regions of the body, such as the spine (Fig. 3), osseous pelvis, hip, shoulder, and facial structures. They are better suited to the assessment of high-density tissues, such as bone, than to those of lower density, such as the soft tissues.

A further refinement of the three-dimensional process is the coupling of the CT data with a numerically controlled milling machine that allows the construction of anatomically accurate plastic models of the area of interest. Utilization of three-dimensional techniques in the design of prosthetic replacements in plastic and orthopaedic surgery remains experimental, although early applications of this technology currently allow the construction of custom-fitted prostheses.

CT is being investigated as a means of studying the motion and mechanics of complex joints, such as the knee and temporomandibular joint. Dynamic displays of normal and abnormal articular movement are produced by cine-CT scanners that allow continuous imaging at high speeds. Of related interest, analysis of joint dynamics can be done by means of MRI in which images are acquired in various stages of articular motion. This technique may prove valuable for investigating patellofemoral or temporomandibular joint abnormalities.

Arthrography

Although advances in MRI have recently decreased the use of arthrography, it remains valuable in the assessment of certain articular disorders. Important uses for arthrography still include the evaluation of internal derangements of the knee (especially in geographic areas where MRI is not yet available), rotator cuff disruption and capsular or labral abnormalities of the shoulder (where MRI is not available), ligamentous or cartilaginous disruption in the

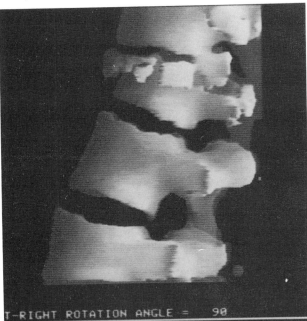

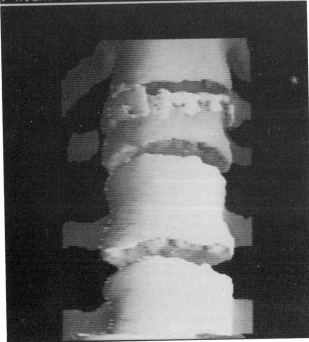

Figure 3

Computed tomography. Three-dimensional image reformation in spinal fracture. Lateral **(top)** and frontal **(bottom)** images derived from transaxial CT data reveal the configuration of this complex fracture of the vertebral body.

scapholunate or lunate-triquetral ligament tears, or of combined tears of both ligaments. Further, recent evidence underscores the importance of the three-compartment injection technique for the arthrographic evaluation of the injured wrist; data indicate that separate injections into the radiocarpal, inferior radioulnar, and midcarpal compartments of the wrist are needed for identification of some abnormalities that would not be detected by injection into one compartment alone.

The combination of arthrography and CT is emerging as a useful procedure in the assessment of soft-tissue abnormalities that accompany subluxations or dislocations of the glenohumeral joint (Fig. 4). This "computed arthrotomography" identifies subtle alterations in the anterior or posterior portion of the glenoid labrum and the superior, middle, or inferior glenohumeral ligament, or in combinations of these structures. Additional indications for computed arthrotomography include the detection of intra-articular cartilaginous or osteocartilaginous bodies and the delineation of the nature and extent of intra-articular masses, although MRI can also be used for these clinical problems.

Arthrography has recently been extended to the evaluation of the apophyseal joints of the cervical spine as well as of the temporomandibular joint. The rationale for injecting contrast material mixed with a corticosteroid preparation or corticosteroid medication alone into the facet joints of the cervical spine is based on the success of a similar procedure in the apophyseal joints of the lumbar spine. Preliminary results indicated a reduction of symptoms and signs after cervical injection in approximately 90% of patients thought to have a facet syndrome, although the rate of recurrent clinical manifestations was high. Arthrography of the temporomandibular joint provides ac

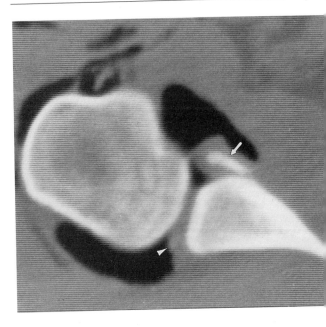

Figure 4

Computed arthrotomography. Multidirectional instability of the glenohumeral joint. Air was introduced into the joint before the CT examination. A single transaxial image reveals an osseous "Bankartian" lesion (arrow) and a subtle fragment of bone posterio (arrowhead).

wrist (because the precise role of MRI in this anatomic area is not clear), masses about any joint, and, when combined with aspiration, painful prostheses.

A digital subtraction technique used in combination with standard arthrography allows careful monitoring of the injection process and subtraction of the bones, so that the location and appearance of the contrast material are augmented. This technique is particularly useful in wrist arthrography, allowing the precise identification of isolated

curate information regarding the position, shape, and integrity of the meniscus. MRI, however, achieves many of these goals and, because it is less invasive, may be preferred for assessing the "temporomandibular joint syndrome."

Other Invasive Techniques

Percutaneous Drainage Percutaneous drainage of intra-articular or paraosseous abscesses has been done with fluoroscopic, computed tomographic, and ultrasonic guidance. In general, this procedure initially requires needle placement within the joint or soft-tissue abscess. A flexible wire then is inserted through the needle, and progressively larger catheters are placed over the wire. Ultimately, a large catheter containing several holes is used for repeated irrigation. There are anecdotal reports of therapeutic success with percutaneous procedures in a limited number of patients with septic arthritis or paraspinal abscesses.

Percutaneous Biopsy Although open biopsy is an accepted surgical procedure in the diagnosis of a variety of skeletal and soft-tissue disorders, this procedure requires considerable time and expense, operating-room space and personnel, and general anesthesia in most cases. Therefore, repeated attempts have been made to devise special instruments for percutaneous needle biopsy of bone and soft tissue. More recently, advances in radiology, including image intensification, biplanar videofluoroscopy, CT, and high-resolution radionuclide bone scanning, have made such percutaneous procedures easier to perform and have increased their accuracy. The bone specimen can be obtained in one of two ways: aspiration by needle or core by trephine. Tissue obtained by needle aspiration is small in quantity and distorted by loss of cellular configuration; tissue obtained by trephine biopsy is greater in quantity and intact, although this technique requires a larger needle. Needle aspiration is most useful for tissue culture to exclude an infection; trephine biopsy is a superior technique for histologic diagnosis.

A variety of needles are available for both trephine and aspiration biopsy. The standard trephine instrument remains the Craig needle, although others, including the Ackermann needle, are frequently used. A recent advance is the development of needles that incorporate power drills affixed to two concentric telescoping stainless-steel tubes containing sawteeth that face in opposite directions. When the tubes are rotated in opposing directions, the passing teeth act like the blades of scissors, providing an adequate core of soft and hard tissues.

Ultrasonography

Diagnostic ultrasound has a central role in the evaluation of many clinical problems in obstetrics, medicine, and surgery. The advent of gray-scale signal processing and the routine use of higher-frequency transducers have broadened the applicability of this technique to encompass assessment of smaller lesions as well as organ parenchymal texture. Real-time scanners have become popular because of their excellent resolution, ease of use, portability, and relatively low cost. Although the role of diagnostic ultrasound in problems related to bone, joint, and soft tissue is limited in scope, this method may be used effectively in certain situations, including the evaluation of the thickness of the articular cartilage of the knee, the detection of intra-articular fluid in the hip or knee, the assessment of the relationship of the unossified femoral head and the acetabulum in infants with congenital hip dysplasia, and the diagnosis of iliopsoas bursitis. Among the traumatic conditions that can be evaluated with ultrasonography are intramuscular hematomas and injuries of tendons (such as the patellar, rotator cuff, and Achilles tendons). Sonography can be used to evaluate masses arising in the soft tissues of the extremity; although the technique easily catalogues these lesions into cystic or solid groupings, little histologic specificity can be obtained from sonographic appearances alone. Because ultrasonography has had negligible success in establishing bone-soft tissue relationships, it has a limited role in the assessment of lesions either arising from bone or involving bone secondarily, whether those lesions are neoplastic or infectious in nature.

Although the sonographic appearance of abscesses varies, overlapping those of hematomas and tumors, a typical abscess contains predominantly fluid but often has debris manifested as fine, low-level echoes within the cystic mass. This material sometimes accumulates in the dependent portion of the abscess, a phenomenon that can be documented by changing the patient's position. Differentiating an abscess from simple cellulitis of the extremity can be accomplished with sonography. Sonographic guidance for percutaneous aspiration of abscesses, as well as neoplasms, is also possible.

Additional clinical applications of sonography are the detection and localization of foreign bodies in the soft tissues, the delineation of synovial cysts, and the demonstration of a variety of intraspinal abnormalities in infants in whom the incompletely ossified posterior arch of the vertebra provides a window for scanning from a posterior approach.

Scintigraphy

Single-photon emission computed tomography (SPECT) is a relatively new diagnostic technique that combines the advantages of scintigraphy with those derived from a tomographic display. When compared with conventional or plain bone imaging, SPECT offers both improved image contrast and more complete spatial information. SPECT essentially removes undesirable noise (but not signal) from the image by removing the radionuclide activity from in front of and behind the tomographic plane being evaluated on each separate image. The major application of SPECT is the evaluation of anatomic regions where two bones, such as the femoral head and acetabulum in the hip, overlap on standard images. Using SPECT in such instances allows the radionuclide activity derived from each of the overlying structures to be determined. In the spine, where activity in the anterior and posterior osseous elements of a single vertebra are not easily separated by standard planar scintigraphy, SPECT can also be useful. Specific situations in which SPECT can provide more diagnostic information include spondylolisthesis, spondylolysis, pseudarthrosis, failed spinal fusion, and osteoarthritis in the apophyseal joints. Other indications for SPECT include ischemic necrosis of the femoral head, patellofemoral disease, and abnormalities of the facial bones. Three-dimensional displays of data derived from SPECT have been evaluated in a preliminary fashion.

The assessment of musculoskeletal infection with radionuclide techniques, including scanning with bone-seeking radionuclides, gallium citrate Ga 67, and leukocytes labeled with indium In 111 has continued to receive considerable attention. In general, technetium Tc 99m methylene diphosphate bone scans become abnormal within hours to days of the onset of osteomyelitis; although initially a photon-deficient area ("cold" spot) related to fulminant infection with thrombosis or vascular compression can be seen, later increased accumulation of the radioisotope ("hot" spot) is typical. Occasional difficulty in interpreting the bone scan in younger patients arises from an inability to differentiate between normal and abnormal activity in the metaphysis. Although high-resolution gamma cameras and magnification techniques may diminish this difficulty, using gallium scans in this situation, even though these are associated with less radionuclide accumulation, may allow more accurate interpretation of the metaphyseal activity. Leukocytic uptake of the radionuclide may explain, at least in part, augmented activity at sites of skeletal infection on gallium scans.

The rationale for the use of gallium as an adjunct to technetium phosphates in evaluating inflammatory lesions of bone is based on several considerations. As technetium accumulation is related to the integrity of the vascular tree, increased intramedullar pressure accompanying osteomyelitis can partially prevent augmented blood flow and also prevent significant accumulation of the radionuclide. Gallium, being less dependent on the vascular flow, may still localize at the site of infection. Unfortunately, as gallium accumulation also occurs in soft-tissue infection, differentiating between cellulitis and osteomyelitis is usually impossible with this agent. In some instances, a gallium scan can be obtained in conjunction with a technetium scan in the same patient, and the information obtained may be even more useful than that from either examination alone. Gallium scans may reveal abnormal accumulation in patients with active osteomyelitis when technetium scans reveal decreased activity ("cold" lesions) or perhaps normal activity (transition period between "cold" and "hot" lesions). Further, gallium accumulation appears to correlate more closely with activity in chronic osteomyelitis than does technetium uptake, and it may be superior in determining the response of acute or chronic osteomyelitis to various therapeutic regimens.

The changing patterns of scintigraphic activity on initial and delayed images after injection of bone-seeking radiopharmaceutical agents underscore possible inaccuracies in the analysis of single-phase bone images alone. In an attempt to improve diagnostic accuracy, considerable attention has been given to the "three-phase" examination in patients with musculoskeletal infection: Serial images are obtained during the first minute after the injection of the technetium-compound bolus (angiographic phase); a postinjection image is then obtained at the end of the first minute or several minutes (blood-pool phase); and further images are obtained two or three hours later (delayed phase). The addition of a fourth phase to the scintigraphic examination, representing a static image obtained 24 hours after the injection of the bone-seeking radiopharmaceutical agent, has been emphasized as a means of improving specificity. As an example, the differentiation of cellulitis alone from cellulitis with accompanying osteomyelitis may depend on the presence of increased activity only on the immediate images in cellulitis and of increased activity on the immediate and delayed images in osteomyelitis.

Investigations of the value of ^{111}In-labeled leukocytes in the diagnosis of musculoskeletal infection have continued in recent years. The success of this technique relies on the migration of the leukocytes to the site of infection. The technique appears to be better suited to assessment of acute infections associated with vigorous leukocyte infiltration than to chronic infections in which such infiltration may be insufficient. Recent attempts to label an increased number of lymphocytes, as opposed to polymorphonuclear leukocytes, with indium have resulted in more successful identification of sites of low-grade musculoskeletal sepsis. Antibiotic administration does not appear to influence the sensitivity of detection. In general, ^{111}In-labeled leukocyte scintigraphy is less sensitive in detecting bone infections than soft-tissue infections and is not helpful in differentiating osteomyelitis from septic arthritis. It can demonstrate soft-tissue extension from an area of bone infection and may be useful in the evaluation of a painful arthroplasty. It is important to remember that positive leukocyte images occur in musculoskeletal conditions other than infection, such as rheumatoid arthritis and primary or secondary tumors in the soft tissues or bone. Additional disadvantages of leukocyte imaging include long preparation time and poor spatial resolution.

Joint Replacement

Considerable attention continues to be given to imaging techniques that may be useful in the evaluation of complications of arthroplasty, particularly prosthetic loosening with or without infection. On conventional radiographs alone, a prosthesis in a patient with infection is rarely distinguishable from a prosthesis that is loosened but not infected. The typical features of osteomyelitis—bone destruction and irregular periosteal new-bone formation—are uncommon manifestations of an infected arthroplasty. The presence of a radiolucent zone at the bone-cement or prosthesis-cement interface signifies a gap that does not uniformly correlate with gross prosthetic loosening that is detected at the time of surgery. A large radiolucent zone generally reflects at least micromotion of the component. Such zones, however, may indicate either aseptic loosening or septic loosening.

Wear Debris

Wear debris is generated from the articulating surfaces of the prosthesis as well as from those surfaces in contact with the bone; this debris results in a tissue reaction and may contribute in a number of ways to implant failure. In general, a routine radiograph does not directly identify the debris itself, but may reveal the effects of the debris such as enlarging radiolucent areas near the interface that may indicate an inflammatory response to the metal, polymethylmethacrylate, polyethylene, or to combinations of the three. The recent use of uncemented, porous-coated prosthetic components has led to the radiographic identification of detached beads in some cases. It has been suggested by some investigators that the presence of detached beads adjacent to a lucent line implies that movement at the corresponding interface has loosened the porous coat, although it is theoretically possible that the beads are detached from the porous coat at the time the prosthesis is inserted.

Conventional radiographic analysis of silicone polymer implants in the wrist, hand, and foot has documented the occurrence in some patients of a distinctive arthritis characterized by deformity and fragmentation of the implant, joint space loss, and cysts and erosions in adjacent bones (Fig. 5). In these instances, histologic evaluation of synovial tissue has revealed hyperplastic synovium and cellular infiltration with lymphocytes, macrophages, and foreign-body giant cells containing silicone particles. These microscopic findings are consistent with an inflammatory response to the Silastic material, although the precise frequency of this complication is not yet clear.

Imaging Techniques

Arthrography Aspiration arthrography remains a popular technique for the analysis of joint prostheses. Although the major purpose of the examination is the recovery of fluid from the articulation, the subsequent injection of radiopaque contrast material is recommended to document the existence of gaps at one or more of the interfaces. It is important to achieve high intracapsular pressure by continuing to inject the contrast agent until there is capsular distension or lymphatic filling. Standard or digitally produced subtraction techniques are useful in the delineation of small collections of the contrast material. Using strict arthrographic criteria, the sensitivity and specificity for demonstrating loosening of the femoral component of a total hip arthroplasty has been reported to be as high as 96% and 92%, respectively, and for loosening of the acetabular component 97% and 68%, respectively.

Radionuclide Imaging Although technetium phosphate bone scans are still used in the evaluation of joint prostheses, the technique is generally unsuccessful in differentiating between aseptic but loose components and infected components. Further, accumulation of the isotope may be a normal finding in the perioperative period. Recent results with cemented implants have indicated that radionuclide activity about the lesser trochanter and pros-

thesis shaft becomes insignificant within six months after total hip arthroplasty, although activity about the acetabulum, greater trochanter, and tip of the femoral prosthesis may persist longer, stabilizing approximately two years after total hip arthroplasty in asymptomatic individuals. Bone scans will be normal in most patients approximately one year after surgery, however. Persistent radionuclide activity about the tibial component after total knee arthroplasty has also been identified in asymptomatic individuals. In some studies, correlation between the degree of isotope uptake and the development of radiolucent lines around the prosthetic components after total knee arthroplasty has been poor. The role of scintigraphy in uncemented prostheses remains to be defined.

Because of problems encountered in the evaluation of bone scans in patients with arthroplasties, attention has been given to other radiopharmaceutical techniques, particularly gallium (Fig. 6) and ^{111}In-labeled leukocyte scintigraphy. In one study of 60 patients with 74 prosthetic joints, all 18 patients with confirmed sepsis had positive indium scans, characterized by migration of granulocytes into the region of the prosthesis. In the same study, 20 of 22 patients with sterile arthroplasties had negative scans. Another investigation also indicated the value of the ^{111}In-labeled leukocyte scan (as well as the erythrocyte sedimentation rate) in predicting infected prostheses.

Arthroscintigraphy, employing a solution containing iodinated contrast material and technetium Tc 99m sulfur colloid injected into the joint, was studied in a preliminary fashion as a method of detecting prosthetic loosening. Results indicated that arthroscintigraphy is potentially more sensitive than conventional arthrography in delineating loosening of the femoral component after total hip arthroplasty, although loosening of the acetabular component cannot be evaluated by scintigraphy alone.

Intraspinal Disorders

Many imaging techniques may be useful in the evaluation of intraspinal disorders. Routine radiography, conventional tomography, CT, MRI, myelography, SPECT, spinal angiography, diskography, epidurography, epidural venography, and ultrasonography can all be applied effectively. Most investigators agree that the initial examination should be conventional radiography, but there is little agreement regarding which method should be used next. The choice of subsequent imaging techniques depends on a number of factors, including the specific clinical situation, the age of the patient, the preference and expertise of the examiner, and the availability of any particular imaging method.

Imaging Techniques

Computed Tomography CT is an effective means of evaluating the spine and its contents, although it is better applied to the assessment of a short spinal segment. When analysis of a long segment of the vertebral column is required, some investigators believe that conventional tomography is preferred, although this method is of little value in the elucidation of nonosseous abnormalities. CT has greater sensitivity than myelography in the detection of disk herniation (Fig. 7) and is superior to routine radiography in the evaluation of osteoarthritis of the facet

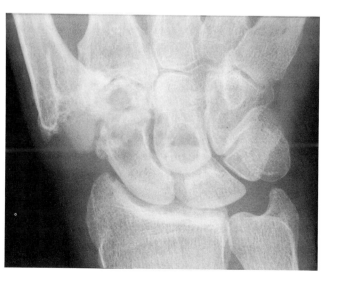

Figure 5

Inflammatory response to Silastic. Observe partial disruption of a Silastic replacement of the trapezium and cystic changes in the bones.

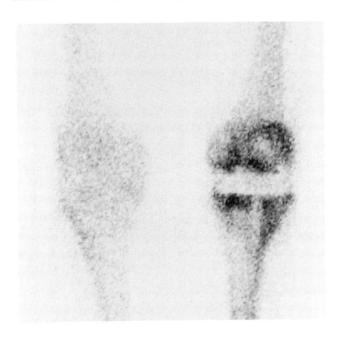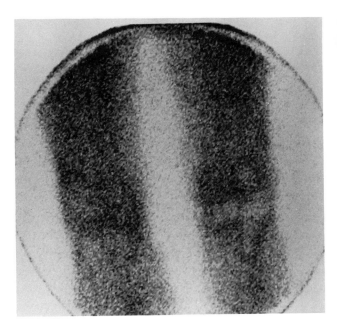

Figure 6
Scintigraphy in total knee arthroplasty shows loose, noninfected prosthesis. **Left,** A technetium scan shows abnormal accumulation of the bone-seeking radiopharmaceutical agent about both the femoral and the tibial components. **Right,** A gallium scan is within normal limits. This combination of findings suggests a loose, noninfected prosthesis.

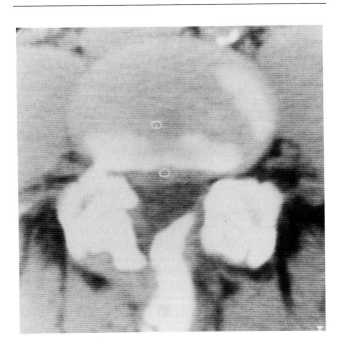

Figure 7
Recurrent disk herniation. In a patient with previous back surgery, a transaxial CT image of a lumbar vertebra shows a soft-tissue density in the spinal canal, posterior to the intervertebral disk. This image was obtained after intravenous administration of contrast material. The lesion did not enhance and is equal in density to the remainder of the disk. This suggests the presence of a recurrent disk herniation rather than a scar, as the latter would be expected to show enhancement after intravenous administration of contrast material.

joints. For cervical radiculopathy, CT is an efficient and effective alternative to myelography, although neither method has a sensitivity sufficiently high to detect small cervical disk fragments. CT complements routine radiography or myelography in the delineation of fractures in patients with spinal trauma. CT can also be used as a primary or supplementary technique in the assessment of congenital, neoplastic, or infectious diseases.

Magnetic Resonance Imaging MRI is currently the best primary diagnostic procedure for spinal intramedullary neoplasms, cysts, and arteriovenous malformations. It is also the examination of choice for the evaluation of extradural processes causing myelopathy, such as skeletal metastasis. The role of MRI in many other clinical situations appears promising, but requires careful prospective studies comparing this method with CT and myelography. Although MRI can be used to detect extramedullary intradural processes, such as a neurofibroma or meningioma, myelography still remains the technique of choice in the evaluation of such lesions. MRI and CT appear to be equally accurate in demonstrating herniated intervertebral disks and osteoarthritis of the apophyseal joints.

Myelography Myelography is a safe and effective method for demonstrating the subarachnoid space, spinal cord, and nerve root sheaths; however, it is more costly and invasive than CT or MRI. Myelography is indicated in patients with cervical radiculopathy, especially if the results of a CT scan of the cervical spine are ambiguous. Myelography is also indicated in the investigation of extramedullary intradural processes, for which the accuracy of MRI is not yet known. Myelography is useful in the detection of cysts within the spinal cord or subarachnoid space because contrast material demonstrates the cystic nature of the lesion and its communication with the subarachnoid space. This technique can be used to assess the cause of persistent low back pain after laminectomy, although other methods are also useful.

Single-Photon Emission Computed Tomography Among the spinal indications for SPECT is the differentiation of healing from nonhealing spondylolytic defects. In general, those patients who have radiographically confirmed spondylolysis without activity on a bone scan have an established nonunion at the site of the defect in the pars interarticularis and healing is unlikely with immobilization alone; and those patients who have spondylolysis and a positive bone scan have a "healing" defect that may progress to union with immobilization.

Arteriography The major indications for spinal arteriography are vascular malformations or tumors involving the spinal cord, dura, spine, or subarachnoid space. Spinal arteriography can be used to evaluate a tumor before surgery or the feasibility of embolizing a vascular malformation. Spinal arteriography, by allowing the identification of the artery of Adamkiewicz, may be useful before certain spinal surgical procedures.

Diskography The value of diskography remains controversial. Although the technique can be useful in assessing clinically significant disk displacements by reproducing the patient's symptoms and signs during injection of contrast material, it is not widely employed for this purpose. Despite previous reports, diskography is contraindicated as a means of documenting the accurate placement of a needle in the nucleus pulposus before the injection of chymopapain.

Diskography combined with CT (CT-diskography) has been reported to be beneficial in the assessment of primary or recurrent disk herniation and, in the view of some investigators, may be more specific than either diskography or CT alone (Fig. 8). After the introduction of contrast material into the disk, transaxial CT images are obtained; the opacification of an extradural mass confirms the diagnosis of a herniated intervertebral disk.

Epidural Venography The primary indication for epidural venography has been a suspected herniated disk or spinal stenosis not detected by myelography; the introduction of CT and MRI has made this relatively invasive method obsolete. Similarly, CT and MRI have replaced epidurography as a means of visualizing the epidural space.

Disk Degeneration

Degenerative diseases of the intervertebral disk lead to characteristic abnormalities on routine radiographs. One of these diseases, spondylosis deformans, relates primarily to disruption of fibers in the outermost portion of the anulus fibrosus and results in bone excrescences, or osteophytes. Two types of osteophytes occurring on the anterior aspect of the lumbar vertebral bodies have been emphasized in the past: the common claw osteophyte that curves at its tip and the less common traction osteophyte that remains horizontal in configuration. Although previous reports indicated that the traction osteophyte may indicate spinal instability, a recent study of 200 cadaveric spines suggested that the two types of osteophytes represent dif-

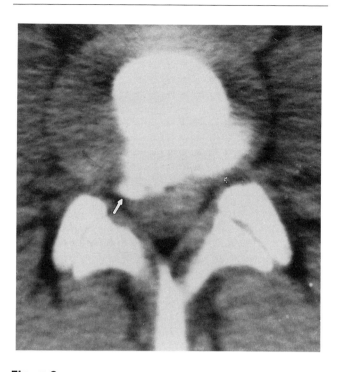

Figure 8

Disk herniation. CT-diskography shows the extension of contrast material into the disk herniation (arrow). (Reproduced with permission from Andrew Deutsch, MD, Los Angeles, California.)

ferent stages of the same pathologic process. This study also confirmed the increased frequency of anterior osteophytes with advancing age (96% of patients older than 70 years had such outgrowths), but the investigators were unable to support or refute a relationship between traction osteophytes and spinal instability.

Computed Tomography Other imaging methods can be used to assess disk degeneration. CT is relatively insensitive to the primary derangement of degeneration when the configuration of the intervertebral disk itself has not changed and may underestimate the severity of the changes within the nucleus pulposus and anulus fibrosus. Secondary manifestations of disk degeneration that can be identified with CT are herniation, anular bulging calcification, vacuum phenomena, and bone sclerosis. The accuracy of CT in the diagnosis of disk herniation has been reported to be 90% or higher; CT appears to be more sensitive than myelography in the detection of disk herniation because of its ability to delineate lateral displacements and herniations at the L5-S1 spinal level. An additional advantage of CT over routine radiography in assessing degenerative disease is its ability to better define ligamentous hypertrophy, osteoarthritis of the facet joints, and other findings of spinal stenosis.

Magnetic Resonance Imaging Recent investigations suggest that MRI is the most accurate means of outlining the morphologic characteristics of disk degeneration. Normally, the region of the vertebral end plate has a low signal intensity on T_1- and T_2-weighted spin-echo images. On T_1-weighted sequences, the central portion of the intervertebral disk normally has a slightly decreased signal intensity

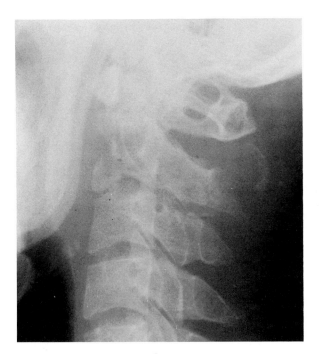

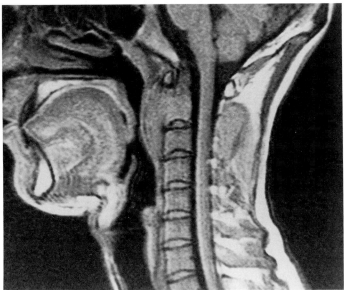

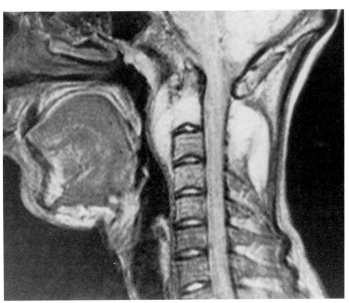

Figure 9

Tuberculosis. A routine radiograph **(left)** reveals destruction of the body of the axis with fragmentation of the spinous process as well. A large soft-tissue mass is present anteriorly. On magnetic resonance imaging, both T_1-weighted **(top right)** and T_2-weighted **(bottom right)** sagittal images reveal the full extent of the process, which involves the body and posterior osseous elements of C2, the posterior elements of C3, and the anterior and posterior paraspinal tissues. Note that the process has an intermediate signal intensity on the T_1-weighted image and a high signal intensity on the T_2-weighted image. (Reproduced with permission from Tor A. Mattsson, MD, Riyadh, Saudi Arabia.)

compared with that in the peripheral portion of the intervertebral disk; the outermost region of the intervertebral disk has a very low signal intensity. On T_2-weighted spin-echo sequences, the normal disk has a high signal intensity in the central portion and a low signal intensity in the peripheral portion. It should be stressed that these MRI characteristics do not indicate a clear separation of the nucleus pulposus and anulus fibrosus; rather, the inner portion corresponds to the nucleus pulposus as well as the innermost fibers of the anulus fibrosus, and the peripheral portion represents the outer layers of the anulus fibrosus and the longitudinal ligaments. Further, on T_2-weighted images, an area of variable size and lesser signal intensity is often visible within the central portion of the intervertebral disk, creating a notch or biconcave appearance similar to that observed with diskography. Histologic studies have indicated that this central area corresponds to a region composed of tissue more fibrous than the surrounding nucleus pulposus and is almost universal in individuals more than 30 years old.

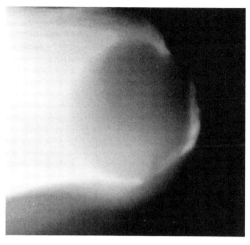
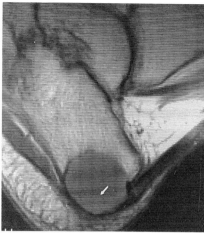
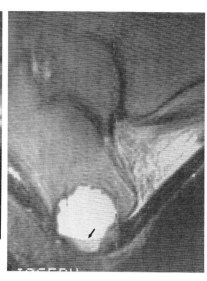

Figure 10

Giant cell tumor. A conventional tomogram **(left)** in the lateral projection reveals a large, osteolytic lesion involving the posterior portion of the calcaneus. On magnetic resonance imaging, T₁-weighted **(center)** and T₂-weighted **(right)** images show the full extent of the neoplasm. A fluid-fluid level appears on both images (arrows). This observation is consistent with a giant cell tumor but is more suggestive of an aneurysmal bone cyst. (Reproduced with permission from Guerdon Greenway, MD, Dallas, Texas.)

Disk degeneration is characterized on MRI sequences by distinct alterations in both the intervertebral disk iself and the adjacent portions of the vertebral body. The dominant change observed within the substance of the intervertebral disk is loss of signal intensity; this is best seen on T_2-weighted images and probably reflects dehydration of disk tissue. The role that specific biochemical changes play in this signal alteration is not yet defined. Vacuum phenomena, representing gaseous collections, and calcification in the disk appear as areas of signal void on all spin-echo images. In the vertebral bone, three patterns of signal change have been identified in patients with disk degeneration: Type I changes, which have been identified in approximately 4% of patients undergoing MRI for lumbar disease, are characterized by decreased signal intensity on the T_1-weighted image and increased signal intensity on the T_2-weighted images within the subchondral bone of the vertebral body and are believed to be related to the presence of vascular fibrous tissue in the bone marrow. Type II changes, seen in approximately 16% of such patients, are characterized by an increased signal intensity on T_1-weighted images and an isointense or slightly hyperintense signal on T_2-weighted images; the changes are indicative of yellow, fatty marrow adjacent to the intervertebral disk. Type III changes are characterized by decreased signal intensity on both T_1- and T_2-weighted image sequences; these changes correlate with radiographically evident bone eburnation or sclerosis. The precise clinical significance of each of these distinct patterns is not known. One of these patterns, type I, resembles that accompanying infectious spondylitis, although in that condition an abnormally high signal intensity within the intervertebral disk and paraspinal tissues on T_2-weighted images usually confirms the diagnosis (Fig. 9).

MRI has been used extensively in the diagnosis of disk herniation. The criteria for the diagnosis of such herniation on MRI are similar to those on CT scans. Disk herniations are characterized by a focal extension of the disk beyond the margins of the adjacent vertebral end plates in a central or lateral direction. On T_1-weighted images, the signal intensity of the herniation is usually similar to that of the parent disk; on T_2-weighted sequences, the signal intensity of the herniated disk may be hypointense relative to the cerebrospinal fluid with small herniations or hyperintense relative to the parent disk with large extrusions or free fragments. In one study of 20 patients with surgically documented sequestered lumbar disks, MRI distinguished sequestered disks from other forms of lumbar disk herniation with 89% sensitivity, 82% specificity, and 85% accuracy.

In experimental situations, MRI has been shown to be effective in the delineation of tears of the anulus fibrosus. One study of 20 cadavers indicated that three distinct types of anular tears could be identified by MRI: radial tears, characterized by rupture of all layers in the anulus fibrosus between the nucleus pulposus and the surface of the disk; concentric tears, characterized by fluid-filled spaces between lamellae; and transverse tears, characterized by rupture of Sharpey's fibers in the periphery of the anulus, near the ring apophysis. Further studies are needed to correlate specific patterns of anular disruption with clinical manifestations.

MRI has also been investigated in the differentiation of epidural scar from herniated disk material. Typically, anterior and lateral recess scars are hypointense or isointense on T_1-weighted sequences and hyperintense on T_2-weighted images relative to the intensity of the major portion of the anulus fibrosus. Free fragments demonstrate a slightly hyperintense signal intensity on T_1-weighted images relative to epidural fibrosis, but demonstrate a hyperintense signal intensity on T_2-weighted sequences similar to that of the recess scars. Prolapsed or extruded disk fragments are hypointense or isointense relative to the parent anulus fibro-

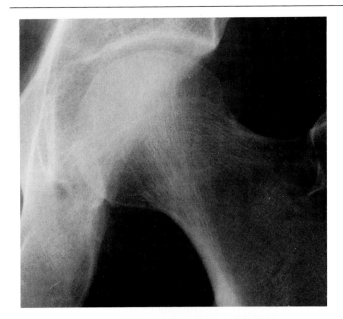

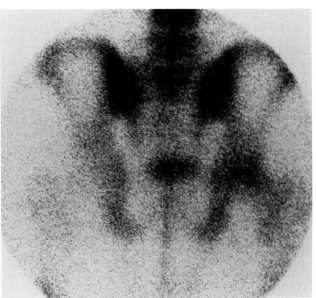

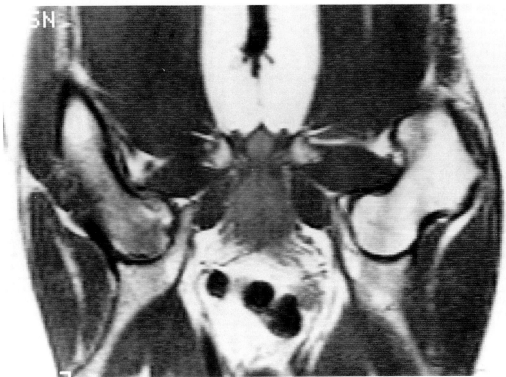

Figure 11

Transient bone marrow edema. **Top left,** A routine radiograph of the hip appears to be normal. **Top right,** A bone scan reveals increased activity in the left femoral head and neck. The findings are compatible with the diagnosis of ischemic necrosis. **Bottom,** A T_1-weighted coronal image shows low signal intensity in the left femoral head and neck. The extent of the process excludes the diagnosis of ischemic necrosis. The clinical and imaging abnormalities lessened during the next six months, consistent with the diagnosis of transient bone marrow edema.

sus on all sequences. Using these criteria, 12 of 14 patients with surgically confirmed scars or herniations, or with both, were correctly identified by MRI. The accuracy of MRI in this clinical situation may increase if paramagnetic contrast agents are employed. With gadolinium-DTPA, there appears to be consistent enhancement of peridiskal fibrosis within 15 minutes after injection and variable en-

hancement of the herniated or degenerative parent disk within 30 minutes after injection.

Bone Marrow Disorders

A variety of disorders affect the bone marrow and a multitude of imaging techniques can be used to evaluate these

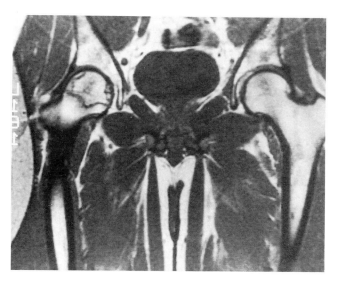

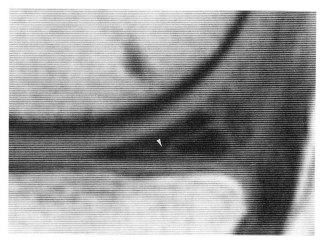

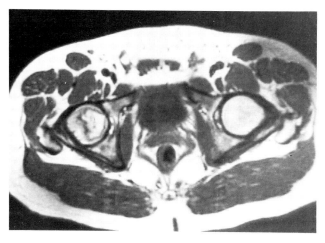

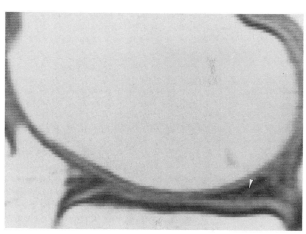

Figure 13

Medial meniscal tear. Two sagittal magnetic resonance images are shown. The first **(top)** employs standard imaging "windows"; the second **(bottom)** employs "windows" that enhance visualization of meniscal abnormalities. Note the oblique tear of the medial meniscus, appearing as a line of intermediate signal intensity (within the low signal intensity meniscus) that extends to the inferior surface of the meniscus (arrowheads).

Figure 12

Ischemic necrosis of the femoral head. Coronal **(top)** and transaxial **(bottom)** T₁-weighted images reveal the characteristic changes of ischemic necrosis of the left femoral head; the right hip is normal. Observe the irregular region of decreased signal intensity surrounding the lesion in the femoral head.

disorders. In normal situations the basic microstructure of bone marrow consists of a trabecular framework housing fat cells covered with hematopoietic cells, both supported by a system of reticulum cells, nerves, and vascular sinuses coursing among them. Two types of marrow have been identified: "red marrow" is considered hematopoietic or active marrow involved in the production of erythrocytes, leukocytes, and platelets; "yellow marrow" is considered hematopoietically inactive and is composed predominantly of fat cells. Red marrow contains approximately 40% water, 40% fat, and 20% protein; yellow marrow contains approximately 15% water, 80% fat, and 5% protein. Conversion of red marrow to yellow marrow normally occurs during growth and development in an orderly fashion. In the fetus, almost the entire marrow space is composed of red marrow; in the postnatal period, conversion from red marrow to yellow marrow begins, starting with the extremities. This conversion progresses from appendicular

toward axial sites with respect to the skeleton as a whole and from diaphyseal to metaphyseal areas in individual long tubular bones. An adult pattern of marrow distribution is normally achieved by the approximate age of 25 years. At this time, red marrow is concentrated in the axial skeleton (skull, vertebrae, ribs, sternum, and pelvis) and in the proximal portions of the appendicular skeleton (proximal femurs and humeri). Alterations in the body's demand for hematopoiesis may provoke a reconversion of yellow marrow to red marrow, a process that follows the initial conversion of red to yellow in reverse, with initial conversion in the axial skeleton and subsequent conversion in the extremities in a proximal to distal direction.

Routine radiography is insensitive to changes in the bone marrow that accompany pathologic states. It has long been known that much bone destruction is required before conventional radiographic findings become abnormal. Radionuclide evaluation of the bone marrow can be accomplished by direct or indirect methods. Direct methods

Computed Tomography

CT can be used to evaluate disorders of bone marrow by measuring the attenuation of the X-ray beam by the marrow elements. The attenuation produced by fat is low, so that CT images of bones that contain predominantly fatty marrow have low-density marrow, on the order of −100 Hounsfield units (HU). With replacement of marrow fat by edema, exudate, or cellular proliferation, X-ray attenuation increases accordingly and the corresponding region in the bone marrow appears denser on the CT examination. It is this change that enables CT to be used to diagnose infectious or neoplastic disorders or other processes in the bone marrow. It should be noted, however, that some variability exists in the attenuation of the X-ray beam in different regions of a bone; therefore, comparison with a patient's opposite (normal) side is required. A difference of 20 HU in the diaphyseal marrow of a long tubular bone between the two sides of the body generally is considered abnormal. Variability is greater in the metaphyseal and epiphyseal regions of the tubular bones, creating some diagnostic difficulty during the interpretation of the examination. Still, the CT analysis of marrow attenuation has many clinical applications, including the evaluation of the osseous extent of neoplastic and infectious disorders.

Magnetic Resonance Imaging

Of all the available imaging methods, MRI has the greatest potential in the assessment of marrow abnormalities. Fat is the major contribution to the marrow signal pattern. Yellow marrow, in which fat predominates, is characterized by a relatively bright signal intensity of T_1-weighted image sequences and by intermediate signal intensity on T_2-weighted sequences. Hematopoietic or red marrow shows different signal characteristics; typically, its signal is less intense than that of fatty marrow but more intense than muscle on T_1-weighted images and is variable in intensity on T_2-weighted images, with the specific signal characteristics being determined by the fractions of fat, water, and protein present.

A recent investigation classified disorders of the bone marrow into five broad groups:

Reconversion The first pattern, designated reconversion, indicates reversal of the process of marrow conversion from red marrow to yellow marrow that normally occurs with advancing age. Reconversion, therefore, is characterized by transformation of yellow marrow to red marrow, which may be related to anemia or marrow replacement disorders, such as myeloma, myelofibrosis, and metastasis. The resultant expansion of red marrow is accompanied by a decreased signal intensity on T_1-weighted images and a variable appearance on T_2-weighted images, changes that may occur in a diffuse or focal distribution. The extent of reconversion is a reflection of the severity of the stimulating process; severe or chronic anemia, such as sickle cell anemia, results in a greater degree of reconversion of marrow. The resultant MRI appearance lacks specificity because it resembles that seen in other processes, including neoplasms.

Marrow Infiltration The second pattern is marrow infiltration or replacement, and generally indicates a tumor (lymphoma, leukemia, multiple myeloma metastasis, and primary bone neoplasms) or infection. Many of these lesions

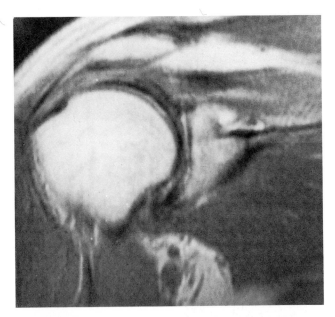

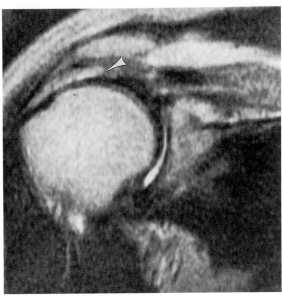

Figure 14

Full-thickness rotator cuff tear. T_1-weighted **(top)** and T_2-weighted **(bottom)** oblique coronal images of the shoulder show disruption of the fibers of the supraspinatus tendon. Fluid in the torn tendon (arrowhead) and joint are readily apparent in the T_2-weighted image. (Reproduced with permission from Michael Zlatkin, MD, Philadelphia, Pennsylvania.)

include physiologic assessment of either hematopoiesis or phagocytosis. In the evaluation of hematopoiesis, active erythroid precursors are targeted and erythropoietic marrow is imaged. Assessment includes the incorporation of a transferrin-bound isotope, such as radioactive iron. To assess phagocytosis, the cells of the reticuloendothelial system are targeted and imaged. One technique assesses the removal of a radioactive colloid from the blood, such as ^{99m}Tc sulfur colloid.

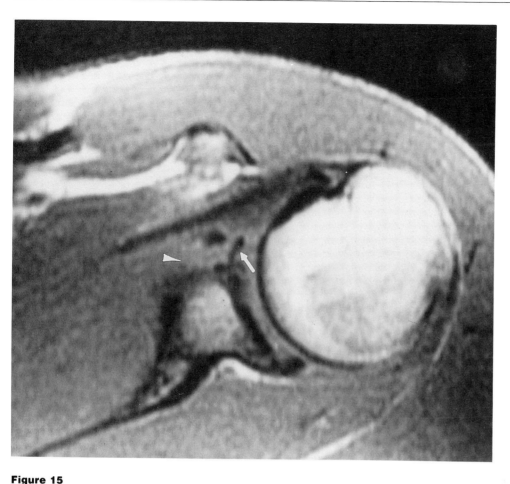

Figure 15
Glenohumeral joint instability. On magnetic resonance imaging, a transaxial T_1-weighted image reveals irregularity of the anterior portion of the glenoid labrum (arrow) and fluid in the subscapular recess (arrowhead). Note the normal appearance of the posterior portion of the glenoid labrum and a Hill-Sachs deformity of the humeral head. (Reproduced with permission from Michael Zlatkin, MD, Philadelphia, Pennsylvania.)

predominate in regions of the skeleton in which red marrow is present. Although the MRI characteristics of these infiltrative lesions are somewhat variable, all demonstrate decreased signal intensity on T_1-weighted images (Fig. 10). Certain of these processes, such as primary bone tumors, metastatic lesions, and infections generally increase signal intensity on T_2-weighted sequences, whereas others, such as leukemia, lymphoma, myelofibrosis, and Gaucher's disease, may be characterized by low or intermediate signal intensity on T_2-weighted sequences.

Myeloid Depletion The third pattern is termed myeloid depletion. Processes that result in depletion of myeloid or hematopoietic cells include aplastic anemia, radiation therapy, and chemotherapy. These disorders produce MRI signal patterns characteristic of fatty marrow on T_1- and T_2-weighted sequences. This fact has obvious clinical significance; for example, it now is possible to differentiate between areas of tumor recurrence and radiation effects, underscoring the importance of this imaging method in monitoring the therapeutic response of neoplasms.

Bone Marrow Edema The fourth pattern is bone marrow edema and may accompany trauma, stress reaction, reflex sympathetic dystrophy syndrome, and transient region os-

teoporosis; it also occurs about regions of tumor, infection, or ischemia (Fig. 11). The common pathophysiologic alteration in these conditions is increased extracellular water in the marrow. This change accounts for decreased signal intensity on T_1-weighted images and increased signal intensity on T_2-weighted images.

Bone Marrow Ischemia in Osteonecrosis The final pattern is the bone marrow ischemia that occurs in subarticular osteonecrosis or metadiaphyseal bone infarction. This pattern has been studied most extensively in patients with osteonecrosis of the femoral head. Osteonecrosis predominates in areas of fatty rather than hematopoietic marrow, perhaps because the blood supply to the yellow marrow is more vulnerable. Interestingly, MRI has identified increased amounts of fatty marrow in the proximal portion of the femur in patients with nontraumatic ischemic necrosis of bone. Although many studies have confirmed the high sensitivity of MRI in the diagnosis of osteonecrosis and its superiority in this regard to routine radiography, CT, planar scintigraphy, and, probably, SPECT, it appears probable that the diagnosis is sometimes delayed even when MRI is used. The signal alterations appear to correspond to changes in marrow fat; it is known that fat cells are more resistant to ischemia than are hematopoietic cells,

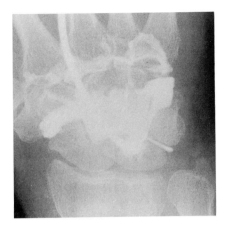 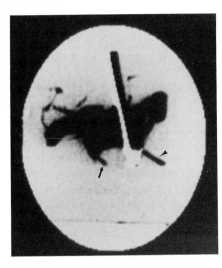 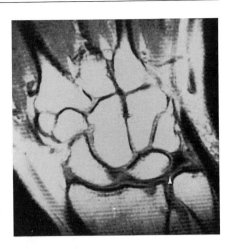

Figure 16

Scapholunate ligament and triangular fibrocartilage disruption. **Left,** A routine radiographic image during the midcarpal compartment injection reveals absence of filling of the scapholunate space (an abnormal finding). Contrast material fills the space between the lunate and triquetrum (a normal finding); absence of filling of the radiocarpal compartment indicates that the lunate-triquetral ligament is intact. **Center,** A digital subtraction arthrogram shows the contrast material in the lunate-triquetral space (arrowhead). Note irregular filling of the scapholunate space (arrow), an abnormal finding consistent with the presence of scar tissue at the site of scapholunate ligament disruption. **Right,** A coronal T_1-weighted magnetic resonance image confirms a tear of the scapholunate ligament with scapholunate widening, or dissociation, and a tear of the triangular fibrocartilage (arrowhead). At surgery, both the scapholunate ligament and triangular fibrocartilage tears were evident.

osteoblasts, osteocytes, and osteoclasts and that fat cells may survive for two to five days after ischemic insult. Further, it is possible that MRI signal abnormalities may not coincide with the death of the fat cells because the signal is derived primarily from depot lipid. These observations may explain why MRI abnormalities are delayed in patients with developing osteonecrosis of the femoral head or elsewhere.

Several different MRI patterns have been described in association with ischemic necrosis of the femoral head, but a finding on the T_1-weighted image that is common to all these patterns is diminished signal intensity within a background of bright signal corresponding to the fatty marrow (Fig. 12). Specific MRI patterns include homogeneous areas of low signal, nonhomogeneous areas of mixed signal, and band and ring-like regions of low signal. Although the appearance of osteonecrosis on T_2-weighted image sequences varies, a distinctive pattern has been designated the double-line sign, in which a band of low signal intensity contains an inner border of brighter signal intensity. It is important to realize that whatever the specific MRI signal pattern, the changes of osteonecrosis are usually localized to the superior portions of the bone. More diffuse regions of low signal intensity that involve large portions of the femoral head on T_1-weighted images are more compatible with alternative diagnoses, including synovitis, transient osteoporosis of the hip, and transient bone marrow edema.

To date, the MRI patterns of osteonecrosis have not been correlated with the accepted classification systems based on routine radiographs. Further, insufficient data exist to determine whether MRI is as effective as plain films or conventional tomography for following the progresson of the disease process.

Internal Derangements of Joints

In no other facet of musculoskeletal disease has MRI imaging had more impact than in the evaluation of internal joint derangements. Indications for arthrography, traditionally considered the primary imaging technique in the analysis of a wide variety of joint abnormalities, have been narrowed cosiderably by MRI; further refinements in MRI technology may lead to the abandonment of arthrographic examinations.

Knee

The first peripheral joint to be studied extensively with MRI was the knee. This technique is both sensitive and specific in the diagnosis of abnormalities of the menisci, cruciate and collateral ligaments, quadriceps mechanism, and, to a lesser extent, articular cartilage. The sensitivity of MRI to alterations in the fibrocartilage of the meniscus has led to the development of a classification system that recognizes three types of signal change. Grade I findings indicate the presence of one or several punctate areas of increased signal intensity within the normally dark signal of the meniscus. These areas of hyperintense signal, which do not violate the surface of the meniscus, correspond to myxoid changes within the substance of the meniscus. Grade II findings represent a linear intrameniscal hyperintense signal intensity that, again, is not associated with disruption of the surface of the meniscus. This finding, too, correlates with myxoid changes in the meniscus. Grade III findings are characterized by an area of increased signal intensity that communicates with at least one meniscal surface (Fig. 13). Although both the clinical significance of grade I and grade II changes and whether or not such changes progress to grade III findings are not known, grade

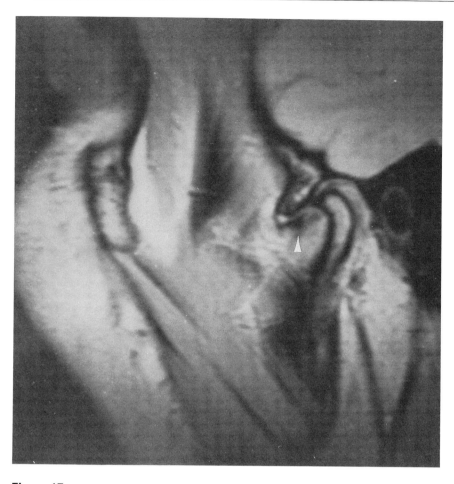

Figure 17

Temporomandibular joint dysfunction. On magnetic resonance imaging, a coronal T_1-weighted image of the closed temporomandibular joint shows that the dark signal of the meniscus (arrowhead) is located abnormally in front of the mandibular condyle. This is diagnostic of a dislocated meniscus.

III alterations do correspond to tears or disruption of the meniscus. Additional signs of meniscal disruption evident on MRI are similar to those delineated by arthrography and include foreshortening, blunting, and irregularity of the meniscal surface. In studies in which only grade III signals were considered consistent with meniscal tears, there was more than 90% agreement between MRI and surgical findings. Further, in those cases in which the MRI findings suggested a tear and arthroscopy did not, the discrepancy may have reflected false-negative arthroscopy rather than false-positive MRI. As in arthrography, diagnostic difficulties occasionally occur during MRI because of obscuration of the posterior portion of the lateral meniscus by the popliteus tendon and sheath.

Although fewer studies have concerned the accuracy of MRI in the detection of abnormalities of the cruciate ligaments, one report indicated an overall accuracy of 95% in the assessment of the anterior cruciate ligament, and another study has shown MRI to be superior to clinical tests in detecting abnormalities of this ligament.

Additional applications of MRI to the knee include the assessment of patellofemoral abnormalities, chondromalacia patellae, osteochondritis dissecans, and synovial or meniscal cysts.

Shoulder

The data describing the effectiveness of MRI in the evaluation of shoulder disorders are less complete, although preliminary reports have indicated that it can delineate full-thickness tears of the rotator cuff with an accuracy of more than 90%. It is sometimes difficult to differentiate between tendinitis and partial tears of the rotator cuff, although further refinements in surface-coil design should make MRI the standard imaging technique for assessment of all problems of the rotator cuff, including the shoulder impingement syndrome (Fig. 14). On the basis of anecdotal reports, it also appears that MRI is capable of defining labral, ligamentous, and capsular alterations that accompany subluxations and dislocations of the glenohumeral joint (Fig. 15).

Other Articular Problems

Other types of articular problems investigated in a preliminary fashion by MRI include the evaluation of the triangular fibrocartilage and interosseous ligaments in the wrist (Fig. 16) and of the ligaments about the elbow and ankle. More extensive data are available concerning the use of MRI in the assessment of temporomandibular joint

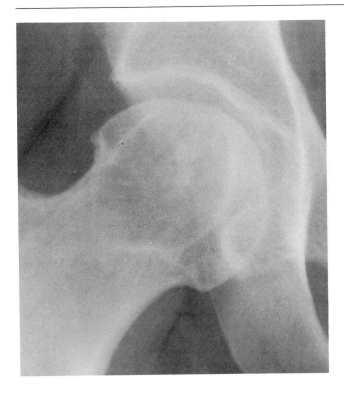 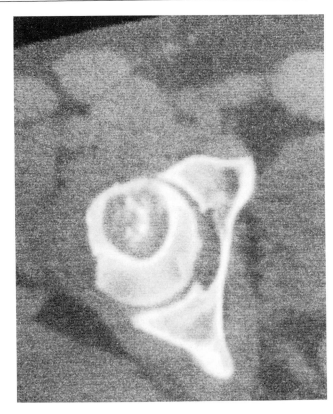

Figure 18

Left, A large, well-defined osteolytic lesion occupies the femoral head. It contains calcifications and is surrounded by a sclerotic margin. **Right,** Transaxial computed tomography exquisitely demonstrates the calcification within the tumor. Although the appearance is similar to that of a chondroblastoma, clear cell chondrosarcoma is a more appropriate diagnosis because the patient is an adult. (Reproduced with permission from Guerdon Greenway, MD, Dallas, Texas.)

dysfunction; the technique has been found to be useful in the diagnosis of displacement of the meniscus and less helpful in defining meniscal perforation (Fig. 17).

Neoplastic Disorders

Most recent radiographic investigations of neoplasms of bone or soft tissue have continued to compare the advantages and disadvantages of available imaging methods in the initial diagnosis of these tumors and in the assessment of their extent and response to treatment. With regard to osseous tumors confined to bone, MRI has been found to be excellent in defining the intraosseous extent of the neoplasm but, in some studies, has not been shown to be significantly better than CT (Fig. 18) or scintigraphy in this regard. Further, MRI is known to be inferior to routine radiography and CT in the evaluation of calcification, ossification, cortical destruction, and endosteal or periosteal reaction (Fig. 19). For soft-tissue tumors and for bone tumors with soft-tissue extension, MRI has been found to be significantly better than other imaging methods (Fig. 20). The interpretation of the MRI findings in soft-tissue involvement is not without difficulty, however; indeed, the detection of areas of high signal intensity in the soft tissues on T_2-weighted images, although consistent with tumor extension, is not specific because this intensity may also be caused by edema. This potential diagnostic pitfall was a significant cause of error in an evaluation of 50 patients

with a variety of musculoskeletal disorders, including malignant neoplasms.

Because of inconsistencies in reports comparing CT, scintigraphy, and MRI in the assessment of neoplastic processes of the bone or soft tissues, further studies are needed to define the role of each of these imaging methods. On the basis of the available data, it seems probable that these further investigations will indicate that the imaging evaluation must be tailored to the specific situation being examined; factors such as the age of the patient and the type and location of the lesion will presumably influence the imaging protocol. What is clear at this time is that MRI characteristics are generally not specific for a single diagnosis in patients with osseous and soft-tissue neoplasms. Routine radiography remains superior in providing a more specific diagnosis in instances of bone neoplasms. CT and MRI are certainly superior to routine radiography in the investigation of soft-tissue tumors, although, in most cases, a specific diagnosis with either of these imaging methods is not possible. Exceptions to this rule include the assessment of lesions containing fat (Figs. 21 and 22), which can be readily identified with CT or MRI, and those containing fibrous tissue or blood, which may be suspected on the basis of the MRI examination.

Contrast-enhanced MRI and positron emission tomography have been investigated in a preliminary fashion in patients with musculoskeletal neoplasms. Preliminary data suggest that these techniques may be helpful in the detection or further delineation of a tumor, but additional investigation of these methods is needed.

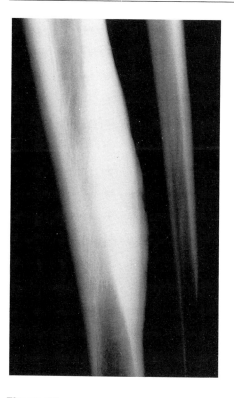 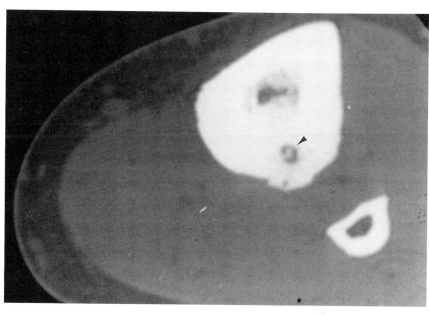

Figure 19

Osteoid osteoma. **Left,** A routine radiograph reveals cortical thickening involving a long segment of the tibia. No nidus is seen. **Right,** Transaxial computed tomography shows the calcified nidus (arrowhead), establishing the correct diagnosis. (Reproduced with permission from Brigette Martin, MD, Paris, France.)

Traumatic Disorders

Recent investigations regarding imaging of traumatic disorders of the musculoskeletal system have emphasized the employment of standard or three-dimensional CT (Figs. 23 and 24). The results of these investigations support the use of this technique, particularly in assessment of fractures or dislocations in anatomically complex regions, such as the spine, shoulder, hip, osseous pelvis, calcaneus, and facial bones.

A variety of techniques have been used to analyze fracture nonunion. Routine radiography and CT may be effective in establishing nonunion in some patients, although the presence of orthopaedic hardware leads to significant degradation of image quality in certain patients. CT with multiplanar reconstruction of the image data represents an effective alternative in such patients, providing a more detailed assessment of malalignment and angular deformities, the magnitude of the gap at the fracture site, and the integrity of the adjacent weightbearing joints. The role of MRI, particularly spectroscopy, in the evaluation of delayed union or nonunion of fractures is not yet clear, although the ability of spectroscopy to measure the pH at the fracture site may prove to be helpful in the evaluation of fracture healing.

Metabolic Disorders

Considerable interest in the quantitative assessment of bone mineral content in recent years has led to many investigations that have produced conflicting results. Controversy continues about the clinical significance of quantitative bone mineral assessment and the best techniques to accomplish this assessment. One method, single-photon absorptiometry (SPA), measures mineral content in the appendicular skeleton and is usually performed on the radius or calcaneus. This technique has been criticized for its tendency to reflect the status of peripheral long bones, which are predominantly cortical and not necessarily the more critical sites of fracture or the entire skeleton.

Unlike SPA, which uses a monoenergetic source such as iodine 125, dual-photon absorptiometry (DPA) uses a radioisotope (gadolinium 153) that emits photons at two different energy levels. This method eliminates the need for a constant soft-tissue thickness across the scan path, allowing its use in areas such as the spine and femur. The radiation does involve a 5 to 15 × 10⁻⁵ Gy exposure. Because DPA integrates compact and cancellous bone, its sensitivity as compared with that of quantitative CT (QCT), which can successfully measure trabecular bone, is believed to be low. Further, density contributed by osteophytes or vascular calcifications may falsely increase DPA determinations. The reliability of this technique in the spine also is reduced by vertebral compression with callus formation, scoliosis, and diskogenic sclerosis. DPA, however, has some desirable characteristics; these include the capability of assessing vertebral, proximal femoral, or total-body bone content independent of the effects of marrow fat and other soft tissues, a relatively low radiation dose, and a 2% to 5% error rate for precision and accuracy.

QCT requires a mineral reference standard such as po-

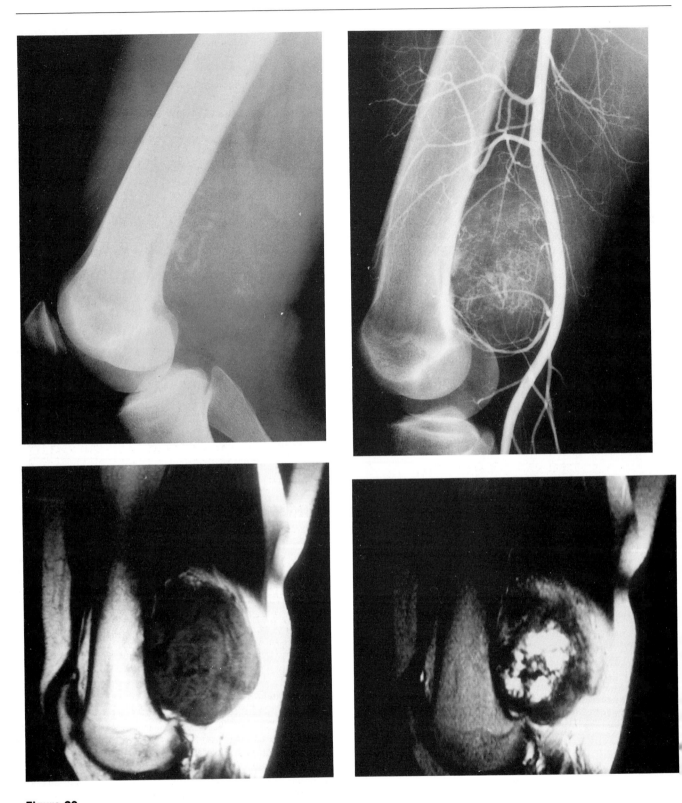

Figure 20

High-grade osteosarcoma of the bone surface. **Top left,** A lateral radiograph reveals a large soft-tissue mass containing ossification and leading to erosion of the posterior surface of the femur. **Top right,** The tumor is hypervascular and contains neoplastic vessels. **Bottom,** Magnetic resonance imaging. T_1-weighted **(bottom left)** and T_2-weighted **(bottom right)** images reveal the full extent of the neoplasm. The signal intensity is low on the T_1-weighted image but areas of high signal intensity appear on the T_2-weighted image. The bone marrow appears to be free of tumor. (Reproduced with permission from Guerdon Greenway, MD, Dallas, Texas.)

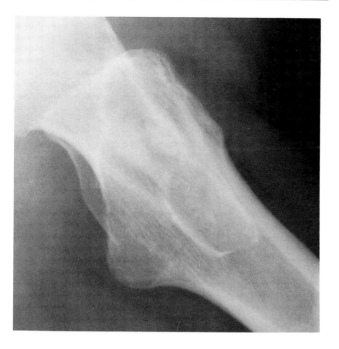

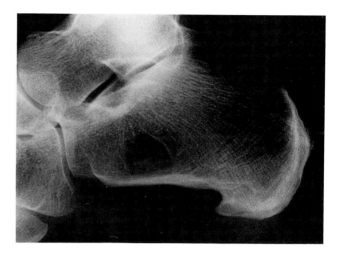

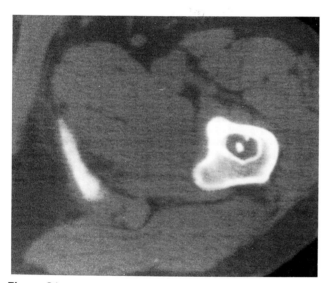

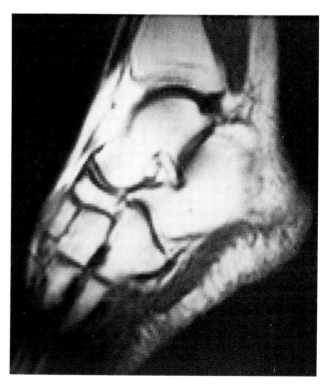

Figure 21

Intraosseous lipoma. **Top,** A lobulated lesion containing calcification is evident in the proximal portion of the femur. **Bottom,** A transaxial computed tomographic scan shows the well-defined lesion and the calcification. Note that the tissue within the tumor is of the same density as the subcutaneous fat, confirming the diagnosis of a lipoma.

Figure 22

Intraosseous lipoma. **Top,** A well-defined lesion is evident in the calcaneus. The appearance is consistent with either a simple cyst or a lipoma. **Bottom,** On a parasagittal T_1-weighted magnetic resonance image, the bright signal in the area of the lesion confirms the presence of fat.

tassium phosphate (K_2HPO_4) for calibration and a scout view for localization. Data derived from scanning the midportion of the vertebral bodies are averaged and used in conjunction with calibration results to calculate mineral equivalent values. The accuracy of single-energy QCT is variable and depends on the amount of fat in the bone marrow. Dual-energy QCT provides more accurate determination of bone mineral content independent of fat and water variation, but at the expense of reduced precision. Radiation exposure from QCT studies of vertebral trabec-

ular bone is variable but significant, on the order of 2 to 2.5×10^{-3} Gy.

QCT can be used to measure cancellous bone, cortical bone, or an integrated sum of both. The selected measurement of cancellous bone is a more sensitive means of quantifying change in metabolic bone diseases. QCT, however, may produce measurements that are falsely lower by 20% to 25% in elderly, osteoporotic persons because the concentration of marrow fat increases with age.

Assessment of trabecular bone density in the proximal

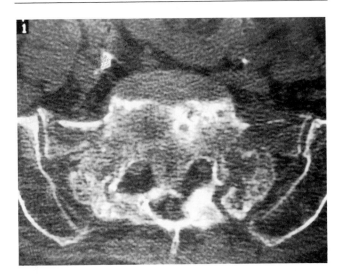

Figure 23

Insufficiency type of stress fracture of the sacrum. Transaxial computed tomography defines a comminuted fracture involving both sides of the sacrum. This is a recognized site of a stress fracture in elderly patients with osteoporosis.

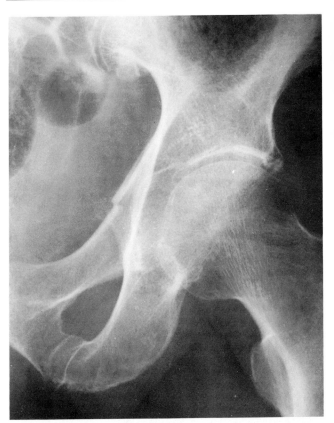

portion of the femur cannot be done with the single-slice CT strategy used for vertebral mineral measurements because of the inherent complexity of the femur's trabecular architecture and geometry. Three-dimensional histographic analysis overcomes this problem but requires expensive software systems that can analyze the CT data further. Although the three-dimensional technique has advantages over the single-slice method in the spine as well, the process is currently too time-consuming to have clinical applications.

A recent and exciting advance in the quantitative assessment of bone mineral content has been the development of an innovative approach that employs dual-energy radiographic absorptiometry (DRA). The technique, which can be used to evaluate the spine, hip, and other sites, is similar in concept to DPA but relies on an X-ray tube rather than a radioisotope source. Because of this modification, DRA can measure a skeletal area with higher resolution and greater speed than existing DPA instruments. More importantly, DRA makes possible a major improvement in precision (Table 1). Further investigation of DRA is needed, but the initial results have been impressive. Additional techniques used in the evaluation of bone mineral content, such as neutron activation analysis and Compton scattering, remain experimental.

Arthritic Disorders

Among the many recent advancements in the area of arthritic disorders, two deserve emphasis. Although the three most common crystalline-induced articular disorders—gout, calcium pyrophosphate dihydrate (CPPD) crystal deposition disease, and calcium hydroxyapatite crystal deposition disease—are easily recognized, the recent attention to coexistence of hydroxyapatite and CPPD crystals in a single joint has led to the designation of mixed calcium phosphate crystal deposition.

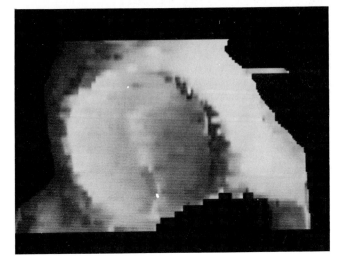

Figure 24

Pelvic fracture with intact acetabulum. **Top,** A routine radiograph shows disruption of the iliopubic line. The lateral extent of the fracture cannot be defined. **Bottom,** A three-dimensional computed tomographic image in which the image data have been manipulated to remove the femoral head so that the lateral portion of the acetabulum can be seen. No acetabular fracture is evident.

Both crystals can cause an inflammatory response and both are associated with cartilage degeneration and a degenerative arthropathy. When the crystals occur together, it is difficult to identify precisely their relative roles in the production of joint damage or, for that matter, to ascertain

Table 1. Bone mineral measurement systems

Measurement	Single-Photon Absorptiometry	Dual-Photon Absorptiometry	Single-Energy Quantitative Computed Tomography	Dual-Energy Radiographic Absorptiometry
Radiation source	^{125}I	^{153}Gd	X-ray	X-ray
Dose (skin exposure)	6 to 18 × 10⁻⁵ Gy	1 to 10 × 10⁻⁵ Gy	1 to 10 × 10⁻³ Gy	3 × 10⁻⁵ Gy
Examination sites	Distal radius, os calcis	Spine, femur	Spine, femur	Spine, femur, total body
Source renewal	6 months	12 to 18 months	Not applicable	Not applicable
Precision				
In vitro (cv*)	1% to 2%	1% to 2%	0.5%	0.4%
In vivo (cv*)	3%	2% to 3%	1.3%	1%
Error rate	1%	1% to 3%	5% to 15%	1%
Type of measurement	Integral	Integral	Trabecular	Integral
Fat error relevant	No	No	Yes	No

*Coefficient of variation.

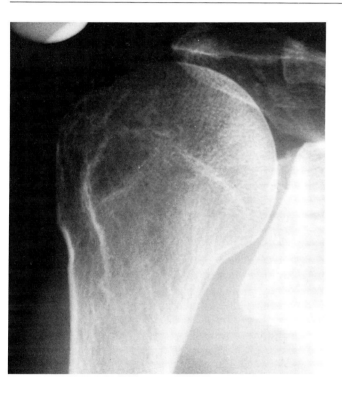
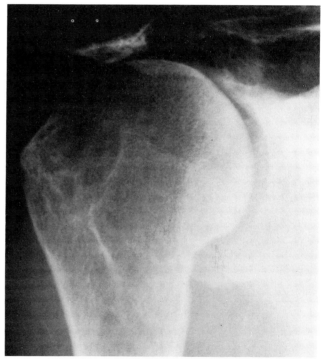

Figure 25

Hydroxyapatite crystal deposition disease in the glenohumeral joint. Two radiographs of the shoulder obtained four years apart reveal a rotator cuff tear with elevation of the humeral head with respect to the glenoid cavity. In the later film **(right),** protrusion of the glenoid cavity is apparent, and erosion, osteophytes, and bone sclerosis are evident. These findings are consistent with intra-articular accumulation of hydroxyapatite crystals. This has been called "Milwaukee shoulder" by rheumatologists and cuff arthropathy by orthopaedic surgeons. (Reproduced with permission from Vinton Vint, MD, San Diego, California.)

whether the combination of these two crystals is more significant than the presence of one alone. The radiographic findings associated with CPPD crystal deposition disease include abnormal calcification, particularly of cartilage (chondrocalcinosis), and destructive joint damage (pyrophosphate arthropathy) that resembles osteoarthritis but affects unusual sites (for example, the compartment of the wrist or the patellofemoral compartment of the knee) and leads to more rapid destructive changes than ordinary osteoarthritis. In hydroxyapatite crystal deposition disease, in addition to calcific tendinitis, a destructive arthropathy, especially in the shoulder (Fig. 25) and knee, may be ev-

ident. Orthopaedic surgeons should be alert to the possibility that crystal deposition disorders may superficially resemble ordinary osteoarthritis.

A destructive spondyloarthropathy was recently observed in a number of patients with chronic renal failure who had been undergoing long-term hemodialysis (Fig. 26). The changes are primarily in the cervical and lumbar segments of the vertebral column and are manifested as subluxation, disk space narrowing and erosion, and sclerosis of subchondral bone in the vertebral body. These findings resemble those of infection. Although interpretation of biopsy specimens from affected sites has been in-

appear to be the most likely cause of this destructive spondyloarthropathy. What appears certain is that infection is not the causative factor in these severe spinal alterations.

Trends

A review of recent advances in musculoskeletal imaging leaves a clear message. We have entered the age of MRI and, with it, of new ways of evaluating bone, joint, and soft-tissue disorders. Although investigations into the clinical applications of this imaging method are in their infancy, the technique is already regarded as the procedure of choice in the assessment of virtually all soft-tissue processes. Further, its impact on imaging of intra-articular and periarticular structures, including ligaments, tendons, hyaline cartilage, and fibrocartilage, will be dramatic. MRI is expected to replace arthrography and related procedures, such as tenography and bursography. MRI, in all likelihood, will become the primary choice for noninvasive assessment of the spine and its contents. It will also be an important tool in the evaluation of bone marrow disorders, including ischemic necrosis, osteomyelitis, and primary and secondary neoplasms.

Despite a certain sense of euphoria during these early years of MRI, the need for other imaging techniques continues, and some of these techniques certainly will survive and even flourish in the years ahead. Routine radiography remains the most specific of available imaging methods for evaluation of many osseous abnormalities, and this will not change in the near future. CT will continue to be used in the assessment of soft-tissue problems, where it possesses clear advantages over conventional radiography. Further, CT, when compared with MRI, can better define areas of calcification and ossification and the bone cortex itself, and this too will not change in the years ahead. Scintigraphy will continue to be valuable, providing physiologic data that cannot be achieved by many other techniques, and ultrasonography, because of its simplicity, availability, and low cost, will be used to investigate superficial musculoskeletal structures.

Still, the impact of MRI has been extraordinary. With refinement in technique and equipment, the cost of MRI will decrease, the time necessary for completion of the examination will shorten, and spatial resolution will improve.

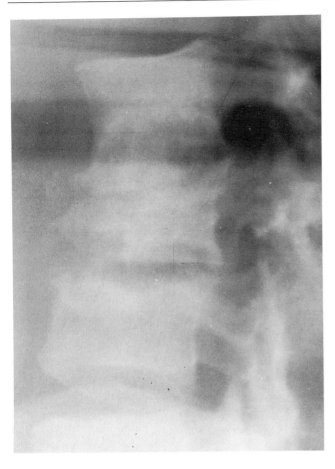

Figure 26
Spondyloarthropathy associated with hemodialysis. A lateral radiograph of the lumbar spine shows the classic features of this recently described disorder. Involvement of three vertebral bodies and two intervertebral disk spaces is evident. Although the appearance is similar to that of infection, the probable cause of the changes appears to be amyloidosis or abnormal crystal deposition.

consistent with regard to the causative agents, leading to the identification of hydroxyapatite, CPPD, or calcium oxalate crystals in some cases, amyloid deposits currently

Annotated Bibliography

Keywords

Absorptiometry; Arteriography; Arthrography; Computed tomography; Diskography; Magnetic resonance imaging; Myelography; Scintigraphy; Ultrasonography

Imaging Techniques

Magnetic Resonance Imaging

Bradley WG Jr: Carmen lecture: Flow phenomena in MR imaging. *AJR* 1988;150:983–994.
This article provides a detailed analysis of flow phenomena encountered during MRI. The author emphasizes that the MRI signal from flowing fluid depends on direction of flow, slice position, slice thickness, and a number of other factors.

Dwyer AJ, Frank JA, Sank VJ, et al: Short-Ti inversion-recovery pulse sequence: Analysis and initial experience in cancer imaging. *Radiology* 1988;168:827–836.
This investigation concerned itself with a description of a pulse sequence that might be useful in the evaluation of tumors, including those of the musculoskeletal system. The

major advantage of this technique is the good contrast achieved between tumor and fat and tumor and muscle in a single image.

Hajek PC, Baker LL, Sartoris DJ, et al: MR arthrography: Anatomic-pathologic investigation. *Radiology* 1987;163:141–147.

The magnetic resonance arthrogram requires that contrast material or saline be placed in the joint before MRI. In this study of 45 fresh cadaveric specimens, some of the created lesions were better detected with magnetic resonance arthrography than with MRI alone.

Konig H, Sauter R, Deimling M, et al: Cartilage disorders: Comparison of spin-echo, CHESS, and FLASH sequence MR images. *Radiology* 1987;164:753–758.

Chemical-shift-selective sequences and fast low-angle shot sequences offer some advantages over the ordinary spin-echo technique. In this investigation, inflammatory, degenerative, and traumatic alterations of the knee, hip, and sacroiliac joint were studied.

Laakman RW, Kaufman B, Han JS, et al: MR imaging in patients with metallic implants. *Radiology* 1985;157:711–714.

This investigation encompassed an analysis of 300 MRI examinations performed in 236 patients with metallic implants. With a low-field-strength magnet, only mild clinical manifestations were evident in individuals with metallic implants, although patients with cardiac pacemakers, electrical implants, prosthetic cardiac valves, and aneurysm clips were excluded from this study.

Pettersson H, Eliasson J, Egund N, et al: Gadolinium-DTPA enhancement of soft tissue tumors in magnetic resonance imaging: Preliminary clinical experience in five patients. *Skeletal Radiol* 1988;17:319–323.

This preliminary report deals with a study of five patients with soft-tissue tumors. Contrast enhancement gave better delineation of the tumor in richly vascularized parts, compressed tissue immediately surrounding the neoplasm, and in atrophic but richly vascularized muscle.

Weiner MW: The promise of magnetic resonance spectroscopy for medical diagnosis. *Invest Radiol* 1988;23:253–261.

This is a detailed analysis of the potential role of spectroscopy in clinical diagnosis.

Computed Tomography

Lobregt S, Kleine Schaars HWG: Three-dimensional imaging and manipulation of CT data: Part I. General principles. *Medicamundi* 1987;32:92–98.

The various phases in the generation of three-dimensional CT images are described, and their clinical usefulness demonstrated by examples from different applications obtained with commercially available systems, as well as with investigational software.

Robertson DD, Walker PS, Granholm JW, et al: Design of custom hip stem prostheses using three-dimensional CT modeling. *J Comput Assist Tomogr* 1987;11:804–809.

The authors describe the methods that allow CT to be used in the design of custom prostheses of the hip. Optimal-fit design was characterized by maximum stem-bone contact while satisfying the requirement that the prosthesis be surgically insertable.

Arthrography

Levinsohn EM, Palmer AK, Coren AB, et al: Wrist arthrography: The value of the three compartment injection technique. *Skeletal Radiol* 1987;16:539–544.

Arthrography employing the three-compartment injection technique was performed in 50 consecutive patients with post-traumatic wrist pain. Many significant abnormalities were identified only when the distal radioulnar and midcarpal joints, in addition to the radiocarpal joint, were injected.

Manaster BJ: Digital wrist arthrography: Precision in determining the site of radiocarpal-midcarpal communication. *AJR* 1986;147:563–566.

The usefulness of digital subtraction arthrography of the wrist was examined. The delineation of scapholunate and lunate-triquetral ligament tears was the major advantage of this technique.

Rafii M, Firooznia H, Golimbu C, et al: CT arthrography of capsular structures of the shoulder. *AJR* 1986;146:361–367.

CT arthrography of the shoulder joint in 45 patients demonstrated the normal and abnormal variations of the joint capsule and particularly the capsular insertions. These CT findings were verified by surgery or arthroscopy in 26 of the cases.

Roy D, Fleury J, Fontaine SB, et al: Clinical evaluation of cervical facet joint infiltration. *J Assoc Can Radiol* 1988;39:118–120.

Twenty-one patients with cervical facet syndrome underwent 39 facet joint injections using corticosteroids. Clinical manifestations were relieved in more than 90% of the patients. Symptoms frequently recurred, however.

Schellhas KP, Wilkes CH, Omlie MR, et al: The diagnosis of temporomandibular joint disease: Two-compartment arthrography and MR. *AJR* 1988;151:341–350.

The reliability and accuracy of two-compartment temporomandibular joint arthrography were compared with those of MRI on the basis of an analysis of surgical findings obtained from joints that had been studied preoperatively with arthrography, MRI or, in some cases, both procedures. The authors recommend MRI as the procedure of choice for the diagnosis of uncomplicated internal derangements of the temporomandibular joint.

Other Invasive Techniques

Gatenby RA, Hartz WH, Rosenblum JS, et al: Percutaneous drainage of intra-articular or paraosseous abscesses in the orthopedic patient. *J Intervent Radiol* 1987;2:69–72.

This is a report of four patients in whom percutaneous drainage was used in the treatment of abscesses involving the disk space, joints, or paraosseous regions.

Onik G, Helms CA, Ginsburg L, et al: Percutaneous lumbar diskectomy using a new aspiration probe. *AJR* 1985;144:1137–1140.

The authors describe a new automated disk-aspiration probe that can be used for percutaneous lumbar diskectomy. A single case report is included to illustrate the clinical application of the technique.

Ultrasonography

Boal DK, Schwenkter EP: The infant hip: Assessment with real-time US. *Radiology* 1985;157:667–672.

Findings of 212 sonograms of infant hips were correlated with those of radiography, orthopaedic examination, or both. There were no false-negative or false-positive results among infants with congenital hip dysplasia. The authors concluded that ultrasonography reveals anatomic detail of the infant hip more accurately than any other currently employed imaging method, including CT.

Harcke HT, Grissom LE, Finkelstein MS: Evaluation of the musculoskeletal system with sonography. *AJR* 1988;150:1253–1261.

This review of the musculoskeletal applications of sonography discusses soft-tissue tumors and tumor-like lesions, foreign bodies, sports injuries, inflammatory conditions, congenital dysplasia of the hip, and other alterations.

Scintigraphy

Collier BD Jr, Hellman RS, Krasnow AZ: Bone SPECT. *Semin Nucl Med* 1987;17:247–266.

The authors present their experience at an institution that has been heavily committed to bone SPECT for more than five years. This information is combined with an analysis of data contained in previous publications. The advantages of SPECT over more routine nuclear tests are reviewed.

Lewin JS, Rosenfield NS, Hoffer PB, et al: Acute osteomyelitis in children: Combined Tc-99m and Ga-67 imaging. *Radiology* 1986;158:795–804.

Thirty-one children were examined for suspected osteomyelitis by a bone scan followed within four days by a gallium scan. Combined gallium and bone scanning increased the accuracy of the scintigraphic diagnosis of acute osteomyelitis. The nonspecificity of both tests, however, is also emphasized.

Maurer AH, Millmond SH, Knight LC, et al: Infection in diabetic osteoarthropathy: Use of indium-labeled leukocytes for diagnosis. *Radiology* 1986;161:221–225.

Imaging of labeled leukocytes was compared with three-phase skeletal scintigraphy as a means of determining whether osteomyelitis was complicating diabetic osteoarthropathy. Abnormal leukocyte localization occurred at all the primary sites of infection in all cases within four hours of injection.

Webb S, Ott RJ, Flower MA, et al: Three-dimensional display of data obtained by single photon emission computed tomography. *Br J Radiol* 1987;60:557–562.

Three-dimensional display of radioactive distributions can be achieved using data generated by SPECT. Computer techniques for constructing these displays are presented.

Wukich DK, Abreu SH, Callaghan JJ, et al: Diagnosis of infection by preoperative scintigraphy with indium-labeled white blood cells. *J Bone Joint Surg* 1987;69A:1353–1360.

This analysis included 50 patients who had suspected osteomyelitis or suspected infection of a total hip prosthesis and who underwent scintigraphy with technetium Tc 99m methylene diphosphate and scintigraphy with indium-labeled leukocytes. The sensitivity and nonspecificity of indium-labeled scintigraphy are emphasized.

Joint Replacement

Bullough PG, DiCarlo EF, Hansraj KK, et al: Pathologic studies of total joint replacement. *Orthop Clin North Am* 1988;19:611–625.

This article reviews some of the important features related to the tissue response to foreign bodies and to prostheses. Debris arising from the polymethylmethacrylate cement was most common; however, fragments of polyethylene or metal were also found within the tissues.

Cheng CL, Gross AE: Loosening of the porous coating in total knee replacement. *J Bone Joint Surg* 1988;70B:377–381.

In a review of 40 cementless knee replacements in 34 pa-

tients, loose beads were identified in 23 knees, more frequently on the tibial side. There was no correlation between the clinical results and the presence of loose beads.

Duus BR, Boeckstyns M, Kjaer L, et al: Radionuclide scanning after total knee replacement: Correlation with pain and radiolucent lines. A prospective study. *Invest Radiol* 1987;22:891–894.

In 35 patients with knee replacements, uptake of the bone-seeking radionuclide was identical in painful and nonpainful knees, and the degree of isotope uptake did not correlate with the development of radiolucent lines around the prosthetic components.

Magnuson JE, Brown ML, Hauser MF, et al: In-111-labeled leukocyte scintigraphy in suspected orthopedic prosthesis infection: Comparison with other imaging modalities. *Radiology* 1988;168:235–239.

In this investigation of 98 patients, positive findings on indium-labeled leukocyte scans and increased erythrocyte sedimentation rates were found to be the most predictive variables in the diagnosis of septic prostheses.

Maus TP, Berquist TH, Bender CE, et al: Arthrographic study of painful total hip arthroplasty: Refined criteria. *Radiology* 1987;162:721–727.

Ninety-seven patients with total hip arthroplasties who had undergone arthrographic study were reviewed. Subtraction arthrography was sensitive in demonstrating loosening of the femoral and acetabular components, but its specificity for demonstrating loosening of the acetabular component was rather low.

Pring DJ, Henderson RG, Rivett AG, et al: Autologous granulocyte scanning of painful prosthetic joints. *J Bone Joint Surg* 1986;68B:647–652.

Autologous indium-labeled granulocyte scanning was used in 60 patients with 74 prosthetic joints. Results indicated that this may be a reliable method of detecting an infected prosthesis.

Resnik CS, Fratkin MJ, Cardea JA: Arthroscintigraphic evaluation of the painful total hip prosthesis. *Clin Nucl Med* 1986;11:242–244.

Arthroscintigraphy was performed in 19 patients with painful total hip prostheses. The advantages and disadvantages of this technique are reviewed.

Rosenthall L, Lepanto L, Raymond F: Radiophosphate uptake in asymptomatic knee arthroplasty. *J Nucl Med* 1987;28:1546–1549.

To characterize the time course of radiophosphate uptake better, bone scans obtained one month to 12 years after surgery were analyzed in 30 asymptomatic patients with 37 total knee replacements. The inadequacies of the scintigraphic examination are emphasized.

Schneider HJ, Weiss MA, Stern PJ: Silicone-induced erosive arthritis: Radiologic features in seven cases. *AJR* 1987;148:923–925.

The authors report seven cases that demonstrated silicone-induced erosive arthritis. Involved joints included the articulations of the hand and foot and the wrist.

Utz JA, Lull RJ, Galvin EG: Asymptomatic total hip prosthesis: Natural history determined using Tc-99m MDP bone scans. *Radiology* 1986;161:509–512.

Technetium bone scans were used in asymptomatic individuals to demonstrate patterns of normal activity that should not be confused with abnormalities.

Intraspinal Disorders

Bundschuh CV, Modic MT, Ross JS, et al: Epidural fibrosis and recurrent disk herniation in the lumbar spine: MR imaging assessment. *AJR* 1988;150:923–932.

Twenty patients were studied prospectively in an evaluation of MRI in epidural scar and herniated intervertebral disks. Morphology, epidural location, mass effect, and signal intensity were important parameters by which scar and disk material could be differentiated with this technique.

Grenier N, Vital J-M, Greselle J-F, et al: CT-diskography in the evaluation of the postoperative lumbar spine: Preliminary results. *Neuroradiology* 1988;30:232–238.

CT-diskography was used successfully in 33 patients with recurrent sciatica after lumbar disk surgery.

Masaryk TJ, Ross JS, Modic MT, et al: High-resolution MR imaging of sequestered lumbar intervertebral disks. *AJR* 1988;150:1155–1162.

The authors reviewed the results of MRI in 20 patients with surgically documented sequestered lumbar disks and concluded that high-resolution MRI is sensitive in detecting disk disease and specifically in characterizing various subtypes of extradural defects.

Modic MT, Masaryk TJ, Ross JS, et al: Imaging of degenerative disk disease. *Radiology* 1988;168:177–186.

This article reviews in great detail the anatomy, biochemistry, and imaging aspects of degenerative disease of the intervertebral disk. Attention is also paid to the accompanying changes within the vertebral body.

Osborn AG, Hood RS, Sherry RG, et al: CT/MR spectrum of far lateral and anterior lumbosacral disk herniations. *AJNR* 1988;9:775–778.

In a study of 48 patients, the authors concluded that MRI and CT are highly accurate, noninvasive methods of delineating extreme lateral lumbar disk herniations.

Pate D, Goobar J, Resnick D, et al: Traction osteophytes of the lumbar spine: Radiographic-pathologic correlation. *Radiology* 1988;166:843–846.

The close correlation between radiographic and pathologic findings allowed the authors to investigate the relationship of claw osteophytes and traction osteophytes occurring on the anterior aspect of the lumbar vertebral bodies.

van den Oever M, Merrick MV, Scott JH: Bone scintigraphy in symptomatic spondylolysis. *J Bone Joint Surg* 1987;69B:453–456.

In a study of 66 patients with back pain and suspected spondylolysis, bone scintigraphy helped to distinguish between those individuals with established nonunion at the spondylolytic defect and those in whom healing was still processing.

Yu SW, Sether LA, Ho PS, et al: Tears of the anulus fibrosus: Correlation between MR and pathologic findings in cadavers. *AJNR* 1988;9:367–370.

The authors correlated MRI with anatomic sections in 20 cadavers to investigate patterns of disruption in the anulus fibrosus. They concluded that MRI is an accurate means of investigating such disruptions.

Bone Marrow Disorders

Mitchell MD, Kundel HL, Steinberg ME, et al: Avascular necrosis of the hip: Comparison of MR, CT, and scintigraphy. *AJR* 1986;147:67–71.

This investigation compared the capabilities of MRI, scintigraphy, and CT in the diagnosis of ischemic necrosis of the femoral head. Evidence is presented that MRI is the most sensitive of these imaging techniques.

Mitchell DG, Rao VM, Dalinka M, et al: Hematopoietic and fatty bone marrow distribution in the normal and

ischemic hip: New observations with 1.5-T MR imaging. *Radiology* 1986;161:199–202.

In an investigation of 50 healthy people and 27 with ischemic necrosis, MRI documented the early conversion to fatty marrow in most patients with ischemic necrosis of the femoral head.

Vogler JB III, Murphy WA: Bone marrow imaging. *Radiology* 1988;168:679–693.

The authors present an extensive review of and classification system for bone marrow disorders. Although many techniques are discussed, MRI is emphasized.

Internal Derangements of Joints

Kneeland JB, Middleton WD, Carrera GF, et al: MR imaging of the shoulder: Diagnosis of rotator cuff tears. *AJR* 1987;149:333–337.

Twenty-five patients with known or suspected tears of the rotator cuff underwent MRI and arthrography or surgery. The results indicated that MRI shows good potential for the diagnosis of rotator cuff disruption.

Mink JH, Levy T, Crues JV III: Tears of the anterior cruciate ligament and menisci of the knee: MR imaging evaluation. *Radiology* 1988;167:769–774.

In a study of a large number of patients with tears of the anterior cruciate ligament or menisci, or both, MRI demonstrated a high degree of accuracy for each of these problems.

Seeger LL, Gold RH, Bassett LW, et al: Shoulder impingement syndrome: MR findings in 53 shoulders. *AJR* 1988;150:343–347.

In an attempt to determine if MRI can be used to depict the abnormalities associated with the impingement syndrome, the authors reviewed 107 scans of painful shoulders. Correlation with arthroscopy or surgery indicated high sensitivity for MRI in such cases.

Stoller DW, Martin C, Crues JV III, et al: Meniscal tears: Pathologic correlation with MR imaging. *Radiology* 1987;163:731–735.

Utilizing material derived from autopsies and amputations, the authors devised an MRI grading system that correlates with the histologic appearance of the menisci.

Neoplastic Disorders

Beltran J, Simon DC, Katz W, et al: Increased MR signal intensity in skeletal muscle adjacent to malignant tumors: Pathologic correlation and clinical relevance. *Radiology* 1987;162:251–255.

The authors evaluated MRI in 50 patients with musculoskeletal disorders. One pattern of abnormality, increased signal on T_2-weighted images, was nonspecific, occurring in both muscular edema and muscular invasion by tumor.

Kern KA, Brunetti A, Norton JA, et al: Metabolic imaging of human extremity musculoskeletal tumors by PET. *J Nucl Med* 1988;29:181–186.

This study indicated that positron emission tomography (PET) can be used to image and evaluate the metabolic activity of human musculoskeletal tumors.

Pettersson H, Gillespy T III, Hamlin DJ, et al: Primary musculoskeletal tumors: Examination with MR imaging compared with conventional modalities. *Radiology* 1987;164:237–241.

This investigation dealt with 176 cases of primary musculoskeletal tumors in which MRI was done. The authors compare the advantages and disadvantages of this technique, CT, and routine radiography.

Traumatic Disorders

Kuhlman JE, Fishman EK, Magid D, et al: Fracture nonunion: CT assessment with multiplanar reconstruction. *Radiology* 1988;167:483–488.

Nineteen patients with suspected or possible fracture nonunion underwent CT with multiplanar reconstruction. The technique demonstrated nonunion in 13 cases. The authors believe it is an important new technique for evaluating fracture nonunion.

Newman RJ, Francis MJ, Duthie RB: Nuclear magnetic resonance studies of experimentally induced delayed fracture union. *Clin Orthop* 1987;216:253–261.

In an experimental study of fracture union in the rat tibia, phosphorus magnetic resonance spectroscopy was used to monitor local pH changes that occurred at the fracture site throughout repair.

Metabolic Disorders

Bhasin S, Sartoris DJ, Fellingham L, et al: Three-dimensional quantitative CT of the proximal femur: Relationship to vertebral trabecular bone density in postmenopausal women. *Radiology* 1988;167:145–149.

As an adjunct to standard quantitative CT in the assessment of vertebral trabecular bone, a three-dimensional technique was introduced. This technique allows analysis of bone mineral content in the proximal portion of the femur and selectively measures cortical, cancellous, and total bone density.

Arthritic Disorders

Halverson PB, McCarty DJ: Patterns of radiographic abnormalities associated with basic calcium phosphate and calcium pyrophosphate dihydrate crystal deposition in the knee. *Ann Rheum Dis* 1986;45:603–605.

Radiographs and synovial fluid collections in 66 knees of patients with osteoarthritis were evaluated to determine the pattern of radiographic abnormalities associated with basic calcium phosphate crystals, calcium pyrophosphate dihydrate crystals, or both crystals together.

Rafto SE, Dalinka MK, Schiebler ML, et al: Spondyloarthropathy of the cervical spine in long-term hemodialysis. *Radiology* 1988;166:201–204.

In five patients with a peculiar pattern of destructive spondyloarthropathy, the cervical spine was involved. Each of the patients was undergoing long-term hemodialysis.

2
Bone Metabolism and Metabolic Bone Disease

Bone metabolism is the study of bone cells, their growth and development, the bone matrix they produce, and how they control mineral metabolism. Calcitropic hormones such as vitamin D, parathyroid hormone, and possibly calcitonin regulate the growth, maturation, and function of bone cells. Therefore, identifying and understanding the roles of these hormones is important to the study of bone metabolism. Ultimately, these studies will elucidate how the functional architecture of bone develops and how structure and function are altered in disease.

Mature bone cells, osteoblasts, and osteocytes originate from local mesenchymal cells, while osteoclasts arise from precursor cells within the marrow. Differentiated bone cells, in close apposition to bone matrix, are responsible for creating, maintaining, and remodeling bone architecture. The resulting structure enables bone to perform its physical, mechanical, and metabolic activities within the body. Hormones, produced outside as well as within bone, regulate the bone cells throughout their ontogeny (growth and differentiation). These signal molecules, along with mechanical stimuli, regulate the day-to-day function of bone cells as they modulate the synthesis, repair, and removal of matrix elements. This ongoing process constitutes bone metabolism.

Cellular Control of Bone Metabolism

The cellular elements of bone respond to a number of "nonspecific" stimuli such as mechanical, electrical, and chemical gradients. Although these stimuli are identified as nonspecific, their direction of application (mechanical and electrical), their intensity and frequency (electric and magnetic fields), and their physicochemical nature (ion gradients) can elicit specific responses from individual classes of bone cells. Bone cells also present specific receptors for a vast array of calcitropic hormones. Therefore, bone cell metabolism can be regulated through the classic sequence of hormone-receptor interaction, followed by membrane or nuclear transduction. The latter sequence causes the activation of intracellular second messengers that produce specific changes or a sequence of changes in cell growth or metabolism. Although the effects of specific molecular signal molecules (hormones) are rapid, the consequences of the nonspecific stimuli (mechanical, electrical, and chemical) factors eventually modify the biomechanical properties of bone. Ultimately, the sum of these stimuli determines bone cell ontogeny and function.

Osteoblasts and Osteocytes

Methods of identifying the mesenchymal or stromal precursor cells that give rise to osteoblasts have not yet been found, so it has been impossible to estimate the number of osteoprogenitor stem cells or to determine whether the pluripotent stem cells are self-renewing. Nor is it known how or by what hormonal stimulus these cells become committed to the bone cell lineage. Much needs to be learned about the ontogeny of these cells. Preliminary studies demonstrate that select populations of committed osteoblasts express specific receptors for calcitropic hormones such as parathyroid hormone. This suggests that cell-to-cell signaling can occur within committed bone cell precursors. The production and release of paracrine substances (locally produced and locally active hormones such as the prostaglandins and cytokines), as well as classic calcitropic hormones, are thought to be responsible for the coupling of osteoblast and osteoclast function.

The more differentiated, tall osteoblasts that line bone surfaces where bone formation is occurring are metabolically active cells dedicated to the synthesis and release of the organic matrix elements of bone. Among the matrix elements produced by osteoblasts are type I collagen, osteocalcin (a Gla-protein), and osteonectin. Important regulatory factors (including endocrine, paracrine, and autocrine regulators) produced by these osteoblasts include alkaline phosphatase, collagenase, collagenase inhibitor, plasminogen activator, interleukin-1, and prostaglandin E_2. Flat, metabolically quiescent cells "lining the resting regions" of bone probably consist of metabolically inactive osteoblasts. These lining cells, along with the entrapped osteocytes, are thought to be important in maintaining the ionic milieu of bone. Lining osteoblasts and osteocytes are connected through a network of slender cell processes that traverse the microcanaliculi of bone and form gap junctions. Rapid fluxes of bone calcium induced by parathyroid hormone are thought to be mediated by these cellular elements.

Activation of mature osteoblasts and osteocytes to states of high metabolic activity can result from a variety of physical and chemical signals. Activation of osteoblasts at specific bone sites is thought to occur after disruption of the lining-cell layer that covers the bone surface. This exposure of the matrix may be caused by contraction of the lining cells, which could be hormonally mediated by parathyroid hormone or prostaglandin E. Subsequent molecular alteration of the underlying matrix may result from osteoblast release of collagenase or enzyme release by mononucleated or multinucleated phagocytic cells (monocytes and osteoclasts) lining the matrix. After cellular activation, signal molecules normally buried within the bone matrix are released. These released signal molecules, which have mitogenic, differentiating, and chemoattractant properties, modulate cellular events at that specific region of bone. Other unreleased matrix molecules serve as anchoring molecules to which effector cells attach and effect local remodeling of bone. Although largely conjectural, this proposed sequence of events is a graphic example of how bone cells and signal molecules converge at a specific bone site to affect bone metabolism.

Osteoclasts

Osteoclasts derive from hematopoietic precursors that also give rise to monocytes and macrophages. Larger multinucleated osteoclasts form from mononuclear cells through fusion in a manner thought to be similar to that of other giant histiocytes. Osteoclasts differ from other mononuclear phagocytes in their specific affinity for bone and unique enzyme profile (tartrate-resistant acid phosphatase). Briefly, monocytes (preosteoclasts) or osteoclasts are attracted to bone regions where there is a gap in lining cells and molecular or macroscopic disruption of the matrix envelope has occurred.

At these sites, the mononuclear osteoclast is able to attach, and may become activated and grow to form giant cells by fusion. Attachment occurs through receptor molecules on the cell surface that recognize a specific sialoprotein that is probably unique to bone. At the site of attachment to the bone matrix, a unique ruffled border forms and is characterized by a redundant folding of the cell membrane. At this site of attachment, an isolated environment is established in which a low pH is achieved through the activation of skeletal carbonic anhydrase. Hydrogen ions produced by carbonic anhydrase are pumped into the resorbing space below the ruffled membrane where the underlying hydroxyapatite is solubilized in the low pH and calcium ions are released. Free calcium ions are moved from bone to the extracellular space by membrane pumps. Lysosomal acid hydrolases, including cathepsin B, are also released, causing the dissociation and degradation of the organic matrix elements of bone, including collagen.

Through these osteoclast-mediated events, the mineral and organic matrix of bone is resorbed, producing Howship lacunae. Only osteoclasts have this capacity to resorb cortical bone; monocytes and macrophages do not. Other cells, such as mast cells, seem to augment bone resorption through the release of heparin, which enhances collagenase activity. Monocytes and lymphocytes appear to modulate bone remodeling through their release of local regulatory factors.

Osteoclastic resorption of bone is a much more rapid process than osteoblast-mediated formation of bone. However, it is the relative rate of the processes, resorption to formation, that are important. In childhood and adolescence, formation exceeds degradation. During the middle years, there is a balance between bone degradation and regeneration. With advancing age, formation fails to keep pace with degradation and there is progressive loss of skeletal mass. The earlier this imbalance occurs and the more extreme it is, the greater the loss of skeletal mass and the more severe the skeletal dysfunction and failure will be.

Bone Matrix

Although it is evident that bone cells are the principal mediators of bone metabolism, synthesis, and degradation, the organic and mineral matrix is more than a passive element in these cell-mediated processes. This matrix consists of inorganic and organic fractions.

Inorganic Matrix The inorganic fraction is composed primarily of calcium phosphate in the form of hydroxyapatite and far lesser amounts of octacalcium phosphate or brushite. The hydroxyapatite in bone is present as plate-like crystals that are 20 to 80 nm long and 2 to 5 nm thick. Crystalline hydroxyapatite found in bone contains small amounts of contaminants such as carbonate, which can replace phosphate or chloride, and fluoride, which can replace hydroxy groups. These contaminants alter the physical properties—such as solubility—of bone hydroxyapatite and thus can alter the biologic characteristics of the bone, including its ability to be degraded. Approximately two thirds of the dry weight of bone consists of its inorganic components. Newly formed bone is not as well mineralized and contains particles with a smaller average crystal size than older, "more mature" bone such as that found in the midportion of cortical bone.

Organic Matrix The organic matrix of bone is made up of proteins, glycosaminoglycan, chondroitin sulfate, lipids, and citrate. Collagen, a ubiquitous protein of extremely low solubility, constitutes 90% to 95% of the organic component of the bone matrix. The collagen molecule consists of three tropocollagen, polypeptide chains composed of approximately 1,000 amino acids. Bone collagen is constructed in the form of a triple helix of two $\alpha 1(I)$ chains and one $\alpha 2$ chain cross-linked by hydrogen bonding through the amide and carboxyl peptide backbone. This produces a linear molecule 300 nm long.

The pro-L1 and L2 precursors are synthesized and released into the extracellular space by osteoblasts and fibroblasts. Much posttranslational and postsecretory processing occurs, yielding mature bone collagen. In particular, the precursor peptides have their amino-terminal sequences enzymatically shortened, and almost one half of the proline and lysine residues are hydroxylated. These modifications have critical effects on facilitating protein transport to the extracellular space, and on the formation of the triple-helix structure. The individual tropocollagen chains can aggregate in such a way that their ends are level with one another or, alternatively, that they are offset by some portion of their length. The manner of aggregation clearly alters the end-to-end association of different collagen molecules; this change is "locked-in" when interchain cross-linking occurs. This cross-linking of the collagen chains decreases their solubility as well as increases their tensile strength. The mineral component of bone is primarily responsible for the compressive strength of bone and the fibrous collagen lattice accounts for the tensile strength of bone. Lamellar bone has a measurable tensile strength of 17,000 N/cm^2 and a compressive strength of 15,000 N/cm^2. These physical properties exceed the strengths of the common structural components used in the building of our homes.

Osteocalcin, the other major bone-specific protein produced by osteoblasts, accounts for 1% to 3% of the organic component of bones. This small (5.8 kd) protein contains three γ-glutamic acid residues produced by a vitamin K-dependent posttranslational modification of the peptide. These residues are necessary for binding to calcium ion. This protein is closely associated with the mineral component of bone, and its levels in bone are positively correlated with the amount of mineral. The spacing of the Gla-protein residues in the osteocalcin molecule aligns with the calcium ions on the hydroxyapatite crystal surface. The function of this protein is not known, but it is thought to have some role in attracting osteoclasts to sites of bone resorption. It may also regulate the rate of mineralization or the final shape assumed by the crystals. Vitamin D can enhance the synthesis of osteocalcin, whereas parathyroid hormone and corticosteroids inhibit it.

Osteonectin is a 32-kd protein secreted by osteoblasts and found in bone. It binds both collagen and hydroxyapatite and contains a phosphoserine residue. Its role in bone is not known, but it may potentiate calcium phosphate nucleation, stabilization, or organization. Other minor protein compounds found in bone matrix include a second Gla-protein that has yet to be named. Sialoproteins, proteoglycans, and other phosphoproteins thought to be synthesized by the osteoblasts have recently been described.

Mineralization of the organic matrix of bone is a complicated process that is not fully understood. Osteoblasts regulate the concentration of calcium ions in the matrix through their release of calcium from intracellular compartments, primarily their mitochondria. Osteoblasts also secrete macromolecules that determine the site and rate of calcification. The list of these regulatory compounds begins with collagen, the major lattice for mineralization. Proteoglycans control the sequence rate and degree to which mineralization occurs. Phosphoproteins and phospholipids are thought to facilitate the nucleation process that initiates mineralization and glycosaminoglycans are thought to be inhibitors of the calcification process. The temporal sequence by which osteoblasts synthesize and release these key building-blocks of bone is largely regulated by local and distally produced factors (such as hormones) that modulate the growth, differentiation, and function of osteoblasts.

Calcium Metabolism

Calcium Balance

Since calcium is a second messenger in almost every cell of the body, tight regulation of intracellular and extracellular levels is constantly maintained. At the macroscopic level, calcium homeostasis is maintained by three organ systems—the intestines, bone, and kidneys. In all three systems, hormones act to modulate organ function with respect to calcium.

In the intestines, calcium is actively absorbed in the duodenum by a calcium-binding protein. With low-calcium diets, most dietary calcium is taken up by this active absorption mechanism. In the jejunum, there is passive diffusion of calcium through the intestines. With calcium-replete diets, most calcium absorbed through the intestines enters passively because active transport is limited by the amount of calcium-binding protein, the pH, and transit time in the duodenum.

Dietary requirements for calcium are increased in both very young patients and in older patients (Table 1). Early in life, the body has a great need for calcium as the growing skeleton is mineralizing. Late in life, it is necessary to coun-

teract the net loss of calcium from the body caused by increased bone resorption. Other specific periods of increased need include child-bearing and nursing. During these times, the recommended intake is approximately 1,500 mg of elemental calcium per day. With an adequate dietary intake, the average adult absorbs 300 to 400 mg of elemental calcium per day. Approximately 100 to 200 mg is secreted back into the intestinal lumen, resulting in a net intake of 200 mg. The normal blood level of calcium is 9 to 10 mg/dl; approximately one half is bound to plasma protein (primarily albumin), a small fraction is tightly coordinated with phosphate or citrate, and about 45% exists in the form of free ions. The kidney filters approximately 10 g of calcium per day, reabsorbing 9.8 g; thus, there is a net urinary loss of 200 mg. By this arithmetic, there is a net balance between total absorption and excretion. This situation characterizes the third and fourth decades of life. In the first to third decades, there is a net positive balance, as the skeleton grows and reaches its peak bone mass, 1,000 to 1,100 g of calcium. This peak bone mass represents the life endowment for the individual. After the fourth decade, bone resorption exceeds formation and there is a net negative calcium balance, leading to an inexorable decline in bone mass. Severe calcium deficiencies during the critical accumulation period adversely affect peak bone mass. Individuals who suffer such deficiencies, and whose peak bone mass is therefore lower, experience skeletal dysfunction sooner.

The large reserve of calcium in bone slowly turns over as bone is remodeled. Approximately 400 mg of calcium is released from the bones each day. Most of this calcium is released as a consequence of osteoclastic remodeling. Some investigators have shown that osteocytes can mobilize calcium from perilacunar spaces. The amount of calcium released by this mechanism is unknown. Calcium approximately equivalent to the amount released (400 mg) is redeposited by osteoblasts as they form bone in response to osteoclast resorption (coupling). Calcium is also thought to reaccumulate in the perilacunar spaces that surround quiescent osteocytes.

Hormones modulate these fluxes in bone calcium by acting on the key cellular components. Parathyroid hormone induces osteoblasts (and possibly mononuclear phagocytes) to produce coupling factors that activate osteoclasts. The consequence of this action is an increase in osteoclast number and activity leading to increased resorption. This results in a concomitant activation of osteoblasts and increased bone formation to complete the remodeling loop. The complete sequence involves activation, resorption, reversal, formation, and a prolonged resting phase. The initial effect is augmented calcium release. This response is slow, taking days to weeks to initiate since cell proliferation, attachment, and fusion are required. By contrast, the ability of osteocytes to mobilize perilacunar calcium stores in response to parathyroid hormone is far more rapid, taking place within minutes. It is for this reason that the minute-to-minute variation in blood calcium level is probably a consequence of osteocyte-mediated fluxes. Calcitonin can briefly decrease osteoclast- and osteocyte-mediated resorption, but it has not been shown that these pharmacologic effects of calcitonin have any physiologic relevance. The formation and resting phases of bone metabolism are very prolonged. In some cases, the resting phase can last for years. There is at pres-

Table 1. Daily calcium requirements

Status and Age	Elemental Calcium (mg/day)
Youth (1 to 10 yrs)	800 to 1,000
Young adult (11 to 25 years)	1,200
Premenopausal (26 to 49 years)	1,000
Postmenopausal (50 years and older)	1,500
Pregnancy	1,500
Lactation	1,500 to 2,000
Fracture healing	1,500

ent no proven role for the various cytokines or endogenous growth factors capable of altering bone metabolism.

Parathyroid hormone can profoundly alter calcium metabolism through its effects on renal function. Although calcium (like sodium) can be absorbed throughout the length of the renal tubule, it is only in the distal tubule that parathyroid hormone, via a mechanism dependent on cyclic adenosine monophosphate (cAMP), enhances active resorption of calcium. The consequences of parathyroid hormone stimulation are a net fractional increase in the absorption of calcium presented to the tubule and an associated net increase in the fractional excretion of phosphorus. A second effect of parathyroid hormone on the kidney is to activate the 1-hydroxylase activity that produces biologically active calcitriol. This results in the induction of calcium-binding protein in the intestine and increased absorption of dietary calcium.

Parathyroid hormone secretion is exquisitely responsive to small changes in serum ionized calcium. This sensitivity to calcium accounts for the rapid feedback by which serum calcium concentration is maintained within a narrow range.

Endocrine Hormones

Regulation of calcium homeostasis is delicately balanced by the three major organ systems (intestine, bone, and kidney). Calcium metabolism is controlled largely through endocrine gland monitoring and secretion of calcitropic hormones. Important endocrine elements in the regulation of calcium include the parathyroid gland, skin, liver, kidney, gonads, adrenal tissues, and the thyroid.

Parathyroid Hormone Parathyroid hormone is an 84-amino acid single-chain peptide produced by the parathyroid glands. It is synthesized as a larger preproparathyroid hormone that is cleaved rapidly to the "intact" 84-amino acid form before being released into the circulation. The rate of synthesis and release of parathyroid hormone is inversely related to extracellular ionized calcium concentration. Transcription does not appear to depend on cytosolic calcium-ion concentration. The intracellular mechanisms by which the external calcium ion concentration regulates transcription or translation is not known. Recent data have demonstrated that the vitamin D metabolite calcitriol can inhibit transcription of parathyroid hormone both in vivo and in vitro.

Intact parathyroid hormone is relatively short-lived once it enters the circulation. The liver and kidney rapidly cleave the circulatory intact molecule at the 33 and 34 or 36 and 37 residues into amino-terminal and carboxy-terminal fractions. Both the biologically active amino-terminal fractions and the intact hormone have a circulating half-life shorter than that of the carboxy-terminal fragments. With renal impairment, clearance of the carboxy fragment is prolonged so that the levels of carboxy-terminal fragments increase, confounding the assessment of circulating, biologically active hormone. Radioimmunoassays using a double-antibody method have recently been developed. These assays detect intact parathyroid hormone and thus should provide an accurate measurement of the biologically active hormone components.

The principal target tissues for parathyroid hormone are bone and kidney. In both tissues, adenyl cyclase and later intracellular protein kinases are activated by specific membrane receptors coupled through proteins that bind guanosine triphosphate. The specific molecular targets and key biochemical pathways affected in the target tissues have not been fully elucidated. A variety of factors and pharmacologic agents known to modulate the guanosine triphosphate-adenyl cyclase pathway can alter the effect of parathyroid hormone on these targets. Interestingly, specific receptors for parathyroid hormone cannot be demonstrated on osteoclasts; rather, they are found on osteoblasts and osteoblast precursors. This implies that osteoblasts must regulate the subsequent proliferation and activation of osteoclasts that follow parathyroid hormone stimulation. The signals from osteoblast to osteoblast have not been elucidated. It is assumed that osteocytes have parathyroid hormone receptors because when stimulated by parathyroid hormone they rapidly mobilize the calcium salts immediately surrounding them. The expansion in osteoclast number that follows parathyroid hormone stimulation is long-lasting and significantly augments bone resorption.

In the kidney, parathyroid hormone activates adenyl cyclases distributed along the length of the renal tubule. In the proximal tubule, parathyroid hormone decreases phosphorus reabsorption. Distally, parathyroid hormone increases the reabsorption of calcium. Consequent to the activation of tubular adenyl cyclase, cAMP content in the urine is augmented. Urinary cAMP reflects total cAMP excreted and represents the sum of the nephrogenous cAMP (that portion derived from the renal tubule) and the cAMP passively filtered from the bone. The normal urinary cAMP value is 3.5 nmol/dl of glomerular filtrate. After parathyroid hormone administration (or stimulated secretion), more than 90% of the cAMP measured in the urine may be of nephrogenous origin. Therefore, nephrogenous cAMP is a good indicator of circulating parathyroid hormone levels; unfortunately, other circulating or locally produced factors can also increase the nephrogenous cAMP level. Recently, putative circulating humeral factors thought to be responsible for cancer-related hypercalcemia have been described. These factors are homologous to the first 11 to 17 amino acids of parathyroid hormone and are known to bind to parathyroid hormone receptors. In many patients with cancer, nephrogenous cAMP levels are increased. However, factors resembling parathyroid hormone are only one cause; prostaglandins can also increase nephrogenous cAMP levels.

Increased levels of parathyroid hormone (indicated by assays for intact, biologically active parathyroid hormone or parathyroid hormone fragments) have been noted in the elderly. Nephrogenous cAMP levels are increased in these subjects, as is tubular excretion of phosphorus. These findings support the conclusion that parathyroid hormone may have an aggravating role (possibly a pathologic one) in the progressive loss of bone mass seen in the aged.

Vitamin D Vitamin D is a unique sterol hormone that can modulate calcium homeostasis directly or through its effects on the differentiation of various calcium-regulating cell systems. Vitamin D_3 (cholecalciferol) can be formed by ultraviolet light in the skin from endogenously synthesized 7-dehydrocholesterol. As little as 15 minutes of bright sunlight may be sufficient to produce the daily requirement of vitamin D_3 in a fair-skinned individual. The other major source is vitamin D_2 (ergocalciferol) in the diet (primarily cod-liver oil, the only significant natural source, and milk to which ergocalciferol has been added).

Vitamin D from the skin undergoes C-25 hydroxylation in the liver to produce the major circulating pro-hormone, calcifediol. Calcitriol is considered to be the physiologically active form of the vitamin. Hydroxylation at the C-1 position is the rate-limiting step in the production of this biologically active form of the vitamin and the hydroxylase enzyme for this reaction, located in the mitochondria of renal cells, is activated by parathyroid hormone. In the presence of low parathyroid hormone levels and high calcitriol levels, alternate hydroxylation of calcifediol occurs at the C-24 position, yielding an inactive metabolite, $24,25(OH)_2D_3$.

A principal target tissue for calcitriol is the intestine. Here, calcitriol induces the production of a critical calcium-binding protein that is responsible for active calcium transport. Like the other sterol hormones, calcitriol binds to a specific receptor protein, which has recently been cloned and resembles the glucocorticoid and estrogen receptors. The receptor-ligand complex is transported to the nucleus where it binds to DNA. If calcitriol is similar to the other sterol hormones, the receptor-ligand complex binds to a promoter region responsible for inducing transcription of the calcium-transporter gene. To date, the promoter region for calcitriol has not been identified. An alternate hypothesis about the mechanism of calcitriol's effect focuses on its capacity to induce cell differentiation. Recent studies suggest that calcitriol is taken up by the differentiating epithelial cells in the lower segments of the villous crypts. Because calcium transport protein is expressed in the more differentiated cells found higher up in the crypt, it has been suggested that calcitriol induces cell differentiation with calcium transport protein expression being a consequence of that differentiation. The ultimate consequences through either pathway would be the same: increased calcium-transport protein resulting in increased calcium absorption through the intestine.

Bone is another target tissue for calcitriol; however, here its physiologic role is not as well understood. On the basis of studies with monocytes and macrophages, calcitriol is thought to promote the differentiation of osteoclasts. At pharmacologic doses, it can induce accelerated bone resorption by increasing the activity and number of osteoclasts. Additionally, calcitriol can alter phospholipid metabolism by osteoblast-like cells. Taken together, these two findings may explain the mechanisms by which calcitriol modulates bone mineralization.

Interestingly, circulating levels of the pro-hormone calcifediol decrease with age. There is no convincing evidence of decreased intestinal absorption or liver metabolism nor have decreased binding-protein levels or increased metabolic clearance of calcifediol been demonstrated. Therefore, the available data suggest that decreased intake and/or skin synthesis may be responsible for the lower circulating levels measured. In the few studies in which it was examined, a matching decrease in calcitriol in the elderly has been reported, but there appears to be less agreement with this observation. Preliminary studies suggest that 1-hydroxylase activity is reduced in the aged. As possible corroborative evidence for calcitriol deficiency in the elderly, it is known that fractional calcium absorption decreases with age.

Estrogen Since the earliest observations that fractures were more common in women after middle age or after oophorectomy, the relationship between endocrine function in females and the integrity of bone has been highlighted. Many studies have now documented the accelerated loss of bone mass after menopause. Conversely, when ovarian hormone production ceases and circulating levels fall to 20% of previous levels, accelerated loss in bone mass can be abrogated by the simultaneous administration of calcium and estrogen. Interestingly, obesity can protect against this postmenopausal bone loss, probably because adrenal androgens, which continue to be produced after ovarian failure, are converted to estrogen and stored by fatty tissues. Although estrogens are known to inhibit bone resorption, the mechanisms responsible for this effect are not understood. Only recently has the presence of specific estrogen receptors in osteoblasts been confirmed. Although the level of such receptors in osteoblasts is quite low, they appear to be functionally active, providing the first real evidence that bone is a target tissue for estrogen action.

Calcitonin The gene for this small peptide hormone is expressed in many different tissues, including the brain. However, only in the parafollicular cells (C-cells) of the thyroid are the newly transcribed mRNA molecules processed to produce an mRNA that when translated yields the biologically active, 32-amino acid peptide chain of calcitonin. In the other tissues, alternate splicing of mRNA results in the synthesis of larger peptides that do not share calcitonin's activities. The function of these alternate products is not known. By the same token, an exact physiologic role for authentic calcitonin is not known.

Calcitonin secretion increases slightly with the postprandial rise in serum calcium. Calcitonin causes osteolytic retraction and inhibits osteoclastic resorption, effects that would be expected to decrease calcium ion release into the perilacunar spaces around these cells. Similarly, osteoclasts have receptor sites for calcitonin and respond to this hormone by decreasing osteoclast activity and number. Bone formation temporarily increases in relationship to bone resorption. In the kidney, supraphysiologic (pharmacologic) levels of calcitonin cause increased secretion of sodium, potassium, and chloride as well as a concomitant increase in calcium excretion. Bone and kidney responses to calcitonin are negligible. Patients with medullary carcinoma of the thyroid (a C-cell cancer) can have circulating levels of calcitonin that are increased a millionfold without any evidence of a lasting biologic effect on bone or kidney function.

Thyroid Hormones Thyroxine (T_4) is the major hormone product (and the major circulating product) of the thyroid gland. Triiodothyroxine (T_3), which is three to four times more active than thyroxine in many tissues, is also secreted by the thyroid. However, more than three fourths of the circulating level of triiodothyroxine results from conversion (deiodination) in the peripheral tissues. Normal circulating levels of thyroxine and triiodothyroxine are 4 to 12 μg/dl and 150 ng/dl, respectively. The thyroid hormones resemble steroid hormones in that they circulate while bound to specific and nonspecific serum proteins. They act on cells after interaction with a specific cell receptor and binding to nuclear DNA.

Thyroxine can increase the rate of bone metabolism, increasing both formation and resorption. It also appears to have a direct effect on inducing bone resorption. A net consequence of supraphysiologic (pharmacologic) levels of thyroxine is loss of bone mass. The actual mechanism for this effect is unknown.

It is now evident that "thyroid-suppressive" doses (that is, 200 μg of thyroxine per day) can accelerate the net loss of bone mineral and have detrimental consequences on the functional integrity of the skeleton. Therefore, when prolonged thyroid suppression is necessary, the potentially detrimental effect of thyroid hormone on skeletal mass in patients susceptible to osteoporosis must be taken into account.

Bone Biomechanics and Microstructure

Bone (the organ) is composed of cortical and cancellous bone and either fatty or hematopoietic marrow tissue. Functionally, it provides mechanical support for the body and acts as a reservoir for elemental ions such as calcium, phosphate, and magnesium. Its separate components and functions are closely interrelated.

Mineralized bone (the tissue) is a composite of an organic matrix (40% of dry weight) and inorganic salts (60% of dry weight). The predominant organic substance consists of type I collagen (94%) and glycosaminoglycans (1%). These provide the tensile strength of cortical bone. The inorganic component is composed primarily of calcium hydroxyapatite.

At the microscopic level, mature cancellous and cortical bone are both composed of lamellar bone. The primary structural subunit of cortical bone is the osteon; for cancellous bone it is the trabeculum. Biomechanical testing of these individual subunits yields similar structural properties for each. It is the macroscopic arrangement of the microscopic subunits that accounts for the markedly different mechanical properties of cortical and cancellous bone. Cortical bone is excellent for resisting torque and bending moments. Cancellous bone is designed to accept compressive and shear forces. Bone is an anisotropic and a viscoelastic material. An anisotropic material has strength and elastic properties that differ depending on the direction in which the structure is loaded. A viscoelastic material has strength and elastic properties that depend on the rate and duration of the applied load. The strength and stiffness of bone doubles as the rate of loading increases from a slow to a rapid rate.

The structural properties of mature bone may be changed by either modeling or remodeling. Modeling can be defined as the appositional growth that occurs on the surface of mature bone in response to increased stresses (Wolff's law). Material properties dictate that bone located furthest from the center of the structure is mechanically best for resisting torque and bending. One theoretical model suggests that the gradual maturation that occurs during bone deposition can have a significant influence on decreasing the time course of surface modeling responses.

Remodeling involves a process of removing existing bone and replacing it with new bone. This new bone is initially weaker than the previous bone. This is why patients with hypermetabolic states such as hyperparathyroidism have a high rate of developing stress fractures. In osteoporosis, the resorption of bone is slightly greater than the formation of new bone; this results in a slight uncoupling of this normally tightly interrelated process.

Interesting new information has become available on the early physiologic events that occur after a bone has been loaded. In an adult avian ulnar model, osteoblasts responded within 24 hours of dynamic loading by increasing their RNA production. Within seven days an active periosteal surface developed on the stressed side of the ulna. The mechanism that couples stress in the bone with the activation of the osteoblasts has yet to be understood.

A canine model has been developed that allows the application of a known stress to a region of cancellous bone. The response of the bone is biphasic, with an initial peak of activity by eight weeks that is characterized by intensive but unorganized bone function. After 18 to 22 weeks, a gradual reorganization of the trabecula allows better acceptance of the transmitted load. The response is closely related to the strain energy density.

It has been hypothesized that mechanical forces strongly influence skeletal morphogenesis, growth, and development beginning with the cartilaginous anlage in the embryo. The natural sequence of events for all cartilage that undergoes endochondral ossification is proliferation, maturation, degeneration, and ossification. This process is accelerated by intermittently applied shear stress and is inhibited by compressive stress. Application of this hypothesis, via a mathematical model, to the differing arrangement of ossification centers in the sternum produced an acceptable correlation.

Osteoporosis and Osteopenia

The National Institutes of Health Consensus Conference defined primary osteoporosis as an age-related disorder characterized by decreased bone mass and increased susceptibility to fractures in the absence of other recognizable causes of bone loss. The consequences of osteoporosis are severe—15 to 20 million people in the United States are currently suffering from osteoporosis and at least 1.2 million fractures (more than 200,000 involving the hip, 538,000 involving the vertebral body, and 172,000 involving the distal forearm) can be attributed to osteoporosis each year. More than one third of all women past the age of 65 years have suffered vertebral crush fractures. Of individuals who live to be 90 years old, 32% of women and 17% of men have also sustained hip fractures. The mortality rate for patients sustaining hip fractures is 12% to 20% higher than that for individuals without hip fractures. Fewer than 30% of patients with hip fractures return to a lifestyle comparable to the one they had before the fracture. It has been estimated that more than $7 billion is spent annually in the United States on the primary care of osteopenic fractures.

Although all individuals lose bone after the fourth decade, certain individuals are at increased risk. The major risk factor appears to be early or surgically induced menopause. Impaired metabolism, long-term calcium deficiency, secondary hyperparathyroidism, and decreased activity levels have all been implicated. Other risk factors include genetic predisposition (individuals who are fair, small, hypermobile, of northwestern European ancestry, or who have scoliosis), cigarette smoking, and excessive alcohol intake. Cigarette smokers have significantly more bone loss and an increased incidence of hip and vertebral fractures. This may in part be related to enhanced degradation of estrogen. Heavy alcohol users have decreased bone density on iliac crest biopsy and decreased bone density of the vertebral bodies and femoral necks. Alcohol directly depresses osteoblast function. There is considerable controversy about the effects of many of these factors.

Often many factors co-exist, blurring the distinction between primary or involutional osteoporosis and secondary osteoporosis. The differential diagnosis of osteopenia includes a number of other entities that may simulate osteoporosis. In addition to involutional or primary osteoporosis, these include endocrinopathy, neoplastic disease, hematologic disorders, mechanical disorders, metabolic collagen disturbances, nutritional aberrations, and osteomalacia (Outline 1). Such conditions must be ruled out before a diagnosis of primary osteoporosis can be made.

Bone mass loss is thought to be a universal phenomenon of aging. Peak mass is achieved in the third and fourth decades of life and is affected by sex, nutrition, race, exercise, and overall health. Peak bone mass is 30% higher in men than in women and 10% higher in blacks than in whites. Once peak mass is attained, a slow phase of bone loss commences at about the age of 35 years. This continues equally in men and women at the rate of 0.3% to 0.5% per year. This loss is directly related to continuous negative calcium balance. The accelerated phase of bone loss, which occurs at the rate of 2% to 3% per year, begins after surgical or natural menopause. This phase lasts for six to ten years, after which bone loss returns to a basal slow phase level of 0.3% to 0.5% per year. Many studies have demonstrated the importance of decreased estrogen level in the accelerated phase of bone loss.

Bone contains both trabecular and cortical components. Trabecular bone has a low volume and a high surface area. Conversely, cortical bone has a high volume and a low surface area. Remodeling of bone takes place on the surface. Consequently, trabecular bone, with its higher surface

area, is the prime target of the accelerated bone loss that takes place after menopause and estrogen deprivation. Bones containing a large trabecular component and dependent on it for structural integrity are, therefore, at higher risk of fracture than cortical bone during the initial stages of skeletal bone loss. The vertebral body, which is composed predominantly of trabecular bone, manifests crush fractures ten to 15 years before the rate of hip fractures increases.

Involutional osteoporosis has been categorized on the basis of these two patterns of fracture and bone loss. Type I, or postmenopausal osteoporosis, occurs in women from the time of menopause to the age of 65 years, involves predominantly trabecular bone, and is characterized by vertebral and Colles' fractures. Decreased estrogen levels play a primary role in type I osteoporosis. In contrast, type II, or senile osteoporosis, occurs both in women and in men, usually after the age of 75 years, involves cortical bone as well as trabecular bone, and is characterized by fractures of the hip, pelvis, proximal humerus, and proximal tibia. The bone loss in type II osteoporosis is related to aging and long-term calcium deficiency.

Exercise and Bone Homeostasis

The natural history of bone mass regulation in women is one of accumulation of bone through the third and fourth decades, followed by a period of homeostasis lasting until menopause, and then a rapid decrease in cortical and especially trabecular bone. Any process that inhibits bone formation early in life or accelerates bone loss later in life can negatively affect the structural integrity of the skeleton with aging.

In young females there is a correlation between amenorrhea associated with exercise and loss of bone mineral content in the lumbar spine. Most studies so far have used amenorrheic runners as their population base. It is apparent that several factors contribute to the development of amenorrhea. Runners who begin training at or before the onset of menarche have a higher rate of amenorrhea. Other possible factors are body-fat composition, nutritional status, and weekly mileage. As many as one third of highly competitive female athletes have some form of eating disorder and there is a correlation between low caloric intake and amenorrhea.

A recent study of elite runners (>65 km/wk) found that the mineral content of the lumbar spine was lower in a group of amenorrheic runners than in female runners without amenorrhea and an age-matched control group. The mineral content was higher in the amenorrheic elite group than in a less competitive group (<65 km/wk) of amenorrheic runners. This implies that running at a very competitive level partially protects the bone against loss caused by amenorrhea. A more practical recommendation is that female athletes who participate in endurance activities should not train to the extent that menstrual function is compromised. It is not known whether estrogen replacement therapy to institute menstrual cycles protects against bone loss in amenorrheic athletes.

The rate of stress fractures also correlates with the presence of amenorrhea in endurance athletes. These fractures occur in as many as 49% of amenorrheic runners compared with 29% of runners with normal menstrual cycles. The most commonly injured bone was the tibia, with the tarsal

Outline 1. Differential diagnosis of osteopenia

Collagen disorder
   Homocystinuria
   Osteogenesis imperfecta
   Scurvy
Endocrine disorder
   Acromegaly (?)
   Cushing's disease
   Diabetes mellitus
   Estrogen deficiency
   Hyperparathyroidism
   Hyperthyroidism
   Hypogonadism
   Iatrogenic glucocorticoid treatment
Hematologic disorder
   Sickle cell anemia
   Thalassemia
Involutional (or primary) osteoporosis
   Type I, postmenopausal
   Type II, senile
Mechanical disorder
   Disuse
   Immobilization
Neoplastic disorder
   Leukemia
   Multiple myeloma
Nutritional disorder
   Alcoholism
   Malnutrition
Osteomalacia
   Aberrant vitamin D metabolism
   Malabsorption syndromes
   Vitamin D-deficiency rickets

bones second. The stress fractures were bilateral in 16% of cases.

Three theories have been proposed to explain stress fractures: The first is that these fractures result from focal areas of structural weakness that occur as bone remodels in response to the application of a new or greater stress. The second is that muscle weakness reduces the shock-absorbing capability of the lower extremity, causing focal areas of increased bone stress. The third is that repetitive muscle pull across a bone creates a stress fracture. Probably all three factors play a role in the development of these fractures.

It is well documented that routine exercise inhibits bone loss from the vertebral body in normal postmenopausal women. The exercise session can be as short as one hour twice weekly. These routines do not significantly affect bone density in the distal radius.

Activity level early in life has not been proven to correlate with increased bone density later in life. It appears that participation in a regular, sustained athletic program throughout life is the best method of producing an adequate bone stock in early years and of preserving bone later in life.

Clinical Presentation and Diagnosis of Osteoporosis

Osteoporosis is a silently progressive disorder that comes to the attention of the physician after an acute painful fracture, the recognition of an asymptomatic thoracic wedge or lumbar compression, a fracture noted on routine radiographic examination, or the observation of generalized osteopenia on plain radiographs. Before bone loss is detectable on radiographs, a 30% reduction in bone mineral content must have occurred. Most thoracic fractures are asymptomatic and unrecognized by the patient. Thus, patients at risk who have documented osteopenia should undergo regular spinal surveys to identify vertebral fractures. The differential diagnosis of osteopenia centers on bone marrow disorders, endocrinopathies, osteoporosis, and osteomalacia (Outline 1).

Diagnostic Techniques

The examination of an individual with osteopenia uses both invasive and noninvasive tests. Noninvasive techniques are used to quantitate bone mass for the purpose of diagnosing osteoporosis and evaluating the efficacy of treatment. The National Osteoporosis Foundation stated that the indications for measuring bone density in the axial skeleton are to decide whether to begin preventive treatment in women at menopause, to screen for low bone mass in persons who are at major risk for osteoporosis (especially postmenopausal women of European or Asian ancestry), to establish the diagnosis of osteoporosis (especially in patients whose spinal-column roentgenograms show only decreased bone radial lucency or minimal vertebral deformities), and to determine the severity of bone loss in newly diagnosed osteoporotic patients with vertebral fractures so that the most appropriate therapy can be selected.

Several radiologic methods are available for evaluation of bone mineral content. Each is useful for measuring specific skeletal sites and specific types of bone. Three commonly used methods are single-photon absorptiometry, dual-photon absorptiometry, and quantitative computed tomography.

Absorptiometry Single-photon absorptiometry uses a single-beam photon source and is preferred for bones with little soft-tissue interference such as the radius or calcaneus. The radiation dose is small (2 to 5×10^{-5} Gy); precision (error rate, 3% to 5%) and accuracy (error rate, 1% to 4%) are good. The limitation of this technique is the difficulty of positioning the examination site exactly. Single-photon absorptiometry has traditionally been used to measure cortical bone, which is the skeleton's least metabolically active bone type. Recent work using the "5-mm site" or the "ultra distal" radius has increased the amount of trabecular bone within the field, apparently improving the correlation with general skeletal bone mass.

Dual-photon absorptiometry, which is a modification of the single-photon technique, uses a radioisotope that emits photons at two energy levels. This modification eliminates soft tissue from the image and allows direct measurement of the apparent bone density of the vertebral body and the femoral neck. All bone is measured within the specific windows. Consequently, measuring the bone density of the vertebral body requires both cortical and cancellous bone of the body and its posterior elements to be measured. This apparent density can be corrected for area measurements. The radiation dose is low (5 to 15×10^{-5} Gy); precision (error rate, 3%) and accuracy (error rate, 4% to 6%) are good. Because this technique directly measures the femoral neck and spine, it more reliably predicts the risk of fracture and the efficacy of treatment at these sites than the single-photon technique does. Limitations of this method include the possibility of falsely increased values in patients with osteophytes or significant deformity that precludes identification of a individual vertebral body. A newly devised instrument using an X-ray source has improved precision to 99% and speeded up the testing to five minutes. The dual-photon and dual-beam X-ray techniques do not underestimate bone mass but may overestimate it because of spurious calcifications within the fields of examination.

Computed Tomography Quantitative computed tomography can measure bone mass by evaluating the density within a clearly defined area window in the anterior third of the vertebral body at mid-height. In carefully controlled applications of this technique, error rates as low as 3% have been reported. However, error rates of 7% to 15% are more common and the radiation dose is appreciably higher (2×10^{-3} Gy) than that of the dual-photon technique. Quantitative computed tomography is, however, the only method that can specifically identify trabecular bone, the most metabolically active component of the skeleton. Thus, it is more sensitive to changes in the skeleton during the course of therapeutic intervention. Artifactually low readings can, however, result from the increased fat within the marrow space that occurs with aging and from variable presentations of venous lakes within the body.

Rationale for Use Quantitative bone-density determinations are useful because of their ability to predict which patients are at high risk for fracture. However, many other factors determine whether a fracture will occur, including the structural geometry of bone, the force (magnitude and direction) of the insult, and the ability of the soft tissues to absorb trauma. Quantitative bone density measurements evaluate only one of these factors. Despite this limitation, studies have demonstrated a significant correlation between bone mineral density and fracture risk. Although a fracture threshold of 1 g/cm² has been described (90% of nontraumatic vertebral fractures occur in patients with bone densities below this level), there is a significant overlap between diseased and healthy populations. Although most recent studies suggest that fracture risk is strongly related to bone mass and age, even among those with the least bone mass some individuals will never experience a spinal or femoral fracture (Tables 2 and 3).

Invasive Studies Invasive studies consist primarily of laboratory analysis to determine the cause and extent of osteopenia. Despite newly developed biochemical indices, the ability to predict which individuals will have the most bone loss is still uncertain. One institution reported that a single determination of body-fat mass, urinary levels of calcium and hydroxyproline, and serum levels of alkaline phosphatase correctly identified 79% of "fast bone-losers" (bone loss more than 3% annually) and 78% of "slow bone-losers." Within this sample, however, a significant number of patients did not fall into either group. Laboratory studies can, however, be helpful in partial segregation of those individuals with documented osteopenia.

An algorithm has been created to differentiate among patients with common forms of primary and secondary osteoporosis (Algorithm 1). Patients with an abnormal complete blood cell count, erythrocyte sedimentation rate, or serum protein electrophoresis findings should undergo bone marrow sampling to test for myeloma, leukemia, and benign bone marrow abnormalities. Patients with abnormal parathyroid or thyroid hormone levels, cortisol levels, or glucose metabolism may have one of the endocrinopathies (hyperparathyroidism, hyperthyroidism, diabetes mellitus, and Cushing's disease). In one study, approximately 8% to 10% of patients with hip fractures had osteomalacia. In this group, serum and urinary calcium levels, serum and urinary phosphorus levels, serum alkaline phosphatase level, renal function, and calcifediol level identified only one half of the true osteomalacia patients. In the others, transilial bone biopsy was needed to identify the milder forms of osteomalacia. The absolute diagnosis of osteomalacia is made from an analysis of the undecalcified bone histomorphometry of double tetracycline-labeled specimens. In osteomalacia there is a relative increase in nonmineralized osteoid, a significant delay in mineralization rate, and smudging of the tetracycline label. Without data from bone histomorphometry, 4% of osteopenia cases will not be diagnosed because the osteomalacia is mild enough that the calcitripic hormones levels are within normal limits.

New laboratory studies evaluate the level of osteocalcin, a noncollagenous Gla-protein, which may correlate with rates of bone formation. It is still too early to state that the osteocalcin level is always increased in augmented bone formation.

Treatment and Prevention of Osteoporosis

Osteoporosis is a heterogeneous disease of multifactorial origin that has only recently become the subject of intensive research efforts. The treatment of this condition is both complex and controversial. There appears to be a consensus in regard to prevention (bone maintenance), but bone augmentation is still under intensive investigation. The general opinion within the medical community is that every effort should be made to maximize peak bone mass and prevent the rapid bone loss that occurs after menopause.

Exercise

A comprehensive general rehabilitation program that stresses spinal extension and strengthening exercises, as well as impact loading activities such as walking, should be part of all treatment programs for osteoporotic patients. Prospective studies have demonstrated that one hour of impact exercise two or three times each week can maintain or slightly increase bone mass in the lumbar spine and the total-body calcium level in postmenopausal women. Conversely, sedentary control groups in these studies continued to lose bone.

Calcium Supplements

The role of calcium supplementation in the treatment of osteoporosis is controversial. There is no evidence that it is beneficial. Several studies have suggested that the average premenopausal woman does not ingest enough calcium in her diet to achieve a net neutral calcium balance, much less achieve the peak bone mass necessary by the middle of the third decade of life. These studies concluded that 1.2 g/day of elemental calcium is necessary to achieve peak bone mass. Once this has been achieved, lower levels of calcium (800 to 1,000 mg/day) can maintain a neutral balance before menopause. Once menopause has begun, approximately 1.5 g of calcium and 400 to 800 IU of vitamin D per day are needed to achieve a neutral balance (Algorithm 2). Calcium is clearly less effective than estrogen in preventing early postmenopausal bone loss. Calcium may have a minor effect on cortical bone loss but appears to have no effect on trabecular bone loss in early menopause. Lack of calcium, however, plays a critical role in senile (type II) osteoporosis. High calcium intake is associated with a significant lower rate of hip and spine fractures in persons more than 65 years old; thus, life-long calcium supplementation has been advocated (Table 1). Most investigators believe that a high calcium intake in the years before menopause may help prevent postmenopausal osteoporosis.

The bioavailability of calcium varies. Many dietary and nondietary factors can affect calcium absorption and excretion (Table 4). Calcium absorption is increased by vi-

Table 2. Bone density values in patients undergoing natural menopause

Spinal Fracture	No. of Patients	Bone Density Values
Yes	81	0.08 ± 0.14 g/cm²
No	225	0.89 ± 0.16 g/cm²
P value		< .001

Table 3. Spinal fractures and bone density values in postmenopausal women

Bone Density Values (g/cm²)	% of Women With Spinal Fractures
0.8 to 0.9	26
0.7 to 0.8	33
0.6 to 0.7	51
0.5 to 0.6	63

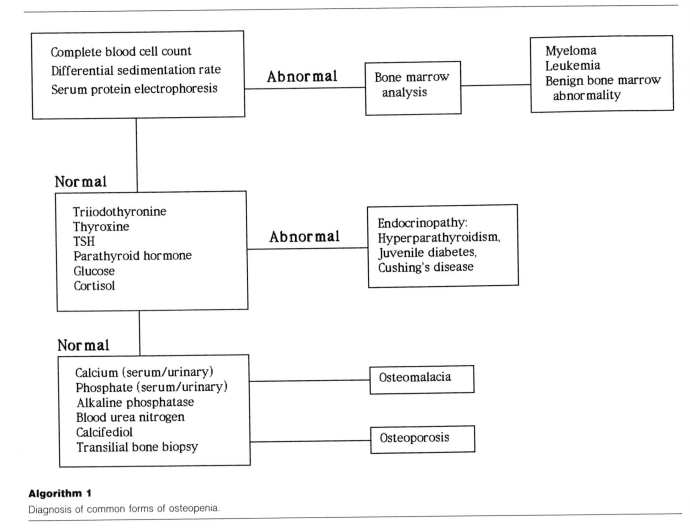

Algorithm 1

Diagnosis of common forms of osteopenia.

tamin D, citric acid, and lactose and decreased by a high concentration of oxalate, which is found in vegetables such as spinach, Swiss chards, sorrels, parsley, and beet greens. Although not all these vegetables have been tested, calcium bioavailability from spinach, for example, appears to be zero.

Calcium absorption requires an acid medium within the stomach (pH 3 or lower). The most common form of calcium supplement is calcium carbonate. Because it does not dissolve in a neutral medium, patients who have undergone vagotomies or who have achlorhydria should use other forms of calcium. Recent studies have suggested that not all generic calcium carbonates are equal. Some do not dissolve enough for solubilization. Calcium carbonate tablets should undergo a "vinegar" test to ensure that the calcium pill in question disintegrates in vinegar within 45 minutes. Excessive packing precludes disintegration in many generic calcium carbonate tablets, making the calcium unavailable.

Recent studies have suggested that calcium citrate offers certain advantages over calcium carbonate. Calcium citrate dissolves in neutral pH, does not produce a carbon dioxide by-product, causes less constipation, and appears to be less likely to lead to kidney stone formation. At this time, each pill contains only 150 to 250 mg of calcium; thus, more pills must be taken to achieve the desired dosage of 1,500 mg. Patient compliance with this increased number of pills may be the limiting factor.

Bone meal is not recommended because of variable levels of contamination with lead, arsenic, and strontium.

Estrogen Supplements

Estrogen replacement therapy is generally believed to prevent postmenopausal acceleration of bone loss and reduce the incidence of hip fracture in aging women. A retrospective study comparing estrogen users with 245 matched controls found that after 17 years the estrogen users had had about half as many vertebral fractures as the controls. Another investigation supported the hypothesis that postmenopausal use of estrogen partially protects against hip fractures. In several studies of bone mineral content in selected bones, including the forearm and the spine, estrogen-treated women demonstrated a maintenance of bone mass. Conversely, bone mass significantly decreased in groups receiving only calcium or placebo. The benefit of estrogen is maximized when treatment begins within the first six years after the onset of menopause, before the major trabecular bone loss occurs. After that time, estrogen has a lesser effect, although several studies have suggested that it still confers a benefit by decreasing the fracture rate well into the eighth decade of life.

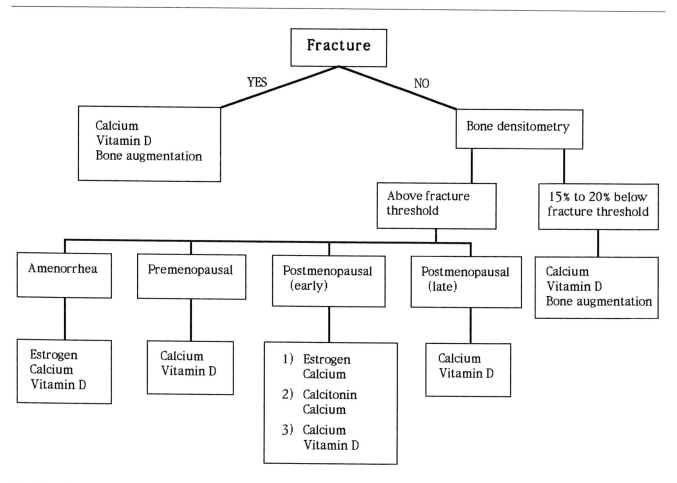

Algorithm 2

Prevention and treatment of osteoporosis.

Table 4. Food components that affect calcium balance

Component	Effect on Calcium
Caffeine	Increases excretion
Fat	Increases absorption
Fiber	Decreases absorption
Lactose	Increases absorption
Oxalates	Decreases absorption
Phosphorus	Probably no significant effect
Phytates	Decreases absorption
Protein	Increases excretion
Sodium	Increases excretion
Vitamin D	Increases absorption

Estrogen has a number of deleterious side effects, including endometrial hyperplasia and carcinoma in patients treated with cyclic estrogen alone, worsening of preexisting breast cancer, aggravation of thrombophlebitis, and potentiation of gallstones. There are no data to suggest that estrogen causes breast cancer but its potential for accelerating preexisting breast cancer makes regular mammographic monitoring necessary. Candidates for estrogen treatment must be carefully screened to exclude those with histories of or existing breast cancer or thrombophlebitis.

Endometrial hyperplasia and carcinoma can be significantly diminished by the concomitant use of progestational agents in a cyclical fashion. The two commonly used programs are (1) estrogen administered for 25 days and 10 mg of progestational agents in the last ten days of the cycle and (2) continuous estrogen supplementation and progesterone administration in the first ten days of each month. The first regimen is associated with the traditional menstrual cycle; the second may preclude menstruation. Patients on the second regimen, however, may require regular endometrial biopsies. The estrogen dermal patch has been demonstrated in limited studies to provide adequate bone protection along with a lesser likelihood of thrombophlebitis and gallstones. However, the progesterone agents are still needed. Conjugated estrogen equivalents at dosages of 0.3 mg or less have failed to demonstrate long-term efficacy. Estrogen is also associated with prevention of cardiovascular disease, but the addition of progesterone appears to diminish this effect. For patients who have undergone hysterectomy for benign disease, estrogen without progesterone may well be the preferred mode of therapy.

Calcitonin

Calcitonin was recently approved by the U.S. Food and Drug Administration for treatment of osteoporosis. Calcitonin is a peptide hormone that inhibits osteoclastic bone resorption and can only be given by injection. Various trials have shown that daily or alternate-day injections of calcitonin in postmenopausal osteoporotic women can increase total-body calcium, iliac crest bone volume, and the bone mineral content of the lumbar vertebrae and femoral diaphysis. A recent study demonstrated that calcitonin can provide the same benefits as estrogen in early menopause. The side effects of calcitonin include nausea (when injected intramuscularly), flushing, and hypersensitivity. Administering antihistamines an hour before the injection and using a subcutaneous injection into fat may eliminate most of these side effects. Dosages as low as 50 units three times a week appear to be as efficacious as 100 units daily. The drug is expensive and the mode of administration is disliked by most patients. However, for those individuals who cannot tolerate an estrogen-progesterone program, calcitonin is clearly a comparable alternative mode of bone maintenance. Calcium supplementation is essential to prevent hypocalcemia and to stabilize the skeleton.

Bone Augmentation

Calcium, vitamin D, estrogen, and calcitonin maintain the skeleton, but the skeleton that is severely depleted or weakened by established osteoporosis requires augmentation of the bone mass. All such bone-augmenting agents are still considered experimental and have not yet been formally approved.

Sodium Fluoride Sodium fluoride stimulates bone formation and increases bone mass in more than 80% of patients with osteoporosis. The bone formed during fluoride therapy is denser but its quality is somewhat compromised. Histomorphometric analysis of fluoridic bone demonstrates an increased number of osteocytes, increased lacunae diameter, slight basophilia about the lacunae, and slight irregularity of the collagen matrix. Trabecular bone (and thus parts of the skeleton, such as the spine, made of trabecular bone) appears to be the primary beneficiary of sodium fluoride. Cortical bone responds much more lowly.

It has been suggested that combinations of fluoride (1 mg/kg/day), estrogen, and calcium reduce fracture recurrence. Several studies have demonstrated bone accretion rates of 8% to 20% per year, a dramatic decrease in spinal fractures, and improvement in general well-being. Fracture rates may increase, however, if fluoride is administered without adequate calcium supplementation. Conversely, one large collaborative investigation indicated that hip fracture rates do not improve despite appropriate combined fluoride and calcium supplementation. Whether or not there is an actual decrease in hip fractures is yet to be determined.

The side effects of fluoride include brittleness of the bone (if calcium and vitamin D supplements are not administered), arthralgias in weightbearing bones (20% of cases), dyspepsia (3% of cases), and rare instances of gastric erosions. Arthralgias can be managed by stopping fluoride administration for two to four weeks and initiating a concurrent course of calcitonin (50 units three times a week). A hypermetabolic state and osteomalacia are direct contraindications; these underlying problems must be treated before fluoride is administered. Government-sponsored random-trial studies are currently underway to determine the ultimate efficacy of fluoride therapy.

Alternative Bone-Augmentation Programs Several other innovative and experimental methods of bone augmentation are currently under investigation. Episodic parathyroid administration produces significant bone augmentation in males. Manipulation of the bone-remodeling sequence so that the bone-resorption phase is shortened and the bone-formation phase is prolonged is theoretically promising. Phosphate and etidronate have been reported to produce significant bone accretion. Local growth factors and cytokines are being studied as initiating agents of selected forms of osteoporosis. Several strategies for strengthening the skeleton with growth factors and prostaglandin inhibitors are under investigation.

All bone-augmentation programs are, however, experimental and the bone that they form does not usually have entirely normal matrix characteristics. None of these methods addresses periosteal bone formation; the stimulated bone appears to be within the marrow canal or on the endosteal surface. Although biomechanical studies suggest that a shift of bone mass farther from the neutral axis may strengthen the bone, none of these augmentation strategies produces such a shift. Thus, the best current strategy for treating osteoporosis is prevention, maximizing peak bone mass, and maintaining bone mass.

Prevention of Osteoporosis

The key factors in preventing osteoporosis are impact exercises and maintenance of physiologic levels of calcium and vitamin D in most premenopausal women, in the 30% of women in early menopause whose peak bone mass was high and who are not now losing bone mass (demonstrated by serial bone density studies), and in women in late menopause (those 65 years of age and older). A cyclical estrogen-progesterone regimen or birth control pills should be used to reestablish the menstrual cycle in oligomenorrheic and amenorrheic premenopausal women. Women in early menopause, especially those with risk factors, should also consider a cyclic estrogen-progesterone regimen. For those who cannot tolerate estrogen, calcitonin is a good alternative.

Osteomalacia

Osteomalacia is a metabolic bone disorder in which there is inadequate mineralization of the newly formed organic matrix (that is, osteoid). This is usually a generalized problem resulting from vitamin D deficiency and/or renal phosphate wasting.

Rickets, osteomalacia of the developing and growing skeleton because of a dietary deficiency of vitamin D, has become rare since the widespread supplementation of dairy products with vitamin D. Clinically evident rickets occurs in children with familial hypophosphatemia, an X-linked genetic disorder characterized as a vitamin D-resistant rickets. Recently, a new hereditary syndrome of hypophosphatemic rickets has been described that is unusual in that symptoms include hypercalciuria and a normal serum calcium level. High calcitriol levels and hyperabsorption of dietary calcium distinguish this new disorder from the more common X-linked familial hypophosphatemic rickets in which defective calcitriol production is the usual feature.

Hypophosphatemic rickets emphasizes the role of phosphate in mediating vitamin D production in humans. It is probable that both the X-linked and the hypophosphatemic forms have a similar renal tubular defect in phosphate reabsorption. In hypophosphatemic rickets there is no apparent defect in calcitriol synthesis or action. Excessive calcifications of tendons, ligaments, and joint capsules of the hand and sacroiliac joints have been reported as late sequelae of rickets.

Osteomalacia may occur in the elderly if their diets are deficient in vitamin D or if they are not exposed to sunlight. Risk factors for osteomalacia are the use of anticonvulsants, gastrectomy, decreased renal function, and malnutrition. Such patients come to medical attention because of fractures (about one third of reported cases) or because biomechanical tests reveal low serum calcium (64%) and phosphate (27%) levels or increased alkaline phosphatase levels (100%). Fractures usually occur in the neck of the femur. Therefore, the physician must look for risk factors that suggest osteomalacia, especially with regard to diet and activities as well as the biochemical profile. In this manner it is possible to distinguish the elderly patient with vitamin D deficiency from the usual cohort of osteoporotics. Replacement with 400 to 1,000 units of vitamin D daily has been recommended in those patients suspected of deficiency. Recently, it has been suggested twice-yearly supplementation with 2.5 mg (100,000 units) of vitamin D is sufficient prophylaxis.

Paget's Disease of Bone

Paget's disease is a relatively common disorder of bone characterized by a hypermetabolic level of bone resorption and remodeling. The incidence varies by geographic location and the age of the population surveyed. Autopsy and radiographic studies have shown an incidence of as much as 4% in an Anglo-Saxon population more than 55 years of age. In other areas of the world it is significantly less common. A recent report discovered a surprisingly high prevalence of 1.3% in the black population of South Africa.

Extensive studies have shown no genetic predisposition and no association with HLA antigen typing. A viral origin was proposed in 1974 when virus-like inclusion bodies were found in osteoclasts from affected bone. Since then, research has focused on a slow virus as the causative agent. Some studies have implicated both the measles virus and the respiratory syncytial virus but conclusive evidence that either is the etiologic agent is lacking.

Diagnosis

The technetium Tc 99m bone scan is an excellent method of screening for additional area of involvement. It detects 8% more lesions than a skeletal survey does.

The initial event histologically is lysis of bone by large numbers of activated osteoclasts; this is followed by activation of osteoblasts that produce pagetic bone. The new bone is produced in abundance and contains widened lamellae and disorganized cement lines yielding the characteristic mosaic appearance of pagetic bone. At the time of osteoblast activation, the normal fatty or hematopoietic marrow is replaced by a loose, highly vascularized fibrous connective tissue. The osteoclastic activity and then the osteoblastic activity decrease, providing the "burned-out" stage with enlarged and deformed bones that are densely sclerotic.

The radiographic pattern closely follows the histologic course. Initially, the resorptive stage is seen as a discrete area of bone lysis, classically described as flame-shaped, in the long bones. This resorptive stage involves the endosteum and the inner layers of the diaphyseal cortex. Subsequent activation of the subperiosteal cortex leads to expansion of the bone with subperiosteal new bone; the activated osteoblasts centrally produce the sclerotic medullary bone. Treatment with calcitonin or a diphosphonate may transform the lytic pagetic bone into dense bone, providing radiographic evidence of therapeutic success.

The high rate of bone turnover produces localized fluxes of calcium and phosphate but the overall control of these two ions is tight, allowing no change in whole-body homeostasis in the absence of any other significant metabolic disorder. The activity of the disease process can be measured by monitoring serum alkaline phosphatase levels. A reduction by 50% in the serum level of this enzyme, which is involved in bone formation, is considered to be a therapeutic response. The enzyme level decreases one to two weeks after initiation of therapy.

The level of increased bone resorption can be monitored by measuring urinary excretion of collagen breakdown products. Hydroxyproline is a major component of type I collagen, the most common form of collagen in bone. Its 24-hour urinary clearance rate gives an excellent indication of the level of activity in Paget's disease. Treatment with calcitonin often results in a rapid (less than 24 hours) decrease in hydroxyproline clearance. Other by-products of bone resorption or formation, such as serum bone Gla-protein and osteocalcin, have not been found to be sensitive markers of the level of activity in Paget's disease.

The treatment of degenerative joint disease of either the hip or the knee is possible with total joint arthroplasty, although most cases respond to conservative management. A ten-year follow-up study of total hip arthroplasty in patients with degenerative coxarthrosis secondary to Paget's disease showed their rate of revision was not statistically higher than that of patients without Paget's disease. Aseptic loosening made revision necessary in approximately 15%.

The polyosteotic form typically involves the pelvis and spine. Pelvic lesions are well tolerated unless the acetabulum is involved. Spinal involvement is not as well tolerated. Low back pain is a frequent complaint and is often associated with symptoms of spinal stenosis. The affected spinal segments become progressively deformed, resulting in a narrowing of static canal measurements. These patients often respond well to pharmacologic therapy. Patients with advanced pagetic spinal involvement with myelopathic changes require surgical decompression after drug therapy has been initiated. These patients typically have multiple medical problems and can be at high risk for surgical complications.

Malignancies

Sarcomatous degeneration occurs in less than 1% of patients with active Paget's disease. Those with the polyosteotic form are most at risk, but it is not uncommon for patients with the monosteotic form to develop malignant degeneration. Osteogenic sarcoma is the most common type of sarcoma but chondrosarcomas, fibrosarcomas, and malignant giant cell tumors also occur.

Any increase in pain secondary to Paget's disease is strongly suggestive of the development of a sarcoma.

Radiographs, combined with a ^{99m}Tc technetium bone scan and gallium scan, are useful in detecting malignant degeneration. The diagnosis is based on a bone scan showing increased uptake in the region of Paget's disease with less uptake in the region of tumor and a gallium scan showing increased uptake only in the region of the tumor. A carefully planned biopsy confirms the diagnosis. Common problems caused by a biopsy include a pathologic fracture through the pagetic bone and excessive bleeding from the tumor or vascular fibrous tissue.

The treatment of a sarcoma is surgery and, if possible, chemotherapy. Many elderly debilitated patients cannot tolerate the aggressive chemotherapy that has improved survival rate for primary osteogenic sarcoma. The survival rate for Enneking stage IIB disease is 15%, with appendicular lesions having the best prognosis.

Treatment

The main indications for treating Paget's disease are significant deformity of the long bones or impending fracture, pain, progressive hearing loss, spinal impingement, medical disorders secondary to the hypermetabolic state, or concurrent treatment for any elective orthopaedic surgical procedure. Currently, there are three pharmacologic modes of treatment—calcitonin, mithramycin, and the diphosphonates.

Calcitonin Calcitonin acts via osteoclast inactivation and causes a rapid decrease in urinary hydroxyproline clearance. In a significant number of cases continued treatment leads to calcitonin resistance secondary to the development of antibodies to the form of calcitonin used or as a result of osteoclast desensitization. Subcutaneous calcitonin is more effective than calcitonin delivered by nasal spray (still experimental), but the spray form causes fewer side effects and is better tolerated.

Mithramycin Mithramycin is a potent agent that blocks bone resorption. Its severe side effects (hepatic and renal) limit its use to impending paraplegia secondary to Paget's disease or malignant hypercalcemia.

The Diphosphonates The diphosphonates are a promising class of drugs. Etidronate is currently the only medication approved for use. It takes several weeks for its clinical effect to become apparent. Combining calcitonin and etidronate decreases urinary hydroxyproline clearance significantly more than either drug alone. Etidronate produces sustained control of bone turnover even after administration is discontinued. Failure to achieve control carries a poor prognosis. Higher doses of etidronate are not effective and often result in osteomalacia.

The new experimental drug, 3-amino-1-hydroxypropylidene-1,1-bios-phosphonate (APD or AHPrBP), is promising. Clinical trials have shown a high rate of response and sustained remission with short courses of therapy. Side effects at therapeutic dosages have been negligible.

Osteopetrosis

Osteopetrosis (Albers-Schönberg disease or marble bone disease) is a rare metabolic bone disease that occurs in several species. It is characterized in humans by a diffuse increase in skeletal density with obliteration of the medullary canal and widening of the metaphyses but no gross alterations in the secondary epiphyses. Histologically, cores of calcified cartilage are surrounded by areas of new bone, indicating no abnormalities in the rate of bone or cartilage formation. A variable number of osteoclasts may be present. Those present lack the characteristic clear zone and ruffled border of osteoclasts actively resorbing bone.

Animal models (rat, rabbit, dog, and chicken) are available for laboratory use and may lead to elucidation of the different pathways by which osteoclastic function can be blocked. In the chicken, a form of osteopetrosis can be induced by infecting embryos with a retrovirus.

In humans, osteopetrosis has traditionally been diagnosed as congenital (juvenile, malignant, or infantile form) or adult (tarda form). This system clearly oversimplified the classification. Osteopetrosis is a genetically heterogeneous group of disease states.

Extreme variation occurs in the congenital form, which is classically characterized by profound anemia, splenohepatomegaly, thrombocytopenia, cranial and optic nerve palsy, and a compromised immune system. Death usually occurs at a young age secondary to overwhelming sepsis.

The congenital form is treated by bone marrow transplantation at a young age if an appropriate HLA-matched donor is available within the family. A successful transplant rapidly resolves the hematologic abnormalities, including the defect in immune function and a gradual restoration of the medullary cavity. HLA-mismatched transplants are less successful (30%) because of rejection or the development of graft versus host disease.

Recently, moderate success has been reported with prednisone and dietary manipulation in young patients for whom no HLA-matched bone marrow donors are available. An alternate form of therapy is high-dose calcitriol treatments and a low-calcium diet. Calcitrol at high dosages induces osteoclasts to form a ruffled border and a clear zone, indicating that they are actively resorbing. Treatment must be instituted at an early age to be effective.

A syndrome composed of osteopetrosis, renal tubular acidosis, cerebral calcifications, and minimal hematologic abnormalities has been described. It is inherited as an autosomal recessive trait and the defect has been traced to a deficiency of an isoenzyme of carbonic anhydrase. Techniques are being developed to screen potential carriers and should be available soon.

The adult (tarda) form of osteopetrosis is typically inherited as an autosomal dominant trait but an autosomal recessive form of the disease has also been described. Usually the adult form is expressed with minimal clinical manifestations, except for higher rates of fracture and cranial nerve palsies. Two distinct phenotypes exist in the adult form. Both are inherited as autosomal dominant traits and show progressive sclerosis of bone. Type I is characterized by sclerosis of the entire skull, minimal involvement of the spine, and a high incidence of conductive hearing loss. Type II shows radiographic evidence of sclerosis, primarily at the base of the skull, increased radiographic densities at the vertebral end plates ("rugger-jersey" spine), and the appearance of a "bone within a bone" in the pelvic ring. Serum acid phosphatase levels are increased in type II patients.

It is now clear that osteopetrosis is caused by several different genetic defects, all of which include the disruption of osteoclast function.

Outline 2. Growth factors involved in the local regulation of bone remodeling

Synthesized by skeletal cells
   Transforming growth factor-β
   Bone-derived growth factor or β_2-microglobulin
   Somatomedin C or insulin-like growth factor 1
   Platelet-derived growth factor
Isolated from bone matrix
   Transforming growth factor-β_1 and β_2
   Bone-derived growth factor
   Somatomedin C
   Platelet-derived growth factor
   Fibroblast-derived growth factors α and β
Synthesized in adjoining tissues
   Cartilage
      Somatomedin C
      Fibroblast-derived growth factor-β
   Monokines
      Interleukin-1
      Tumor necrosis factor-α
      Macrophage-derived growth factor
      Platelet-derived growth factor
   Lymphokines
      Lymphotoxin or tumor necrosis factor-α
      Interferon-γ

Growth Factors

Growth factors have a profound effect on injuries to and repair of bone, cartilage, and soft tissues. At this juncture, most investigative efforts have been directed toward isolation and characterization of growth factors in cell cultures and organic systems. These factors, exported into the matrix by local indigenous cells, or provided by cells recruited to the site of injury, manifest a broad spectrum of functions. These activities include chemotaxis, mitogenic activities, regulation of differentiation and maturation, and control of matrix synthesis. Growth factors can be endocrine, paracrine, or autocrine. Insulin-like growth factor (1 and 2) is delivered via the blood to a distant site of action in an endocrine manner of action. Platelet-derived growth factor and transforming growth factors (TGF-α and TGF-β) are synthesized at the site by one cell and used by another neighboring cell, a paracrine action. Other growth factors are produced and utilized by the same cell in an autocrine or self-stimulatory fashion. Bone morphogenic protein and other osteoinductive factors are currently being studied by classic biochemical techniques. Other factors that affect mesenchymal and epithelial cells and have been clinically defined are shown in Outline 2.

Trends

Significant advances in the understanding and treatment of metabolic bone diseases can be anticipated. Knowledge is rapidly expanding, particularly with regard to paracrine and autocrine factors that affect bone and the ontogeny and function of bone cells. New therapeutic agents that alter bone matrix are being developed. For several years, attention has focused on identifying, isolating, and testing autocrine and paracrine sustances produced in bone. These factors alter the local milieu through their modulation of the ontogeny and function of osteoprogenitor and differentiated bone cells. The usefulness of modulating local production or therapeutically applying these factors in the treatment of metabolic bone disorders is under active study. Significant advances are being made in the characterization of cell surface antigens and the identification of functional subclasses among committed osteoprogenitors. The possibility of carrying out cellular engineering, that is, the isolation, expansion, and administration of autologous bone cells to improve bone repair or function could one day become a reality. Finally, a greater understanding of the changes in bone matrix caused by specific therapies will provide more accurate end points for therapeutic trials. Ultimately, this new information will lead to intervention with recombinant cytokine material, autologous cell transplants, and matrix conditioning to prevent or repair skeletal damage resulting from metabolic bone disorders.

Annotated Bibliography

Keywords

Bone; Calcitonin; Estrogen; Matrix; Osteoblast; Osteoclast; Osteomalacia; Osteopenia; Osteoporosis; Paget's disease; Parathyroid hormone; Vitamin D

Cellular Control of Bone Metabolism

Centrella M, Canalis E: Local regulators of skeletal growth: A perspective. *Endocrinol Rev* 1985;6:544–551.
   Paracrine and autocrine regulators of bone growth, differentiation, and function.

Conn KM, Termine JD: Matrix protein profiles in calf bone development. *Bone* 1985;6:33–36.
   Profiles of matrix proteins during development.

Owen M: Lineage of osteogenic cells and their relationship to the stromal system, in Peck WA (ed): *Bone and Mineral Research.* Amsterdam, Elsevier, 1985, vol 3, pp 1–25.
   Origins of bone cells and review of bone cell ontogeny.

Pacifici R, Rifas L, Teitelbaum S, et al: Spontaneous release of interleukin 1 from human blood monocytes reflects bone formation in idiopathic osteoporosis. *Proc Natl Acad Sci USA* 1987;84:4616–4620.
   Examination of cytokine activity and skeletal dynamics.

Vaes G: Cellular biology and biochemical mechanism of bone resorption: A review of recent developments on the formation, activation, and mode of action of osteoclasts. *Clin Orthop* 1988;231:239–271.
   Review of recent literature on osteoclast-mediated resorption and the factors and cells that regulate osteoclasts.

Calcium Metabolism

Audran M, Kumar R: The physiology and pathophysiology of vitamin D. *Mayo Clin Proc* 1985;60:851–866.
Review of vitamin D physiology.

Auwerx J, Bouillon R: Mineral and bone metabolism in thyroid disease: A review. *Q J Med* 1986;60:737–752.
Effect of thyroid hormone on bone calcium metabolism.

Brommage R, DeLuca HF: Evidence that 1,25-dihydroxyvitamin D3 is the physiologically active metabolite of vitamin D3. *Endocrinol Rev* 1985;6:491–511.
Review of vitamin D endrocrinology.

Coindre JM, David J-P, Riviere L, et al: Bone loss in hypothyroidism with hormone replacement: A histomorphometric study. *Arch Intern Med* 1986;146:48–53.
Effects of thyroid hormone on bone loss.

Cooper DS: Thyroid hormone and the skeleton: A bone of contention, editorial. *JAMA* 1988;259:3175.
This editorial outlines a role for iatrogenic thyroid-induced osteoporosis.

Eastell R, Riggs BL: Calcium homeostasis and osteoporosis. *Endocrinol Metab Clin North Am* 1987;16:829–842.
Recent review of calcium homeostasis as it relates to osteoporosis.

Fischer JA, Born W: Calcitonin gene products: Evolution, expression and biological targets. *Bone Mineral* 1987;2:347–359.
Alternate mRNA splicing products from the calcitonin gene.

Forero MS, Klein RF, Nissenson RA, et al: Effect of age on circulating immunoreactive and bioactive parathyroid hormone levels in women. *J Bone Mineral Res* 1987;2:363–366.
Measurements of immunoreactive and bioactive parathyroid hormone show an increase with age.

Hurley DL, Tiegs RD, Wahner HW, et al: Axial and appendicular bone mineral density in patients with long-term deficiency or excess of calcitonin. *N Engl J Med* 1987;317:537–541.
The non-role of calcitonin in calcium homeostasis is examined through patient studies.

McSheehy PM, Chambers TJ: 1,25-Dihydroxyvitamin D3 stimulates rat osteoblastic cells to release a soluble factor that increases osteoclastic bone resorption. *J Clin Invest* 1987;80:425–429.
Role of soluble factors in coupling osteoblasts and osteoclasts.

Bone Biomechanics and Microstructure

Carter DR, Spengler DM: Mechanical properties and composition of cortical bone. *Clin Orthop* 1978;135:192–217.
A well-written and easily understood review of the basic biomechanics and biochemistry of bone that forms the basis of work currently being performed.

Frost HM: The mechanostat: A proposed pathogenic mechanism of osteoporoses and the bone mass effects of mechanical and nonmechanical agents. *Bone Mineral* 1987;2:73–85.
Role of mechanical signals in bone metabolism.

Goldstein SA, Ku JL, Hollister S, et al: Experimentally controlled trabecular bone remodeling: Effects of applied stress. *Trans Orthop Res Soc* 1987;12:461.
A model developed in the dog allows for the application of known stress to a portion of bone. Trabecular rearrangement occurs rapidly (within 22 weeks) to accept these new stresses.

Hart RT, Cowin SC, Davy DT, et al: The influence of bone maturation rates on surface bone remodeling. *Trans Orthop Res Soc* 1986;11:435.
A mathematical model is proposed for evaluating rates of bone maturation in newly remodeled areas.

Skerry TM, Pead MJ, Suswillo R, et al: Strain-related remodeling in bone tissue: Early stages of the cellular response to bone loading in vivo. *Trans Orthop Res Soc* 1988;13:97.
Interesting new information on the early physiologic events that occur after a bone is loaded.

Wong M, Carter DR: Mechanical stress and morphogenetic endochondral ossification of the sternum. *J Bone Joint Surg* 1988;70A:992–1000.
An interesting hypothesis about the possible role of mechanical stress in determining the pattern of endochondral ossification.

Osteoporosis and Osteopenia

Barth RW, Lane JM: Osteoporosis. *Orthop Clin North Am* 1988;19:845–858.
A comprehensive review of osteoporosis with 86 references.

Lane JM, Werntz JR, Healey JH, et al: Metabolic bone disease and Paget's disease in the elderly: Part I. Metabolic bone disease. *Clin Rheum Dis* 1986;12:49–70.
A thorough discussion of the diagnosis, treatment, and prevention of osteoporosis.

Raisz LG: Local and systemic factors in the pathogenesis of osteoporosis. *N Engl J Med* 1988;318:818–828.
An excellent review of the role of local bone factors in the etiology of the metabolic bone disorders of osteopenia.

Riggs BL, Melton LJ III: Evidence for two distinct syndromes of involutional osteoporosis. *Am J Med* 1983;75:899–901.
The first description of the two forms of osteoporosis.

Riggs BL, Melton LJ III: Involutional osteoporosis. *N Engl J Med* 1986;314:1676–1686.
This is a superb overview of osteoporosis with 124 references.

Exercise and Bone Homeostasis

Barrow GW, Saha S: Menstrual irregularity and stress fractures in collegiate female distance runners. *Am J Sports Med* 1988;16:209–216.
A strong correlation was found between severity of menstrual irregularity and the occurrence of stress fractures. The tibia was the most commonly involved bone.

Lester GE, Dutrow KD, Sutton WR, et al: Relationship between physical activity and bone density in Caucasian women: A 1–2 year follow-up. *Trans Orthop Res Soc* 1987;12:464.
This study correlates preservation of bone stock with regular exercise. No correlation was found between bone density and exercise level early in life.

Marcus R, Cann C, Madvig P, et al: Menstrual function and bone mass in elite women distance runners: Endocrine and metabolic features. *Ann Intern Med* 1985;102:158–163.

A well-designed study showing that the mineral density in the lumbar spines of amenorrheic runners is decreased when compared with control runners but increased when compared with less physically active amenorrheic runners.

Matheson GO, Clement DB, McKenzie DC, et al: Stress fractures in athletes: A study of 320 cases. *Am J Sports Med* 1987;15:46–58.

A detailed review of the findings in 320 cases of stress fractures.

Clinical Presentation and Diagnosis of Osteoporosis

Christiansen C, Riis BJ, Rodbro P: Prediction of rapid bone loss in postmenopausal women. *Lancet* 1987;1:1105–1108.

The authors present an approach to biochemical evaluation of bone losers.

Ott SM, Kilcoyne RF, Chestnut CH: Ability of four different techniques of measuring bone mass to diagnose vertebrae fractures in postmenopausal women. *J Bone Mineral Res* 1987;2:201–210.

A comparative study of the various noninvasive bone density determinations.

Riggs BL, Wahner HW: Bone densitometry and clinical decision-making in osteoporosis, editorial. *Ann Intern Med* 1988;108:293–295.

Guidelines for noninvasive densitometry.

Treatment and Prevention of Osteoporosis

Prevention and treatment of postmenopausal osteoporosis. *Med Lett* 1987;29:75–77.

A superb summary of treatment modalities for osteoporosis.

Kiel DP, Felson DT, Anderson JJ, et al: Hip fracture and the use of estrogens in postmenopausal women: The Framingham study. *N Engl J Med* 1987;317:1169–1174.

Estrogen supplementation affected the hip fracture rate in the Framingham study.

Lindsay R: Managing osteoporosis: Current trends, future possibilities. *Geriatrics* 1987;42:35–40.

A summary of the pathogenesis of and prevention programs for osteoporosis.

MacIntyre I, Stevenson JC, Whitehead MI, et al: Calcitonin for prevention of postmenopausal bone loss. *Lancet* 1988;1:900–902.

A random study demonstrating parity for estrogen and calcitonin in preventing bone loss.

Riis B, Thomsen K, Christiansen C: Does calcium supplementation prevent postmenopausal bone loss? A double-blind, controlled clinical study. *N Engl J Med* 1987;316:173–177.

Calcium may have had a minor effect on the loss of cortical bone but it had no effect on the trabecular bone.

Schnitzler CM, Sweet MB, Blumenfeld TS, et al: Radiographic features of the spine in fluoride therapy for osteoporosis. *J Bone Joint Surg* 1987;69B:190–194.

A detailed description of fluoride bone augmentation and its effect on the skeleton.

Slovik DM, Rosenthal DI, Doppelt SH, et al: Restoration of spinal bone in osteoporotic men by treatment with human parathyroid hormone (1–34) and 1,25-dihydroxyvitamin D. *J Bone Min Res* 1986;1:377–384.

The study documented the efficacy of parathyroid hormone in a program of bone augmentation.

Osteomalacia

Borrie MJ, Campbell AG, Carodoc-Davies TH: Osteomalacia in the elderly. *N Engl J Med* 1985;98:989–991.

Prevalence and clinical manifestations of osteomalacia in the elderly.

Paget's Disease of Bone

Maldague B, Malghem J: Dynamic radiologic patterns of Paget's disease of bone. *Clin Orthop* 1987;217:126–151.

A description of the radiographic patterns in the different stages of Paget's disease and their appearance after treatment.

McDonald DJ, Sim FH: Total hip arthroplasty in Paget's disease: A follow-up note. *J Bone Joint Surg* 1987;69A:766–772.

A presentation of the long-term follow-up of total hip arthroplasty in patients with Paget's disease.

Merkow RL, Lane JM: Metabolic bone disease and Paget's disease in the elderly: Part II. Paget's disease. *Clin Rheum Dis* 1986;12:70–96.

A review of the pathogenesis, diagnosis, and treatment of Paget's disease.

Thiebaud D, Jaeger P, Gobelet C, et al: A single infusion of the bisphosphonate AHPrBP (APD) as treatment of Paget's disease of bone. *Am J Med* 1988;85:207–212.

A promising new therapy for the treatment of mild or moderate Paget's disease.

Weisz GM: Lumbar canal stenosis in Paget's disease: The staging of the clinical syndrome, its diagnosis, and treatment. *Clin Orthop* 1986;206:223–227.

An article on the diagnosis, etiology, staging, and treatment of stenosis of the lumbar canal in patients with Paget's disease.

Osteopetrosis

Bullerslev J, Andersen PE Jr: Radiological, biochemical and hereditary evidence of two types of autosomal dominant osteopetrosis. *Bone* 1988;9:7–13.

An excellent review of the function and origin of the osteoclast and its role in osteopetrosis. The heterogeneity of the osteopetrotic lesion is discussed.

Dorantes LM, Mejia AM, Dorantes S: Juvenile osteopetrosis: Effects on blood and bone of prednisone and a low calcium, high phosphate diet. *Arch Dis Child* 1986;61:666–670.

A promising new treatment regimen using prednisone and dietary manipulation is proposed as an alternative for patients without appropriately matched bone marrow.

Fischer A, Griscelli C, Friedrich W, et al: Bone-marrow transplantation for immunodeficiencies and osteopetrosis: European survey, 1968–1985. *Lancet* 1986;2:1080–1084.

The results from a multicenter study show that HLA type is important for graft survival (47% for HLA-matched grafts compared with 29% for HLA-mismatched grafts).

Kaplan FS, August CS, Fallon MD, et al: Successful treatment of infantile malignant osteopetrosis by bone-marrow transplantation: A case report. *J Bone Joint Surg* 1988;70A:617–623.

Five-year follow-up data for a patient who received a bone

marrow transplant for osteopetrosis and a review of the subject.

Marks SC Jr: Congenital osteopetrotic mutations as probes of the origin, structure, and function of osteoclasts. *Clin Orthop* 1984;189:239–263.

An excellent review of the function and origin of the osteoclast and its role in osteopetrosis. The heterogeneity of the osteopetrotic lesion is discussed.

Growth Factors

Canalis E, McCarthy T, Centrella M: Growth factors and the regulation of bone remodeling. *J Clin Invest* 1988;81:277–281.

A detailed discussion of the effect of growth factors on bone.

Hauschka PV, Mavrakos AE, Iafrati MD, et al: Growth factors in bone matrix: Isolation of multiple types by affinity chromatography on heparin-sepharose. *J Biol Chem* 1986;261:12665–12674.

A thorough review of growth factors.

Nemeth GG, Bolander ME, Martin GR: Growth factors and their role in wound and fracture healing. *Prog Clin Biol Res* 1988;266:1–17.

A discussion of growth factors and cell activation.

3
Exercise and Athletic Conditioning

The orthopaedic surgeon is not only becoming increasingly involved in many aspects of sports medicine, but is applying knowledge of muscle physiology, rehabilitation, and the effects of exercise to general orthopaedic patients.

Effect of Warm-up Activities

Warm-up activities before athletic training and competition serve to increase muscle tone, increase blood flow, and increase flexibility. Stretching and the warm-up activity itself increase body temperature directly and increase the flexibility of the connective tissue so that it becomes more elastic. Motor nerve conduction velocity is increased after five minutes of exercise on a bicycle ergometer.

The value of muscle stretching in preventing athletic injury is still controversial. A significant increase in knee laxity after fatigue of the quadriceps and hamstrings was noted in one study. This may increase the risk of ligamentous injury. In another study, the effects of stretching were evaluated in 12 boys with an average age of 15.3 years. These boys participated in a rigorous protocol for stretching the knee and hip joints three times a week for seven weeks. The protocol included passive slow stretching and range-of-motion flexibility exercises. After the protocol was completed, evaluation showed increased flexibility, increased stride frequency, better relaxation time, improved fast isometric force development, and increased speed of concentric contractions. It was concluded that stretching positively influenced intrinsic muscle mechanics. Stretching has a positive effect on range of motion. Tensile force applied to a muscle increases its range of motion and its strength at the myotendinous junction.

Muscle Soreness

The cause of muscle soreness, or postexercise muscle pain, is being elucidated. Eccentric muscle contractions lead to a much greater degree of muscle pain than the more common concentric muscle contraction. Recent studies indicate that selective injury to type II or glycolytic muscle fibers in eccentric muscle contraction occurs at the myotendinous junction. (Eccentric contractions represent resisted lengthening of a contracted muscle.) Exhausting exercises, as in endurance sports such as long distance running and swimming, increase serum levels of muscle enzymes and indicate that muscle damage has occurred. An associated increase in hydroxyproline levels in the urine points to involvement of both muscle and connective tissue; again this probably occurs at the myotendinous junction.

Rehabilitation After Injury

Rehabilitation after muscle injury has been described with respect to overuse syndromes. Most authors advocate early, gentle range of motion. When to begin range of motion depends on whether or not the injured extremity requires splinting. After early range of motion is begun, isometric exercises should be started with flexibility exercises. Next, progressive resistance and dynamic exercises, including both isotonic and isokinetic exercises, may be started. When the patient reaches this activity level with minimal pain, athletic reconditioning can begin. If the injured muscle is one that is greatly stressed in the patient's particular sport, other conditioning exercises may be used. Cross-training has recently gained popularity. For example, injured runners can swim or bicycle for conditioning if they cannot run.

Nonsteroidal Medication After Muscle Injury

The use of nonsteroidal anti-inflammatory agents to treat soft-tissue injuries has been debated. One trial showed that they were not helpful in rehabilitation. Most authors indicate that they are helpful in reducing pain and inflammation during the first three days after injury. When muscles were immobilized and treated with piroxicam, a slight improvement was noted in the maximum load to failure compared with untreated controls. Nonsteroidal anti-inflammatory agents all inhibit prostaglandin synthesis. They are thought to act by mediating acute inflammation, changing the local and systemic concentrations of prostaglandins, vascular permeability, and the influx of polymorphonucleocytes. In adults, no one specific nonsteroidal agent is thought to be better than the next for the treatment of muscle injury. Nonsteroidal agents can be chosen for other properties such as frequency or dose, effects on gastric mucosa, cost, and the like. The Food and Drug Administration has approved the following nonsteroidal agents as analgesics: ibuprofen, naproxen, diflunisal, fenoprofen, suprofen, and mefenamic acid.

Exercise and Rehabilitation

The use of exercise in the rehabilitation of muscle injuries requires a knowledge of the different types of exercise (eccentric, concentric, isometric, isotonic, isokinetic). The duration of exercise and training for a specific task are important. Most studies indicate that eccentric exercise is more disruptive to muscle undergoing rehabilitation than concentric exercise. There appears to be increased mechanical destruction of the fibers and local tension with eccentric exercise protocols. Eccentric contractions are also associated with increased cellular damage and decreased motor performance.

Although training can decrease postexercise muscle soreness, even trained athletes become sore after using untrained muscle groups. Muscle training and adaptation is specific to the exercise performed. For this reason, a trained runner may have great difficulty swimming efficiently although equal amounts of energy are expended. These considerations must be taken into account when prescribing a muscle rehabilitation program. In rehabilitating muscle, the practitioner should consider which fiber types are involved. Endurance exercise is prescribed to recondition slow-twitch fibers, whereas speed and strength exercises should be prescribed for fast-twitch muscle fiber rehabilitation.

Preventing Reinjury

The management of hamstring injury has been reviewed in a retrospective study in which football injuries were evaluated. The players were treated with stretching, running, and resistance exercises. A second group of players underwent testing to determine the relative ratio of hamstring to quadriceps strength. If a deficiency was noted, strength was corrected to a quadriceps-hamstring ratio of 0.6. Reinjury was greatly decreased in the second group, in whom objective testing of hamstring strength after injury indicated normal quadriceps-hamstring ratios. It was concluded that players should not return to full competition and training until normal quadriceps-hamstring strength has been established.

Continuous Passive Motion

The use of continuous passive motion (CPM) was first investigated in a study in which lesions were created in the articular cartilage of rabbits. The joints were then immobilized in plaster or immediately mobilized with CPM. It was noted that improved joint surface regeneration occurred in the limbs treated with CPM. Subsequent studies indicated that regenerated cartilage is represented by newly formed fibrocartilage. More recently, CPM has been widely applied in orthopaedic rehabilitation. It is used in a variety of conditions. Its most common applications are postoperatively after total joint arthroplasty and intra-articular surgery on the knee.

The general effect of CPM on joint physiology is the stimulation of healing of articular fibrocartilage (type II collagen). Improved joint range of motion results. CPM prevents contracture of connective tissue after surgical intervention.

Advocates of CPM state that there is no increase in joint effusion or edema, hemarthrosis, or wound complications when it is used after surgery. The indications for CPM include open reduction and internal fixation of intra-articular fractures, arthrotomy, arthrolysis, metaphyseal osteotomy, free autogenous periosteal grafts for biologic resurfacing, and total joint replacement. In general, CPM has been used whenever there is a risk of diminished range of motion.

Diseases or conditions associated with joint ankylosis and contractures appear to be particularly well suited for treatment with CPM. CPM has been used in the treatment of arthrogryposis. This regimen, combined with stretching and splinting, decreased the need for tendon-lengthening procedures in selected patients. CPM is indicated in resolved joint infections when there is a potential for flexion contractures or ankylosis.

In patients requiring synovectomy, CPM may prove helpful. It has been used successfully in patients with rheumatoid arthritis and hemophilia after this type of surgery.

Various CPM protocols have been compared. In one study of 23 patients undergoing two CPM protocols after total knee replacement (20 hours of CPM per day in one group and five hours per day in the other), there was no difference between the two groups in total range of motion, hospital stay, edema, and number of physical therapy treatments required. Patients treated for five hours per day had better knee extension at day 6. Other studies have suggested that six to eight hours of CPM per day is as effective as CPM for longer periods.

Although CPM is in wide clinical use, many questions remain about its efficacy. Unresolved issues include optimal protocols in specific surgical procedures, its value in association with other treatments such as electrical stimulation, its role in preventing deep venous thrombosis, and its cost-effectiveness. These issues are now being addressed in clinical studies.

Psychological Disorders in Athletes

Appetite Disorders

The strict diagnostic criteria for appetite disorders include psychiatric as well as physiologic factors. Appetite disorders include anorexia nervosa, bulimia, pica, rumination disorder, and atypical eating disorders. The most common eating disorders seen in athletes are anorexia nervosa, bulimia, and atypical eating disorders. Appetite disorders are usually first evident in infancy, childhood, or adolescence.

The athletes most at risk for appetite disorders are runners, cheerleaders, gymnasts, and dancers.

Anorexia Nervosa Anorexia nervosa is characterized by intense fear of becoming obese, a disturbed body image, significant weight loss, and refusal to maintain minimal normal body weight. In women, amenorrhea occurs early in the course of the disease. The physical characteristics associated with this condition include a body fat of less than 12% in women and 6% in men. Often, there is a history of weight loss of more than 25% of the body weight.

Patients generally lose weight by decreasing their caloric intake, vomiting, taking diuretics and/or laxatives, and exercising to remarkable extremes. Death occurs in 15% to 21% of those afflicted. The most common cause of death is cardiac arrhythmia. Ninety-five percent of those affected are females. Approximately one in 250 females is thought to have this disorder to some degree. One third were mildly overweight before the onset of the illness. A close relative has often suffered from this disorder.

Medical intervention is imperative once the diagnosis of anorexia nervosa is made. Psychiatric and other appropriate medical help should be sought because of the high mortality rate associated with this disorder.

Bulimia Bulimia is associated with recurrent episodes of binge eating. Three of the following criteria must be met before the diagnosis is made: eating foods high in calories, inconspicuous eating during binging, termination of the binge by abdominal pain, and a change in sleep pattern. Repeated attempts to lose weight by severe dietary restrictions, self-induced vomiting, and use of laxatives or diuretics are common. Repeated weight fluctuations of 4.5

kg (10 lb) or more as a result of alternating binges and fasting are often noted. Most patients are aware that their eating pattern is abnormal. They have an intense fear of not being able to terminate eating voluntarily. They report depression and self-deprecating thoughts. Commonly, these patients are moderately obese; however, some are thin. The bulimic is concerned about body image. This is often related to a perceived loss of sexual attractiveness. Bulimics are subject to intermittent substance abuse disorders. Onset is usually in adolescence or early adulthood. Many patients first manifest signs of a disorder in college. Women are more often affected. Bulimia can be associated with electrolyte disturbances and dehydration secondary to the use of laxatives, diuretics, or self-induced vomiting. The differential diagnosis includes central nervous system tumors, seizure disorders, Klein-Levin syndrome, and Kluver-Bucy syndrome, all of which should be considered before a patient is diagnosed as having bulimia.

Atypical Eating Disorders An atypical eating disorder is usually seen as a single episode but it may appear in a chronic form in patients who steadfastly adhere to bizarre diets. Atypical eating disorder is defined as a disorder that cannot be classified as anorexia nervosa, bulimia, pica, or rumination disorder of infancy. For example, one atypical eating disorder can be diagnosed in a patient who eats massive quantities of bran. Diets such as this can result in hypocalcemia secondary to bran adsorption of calcium in the gut. This can induce secondary osteomalacia and stress factors.

Exercise as an Obligation

Several psychological effects that accompany exercise have medical significance. In particular, decreased somatic tension and anxiety are most common. Chronic exercise decreases the psychological symptoms of moderate depression. Although biologic adaptations are known to follow exercise training and to subside with diminished activity, there is currently no objective evidence that habitual exercise leads to psychological dependence. No direct relationships have been shown between exercise-induced mood swings and endorphin release or biogenic amines. Although habitual runners have reported euphoric states during or after exercise, this remains a subjective and unpredictable event.

The basis of obligatory exercise is both physiologic and psychological. Physiologic explanations include the release of β-endorphins and the overall improvement in fitness associated with athletic activity. The psychological aspects of this phenomenon include improved self-esteem. These effects can be so profound that the patient uses exercise regimens to cope with psychological, emotional, and personal problems.

Circadian Rhythms

Circadian rhythms include both behavioral and physiologic factors related to daily biologic cycles. Neuromuscular, cardiovascular, and metabolic factors are influenced by the circadian rhythm. Circadian rhythms affect the levels of performance capacity. The modulators of circadian rhythm include work load and psychological and physical stresses. Time of day, social interaction, lighting, sleep, altitude, diet, and age all affect circadian cycles. Circadian

dysrhythmia is characterized by sudden changes in chronologically associated activities. Abrupt changes in circadian rhythm adversely affect physical and mental performance. Abrupt circadian changes are induced by changing sleeping patterns (as happens in jet lag). For maximal physical and mental performance, circadian cycles must be adjusted by reestablishing normal sleep and activity patterns in a new time zone.

Drug Use

The use of drugs to enhance athletic performance is associated with increased risk for sudden death. In particular, centrally acting stimulants, such as amphetamines and cocaine, cause tachycardia that can lead to arrhythmia and cardiac arrest. Stimulants are also associated with an increased risk for cerebral vascular accidents secondary to acutely increased blood pressure. Anabolic steroids can cause sudden death from electrolyte imbalance and secondary cardiac arrhythmia. They may increase aggressiveness, leading to fatal confrontational situations. Depressants such as narcotics and barbiturates can also impair judgment. For example, divers taking a depressant may become unconscious while submerged because of cerebral hypoxia following hypoventilation induced by the drug. Diuretics, phenothiazines, and anticholinergics impair the thermoregulatory response and thereby increase the risk of hyperthermia.

Athletic Competition and Doping

Drug use is common in high-school, college, and professional athletes. No age group is free of this problem.

The International Olympic Committee defines doping as:

> The administration of or use by a competing athlete of any substance foreign to the body or of any physiologic substance taken in abnormal quantity or taken by an abnormal route of entry into the body with the sole intention of increasing in an artificial and unfair manner his/her performance in competition. When necessity demands medical treatment with any substance which because of its nature, dosage, or application is able to boost the athlete's performance in competition in an artificial and unfair manner, this too is regarded by the IOC as doping ... The presence of the drug in the urine constitutes an offense, irrespective of the route of administration.

Banned drugs include all medications or substances that enhance performance. The International Olympic Committee bans (1) stimulants, (2) narcotic analgesics, (3) anabolic steroids and human growth hormones, (4) β-blockers and (5) diuretics.

Stimulants Stimulants are a class of drugs that decrease fatigue, increase alertness, and may increase competitiveness and hostility. The effects of these drugs are both psychological and physiologic. They increase blood pressure, heart rate, and sympathetic tone. They are associated with anxiety, tremor, aggressiveness, and dehydration. The complications of using these drugs during athletic competition include increased risk for intracranial hemorrhage, stroke, arrhythmia, and cardiac arrest.

Narcotics Narcotics are drugs used to increase pain threshold and sometimes to decrease ventilation rate. The psychological effects of euphoria, stimulation, and a false feeling of invincibility are sometimes sought by athletes. Examples of these drugs include the opiates, such as morphine, cocaine, and codeine.

Anabolic Steroids Anabolic steroids are probably the most commonly abused drugs in athletics.

Anabolic steroids increase lean tissue mass and induce muscular hypertrophy. Whether or not they improve athletic performance is somewhat controversial. There is evidence that vigorous power training in combination with the ingestion of anabolic steroids may enhance the development of muscle strength. Significant performance improvement attributed to the use of anabolic steroids may actually result from behavior modification induced by these substances. Increased aggressiveness and euphoria may stimulate more intensive individual training. Anabolic steroids may create an illusion of performance that is not substantiated by careful measurement. Anabolic steroids also affect the libido, kidney, and liver. Musculoskeletal injuries induced by steroids include spontaneous tendon ruptures. Long-term use increases the risk of liver carcinoma, arteriosclerotic heart disease secondary to hyperlipidemia, stress fractures, and hyperglycemia. Impotence, testicular atrophy, decreased sperm production, breast enlargement, premature male baldness, enlarged prostate, and prostatitis are common. Adolescents may develop severe facial and body acne and premature closure of the physes, leading to short stature.

Female athletes who use these drugs to enhance performance are subject to masculinization and abnormal menstrual cycles. Additional changes noted in women, which may be permanent, include excess facial and body hair, an enlarged clitoris, and deepened voice.

These serious effects appear to have had little impact on the use of anabolic steroids among overly competitive athletes. The potential changes in sexual characteristics and possible impotence are generally more effective in convincing athletes to stop taking these drugs.

Human Growth Hormone Although the International Olympic Committee currently lists human growth hormone as a subgroup of anabolic steroids, it is a hormone secreted by the pituitary gland. It is a prohibited drug, but no test for its abuse is yet available. Human growth hormone affects all musculoskeletal tissues. Muscle growth is enhanced. The normal serum concentration of human growth hormone depends on the age, sex, body composition, and fitness of the athlete. Administration of growth hormone in animals induces muscle hypertrophy but produces no concomitant increase in strength. In humans, administration of growth hormone eventually leads to acromegaly, which is associated with myopathy and weakness. Because the supply from cadaveric sources has been limited, this drug has not been widely abused. The use of growth hormone may, however, become more prevalent as the genetically synthesized form becomes more readily available.

β-Blockers β-Blockers are compounds that affect the sympathetic nervous system by blocking the b-adrenergic response. They decrease blood pressure and heart rate and block the sympathetic cascade. These medications are abused in sports, such as shooting and archery, in which fine motor control and steadiness of hand are at a premium. Their side effects include hyperglycemia, wheezing, precipitation of congestive heart failure, headache, and impotence. Renal function may also be impaired.

Diuretics Diuretics are a class of drugs that increase renal excretion of fluid. Each of these drugs has specific effects on the kidney and may act at the proximal tubule, the glomerulus, the collecting tubules, or the loop of Henle. There may be potassium sparing or wasting. Certain electrolytes are preferentially excreted over others, depending on the diuretic used. Because they decrease weight by inducing water loss, diuretics are used primarily in sports with weight classifications such as wrestling and boxing. Side effects include electrolyte imbalance, metabolic alkalosis or acidosis, dehydration, and renal impairment.

The International Olympic Committee imposes different penalties for different drugs. Use of anabolic steroids, amphetamine-related and other stimulants, caffeine, diuretics, β-blockers, narcotic analgesics, and "designer" drugs results in a two-year ban for the first offense and a life ban for the second offense. Athletes using ephedrine, phenopropanolamine, codeine, and similar drugs as a cough suppressant or analgesic are suspended for a maximum of three months for the first offense and two years for the second offense and are banned for life for the third offense. Those who aid the athlete in the procurement or administration of these drugs are also subject to penalties.

Blood Doping Blood doping is the administration of blood or related erythrocyte products to an athlete for other than legitimate medical treatment. This is done in the unconfirmed belief that improving the oxygen-carrying capacity of the blood will improve aerobic performance. The complications of this abuse include transfusion reactions, such as rash or fever, delayed transfusion reaction, including fever or jaundice, and acute hemolytic reactions with kidney damage. Transmission of infections is a real risk. Overloading the circulation may lead to congestive heart failure or metabolic shock.

Sudden Death in Athletes

The causes of sudden death in athletes range from those of cardiac origin, thermoregulatory aberrations, dietary deficiencies, infection, illicit drugs, and chronic disease.

The reasons for sudden death from cardiovascular disease vary with age. Exercise-related deaths in older adults participating in various sports generally indicate that underlying cardiovascular disease was responsible for death in most cases. In patients less than 35 years old, unrecognized congenital cardiac abnormalities were frequently responsible and heart disease was diagnosed in only 25% of cases. These abnormalities include hypertrophic cardiomyopathy, congenital coronary artery anomalies, and ventricular abnormalities. Congenital conduction disturbances resulting in fatal cardiac arrhythmias were also noted. Uncommon cardiac problems in this young group include viral myocarditis, mitral valve prolapse, aortic stenosis, Marfan's syndrome, and sarcoidosis.

Studies have identified arteriosclerotic cardiovascular diseases in a majority of patients more than 35 years old who died suddenly while participating in sports. In one autopsy study of 60 athletes who died while playing squash,

58 deaths were attributed to cardiac causes. Fifty-one of the athletes had coronary artery disease, four had valvular heart disease, two had cardiac arrhythmia, and one had hypertrophic cardiomyopathy. The athletes included 59 men and one woman and the average age was 46 years (range, 22 to 66 years).

In another review of exercise-related deaths, 23% occurred during golfing, 20% during jogging, and 11% during swimming. The cause of death was arteriosclerotic heart disease in 88%. Only 7% of these recreational athletes were considered to be healthy before they died. Six patients were 29 years old or younger at the time of death. Congenital cardiovascular disease, valvular heart disease, hemorrhagic gastritis, and hypertrophic cardiomyopathy were the causes of death in these young individuals.

Environmental Risks

Environmental risks associated with athletic morbidity include temperature-related phenomena and lightning accidents.

Hyperthermia is a common problem associated with sudden death during exercise. Symptoms of hyperthermia include core temperature above 40 C, decreased sweating, confusion, cramping, cardiac arrhythmia, and headache. Hyperthermia is a medical emergency and should be suspected in any person who shows unusual behavioral or psychological changes during vigorous physical activity. Hyperthermia is the second most common cause of exercise-related deaths. Hyperthermia is more common in people more than 50 years old. Rectal temperatures of 41 C or above are associated with a 50% mortality rate.

This condition is often associated with a preexisting medical condition such as atherosclerosis, diabetes, obesity, or alcoholism. Certain drugs, such as diuretics, nonsteroidal anti-inflammatories, phenothiazines, sedatives, and anticholinergic drugs, affect the thermoregulatory system. All these medications should be considered risk factors for hyperthermia. Treatment of hyperthermia consists of lowering body temperature as rapidly as possible by any means available. Vigorous hydration, usually by intravenous infusion, should be initiated.

Athletes may become hypothermic during competition. This is most common in water sports. Rapid heat loss from both conduction and convection occurs in cold water. In general, cold environments in which athletes are improperly clothed predispose to hypothermia. A patient whose core temperature is less than 35 C is suffering from hypothermia. Hypothermia should also be suspected in any person who shows behavioral or psychological changes during cold exposure. Athletes who have arteriolosclerotic disease and/or who drink alcohol before participating in sports are predisposed to hypothermia. Alcohol decreases core temperature by inducing inappropriate peripheral vasodilitation and a decreased shivering response to the cold.

Proper acclimatization to temperature extremes is an important factor in preventing temperature-related morbidity and mortality.

Lightning is also responsible for a significant number of sports-related deaths. Open-air competition and training should be halted during lightning storms.

Exercise Prescriptions

Exercise prescriptions help maintain a general level of fitness and health. Exercise can also be used to maintain an optimal functional level in chronic disease. Exercise prescriptions must take into account the health status of the individual. A general health screening examination can serve to identify patients at risk for exercise-related injury and potential cardiovascular problems. The goals of such screening are to identify major medical problems, such as hypertension or diabetes, and to detect previously unsuspected cardiac disease. In young patients, hypertrophic cardiomyopathy, arrhythmia, aortic disease, Marfan's syndrome, and anomalous left coronary artery are the most important conditions.

Exercise screening in children has been reviewed extensively. It has been noted that the routine physical examination seldom identifies serious health problems in healthy children. A family history should be taken to document any instances of premature or sudden death. This information may indicate congenital risk factors such as hyperlipidemia, arrhythmias, or coronary anomalies requiring further evaluation.

In adults, the primary risk of dying during exercise-related activity is from cardiovascular disease. An electrocardiographic stress test is considered the best general screening method for identifying previously undiagnosed asymptomatic cardiovascular problems. Exertional hypotension has also been implicated as a risk factor for cardiac death during exercise.

General recommendations for exercise prescriptions should first identify the goals to be accomplished. Next, the type of exercise, its intensity and frequency, and monitoring of intensity, fitness, and strength should be determined before a program is begun. For endurance development, the exercise should be continued for 20 to 30 minutes three to four times a week. For maximal aerobic effect, heart rate should be increased to 80% of age-level maximum. Walking, running, cycling, swimming, cross-country skiing, jumping rope, and the like can all be good endurance-enhancing exercises.

Exercise and Pregnancy

Pregnant women can safely participate in many sports such as cycling, swimming, walking, and jogging. If a pregnant woman plans any extreme physical exertion, fetal heart monitoring should be done at regular intervals to assess the effect the sports activity has on the fetus. In particular, the placental steal syndrome should be looked for during physical activity. This condition involves shunting of blood away from the placenta during extreme exertion. Patients with uteroplacental insufficiency are more likely to have fetal stress changes during exercises secondary to an already compromised blood flow to the placenta. In general, aerobic work capacity during pregnancy should maintain the level of fitness already established before the onset of pregnancy. Fetal metabolism studies in animals show no adverse effects of exercise if exertion is mild to moderate.

Exercise and the Disabled

Disabled patients may need special provisions when participating in sports. The blind, for example, can use monitors that help guide them during exercise. This allows the blind to participate in sports such as cross-country skiing, cycling, and track and field. Athletes who participate in wheelchair sports can successfully compete and train in graded programs. However, paraplegic patients have impaired heat-regulatory mechanisms; because of loss of sympathetic control, they must be closely monitored for hyperthemia. Those who have not participated in exercise programs previously may be overweight and, therefore, at increased risk for cardiovascular disease. Before vigorous training begins, they should undergo careful cardiovascular screening.

Exercise and Cardiovascular Disease

Aerobic exercise is an excellent way of conditioning the cardiovascular system, one that uses both fatty acids and carbohydrates for energy. Endurance athletes usually have a slow resting pulse and a high maximal oxygen consumption. Their left ventricles are larger and thicker than those of sedentary persons and their hearts are more efficient. Being aerobically unfit is associated with impaired left ventricular efficiency. Decreased sympathetic nervous system tone accompanies aerobic training. This is represented by slower resting heart rates and increased efficiency of cardiac muscle. Aerobic activities are preferable to anaerobic activities such as weight-lifting for hypertensive patients. Aerobic training can decrease resting heart rate and moderate elevated blood pressure. Strength training can significantly increase systolic blood pressure during heavy-resistance weight-training.

Myocardial Infarction After myocardial infarction, typical and atypical angina should be documented and its severity should limit the patient's participation in exercise. The electrocardiogram should be carefully monitored and patients should stop their activity if they develop symptoms. In general, patients can recover cardiovascular tolerance to strenuous aerobic exercise, but this requires a well-supervised program of progressive aerobic training monitored by experienced personnel.

One study of a two-year walking-jogging program described 36 men, 21 to 57 years old, who had received heart transplants. The group's average weekly training distance was 24 km. After training, lean tissue increased and dia-

Table 1. Modifiable aspects of aging*

Aging Marker	Decisions Required†
Cardiac reserve	Exercise, nonsmoking
Dental decay	Prophylaxis, diet
Glucose tolerance	Weight control, exercise, diet
Intelligence tests	Training, practice
Memory	Training, practice
Osteoporosis	Weightbearing exercise, diet
Physical endurance	Exercise, weight control
Physical strength	Exercise
Pulmonary reserve	Exercise, nonsmoking
Reaction time	Training, practice
Serum cholesterol	Diet, weight control, exercise
Social ability	Practice
Skin aging	Sun avoidance
Systolic blood pressure	Salt limitation, weight control, exercise

*Reproduced with permission from Fries, JF, Crapo LM: *Vitality and Aging.* New York, WH Freeman, 1981, p 125.
†These decisions to change environment or lifestyle may decrease the severity and impact of many age-related physiologic changes.

stolic blood pressure and resting heart rate decreased. There is one report of a heart transplant patient who ran a 20-km race nine months after surgery. This transplant patient responded to most registered physiologic variables in the same manner as normal controls. There were some differences in renal function because the patient was taking immunosuppressive drugs.

Exercise and Chronic Disease

Patients with renal disease can benefit from physical activity that decreases depression and increases fitness. The effect of exercise on endocrine diseases, in particular, can help control the blood glucose level in diabetes mellitus. The effect of exercise is to decrease the amount of insulin required by insulin-dependent diabetics. Any aerobic activity has this effect.

For patients who have degenerative joint disease, sports activities should be selected to prevent further deterioration of damaged joints. For example, for patients with lower-extremity arthritis, swimming is an excellent aerobic activity. This type of exercise prescription encourages activity while increasing caloric consumption. Increased fitness and decreased weight generally have positive effects on this group of patients.

Exercise and Age

Approximately 44% of the population more than 65 years old have some degree of physical disability. Disuse atrophy is responsible for a major proportion of the functional decline associated with aging. The physiologic response to training, however, occurs at any age. There is evidence that exercise can improve physiologic function and decrease the impact of chronic disease in the elderly. Reported benefits include improved cardiovascular and respiratory function, reduced risk of coronary artery disease, decreased body fat, and increased lean body mass. There is increased bone mass, increased work capacity, greater flexibility, reduced susceptibility to depression, improved self-esteem, and greater independence.

Social sports and group activities are popular among the elderly. Exercise prescriptions should also take into account the patient's particular interests. The effects of physical activity on the aging process can, in general, be summed up as preventing many of the factors that we associate with aging (Table 1). Because regular physical activity maintains bone mass, it is important in the treatment of osteoporosis. Bone resorption and muscle atrophy can be minimized by regular physical activity.

Trends

An important trend in recent years has been the application of rehabilitation techniques and physiologic knowledge to a broader spectrum of orthopaedic patients. Further, there is an increasing interest on the part of the orthopaedic research community in providing a scientific basis for clinical practice. Other goals will be improved management of the apparently increasing incidence of eating or nutritional disorders and drug use, particularly anabolic steroids. Both problems appear to reflect the public's preoccupation with body image.

Annotated Bibliography

Keywords

Anabolic steroids; Anorexia nervosa; Biorhythms; Bulimia; Cardiovascular disease; Continuous passive motion; Exercise; Human growth hormone; Muscle; Pregnancy; Rehabilitation; Sports medicine

Effect of Warm-up Activities

Hortobágyi T, Faludi J, Tihanyi J, et al: Effects of intense "stretching"-flexibility training on the mechanical profile of the knee extensors and on the range of motion of the hip joint. *Int J Sports Med* 1985;6:317–321.
The authors review the effects of stretching on intrinsic muscle mechanics and range of motion.

Skinner HB, Wyatt MP, Stone ML, et al: Exercise-related knee joint laxity. *Am J Sports Med* 1986;14:30–34.
This study shows how exercise and muscle fatigue are related to knee joint laxity and subsequent injury.

Muscle Soreness

Byrnes WC, Clarkson PM: Delayed onset muscle soreness and training. *Clin Sports Med* 1986;5:605–614.
Training specificity and eccentric contractions are cited as reasons for poor motor performance in this review article. The authors also discuss the perception of muscle soreness.

Lieber RL, Fridén JO, McKee-Woodburn TG: Selective damage of fast glycolytic muscle fibers with eccentric exercise of the rabbit tibialis anterior. *Trans Orthop Res Soc* 1988;13:337.
This abstract clearly delineates selective damage to type II muscle fibers from eccentric exercise.

Rehabilitation After Injury

Heiser TM, Weber J, Sullivan G, et al: Prophylaxis and management of hamstring muscle injuries in intercollegiate football players. *Am J Sports Med* 1984;12:368–370.
This retrospective study found that athletes had fewer reinjuries if they achieved a normal quadriceps-hamstring ratio before returning to competition.

Kellett J: Acute soft tissue injuries: A review of the literature. *Med Sci Sports Exerc* 1986;18:489–500.
The author classifies and describes acute soft-tissue injuries and discusses a comprehensive rehabilitation program.

Renström P, Johnson RJ: Overuse injuries in sports: A review. *Sports Med* 1985;2:316–333.
The authors discuss different types of overuse syndromes and present guidelines for their treatment.

Continuous Passive Motion

Basso DM, Knapp L: Comparison of two continuous passive motion protocols for patients with total knee implants. *Phys Ther* 1987;67:360–363 [erratum, 1987;67:979].
Fifteen of 23 patients who underwent total knee replacement were treated with continuous passive motion for 20 hours a day. The other eight were treated for five hours a day. On postoperative days 3 and 6, there were no differences between the two groups in terms of total range of motion, length of hospital stay, presence of edema, and number of physical therapy sessions. The group treated for five hours a day, however, had better knee extension on day 6.

Limbird TJ, Dennis SC: Synovectomy and continuous passive motion (CPM) in hemophiliac patients. *Arthroscopy* 1987;3:74–79.
Five hemophiliacs treated with immediate postoperative continuous passive motion had regained their preoperative range of motion by six months after synovectomy.

Lynch AF, Bourne RB, Rorabeck CH, et al: Deep-vein thrombosis and continuous passive motion after total knee arthroplasty. *J Bone Joint Surg* 1988;70A:11–14.
A prospective study critically examining the use of continuous passive motion in 150 consecutive patients divided into two equal groups demonstrated no difference in the incidence of deep venous thrombosis.

Videman T: Connective tissue and immobilization: Key factors in musculoskeletal degeneration? *Clin Orthop* 1987;221:26–32.
The role of various therapies in immobilized limbs is discussed.

Vince KG, Kelly MA, Beck J, et al: Continuous passive motion after total knee arthroplasty. *J Arthrop* 1987;2:281–284.
Of the 62 patients who underwent total knee replacement, those who had postoperative continuous passive motion had a lower incidence of deep venous thrombosis on venogram.

Psychological Disorders in Athletes

Diagnostic and Statistical Manual of Mental Disorders, ed 3. Washington, DC, American Psychiatric Association, 1980, pp 67–73.
This comprehensive text provides the diagnostic criteria, descriptions, predisposing factors, prevalence, and differential diagnosis for psychiatric disorders.

Blumenthal JA, O'Toole LC, Chang JL: Is running an analogue of anorexia nervosa? An empirical study of obligatory running and anorexia nervosa. *JAMA* 1984;252:520–523.
In this study, 43 runners and 23 anorexics took the Minnesota Multiphasic Personality Inventory. The conclusion was that obligatory runners do not suffer from the same degree of psychopathology as anorexics.

Dishman RK: Medical psychology in exercise and sport. *Med Clin North Am* 1985;69:123–143.
This excellent review article details the psychological outcomes that accompany short- and long-term exercise. Cognitive and perceptual changes associated with exercise and the possible relation to biochemical events are presented.

Hatfield BD, Goldfarb AH, Sforzo GA, et al: Serum beta-endorphin and affective responses to graded exercise in young and elderly men. *J Gerontol* 1987;42:429–431.
No changes in β-endorphin were noted after exercise. Serum levels were the same in young and in elderly men.

Lundholm JK, Littrell JM: Desire for thinness among high school cheerleaders: Relationship to disordered eating and weight control behaviors. *Adolescence* 1986;21: 573–579.

A strong desire for thinness was associated with an increased rate of eating disorders in this study of 751 high-school cheerleaders.

Wheeler GD, Wall SR, Belcastro AN, et al: Are anorexic tendencies prevalent in the habitual runner? *Br J Sports Med* 1986;20:77–81.

No significant increase in anorexia nervosa was found in 49 runners compared with 18 controls but there was a high prevalence of distorted body image among runners.

Circadian Rhythms

McMurray RG, Fafrowicz JF, Berry M: The endorphin response of women to sleep loss and exercise. *Aviat Space Environ Med* 1988;59:129–132.

Seven women ran one hour on a treadmill at 80% of Vo_2 maximum after normal sleep and after 36 hours of sleep deprivation. Venous blood samples of β-endorphins, oxygen uptake, heart rate, blood pressure, and perceived exertion were the same after both tests.

Winget CM, DeRoshia CW, Holley DC: Circadian rhythms and athletic performance. *Med Sci Sports Exerc* 1985;17:498–516.

Excellent review article that discusses the effect of circadian rhythm on physiology and behavior important to athletic performance. The authors explain disturbance of circadian rhythm (jet-lag) and delineate how it can result in poor performance.

Drug Use

American College of Sports Medicine: Position stand on the use of anabolic-androgenic steroids in sports. *Med Sci Sports Exerc* 1987;19:534–539.

This statement reviews the literature and condemns the use of steroids.

Ballarin E, Guglielmini C, Martinelli S, et al: Unmodified performance in runners following anabolic steroid administration. *Int J Sports Med* 1986;7:302–306.

Low-dose steroid use was studied in ten well-trained runners over six weeks. Serum tests documented the effects of steroid use. No improvements in running times or Vo_2 maximum were found.

Haupt HA, Rovere GD: Anabolic steroids: A review of the literature. *Am J Sports Med* 1984;12:469–484.

The authors discuss why the use of steroids is controversial. A detailed review of the literature is thoughtfully presented.

Kibble MW, Ross MB: Adverse effects of anabolic steroids in athletes. *Clin Pharm* 1987;6:686–692.

This review of the literature discusses the effects of steroids on performance and their adverse effects on the body.

Macintyre JG: Growth hormone and athletes. *Sports Med* 1987;4:129–142.

This review of the literature presents the action and side effects of growth hormone in animals and humans.

McKillop G, Ballantyne D: Liproprotein analysis in bodybuilders. *Int J Cardiol* 1987;17:281–288.

Twenty-four subjects were studied with respect to steroid use and bodybuilding. Those subjects using steroids were found to have higher levels of serum liproproteins associated with a greater risk for arteriosclerotic cardiovascular disease.

USOC Division of Sports Medicine and Science: *Guide to Banned Medications*. United States Olympic Committee, 1988.

The guide lists all banned medications and includes the official definition of "doping."

Sudden Death in Athletes

Amsterdam EA, Laslett L, Holly R: Exercise and sudden death. *Cardiol Clin* 1987;5:337–343.

Mechanisms of sudden death and the screening of asymptomatic patients.

Driscoll DJ: Cardiovascular evaluation of the child and adolescent before participation in sports. *Mayo Clin Proc* 1985;60:867–873.

Excellent article details the cardiovascular evaluation of children and adolescents before sports participation. The authors review the causes of cardiovascular disease and how to diagnose them in this population.

Epstein SE, Maron BJ: Sudden death and the competitive athlete: Perspectives on preparticipation screening studies. *J Am Coll Cardiol* 1986;7:220–230.

Sudden death usually results from cardiovascular disease and the specific causes are age-dependent. This article reviews the place of screening for age-specific cardiovascular disease and discusses how to design screening programs.

Maron BJ, Epstein SE, Roberts WC: Causes of sudden death in competitive athletes. *J Am Coll Cardiol* 1986;7:204–214.

Common and uncommon cardiovascular diseases responsible for sudden death are presented in this comprehensive article.

Maron BJ, Bodison SA, Wesley YE, et al: Results of screening a large group of intercollegiate competitive athletes for cardiovascular disease. *J Am Coll Cardiol* 1987;10:1214–1221.

Of 501 patients screened for cardiovascular disease, 84% had no evidence of cardiovascular disease and 15% had positive echocardiographic findings with mitral valve prolapse. One patient had mild systolic hypertension.

Northcote RJ, Flannigan C, Ballantyne D: Sudden death and vigorous exercise: A study of 60 deaths associated with squash. *Br Heart J* 1986;55:198–203.

The authors describe 60 persons who died suddenly while playing squash. Autopsy reports were available for 51 patients. There were only two deaths for noncardiac reasons. Twenty-two patients had at least one medical condition related to the cardiovascular system before death.

Environmental Risks

Appenzeller O, Atkinson R (eds): *Sports Medicine: Fitness, Training, Injuries*. Baltimore, Urban & Schwarzenberg, 1981, pp 13–40.

A basic review of thermoregulatory disorders in athletics.

Exercise Prescriptions

Cantwell JD: Cardiovascular aspects of running. *Clin Sports Med* 1985;4:627–640.

Running provides excellent conditioning of the cardiovascular system. The authors evaluate its physiologic consequences.

Cantwell JD: The athlete's heart. *Compr Ther* 1985;11: 26–38.

The author discusses exercise and its effect on myocardial metabolism, including changes in the autonomic nervous system. Cardiovascular screening is also examined.

Carney RM, Wetzel RD, Hagberg J, et al: The relationship between depression and aerobic capacity in hemodialysis patients. *Psychosom Med* 1986;48:143–147.

The authors cite their reasons for encouraging exercise in hemodialysis patients.

Colt EW, Hashim S: Effect of exercise and diet on lipids and cardiovascular disease. *Curr Concepts Nutr* 1986;15: 117–143.

A review article addressing exercise, lipids, and cardiovascular disease.

Gorski J: Exercise during pregnancy: Maternal and fetal responses. A brief review. *Med Sci Sports Exerc* 1985;17: 407–416.

An excellent, comprehensive article that reviews the physiologic effects of exercise on pregnancy and on the fetus. Training adaptations, hypoglycemia, veteroplacental insufficiency, and hyperthermia are discussed.

Kavanagh T: Distance running and cardiac rehabilitation: Physiologic and psychosocial considerations. *Clin Sports Med* 1984;3:513–526.

The author reviews how long-distance running can improve hemodynamic performance, alter lipid profile, and alleviate depression.

Kavanagh T, Yacoub MH, Mertens DJ, et al: Cardiorespiratory responses to exercise training after orthotopic cardiac transplantation. *Circulation* 1988;77:162–171.

In 36 men who were tested in a two-year program after surgery, fitness was improved. The physiologic responses are discussed.

Landin RJ, Linnemeier TJ, Rothbaum DA, et al: Exercise testing and training of the elderly patient. *Cardiovasc Clin* 1985;15:201–218.

The authors show how disuse atrophy or inactivity is responsible for the functional decline typical of aging.

Lehmann M, Schmid P, Keul J: Age- and exercise-related sympathetic activity in untrained volunteers, trained athletes and patients with impaired left-ventricular contractility. *Eur Heart J* 1984;5(suppl E):1–7.

The influence of training on aging, left ventricular contractility, and the sympathetic nervous system was studied in a variety of patients.

Meusel H: Developing physical fitness for the elderly through sport and exercise. *Br J Sports Med* 1984;18:4–12.

The authors reviews the means by which the elderly can maintain fitness and avoid many of the consequences traditionally associated with aging but actually resulting from poor fitness.

Opasich C, Cobelli F, Assandri J, et al: Is old age a contraindication to cardiac rehabilitation after acute myocardial infarction? *Eur Heart J* 1984;5(suppl E):105–107.

Fifty men older than 65 years of age were tested and then placed on a program of fitness after myocardial infarctions. The recovery of fitness was documented.

Risser WL, Hoffman HM, Bellah GG Jr, et al: A cost-benefit analysis of preparticipation sports examinations of adolescent athletes. *J Sch Health* 1985;55:270–273.

This article discusses the costs of screening compared with its benefits.

Rowland TW: Preparticipation sports examination of the child and adolescent athlete: Changing views of an old ritual. *Pediatrician* 1986;13:3–9.

This article reviews physiologic changes occurring with exercise in young people and discusses health screening for participation in sports.

Ungerman-deMent P, Bemis A, Siebens A: Exercise program for patients after cardiac surgery. *Arch Phys Med Rehabil* 1986;67:463–466.

The effects of an exercise program on patients are described with respect to fitness and hospital morbidity and hospital stay.

Vallbona C, Baker SB: Physical fitness prospects in the elderly. *Arch Phys Med Rehabil* 1984;65:194–200.

The prevalence of physical disability and the impact of fitness programs are discussed with respect to the elderly.

4
Arthritis

Advances in our knowledge and treatment of arthritis include new concepts of normal joint structure and function and a better understanding of the pathophysiology of osteoarthritis and the inflammatory arthropathies. A notable development of the past ten years in arthritis treatment has been the improvement, implementation, and widespread use of arthroscopy. Arthroscopy is helpful in the diagnosis and treatment of moderate traumatic injuries, in synovectomy for rheumatoid arthritis, and in debridement for infection. The continuing evolution of and improvements in total joint replacement for all forms of end-stage arthritis continue to be of importance. In 1986 when 10% of the American Rheumatism Association was polled with respect to the most important advances in the management of rheumatic diseases during the preceding 20 years, total joint replacement outscored all other advances (Table 1).

Normal Joint Physiology

Articular cartilage is avascular, aneural, and alymphatic tissue made up of a small number of chondrocytes surrounded by a large quantity of extracellular matrix. The matrix, which is a superhydrated material (approximately 72% water), is composed predominantly of proteoglycans and collagen and provides articular cartilage with its material properties and many of its characteristics.

Chondrocytes

The cells in articular cartilage constitute 5% or less of its volume and are found as individual cells or cell nests. Chondrocytes are nourished principally by diffusion of the smaller (<100 kd) molecules, which enter the synovial fluid as a transudate of plasma through the vessels in the synovium. A lesser amount of nourishment comes through the subchondral bone plate. Because all nourishment, oxygenation, and communication must diffuse through the matrix to reach the cartilage cells, the microenvironment of the chondrocytes is different from those of most other

Table 1. Important recent advances*

Advance	Clinical Impact Score†
Total joint replacement	1.47
Methotrexate treatment	2.10
Early aggressive treatment	2.16
Cytotoxic treatment	2.38
Emphasis on functional outcomes	2.40
Penicillamine treatment	2.87
Advent of arthritis professionals	2.88
Patient self-management programs	2.89

*Reproduced with permission from Fries JF: Milestones in rheumatologic care (1965–1985), in Fries JF (ed): *Milestones in Management: Rheumatoid Arthritis.* Puerto Rico, Syntex, 1988.
†On a scale of 1 to 5, with 1 being critically important.

cells in the body. There is a higher level of carbon dioxide and the cells can tolerate a lower level of oxygenation. Articular cartilage cells survive for 48 hours or longer after the death of the organism. Chondrocytes, embedded in their matrix, rely on the diffusion of small messenger molecules for communication. Histamine activates chondrocyte adenylate cyclase through a histamine$_2$ (H$_2$) receptor. Cartilage cells are actually more responsive to histamine than are synovial fibroblasts. Interleukin-1, a small molecular messenger synthesized by macrophages and leukocytes, stimulates chondrocytes to degrade their own matrix by releasing a variety of collagenolytic and proteoglycanase products. Other mediators such as insulin, estrogen, thyroid-derived factors, and a variety of growth factors by themselves or in combination have trophic effects on cartilage cells (Table 2). Cartilage-derived growth factor can increase hyaluronate synthesis while decreasing synthesis of sulfate glycosaminoglycans. Cell density increases with age. Insulin-like growth factor 1 stimulates clonal growth of postnatal chondrocytes to a greater extent than it does fetal chondrocytes.

The pH surrounding the chondrocytes is normally at or just below 7.4. When the pH is artificially increased or decreased, a variety of disruptive ultrastructural changes are observed.

The four zones of the articular cartilage are the superficial zone, the transitional zone, the deep (or radial) zone, and the calcified zone. The tidemark separates the calcified from the noncalcified zones. On scanning microscopy, the normal articular surfaces show distinct elevations at the microscopic level; these represent the outlines of the superficial chondrocytes. Cells in the superficial zone are densely packed and, unlike those in the deeper layers, are organized tangential to the surface, providing a "skin"-like interface. The chondrocytes have increasing amounts of endoplasmic reticulum, Golgi apparatus, mitochondria, and lysosomes from the superficial zone through the top half of the calcified zone. In the bottom half of the calcified zone these organelles decrease. Thus, chondrocytes are metabolically active in all zones but show signs of less activity in the calcified zone. The amount of rough endoplasmic reticulum area per unit volume is also greater in the superficial zone than in the deeper layers. The deeper layers of chondrocytes show a marked increase in intraplasmic filaments compared with the superficial zone; this increase is thought to be associated with degenerating cells.

Chondrocyte synthesis of glycosaminoglycans under intermittent compressive forces differs from that under static compressive forces or no compressive force. The compressive forces tested thus far are only slightly greater than normal atmospheric forces, whereas articular cartilage cells are normally subjected to regular stresses of 7 to 10 atm with each cycle of active joint motion. Normal joint hydrostatic forces may be important in preserving articular

Table 2. Influence of growth factors on articular cartilage

Growth Factor	Extracellular Matrix		Cell Proliferation
	Glycosaminoglycan Synthesis	Collagen Synthesis	
Transforming growth factor-β	Stimulates	Stimulates	Stimulates
Tumor necrosis factor-α	Inhibits	Not tested	Stimulates
Insulin-like growth factor 1	Stimulates	Stimulates	Stimulates
Fibroblast growth factor-α	Stimulates	Not tested	Stimulates
Fibroblast growth factor-β	Stimulates	Not tested	Stimulates
Platelet-derived growth factor*	Stimulates	Not tested	Stimulates
Insulin	Stimulates	Not tested	Stimulates
Epidermal growth factor*	Stimulates	Not tested	Stimulates

*Tested with 1% serum.

cartilage from the invasion of blood vessels. Cartilage disruption is closely associated with vascular invasion in a wide spectrum of diseases.

Matrix

The extracellular chondrocyte products that form the matrix are collagen, a triple-helix molecule with excellent tensile strength, proteoglycans, anionic macromolecules that aggregate on long chains of hyaluronic acid, and water, which is trapped within the collagen-proteoglycan complex by hydrostatic forces.

The fibrillar network of cartilage is largely composed of type II collagen. Type II collagen is known to appear in all hyaline cartilages and represents about 90% to 95% of the total cartilage collagen. Collagen types IX and XII are also present in all hyaline cartilage. Type I is present in the superficial layers of articular cartilage and types V and VI have recently been identified in bovine cartilage.

Proteoglycans are made up of repeating units or monomers held by a small segment, called link protein, that stabilizes the monomers to a long hyaluronic acid chain woven throughout the cartilage matrix. The proteoglycan monomers themselves are soluble when not stabilized to the hyaluronic acid and can diffuse out into the synovial fluid and then into the bloodstream. Hyaluronic acid chains with multiple monomers linked to them are referred to as aggregates and are insoluble. The proteoglycan monomer (subunit) has a core protein surrounded by glycosaminoglycans (principally chondroitin sulfate or keratan sulfate). The end of the core protein farthest from its link to the hyaluronic acid is made up of a C-terminal globular domain. Proximal to this, there is a large region of the core protein to which chondroitin sulfate attaches at right angles; next, there is a region to which keratan sulfate attaches; finally, there is a small, 50-kd hyaluronate-binding region. This region has few or no glycosaminoglycan chains and is a globular domain that mediates binding to the hyaluronic acid along with link protein.

There are two major populations of aggregating proteoglycans in cartilage. They differ in the size of their protein cores and in the relative proportions of their side chains. Articular chondrocytes appear to have an inherent program that determines the specific nature of proteoglycans synthesized at different ages. Early in life, only one type of aggregating proteoglycan is found in cartilage—the larger, slower, migrating proteoglycan. The proteoglycan monomer is synthesized as a precursor that has a low affinity for hyaluronic acid. There is no age-related change in the size of newly synthesized hyaluronic acid but there

is a decrease in the size of the proteoglycan aggregate with age.

Proteoglycan aggregates typically stimulate the formation of type II collagen fibrils. Nonaggregating proteoglycans retard the formation of type II collagen fibrils except early in life when they strongly stimulate fibril formation in cartilage.

The extracellular matrix is in constant turnover. Under normal circumstances, the chondrocyte controls the turnover in the matrix by both synthesis and degradation. Chondrocytes degrade the matrix by the manufacture and release of proteases. Chondrocytes also produce protease inhibitors that are normally found in excess. The chief neutral protease may be a metal-dependent proteoglycanase. This enzyme exists mostly in latent form and is activated when a 10-kd fragment is removed from the molecule. Inhibitors of proteoglycan-degrading enzymes are plentiful throughout the synovial fluid and articular cartilage. The chondrocyte governs the homeostasis of matrix turnover and, in turn, responds to a variety of mediators and monokines diffusing through the articular cartilage.

Biomechanics

The chondro-osseous skeleton undergoes repetitive intermittent loading. The mechanical stresses on these tissues to some extent control skeletal morphogenesis, growth, regeneration, maintenance, and degeneration. Stress analyses indicate that the local tissue-stress history plays a major role in controlling the biologic features of connective tissue throughout life. The influence of mechanical forces on cartilage is incompletely understood, but recent—although largely theoretical—insights suggest exciting possibilities.

Intermittent mechanical loading of skeletal tissues is often expressed in terms of applied cyclic stress. Stress is a tensor quantity, which must be defined by specifying six stress components or three principal stresses with their orientation angles for a three-dimensional analysis. Stress descriptions can, however, be somewhat simplified by using two stress invariants: hydrostatic stress and octahedral shear stress. If cartilage is exposed to equal compressive stress from all directions, a state of pure hydrostatic stress is present. If the stresses are not equal from all directions, shear stresses are present in addition to hydrostatic stresses. Shear in articular cartilage occurs when tensile strain is perpendicular to the primary direction in which the cartilage is being compressed.

On the basis of stress analyses of the ossifying femoral anlage and of the pathogenesis of osteoarthritis in the adult hip joint, it has been proposed that cartilage degeneration and ossification are promoted by intermittently applied shear stresses and inhibited or prevented by intermittently applied hydrostatic compressive stresses.

The very existence of articular cartilage in a mature human diarthrodial joint can thus be ascribed to the absence of significant shear stress and the inability of the subchondral ossification front to advance into areas of intermittent high-magnitude hydrostatic pressure.

The magnitude of compressive hydrostatic stress in subchondral bone correlates with cartilage thickness and is highest in the superior femoral head and moderate at the acetabular roof, as determined by finite-element analysis. The surfaces of the medial-inferior and the peripheral areas of the femoral head and the roof of the acetabulum have lower hydrostatic compression and higher subchondral bone tensile strains tangential to the joint surface. Initial cartilage fibrillation and osteophyte formation often occur in these areas. The intermittent hydrostatic pressure to which normal articular cartilage is subjected (7 to 10 atm) appears to inhibit vascular invasion and prevent the degeneration and ossification of articular cartilage. The generation of tensile strain may promote the degenerative process by direct mechanical mechanisms. Additionally, since tensile strains are associated with a reduction in the compressive hydrostatic stresses in the cartilage and an increase in shear stresses, their presence may permit or promote vascular invasion, cartilage degeneration, and osteophyte formation.

The same mechanical principles important in explaining degenerative arthritis (arthrosis) appear to guide the degeneration and ossification of cartilage primordium during skeletal morphogenesis (Fig. 1). In this sense, arthrosis can be considered the final stage in the degeneration and ossification of the cartilage anlage.

Osteoarthritis

Osteoarthritis is the most common form of articular cartilage degeneration. Its prevalence generally increases with age. In the Framingham study of 1,424 patients between the ages of 63 and 94 years, knee radiographs demonstrated that 27% of those 65 to 69 years old and 51% of those 85 years old or older had osteoarthritis. There was no significant difference in incidence between men and women but women were more symptomatic.

Osteoarthritis is usually described as primary (idiopathic) or secondary. This distinction has historically been based on demonstrable local or systemic etiologic factors. Such rigid classifications are probably artificial as certain conditions previously thought to be primary are now considered to be examples of secondary osteoarthritis (for example, adult-onset osteoarthritis of the hip secondary to a childhood developmental abnormality such as congenital hip dysplasia). Secondary osteoarthritis indicates that a specific, known factor induces the arthritis. Frequently this factor is trauma, but many other secondary types of osteoarthritis are known. These include such conditions as congenital epiphyseal dysplasia, postinflammatory arthritis (as in rheumatoid arthritis or after septic arthritis), endocrine disorders such as acromegaly, and metabolic disorders such as hemachromatosis, ochronosis, and hyperparathyroidism.

Many hypotheses have been advanced to explain osteoarthritis (Fig. 2). These theories can be grouped into two basic categories: (1) excessive stresses on normal tissues and (2) an inadequate chondrocyte response to normal forces. Excessive stresses can occur from direct trauma, developmental abnormalities leading to altered patterns of joint stress, and changes in joint biomechanics such as follow disruption of a ligament. It is believed that enzymes synthesized by the chondrocytes may be early mediators in the pathogenesis of cartilage breakdown from osteoarthritis. The fatigue strength of articular cartilage has been shown to decrease with age. Genetic and constitutional factors that subtly change the distribution of stresses across joints, the strength of the articular cartilage, and the biochemical responses of articular cartilage to various external

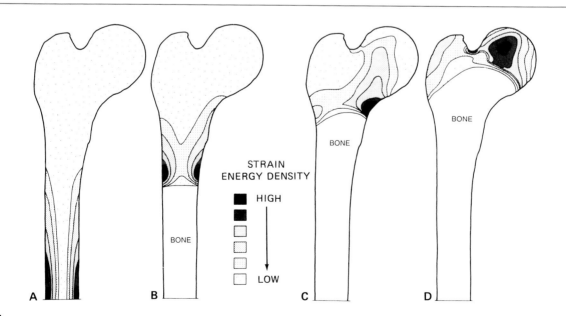

STRAIN ENERGY DENSITY

HIGH

LOW

BONE

Figure 1

Degeneration and ossification of cartilage primordium during skeletal morphogenesis. (Reproduced with permission from Carter DR: Mechanical loading history and skeletal biology. *J Biomech* 1987;20:1095–1109.)

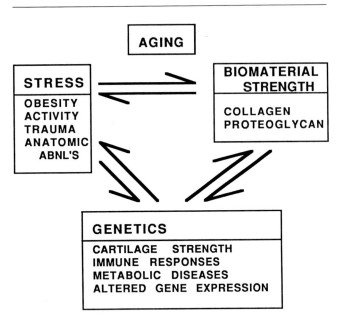

Figure 2

Etiology of osteoarthritis. Aging potentially results in cumulative failures of multiple systems. These failures interact to produce progressive damage to the articular cartilage.

stimuli underlie the pathologic characteristics and causes of osteoarthritis.

Experimental Osteoarthritis

The most widely used model for degenerative arthritis involves transection of the anterior cruciate ligament in an animal. Overt fibrillation can occur in the articular cartilage within six weeks, although in some cases only mild cartilage changes have been reported after almost four years. The onset and severity of the lesions in the cartilage are sensitive to factors such as the specific breed of the dog, its age and weight, the amount of exercise, and the surgical technique.

In a rabbit model, 12 weeks after the anterior cruciate ligament was severed, water content and fixed-charge density correlated with the surface area of induced cartilage fibrillation. Before fibrillation began, cartilage hypertrophy, reduced cell density, cystic lesions, and enlarged periochondrocytic lacunae were observed histologically. In a similar canine model, cartilage in the weightbearing areas of the knees displayed a progressive and significant decrease in hyaluronic acid content seven to 14 weeks postoperatively.

The loss of hyaluronic acid early in the course of this type of osteoarthritis may promote further alterations in proteoglycan aggregation. In adult articular cartilage there are at least two types of proteoglycans that aggregate with hyaluronate. The larger proteoglycan is richer in chondroitin sulfate and the smaller proteoglycan is richer in keratan sulfate. Keratan sulfate may be entirely absent in neonatal cartilage. With maturation, the number of proteoglycans containing keratan sulfate increases. Osteoarthritic cartilage resulting from anterior cruciate ligament disruption contains a much larger proportion of the large, chondroitin sulfate-rich proteoglycans than sites not involved with osteoarthritis. In a canine model of anterior cruciate ligament

disruption, newly synthesized proteoglycans extracted from cartilage from osteoarthritic joints were larger than those from normal cartilage three weeks, three months, and six months after surgery. An investigation of the chondroitin sulfate-rich proteoglycan region from joints with experimentally induced osteoarthritis demonstrated that it was slightly larger hydrodynamically than normal control tissue and had higher uronate-protein and galactosamine-glucosamine ratios.

Proteoglycan synthesis is increased in early experimental osteoarthritis but much of the proteoglycan produced diffuses away without being incorporated into the cartilage matrix. A comparison of the capacities of immature and mature chondrocytes in culture to synthesize link protein and to assemble proteoglycan aggregates showed markedly decreased capacity in the mature chondrocytes. Because of its relative insufficiency of link protein, it was hypothesized, mature cartilage with osteoarthritis may not be able to take advantage of the increased synthesis of proteoglycan subunits by stabilizing them as aggregates and thereby incorporating them into a reparative matrix.

Interleukin-1, also referred to as catabolin, is released by a variety of cells, including synoviocytes, monocytes, and perhaps chondrocytes themselves. This multifunctional monokine stimulates chondrocyte release of degradative enzymes that affect cartilage matrix. Interleukin-1 was formerly believed to be primarily a mediator of normal matrix maintenance. Because it is extremely abundant in inflammatory arthritis, particularly rheumatoid arthritis, and because even traumatic osteoarthritis has some inflammatory aspects, it is likely that interleukin-1 plays some role in degenerative phenomena.

A survey of degradative enzymes present in fibrillated cartilage in a rabbit model of anterior cruciate ligament deficiency showed unmodified collagenolytic activity but significantly increased acid phosphatase, glycosidase, and neutral protease activity. Neutral metalloproteoglycanases are found in both active and latent forms in experimental osteoarthritis. This enzyme degrades proteoglycan, reducing its hydrodynamic size and preventing reaggregation with hyaluronic acid. There are indications that this enzyme works at the hyaluronate-binding region of the proteoglycan as well as at the chondroitin sulfate-rich region of the core protein.

Cartilage appears to be sensitive to sex hormones. In rabbits with meniscectomy-induced osteoarthritis, estradiol increased erosive changes in the cartilage and tamoxifen, an estrogen antagonist, reduced erosive changes. In a similar study in both rabbits and dogs, fibronectin was increased tenfold to 40-fold throughout the matrix of degenerated cartilage.

Immobilization of a rabbit leg in extension initially produces aseptic inflammation, synovial effusion, and stiffening; osteoarthritis of the knee then develops. Measurement of hydrostatic pressures in the femoral metaphysis and diaphysis demonstrated increased pressures. These were maximal at two days and slowly decreased during the next two weeks.

A comparison of the effects of anterior cruciate ligament instability and repetitive impulse loading showed that synovial inflammation preceded cartilage destruction in both cases and appeared as soon as three days postoperatively but only after the eighth week of impulse loading. In a similar model of impulse loading in rabbits, vascular alterations in the subchondral bone were observed within three weeks and were believed to be a function of both the magnitude and the rate of loading.

In dogs with transected anterior cruciate ligaments, neutral metalloproteoglycan-degrading enzyme activity increases in the osteoarthritic cartilage between two and 12 weeks after transection. Treatment with prednisone (0.2 mg/kg/day for four weeks) blocks the increased activity of these enzymes. In a rabbit model of meniscectomy, glycosaminoglycan polysulfuric acid ester retarded the development of erosions and improved the histologic appearance of the lesions. Thus, it appears to prevent lesions and to treat those that already exist.

Drug Treatment

Many anti-inflammatory prescription drugs are available. Because their pharmacologic properties, efficacy in clinical trials, and toxicity profiles are similar, no one drug has been shown to be consistently better than the others. Nonetheless, because patients respond differently to different drugs, one of the nonsteroidal anti-inflammatory drugs (NSAIDs) may be more beneficial in a particular case. Peptic ulcers develop in approximately 1% of patients taking NSAIDs. Discontinuing the NSAID and treating the patient with ranitidine or sucralfate produces healing in 90% of these patients (mean time to healing, 4.6 weeks), whereas healing occurred in only 76% of patients treated with anti-ulcer therapy but continuing to take NSAIDs. Treatment continued for 12 to 15 weeks in both groups and time to healing was the same for both groups.

A new NSAID, S-adenosylmethionine, is well tolerated in human patients and its results are equivalent to those of other NSAIDs. S-Adenosylmethionine reduced gastric mucosal injury induced by aspirin, ethanol, or stress in a rat model. Human studies (22,000 patients with osteoarthritis in countries other than the United States) suggest that the therapeutic activity of S-adenosylmethionine against osteoarthritis is similar to those of other NSAIDs.

Education

An educational program about self-care for osteoarthritis was tested on a group of senior citizens. There were statistically significant changes in behavior and the patients' knowledge increased.

Surgical Treatment

Knee In one study, 14 of 15 valgus knees with osteoarthritis of the lateral compartment were successfully treated by femoral supracondylar varus osteotomy. The average follow-up was four years. Femoral supracondylar varus osteotomy is not recommended when the knee has inadequate motion or in patients with rheumatoid arthritis.

Hip As many as 5% of individuals with Down's syndrome have subluxation of the hip. In many cases this progresses to coxarthrosis in adulthood. Total hip replacement has been reported to be successful in such circumstances.

Trapeziometacarpal Joint Osteoarthritis of the trapeziometacarpal joint severe enough to require arthroplasty is frequently associated with other problems. Of patients undergoing arthroplasty, 75% require treatment for a variety of other problems in the same anatomic area. These include carpal tunnel syndrome, tenosynovitis, and arthritis of other carpal joints. In one study, 65% of patients treated with trapezium arthroplasty had at least one other surgical procedure.

Thumb Helium-neon laser treatment for osteoarthritis of the thumb was found to be ineffective in a masked, randomized, and controlled study.

Inflammatory Arthropathies

Etiology and Genetics

Immune response genes appear to be critically involved in an individual's susceptibility to a number of rheumatic diseases. The most striking example is the association of HLA-B27 with ankylosing spondylitis. Evidence suggests that rheumatoid arthritis and other rheumatic diseases may be associated with a specific genetic predisposition. Specific gene identification is becoming increasingly sophisticated and is likely to furnish major new insights in the future.

Immune response genes are congregated on the short arm of chromosome 6 in a segment called the major histocompatibility complex. Human leukocyte antigens (HLA) used as serologic alloantigens are the products of genes in the major histocompatibility complex and hence were used to map and sort the complex. The entire HLA complex spans approximately 1,000 kilobase on chromosome 6. It is divided into three regions: class I, class II, and class III loci. HLA typing of parents and offspring is required to determine the specific alleles that produce a particular individual expression.

Class I antigens are expressed on all cells and identify the cells as "self." Class I antigens evoke strong graft rejection responses. Class II antigens are present on B cells, macrophages, and activated T-helper or T-killer cells. Aberrant induction of class II antigen expression on cells that normally do not express these molecules is associated with inflammation in some autoimmune diseases. Class III antigens are located between the class I and class II regions and code for soluble proteins primarily involved in the complement cascade.

Rheumatic diseases associated with class I antigens include arthropathies of the axial skeleton (for example, ankylosing spondylitis) and Reiter's syndrome. Class II antigens have been associated with rheumatoid arthritis, Sjögren's syndrome, juvenile rheumatoid arthritis, and systemic lupus erythematosus.

The application of recombinant DNA technology in the past few years is leading to better understanding of diseases associated with HLA antigens. Rheumatoid arthritis is associated with a class II HLA-DR4. Some 60% to 80% of patients with rheumatoid arthritis are serologically type HLA-DR4 compared with approximately 20% of the general population. Of the five subtypes of HLA-DR4, the ones with which rheumatoid arthritis is most closely associated are subtypes Dw4 and Dw14. The HLA-DR4 subtypes can be defined at the DNA sequence level. A particular area known as the third hypervariable region is especially subject to polymorphisms that may arise as a result of gene conversion. Gene conversion means the shuffling of the hypervariable segments of regional exons (nucleotide segments that code for amino acids) into alternative frameworks. These new frameworks lose their normal ability to be typed by conventional allosera but the newly shuffled genes can still be recognized by T cells. Reshuffling the hypervariable segments is one manner in which genes undergo change or conversion. The reshuffled gene segments remain potential functional units. The functional unit has been referred to as a "shared epitope." Alloreactive T-cell clones can find these reshuffled genes even when the standard typing allosera are masked. In one study, investigators were able to demonstrate "shared epitopes" on the cells of all tested patients with seropositive rheumatoid arthritis regardless of their HLA-D or HLA-DR type (determined by allosera). This promising technology may be able to define the risks for clinical diseases with increasing specificity.

Rheumatoid Arthritis

When synovial cells from patients with rheumatoid arthritis are exposed to interleukin-1, phospholipase A_2 is secreted by the cells in a dose-dependent fashion. Prostaglandin E_2 and plasminogen activator are stimulated in a similar fashion by interleukin-1. The response is measurable within six hours. When interleukin-1 is added to articular cartilage slices, the cartilage is depleted of proteoglycan. Evaluation of the proteoglycans released into the medium shows limited cleavage near the haluronate-binding region and release of the remainder of the subunit. The medium contains increased amounts of latent neutral metalloproteases and acid proteinase. The effect of interleukin-1 stops 24 hours after it is removed. When synovium is co-cultured with articular cartilage, the effect can be blocked by early administration of cortisone. However, later administration of cortisone has little effect on the ongoing production of a factor similar to interleukin-1 and does not prevent cartilage breakdown.

When human polymorphonuclear leukocytes are stimulated and added to articular cartilage, proteoglycan synthesis is inhibited and existing matrix proteoglycans are degraded. An inhibitor of both serine protease and elastase prevents this action. In cartilage taken from rheumatoid knees, the neutral metalloprotease with proteoglycan-degrading activity is eight times more abundant than in normal cadaver cartilage.

Pannus ingrowth occurs in four stages, starting with simple hypertrophy of the synovial cells and ending in loss (digestion) of the meniscus and denudation of the articular cartilage. Articular cartilage destruction occurs only after meniscal involvement.

Immunoglobulins are far more abundant in articular cartilage from joints with rheumatoid arthritis than in cartilage from joints with osteoarthritis. In turn, osteoarthritic cartilage contains considerably more immunoglobulin than does normal cartilage. Whole pieces or extracts, including immune complexes, from rheumatoid arthritic articular cartilage fail to stimulate autologous or allogeneic lymphocytes. Thus, even though rheumatoid cartilage contains immune complexes, the complexes have not yet been shown to stimulate inflammatory reactions in peripheral blood lymphocytes or monocytes. Immune complexes are found at the sites of cartilage fragmentation in a rabbit model. It remains to be proven whether immune complexes are a cause or a result of cartilage degradation in rheumatoid arthritis.

The pH of inflamed joints decreases in direct proportion to the density of the inflammatory cells. In a rabbit model,

lowering the pH to 4 by means of buffered solutions makes it possible for scanning electron microscopy to demonstrate a fibrillation network parallel to the surface of the cartilage. These fibrillations can heal in immature animals but not in adults. A model of murine antigen-induced arthritis demonstrated that chondrocyte death is associated with both the severity and the chronicity of inflammation. Chondrocyte death, a pathogenic finding in rheumatoid arthritis, augments the process of irreversible joint destruction. The specific causes of chondrocyte death are still speculative.

Treatment The many new drugs being introduced for the treatment of rheumatoid arthritis typically reduce symptoms but fail to alter the course of the disease. Although these drugs are important and useful, even these agents, which are designed to induce remission, have not been proven to alter the final course of the disease nor to change the rate of joint destruction.

In a specific joint that has not responded to systemic therapy, synovectomy can decrease symptoms and retard disease progression. In a controlled clinical trial, dysprosium Dy 165 ferric hydroxide macroaggregates produced good results in two thirds of the cases for two years after treatment. This radiation synovectomy works best in the earlier stages of rheumatoid arthritis. The treatment can be repeated; 50% of a group of initially failed radiation synovectomies responded to a repeat treatment with good results after one year of follow-up. Radiation synovectomy is still available only under experimental protocols in the United States despite its great popularity in other countries. Leakage of radioactivity into regional and distal lymph nodes is a major concern. Radiation leakage from the involved joint has been minimized by the use of ferric hydroxide macroaggregates linked to an isotope (dysprosium) with a short half-life (139 minutes). Although promising, radiation synovectomy is still investigational and its toxicity and benefits must be clarified further before it is released for general use.

Historically, surgical synovectomy appeared to offer significant benefits for a few years after the procedure. A prolonged postoperative recovery was not uncommon and for that reason acceptance of the procedure remained limited. A comparison of arthroscopic synovectomy and open synovectomy showed no significant differences between the two procedures after the first few months, although, as expected, the postoperative management of open synovectomy was more difficult. Arthroscopic synovectomy is most often used for the knee and the results are best when the remaining articular cartilage is good. Range of motion often improves by 20 degrees. Arthroscopic synovectomy has also been used in many other joints, including the shoulder and the elbow, with favorable outcomes.

Juvenile Rheumatoid Arthritis

The three types of juvenile arthritis are categorized according to clinical symptoms in the first three months of the disease. The systemic type constitutes 20% of the total number of cases, the polyarticular type constitutes 50%, and the pauciarticular type constitutes 30%. Rheumatoid factor is not usually present, although it can be found in as many as 15% of patients with the polyarticular type. The pauciarticular and polyarticular types affect females more than males; the two sexes are equally affected in the systemic type. In the pauciarticular type, three or fewer joints are involved; in the systemic type, symptoms include fever, rash, leukocytosis, and hepatosplenomegaly.

Proteoglycans are released from articular cartilage when synovial fluid from the joints of patients with polyarticular or pauciarticular juvenile arthritis or from children with ankylosing spondylitis is added to articular cartilage slices in culture. However, proteoglycan is not released when synovial fluid from juvenile traumatic joint effusions is added. There is no effect on collagen release. If peripheral blood mononuclear cells from patients with systemic juvenile arthritis and some patients with polyarticular juvenile arthritis are incubated in culture medium for several days, adding the cell-free medium to cartilage culture releases both proteoglycan and collagen. This phenomenon does not occur with peripheral blood mononuclear cells from patients with pauciarticular or, in some cases, polyarticular juvenile arthritis.

Ankylosing Spondylitis

This form of arthritis is closely associated with the leukocyte antigen serum test for HLA-B27. This is a marker for a specific haplotype of the class I antigens of the major histocompatibility complex of genes. The presence of HLA-B27 is a widely used blood test that confirms the likelihood of ankylosing spondylitis in patients with signs and symptoms of the illness. Ankylosing spondylitis actually develops in only a small percentage of patients with this haplotype, but almost all Caucasian patients in whom ankylosing spondylitis does develop have this haplotype. The diagnosis may be elusive early in the course of the disease when young patients first experience involvement of the axial skeleton (for example, morning stiffness of the spine). Radiographic changes of the spine or sacroiliac joints may be minimal or absent. Under these circumstances, the HLA-B27 blood test can be highly useful in the diagnosis.

Animal models of adjuvant arthritis typically involve spondylitis. Classic adjuvant arthritis frequently affects primarily the spine and affects the peripheral joints to a much lesser degree. One new animal model of spondylitis is especially interesting. If female BALB/c mice are given human fetal cartilage proteoglycan (treated with chondroitinase ABC to remove the glycosaminoglycan side chains) in adjuvant arthritis, spondylitis and erosive polyarthritis develop. The animal model is specific to the strain of mouse, but the specific genes responsible have not been isolated. Antibodies to the immunizing human proteoglycan as well as antibodies to native mouse proteoglycan develop in animals with arthritis but not in those without arthritis.

Crystal Arthritis

Gout

Monosodium urate crystals are easily identified in synovial fluid. Their presence is diagnostic of gout. The needle-like crystals are negatively birefringent when viewed with a polarized microscope and a first-order red compensator. Other crystal-induced disorders may exist concomitantly in the same joint. Gout may resemble many other forms of arthritis. Because its definitive diagnosis is straightforward and its treatment so successful, it is important to

maintain a high index of suspicion. With the onset of a gout attack, all of the following values may be elevated: leukocyte count, platelet count, erythrocyte sedimentation rate, and acute phase reactants such as C-reactive protein. Urate crystals cause the release of interleukin-1 from human blood monocytes and synovial fluid mononuclear cells. Hydroxyapatite crystals stimulate human monocytes to a much lesser extent and calcium pyrophosphate dihydrate does not stimulate interleukin-1 release.

Although gout is most commonly associated wih podagra (pain in the first metatarsophalangeal joint), attacks may occur in almost any joint. Tenosynovitis may result from an acute gouty attack.

NSAIDs are commonly recommended in preference to colchicine for both treatment and prevention of acute attacks. If given in adequate dosages early in the course of an attack, NSAIDs, including piroxicam, naproxen, ketoprofen, diclofenac, indomethacin, and phenylbutazone, are effective. Recently, 100 patients were prospectively treated for a one-year period with either a single intramuscular injection of corticotropin (40 IU) or oral indomethacin (50 mg four times daily with meals) until pain subsided for any acute attack. On the average, corticotropin produced relief within three hours, whereas indomethacin took 24 hours. Moreover, none of the patients receiving corticotropin reported side effects, whereas more than one half of those receiving indomethacin had gastrointestinal disturbances and almost as many had headaches or other central nervous system symptoms.

Diet is an important factor in the prevention of gouty attacks. In nutritional experiments with formula diets, the same quantity of DNA taken orally increased the serum uric acid concentration only half as much as did RNA.

Chondrocalcinosis

In this condition, calcium pyrophosphate crystals are deposited in articular cartilage, menisci, or synovium. Chondrocalcinosis may be asymptomatic or symptomatic. The condition is usually diagnosed by radiographic findings of calcification in the articular cartilage but can be diagnosed from tissue removed at arthroscopy. Symptomatic chondrocalcinosis may be indistinguishable from osteoarthritis or manifest as acute, inflammatory joint swelling similar to attacks of gout (sometimes called pseudogout). In one study of pseudogout, 14 of 93 acute inflammatory arthritic attacks were misdiagnosed as septic arthritis. Typical pseudogout attacks are associated with fever.

Pseudogout can be classified as sporadic, hereditary, or associated with metabolic diseases. The metabolic diseases include hemochromatosis (in which pseudogout is a late manifestation), hyperparathyroidism, hypothyroidism, and hypomagnesemia. Calcium pyrophosphate crystals can also be found in patients with rheumatoid arthritis, osteoarthritis, and gout.

The hereditary form of the disease is usually autosomal dominant. Most patients have symptoms indistinguishable from those of the sporadic form of the disease. Thus far there has been no linkage of chondrocalcinosis to HLA typing.

A radiographic comparison of 74 patients with pseudogout and 68 patients with osteoarthritis showed no significant differences in the severity of radiographic changes or in distribution. Electron microscopy demonstrates great variation in crystal size and shape with most of the pyrophosphate crystal being phagocytized by polymorphonuclear leukocytes. In patients with pseudogout, each crystal measures 1 μ or less. The crystals are often adjacent to chondrocytes and large numbers of polymorphonuclear leukocytes are attached to the eroded articular cartilage.

NSAIDs are useful in the treatment of pseudogout. In one study, ten patients who had had 32 attacks of pseudogout during the previous year were given 0.6 mg of colchicine twice a day. During the next year the total number of attacks decreased to ten, and nine of the ten patients had fewer attacks.

Infection

Acute septic arthritis caused by *Staphylococcus aureus* was studied in the chicken knee (hock) joint. After direct bacterial inoculation into the joint, the numbers of bacteria initially decreased and then hours later began to multiply rapidly. The leukocyte count began to rise within 90 minutes. Gross destruction of the articular cartilage was observed at four days, by which time the staphylococci had adhered to the cartilage surface. Extensive erosions were evident by the 14th day. Transmission and scanning electron microscopic studies of staphylococci in both rabbits and humans demonstrated bacteria in intimate contact with the cartilage matrix surface. The staphylococci appeared to have a special affinity to exposed collagen matrix and a binding assay further demonstrated preferential binding to cartilage matrix in some instances. A rabbit model using *S aureus* demonstrated that juxta-articular marginal erosions began by the fifth day and that there was total joint destruction by five weeks. Loss of glycosaminoglycans from rabbit knees infected with *S aureus* was first evident four hours after the onset of infection. The sooner antibiotics were started, the smaller was the loss of glycosaminoglycans and collagen three weeks later. Prophylactic use of antibiotics completely prevented any cartilage degradation.

Antigen-induced arthritis in the rabbit was compared with infection induced by *S aureus* and followed histologically for two weeks. The histologic changes were more severe in the infected joints.

In infected joints, the subchondral bone becomes infected with abscesses at the juxta-articular margin and at the intra-articular attachments of the ligaments and precedes involvement of bone in the areas covered by articular cartilage. A comparison of *S aureus* and *Escherichia coli* infections and a severe form of antigen arthritis in a rabbit model showed progressive loss of glycosaminoglycans and collagen in all three conditions. By 48 hours, knees with *E coli* infection lost 20% of their glycosaminoglycans, whereas those infected with *S aureus* lost 42%. Collagen losses were not significant until the third week, at which time about 40% depletion was noted (Table 3). Killed *Mycobacterium butyricum* with adjuvant produced equally severe destruction and a histologic pattern of granulomas. The biochemical studies indicated that proteoglycan subunits are lost as whole pieces and that the glycosaminoglycan chains are not attacked specifically. Moreover, there is a rapid initial loss of proteoglycan subunits that precedes collagen loss.

The usefulness of leukocyte scans was reported in several human studies. Pooled results for the total of 70 cases in

Table 3. *Staphylococcus aureus* infection of the knee*

Antibiotic Therapy Begun	Glycosaminoglycan Loss (%)	Collagen Loss (%)
After 48 Hours		
None	32	0
At 4 hours	12	0
At 8 hours	18	0
At 12 hours	24	0
After 21 days		
Before injection	0	0
On day 1	55	29
On day 2	71	37
On day 7	82	89
None	82	89

*Reproduced with permission from Schurman DJ, Smith RL: Surgical approach to management of septic arthritis. *Orthop Rev* 1987;16:241–245.

which bacterial infection was confirmed by surgery showed false-positive findings in 10% and false-negative findings in 1%. Thus, sensitivity was excellent, but the specificity was less than 90%.

At least four studies have described the use of arthroscopy for lavage and debridement of septic arthritis and it has been recommended for both pediatric and adult problems. Low morbidity and rapid return of function were consistently reported. In addition, complete visualization, ease of drain placement, rapid return of range of motion, and good to excellent follow-up results were reported. The studies did not directly compare arthroscopy with needle aspiration or surgery.

A study of 150 consecutive patients treated at an acute arthritis clinic during a one-year period surveyed the diagnoses in this group. Ten patients had septic arthritis. (Eight of these patients had concomitant rheumatoid arthritis; one of the eight died of septic arthritis. Of the remaining two patients, one also died of sepsis.) The most common diagnosis was gout, a condition often confused with septic arthritis. Interestingly, rheumatoid arthritis accounted for only 19 of the 150 patients. A high index of suspicion must be maintained for both septic arthritis and gout as they are easily diagnosed and the most readily treatable and reversible forms of arthritis.

Trends

Total joint arthroplasty remains the single most effective treatment for joints in which the articular cartilage has been destroyed. Joint replacement with osteocartilaginous transplants gained advocates in the early 1980s and further experience will be gained in the 1990s.

No medical advance in the 1980s equaled the introduction of allopurinol for the treatment of gout several decades ago, although NSAIDs have replaced aspirin because they were more convenient and had somewhat fewer side effects.

The past decade was probably most notable for scientific accomplishments that have yet to be translated into important clinically useful strategies. Immunology, biochemistry, molecular biology, and genetic engineering all progressed, and in the next decade may produce clinically applicable advances.

Annotated Bibliography

Keywords

Ankylosing spondylitis; Arthritis; Articular cartilage; Chondrocalcinosis; Chondrocyte; Collagen; Gout; Immunology; Infection; Osteoarthritis; Rheumatoid arthritis; Septic arthritis

Normal Joint Physiology

Hamerman D, Sasse J, Klagsbrun M: A cartilage-derived growth factor enhances hyaluronate synthesis and diminishes sulfated glycosaminoglycan synthesis in chondrocytes. *J Cell Physiol* 1986;127:317–322.
  A cartilage-derived growth factor purified using affinity chromatography on columns of heparin-sepharose is mitogenic for bovine fetal chondrocytes. Hyaluronate synthesis increased as did chondrocyte proliferation, whereas sulfated glycosaminoglycans decreased. It was concluded that this growth factor differs from somatomedins.

Paukkonen K, Helminen HJ: Rough endoplasmic reticulum and fine intracytoplasmic filaments in articular cartilage chondrocytes of young rabbits: A stereological morphometric study using transmission electron microscopy. *J Anat* 1987;152:47–54.
  A simple and rapid stereologic method was designed for quantifying the synthetic activity of the chondrocytes in the different zones of uncalcified articular cartilage by measuring the amount of rough endoplasmic reticulum on electron micrographs. The authors determined the surface area of the rough endoplasmic reticulum per unit volume of the chondrocyte cytoplasm, of cartilage, and per chondrocyte. Chondrocytes containing filaments are associated with diminished amounts of rough endoplasmic reticulum and are probably degenerating cells.

Sapolsky A, Malemud C, Sheff M: The proteoglycanase from human cartilage and cultured rabbit chondrocytes and its relation to osteoarthritis. *J Rheumatol* 1987;14(suppl 14):33–35.
  The predominant neutral protease present in patellar cartilage and cultured rabbit chondrocytes is a metal-dependent proteoglycanase. The protease exists predominantly in latent form and occurs in two molecular weights.

Thonar EJ, Buckwalter JA, Kuettner KE: Maturation-related differences in the structure and composition of proteoglycans synthesized by chondrocytes from bovine articular cartilage. *J Biol Chem* 1986;261:2467–2474.
  Bovine articular chondrocytes were isolated and cultured as high-density monolayers from 2- to 3-month-old calves and 18-month-old steers. Fractions of proteoglycan were analyzed on day 5 during a 15-hour period of labeling sulfate and glucosamine. Maturation differences were observed between the cartilage cells of the calves and those of the older steers. In the calf, buoyant high-density fractions of proteoglycans were larger, had longer chondroitin sulfate chains, and had lower ratios of keratan sulfate.

Osteoarthritis

Adams ME, Grant MD, Ho A: Cartilage proteoglycan changes in experimental canine osteoarthritis. *J Rheumatol* 1987;14(suppl 14):107–109.
  Experimental osteoarthritis was induced in 11 dogs by transection of the anterior cruciate ligament. The osteoarthritic cartilage had more proteoglycan and an increased amount of large proteoglycans that were richer in chondroitin sulfate than the normal controls. These data support the hypothesis that reactive osteoarthritic cartilage contains an increased amount of the proteoglycans characteristic of immature cartilage.

Burton-Wurster N, Butler M, Harter S, et al: Presence of fibronectin in articular cartilage in two animal models of osteoarthritis. *J Rheumatol* 1986;13:175–182.
  In a rabbit meniscectomy model and a canine spontaneous model of osteoarthritis, fibronectin content was determined by urea extracts from articular cartilage. Immunosorbent assay demonstrated that osteoarthritic cartilage had ten to 40 times the amount of fibronectin present in normal cartilage in both animal models. The fibronectin was distributed throughout the martrix in both normal and osteoarthritic cartilage.

Carter DR, Rapperport DJ, Fyhrie DP, et al: Relation of coxarthrosis to stresses and morphogenesis: A finite element analysis. *Acta Orthop Scand* 1987;58:611–619.
  Subchondral deformations and stresses in the femoral head and the acetabulum during weightbearing were calculated by means of finite-element models. The mechanical principles in arthrosis are the same as those that have been previously demonstrated to guide the degeneration and ossification of the cartilage primordium during skeletal morphogenesis. Arthrosis may be viewed as the final stage in the degeneration and ossification of the cartilage anlage.

Rosner IA, Goldberg VM, Moskowitz RW: Estrogens and osteoarthritis. *Clin Orthop* 1986;213:77–83.
  In a meniscectomy-induced osteoarthritis produced in rabbits, estradiol accentuated the arthritic findings, whereas tamoxifen and estrogen antagonist decreased the erosive changes. These findings suggested that cartilage is a tissue sensitive to sex hormones.

Inflammatory Arthropathies

Goronzy J, Weyand CM, Fathman CG: Shared T cell recognition sites on human histocompatibility leukocyte antigen class II molecules of patients with seropositive rheumatoid arthritis. *J Clin Invest* 1986;77:1042–1049.
  Alloreactive human T-cell clones were developed by stimulating peripheral blood lymphocytes of normal donors against a lymphoblastoid cell line from a patient with seropositive rheumatoid arthritis. Using T-cell clones with specificities for determinants expressed on Dw14 homozygous typing lines, shared epitopes were demonstrated on cells of all patients tested with seropositive rheumatoid arthritis regardless of their HLA-D or HLA-DR type.

Schurman DJ, Palathumpat MV, DeSilva A, et al: Biochemistry and antigenicity of osteoarthritic and rheumatoid cartilage. *J Orthop Res* 1986;4:255–262.
  Articular cartilage samples were obtained from patients with rheumatoid arthritis, osteoarthritis, and ankylosing spondylitis. Samples were characterized with respect to their content of immunoglobulins, collagen, and proteoglycan. Lymphocyte proliferation quantified by uptake of tritiated thymidine was unaltered by the addition of cartilage fragments, low and high salt extracts, or cartilage residues. These techniques failed to demonstrate any cartilage factors in these forms of arthritis that would stimulate peripheral blood lymphocytes.

Shibata T, Shiraoka K, Takubo N: Comparison between arthroscopic and open synovectomy for the knee in rheumatoid arthritis. *Arch Orthop Trauma Surg* 1986;105:257–262.

Ten surgical synovectomies and 14 arthroscopic synovectomies were evaluated for their early postoperative results. Although postoperative management was more difficult and complex in the surgical group at two months, the results in both groups were similar.

Silverman ED, Smith RL, Schurman DJ, et al: Spontaneous secretion of a proteoglycan releasing factor by mononuclear cells in juvenile arthritis. *J Rheumatol* 1987;14:540–547.

Joint fluid from knees of patients with polyarticular juvenile rheumatoid arthritis and systemic juvenile rheumatoid arthritis were cultured with conditioned media of peripheral blood mononuclear cells from patients with juvenile rheumatoid arthritis. When these media were added to organ cultures of bovine articular cartilage, there was, with few exceptions, an increased release of proteoglycan from the cartilage. This was not true when the peripheral blood mononuclear cells of normal children were used unless the cells were first stimulated with mitogens. These findings indicate that, in general, the synovial fluid of patients with juvenile rheumatoid arthritis stimulates peripheral blood mononuclear cells to produce a factor that resorbs articular cartilage matrix.

Sledge CB, Zuckerman JD, Shortkroff S, et al: Synovectomy of the rheumatoid knee using intra-articular injection of dysprosium-165-ferric hydroxide macroaggregates. *J Bone Joint Surg* 1987;69A:970–975.

A group of 111 patients with seropositive rheumatoid arthritis with persistent synovitis of the knee were treated with intra-articular injections of 270 mCi of dysprosium Dy 165 bound to ferric hydroxide macroaggregates. A two-year follow-up of 59 patients demonstrated that this technique was as effective as radiation synovectomy, especially in the presence of the earliest roentgenographic changes.

Crystal Arthritis

Axelrod D, Preston S: Comparison of parenteral adrenocorticotropic hormone with oral indomethacin in the treatment of acute gout. *Arthritis Rheum* 1988;31:803–805.

The authors conducted a randomized prospective study of 100 consecutive male patients with gout treated with either corticotropin or oral indomethacin (50 mg four times daily). For the corticotropin group, the mean pain relief interval was three hours and there were no side effects. For the indomethacin group, the mean pain relief interval was 24 hours and more than 50% had side effects.

Di Giovine FS, Malawista SE, Nuki G, et al: Interleukin 1 (IL 1) as a mediator of crystal arthritis: Stimulation of T cell and synovial fibroblast mitogenesis by urate crystal-induced IL 1. *J Immunol* 1987;138:3213–3218.

The release of interleukin-1 activity from human blood monocytes and synovial fluid mononuclear cells was found after stimulation with monosodium urate crystals. Hydroxyapatite was a much less potent stimulus than the monosodium urate crystals and calcium pyrophosphate dihydrate failed to stimulate the release of interleukin-1.

Rodriguez-Valverde V, Zuniga M, Casanueva B, et al: Hereditary articular chondrocalcinosis: Clinical and genetic features in 13 pedigrees. *Am J Med* 1988;84:101–106.

Thirteen pedigrees with familial articular chondrocalcinosis were identified and studied. Examination of first-degree blood relatives (mean age, 65 years), showed that the pattern of involvement supported an autosomal dominant model of inheritance. There was no way to distinguish early vs late onset of illness by inheritance. The data also failed to distinguish between the sporadic form of the disease and the inheritable form. Pseudogout was reported in 17% of these family members but in other studies has been as high as 28%.

Roseff R, Wohlgethan JR, Sipe JD, et al: The acute phase response in gout. *J Rheumatol* 1987;14:974–977.

Temperature, leukocyte count, platelet count, erythrocyte sedimentation rate, and serum levels of amyloid α-protein and C-reactive protein all tended to be increased during a gouty attack. The acute phase response resolved rapidly with treatment. The importance of these findings is that gout may occasionally be misdiagnosed as infection and treated inappropriately.

Infection

Alderson M, Nade S: Natural history of acute septic arthritis in an avian model. *J Orthop Res* 1987;5:261–274.

Staphylococcus aureus was injected into chicken hock joints and monitored for the first 14 days. Leukocyte counts in joint fluid rose rapidly, starting within 90 minutes of bacterial injection. Gross articular destruction was observed at four days. Staphylococcal adherence to the articular cartilage surface appeared to be an integral mechanism in the destructive process.

Mahowald ML, Peterson L, Raskind J, et al: Antigen-induced experimental septic arthritis in rabbits after intraarticular injection of *Staphylococcus aureus*. *J Infect Dis* 1986;154:273–282.

Infection in this model produced subsynovial abscesses extending into the subchondral bone around the juxta-articular margins of the articular cartilage. Infection rapidly entered around the base of the cruciate ligaments as well. Osteomyelitis is an early secondary event in septic arthritis.

Petty W, Spanier S, Shuster JJ: Prevention of infection after total joint replacement: Experiments with a canine model. *J Bone Joint Surg* 1988;70A:536–539.

Three types of antibiotic administration (intraoperative irrigation, perioperative systemic administration, and addition to bone cement) were compared in dogs undergoing joint replacement. Gentamicin alone in bone cement prevented infection from *Staphylococcus epidermidis*, *Staphylococcus aureus*, and *Escherichia coli* better than either of the other methods.

Smith RL, Schurman DJ, Kajiyama G, et al: The effect of antibiotics on the destruction of cartilage in experimental infectious arthritis. *J Bone Joint Surg* 1987;69A:1063–1068.

The authors serially measured the extent to which early therapy with long-acting cephalosporin altered degeneration of the cartilage after arthritis caused by *Staphylococcus aureus* injected into rabbit knee joints. To prevent any loss of proteoglycan, antibiotics had to be given within the first few hours after the onset of infection. Proteoglycan loss is rapid with early onset. Significant collagen loss does not occur for at least some days and lags significantly behind proteoglycan loss.

5
Child Abuse: Trauma

Maltreatment of children remains an abhorrent social problem. Because many cases of child abuse are seen first by a physician, physicians have a pivotal role with regard to differential diagnosis and subsequent intervention.

History and Epidemiology

The maltreatment of children by their caretakers has been documented throughout history. In the late 20th century, increased awareness has allowed us to detect child abuse more precisely. We now know that its magnitude and consequences are substantial.

In 1962, the term "the battered child syndrome" was coined to describe the constellation of findings associated with serious physical abuse, including skeletal fractures, subdural hematomas, failure to thrive, soft-tissue swellings, and bruises. The degree and the type of injury were often at variance with the history regarding the occurrence of the trauma. This early report stimulated a wider recognition in the medical community of the reality of child abuse, as well as an enormous increase in published reports of child maltreatment.

By 1967, all 50 states had enacted mandatory reporting laws. In 1974 the Federal Child Abuse Prevention and Treatment Act (Public Law 93-247) created the National Center on Child Abuse and Neglect, with a mandate to conduct research, compile statistics, and provide assistance to local agencies. In the years since the passage of state and federal child protection legislation, the number of reported cases has increased 100-fold. Unfortunately, data on the prevalence and incidence of child abuse still remain poor. Epidemiologic studies have used varying definitions, which have made comparisons over years and across types of abuse unreliable. Case report estimates suggest a range of 350,000 to 850,000 cases of physical abuse per year. Most informed observers believe these estimates are low. It has been estimated that orthopaedic surgeons may see 30% to 50% of the physically abused children who come to the attention of a physician.

Family Characteristics

A number of characteristics of the families of abused children bear mentioning. Abuse is often intergenerational, that is, the parents of abused children were often abused during their own childhoods. It is estimated that an abused child has a 50% chance of becoming an abusive parent. Child abuse and abuse of women are connected: there is a high likelihood that an abused child's mother is a battered woman. Abuse occurs in all socioeconomic strata. Although the problem appears to be more prevalent in impoverished families, it is quite clear that middle-and upper-income families are in no way immune to family violence. Cases are far less likely to be diagnosed and reported in higher-income families. Abuse often occurs in the setting of social isolation—in families that move frequently and have few connections to friends and other family members. Abuse is also frequently associated with increased social stress. Drug and alcohol abuse are present in many cases.

Etiology

Since the original description of the battered child syndrome in 1962, both the definition and our understanding of the causes of abuse have broadened. The initial focus was on what social scientists call a perpetrator-victim model. A mentally deranged adult was seen as willfully inflicting violence on a defenseless child. This position was challenged by data suggesting that severe psychopathology is no more prevalent among abusive parents than it is in the general population. In the 1970s the definition of child abuse evolved to include broader concepts of family dysfunction. Three key variables were proposed: a child with provocative qualities, a parent with the psychological potential to abuse, and a stressful event that acts as a trigger. Continuing to expand on this interactional concept, current thinking centers on what has come to be known as the ecologic theory of etiology. Child maltreatment is still seen as a symptom of family dysfunction. The interrelationships among attributes of child, parent, family, community, and society together result in the family dysfunction that expresses itself in one of its manifestations as child maltreatment. In this theory, simply specifying a particular "perpetrator" may not help in developing understanding and guiding a sound intervention plan.

Legal Issues

Every state now obligates physicians to report suspected child abuse or neglect. Neither definite knowledge that a child is abused or neglected nor specific diagnosis is required, and physicians increasingly are being held to a high standard with regard to reporting child abuse. Physicians who treat children should be familiar with the reporting requirements and procedures in their states. Most jurisdictions have 24-hour reporting hotlines.

If possible, it is best to have a social worker meet with the child's family before the case is reported; the social worker and the history gathered in the interview are often valuable in eliciting the best response from the child protection agency and in allaying the family's fears. Most jurisdictions allow reports to be made anonymously, but because families expect confidentiality from the physician and because the informed consent doctrine must be respected, it is well to inform the parents of the need to make the report. It is often helpful to emphasize the legal requirement to do so.

This legal requirement has been enforced in many ways since the reporting laws came into being in the 1960s. Most states now include sanctions for not reporting, including fines. Failure to report has been seen as an intervening cause of subsequent injury to the child in what has become a whole body of malpractice law. Fines of many hundreds of thousands of dollars have been sustained by the courts, and physicians who ignore reporting requirements may imperil their liability protection.

All states include in their reporting laws exemptions against liability in criminal actions or such civil actions as defamation or invasion of privacy for professionals filing mandatory reports. It is preferable to err on the side of making the report if the clinical circumstances are ambiguous. It is always a good idea to discuss the reporting obligation with the child's primary physician. Pediatricians are especially alert to the requirements and nuances of reporting cases of child abuse.

Diagnosis

A strong working knowledge of the signs and symptoms of child maltreatment and a high index of suspicion are necessary for the recognition of child abuse. Outline 1 lists the differential diagnosis of physical findings in child maltreatment.

Orthopaedic Manifestations of Abuse

Multiple unexplained fractures in different stages of healing in a child without an ongoing pertinent disease process are pathognomonic of abuse (Fig. 1). Fractures of the extremities are most common, followed by fractures of the skull and then the rib cage. Fractures in children less than 2 years of age are commonly associated with abuse whereas fractures in children older than 5 years are rarely inflicted.

Epiphyseal-metaphyseal injuries in infants are also considered virtually pathognomonic of abuse because the direct pulling or twisting forces necessary to produce these injuries are rarely generated by the usual accidental trauma in this age group. Epiphyseal plate injuries involving only cartilage may be difficult to diagnose radiographically before the signs of healing. Periosteal hematomas, which may be the only result of epiphyseal-metaphyseal trauma, are not visible until five to 14 days after the injury when periosteal ossification begins. Although epiphyseal-metaphyseal fractures and multiple fractures at different stages of healing are more specifically diagnostic of abuse, single

Outline 1. Clinical findings in child abuse*

Osseous lesions
  Diaphyseal fracture (multiple or in various stages of healing)
  Metaphyseal and/or epiphyseal lesions
  Subperiosteal ossification
Cutaneous lesions
  Bruising
  Local erythema or bullae
Ocular findings
  Retinal hemorrhage
  Conjunctival hemorrhage
  Orbital swelling
Hematuria
Acute abdominal signs

*In each category, child abuse is part of a large differential diagnosis. The presence of more than one category in a given patient makes the diagnosis of child abuse more likely.

fresh diaphyseal fractures are much more common. A spiral fracture of the long bones in an infant is especially suggestive of abuse. In contrast, in children who can walk, spiral fractures of the long bones can be caused by accidental trauma ("toddler's fracture" of the tibia) as well as assaults. Transverse fractures are the most common type of fracture resulting from abuse, although again they are not specifically diagnostic of abuse. Diaphyseal fractures occur approximately four times more often than the typical epiphyseal-metaphyseal injury. The most common fractures in abused children occur in the humerus, tibia, and femur, in that order. Because of the nonspecificity of diaphyseal injuries, the history, other physical findings, and characteristics of the child and caregiver are particularly important in the diagnostic process.

Direct blows or squeezing of a child's thorax can result in rib fractures. Accidental injuries to the rib cage are rare in infants and young children. Although common as a result of cardiopulmonary resuscitation in adults, these injuries are almost never caused by resuscitative efforts in the young pediatric population. Rib fractures secondary to inflicted injury tend to be multiple and to occur posteriorly, adjacent to the costovertebral junction.

Clavicular fractures are a common result of accidental injury in childhood and usually occur at midshaft. When they occur as avulsion fractures at the ends of the clavicle, they should be considered possible manifestations of inflicted injury.

Imaging

The usual radiographic skeletal survey includes an anteroposterior projection of the trunk and extremities, plus anteroposterior and lateral views of the skull. Radiographs of the hands and feet should be specifically requested so that other signs of osseous trauma can be identified. Adequate penetration of the thorax for visualization of the posterior ribs is necessary.

Complete skeletal surveys should be obtained for most children less than 2 years of age when evidence of physical abuse is present. For children more than 2 years old, the number of positive findings on a skeletal survey diminishes. A more selective approach is required. In children between 2 and 5 years of age who have histories of frequent trauma and/or in whom abuse is strongly suspected, a skeletal survey should be completed after the initial radiographic evaluation of the manifest locus of injury. In children more than 5 years old, skeletal surveys are rarely helpful, and radiographic evaluation should be limited to specific examinations based on the physical findings.

Whether to use conventional skeletal radiographs and/or a radionuclide bone scan in the diagnosis of suspected child abuse is a matter of continuing debate. Conventional radiographs are able to define both the anatomy and the age of osseous lesions. Bone scans cannot. A bone scan does, however, have the advantage of detecting fractures sooner than radiography. It shows increased radionuclide uptake at the site of fracture within 24 to 48 hours of the injury. Radionuclide studies are particularly useful in detecting fractures, such as vertebral, rib, and subtle nondisplaced fractures of the long bones, that are difficult to recognize on plain radiographs. Nondisplaced fractures and isolated periosteal hematomas may not be apparent on plain radiographs for five to 14 days when periosteal new bone begins to form. Bone scans lack sensitivity, however,

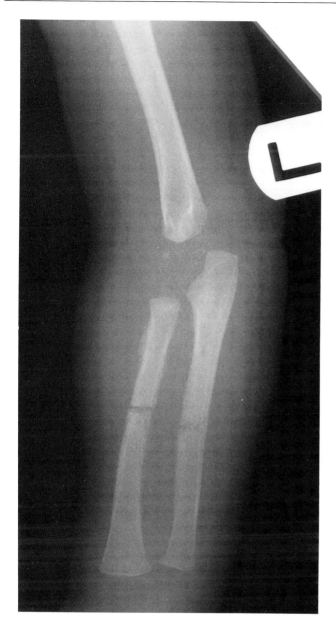 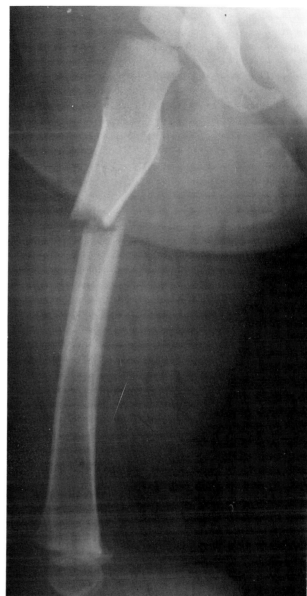

Figure 1
A 4-month-old child was brought to the emergency room after his mother noted tenderness of his left forearm during bathing. No explanation was given. **Left**, Transverse fractures at the midshaft of the left radius and ulna. A skeletal survey completed one day later also showed bucket-handle fractures of the distal left femur and distal left tibia and bilateral periosteal reactions over the proximal tibias. These findings are virtually pathognomonic of child abuse. **Right**, Eight months later, with the child still in the custody of his parents, he sustained a transverse fracture of the proximal femur after "falling and catching his leg between the rungs of a bannister." The child was subsequently placed in foster care.

in identifying injury at the growth plates because of the normal increase in radionuclide uptake in these areas. Bone scans also cannot differentiate infectious and malignant lesions from lesions of traumatic origin.

Because neither conventional radiographs nor radionuclide bone scans approach 100% sensitivity, these tests should be seen as complementary. A radiographic skeletal survey is usually the initial diagnostic study. If the result is either noncontributory or not sufficiently supportive of the diagnosis, and significant evidence of physical abuse is present, then a radionuclide bone scan can be performed.

Nonorthopaedic Manifestations of Abuse

Soft-tissue injuries (ecchymoses, hematomas, abrasions, and contusions) are the most common injuries in abused children. Because these injuries often occur in nonabused children as well, a number of differentiating features are important. Injuries over the bony prominences of the trunk and extremities and injuries over the malar region of the face and other parts of the head can be accidental. In contrast, injury to the soft parts of the body, such as the buttocks, genitals, thighs, back, cheek, and neck are more typical of inflicted trauma. Lesions over different body planes, when not associated with a tumbling fall, are also suggestive of abuse.

Bruises The colors and approximate ages of bruises should be noted: bruises turn from red-purple-blue during the first 24 hours to blue-brown on days 1 to 3, greenish on days 5 to 7, yellow by day 10, and brownish after two to four weeks. The child's complexion and peripheral perfusion affect the interpretation of the ages of bruises.

The age of the bruises should be compared for consistency with the history given. Patterns should be noted. Ecchymoses in the shape of a handprint or abrasions or ecchymoses in the shape of a looped cord or belt are highly suggestive of abuse. Linear bruises, crescentic bite marks, alopecia, or subgaleal hematoma from hair pulling are common manifestations. Circumferential marks around the neck, wrist, or ankles suggest restraints.

Burns Burns are a frequent manifestation of child abuse. Four basic patterns of inflicted burns have been described. Immersion burns are produced when a child is forcibly dipped into a hot liquid. This usually results in a uniform burn with clear lines of demarcation between burned and unburned areas. Stocking or glove distributions are typical. Occasionally, an area is spared as a result of the body's contact with the cooler surfaces of the container such as the enamalized steel of a bathtub; this leaves a doughnut-shaped burn. Marked flexion of the body when immersed can result in a striped pattern, sparing the skinfolds of the thorax and abdomen. Splash burns may produce multiple, noncontiguous burn areas of nonuniform depth. Contact with hot objects such as an iron or radiator may leave burns, usually at least second-degree, in the shape of the implement used to hurt the child.

Lesions Several lesions can be mistaken for bruises. A "mongolian spot" is a birthmark that occurs in most black, Asian, Native American, and Latino babies as well as in approximately 10% of white children. These spots are gray-blue, usually occur on the back or buttocks, have clearcut margins, are uniformly pigmented, and may last from two to five years. Phytophotodermatitis consists of brown macules that occur when the skin comes into contact with certain foods, such as limes, lemons, celery, figs, or parsnips. Buccal cellulitis caused by *Hemophilus influenzae* can produce a bluish discoloration of the cheek.

Periorbital cellulitis can produce marked swelling and redness around the eyes and involving the eye lids. In both buccal and periorbital cellulitis the child is usually febrile and can appear quite ill.

Head Injuries Head injuries are believed to be the leading cause of morbidity and mortality in abused children. Intracranial injury is highly associated with inflicted trauma in children less than 2 years of age in the absence of a history of significant, verifiable, accidental injury. Skull fractures are infrequently a result of falls from a standard bed to the floor. They do not occur when an infant or toddler falls from a standing or sitting position to the ground. Attempts to identify radiographic features of skull fractures characteristic of abuse have been unproductive, although multiple fractures, bilateral fractures, and fractures crossing suture lines are apparently more common in nonaccidental injury. Linear fractures are common in both nonaccidental and accidental injuries. Intracranial in-

juries resulting from abuse include subarachnoid hemorrhage, cerebral edema, cerebral hemorrhage, and subdural hematoma. Craniocerebral computed tomography and magnetic resonance imaging play major roles in the diagnosis of these lesions.

Because intracranial trauma is clearly associated with skeletal injury in cases of child abuse, the orthopaedic surgeon should be especially attentive to signs and symptoms suggesting cerebral injury. In an infant with head trauma, these include lethargy, vomiting, irritability, a high-pitched cry, respiratory difficulty, or a bulging fontanelle. Often, these injuries are not associated with skull fractures or other external evidence of abuse. Such injuries occur in the "shaken baby syndrome," in which violent shaking of the baby's trunk results in a whiplash motion of the head and neck. The bridging cerebral veins tear, typically leading to subdural or subarachnoid bleeding along the interhemispheric parieto-occipital cortex. The significant acceleration-deceleration forces also result in telltale retinal hemorrhages, spinal injuries, and epiphyseal-metaphyseal injury to the long bones. Full ophthalmologic and skeletal evaluations, in addition to the general examination, are mandatory in any child with unexplained head trauma.

Ocular injuries from both direct and indirect forces include subconjunctival hemorrhage, corneal abrasion, hyphema, dislocated lens, retinal detachment, and retinal hemorrhage. Other injuries from head trauma include a ruptured tympanic membrane from blows to the side of the head, or from a basilar skull fracture; loosened, fractured, or avulsed teeth from blows to the mouth; and maxillary or mandibular fractures from a blow to the face or jaw. Mandibular fractures are common in accidental injury and occur relatively easily. Maxillary fractures, conversely, require extreme force and are quite unusual in childhood.

Abdominal Injuries Intra-abdominal injuries are believed to be the second most common cause of death in abused children. Injuries include rupture of the liver or spleen, duodenal or jejunal hematoma, traumatic pancreatitis and pseudocyst formation, intestinal perforation, renal, bladder or ureteral injury, ruptured blood vessels, and ruptured lymphatic vessels resulting in chylous ascites. Bruises of the abdominal wall or flank can help to establish the diagnosis but there are no discernible marks in more than 50% of children with intra-abdominal trauma because of the distensibility of the overlying skin.

General Characteristics

A number of questions must be answered whenever there is any possibility of abuse, regardless of the exact nature of the injury.

The History Is the injury consistent with the explanation given? Is the parent reluctant to give an explanation? Is the explanation consistent with the child's level of development (for example, a 6-month-old cannot reach a pot of hot liquid on the stove while sitting on the floor)? Is the story reliable or does it vary among different caregivers at different times? Is the child alleged to have injured himself or is the child's sibling alleged to have inflicted the injury? Was there a significant delay in seeking medical care?

Physical Findings Are there multiple injuries? Did the injuries occur at different times (that is, are some older than others)? Does the pattern of injuries suggest abuse?

Characteristics of the Caregiver Does the caregiver display critical or angry behavior toward the child? Is the affect inappropriate (that is, a lack of concern about a significant injury or overconcern about a minor one)? Does the caregiver respond inappropriately or not at all to a distressed child? Is there evidence of alcohol or drug use?

Characteristics of the Child Does the child indiscriminately seek contact with unfamiliar adults or, conversely, appear extremely frightened of strangers? Is the child unable to separate from the caregiver or, conversely, unable to look to the caregiver for reassurance? Is the child hyperalert or, conversely, extremely passive and/or emotionally constricted?

In addition to the problem leading to treatment in cases of suspected abuse, information about the child's medical and family histories is essential. Chronic and acute illness, lack of appropriate immunizations or other well-child care, and a history of recurrent accidents or unexplained injuries are all associated with a greater risk of abuse. A family history of blood dyscrasias, skeletal abnormalities, or metabolic disease may be helpful in making the differential diagnosis but does not rule out abuse. If the child is being treated in a medical setting in which other physicians or providers have previously seen the family, it is important to review the child's medical record. Discrepancies between the medical record and the history given by the family should raise concern.

Management

The role of the orthopaedist in cases of child abuse involves recognition and early case management. The physician may take the initial steps independently or, preferably, with the help of an interdisciplinary child protection team. The following is a guide to initial management:

It is important to elicit a detailed history of the injury and to record this information meticulously in the medical record. If the child is old enough to give a history, this should be done in private. It is important not to make any attempt to elicit a confession from the caregivers if one is not readily offered. Confrontation often results in angry outbursts and refusals to talk, which may severely limit the ongoing assessment process and possibly further endanger the child. It is more important to gain the trust of the parents. Attempts to determine precisely who injured a child and why may limit this process.

Perform a thorough physical examination. If a pediatrician is available for a consultation, this should be requested. Ideally, the child's own doctor should perform the examination.

Perform radiographic examinations as indicated.

If the child has ecchymoses or other signs of hemorrhage, and if there are no other obvious signs of trauma, a platelet count, bleeding time, partial thromboplastin time, and prothrombin time should be done to rule out a bleeding disorder.

Ask the parents for their permission to contact the family's pediatrician. Explain that the pediatrician should be involved in the ongoing care of the child and that you hope to get information that will allow you to better understand the family and help the child.

Make a report to the local child protection agency. Explain to the family your legal obligation to report the case and emphasize your concern for the child's well-being and protection from harm.

Photographic documentation of some injuries may be useful. Photographs are required by law in some states. It is important that the photograph not be used to exaggerate trauma but depicts it as realistically as possible. In many states photographs can be taken only after informed consent is given by the child's parents. The need for these photographs must be explained openly and honestly. At times it may be better to forgo photography in the interest of developing a positive relationship with the family.

After the initial telephone report is received by the local child protection agency, a plan should be made for immediate disposition of the case. The physician's input is integral to this decision. If it is considered safe for the child to go home with the family, evaluation may be continued on an outpatient basis. In some cases, the child may be placed in a temporary emergency shelter or foster home while the evaluation proceeds. If there are questions about the safe disposition of the case or if timely emergency placement cannot be arranged through the local child protection agency, hospitalization is a safe interim step. This is especially important because, once child abuse is diagnosed, the child is at great risk of reinjury unless intervention occurs.

Ongoing management of child abuse cases should be coordinated by a multidisciplinary group that includes a social worker, pediatrician, nurse, psychologist and/or psychiatrist, and legal counsel. Public social service agencies vary in their ability to ensure that a child remains safe and to provide ongoing treatment and resources for families. Physicians who routinely see children should be aware of the child protection teams in their communities and consult them without hesitation. If a team is not available, a pediatrician should be asked for help in the initial management and follow-up of these cases.

Trends

Child abuse is no longer perceived as a rare problem. Professional obligations to protect children have been mandated by legislation. The evolution of the child abuse reporting laws suggests that the physician's responsibilities in regard to diagnosis and intervention are an integral part of addressing these problems.

Unfortunately, however, the obligations of physicians to diagnose and report the various manifestations of child abuse have not been met by a concomitant increase in the resources, or the competency, of the agencies of the state to which the case reports are made. In the face of federal, state, and local fiscal retrenchments, child welfare and child protection agencies are increasingly overburdened, and sometimes one must wonder whether one will do more harm than good by identifying and reporting a case. Experience suggests, however, that a physician's report, especially when accompanied by an indication of the physician's concern about the quality of the service to be provided to the family, can produce an appropriate response from the protective service personnel. It is always a good idea to identify someone to act as an advocate at the time that a case report is made. Often, the child's own primary care physician can serve this role.

Many child abuse cases are now brought before the criminal courts for prosecution. Most states in the last decade have obliged social welfare agencies to report serious cases of child abuse and almost all cases of sexual offenses to the local prosecuting attorney. This can have vexing consequences for the physician when expert testimony is required. It is important to keep excellent records of the clinical and laboratory findings and all contacts with the child, family, and outside providers and agencies. When the call to serve is received, it is best to review these materials in advance of the court appearance both with the prosecutor, who will nearly always be willing to come to a physician's office for preparation, and with one's own counsel. In many jurisdictions, an interdisciplinary child abuse consultation team is available to give guidance in matters of this kind; several national professional organizations, including the American Academy of Pediatrics and the American Medical Association, are establishing consultative committees or resource centers to assist physicians involved in child abuse cases.

Annotated Bibliography

Keywords

Abdominal injury; Bruises; Burns; Child abuse; Diaphyseal fracture; Epiphyseal fracture; Fracture; Head injury; Law and medicine; Metaphyseal fracture

General Considerations

Helfer RE, Kempe RS (eds): *The Battered Child*, ed 4. Chicago, University of Chicago Press, 1987.
This updated version of the original text on child abuse covers most aspects of the subject.

History and Epidemiology

Bloch H: Abandonment, infanticide, and filicide: An overview of inhumanity to children. *Am J Dis Child* 1988;142:1058–1060.
A succinct chronology of the cultural and religious underpinnings of child maltreatment from prehistory to the present.

Gelles RJ: Family violence: What we know and can do, in Newberger E, Bourne R (eds): *Unhappy Families: Clinical and Research Perspectives on Family Violence*. Littleton, PSG Publishing Co, 1985.
Describes one method of arriving at incidence and prevalence data using interview and population-sampling techniques. The author points out that if abused children were distributed through the population evenly, one of every 22 children seen by a physician would have experienced abuse. Labeling bias and characteristics of families that correlate with child abuse are discussed.

Etiology

Newberger CM, Newberger EH: The etiology of child abuse, in Ellerstein NS (ed): *Child Abuse and Neglect: A Medical Reference*. New York, John Wiley & Sons, 1981.
A look at the different etiologic theories of child abuse and a discussion of the relationships among them.

Legal Issues

Bross DC: Liability of agencies, child protection teams, and individuals, in Bross DC, Krugman RD, Lenherr MR, et al (eds): *The New Child Protection Team Handbook*. New York, Garland Publishing, 1988.
A discussion of liability and confidentiality issues pertinent to those involved in the care of abused children.

Page SP: The law, the lawyer, and medical aspects of child abuse, in Newberger EH (ed): *Child Abuse*. Boston, Little, Brown & Co, 1982.
An in-depth discussion of the history of child protection legislation, the meaning of this legislation for medical practice, and the criminal civil processes involved in child protection.

Diagnosis

Ellerstein NS (ed): *Child Abuse and Neglect: A Medical Reference*. New York, John Wiley & Sons, 1981.
The most comprehensive text on the medical diagnosis of child abuse. Orthopaedic and nonorthopaedic manifestations are discussed in detail.

Orthopaedic Manifestations of Abuse

Feldman KW, Brewer DK: Child abuse, cardiopulmonary resuscitation, and rib fractures. *Pediatrics* 1984;73:339–342.
In this analysis of 41 cases of child abuse, 50 patients who underwent cardiopulmonary resuscitation, and 22 patients with clinically undetected rib fractures noted on chest radiographs, no fractures could be attributed to cardiopulmonary resuscitation. In contrast, rib fractures occurred in 15% of the abused children.

Helfer RE, Slovis TL, Black M: Injuries resulting when small children fall out of bed. *Pediatrics* 1977;60:533–535.
The authors review the cases of 246 children aged 5 years or less who fell from a height of approximately 90 cm (the height of a bed) to the floor. There were three fractured clavicles, three skull fractures, and one fractured humerus. No serious, life-threatening injuries occurred.

King J, Diefendorf D, Apthorp J, et al: Analysis of 429 fractures in 189 battered children. *J Pediatr Orthop* 1988;8:585–589.
In a retrospective analysis of 189 abused children with fractures, it was found that 50% had only one fracture, of which 48% were transverse, 26% were spiral, and 16% were avulsion fractures. Fractures of the humerus, femur, and tibia were most common. The authors emphasize that the possibility of child abuse should not be discounted when only a single fresh diaphyseal fracture is present.

Mellick LB, Reesor K, Demers D, et al: Tibial fractures of young children. *Pediatr Emerg Care* 1988;4:97–101.

The records of 30 children 5 years of age or younger with tibial fractures were reviewed and no features distinguishing accidental from inflicted injury were identified. The authors also noted that nondisplaced (toddler's fracture) or minimally displaced spiral fractures of the mid or distal tibia can occur with relatively weak rotational forces during accidental injury but also occurred as a result of abuse in their sample.

Worlock P, Stower M, Barbor P: Patterns of fractures in accidental and non-accidental injury in children: A comparative study. *Br Med J* 1986;293:100–102.

In this population-based retrospective analysis of 35 abused and 826 nonabused children with fractures, the authors found that among children less than 18 months of age, one child in eight who sustains a fracture may be a victim of child abuse. They also noted that abused children had more frequent multiple fractures, rib fractures, spiral fractures of the humeral shaft, and bruising of the head and neck than did controls.

Imaging

Kleinman PK: *Diagnostic Imaging of Child Abuse.* Baltimore, Williams & Wilkins, 1987.

A comprehensive and up-to-date text on diagnostic imaging of abuse, including an excellent chapter on differential diagnosis.

Merten DF, Radkowski MA, Leonidas JC: The abused child: A radiological reappraisal. *Radiology* 1983;146: 377–381.

The appropriate use of radiographic examination in the evaluation of suspected child abuse is discussed in this retrospective analysis of 563 abused infants and children.

Nonorthopaedic Manifestations of Abuse

Alexander RC, Schor DP, Smith WL Jr: Magnetic resonance imaging of intracranial injuries from child abuse. *J Pediatr* 1986;109:975–979.

Magnetic resonance imaging was better than computed tomography for detection of intracranial injury in the "shaken baby syndrome" in four cases that occurred during a one-year interval.

Schmitt BD: The child with nonaccidental trauma, in Helfer RE, Kempe RS (eds): *The Battered Child,* ed 4. Chicago, University of Chicago Press, 1987.

A thorough discussion of the nonorthopaedic manifestations of inflicted injury as well as suggestions for early management.

Management

Bittner S, Newberger EH: Pediatric understanding of child abuse and neglect. *Pediatr Rev* 1981;2:197–207.

A general discussion of the interdisciplinary management of child abuse is presented.

6
Hard-Tissue Trauma

In recent years there has been an increasing amount of research related to the basic science of fracture occurrence and healing. The significant expense associated with trauma in general and fractures in particular is receiving more attention, as are the factors related to pathologic fractures. Information about fracture healing is of particular value because it can be extrapolated to the clinical setting and the use of autografts and allografts in reconstructive surgery.

Epidemiology

In 1983, the total health-care costs of fractures attributable to osteoporosis in the United States was estimated to be $6 billion. According to recent reports, the incidence of age-adjusted fractures of the proximal femur is rising. This increase of 6% per year affects primarily men and women more than 75 years old. Most proximal femoral fractures are caused by minimal to moderate trauma. The incidence of greater trochanteric fractures is increasing more steeply than that of fractures of the femoral neck. This has led to speculation that bone fragility has increased because of the deteriorating bone quality that accompanies aging. The incidence of diaphyseal femoral fracture caused by moderate trauma is increasing at a rate of 10% per year in women 75 years of age and older. In some studies, a metal implant or a neuromuscular disorder that causes disuse osteoporosis was associated with one third of the femoral diaphyseal fractures. A higher age-specific incidence of distal forearm fractures in men and women more than 50 years old has been reported. This increase paralleled an increase in the number of hip fractures in both men and women.

Fractures of the hip are associated with more deaths, disability, and medical costs than all other osteoporotic fractures combined. A total of 210,000 hip fractures occur in the United States each year. After the age of 50 years, the incidence of hip fracture rises dramatically; at all ages it is about twice as high for white women as for white men. Approximately 32% of women and 17% of men will sustain a hip fracture by the age of 90 years. About 75% to 80% of all hip fractures occur in women, and almost 50% occur in persons 80 years of age or older. The average hospital stay is three weeks. The mortality rate in patients with hip fractures is 12% to 20% higher than in persons of similar age and gender who do not have fractures. Even with adequate care, 40% of patients who sustain a hip fracture will not survive two years; of those who reside in a nursing home at the time of fracture, 70% will not survive one year. Most of these deaths occur in the first four months after fracture.

Blacks in the United States have more bone mass, greater bone density, thicker bone cortex, and greater vertebral density than whites. Age-specific incidence rates of hip fractures are about twice as high in white women as in black women. Low body weight is a significant risk factor for hip fractures in black and white women. These findings, coupled wih the known higher prevalence of obesity in older black women, suggest that differences in body weight may play a significant role in the lower incidence of hip fracture among black women.

The incidence of fractures in the elderly is increasing. Osteoporosis has been the predisposing condition for this problem. Alcohol is a leading cause of osteoporosis in men, and menopause is associated with an increased incidence in women. Smoking, inactivity, and certain medications (phenytoin, tranquilizers, steroids) all contribute to decreased bone mass. Treatment with vitamin D and calcium supplements, in addition to a gentle exercise program, may decrease the progression of the disease. All elderly patients taking phenytoin for a seizure disorder should receive vitamin D and calcium supplementation.

Age is a much more reliable predictor of hip fractures than is bone mass, particularly when mass is measured in the distal radius. Age-related risk factors for fracture need to be identified. Elderly patients with hip pain or suspected hip fracture should undergo isotope bone scanning if routine radiographs appear to be normal. Thirty percent of such patients will have nondisplaced fractures that can become displaced.

Maintenance of a skeleton capable of resisting the stresses of everyday life depends on the mechanical forces applied to the skeleton during normal activity in the 1g environment. When the effects of gravity on the longitudinal skeleton are removed, as happens in space travel or inactivity, bone and bone mineral are lost because bone resorption is greater than bone formation. Attempts to prevent disuse osteoporosis by mechanical loading or biochemical manipulations, skeletal compression, increased hydrostatic pressure, supplemental calcium, and/or phosphorus, calcitonin, or etidronate, have not been successful to date.

Recent reports have indicated an increasing incidence of musculoskeletal injuries from motorcycles and recreational vehicles, including three- and four-wheel all-terrain vehicles, dirt bikes, and snowmobiles. All three-wheel and some four-wheel all-terrain vehicles are inherently unstable. Death or significant injuries to children under the legal driving age have occurred in more than 30% of reported cases. Lack of supervision, failure to use a helmet, and alcohol abuse are major contributing factors to these severe injuries. Legislated helmet use would lessen the direct and indirect costs of motorcycle accidents. Motorcyclists sustaining head injuries use more health care dollars ($21,945 with head injury and $11,941 without head injury) and are more likely to be permanently impaired.

Stress Fractures

A prospective study of Israeli military recruits showed a 31% incidence of stress fractures, significantly higher than reported incidences in American recruits (2% to 12%). The distribution of fractures in the Israeli recruits approximated that seen in runners and joggers and may be a more relevant model for civilian stress fractures than that in American military recruits. Bone scans used to diagnose the stress fractures showed that 90% occurred in the femur (34%) and tibia (56%) and only 9% occurred in the tarsus and metatarsus. Femoral stress fractures were asymptomatic more often than were tibial fractures (69% vs 8%). Displacement of these fractures is a potential problem. Exertional bone pain in a recruit or a runner should be evaluated, because more than 50% will have a stress fracture.

Stress fractures recurred in 10.6% of the recruits by one year after the original diagnosis. All patients with recurrent fracture had at least one original stress fracture in the femur, for an incidence of 25% in patients with stress fractures of the femur. No recurrence occurred at the original anatomic site.

Four factors have been shown to predispose to stress fracture: sex (women are more susceptible than men), race (white more than black), age (older persons more than younger), and underlying metabolic bone disease (rickets, osteomalacia, hyperparathyroidism, or osteoporosis). In a symptomatic, high-risk patient, a technetium bone scan is necessary to rule out a stress fracture. Limitation of activity is adequate treatment for most stress fractures, but overt nonunion may still occur.

Metabolism of Fracture Healing

Growth hormone, thyroid hormone, anabolic agents, and vitamin D all have beneficial effects on the process of fracture repair. Conversely, steroids have a negative effect. Callus formation is an active process that consumes local calcium. Because calcium homeostasis is regulated by parathyroid hormone, calcitonin, and vitamin D metabolites, it is important to understand their function in fracture repair. Recent studies in dogs and in humans have investigated their roles in normal fracture healing.

In the dog, a bridging callus is usually present at a fracture site by three to four weeks. Callus is apparent clinically and radiographically by three weeks. Hypocalcemia and reciprocal hyperphosphatemia develop four hours after the fracture in the canine model. The serum level of magnesium parallels that of calcium, but the changes are less obvious. These changes represent an immediate, nonspecific posttraumatic reaction (acute-phase reaction) to the injury.

During fracture healing, there is an increase in serum levels of calcitonin, $24,25(OH)_2D_3$, and parathyroid hormone. Calcitonin is a calcium-preserving hormone and an antagonist to most of the actions of parathyroid hormone. It inhibits bone resorption by direct inhibition of the osteoclast. In the canine model, serum calcitonin levels increase during the bone healing process, confirming observations in humans. This supports the suggestion that calcitonin plays an important positive role in bone repair.

In the kidney, two active end-metabolites of vitamin D are formed—calcitriol and $24,25(OH)_2D_3$. These metabolites are formed from the common precursor calcifediol.

Calcitriol is the principal factor governing calcium and phosphorus absorption from the gastrointestinal tract and regulates calcium and phosphorus concentrations in the extracellular fluid. Some investigators suggest that $24,25(OH)_2D_3$ may act directly on bone cells. However, all investigators agree that it is in part an inactive metabolite of vitamin D. In the canine model, serum levels of $24,25(OH)_2D_3$ are increased during fracture healing. The conversion of the precursor to $24,25(OH)_2D_3$ explains the persistently low concentrations of calcifediol during the fracture healing period. Obviously, vitamin D is a prerequisite for normal fracture healing. An increase in serum levels of parathyroid hormone during regular fracture healing is explained by the body's effort to mobilize calcium and increase its availability for callus calcification.

Patients with fractures have been tested for parathyroid hormone, calcitonin, and vitamin D metabolites during fracture healing. The plasma calcium level on the day of fracture was significantly decreased compared with that in a group of healthy volunteers of similar age and sex. Serum calcitonin level on the day of fracture was significantly increased and it continued to increase during the healing period. A significant increase was noted in the plasma level of $24,25(OH)_2D_3$ on the day of fracture, and this continued to increase for as long as six weeks. No significant changes were found in serum parathyroid hormone levels on the day of fracture or during the healing process. The results suggest a possible active role of calcitonin. The changes in $24,25(OH)_2D_3$ during fracture healing in humans may reflect inactive byproducts of vitamin D metabolism or a product that has a specific function.

Steroid Effects

The administration of high doses of cortical glucocorticoids has been associated with osteoporosis and pathologic fractures. Systemic corticosteroids affect bone in a characteristic distribution, with predominant loss of trabecular bone density in the axial skeleton such as the ribs and vertebrae. These areas are known to have a high content of trabecular bone with a rapid turnover rate. This is in contrast to the less dramatic changes in bone density and less frequent fractures that occur in the appendicular skeleton, where cortical bone predominates.

A rough but statistically significant relationship has been demonstrated between duration of steroid therapy and loss of trabecular mass in patients with various disorders (primarily rheumatoid arthritis). Rheumatoid arthritis is associated with osteopenia. Concomitant steroid therapy, therefore, may have a further detrimental effect on bone mass in these patients. If long-term steroid therapy is required for asthma or other medical conditions, the bone loss that may result should be treated.

A recent study investigated the possibility of preventing prednisone-induced protein wasting by regular physical activity. Healthy, untrained volunteers were subjected to a four-week regimen of prednisone therapy (30 mg/day) during an exercise program (jogging 2.5 miles four times per week) and again without exercise. Whole-body protein synthesis and breakdown were measured (nitrogen flux, nitrogen intake, and urinary nitrogen elimination), as was bone protein metabolism (serum bone Gla-protein and urinary hydroxyproline). The data suggested that moderate exercise training can prevent, at least in part, the protein loss induced by prednisone.

Replacement of Bone Defects

Bone grafts serve one or both of two main functions: they provide a source of bone inductive material and they serve as a mechanical support. Autografts, both cancellous and cortical, are implanted fresh and are osteogenic (either as a source of osteoprogenitor cells or by being osteoinductive). All bone grafts undergo resorption; cancellous grafts are completely replaced in time by creeping substitution, whereas cortical grafts remain a mixture of necrotic and viable bone for prolonged periods.

Autogenous cancellous bone remains the most osteogenic and reliable bone grafting material even after 30 years of experimental research on alternative materials. Because of problems associated with the availability and acquisition (pain, blood loss, time) of autogenous grafts, alternative materials continue to be investigated.

Allograft bone, both fresh and preserved, is increasingly being used for longer bone defects. Porous ceramic materials (tricalcium phosphate and hydroxyapatite) have shown promise as osteoconductive materials. They have been particularly useful in areas involving cancellous bone (metaphyseal defects). The materials are quite similar, with the exception that tricalcium phosphate appears to resorb consistently while hydroxyapatite does not.

The use of bone marrow obtained by percutaneous aspiration as graft material has been proposed as well. Favorable outcomes have been obtained when bone marrow aspirate and bone morphogenic protein (used as osteoinductive material) are combined with tricalcium phosphate or hydroxyapatite (osteoconductive materials). In a recent study in rats, demineralized bone powder used as an osteoinductive substance in large segmental defects was as effective as autologous bone in bridging the gap. Clearly, more research is necessary in this area.

Bioelectricity

There is much controversy about the use of electrical impulses to heal fractures and nonunions. Electrical impulses do not hasten normal fracture healing. The method has been reported to be effective (70% to 90% success) in treating delayed union and nonunion.

Electricity may be applied to bone by one of three methods: direct current, inductive coupling, and capacitive coupling. Direct current is invasive and involves the direct insertion of wire electrodes into the area of application. Power to the electrodes can be applied by a power pack outside the skin, which requires wires through the skin, or by an implantable battery pack. Inductive coupling is noninvasive and uses a pair of coils outside the skin to generate a pulsed electromagnetic field through the affected bone. This method requires a large power source using household current or a bulky battery pack. Capacitive coupling is noninvasive, uses portable equipment, allows full weight-bearing in a cast, is easy to apply, and does not require precise location of the capacitor plates on the skin. Because of these advantages, this method may be preferable to the others. Reported rates of union are similar with all three methods.

Unfortunately, no large prospective double-blind study using any of these systems has been reported. Therefore, the actual union rates are unknown. A great deal of basic research has been conducted in electrical stimulation and demonstrates a definite effect on osteogenesis. Application of this research in clinical practice has been controversial. Many variables need to be evaluated when considering use of the technique. These include presence of infection, synovial pseudarthrosis, the size of the bone gap, ability to immobilize the nonunion, patient cooperation, nutritional status, previous treatment, and others. The only prospective randomized study reported in humans was small and showed no effectiveness of the method.

The method appears to be highly effective for treatment of scaphoid nonunion, but less effective for humeral nonunion. Published reports regarding effectiveness of the methods offer conflicting data.

Recent animal studies have shown that electrical stimulation has no significant effect on healing of bone defects in the dog with or without bone graft. The method is being evaluated in animals as a potential treatment for osteonecrosis, disuse osteoporosis, castration-induced osteoporosis, and nerve injuries. The method may have application as an osteoinducer to be used in conjunction with osteoconductive material (tricalcium phosphate, hydroxyapatite) for bone grafting.

Trends

There will be heightened interest in the economic implications of osteoporosis and fracture occurrence, particularly in the older population. There will be increased research into the prevention and diagnosis of this family of diseases, particularly because the age group most at risk, the elderly, constitutes an increasingly large segment of the population.

Genetic engineering and the expanding understanding of various growth factors will be significant in fracture healing. It is anticipated that the next several years will see a markedly increased application of such technology to clinical practice.

Annotated Bibliography

Keywords

Bioelectricity; Bone graft; Calcium; Corticosteroids; Estrogen; Fracture; Osteoporosis; Parathyroid hormone; Vitamin D

Epidemiology

Arneson TJ, Melton LJ III, Lewallen DG, et al: Epidemiology of diaphyseal and distal femoral fractures in Rochester, Minnesota, 1965–1984. *Clin Orthop* 1988;234:188–194.

One third of the fractures were associated with moderate trauma and were responsible for the rising incidence rates at all three fracture sites. These increases were greater in women.

Bried JM, Cordasco FA, Volz RG: Medical and economic parameters of motorcycle-induced trauma. *Clin Orthop* 1987;223:252–256.

A retrospective review of all patients injured in motorcycle accidents who were admitted to a single institution and studied over a one-year period. The 71 patients averaged 26 years of age; 79% were men, 75% were not wearing helmets, and 24% were legally intoxicated. The cost of care was significantly higher for patients who sustained head injuries.

Cummings SR, Kelsey JL, Nevitt MC, et al: Epidemiology of osteoporosis and osteoporotic fractures. *Epidemiol Rev* 1985;7:178–208.

This comprehensive review of osteoporotic fractures discusses methods of measuring the degree of osteoporosis. Risk factors such as age, sex, race, geography, reproductive history, dietary factors, physical activity, alcohol, and others are related.

Hedlund R, Ahlbom A, Lindgren U: Hip fracture incidence in Stockholm, 1972–1981. *Acta Orthop Scand* 1986;57:30–34.

The incidences of cervical and trochanteric fractures were studied. Moderate trauma caused hip fractures that increased at an annual rate of 6% in both males and females.

Hedlund R, Lindgren U: Epidemiology of diaphyseal femoral fracture. *Acta Orthop Scand* 1986;57:423–427.

The incidence of diaphyseal femoral fracture decreased from the age of 20 years to middle age, after which it increased into old age. The incidence of diaphyseal femoral fracture caused by moderate trauma increased annually by 10% in women 75 years of age and older.

Holmberg S, Conradi P, Kalen R, et al: Mortality after cervical hip fracture: 3002 patients followed for 6 years. *Acta Orthop Scand* 1986;57:8–11.

Patients admitted from institutions had a mortality rate three to four times higher than those coming from home. After six years, 54% of the patients admitted from home were alive compared with only 16% of those admitted from institutions.

Ruff CB, Hayes WC: Sex differences in age-related remodeling of the femur and tibia. *J Orthop Res* 1988;6:886–896.

Only men tend to remodel bone in a way that tends to compensate for loss of bone strength with aging.

Schneider VS, McDonald J: Skeletal calcium homeostasis and countermeasures to prevent disuse osteoporosis. *Calcif Tissue Int* 1984;36(suppl 1):S151–S154.

Attempts to prevent disuse osteoporosis with biomechanical and biochemical means, including exercise, skeletal compression, increased hydrostatic pressure to the lower body, supplemental calcium, and/or phosphorus, calcitonin, or etidronate, were not successful.

Stress Fractures

Giladi M, Milgrom C, Kashtan H, et al: Recurrent stress fractures in military recruits: One-year follow-up of 66 recruits. *J Bone Joint Surg* 1986;68B:439–441.

Of 66 recruits who sustained stress fractures during basic training and returned to training after a period of rest, seven (10.6%) sustained a recurrent stress fracture within one year. None of the recurrences was at the original anatomic site.

Matheson GO, Clement DB, McKenzie DC, et al: Scintigraphic uptake of 99mTc at non-painful sites in athletes with stress fractures: The concept of bone strain. *Sports Med* 1987;4:65–75.

Asymptomatic uptake of ^{99m}Tc occurs frequently in athletes with stress fractures, and there are no significant clinical differences between those with asymptomatic uptake and those without.

Milgrom C, Giladi M, Stein M, et al: Stress fractures in military recruits: A prospective study showing an unusually high incidence. *J Bone Joint Surg* 1985;67B:732–735.

A prospective study of 295 male Israeli recruits demonstrated a 31% incidence of stress fracture. Eighty percent of fractures were in the tibia or femoral shaft, and only 8% occurred in the tarsus and metatarsus.

Metabolism of Fracture Healing

Ettinger B, Genant HK, Cann CE: Long-term estrogen replacement therapy prevents bone loss and fractures. *Ann Intern Med* 1985;102:319–324.

The incidence of osteoporotic fracture in estrogen users was 50% of that in controls (P < .01). Estrogen users had significantly more bone mineral. Long-term estrogen replacement therapy confers significant protection against bone loss and fracture.

McKenna MJ, Frame B: Hormonal influences on osteoporosis. *Am J Med* 1987;82:61–67.

Estrogen is known to have a protective effect on the female skeleton. Calcitonin levels, which decrease after menopause, return to normal with estrogen; other hormones may also play important roles.

Steroid Effects

Garrel DR, Delmas PD, Welsh C, et al: Effects of moderate physical training on prednisone-induced protein wasting: A study of whole-body and bone protein metabolism. *Metabolism* 1988;37:257–262.

A well-controlled study of the effect of physical activity on protein wasting in healthy volunteers demonstrated that moderate exercise training can prevent the protein loss induced by prednisone.

Replacement of Bone Defects

Gepstein R, Weiss RE, Hallel T: Bridging large defects in bone by demineralized bone matrix in the form of a powder: A radiographic, histological, and radioisotope-uptake study in rats. *J Bone Joint Surg* 1987;69A:984–992.

Demineralized bone powder was used as an osteoinductive substance to bridge large defects (50% of total bone length) in rats. Results with the bone powder compared favorably to those with autogenous bone graft.

Holmes RE, Bucholz RW, Mooney V: Porous hydroxyapatite as a bone-graft substitute in metaphyseal defects: A histometric study. *J Bone Joint Surg* 1986;68A:904–911.

Porous hydroxyapatite was incorporated into the skeleton of dogs when placed into a metaphyseal defect, with bone forming well within the substance of the synthetic graft material.

Lange TA, Zerwekh JE, Peek RD, et al: Granular tricalcium phosphate in large cancellous defects. *Ann Clin Lab Sci* 1986;16:467–472.

Tricalcium phosphate was placed into large metaphyseal defects (12 cm³) in pigs. After four months the specimens showed no inflammation and the tricalcium phosphate was surrounded by viable trabecular bone. Tricalcium phosphate appeared to absorb completely by nine months.

Paley D, Young MC, Wiley AM, et al: Percutaneous bone marrow grafting of fractures and bony defects: An experimental study in rabbits. *Clin Orthop* 1986;208:300–312.

Bone defects grafted with bone marrow united by means of a bony bridge, whereas those grafted with saline controls did not. Percutaneous bone marrow grafting is a simple, semi-invasive technique that may have potential clinical applications.

Bioelectricity

Barker AT, Dixon RA, Sharrard WJ, et al: Pulsed magnetic field therapy for tibial non-union: Interim results of a double-blind trial. *Lancet* 1984;1:994–996.

Patients with tibial fractures that had not united after at least 52 weeks were randomly assigned to either active or sham pulsed magnetic field stimulators and treated in casts for 24 weeks with nonweightbearing. Five of nine fractures given active treatment united and five of seven given sham treatment united. The high proportion of fractures uniting in the control group suggests that conservative management of nonunion is effective.

Brighton CT, Luessenhop CP, Pollack SR, et al: Treatment of castration-induced osteoporosis by a capacitively coupled electrical signal in rat vertebrae. *J Bone Joint Surg* 1989;71A:228–236.

Castrated rats were subjected to capacitively coupled electrical fields. The signal used significantly reversed the castration-induced osteoporosis in the lumbar vertebrae.

Brighton CT, Pollack SR: Treatment of recalcitrant nonunion with a capacitively coupled electrical field: A preliminary report. *J Bone Joint Surg* 1985;67A:577–585.

Seventeen of 22 ununited fractures (77%) achieved solid osseous union after an average of 22.5 weeks of treatment with capacitive coupling.

Miller GJ, Burchardt H, Enneking WF, et al: Electromagnetic stimulation of canine bone grafts. *J Bone Joint Surg* 1984;66A:693–698.

No significant effect was noted on the biomechanical strength, histologic presentation, or time to union with either two months or six months of pulsed electromagnetic field stimulation in segmental, autogenous cortical bone grafts in dogs.

7
Polytrauma

Accidents, which have been characterized as the neglected disease of modern society, are the leading cause of death for persons 1 through 39 years old and the third leading cause of death for all age groups. Trauma deaths exceed those from heart disease, stroke, and cancer combined.

In the past decade, trauma care has emerged as a specialty. Mortality and morbidity have been reduced through improved field resuscitation, rapid transport to trauma centers, and earlier surgical intervention, while a greater knowledge and understanding of the metabolic response to trauma has reduced late deaths from multiple organ system failure. In addition, the fat embolism syndrome has almost been eliminated through a greater understanding of respiratory failure, improved resuscitation, endotracheal intubation, ventilatory support, and early fracture stabilization. Perhaps the most significant contribution to the decrease in trauma morbidity and mortality has been the establishment of regionalized trauma centers.

Many studies have provided evidence that regionalization of trauma care and the establishment of trauma centers significantly reduce treatment delay, suboptimal care, and preventable trauma deaths. Audits of trauma care in San Diego County, for example, done before and after the implementation of a regionalized trauma system (Table 1), showed significant and dramatic improvements in the following areas: suboptimal care of multiple trauma victims declined from 32% to 4.2%; delay in evaluation, from 41% to 10%; delay in disposition, from 53% to 7%; suboptimal assessment, from 22% to 1%; multiple trauma mortality, from 26.4% to 8.2%. The ultimate proof of the benefit of a trauma center, however, is the reduction of preventable

deaths; the implementation of a trauma care system reduced the preventable death rate from 13.6% to 2.7%. These data must be regarded as the standards by which community and regional prehospital, emergency department, and in-hospital care systems are evaluated.

Resuscitation

Triage

Advanced life-support techniques used by emergency medical technicians in the prehospital care of critically injured patients have reduced the mortality rate from penetrating and blunt trauma and have improved the hemodynamic status of these patients.

With the increasing success of the nationwide effort to designate specific hospitals as trauma centers, the major problem of prehospital trauma triage has become the identification of patients who should be taken to trauma centers. Several field triage scales and a checklist (Outline 1) have been developed to help in this assessment. (The presence of any of the checklist items mandates transport to a trauma center.) The primary goal of triage, to identify most trauma victims whose injuries are life-threatening, must be accomplished quickly. An important contribution to practical triage criteria is the Trauma Score, which is based solely on physiologic assessment. The Trauma Score (Table 2), when combined with anatomic injuries and other criteria (Outline 1), is sufficiently sensitive to accomplish the triage objectives. The major cause of early death is head injury and the level of consciousness is the most sensitive indicator of a fatal prognosis.

Table 1. Results of audits done before and after implementation of a trauma system*

Data	1982 Study†		1984 Study†		P Value
	No.	%	No.	%	
Delays					
Total number	341	—	1,366	—	
Initial evaluation	134	41.3	137	10.6	< .01
Disposition	192	53.6	103	7.5	< .01
Suboptimal assessment on treatment					
Total number	341	—	1,366	—	
Initial hospital phase	113	32.0	23	1.7	< .01
All hospital phases	113	32.0	40	2.9	< .01
Deaths					
Total number	90	26.4	112	8.2	< .01
Nonpreventable	69	78.5	101	90.2	< .05
Potentially salvageable	7	7.9	8	7.1	NS
Clearly preventable	12	13.6	3	2.7	< .01

*Reproduced with permission from Shackford SR, Hollingworth-Fridlund, P, Cooper GF, et al: The effect of regionalization upon the quality of trauma care as assessed by concurrent audit before and after institution of a trauma system: A preliminary report. *J Trauma* 1986;26:812–820.

†The data for 1982 were accrued over a three-month period and those for 1984 over a five-month period.

Outline 1. Triage checklist*†

No spontaneous eye opening
Abnormal capillary refill
Penetrating injuries
 Cranial
 Neck
 Chest
 Abdominal
Blunt thoracic trauma with systolic blood pressure < 90 mm Hg
Flail chest
Blunt abdominal trauma
 In a pedestrian struck by a motor vehicle
 In a motorcyclist
Fall of more than 15 ft
Age < 5 years or > 65 years

*Adapted from Kane G: Empirical development and evaluation of prehospital trauma triage instruments. *J Trauma* 1985;25:482–489.
†A patient with any listed condition should be taken to a trauma center.

Airway

Maintaining the airway of a trauma victim is essential. Properly trained paramedics have performed endotracheal intubation in the field with a 96% success rate but, because this procedure requires special training, the esophageal ob-turator airway was developed to improve ventilation and oxygenation and to help prevent aspiration of gastric contents. The esophageal obturator airway is no longer recommended, however, because inadvertent tracheal intubation can be life-threatening and because other possible complications include esophageal rupture and laceration, gastric rupture, and tracheal occlusion.

Pneumatic Antishock Garments

Pneumatic antishock garments have been recommended for the treatment of hypovolemic hypotension and for long-term control of retroperitoneal and intraperitoneal hemorrhages. During the last few years, there have been several reports of compartment syndrome after their use. One recent study has shown that a pressure of 30 mm Hg or more applied to the whole limb stops microcirculation and results in tissue anoxia. Therefore, pneumatic anti-shock garments should not be used if there are major ex-tremity fractures. When they are used for longer than 90 minutes, the pressure should not exceed 20 mm Hg.

The authors of a prospective, randomized evaluation of pneumatic antishock garments concluded that, for pene-

Table 2. The Trauma Score*

Assessment	Response	Code	Score
A. Respiratory rate	10 to 24	4	A. _____
	25 to 35	3	
	35	2	
	10	1	
	0	0	
B. Respiratory effort	Normal	1	B. _____
	Retractive	0	
	≥ 90	4	
C. Systolic blood pressure	70 to 89	3	C. _____
	50 to 69	2	
	< 50	1	
No carotid pulse	0	0	
D. Capillary refill			D. _____
Normal	≤ 2 sec	2	
Delayed	> 2 sec	1	
None	——	0	
E. Glascow Coma Scale Eye opening	Spontaneous	4	E. _____
	To voice	3	
	To pain	2	
	None	1	
	Oriented	5	
Verbal response	Confused	4	
	Inappropriate	3	
	Incomprehensible	2	
	None	1	
Motor response and response to pain	Obeys commands	6	
	Purposeful	5	
	Withdraws	4	
	Flexion	3	
	None	1	
Coma Scale Points	14 to 15	5	
	11 to 13	4	
	8 to 10	3	
	5 to 7	2	
	3 to 4	1	
Trauma Score (A + B + C + D + E)			_____

*The Trauma Score ranges from 1 (worst prognosis) to 16 (best prognosis). A score of 12 indicates an 87% survival rate, 10 indicates a 60% rate, 8 indicates a 26% rate, 6 indicates an 8% rate, and 1 indicates a 1% rate.

trating trauma with a prehospital time of 30 minutes or less, they provided no advantage with regard to survival, length of hospital stay, or reduction in hospital cost.

Shock

Fluid Resuscitation

One half of civilian trauma deaths occur within one hour of injury as a result of exsanguination or damage to the central nervous system. An additional 30% of trauma victims die within two or three hours from major internal hemorrhage.

In an animal model of fatal hemorrhage, Ringer's lactate provided better survival than normal saline, Plasmalyte-A, or Plasmalyte-R, probably because this crystalloid solution contains less chloride and no acetate or magnesium.

A similar model was used to compare colloid solutions. Blood was replaced in a 1:1 ratio with autologous whole blood, untyped fresh-frozen plasma, typed fresh-frozen plasma, 5% human serum albumin, or normal saline. Analysis indicated that whole blood provided significantly better survival than untyped fresh-frozen plasma, albumin, or normal saline but not typed fresh-frozen plasma. Data from hemodynamic, arterial blood gases, and acid-base analyses indicated that whole blood and fresh-frozen plasma provided a better acid-buffering capacity in surviving animals. When typed blood is not available, type-specific fresh-frozen plasma appears to be an adequate alternative.

Transfusion

The ideal fluid for trauma resuscitation has not yet been perfected. Controversy still exists as to whether type O uncrossmatched blood or type-specific blood should be used in the acute resuscitation of the trauma patient. A two-year study found type O uncrossmatched packed erythrocytes to be safe and effective in acute resuscitation. The advantages include immediate availability, suitability for all recipients, and the fact that there is no risk of transfusing high-titer plasma. In addition, using type O blood avoids possible typing errors in urgent situations, especially if several patients are being treated.

Hemorrhagic shock is characterized by the loss of erythrocyte mass and intravascular volume, which results in tissue ischemia. The optimal hematocrit after shock and trauma is somewhat controversial. A recent prospective study randomly assigned patients to either a 0.30 (30%) hematocrit group or a 0.40 (40%) hematocrit group. The higher level appeared to offer no advantage. In the 0.30 (30%) group, oxygen consumption was correlated with oxygen delivery. In addition, there was a decreased incidence of intrapulmonary shunting.

Hemorrhagic Shock

Life-threatening hemorrhage is a frequent complication of major pelvic fractures, and definitive treatment mandates an organized multispecialty team approach. Although there has been recent support for using pneumatic antishock garments for pelvic compression, the use of external skeletal fixation for reduction and bone stabilization appears to be superior. Hemorrhaging was controlled in 71% of patients treated with the antishock garments alone but in 95% of

patients treated with external skeletal fixation. External skeletal bone fixation is superior to antishock garments in that it reduces the compression of abdominal contents (which impairs ventilation), reduces the risk of lower-extremity compartment syndromes, and allows better access to the abdomen. A few patients require selective embolization with pelvic angiography to control pelvic hemorrhage. Arteriography demonstrates that hemorrhage from pelvic arteries is not a frequent problem. Autopsy studies have suggested that the most common sources of hemorrhage are the bony edges.

Shock and blood loss have been found to be major risk factors for postoperative infection. The incidence of wound infection is almost doubled when shock occurs. Shock depresses the immune system, which may explain its causal relationship to increased infection rates.

Diagnostic Techniques

Peritoneal Lavage

The accuracy of clinical evaluation alone in diagnosing significant intra-abdominal injuries in patients with blunt abdominal trauma has been reported to range from 42% to 84%. The use of diagnostic peritoneal lavage has greatly improved this accuracy. In a prospective study of patients with significant intra-abdominal injuries secondary to blunt abdominal trauma, positive findings included blood cell count criteria (Outline 2) (erythrocyte count, $> 0.1 \times 10^{12}$/L; leukocyte count, $\geq 0.5 \times 10^9$/L), free aspiration of blood, increased amylase levels in the presence of bile, or bacteria in the lavage fluid. The overall accuracy rate was 97.8%, the false-positive rate was 3.4%. Diagnostic peritoneal lavage is controversial in cases in which the erythrocyte count is lower than 0.1×10^{12}/L. Several studies have shown that significant intra-abdominal abnormalities may occur with isolated erythrocyte counts between 0.02 and 0.1×10^{12}/L. In such cases, reexamination and/or relavage may be indicated as well as computed tomographic scans and/or ultrasonography.

Outline 2. "Standard" criteria for interpreting lavage data*

Positive
  Aspiration of 10 ml of free-flowing, unclotting blood
  Grossly bloody lavage return
  Lavage fluid exits via Foley catheter or chest tube
  Evidence of food, foreign particles, or bile
  Erythrocyte count > 100,000/mm³ (> 0.1×10^{12}/L)
  Leukocyte count > 500/mm³ (> 0.5×10^9/L)
  Amylase level > 175 U/dl (> 1,750 U/L)
Intermediate
  Aspiration of < 10 ml of free-flowing, unclotting blood
  Erythrocyte count between 50,000 and 100,000/mm³ (0.5×10^{11} and 0.1×10^{12}/L)
  Leukocyte count between 100 and 500/mm³ (0.1×10^9 and 0.5×10^9/L)
  Amylase level between 75 and 175 U/dl (750 and 1,750 U/L)
Negative
  Erythrocyte count < 50,000/mm³ (0.5×10^{11}/L)
  Leukocyte count < 100/mm³ (< 0.1×10^9/L)
  Amylase level < 75 U/dl (< 750 U/L)

---

*Adapted with permission from McLellen BA, Hanna SS, Montoya DR, et al: Analysis of peritoneal lavage parameters in blunt abdominal trauma. *J Trauma* 1985; 25:394.

Computed Tomography

Although computed tomography has been used to diagnose both intra-abdominal and retroperitoneal injuries in recent years, peritoneal lavage remains a superior diagnostic technique. In one study, using both oral and intravenous contrast media, the results of computed tomography and diagnostic peritoneal lavage were compared to the findings at laparotomy or to the clinical course of patients who did not undergo exploratory surgery. The sensitivity, specificity, and accuracy of peritoneal lavage were 90%, 100%, and 98%, respectively. For computed tomography, these values were 85%, 100%, and 97%. Thus, even with experienced examiners, computed tomography offers no diagnostic advantage over peritoneal lavage in blunt trauma.

Computed tomography is, however, a reliable alternative when circumstances do not allow peritoneal lavage or when the peritoneal lavage data are questionable. Computed tomography is, for example, valuable for pregnant patients and patients who have undergone abdominal explorations previously. Computed tomography also has certain advantages in evaluating bowel and mesenteric injuries and has been helpful in distinguishing injuries that require surgical repair from those that can be safely monitored and observed. Computed tomography is also appropriate for stable patients with equivocal abdominal findings, stable patients with closed head injury, and patients with spinal cord injuries, hematuria, or pelvic fractures accompanied by significant bleeding. In addition, it can be used in stable patients who cannot undergo physical examination, such as those requiring surgical fixation of extensive orthopaedic injuries. Algorithm 1 gives general guidelines.

Arteriography

Arteriography is a widely used diagnostic tool in the management of suspected vascular injuries of the extremity. However, the routine use of arteriography in the evaluation of patients without clinical findings of vascular trauma has resulted in a high percentage of negative arteriograms. Its use is controversial in patients who undergo arteriography only because of penetrating injury in the proximity of a major vessel. Because arteriography in such cases identifies few vascular injuries (range, 0% to 20%) that are later confirmed by surgery, recent studies conclude that routine arteriography for isolated penetrating trauma in the proximity of a major vessel (that is, when such trauma is the only injury) is unnecessary. Instead, the patient is admitted to the hospital for a 24-hour period of observation and repeat physical examination.

Intravenous Pyelogram

Emergency intravenous pyelogram is commonly used to evaluate blunt abdominal trauma. Traditionally, it has been ordered in all cases of hematuria, whether microscopic or gross. More recently, it has been suggested that an emergency intravenous pyelogram be performed only on trauma patients with gross hematuria and that those with lesser degrees of hematuria be observed. Retrospective evaluation of this practice has confirmed its usefulness. Although any degree of hematuria after trauma demands attention, microscopic hematuria alone after blunt abdominal trauma does not mandate an emergency intravenous pyelogram. Radiologic evaluation can be safely reserved for patients in whom hematuria does not resolve within 24 hours.

Treatment

Head Injuries

The most common cause of death in the first few hours after trauma is head injuries. In a severe closed injury, acute subdural hematoma is the most common sign of the need for surgery. An acute subdural hematoma is a collection of blood under the dura mater of sufficient size to compress the brain; it requires surgery as soon as possible if life and function are to be preserved. Because surgical decompression is urgent, direct admission to trauma centers for patients with acute subdural hematoma has improved survival. A comparison of patients with acute subdural hematoma admitted directly to a trauma center with those transferred to the trauma center from another institution (involving a delay of several hours) showed that the former fared significantly better: mortality rates were 50% and 76%, respectively.

On the Glasgow Coma Scale (Table 2), a score of 8 or less represents a patient with severe head injury. Preoperative clinical signs associated with a high mortality rate include midzone fixed pupils, flaccidity, and unresponsiveness; bilaterally dilated and fixed pupils; apnea or irregular respiration; absent pupillary light reaction bilaterally; and decerebrate posturing. The best results occurred in patients who were lucid and admitted directly to a trauma center where surgery was performed within the first four hours. These patients had a 30% mortality rate compared with 90% for patients undergoing surgery after four hours.

Outcome in such cases has been improved by means of early diagnosis and intensive management. Besides the evacuation of intracranial mass lesions, management should include artificial ventilation to help lower Pco_2. Secondary cerebral insults detected by means of hypoxia or brain swelling should be treated with artificial ventilation along with continuous monitoring of intracranial pressure and control of intracranial hypertension by mannitol and pentobarbital or drainage of cerebrospinal fluid. These techniques and intraventricular pressure monitors have improved the outcome in patients with severe head injuries.

Thoracoabdominal Injuries

Myocardial Contusion Blunt chest trauma causes myocardial damage ranging from insignificant contusion to overt myocardial rupture. The diagnosis and clinical relevance of myocardial contusion, however, are a problem in the clinical setting. At autopsy, myocardial contusion has been found to be present in 15% of patients with blunt trauma; this figure increases to 40% when there is direct anterior chest trauma. Myocardial contusion can be diagnosed on the basis of increased serum levels of the isoenzyme creatine kinase. However, since this enzyme disappears within 24 hours, levels need to be obtained at admission and every six hours thereafter for a 24-hour period. Although a creatine kinase level above 5% is an indication of a myocardial contusion, no correlation has been found between enzyme level and myocardial damage. Two-dimensional echocardiography is useful in assessing the severity of a myocardial

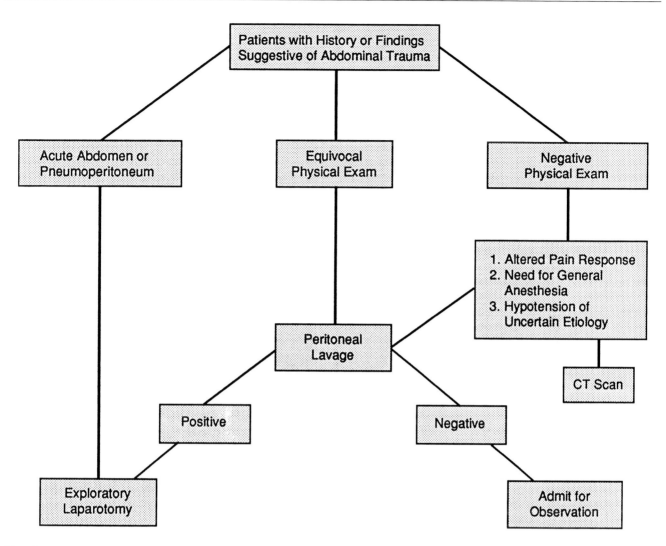

Algorithm 1

Guidelines for the management of blunt abdominal trauma. (Reproduced with permission from Gomez GA, Alvarez R, Plasencia G, et al: Diagnostic peritoneal lavage in the management of blunt abdominal trauma: A reassessment. *J Trauma* 1987;27:1–5.)

injury. Posttraumatic cardiac monitoring is needed because fatal arrhythmias, severe heart failure, myocardial infarction, and death have occurred after cardiac contusion.

Considerable trepidation has been expressed regarding general anesthesia for a patient with a cardiac contusion. Treatment similar to that for acute myocardial infarction has been suggested. However, when proper physiologic monitoring is performed during surgical procedures, myocardial contusion does not constitute an absolute contraindication to needed surgery for the patient with multiple injuries.

Bronchial Rupture Disruption of major bronchi or the intrathoracic trachea secondary to blunt thoracic trauma is a formerly rare injury that has been reported with increasing frequency in recent years. Major tracheal and bronchial injuries present special problems in the context of multiple system trauma. Subcutaneous emphysema, especially with persisting pneumothorax or a significant air leak, suggests this diagnosis. Bronchoscopy should be performed before thoracotomy. Celiotomy may be needed if an adequately oxygenated patient is hemodynamically unstable.

Splenic Rupture The spleen is the organ most frequently injured by blunt abdominal trauma. Considerable controversy has arisen in recent years regarding the most appropriate method of managing trauma to the spleen. Splenectomy, once routine, is now being challenged because of a better appreciation of the physiologic importance of the spleen. Although the risk of postsplenectomy sepsis may be slight, it represents a possibly lethal complication. Selective criteria for nonsurgical management of splenic injuries have been developed; these include absolute hemodynamic stability, minimal or no peritoneal findings, and a maximal transfusion requirement of 2 units. If abdominal surgery is necessary, the spleen should be repaired if at all possible. However, attempts at repair should be abandoned if, in the surgeon's judgment, hemostasis is inadequate, less than one third of the remaining splenic tissue functions, or associated life-threatening injuries take precedence.

There has been concern that selective use of nonsurgical management of splenic injuries may lead to an intra-abdominal injury being overlooked. Although diaphragmatic or major bowel injuries are associated with blunt splenic or liver trauma in about 10% of cases, their incidence is low in the minor splenic injuries that can be managed nonsurgically.

Liver Injury After the spleen, the liver is the organ most commonly injured by blunt abdominal trauma. Liver injury is associated with injury to multiple organs in a high percentage of cases. The mortality rate from liver injury is 10% to 20% in most series. The major cause of death from liver injury is exsanguinating hemorrhage. Control of hemorrhage at the time of surgery can be extremely difficult. Packing the liver to control the hemorrhage, with later relaparotomy for removal of packs and definitive treatment, has recently been advocated; this provides hemodynamic stability and allows the associated coagulopathies to be treated.

Diaphragmatic Rupture Traumatic rupture of the diaphragm is relatively uncommon in blunt abdominal trauma (about 5% of cases) and the diagnosis is difficult. Only 50% of ruptured diaphragms are diagnosed preoperatively, 25% of those via an upright chest radiograph that shows loops of hollow viscus in the chest or the presence of a nasogastric tube in the hemithorax. Because most ruptured diaphragms are discovered at the time of abdominal exploration, the clinician must have a high index of suspicion for this injury and thoroughly investigate the upper abdomen at the time of surgery.

Urologic Trauma Approximately 80% of patients with severe renal injuries manifest gross hematuria, but the use of excretory urograms, cystograms, and urethrograms allows prompt detection of major injuries in nearly all patients. The nonvisualization of a kidney by excretory urography suggests a major renal arterial injury until proven otherwise. Most renal injuries (85%) are minor and do not require surgery, but 5% result in severely damaged kidneys that must be removed.

Renal injury may be discovered during laparotomy for intra-abdominal injuries. Surgical management prolongs the time required for the laparotomy, but may preserve renal tissue. Immediate surgical management of more severe renal injuries slightly increases salvage of the kidney and markedly decreases morbidity. Fifteen percent of patients with major fractures of the pelvic ring have an associated injury to the bladder, most commonly anterior extraperitoneal disruption. Hematuria is usually present and the injury is diagnosed by means of a cystogram.

A urethral injury should be suspected in a trauma patient who is unable to void and who has hematuria or blood at the external meatus. A retrograde urethrogram should be performed. Catheterization is not advisable since it may convert a partial rupture to a complete one and cause infection. Urinary diversion through a suprapubic cystostomy tube is usually indicated before repair.

Skin Loss Therapy for patients with major burns has changed significantly during the past decade, resulting in improved survival, better function, and better cosmetic results. Major emphasis has been placed on early sequential (tangential or full-thickness) excision of all deep and partial-thickness burns as well as areas of full-thickness thermal injury. However, excision must be followed by wound closure to avoid infection and unacceptable scar formation. When conventional split-thickness skin grafting is not possible, these wounds can be covered with a biosynthetic skin substitute. A promising prototype is a biolayer artificial skin composed of a temporary Silastic epidermis and a porous, biodegradable dermis of fibrillar collagen. It provides a vapor barrier and prevents wound desiccation. A comparison of the clinical results with the artificial skin and with conventional wound closure using split-thickness skin grafting showed that the areas covered with artificial skin were rated equal or better by patients and physicians. No evidence of antibody production to the collagen was noted and a histologic review of the cutaneous biopsy specimens revealed near-normal dermal architecture.

Free-flap reconstruction after trauma minimizes the duration of hospitalization and the number of surgical procedures required to achieve soft-tissue coverage, thus accelerating the process of recovery and rehabilitation. Its advantages include closure of large wounds in a single procedure, enhanced rehabilitation through early range of motion, flap survival in avascular areas, and enhanced vascularity of the traumatized region (which may increase the potential for fracture healing). The best time to perform microvascular reconstruction of complex trauma is within the first 72 hours. When compared with reconstructions done three days to three months after injury, early reconstructive procedures significantly decreased flap failure, the incidence of infection, bone healing time, length of hospital stay, and number of operations. These findings were thought to result from removal of devitalized tissue and provision of a vascularized soft-tissue envelope before wound colonization. Flap coverage of a colonized wound is subject to invasive infection with additional soft-tissue loss.

Adult Respiratory Distress Syndrome

Lung parenchymal damage resulting from severe systemic insults by means of multiple chemical mediators has recently been called acute lung injury. Acute lung injury thus refers to a clinical spectrum ranging from mild disease (pulmonary edema) to severe illness (adult respiratory distress syndrome). The adult respiratory distress syndrome represents a final common designation of many different clinical states resulting from direct or indirect damage to the alveolar capillary membrane. Morphologically, the syndrome involves diffuse cellular damage to both the endothelium and the epithelium. Altered endothelial cell permeability is commonly the first identifiable abnormality and results in an increased movement of water and colloid into the lung interstitium. This movement commonly results in noncardiogenic edema.

Among the causes of direct damage are aspiration of gastric contents, drug injury, inhalation of toxic substances, smoke, and water (near-drowning), lung contusion, and pneumonia. Indirect causes include sepsis, trauma with severe shock, and multiple blood transfusions. Trauma and shock by themselves have not been demonstrated to cause adult respiratory distress syndrome if they are not accompanied by massive blood transfusion or severe tissue damage. These indirect causes of damage are thought to be mediated by cellular and/or humoral mechanisms. This results in injury to the capillary endothelium in the lungs. It has been suggested that complement-mediated pulmonary sequestration of neutrophils occurs and that the release of toxic substances from these cells results in the endothelial damage. Prolonged hypovolemia and reduced left ventricular performance have been found to have an additive affect on adult respiratory distress syndrome in trauma patients after hemorrhage. Low platelet counts and antiplasmin levels, as well as a tendency to decrease antithrombin III, fibrinogen, and plasminogen levels, appear to be somewhat predictive for the development of adult respiratory distress syndrome. Patients with adult respiratory distress syndrome also have significantly higher complement (C3a and C5a) values. The amount of complement activated in patients with incipient respiratory failure correlates with the severity of eventual pulmonary insult. Whatever the cause, adult respiratory distress syndrome increases intrapulmonary shunting and decreases pulmonary compliance and functional residual capacity.

Adult respiratory distress syndrome is readily identified by the following criteria: (1) Compatible clinical history and physical findings. The clinical pattern is that of a patient who develops difficulties in breathing after trauma or surgery. The patient is initially tachypneic and restless and, as the hypoxia increases, may become disoriented. If this condition is not treated, severe hypoxemia and death ensue. (2) Refractory hypoxemia (arterial Po_2 of less than 60 mm Hg at an Fio_2 of 0.5 or higher). Blood gas analysis, which is the best tool for the diagnosis and evaluation of adult respiratory distress syndrome, will demonstrate hypoxemia (decreased Pao_2) accompanied by hypocapnia (decreased $Paco_2$). This hypoxemia, which is caused by shunting, is refractory to oxygen enrichment by mask. (3) Markedly diminished pulmonary compliance. (4) A chest roentgenogram with diffuse bilateral parenchymal infiltrates. The chest roentgenogram may at first be normal but will later show the characteristic findings. Although the roentgenographic findings resemble those of cardiac pulmonary edema, this condition can be differentiated by the presence of a low pulmonary wedge pressure; therefore, the syndrome is also called low-pressure pulmonary edema.

A great deal of research has recently been devoted to the pathophysiology of adult respiratory distress syndrome. Two theories are currently favored: (1) the central nervous system derangement theory and (2) the cellular humoral theory. The first theory suggests that shock and sepsis cause microchanges in the hypothalamic adaptive centers of the brain, producing cell hypoxic damage with a secondary cybernetic derangement of the functional aspects of the stress-adaptation center. This may eventually lead to adult respiratory distress syndrome through overactivity of the stress mechanism. This theory is strengthened by the prophylactic effect of neurodepressant agents against adult respiratory distress syndrome in trauma models. The second theory focuses on the neutrophil mediators of tissue injury or, alternatively, on superoxide radicals, hydroxyl ions, lysosomal enzymes, and humoral factors such as histamine, serotonin, kinins, and prostaglandins thought to play a role in the pathogenesis of adult respiratory distress syndrome.

It is believed that adult respiratory distress syndrome is responsible for 75,000 deaths per year in the United States. In addition, it is estimated that 150,000 people per year have the disease and that the median cost of hospitalization for each patient is about $54,000. There is as yet no direct treatment for adult respiratory distress syndrome; there-

fore, therapy is aimed at treating the underlying disease and maintaining oxygenation so as to create the best conditions for the damaged lung to heal.

Because hypoxemia is the most dangerous alteration in adult respiratory distress syndrome, it must be corrected as quickly and vigorously as possible. Because this hypoxemia is refractory to oxygen administered by mask, artificial mechanical ventilation should be instituted, keeping the patient's Pao_2 above 60 mm Hg with the lowest possible Fio_2. These goals can seldom be achieved without applying positive end expiratory pressure (PEEP) therapy. The PEEP level at which a Pao_2 of 60 mm Hg is achieved with an Fio_2 of 0.4 or less corresponds to the classic "optimal" or "best" PEEP.

In some cases, very high PEEP (super-PEEP) must be applied to maintain a Pao_2 compatible with life. Patients with noncardiogenic edema usually show significant improvement in gas exchange with a PEEP of 5 to 15 cm H_2O. Others improve with a PEEP of 10 to 30 cm H_2O; most of these patients respond optimally with a PEEP between 10 and 20 cm H_2O. It is important to remember that most treated patients with adult respiratory distress syndrome do not die of hypoxemia but as a result of treatment complications or the primary disease. Most deaths are caused by sepsis, multisystem organ failure, or severe, irreversible cerebral damage.

Patients with adult respiratory distress syndrome should receive a sufficient caloric intake. Intensive nursing is needed to avoid bedsores and to prevent infections from indwelling catheters. General sepsis, and lung infection in particular, is a real hazard. Prophylactic antibiotic therapy has no place in the prevention of sepsis in patients with adult respiratory distress syndrome. Corticosteroids are at best controversial, and other drugs (such as neurodepressant agents, β-adrenergic blockers, prostacyclin, antiplatelet agents, serotonin antagonists, and specific inhibitors of prostaglandin and leukotriene biosynthesis) have yet to prove their value.

As in every disease, prevention is better than treatment. If shock and bleeding are dealt with in time, multiple blood transfusions and overhydration can be avoided, and adult respiratory distress syndrome can to some extent be prevented. It has recently been established that, in traumatized patients, early rigid fixation of long-bone fractures decreases the incidence of adult respiratory distress syndrome (Table 3). In a group of 132 patients with fractures of the long bones whose injury severity scores were 18 or more, a delay of more than 24 hours in fixation of femoral fractures was associated with a fivefold increase in adult respiratory distress syndrome. In the same study, it was

Table 3. Effect of early stabilization of femoral fractures

Data	Stabilization	
	Early	Late
No. of patients	45	37
Age (years)	27.9	29.4
Injury severity score*	31.0	31.3
Ventilation (days)	2.4	6.9
Intensive care unit (days)	2.7	7.6
Hospital stay (days)	17.5	26.6
Pulmonary complications	1 case (2.2%)	14 cases (37.8%)
Cost	$19,492	$32,915

*Described in Civil ID, Schwab CW: The abbreviated Injury Scale, 1985 revision: A condensed chart for clinical use. *J Trauma* 1988;28:87–90.

demonstrated that patients with injury severity scores above 20 who underwent early fracture fixation had an incidence of adult respiratory distress syndrome of 17%; that of patients who had late surgery was 75%. Additionally, early prophylactic mechanical ventilation for 24 hours can reduce the incidence of adult respiratory distress syndrome in patients with multiple trauma.

Fat Embolism

Fat embolism is a syndrome that usually occurs 24 to 72 hours after injury. It is fatal in 10% to 15% of cases. Its manifestations include fever, tachycardia, acute respiratory distress with tachypnea, arterial hypoxemia (decrease in Po_2), and low Pco_2. There are also mental manifestations, such as restlessness, incoherency, and confusion. Chest radiographic findings are identical to those seen in adult respiratory distress syndrome, with bilateral patchy infiltrations. Petechiae appear on the conjunctiva, the chest, and the anterior fold of the axilla. Blood tests show thrombocytopenia. Fat embolism is commonly associated with trauma, especially with long-bone fractures. It has also been described in severe trauma without bone involvement and after total hip replacement and, to a lesser extent, total knee replacement.

Many researchers have investigated the pathophysiology of fat embolism but it remains unclear. There are two theories. According to the embolization theory, fat from the bone marrow, after a fracture or installation of total hip stems, forces its way into the ruptured blood vessels (veins) and forms an embolism in the lung. There the fat globules are degraded by pneumocytes to free fatty acids, which are toxic to the lung parenchyma. This theory is supported by bone spicules and bone marrow elements sometimes found in the lung vessels at autopsy.

The second theory holds that the fat embolism is non-traumatic in origin. According to this theory, changes in the stability of chylomicra in the blood are caused by stress. This results in the release of free fatty acids that damage the lung parenchyma.

Treatment of fat embolism should be designed to avoid hypoxemia and should consist of the same measures used in adult respiratory distress syndrome, that is, oxygenation and artificial ventilation whenever necessary. PEEP should be used to reach a Pao_2 of 60 mm Hg. Aggressive chest physiotherapy helps prevent atelectasis and infection. The patient should be provided with a sufficient caloric intake. Bedsores should be avoided. A recent study showed that 9 mg/kg of methylprednisolone given to patients after trauma had a prophylactic effect against fat embolism. Only 2.5% of the treated group developed fat embolism compared with 28.8% of the untreated group.

Specific medications such as low molecular dextran, heparin, ethanol, and corticosteroids show no beneficial influence on the outcome and should not play a role in the treatment of fat embolism.

The most important step is prevention. It has been found that early stabilization of fractures can reduce the incidence of fat embolism in trauma. Once fat embolism has been diagnosed, guidelines for treatment are the same as those for adult respiratory distress syndrome.

Trends

Although regionalization and the other improvements in care delivery have reduced morbidity and mortality from trauma, the key to reducing the number of victims is trauma prevention: increased use of seat belts, control of alcohol-impaired drivers, and the regulation of the availability of handguns. Analysis of injuries sustained in relation to their average crash severity has shown that for frontal motor-vehicle impacts, seat belts have a major protective effect, dramatically reducing the incidence of serious and fatal injuries. There was an impressive reduction in the highway fatality rate from 3.34 to 2.59 per 100,000 vehicle miles traveled after the institution of a seat-belt law. However, even with these impressive figures, seat-belt use is only approximately 45%. Greater public awareness of the beneficial effect of seat belts must be created.

Prevention, however, is also applicable to trauma care, particularly in terms of the prevention of debilitating systemic consequences such as adult respiratory distress syndrome, pulmonary and organ failure, sepsis, and the like. Through a better understanding of the pathophysiology of trauma, we are slowly beginning to understand the cause of organ failure and death. What was perceived as isolated organ failure, such as adult respiratory distress syndrome, is now seen as part of a systemic response to injury and repair.

Early stabilization of musculoskeletal injury in the patient with multiple trauma has reduced pulmonary failure and adult respiratory distress syndrome. Although there appears to be a significant benefit in allowing the patient to be mobilized and to begin eating earlier, fracture stabilization also has a beneficial effect on the traumatic wound. Further research into wound management and regulation of wound mediators and their influence on the systemic effect of trauma is underway. Cyclo-oxygenase inhibitors, such as indomethacin, ibuprofen, and sulindac, have effectively treated hypoxia, interpulmonary shunting, pulmonary hypertension, and pulmonary vasoconstriction in an animal model of trauma. Through modification of mediators, such as leukotrienes, histamines, and oxygen free radicals, capillary leakage with pulmonary failure can be reduced. Improved understanding of granulocyte and macrophage production in the wound, the liver, and the lung will improve our ability to modify these mediators and alter the physiologic and metabolic response to trauma.

In conclusion, since the best "treatment" is prevention, trauma care for the next decade will be aimed at reducing the number of trauma victims, obtaining optimal care through regionalization of trauma centers, and managing injuries not only through surgery but through modification of the physiologic and metabolic responses to trauma.

Annotated Bibliography

Keywords

Abdominal injury; Adult respiratory distress syndrome; Arteriography; Computed tomography; Fat embolism; Head injury; Hemorrhage; Intravenous pyelogram; Peritoneal lavage; Polytrauma; Resuscitation; Shock; Thoracic injury

Baker SP: Injuries: The neglected epidemic. *J Trauma* 1987;27:343–348.
Injuries are the most serious but most preventable of all major health problems in the United States. More than 150,000 deaths result from trauma each year. Motor-vehicle accidents are the leading cause of death in persons 1 to 34 years old.

Resuscitation

Christensen KS: Pneumatic antishock garments (PASG): Do they precipitate lower-extremity compartment syndromes? *J Trauma* 1986;26:1102–1105.
Transcutaneous oxygen tension beneath a full-length pneumatic splint was measured in 12 normotensive subjects. The author concluded that Pneumatic Antishock Garment pressures of 30 mm Hg or more applied to a whole limb stop microcirculation and produce tissue anoxia.

Hervé C, Gaillard M, Huguenard P: Early medical care and mortality in polytrauma. *J Trauma* 1987;27:1279–1285.
The establishment of an emergency medical aid service that provided early care at accident sites substantially decreased cardiac arrests. Mortality from spinal, chest, abdominal, and pelvic trauma was also decreased.

Mattox KL, Bickell WH, Pepe PE, et al: Prospective randomized evaluation of antishock MAST in post-traumatic hypotension. *J Trauma* 1986;26:779–786.
A total of 352 hypotensive patients were randomly assigned to treatment groups with and without Military Anti-Shock Trousers. The authors found that the garment had no effect on survival, length of hospital stay, or hospital costs provided that the patient reached the hospital within 30 minutes.

Shackford SR, Hollingworth-Fridlund P, Cooper GF, et al: The effect of regionalization upon the quality of trauma care as assessed by concurrent audit before and after institution of a trauma system: A preliminary report. *J Trauma* 1986;26:812–820.
Institution of a regional trauma system decreased preventable deaths from 13.6% of all fatalities to 2.7% and significantly reduced delays and the incidence of inadequate care.

Shock

Fortune JB, Feustel PJ, Saifi J, et al: Influence of hematocrit on cardiopulmonary function after acute hemorrhage. *J Trauma* 1987;27:243–249.
A comparison of patients whose hematocrit levels were raised to 0.30 with patients whose hematocrit levels were raised to 0.40 showed that the higher value offered no advantage. Additionally, the higher value may increase intrapulmonary shunting, which can be detrimental.

Schwab CW, Shayne JP, Turner J: Immediate trauma resuscitation with type O uncrossmatched blood: A two-year prospective experience. *J Trauma* 1986;26:897–902.
The authors found that type O erythrocytes are safe to use for immediate trauma resuscitation and have several advantages over typed blood and type O whole blood. Among these are immediate availability, universal application, and elimination of the risk of transfusing "high-titer" plasma.

Traverso LW, Hollenbach SJ, Bolin RB, et al: Fluid resuscitation after an otherwise fatal hemorrhage: II. Colloid solutions. *J Trauma* 1986;26:176–182.
In a porcine model of hemorrhage, whole blood with compatible fresh-frozen plasma was superior to human serum albumin, normal saline, and untyped fresh-frozen plasma as a resuscitation agent.

Traverso LW, Lee WP, Langford MJ: Fluid resuscitation after an otherwise fatal hemorrhage: I. Crystalloid solutions. *J Trauma* 1986;26:168–175.
Using a swine model of hemorrhage, the authors compared the abilities of crystalloid solutions to prevent death after a hemorrhage that would otherwise have been fatal. Ringer's lactate had the highest survival rate (67%), followed by normal saline (50%), Plasmalyte-R (40%), and Plasmalyte-A (30%).

Diagnostic Techniques

Donohue JH, Federle MP, Griffiths BG, et al: Computed tomography in the diagnosis of blunt intestinal and mesenteric injuries. *J Trauma* 1987;27:11–17.
Twenty-four patients with computed tomographic signs of mesenteric or intestinal injuries were treated during a five-year period. Computed tomography appeared to have advantages over peritoneal lavage in the evaluation of bowel and mesenteric injuries and to distinguish injuries that required surgery from those that required only monitoring.

Fabian TC, Mangiante EC, White TJ, et al: A prospective study of 91 patients undergoing both computed tomography and peritoneal lavage following blunt abdominal trauma. *J Trauma* 1986;26:602–608.
On the basis of findings at laparotomy, computed tomography offered no diagnostic advantage over peritoneal lavage in blunt trauma but proved to be a reliable alternative when peritoneal lavage could not be performed. The sensitivity, specificity, and accuracy of computed tomography were 85%, 100%, and 79%, respectively. The corresponding figures for peritoneal lavage were 90%, 100%, and 98%.

Gomez GA, Alvarez R, Plasencia G, et al: Diagnostic peritoneal lavage in the management of blunt abdominal trauma: A reassessment. *J Trauma* 1987;27:1–5.
A prospective study undertaken to evaluate the diagnostic accuracy of peritoneal lavage demonstrated that 28 of 29 patients with positive findings had significant intra-abdominal injuries, confirming the accuracy of peritoneal lavage in blunt abdominal trauma.

Gomez GA, Kreis DJ Jr, Ratner L, et al: Suspected vascular trauma of the extremities: The role of arteriography in proximity injuries. *J Trauma* 1986;26:1005–1008.
A review of 72 patients who underwent arteriography because of penetrating proximity injuries showed no evidence of vascular trauma. No vascular injury was found in the one patient who underwent arteriography because of popliteal artery spasm. Thus, routine arteriography may be unnecessary in such cases. A 24-hour observation period may be a safe alternative.

Kisa E, Schenk WG III: Indications for emergency intravenous pyelography (IVP) in blunt abdominal trauma: A reappraisal. *J Trauma* 1986;26:1086–1089.
Emergency intravenous pyelography is useful in patients

with specific indications and gross hematuria but unnecessary in patients whose posttraumatic hematuria is detected only microscopically. Computed tomography appears to be more useful than intravenous pyelography for renal imaging in patients who have blunt abdominal trauma but who are in a stable condition.

Peitzman AB, Makaroun MS, Slasky BS, et al: Prospective study of computed tomography in initial management of blunt abdominal trauma. *J Trauma* 1986;26: 585–592.

In this prospective study, the indications for emergency computed tomography in blunt abdominal trauma were equivocal abdominal findings, closed head injury, spinal cord injury, hematuria, or pelvic fractures. Used in conjunction with close clinical monitoring, computed tomography reliably evaluated blunt abdominal trauma in this selected group of stable patients.

Treatment

Head Injuries

Baxt WG, Moody P: The impact of advanced prehospital emergency care on the mortality of severely brain-injured patients. *J Trauma* 1987;27:365–369.

The authors compared the mortality rates for two groups of patients with severe brain injuries who received advanced support before being transported to a trauma center. The 128 consecutive patients given land-based treatment had a mortality rate of 40% whereas the 104 consecutive patients given helicopter-based treatment had a mortality rate of 31%, confirming the importance of early transport to a trauma center.

Stone JL, Lowe RJ, Jonasson O, et al: Acute subdural hematoma: Direct admission to a trauma center yields improved results. *J Trauma* 1986;26:445–450.

Of 128 patients with acute subdural hematomas entering a hospital trauma unit, 82 were admitted directly and 46 were transferred from another hospital. The transferred patients had a mortality rate of 76% whereas that of the direct-admission patients was only 50%.

Thoracoabdominal Injuries

Fabian TC, Mangiante EC, Patterson CR, et al: Myocardial contusion in blunt trauma: Clinical characteristics, means of diagnosis, and implications for patient management. *J Trauma* 1988;28:50–57.

Myocardial contusion is probable when the MB isoenzyme of creatine phosphokinase is 5% or less of the total creatine phosphokinase and an abnormal electrocardiogram at admission becomes normal before the patient is discharged. In 37 patients with positive findings, surgical procedures requiring general anesthesia produced no cases of significant arrhythmia.

Flancbaum L, Wright J, Siegel JH: Emergency surgery in patients with post-traumatic myocardial contusion. *J Trauma* 1986;26:795–803.

Myocardial contusion was diagnosed in 19 patients with major blunt thoracic trauma on the basis of clinical findings, serial electrocardiograms, and determinations of the MB isoenzyme of creatine phosphokinase. All 19 required surgery for associated injuries. Eleven required perioperative inotropic cardiac support but there were no related deaths. Thus, emergency surgery can be performed in such patients as long as careful hemodynamic monitoring is maintained.

Hanna SS, Gorman PR, Harrison AW, et al: Blunt liver trauma at Sunnybrook Medical Centre. *J Trauma* 1987; 27:965–969.

Patients with liver injuries constituted 11% of all patients admitted to this medical center. The mortality rate was 6%. Only minor surgery was required in 62%.

Morgan AS, Flancbaum L, Esposito T, et al: Blunt injury to the diaphragm: An analysis of 44 patients. *J Trauma* 1986;26:565–568.

Of 44 patients with blunt abdominal trauma that resulted in a ruptured diaphragm, 93% received the correct diagnosis within six hours of admission. The most useful diagnostic aids were the admission chest radiograph, peritoneal lavage, upper gastrointestinal tract contrast studies, and computed tomography.

Mucha P Jr, Daly RC, Farnell MB: Selective management of blunt splenic trauma. *J Trauma* 1986;26:970–979.

After an eight-year study of patients with blunt splenic trauma, the following criteria were established for nonsurgical management: (1) absolute hemodynamic stability; (2) minimal or no perioneal findings; and (3) a transfusion requirement for splenic injury of no more than 2 units.

Genitourinary Injuries

Barbagli G, Selli C, Stomaci N, et al: Urethral trauma: Radiological aspects and treatment options. *J Trauma* 1987;27:256–261.

A retrograde urethrogram should be performed whenever urethral injury is suspected. This applies to all trauma patients who are unable to void, who have hematuria, or who have blood at the external meatus. An excretory urethrogram is advisable in all cases of pelvic trauma to evaluate the upper urinary tract and to define exactly any bladder tears or pelvic hematomas that may be present.

Skin Injuries

Gerding RL, Imbembo AL, Fratianne RB: Biosynthetic skin substitute vs. 1% silver sulfadiazine for treatment of inpatient partial-thickness thermal burns. *J Trauma* 1988;28:1265–1269.

A biosynthetic skin substitute significantly decreased the time to healing and the pain of superficial or moderately deep partial-thickness burns when compared with 1% silver sulfadiazine cream. It also reduced nursing time and cost.

Godina M: Early microsurgical reconstruction of complex trauma of the extremities. *Plast Reconstr Surg* 1986; 78:285–292.

After reviewing 532 patients who underwent microsurgical reconstruction after trauma to the lower extremities, the author found that results were best in patients treated by free flap transfers within 72 hours of injury.

Adult Respiratory Distress Syndrome

Alberts KA, Norén I, Rubin M, et al: Respiratory distress following major trauma: Predictive value of blood coagulations tests. *Acta Orthop Scand* 1986;57:158–162.

The most sensitive indicator of adult respiratory distress syndrome in trauma patients is the platelet count; tentative laboratory values are suggested to indicate risk levels for developing adult respiratory distress syndrome.

Bone L, Bucholz R: The management of fractures in the patient with multiple trauma. *J Bone Joint Surg* 1986; 68A:945–949.

A review of the evaluation, resuscitation, and early management of multiple trauma including fractures.

Bone LB, Johnson KD, Weigelt J, et al: Early versus delayed stabilization of femoral fractures: A prospective randomized study. *J Bone Joint Surg* 1989;71A:336–340.

This study of the effect of early stabilization on pulmonary failure included 177 patients. Early stabilization (within 24 hours) significantly decreased the incidences of adult respiratory distress syndrome, pulmonary dysfunction, fat embolism syndrome, pulmonary emboli, and pneumonia. These developed in only 2.2% of the early-treated group compared with 38% of the group whose fractures were stabilized more than 48 hours after injury. Thus, there is no doubt that early management of long-bone fractures is beneficial to patients with multiple injuries.

Carroll GC, Tuman KJ, Braverman B, et al: Minimal positive end-expiratory pressure (PEEP) may be "best PEEP." *Chest* 1988;93:1020–1025.
Using lower PEEP may improve the 20% rate of pneumothorax and 27% mortality in ventilated patients with adult respiratory distress syndrome.

de Oliveira GG, Shimano LT, de Oliveira Antonio MP: Acute respiratory distress syndrome (ARDS): The prophylactic effect of neurodepressant agents. *J Trauma* 1986;26:451–457.
Neurodepressant agents such as morphine, pentobarbital sodium, diazepam, and others were found to prevent adult respiratory distress syndrome in rats sustaining central and peripheral trauma.

Herala M, Gislason T: Chest physiotherapy: Evaluation by transcutaneous blood gas monitoring. *Chest* 1988;93:880–802.
Chest physiotherapy, either thoracic compression or positive expiratory pressure, may improve blood gases.

Julien M, Lemoyne B, Denis R, et al: Mortality and morbidity related to severe intrapulmonary shunting in multiple trauma patients. *J Trauma* 1987;27:970–973.
In patients with multiple trauma, death is seldom related to respiratory failure itself. Severe hypoxemic respiratory failure in trauma patients usually results from a combination of causes.

Loder TT: Pediatric polytrauma: Orthopaedic care and hospital course. *J Orthop Trauma* 1987;1:48–54.
This study included 78 children who had sustained one major musculoskeletal injury and at least one other major injury. Early osteosynthesis shortened the time of the hospital stay, the time spent in intensive care, and the time ventilatory support was needed. Early surgical stabilization also produced fewer complications.

Norwood SH, Civetta JM: The adult respiratory syndrome. *Surg Gynecol Obstet* 1985;161:497–508.
An up-to-date review of adult respiratory distress syndrome, with 116 references.

Pretorius JP, Schlag G, Redl H, et al: The "lung in shock" as a result of hypovolemic-traumatic shock in baboons. *J Trauma* 1987;27:1344–1353.
Hypovolemic traumatic shock produced morphologic evidence of endothelial and interstitial edema associated with a significant increase in lung water. Other striking histologic findings included significant cellular infiltration of lung tissue, especially by leukocytes showing evidence of deep granulation.

Slotman GJ, Burchard KW, D'Abrezzo A, et al: Keto-

conazole prevents acute respiratory failure in critically ill surgical patients. *J Trauma* 1988;28:648–654.
The incidence of adult respiratory distress syndrome was decreased in patients receiving ketoconazole compared with placebo (6% vs 31%), as was the median intensive-care stay and cost.

Fat Embolism

Hulman G: Pathogenesis of non-traumatic fat embolism. *Lancet* 1988;1:1366–1367.
Nontraumatic explanation of the pathophysiology of fat emulsion.

Kallenbach J, Lewis M, Zaltzman M, et al: "Low-dose" corticosteroid prophylaxis against fat embolism. *J Trauma* 1987;27:1173–1176.
Methylprednisolone in relatively low doses protects against fat embolism and pulmonary dysfunction after skeletal trauma. The safety of this therapy requires further evaluation.

Johnson KD, Cadambi A, Seibert GB: Incidence of adult respiratory distress syndrome in patients with multiple musculoskeletal injuries: Effect of early operative stabilization of fractures. *J Trauma* 1985;24:375–384.
A significant reduction in the incidences of fat embolism and adult respiratory distress syndrome was found in trauma patients when stabilization of fractured bone was achieved within the first 24 hours.

Schnaid E, Lamprey JM, Viljoen MJ, et al: The early biochemical and hormonal profile of patients with long bone fractures at risk of fat embolism syndrome. *J Trauma* 1987;27:309–311.
Mobilized free fatty acids from peripheral adipose tissue are not important in the genesis of fat embolism.

ten Duis HJ, Nijsten MWN, Klausen HJ, et al: Fat embolism in patients with an isolated fracture of the femoral shaft. *J Trauma* 1988;28:383–390.
A series of 172 patients with isolated fractures of the femoral shaft was divided into two groups: decompressed (open fractures, surgically treated) and nondecompressed (conservatively treated fractures). In the second group, the incidence of fat embolism was 3.5% compared with 0% in the first group.

Trends

Petrucelli E: Seat belt laws: The New York experience—preliminary data and some observations. *J Trauma* 1987;27:706–710.
Preliminary data showed that seat-belt use reduced fatalities and serious injuries. The mortality rate declined 7.5% compared with the previous year and 16.9% compared with the average for the previous five years. The frequency of insurance claims for injuries also decreased 5%.

Steinberg S, Dehring D, Martin D, et al: Amelioration of pulmonary pathophysiology of adult respiratory distress syndrome by sulindac, a cyclo-oxygenase inhibitor. *J Trauma* 1987;27:1323–1331.
In a bacteremic porcine model of acute respiratory failure produced by *Pseudomonas aeruginosa*, a cyclo-oxygenase inhibitor reversed the pulmonary hypertension and hypoxia, increased intrapulmonary shunting, and prevented systemic hypotension.

8
Soft-Tissue Trauma

The musculoskeletal soft tissues include muscles, tendons, ligaments, and their connections. In the last several years, much has been learned about their injury and repair and, it is hoped, ongoing clinical and basic science studies will continue to add to our knowledge.

Muscle

Fiber Types

Muscle fiber types are genetically determined. Maintenance of muscle fiber types appears to depend on the specificity of innervation. Muscle fibers are divided into five types or categories: types I, IIA, IIB, IIC, and IIM. Type I is a slow-twitch fiber with low glycogen content and low concentration of glycolytic enzymes. It has high concentrations of mitochondria and associated oxidative phosphorylation enzymes. Type I fibers also have a high myoglobin content. These fibers specialize in high-repetition and low-load endurance activities.

Type IIA and type IIB fibers are found in fast-twitch oxidative muscle. They differ from each other in that type IIA fibers have a higher concentration of oxidative enzymes. In addition, types IIA and IIB fibers have genetically distinct myosin heavy chains, indicating that their proteins are derived from different gene loci. Type IIC fibers contain both these myosin heavy chains. Type IIM fibers, the fastest-contracting fibers, have a third genetically distinctive myosin heavy-chain protein. Type II muscles are generally involved in power and speed activities.

Response to Training

Skeletal muscles increase their functional capability in direct response to overloading. Type I muscle fibers require endurance training, that is, high-repetition and low-load tension activity for a minimum of 30 to 60 minutes. Endurance training enhances the muscle's oxidative capacity. Other general effects of endurance training include an increased oxidative capacity in type II fibers. Capillary density increases in muscle exposed to endurance training.

Type II muscle fibers adapt rapidly to resistance training programs. Unless loads are progressively increased, the adaptation of muscle fibers to strength training reaches a plateau. The effects of training on muscle are rapidly reversible once specific resistance demands are no longer placed on the muscle fibers, and the fibers atrophy.

Some studies have evaluated multiple cycles of eccentric contractions within the normal motion range of animal muscles. These studies mimic the clinical syndrome of exercise-induced muscle soreness (muscle pain 12 to 48 hours after heavy exercise, usually with a high component of eccentric exercise). Research has shown that transient muscle weakness and damage accompany exercise-induced

muscle soreness. Recently, excellent experimental studies have added to our understanding. Histologic evidence of muscle injury was present in more than one third of muscle fibers after a controlled series of eccentric contractions in rabbit muscles. Maximum isometric force production was reduced to less than 25% of normal three days after the eccentric contractions. Compared with eccentric contractions, isometric and concentric (shortening) contractions caused relatively minor fiber changes. It has also been shown that the extent of the injury was proportional to the peak force developed during the contractions.

Clinical studies have focused attention on changes in muscle after high-tension eccentric exercises. Muscle fibers of runners were damaged after marathon races. The ultrastructural changes were consistent with cell damage and an inflammatory response. High-intensity exercises, such as sprinting, also had significant effects on muscle. Many changes were apparent in ultrastructural studies, although changes were less evident on light microscopy. The changes were diffuse and occurred along the length of the muscle. It is important to note that eccentric exercises are not necessarily harmful to muscle in the long-term despite the structural and functional short-term changes. Muscle tissue is obviously highly stressed during high-intensity or long-duration exercises and these changes may be part of the normal injury-repair cycle. In general, clinical experience documents long-term improvement in muscle capacity in response to appropriate exercise. These diffuse changes do not necessarily indicate a clinical muscle injury or "strain."

Hypertrophy Muscle hypertrophy represents a type II fiber response secondary to high-tension and low-frequency loading of muscle. To obtain the maximal benefit from strength training, type II muscle needs 48 hours to recover from exposure to a high-tension workload. Muscle hypertrophy represents primarily an increase in the cross-sectional area of individual muscle cells. This is secondary to an increase in the number of myofibrils per fiber in each muscle cell. Type II muscle fibers tend to increase in volume and size to a much greater degree than type I endurance muscle fibers. Strength training does little to increase capillary density or blood flow to muscles. Strength training also does little to increase oxidative capacity. A controversial area is the possibility that high-intensity, high-tension muscle training causes fiber hyperplasia. There is some indication that fiber hyperplasia may occur, but this certainly makes no more than a minimal contribution to the overall hypertrophy.

Indirect Injury (Strain)

Clinical muscle strains account for the largest number of injuries reported in most epidemiologic studies of sports injuries. Most muscle strains are considered to be partial disruptions of the muscle-tendon unit in response to powerful eccentric contractions. Our basic understanding of these injuries is limited. New imaging techniques such as computed tomography and magnetic resonance imaging are able to localize some significant muscle strains (for example, hamstring injuries). The radiographic appearance of these acute injuries usually consists of an inflammatory reaction within the involved muscle, usually near the myotendinous junction.

In one experimental study, rabbit muscles were stretched into the plastic region of the load-deformation curve. The muscle fibers were disrupted near the myotendinous junction. An intense inflammatory reaction followed, with subsequent fibrosis near the myotendinous junction (Figs. 1 and 2). Active muscle force production fell initially but recovered to near-normal within one week.

In other biomechanical studies, muscles were stretched to failure and relaxed muscle, tetanically stimulated muscle, and submaximally stimulated muscle were compared. The presence of muscle activation did not change the length at which muscle failed. There was a small (15%) increase in force at failure. The most significant difference was the energy absorption before failure. Muscle activation and active force production allow the muscle to absorb twice as much energy as relaxed muscle with no change in length to failure and only a small change in force at failure (Fig. 3).

These data help explain several common clinical per-

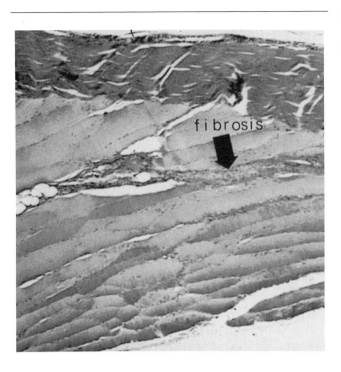

Figure 2

This histologic section of a specimen similar to that in Figure 1 shows the histology of injured muscle seven days after a strain injury. The edema, hemorrhage, and inflammatory reaction have improved and there is a marked amount of fibrosis localized to the injury site. (Reproduced with permission from Nikolaou PK, Macdonald BL, Glisson RR, et al: Biomechanical and histological evaluation of muscle after controlled strain injury. *Am J Sports Med* 1987;15:9–14.)

ceptions regarding muscle injuries. It is thought that muscle weakness and fatigue predispose muscle to injury. Weakness and fatigue are characterized by diminished active force in muscle and, therefore, should result in less energy absorption before failure. Most injuries occur in muscles that are actively decelerating or controlling joint motion by absorbing energy. A muscle can absorb more energy if it has higher active force production while it is being stretched. More active force production allows for a given amount of energy to be absorbed with less stretch. When energy is absorbed through eccentric muscular contraction, less change in length or deformation is necessary.

Injury Prevention There are many unanswered questions about the prevention of muscle injury. One common practice is the use of a "warm-up" period for the working muscles. Clinical studies have indicated performance improves after such warm-ups, but no studies are available that document an influence on injury rate. Animal studies, however, have demonstrated that an isometric warm-up period may offer some benefits. A single maximal isometric contraction in several rabbit muscles led to alterations in the characteristics of the muscles when they were strained to failure; greater lengths and higher forces were present in muscles that underwent a single maximal contraction lasting ten to 15 seconds.

Repair After a severe injury, muscle repair requires the intricate interplay of two distinct cell types. These are the

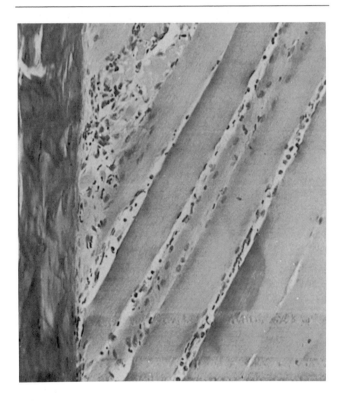

Figure 1

Appearance of injured rabbit skeletal muscle 48 hours after a strain injury with partial disruption of some of the muscle fibers near the myotendinous junction. This section near the myotendinous junction shows an intense inflammatory reaction with cell necrosis, edema, and inflammatory cells. (Reproduced with permission from Nikolaou PK, Macdonald BL, Glisson RR, et al: Biomechanical and histological evaluation of muscle after controlled strain injury. *Am J Sports Med* 1987;15:9–14.)

muscle cell itself and the connective tissue fibroblasts surrounding each individual muscle cell. Connective tissue cells come from a mesenchymal cell lineage. These mesenchymal cells are known to be pleuripotential and can form bone, cartilage, ligament, tendon, and other connective tissues under specific environmental conditions. Many of these conditions have not yet been elucidated.

The ultrastructural sequence of muscle degeneration after an ischemic episode shows early damage to muscle membrane and loss of sarcomeres and Z-bands. There is mitochondrial swelling and nuclear pyknosis. After these early changes, phagocytic cells (macrophages) penetrate the basal lamina of the muscle cells and phagocytize the necrotic muscle fibers. The presence of these phagocytic cells depends on an intact circulation in the damaged muscle tissue. The next cells to enter the muscle cell are the myoblasts, primitive muscle cells that appear within the remaining cell membrane to form a new myotube containing muscle fibers. When the central myoblastic cells migrate to the periphery of the newly formed muscle fiber, regeneration has been completed (Fig. 4).

The type of muscle fiber formed during regeneration is determined by the remaining innervation in the injured muscle tissue. Type II or fast-twitch muscle regeneration occurs in tissues innervated by muscles with type II motor nerves. Similarly, type I slow-twitch fiber regeneration depends on type I motor nerve fibers. Muscle that is reinnervated after nerve injury takes on the fiber type characteristics determined by the innervation entering the regenerated muscle tissue.

The mesenchymal cells form the extracellular matrix that surrounds each myofiber, and they also form the basement membrane around each muscle cell. Failure of muscle to regenerate after injury is primarily associated with overgrowth of fibrous connective tissue. This occurs at the damage site and prevents further regeneration and reformation of muscle tubules.

Effects of Immobilization

The effects of immobilization are many and involve changes in cartilage, tendon, the myotendinous junction, ligament, and bone. These changes are primarily those of deterioration and include changes in tissue morphology, biochemistry, and biomechanics. In soft tissues, the result is to increase joint stiffness and contracture. Long-term immobilization in a flexed or extended position causes a readjustment in sarcomere number. Sarcomeres are added or deleted until sarcomere length accommodates muscle length in the position of immobilization. The addition or loss of sarcomeres occurs primarily at the myotendinous junction. A similar mechanism of sarcomere growth may occur with increased length of muscle as it is stretched by growing bones. In animal studies, immobilization accelerated the production of granulation tissue in injured muscle. Continuing this immobilization for more than five days produced a contracting scar. Poor structural reorganization of muscle and scarring occurred after this critical period of immobilization.

An important factor in determining strength of the myotendinous junction is the position of the immobilized limb. With the limb in a lengthened position, both active and passive components of muscle tension are reorganized. Reorganization of connective tissue components of muscle to accommodate the lengthened or shortened muscle also

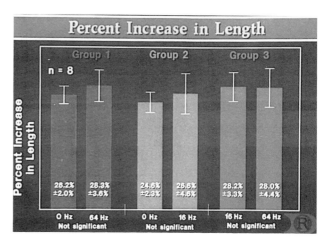

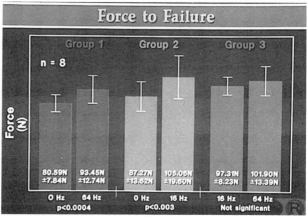

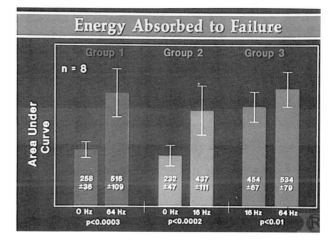

Figure 3

Changes in muscle stretched to failure with and without activation. **Top**, There is no significant change in length. **Center**, Maximal force is slightly increased at the point of failure. **Bottom**, Fully activated muscle absorbs twice as much energy as relaxed muscle when strained to failure, pointing to the important role of muscle as an energy absorber. (Reproduced with permission from Garrett WE Jr, Safran MR, Seaber AV, et al: Biomechanical comparison of stimulated and nonstimulated skeletal muscle pulled to failure. *Am J Sports Med* 1987;15:448–454.)

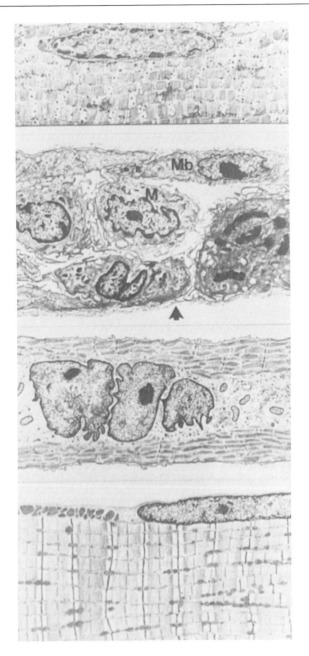

Figure 4

Sequential changes in muscle after ischemic damage. **Top,** Early ischemic changes in muscle cell represented by pyknotic degeneration of the nucleus. The contractile fibrils show disorganization. Mitochondrial swelling is evident. **Top center,** Invasion of the macrophages (M) in the active stages of phagocytizing and removing degenerate muscle fibers. Primitive myoblasts (Mb) are seen on the periphery of the regenerating muscle cell membrane. This cell will eventually participate in the regeneration of the muscle cell fibers. **Bottom center,** Newly forming myotube in a centrally located multinucleated cell. On the periphery are newly formed contractile filaments. **Bottom,** Reformed muscle fiber with the nucleus taking a peripheral position adjacent to the basilar membrane. Regeneration is essentially completed. (Reproduced with permission from Caplan A, Carlson B, Faulkner J, et al: Skeletal muscle, in Woo SL-Y, Buckwalter JA (eds): *Injury and Repair of the Musculoskeletal Soft Tissues.* Park Ridge, American Academy of Orthopaedic Surgeons, 1988, pp 213–291.)

occurs. There is probably less susceptibility to reinjury if muscle fibers heal in a lengthened position.

If a limb is positioned in a shortened attitude, less force is needed to injure the muscle. Rabbit limbs held in a shortened position required less force before tearing than did nonimmobilized contralateral control muscles. It was noted in this study that muscles immobilized in a lengthened position required more tensile force to tear. Of interest is the finding of spontaneous muscle hypertrophy when muscles are immobilized in the lengthened position.

Effects of Electrical Stimulation

There are also effects of trauma on muscle that are separate from the effects of immobilization. Sensory receptors and pain receptors may be a source of muscle inhibition. In many cases, the maximal force exhibited with muscle testing after joint injury or surgery is less related to inherent muscle strength than to the ability of the nervous system to control the muscle and to recruit all the muscle fibers effectively. For instance, after arthroscopic knee surgery there is a pronounced reduction in tested maximal muscle force that persists for days. It is unlikely that disuse atrophy in the muscle can account for this weakness. It has been demonstrated that the injection of saline into normal knee joints to simulate an effusion results in a reproducible decrease in the ability of the quadriceps to produce force. These changes are thought to be secondary to nociceptors and other sensory receptors about the joint.

Long-term electrical stimulation increases the capillary supply in immobilized muscle. In one study, transcutaneous electrical stimulation was applied to the triceps surae in human subjects for 21 days. One group received stimulation at 50 Hz and the other at 2 kHz. At the end of the study, both groups had increases in capillary number and capillary density, a decreased intercapillary distance, and an increase in the ratio of capillaries to muscle fibers. Other studies have demonstrated that electrical stimulation increases muscle weight, fiber diameter, and ratio changes in fiber type in the immobilized limb. Artificial stimulation of muscle, however, does not develop muscle function as well as conventional isotonic contractions.

Thus, there may be two very different effects on the muscle associated with immobilization and injury: an effect caused by immobilization or disuse and an effect caused by altered nervous system recruitment. These two effects may be relatively independent. For example, it has been shown that immobilization of normal limbs in animals does not block recruitment and the electromyographic pattern is normal in immobilized muscles.

Compartment Syndromes

Acute There remains great interest in defining the threshold of muscle and limb injury in the presence of increased compartment pressures. Many investigators believe that absolute measurements of compartment pressures are less reliable than the relative values of intracompartmental pressures and perfusion pressures. Diastolic and mean arterial pressures have been used as an indirect measure of perfusion pressure. A pressure difference of less than 30 mm Hg between the compartment pressure and the mean arterial pressure was associated with the inability of muscle to maintain a normal metabolic state (Fig. 5). After moderate trauma to muscle, a larger pressure differential (at

ANALYSIS OF pH vs. TIME

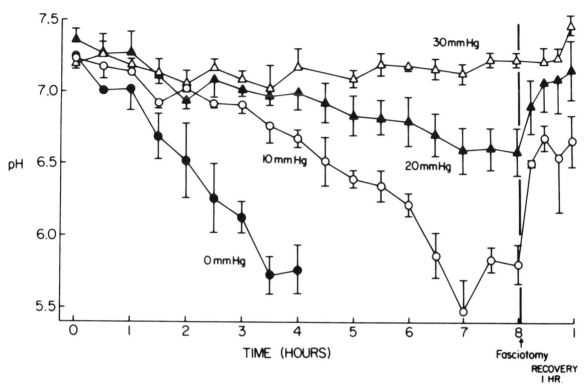

Figure 5

The mean intracellular pH is plotted as a function of time in groups with differences between mean arterial blood pressure and the compartment pressure. It is clear that with a pressure differential of 30 mm Hg, there is little effect on intracellular pH. The effect increases as the pressure differential is smaller. (Reproduced with permission from Heppenstall RB, Sapega AA, Scott R, et al: The compartment syndrome: An experimental and clinical study of muscular energy metabolism using phosphorus nuclear magnetic resonance spectroscopy. *Clin Orthop* 1988;226:138–155.)

least 40 mm Hg) was required to maintain normal muscle metabolism.

Ischemia and increased pressures combined produced more severe muscle damage than ischemia alone. These data indicate the importance of factors other than ischemia in producing muscle injury. Both blunt muscle damage and increased compartment pressures must be considered in the treatment of trauma to muscle in enclosed compartments. Decision-making concerning surgical decompression in acute compartment syndromes would be much easier if absolute pressure thresholds were established. Although intracompartmental pressures of 30 to 45 mm Hg are often mentioned as a threshold, it is apparent that other factors must be considered. Ischemia, muscle damage from blunt trauma, and the diastolic or mean arterial pressure are also important considerations.

Exertional The painful condition in some muscle compartments after exercise may be associated with increased intracompartmental pressures and, therefore, has been considered analogous to the acute compartment syndrome. It is not at all clear whether there are similar metabolic changes and potential catastrophic results in exertional compartment syndromes. The diagnosis and treatment of this disorder are matters of current debate.

The diagnosis of exertional compartment syndrome has been based on various pressure criteria. Increased pressures before, during, and after exercise have all been pro-

posed. Of patients examined because of a possible diagnosis of chronic compartment syndrome, only 25% met appropriate criteria for the condition. Among other diagnoses, periostitis, superficial peroneal nerve compression, medial tibial syndrome, and muscle hernias have been prominent. It is important to realize that leg pain after exercise is not uncommon and increased compartment pressures are not always the cause of this pain.

Studies have shown that pressures may be increased in each of the compartments in the leg. In addition, the deep posterior compartment may actually have a separate fascial covering for the tibialis posterior muscle. The anterior compartment is most frequently involved and the deep posterior compartment and the lateral compartment are less frequently involved. The superficial posterior compartment is least often involved. A fascial defect and an associated muscle hernia or superficial peroneal nerve entrapment have been reported to be a part of the complex of chronic compartment syndromes. The fascial defect may be present in as many as 40% of patients with this condition and occurs anteriorly over the distal compartment where a branch of the superficial peroneal nerve penetrates the fascia.

Correct treatment of exercise-related compartment syndrome requires an accurate diagnosis based on objective pressure measurements. When conservative measures fail and activity modification is inadequate, surgical fasciotomy of the involved compartments is generally successful

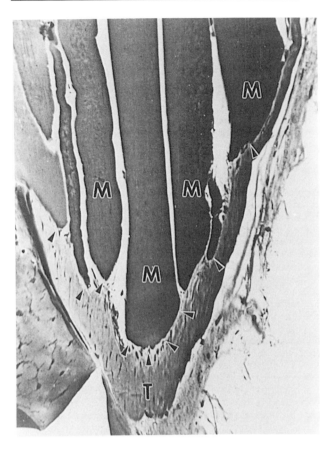

Figure 6

Myotendinous junction in a section of frog semitendinosus showing insertion of the muscle cells (M) into the tendon (T). (Reproduced with permission from Garrett W Jr, Tidball J: Myotendinous junction: Structure, function, and failure, in Woo SL-Y, Buckwalter JA (eds): *Injury and Repair of the Musculoskeletal Soft Tissues.* Park Ridge, American Academy of Orthopaedic Surgeons, 1988, pp 171–207.)

in returning the athletes to their desired activity level. The success rate is lower when the deep posterior compartment is involved than when the anterior compartment is involved. Complete surgical release of the posterior compartment fascia and the fascial covering of the tibialis posterior is required. In addition, the nerve must be decompressed at the site of any fascial hernia. Fascial defects should never be repaired because an acute compartment syndrome may develop, leading to catastrophic consequences.

The pressure increases usually cause enough pain to stop exercise, thus returning the pressure measurements to normal. It has been shown that muscle blood flow decreases with exercise in patients with chronic compartment syndrome. This decrease in flow is associated with an increase in the intramuscular pressure during relaxation of the muscle. Intramuscular pressures increase with muscle contraction and reduce blood flow; most perfusion occurs when the muscle is relaxed. Increased relaxation pressures could certainly diminish blood flow to the muscle at the time when it usually receives most of its perfusion. In one group of patients, fasciotomy resulted in symptomatic relief and normalization of relaxation pressures.

Myositis Ossificans

Ectopic ossification occurs in many locations; when this happens in a muscle, the process is termed myositis ossificans. In an acutely injured muscle, this process causes intense pain, swelling, and, sometimes, erythema. Traumatic myositis ossificans is self-limiting and is treated by rest and protection of the extremity. The usefulness of adjunctive administration of nonsteroidal agents to retard bone formation has been reported after total hip replacement. Radiation therapy has also been found to be effective after acetabular fracture and total hip replacement.

The Myotendinous Junction

The myotendinous junction is the microscopic and ultrastructural connection of muscle fiber to tendon. It is also the biomechanical region in which contractile forces produced by the muscle are transmitted to the tendon and subsequently to its bony attachment.

Electron microscopic visualization of this morphologic region has shown the myotendinous junctional region to be a highly specialized area. The muscle cell is extensively involuted and folded at the myotendinous junction to give maximal surface area for attachment. This allows for greater fixation and transmission of forces (Fig. 6).

There may be additional specialization of the myotendinous junctional architecture according to muscle function. This is exemplified by muscles specializing in static contraction compared with those involved in fast or repetitive movements. Interestingly, the sarcomeres directly adjacent to the myotendinous junction of fast-contracting muscles are shortened in length. This may represent an adaptation of the muscle cell to decrease the intensity of forces generated directly adjacent to this junctional area.

Specific linking proteins are found at the myotendinous junctions. These include actinin, vinculin, and talin. Preliminary studies suggest that these linking proteins are associated with the various fiber types.

A complex intracellular and extracellular transmitting membrane consisting of a glycoprotein has been found at this junctional region. This protein, call vetronectin, links the contractile intracelluar proteins to the extracellular protein connective tissue.

It is becoming evident from animal and clinical studies that the major site of injury in so-called "muscle strains" and complete muscle tears or disruption is the myotendinous junction. Even so-called mid-belly muscle strains still represent myotendinous junctional injuries occurring in central muscle myotendinous attachments (Fig. 7).

Tendon

New information regarding injury to tendon comes primarily from research into flexor and extensor tendons of the hand. Much less information is available about larger tendons such as the Achilles tendon or the rotator cuff although these tendons also have much clinical significance. Tendons transmit the forces and motions generated by muscles to their attachments on bone. Their ability to withstand stress and their ability to move are both important, sometimes leading to contradictory requirements in the treatment of tendon injuries.

Research models for tendon injury usually involve digital flexor tendons, which are lacerated and then surgically repaired. The initial repair response involves the tendon and most of the surrounding structures. When a tendon is immobilized, the tendon healing is a part of the overall scar formation involving all the surrounding structures. Granulation tissue unites the tendon with the other injured structures. This allows healing and recovery of tensile strength but can obviously compromise the motion requirements of tendon. Early motion allows a reparative response from the tendon apart from the overall scar formation. This may allow motion but may sacrifice tensile strength.

The early cellular response when healing occurs in mobilized tendons comes primarily from fibroblasts from the epitenon. Proliferating cells from the epitenon bridge the external gap and fill in the gap between the lacerated ends. Macrophages follow the fibroblasts and healing and remodeling occur. When the synovial sheath is injured and the tendon is immobilized after repair, fibroblasts from the tendon sheath are prominent and result in adhesions between the tendon and the fibrous sheath. These adhesions must be broken or they will limit motion.

New studies are adding further support to the concept that tendons have the ability to repair themselves. Tendon healing can occur in vitro in tissue culture. Epitenon cells proliferate two days after injury and produce collagen after four days. Cells from the endotenon become active but only after a two- to three-week delay. Canine studies have also demonstrated that, when early protected motion was allowed, healing occurred primarily from the epitenon layer without the adhesions seen in immobilized tendons. Studies have also shown that limited early mobilization resulted in higher tensile strength in the repaired tendons. Of course, there remains the problem of exactly how much motion and force the repair can be subjected to before failure.

Repair of tendon lacerations requires a source of cellular nutrition. Diffusion is as effective or more effective than perfusion in the supply of nutrients to tendons. Tendon healing can proceed in avascular areas of tendon via diffusion. Obliteration of the blood supply to avian tendons does not alter the synthesis of collagen in the healing response. This raises the question of whether nutrient diffusion during healing might proceed better if the flexor sheath was intact. Tendons can obtain nourishment from extracellular tissue fluid as well as from synovial fluid.

An experimental study in primates investigated collagen production in profundus tendons in zone II lacerations after repair with and without sheath closure. No beneficial effect of sheath closure was apparent after three and seven days, suggesting that healing may not benefit from sheath repair. In a prospective clinical trial evaluating healing with and without sheath repair in zone II flexor tendon repairs, there were no significant differences in the total active motion in the proximal and distal interphalangeal joints.

Most studies have emphasized tendon production of collagen and mucopolysaccharidase. Other molecules are being investigated in the tendon. For example, the production of fibronectin has been investigated. This molecule is important in the attachment of cells to their substrate. Fibronectin can be found on the external surface of tendons. It appears that this molecule is involved in the attachment of synovial cells to the tendon surface. This molecule may be important in the binding of cells to the tendon

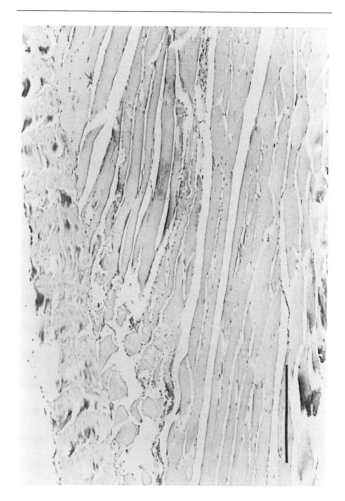

Figure 7

Partial tear of the muscle at its insertion at the myotendinous junction. This acute tear shows some hemorrhage and leukocyte infiltration at the junction. (Reproduced with permission from Garrett W Jr, Tidball J: Myotendinous junction: Structure, function, and failure, in Woo SL-Y, Buckwalter JA (eds): *Injury and Repair of the Musculoskeletal Soft Tissues*. Park Ridge, American Academy of Orthopaedic Surgeons, 1988, pp 171–207.)

surface to avoid detachment with motion. Fibronectin is also present at the surface of fibrocytes in the tendon interior.

Ligament

The basic processes involved in ligament injury and repair have received significant experimental attention in recent years. Most studies have involved the ligaments of the knee because of their clinical significance.

The Effect of Repair

The medial collateral ligament has received a great deal of attention in clinical and laboratory studies. Isolated injuries to the medial collateral ligament in canine and rat models recover well without surgery; in fact, results in surgically treated groups were not as good as results obtained without surgery or immobilization (Fig. 8). The secondary restraints, especially the anterior cruciate ligament, were

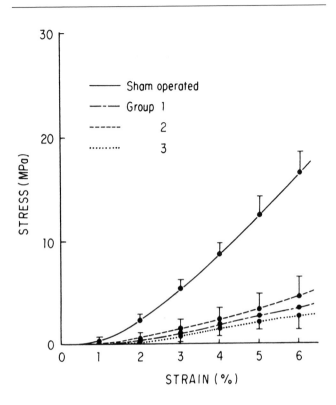

Figure 8

The stress-strain relationship for healing canine medial collateral ligaments. Group 1 had no surgical repair and immobilization. Group 2 had surgical repair with three weeks of immobilization and group 3 had surgical repair with six weeks of immobilization. It can be seen that group 1 ligaments are stiffer than those in the other two groups. (Reproduced with permission from Woo SL-Y, Gomez MA, Inoue M, et al: New experimental procedures to evaluate the biomechanical properties of healing canine medial collateral ligaments. *J Orthop Res* 1987;5:425–432.)

sufficient to retain knee stability and to allow healing with unrestricted knee motion. When the secondary restraints were injured, the medial collateral ligament recovery was not as successful. In any tissue injury, the recovering ligament must be protected from reinjury while healing. In the knee, the secondary restraints help protect the medial ligament.

The Effect of Stress and Strain

Ligament repair progresses more rapidly and to a better recovery if the repair is subjected to controlled stresses and strains during the healing process. A number of studies have demonstrated the beneficial effect of stress and strain on the actual recovery of the injured ligaments. It was once thought that early motion might benefit the articular cartilage, bone strength, muscle function, and other factors but that it would compromise the actual repair of the injured ligament. At present, the bulk of the evidence indicates that the ligament repair itself benefits from early exposures to stress and strain. These data require careful balancing by the clinician. Obviously, a healing ligament needs some protection. At present there is much interest in determining how aggressive rehabilitation should be to obtain quicker and better healing without a high risk of reinjury to the repaired or reconstructed ligament.

The effects of immobilization without injury have been studied recently with regard to ligament biomechanics. Immobilization significantly decreased the strength and energy-absorbing capacity of rabbit bone-ligament-bone preparations. The effect was most obvious at the ligament-bone junction (Fig. 9). A period of immobilization led to an increased likelihood that failure in response to strain would occur at the junction. Histologically, there was increased osteoclastic activity at the junctional region of bone. Stress deprivation decreased strength in the ligament and in the junction. The effects were more pronounced at the junction, however, with functional failure becoming more likely with increased immobilization. This effect is reversible. After immobilization the junction regains its strength, although relatively slowly. Studies have shown that four to 12 months of recovery may be needed before the junction recovers its normal biomechanical characteristics. The age of the animal was also important. In immature animals, failure occurred preferentially at the bone-ligament junction. After epiphyseal closure in rabbits, the site of injury shifted from the junction to the ligament substance. Aging led to increased strength of the ligament substance and the junction. Near the time of epiphyseal closure, junction strength exceeded that of the ligament substance. The strengths of both then leveled off soon after skeletal maturity was reached.

Activity level and exercise have been shown to be important in ligament and junction biomechanics. Exercise has significant effects on the strength of bone-ligament-bone preparations. Ultrastructurally, these changes correlate with differences in the collagen fibrils. Rats subjected to intensive training demonstrated a decrease in the size of collagen fibrils and an increase in the number of fibrils. These changes were associated with little change in the tensile strength of the ligaments; however, the exercised ligaments were less stiff than controls.

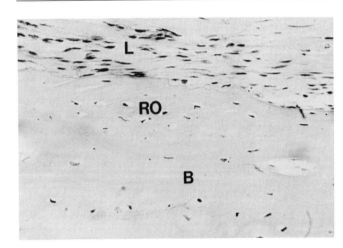

Figure 9

The tibial insertion of the medial collateral ligament of a rabbit after 12 weeks of immobilization and nine weeks of remobilization. Previously resorbed bone has been reossified (RO) and has established continuity with the deeper ligament fibrils (L), overlying more mature bone (B). (Reproduced with permission from Woo SL-Y, Gomez MA, Sites TJ, et al: The biomechanical and morphological changes in the medial collateral ligament of the rabbit after immobilization and remobilization. *J Bone Joint Surg* 1987;69A:1200–1211.)

The Biochemistry of Repair

After injury a ligament undergoes a reparative process similar to those of other healing tisues. The initial clot with fibrin causes the associated blood-borne cells and tissue cells to secrete a number of active substances leading to inflammation. Capillary permeability and increased cellularity are the result of substances such as serotonin, histamine, and prostaglandins. Growth factors must also play a role in the stimulation and chemotaxis of the incoming cells. Collagen synthesis and degradation proceed simultaneously. Throughout the repair process there is increased tissue water or edema. Collagen content increases throughout early healing. The initial collagen is type III, although later the composition changes to predominantly type I collagen. Collagen concentration is low even though the absolute amount is high because of the increased volume and edema. Glycosaminoglycans also increase early. With remodeling and maturation, the contents return toward normal.

Ligaments have the ability to contract or to "tighten up." This factor has been observed clinically for years and there are new experimental data supporting this impression. Rat medial collateral ligaments were Z-lengthened and were able to contract to normal tightness in three weeks. There was an associated increase in the amount of actin as measured by immunofluorescent staining. Actin is the same contractile protein found in the thin filaments of muscle sarcomeres and in the cytoplasm of mobile cells. It is interesting to consider that the repairing tissue has the ability to contract by a mechanism involving proteins and mechanisms similar to those in the contractile process of muscle.

Sensory Functions

Ligament injury has many documented effects on the stability of joints. Recently, more attention has been focused on the possibility that ligaments provide sensory data to the nervous system and may have a significant functional role in the detection of motion and pressure. Human anterior cruciate ligaments contain three morphologic types of mechanoreceptors and free nerve endings (Fig. 10). Ligament and joint capsule receptors have been shown to have significant reflex actions in animals, particularly in the cat. Joint motion leads to afferent signals from the receptors with a corresponding reflex muscular effect. The absence of sensory input can impair motor function in a manner separate from the effect on joint stability.

There are facts that make this concept more interesting. Data have shown that the loads transmitted within the ligament were quite small with most activities and certainly much smaller than the ultimate tensile load. It may be that joint geometry and muscular control are more important than previously believed and ligament restraints may be less important. There is much current interest in

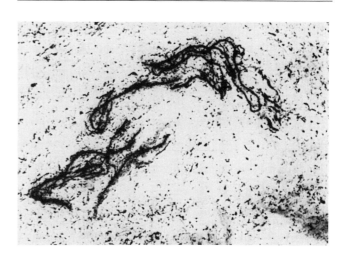

Figure 10

Light micrograph showing a free nerve ending in the anterior cruciate ligament. (Reproduced with permission from Schutte MJ, Dabezies EJ, Zimny ML, et al: Neural anatomy of the human anterior cruciate ligament. *J Bone Joint Surg* 1987;69A:243–247.)

the importance of mechanoreceptors in ligaments. Present surgical treatment is based on restoring gross stability. It may be that procedures or rehabilitation protocols should be developed that are better able to improve proprioception or other sensory data.

Trends

New imaging techniques such as magnetic resonance imaging, computed tomography, and diagnostic ultrasound are being used in the evaluation of soft-tissue injuries. This trend is likely to continue for soft-tissue injuries around joints and to expand for soft-tissue injuries that involve direct or indirect muscle injuries.

Treatment regimens are undergoing evaluation. Rest and immobilization are being emphasized less and early, controlled return to activity is being stressed. In addition, more functional and objective techniques are being applied to recovery and rehabilitation. For example, objective testing of lower-limb functions such as strength, power, and endurance are being used to assess recovery.

Research efforts continue to define the effect of immobilization vs controlled mobilization on healing of soft tissues, especially ligament and tendon. Research is defining the nature and causes of delayed muscle soreness. Laboratory models of acute strains are helping to define factors, such as stretching, strengthening, and temperature, that may protect muscle from injury.

Annotated Bibliography

Keywords

Compartment syndrome; Electrical stimulation; Ligament; Muscle; Myositis ossificans; Myotendinous junction; Tendon

Muscle

Fiber Types

Caplan A, Carlson B, Faulkner J, et al: Skeletal muscle, in Woo SL-Y, Buckwalter JA (eds): *Injury and Repair of the Musculoskeletal Soft Tissues.* Park Ridge, American Academy of Orthopaedic Surgeons, 1988, pp 213–291.

This is the definitive review of the nature of muscle injury and repair, summarizing current knowledge of muscle types and regeneration.

Response to Training

Armstrong RB: Muscle damage and endurance events. *Sports Med* 1986;3:370–381.

This comprehensive review article discusses the relationship between eccentric contractions and damage to muscle.

Indirect Injury (Strain)

Garrett WE Jr, Nikolaou PK, Ribbeck BM, et al: The effect of muscle architecture on the biomechanical failure properties of skeletal muscle under passive extension. *Am J Sports Med* 1988;16:7–12.

This study demonstrated the mechanism of failure of muscle in response to passive stretch. Failure occurred routinely near the myotendinous junction.

Garrett WE Jr, Safran MR, Seaber AV, et al: Biomechanical comparison of stimulated and nonstimulated skeletal muscle pulled to failure. *Am J Sports Med* 1987;15:448–454.

Rabbit hindlimb muscles were strained to failure while the motor nerve was maximally stimulated to provide a model of eccentric contraction. The muscle did not tear at a significantly different length; its maximal force was slightly increased, but the energy absorbed before failure was much higher in contracting muscles than in passively stretched muscle.

Nikolaou PK, Macdonald BL, Glisson RR, et al: Biomechanical and histological evaluation of muscle after controlled strain injury. *Am J Sports Med* 1987;15:9–14.

Rabbit muscles were stretched to a point of nondisruptive tissue injury and the clinical recovery was monitored. Histologic changes showed an intense early inflammatory reaction followed by progressive fibrosis at the region of the distal myotendinous junction. Active force generation recovered after approximately one week.

Effects of Immobilization

Arvidsson I, Eriksson E, Knutsson E, et al: Reduction of pain inhibition on voluntary muscle activation by epidural analgesia. *Orthopedics* 1986;9:1415–1419.

This study demonstrates that failure to achieve muscle force in the postoperative or postinjury period is highly correlated with pain or reflex inhibition. Epidural analgesia was effective in allowing quadriceps muscle activity as measured by integrated electromyographic studies.

Booth FW: Physiologic and biochemical effects of immobilization on muscle. *Clin Orthop* 1987;219:15–20.

There are profound changes in muscle strength and in muscle fatigability after immobilization. The course is reviewed along with ideas to prevent these changes.

Jokl P, Konstadt S: The effects of limb immobilization on muscle function and protein composition. *Clin Orthop* 1983;174:222–229.

This article reviews the effects of the position in which muscle is immobilized on disuse atrophy. Loss of muscle strength and atrophy were lessened in limbs immobilized with the muscles in a stretched position.

Lehto M, Duance VC, Restall D: Collagen and fibronectin in a healing skeletal muscle injury: An immunohistological study of the effects of physical activity on the repair of injured gastrocnemius muscle in the rat. *J Bone Joint Surg* 1985;67B:820–828.

This study reviewed the properties of a healing injury in rat muscle with specific emphasis on how immobilization affects granulation tissue and scar production.

Effects of Electrical Stimulation

Cabric M, Appell HJ, Resic A: Stereological analysis of capillaries in electrostimulated human muscles. *Int J Sports Med* 1987;8:327–330.

The effects of two different electrical stimulation protocols (50 Hz or 2 kHz, each for 21 days) were investigated by means of biopsy specimens taken before and after the study.

Compartment Syndromes

Fronek J, Mubarak SJ, Hargens AR, et al: Management of chronic exertional anterior compartment syndrome of the lower extremity. *Clin Orthop* 1987;220:221–227.

Intramuscular pressures of 10 mm Hg or more at rest and/or 25 mm Hg or more five minutes after exercise were defined as abnormally increased in 18 patients with chronic compartment syndrome. Fasciotomy or reduction of exertional activities was found to be an effective treatment.

Heppenstall RB, Sapega AA, Scott R, et al: The compartment syndrome: An experimental and clinical study of muscular energy metabolism using phosphorus nuclear magnetic resonance spectroscopy. *Clin Orthop* 1988;226:138–155.

Experimental ischemic compartment syndrome was studied in dogs using nuclear magnetic resonance spectroscopy. The injury threshold was defined in terms of a pressure difference between the mean arterial blood pressure and the compartment pressure.

Rorabeck CH, Fowler PJ, Nott L: The results of faciotomy in the management of chronic exertional compartment syndrome. *Am J Sports Med* 1988;16:224–227.

Fasciotomy of the anterior compartment gave excellent relief of pain in 22 of 25 patients who had resting pressures in excess of 15 mm Hg and increased pressures after exercise with delayed normalization.

Styf J: Diagnosis of exercise-induced pain in the anterior aspect of the lower leg. *Am J Sports Med* 1988;16:165–169.

Chronic compartment syndrome was found to be an uncommon cause of chronic exercise-induced pain in the anterior compartment of the lower leg in a series of 98 patients.

Myositis Ossificans

Bosse MJ, Poka A, Reinert CM, et al: Heterotopic ossification as a complication of acetabular fracture: Prophylaxis with low-dose irradiation. *J Bone Joint Surg* 1988; 70A:1231–1237.

A retrospective review of 37 patients was performed to evaluate the effect of postoperative low-dose irradiation. Most of the patients received 10 Gy beginning on postoperative day 3. The incidence of heterotopic ossification was lower in irradiated limbs. In addition, severe heterotopic ossification was also diminished by irradiation.

Schmidt SA, Kjaersgaard-Andersen P, Pedersen NW, et al: The use of indomethacin to prevent the formation of heterotopic bone after total hip replacement: A randomized, double-blind clinical trial. *J Bone Joint Surg* 1988; 70A:834–838.

A clinical trial involving 201 patients was performed to demonstrate the effect of indomethacin on the prevention of heterotopic bone after total hip replacement. Fewer patients who had received indomethacin developed heterotopic bone.

The Myotendinous Junction

Chammout MO, Skinner HB: The clinical anatomy of injured muscle bellies. *J Trauma* 1986;26:549–552.

The authors discuss the site of muscle injury and optimal surgical repair.

Tendon

Banes AJ, Link GW, Bevin AG, et al: Tendon synovial cells secrete fibronectin in vivo and in vitro. *J Orthop Res* 1988;6:73–82.

Secretion of fibronectin in tendon synovial cells was examined in this study. The external surface of flexor tendons was stained with antibody to fibronectin. The authors postulate that fibronectin at the tendon surface may play a role in cell attachment to prevent cell removal by the friction of gliding.

Garner WL, McDonald JA, Kuhn C III, et al: Autono-

mous healing of chicken flexor tendons in vitro. *J Hand Surg* 1988;13A:697–700.

Chicken flexor tendon healing was studied with monoclonal antibodies to type I procollagen. This antibody specifically stained cells secreting collagen. It was shown that tendons have the ability to heal in vitro. Initial healing comes from epitenon cells that give the tendon the capacity for autonomous repair.

Kain CC, Russell JE, Burri R, et al: The effect of vascularization on avian flexor tendon repair: A biochemical study. *Clin Orthop* 1988;233:295–303.

Avian flexor tendon repair was evaluated with and without the blood supply present. It was demonstrated that the absence of a vascular supply did not alter the collagen synthetic activity of the healing flexor tendon. These results support the concept of intrinsic repair capability of tendon.

Peterson WW, Manske PR, Lesker PA: The effect of flexor sheath integrity on nutrient uptake by primate flexor tendons. *J Hand Surg* 1986;11A:413–416.

The healing of tendons with and without a flexor sheath was examined by monitoring the uptake of labeled proline by profundus tendons in zone II in primates. It was found that the uptake of labeled proline was not improved with sheath closure, implying that extracellular tissue fluid was capable of providing nutrients to the tendon in amounts equal to the synovial fluid.

Ligament

Woo SL-Y, Gomez MA, Inoue M, et al: New experimental procedures to evaluate the biomechanical properties of healing canine medial collateral ligaments. *J Orthop Res* 1987;5:425–432.

Canine medial collateral ligaments were transected and treated by no surgical repair with immobilization or surgical repair with varying times of immobilization. It was found that varus-valgus laxity was increased for all experimental knees, but that early immobilization enhanced joint stability.

9

Perioperative Considerations

Advances in orthopaedic surgery and in the treatment of trauma during the last decade have enabled older and more severely traumatized patients to undergo longer and more sophisticated operations. To avoid postoperative complications and ensure successful recovery, greater attention must be paid to perioperative considerations and special care taken in preparing patients for surgery.

Nutritional Support

General Considerations

The presence and prevalence of malnutrition in hospitalized patients has been extensively documented in the past decade. In a survey that utilized anthropometric measurements as well as weight loss and serum albumin levels, approximately 50% of patients in the surgical ward of a major general urban hospital were found to be moderately to severely malnourished. Despite these disturbing figures, not all clinicians approve of the institution of preoperative total parenteral nutrition in malnourished surgical patients.

Of course, there are differences between elective surgery and emergency procedures. In an emergency, the exigencies of the situation must have priority. Conversely, present evidence suggests that elective procedures be postponed until the patient's nutritional condition is satisfactory.

The relationship between abnormalities in various objective measures of nutritional status and postoperative morbidity and mortality is well established. In recent years, investigators have reported relationships among weight loss, serum levels of albumin, prealbumin, and protein total iron-binding capacity, skin test anergy, lymphocyte count, triceps skinfold, and increased rates of postoperative complications. Although these predictive indexes have effectively identified patients at risk, their validity as quantitive measures of nutritional deficit has yet to be established in clinical practice. Taken individually, probably no one of these parameters can be designated as the "prognostic nutritional marker" per se. Anergy is not always attributable to malnutrition, as a variety of nonnutritional factors can produce an anergic state. Significant trauma can lead to the production of serum inhibitors and the development of abnormalities of neutrophil function. There is little doubt, however, that modification of these variables as a group toward the lower range of normal adversely affects surgical outcome. Among the postoperative complications affected by the patient's nutritional status are wound dehiscence and infection, penumonia, and generalized sepsis.

Metabolic Effects of Stress

Injured, traumatized, and infected patients and those who have undergone surgery are hypermetabolic, hypercata-

bolic, and glucose- and insulin-resistant. Such patients oxidize less carbohydrate and more fat than normal and gluconeogenesis continues despite high exogenous carbohydrate intake. Norepinephrine concentrations are high, indicating increased sympathetic activity, as are concentrations of glucagon and cortisol. Nitrogen excretion is more than twice normal and can reach 600 mg/kg/day. Because of these metabolic changes, stressed patients require an increased flow of nutrients, which must be obtained from body stores. It has been suggested that protein breakdown in the muscles of these patients increases to supply this greater need for energy. However, even when stress is severe, endogenous protein accounts for less than 25% of total energy requirements.

The metabolic key during stress is apparently the maintenance of hyperglycemia, even in the absence of exogenous carbohydrate intake. It is the brain's oxidation of large amounts of glucose, far more than the glucose requirement of wounds, that determines the amount of muscle protein that must be catabolized for gluconeogenic purposes in the stressed paient.

Nutritional Requirements

For previously well-nourished patients who have suffered injury or burns, who have undergone elective surgery, or those with sepsis, the goal of nutritional therapy is to prevent or minimize loss of lean body mass. Since nitrogen losses can reach levels of 15 to 40 g/day in severely stressed patients, full enteral or parenteral nutrition should be provided for patients who are not expected to return to adequate oral intake within a few days. Approximately 200 mg/kg/day of nitrogen should be provided. Equal amounts of fat and carbohydrate should constitute the nonprotein energy sources. When the patient becomes less hypermetabolic and hypercatabolic, both energy and nitrogen intakes can be increased to make up for previous losses.

A particularly difficult problem is posed by severely stressed patients who are also malnourished. Nutritional support must be instituted with the hope of minimizing losses rather than achieving equilibrium or repletion, at least at the beginning of treatment.

Although the need to maintain nutritional integrity in the severely traumatized patient is widely accepted, debate persists over the appropriate method of nutritional support and its timing. A number of investigations have demonstrated that function in the small bowel returns to normal within a few hours after surgery. In contrast, stomach and colonic function returns one to two days and three to five days postoperatively, respectively. The earlier return of small-bowel function allows very early tube enteral feeding with elemental formulas.

Early postoperative jejunostomy feeding is a safe and efficacious choice for the patient with multiple trauma who undergoes laparotomy. Patients likely to need nutritional support for more than ten days should have feeding jejunostomy tubes placed at the time of laparotomy. The elemental diet can begin between six and 18 hours postoperatively. The initial amount can be increased to 12,600 kj with 20 g of nitrogen within 72 hours. Clinical experience has demonstrated the feasibility of immediate postoperative enteral feeding after major abdominal trauma and suggests that this early nutrition reduces septic complications in the critically ill patient. This decrease in septic complications appears to be a result of a reduction in jejunal mucosal atrophy when the gut is fed. In animal models, a lack of enteral nutrition for only 24 hours can result in a 50% reduction in the jejunal mucosal mass. This loss can be prevented by immediate enteral feeding. If the gut is not fed, mucosal atrophy will occur and gut endotoxins are able to enter the systemic system, accentuating the systemic septic state.

Pulmonary Function

Both thoracic and abdominal surgical incisions are associated with marked postoperative decreases in lung compartment volumes, with changes most evident in forced vital capacity (FVC) and functional residual capacity (FRC). After upper abdominal surgery, FVC may decline to 40% of its preoperative value on the day after surgery, returning to baseline during the next ten to 14 days. FRC may decline to 60% of preoperative value, with gradual restoration to baseline by the seventh postoperative day. The decline in FRC is especially important because the resulting atelectasis produces physiologic shunting and associated declines in oxygenation.

This decline in postoperative pulmonary function is only one of several risk factors for the development of postoperative pulmonary complications. Other clinical features that increase the patient's risk include obesity, advanced age, the type of anesthesia (general vs spinal), the duration of surgery, baseline pulmonary dysfunction, and, in high-risk patients, the lack of preoperative pulmonary treatment.

In evaluating and treating trauma, early attention should be given to the basic principles of resuscitation, that is, airway, ventilatory, and respiratory function. The patient with an inadequate airway is a common problem in trauma and requires immediate attention. In such patients, treatment can be complicated by major facial injuries that produce edema and bloody secretions in the oropharynx or by spinal cord injury that limits ability to manipulate the head and neck, adding to the problem of airway access. Therefore, when a compromised airway is suspected, it is wise to intervene early and establish an artificial airway before significant cardiovascular instability ensues. Radiographs of the chest should always be done to exclude pneumothorax and atelectasis. Both these complications can jeopardize respiratory status, especially in the severely injured.

Ensuring ventilatory and respiratory function requires an assessment of mechanical and alveolar ventilation and oxygenation status. Spirometric measurements of the patient's ventilatory pattern provide a quantitative assessment of the energy expenditure related to the mechanical work of breathing. In cooperative patients, FVC gives some indication of mechanical ventilatory reserve. The presence

of diaphragmatic breathing, use of accessory muscles, forced exhalation, and discoordinate breathing pattern or paradoxic chest-wall movement must be documented and correlated with the other injuries. Assessing the adequacy of alveolar (effective) ventilation requires that a Pco_2 value be obtained from arterial blood gas analysis. The status of alveolar ventilation is of major importance in patients with head injuries because hypercapnia increases cerebral blood flow, increasing intracranial pressure. The patient's oxygenation status requires an assessment of arterial Po_2 and oxygen content. These primarily reflect hemoglobin content and Fio_2. It is then possible to correlate changes in arterial oxygen tensions with the patient's clinical status.

Thromboembolism

Venous thromboembolism remains a major cause of morbidity and mortality after lower-extremity orthopaedic surgery in the adult. Patients undergoing hip surgery have the highest risk: according to the NIH Consensus Conference (1986), without anticoagulation therapy as many as 70% will display deep venous thrombosis by radiographic criteria and as many as 20% will develop clinically significant pulmonary embolism with a mortality of 1% to 3%. Patients undergoing knee surgery are at significant risk as well: without anticoagulation therapy as many as 80% will display deep venous thrombosis by radiographic criteria and pulmonary embolism will develop in approximately 8% of cases. Fatal pulmonary embolism is less frequent after knee surgery, occurring in less than 1% of these patients.

Obesity, malignancy, older age, pregnancy, and oral contraceptive use all increase the risk of thrombosis. Patients with rheumatoid arthritis are at risk as well, although the incidence following hip surgery may be somewhat lower than in patients with osteoarthritis. Of patients with "idiopathic" pulmonary embolism or deep venous thrombosis (no apparent precipitating event), one third may have defective fibrinolysis or an identifiable disorder in the regulation of the coagulation cascade: deficiency of protein C or protein S (regulators of factors Va and VIIIa and stimulators of fibrinolysis), or antithrombin III (the major inhibitor of thrombin).

Deep Venous Thrombosis

Deep venous thrombosis can occur without any clinical symptoms or signs. In addition, the classic findings of pain, swelling, tenderness, discomfort with passive dorsiflexion of the ankle (Homan's sign), or palpable cord in the thigh or calf are not specific for deep venous thrombosis. Therefore, clinical suspicion of deep venous thrombosis should prompt definitive radiologic evaluation.

Radiocontrast Venography The diagnostic standard for the localization and characterization of deep venous thrombosis in the calf and thigh continues to be radiocontrast venography. Visualization of clots in the iliac veins is less helpful, with accuracy decreasing to approximately 70%. Venography has certain drawbacks. Radiologists occasionally disagree about the interpretation of a venogram. Also, about 5% of patients are not suitable candidates for venography because of lack of venous access or other technical problems. Venography is often uncomfortable for the patient, and clots are induced by the contrast material in approximately 1% of cases. An allergic reaction occurs in 0.02% of cases.

Radioactive Fibrinogen Radioactive fibrinogen (labeled with iodine 125) has been shown to be highly accurate in detecting thrombosis in the calf after total hip replacement. However, the technique has significant drawbacks. Because of the presence of fibrin, the scan is positive in any area close to the site of surgery or trauma and is not, therefore, usful for detecting deep venous thrombosis in the thigh after hip surgery or in the calf after knee surgery. Secondly, because this test uses a product of human serum, concerns exist regarding the potential transmission of viral disease.

Impedance Plethysmography This technique assesses venous hemodynamics in the limb by detecting a gradient in venous flow secondary to occlusion of a major extremity vein. Although impedance plethysmography has been shown to be useful in detecting thigh clots after hip surgery, a significant percentage of clots may be missed with this method, especially in orthopaedic surgery. In a prospective study of patients undergoing elective hip surgery, impedance plethysmography detected only 30% of the large thigh thrombi demonstrated by routine venography. The sensitivity of impedance plethysmography is further reduced in the smaller thrombi in the thigh and calf by the correspondingly small gradient in venous flow. This method also failed to detect iliac thrombi.

Ultrasonography A recent advance in noninvasive testing for proximal deep venous thrombosis is the detection of lack of venous compressibility by high-resolution B-mode ultrasonography. In seven recent trials, compression ultrasonography demonstrated a sensitivity of 90% to 100% and a specificity of 97% to 100% in diagnosing deep venous thrombosis proximal to the trifurcation. The reported accuracy in deep venous thrombosis of the calf was significantly less, approximately 40%. The test has the advantage of being painless, repeatable, and relatively easy and quick to perform.

Prophylaxis Against Deep Venous Thrombosis

The most important reason for preventing deep venous thrombosis is the prevention of potentially life-threatening pulmonary emboli. (A secondary consideration is the prevention of chronic venous insufficiency.) Although patients undergoing hip surgery are more likely to have high-risk thigh thrombi than patients undergoing knee surgery (approximately 80% of clots after hip surgery are above the knee), thrombi isolated to the calf present significant risk for embolization as well. Of patients with isolated calf-vein thrombosis, 20% to 33% demonstrate high-probability changes on ventilation-perfusion scanning, compared with 50% to 55% of patients with proximal venous thrombi.

Various agents have been used to prevent deep venous thrombosis after lower-extremity surgery. These rely on the pharmacologic inducement of a relative state of anticoagulation, the mechanical prevention (for example, by intermittent pneumatic compression) of venous stasis, or both. One mechanical means, continuous passive motion, has not been shown to affect the incidence of calf-vein thrombosis after total knee replacement. In one prospective trial of patients undergoing total knee arthroplasty, the incidence of calf-vein thrombosis was about 40% and the incidence of proximal thrombosis was 5% whether continuous passive motion was administered or not.

Heparin Heparin inhibits thrombosis by enhancing the action of antithrombin III to inhibit factor Xa and thrombin (Fig. 1). Less heparin is required to neutralize factor Xa (and thus prevent thrombin formation) than to neutralize the thrombin produced once the thrombotic process is under way. This is the rationale for the prophylactic antithrombotic regimens in which heparin is administered subcutaneously in very low doses. Although the efficacy of fixed low dosages (such as 500 units subcutaneously twice or three times daily) has been shown in thoracic, abdominal, and pelvic surgery, adjusted dosages providing a higher level of anticoagulation are required for adequate prophylaxis after lower-extremity surgery. After total hip replacement, heparin in adjusted dosages (activated partial thromboplastin time, 31 to 35 seconds) reduced the incidence of deep venous thrombosis threefold compared with fixed low dosages (P < .01). Also, heparin in adjusted dosages was not associated with a higher risk of perioperative blood loss than heparin in fixed low dosages.

The overall incidence of postoperative wound hematoma or remote bleeding with heparin is approximately 8%. In the case of severe hemorrhage, reversal can be achieved by slow infusion of protamine sulfate. Because heparin acts as a circulating inhibitor of the coagulation pathway, transfusions of fresh-frozen plasma or whole blood may not effectively restore coagulation. Paradoxically, conventional heparin preparations have the potential to stimulate platelet aggregation and are associated with a small (usually clinically unimportant) decrease in the platelet count in 30% of cases. More significant heparin-associated thrombocytopenia and arterial thrombosis are extremely rare complications. Treatment consists of stopping the heparin and substituting intravenous dextran or oral warfarin, and, if necessary, surgical removal of the thrombus.

The combination of a venous vasoconstrictor, dihydroergotamine, and fixed low dosages of heparin was shown to reduce the risk of deep venous thrombosis after hip surgery by 50% compared with fixed low dosages of heparin alone. Dihydroergotamine is not currently available for clinical use.

Warfarin An alternative to heparin is anticoagulation with warfarin. Warfarin acts by inhibiting the production of the vitamin K-dependent clotting factors: II, VII, IX, and X (Fig. 2). Factor VII has the shortest half-life, and is the first to be affected by warfarin therapy. The prothrombin time, primarily an assay of the integrity of the extrinsic clotting pathway, is directly prolonged by factor VII depletion and is affected in the early stages of warfarin therapy, before the common clotting pathway is inhibited. Thus, the clinician must be aware that warfarin therapy creates a "window" of vulnerability during the first three to five days, when the prothrombin time may be prolonged but no true anticoagulation exists. Oral warfarin is rapidly absorbed from the alimentary tract and is almost entirely bound to albumin in plasma. It is metabolized in the hepatic microsomes. The presence of one of the various agents that potentiate or antagonize warfarin activity must be suspected whenever oral anticoagulation is difficult to control (Outline 1).

Of all the alternatives available, anticoagulation therapy

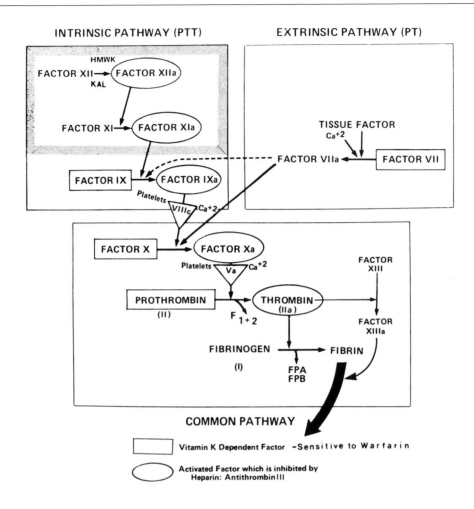

INTRINSIC PATHWAY (PTT)

EXTRINSIC PATHWAY (PT)

COMMON PATHWAY

Vitamin K Dependent Factor -Sensitive to Warfarin

Activated Factor which is inhibited by
Heparin: Antithrombin III

Figure 1

The coagulation pathways. Important features include the contact activation phase, vitamin K-dependent factors (affected by warfarin), and the activated serine proteases that are inhibited by heparin-antithrombin III. Prothrombin time measures the function of the extrinsic and common pathways; the partial thromboplastin time measures the function of the intrinsic and common pathways. (Reprinted with permission from Stead RB: Regulation of hemostasis, in Goldhaber SZ (ed): *Pulmonary Embolism and Deep Venous Thromboembolism*. Philadelphia, WB Saunders, 1985, p 32.)

with warfarin has the best documented efficacy. Five randomized, prospective trials have demonstrated that warfarin decreases the incidence of deep venous thrombosis by twofold to fourfold while decreasing the incidence of fatal pulmonary embolism to less than 1%. Despite its recognized efficacy, warfarin continues to be the agent of choice in less than one third of orthopaedic procedures, primarily because of the known risk of major hemorrhagic complications (as many as 14% of cases). This risk is directly proportional to the dosage and to the elevation of the prothrombin time. Recent researchers have attempted to expand the use of warfarin prophylaxis by limiting the target prothrombin time to 1.3 to 1.5 that of control values. Efficacy appears to be maintained and the incidence of attendant bleeding reduced to approximately 4%. If major bleeding occurs with warfarin, anticoagulation can be reversed within hours with parenteral vitamin K_1 or more quickly when necessary with transfusions of fresh-frozen plasma. Warfarin use is contraindicated during pregnancy, because it crosses the placenta and is highly teratogenic during the first trimester.

Aspirin Aspirin, an agent that inhibits the aggregation of

platelets, has not been found to be effective in preventing deep venous thrombosis after hip and knee surgery. In one recent randomized trial, 1.2 or 0.3 g of aspirin per day was associated with a 60% incidence of new-onset deep venous thrombosis after total hip replacement.

Dextran Low-molecular-weight dextran appears to be approximately as effective as warfarin, with clinically evident deep venous thrombosis reduced to approximately 6% of cases. It is an alernative to heparin for patients who develop complications related to heparin therapy. Dextran has several major drawbacks. Bleeding is dose-dependent and occurs in 7% to 8% of cases. Induced fluid overload with pulmonary edema is a potential complication, as is an anaphylactic reaction.

Intermittent Pneumatic Compression Intermittent pneumatic compression is a nonpharmologic prophylactic technique. The beneficial effects of intermittent pneumatic compression have been attributed to the prevention of venous stasis and an increase in plasma fibrinolytic activity. Intermittent pneumatic compression has the advantages of

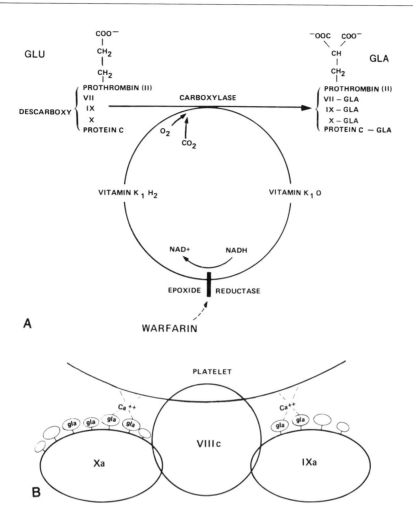

Figure 2

The mechanism of action of warfarin. Warfarin inhibits the reduction of the oxidized storage form of vitamin K_1. The reduced form (K_1H_2) functions as a co-enzyme in the carboxylation of factors II, VII, IX, and X and proteins C and S. Carboxylation of the glutamic acid residues of the vitamin K-dependent factors must occur for effective coagulation of platelet and endothelial phospholipid templates. (Reprinted with permission from Stead RB: Clinical pharmacology, in Goldhaber SZ (ed): *Pulmonary Embolism and Deep Venours Thromboembolism.* Philadelphia, WB Saunders, 1985, p 107.)

Outline 1. Pharmacologic agents that interact with warfarin anticoagulation

Potentiating agents
   Cefamandole
   Cimetidine
   Disulfiram
   Moxalactam
   Phenylbutazone
   Phenytoin
   Trimethoprim
Antagonists
   Cholestyramine
   Griseofulvin
   Phenobarbital
   Rifampin
   Vitamin K-rich foods

being inexpensive and unassociated with bleeding complications. In a randomized trial of 310 patients undergoing elective hip surgery, intermittent pneumatic compression reduced the rate of deep venous thrombosis twofold compared with that of controls (24% vs 49%, P < .001). Another study found intermittent pneumatic compression to be comparable to warfarin for the effective prevention of deep venous thrombosis in patients undergoing total hip arthroplasty. Because the beneficial effect of intermittent pneumatic compression is obtained at the time of application, it is useful for providing early prophylaxis while a pharmacologic agent is taking effect.

Treatment of Deep Venous Thrombosis

Symptomatic deep venous thrombosis, including symptomatic calf-vein thrombosis, should be treated with in-hospital heparin therapy followed by prolonged outpatient oral anticoagulation therapy to prevent propagation of the thrombus and embolization. Isolated calf-vein thrombi produce changes in pulmonary ventilation-perfusion scans in 20% to 33% of cases. In a study of 51 patients with documented calf-vein deep venous thrombosis, 23 patients who took warfarin for three months had no recurrences,

Table 1. Relative frequency of clinical signs and symptoms in pulmonary embolism

Clinical Findings	% of Cases
Symptoms	
Pleuritic pain	74
Apprehension	59
Cough	53
Hemoptysis	30
Signs	
Tachypnea (> 16 breaths/min)	90
Tachycardia (> 100 beats/min)	49
Rales	58
Fever (> 37.8 C)	43

whereas the 28 patients who received no anticoagulation therapy had a 38% recurrence rate and 25% extension rate. Therapy for symptomatic deep venous thrombosis is usually initiated with a continuous intravenous infusion of heparin, because this appears to be more efficacious than intermittent subcutaneous administration. The time for which subsequent oral anticoagulation is needed is more controversial, but a three- to six-month period appears to be effective. For patients with known long-term risk factors for deep venous thrombosis (such as morbid obesity, malignancy, or previous deep venous thrombosis, anticoagulants are given for an indefinite period.

Pulmonary Embolism

Pulmonary embolism can involve any combination of a broad spectrum of nonspecific associated symptoms and signs (Table 1). Dependence on clinical findings alone can lead to both overdiagnosis and underdiagnosis. Confirmatory radiologic tests are also needed.

Diagnosis An electrocardiogram must be obtained to investigate the possibility of concomitant myocardial infarction. The electrocardiogram tends to show abnormalities characteristic of pulmonary embolism only in patients with extensive embolization (massive or submassive). These changes, such as an $S_1Q_3T_3$, right bundle-branch block or right-axis deviation, occur in only 25% of patients with documented pulmonary embolism. A chest radiograph must be obtained; one that is normal in a severely dyspneic patient is strongly suggestive of pulmonary embolism. Classic radiographic abnormalities associated with massive pulmonary embolism include a relative local hyperlucency in a region of segmental arterial occlusion or an engorged major hilar artery. More commonly seen abnormalities, which are highly nonspecific, include pleural effusion, infiltrate atelectasis, or an elevated hemidiaphragm.

Arterial blood gas analysis can occasionally be helpful in the management of patients with suspected pulmonary embolism, but it is not useful for the diagnosis of pulmonary embolism, as the findings are nonspecific in patients who may have a preexisting or concomitant reason for decreased arterial oxygenation. In addition, a normal Po_2 does not exclude the diagnosis of pulmonary embolism. Approximately 15% of patients with angiographically documented pulmonary embolism have a mean arterial Po_2 higher than 85 mm Hg. Therefore, arterial blood gas analysis should not be used as a screening test for pulmonary embolism.

Radionuclide Lung Scanning Radionuclide ventilation-per-fusion lung scanning is the key diagnostic test for pulmonary embolism. False-negative perfusion scanning is exceedingly rare; a normal scan almost excludes any but tiny emboli and directs clinical attention to other diagnostic possibilities. Positive (abnormal) perfusion scans are categorized as of low, moderate, or high probability on the basis of the configuration and conformity of the vascular pattern to the ventilation pattern (ventilation-perfusion mismatch). False-positive perfusion scans are more common than false-negative scans. Of patients with high-probability scans (segmental perfusion defect with normal ventilation pattern), approximately 90% show confirmatory evidence of pulmonary embolism by angiography. Of those with low-probability scans, 15% to 30% have pulmonary embolism confirmed by angiography. Given these limitations, the physician should not defer pulmonary angiography in favor of the results of lung scanning when the results of scanning differ from the clinical presentation. Pulmonary angiography remains the definitive diagnostic step.

Pulmonary Angiography In general, pulmonary angiography should be reserved for patients with low- or moderate-probability lung scans when the clinical suspicion of pulmonary embolism is high. In addition, angiographic confirmation and characterization of the pulmonary embolism may be indicated in the patient with a high-probability scan when thrombolytic therapy or inferior vena cava interruption is being considered. When the lung scan is normal, there is generally no indication to pursue pulmonary angiography. Because of recent advances in contrast materials and flexible catheter materials, the morbidity associated with pulmonary angiography is currently less than 0.5%.

Anticoagulation Treatment Patients with pulmonary embolism should receive anticoagulation to prevent further clot deposition and to allow the body's natural fibrinolytic mechanism to lyse a clot that has already formed. Continuous infusion of heparin appears to be superior to intermittent heparin infusion, providing a more uniform increase in the partial thromboplastin time. Long-term anticoagulation is achieved by oral warfarin, which prevents recurrent venous thromboembolism. In one randomized trial, early recurrence of pulmonary embolism was noted in 20% of patients and seemed to correlate with a subtherapeutic level of anticoagulation. The required duration of anticoagulation after pulmonary embolism is not well defined. However, in patients with transient risk factors (most postoperative orthopaedic patients), the prothrombin time should be kept in the range of 16 to 20 seconds for six to 12 months.

Thrombolytic Therapy Whereas anticoagulation acts primarily to prevent the extension of thrombi, thrombolytic agents promote dissolution of recently formed clots. Relatively few clinical trials have evaluated the various agents available for thrombolysis (streptokinase, urokinase, tissue-plasminogen activator), and the indications for their use are still being defined. Because of an associated increased risk of hemorrhage, thrombolytic agents are generally contraindicated in a patient who has intracranial disease or major trauma or has undergone recent (within ten days) surgery.

Vena Cava Interruption Interruption of the inferior vena cava (usually by means of a percutaneously inserted filter device) is indicated in patients with pulmonary embolism who cannot tolerate anticoagulation or in whom anticoagulation does not prevent recurrence. The disadvantages of these filter devices are that (1) anticoagulation is still recommended to prevent thrombosis at the site of the filter device, (2) the device may become occluded with a thrombus, with large paravertebral venous collaterals then serving as a source of recurrent emboli, and (3) current models can migrate within the venous channel, possibly necessitating surgical removal.

Urinary Tract Infections

The term urinary tract infection implies a bacterial invasion of urinary tract tissue with an associated inflammatory response. The term bacteriuria indicates bacterial colonization of the urinary tract with or without associated clinical symptoms. Bacteriuria is quantitated by the number of bacterial colony-forming units (CFU) per milliliter of urine cultured. Urinary tract infection has traditionally been associated with more than 10^5 CFU/ml of urine. However, lower concentrations of bacteria may be clinically relevant, especially when samples are obtained from sterile aspirates of the urinary tract. In one study, 50% of patients with clinical symptoms of urinary tract infection had less than 10^5 CFU/ml.

Of more significance to the orthopaedic surgeon, especially in joint replacement surgery, is the presence of bacteremia with a risk for subsequent hematogenous seeding of the arthroplasty site.

Although urinary tract infection has been associated with an increased risk for joint sepsis after total joint replacement, documented cases of direct joint seeding are uncommon. In one long-term review of 149 total hip arthroplasties, perioperative or postoperative urinary tract infections developed in 32% of patients but joint sepsis from the same organism cultured from the urinary tract occurred in only one case. In another review of 277 patients, urinary tract infections developed in 12.6%, but none of the three postoperative joint infections could be related to any primary urinary tract organism. Although patients with established urinary tract infections should be treated for the infection before joint replacement, patients with asymptomatic bacteriuria can probably undergo surgery safely as long as appropriate perioperative antibiotic coverage is used.

Catheterization   Some 15% to 60% of patients undergoing hip or knee replacement require perioperative catheterization because of acute urinary retention. The patient's risk of acquiring a urinary tract infection (10^3 to 10^5 CFU/ml) depends on the duration of catheterization and ranges from 4% to 7.5% per day for the first ten days. Because of the associated risk of urinary tract infection, any strategy that enables the physician to reduce the frequency and duration of postoperative catheterization is beneficial. There is evidence that the period of acute bladder distention occurs intraoperatively rather than in the recovery period, and that preventing intraoperative distention may reduce the need for extended postoperative catheterization. In one prospective study, patients who underwent 24 hours of indwelling catheterization at the time of joint arthroplasty surgery had a lower incidence of urinary retention than patients who received postoperative intermittent cathet-

erization (27% vs 52%; $P < .01$). In another prospective study, perioperative indwelling catheterization was associated with a decreased risk of urinary tract infection (4% vs 16%) and postoperative retention (0% vs 65%) compared with intermittent catheterization.

In patients with long-term indwelling catheters, such as those with spinal cord injuries, the incidence of catheter-associated bacteriuria can be reduced by keeping the drainage bag sterile by the addition of a bactericidal agent such as povidone solution or hydrogen peroxide. Prophylactic antibiotics appear to decrease the incidence of urinary tract infections only during shorter periods of catheterization (less than four days).

Prostatic Hypertrophy

Neither the urologic history nor the physical examination of the prostate reliably predicts which patients are most likely to experience urinary retention after total hip arthroplasty. In one prospective study, retention developed in 10% of patients with normal prostatic findings on rectal examination but in 29% of those with enlarged prostates. In the same study, a peak urinary flow rate of less than 17 ml/sec was the only finding statistically associated with the subsequent development of urinary retention. Using a combination of the patient's history, the physical findings, and urine flow studies, the clinician can identify the patients at highest risk for urinary retention, thus making possible preoperative urologic evaluation and treatment.

In one retrospective review of 28 patients undergoing total hip arthroplasty who required transurethral prostatectomy seven to ten days postoperatively, only one patient had a urinary tract infection and none had joint sepsis. All patients were treated at the time of prostatectomy with an eight-day course of antibiotics specific for the urinary culture. This contrasted sharply with an earlier retrospective review that reported that prostatectomy (transurethral or open) in the early postoperative period (eight to 40 days) was associated with a twofold increase in mortality.

Skin Ulcers

Decubitus ulcers, or bedsores, are likely to become a greater problem as the population ages and longer and more complicated operations are performed. About 3% to 10% of all hospitalized patients develop bedsores; this number may be as high as 20% to 30% in the elderly. In one report, 6% of patients with hip fractures developed bedsores; only 10% were less than 70 years of age.

Factors contributing to the formation of bedsores are advanced age, paralysis, sensory impairment, coma, malnutrition, incontinence, anemia, and sepsis. Therefore, the patients most likely to develop bedsores are the aged, the critically ill, and the neurologically impaired. Once an ulcer is established, it is difficult to heal. If it is not treated successfully, morbidity increases.

Skin ulcers can be a source of infection. It has been shown that total knee replacement performed in the presence of skin ulceration carries a higher risk of an infected prosthesis. The estimated cost of healing each ulcer ranges from $5,000 to $40,000.

Prevention should be the main goal. Frequent changing of the position of the bedridden patient is the most important measure. This is a time-consuming task and requires a vigilant nursing staff. There are mechanically and electrically controlled beds that change position periodically. These devices are useful but expensive. Also useful are beds and mattresses that help distribute the pressure more evenly. Among these are waterbeds and mattresses, special foam cushions, and the air-fluidized bed. The latter is promising but very expensive.

In the last five years more attention has been directed to metabolic factors. Such conditions as edema, malnutrition, and, especially, hypoalbuminemia and sepsis must be corrected.

Treatment is difficult. First, debridement should be performed either by surgery or by chemical agents until the wound is clear. It should then be covered by skin. Because bedsores occur over bony prominences exposing the bone, a split-thickness skin graft cannot be used. Encouraging results were obtained with myocutaneous flaps and pedicle grafts.

The Use of Tourniquets

Tourniquet control of blood loss has become routine for many upper-and lower-extremity procedures. Tourniquets are of two types. The pneumatic device with in-line pressure gauge often consists of a wide cuff with variable lengths to accommodate limb circumference. The Esmarch tourniquet is an elastic bandage wrapped in a retrograde fashion to exsanguinate and prevent arterial flow. A disadvantage of the Esmarch tourniquet is that inappropriately high and unmonitored pressures may be generated. Although the use of modern pneumatic cuffs more accurately controls and monitors the generated cuff pressure, certain guidelines for safe use must still be considered.

Tourniquets can be associated with clinically important nerve and muscle damage. Two regions are of concern: tissues distal to the cuff (ischemic zone) and tissues beneath the cuff (compression zone). The region distal to the tourniquet is subjected to ischemia and the resultant metabolic effects of acidosis and anaerobic metabolism. Studies have shown that abnormalities in tissues distal to the tourniquet are reversible after as much as three hours of ischemia. The local acid-base changes within the limb have been shown to recover within 20 to 40 minutes. Further, when tourniquet pressure is decreased, the accumulated ischemic metabolites have been found to have little impact on cardiac function in both animal and human models. Tissues in the ischemic zone, therefore, appear to tolerate tourniquet times of as long as three hours with few local or systemic complications.

Tissues in the zone beneath the cuff are subjected to compression and shear forces as well as ischemia. The area at the cuff-limb interface has the highest shear stress; nerve damage can result from internal disruption of the axonal anatomy with paranodal demyelination. Irreversible nerve damage can occur in as little as two hours if the cuff is improperly applied. In addition, irreversible muscle damage occurs in the region directly beneath the cuff earlier than in the distal zone, indicating that the effect of direct compression may be additive to the effect of ischemia.

Careful application of the tourniquet is neessary to avoid complications. The tourniquet cuff should be as wide as the exposure and procedure allow. The cuff margins must be well padded to minimize shear, especially in a limb that is sharply tapered. The lowest pressure that will prevent capillary flow should be used. In an average-sized, normotensive patient, pressures of 200 mm Hg in the upper limb and 250 mm Hg in the lower limb reliably produce a bloodless field. A wide cuff (15 cm) consistently stops blood flow at lower pressures (systolic); smaller cuffs require suprasystolic pressures. Recently, double tourniquet cuffs in upper-extremity surgery have permitted alternative inflation at hourly intervals. With this technique, safe tourniquet times have been extended to 3½ hours with no instances of permanent nerve palsy. The amount of reperfusion time needed to restore metabolic equilibrium after tourniquet inflation increases with longer inflation time. Magnetic resonance imaging has shown five minutes to be adequate after 90 minutes of ischemia, but 15 minutes appears to be required after three hours.

Trends

The modern orthopaedic patient has benefited from advances in the level of perioperative patient monitoring, postoperative intensive care, and improved techniques of regional anesthesia. High-risk patients who previously would have been ineligible for surgery may today be considered reasonable candidates for elective procedures.

Guiding the high-risk patient safely through the perioperative period presents a great challenge to the orthopaedic surgeon, especially because of increasing pressures to provide high-quality service during shorter and shorter hospital stays. Future advances in the perioperative care of the orthopaedic patient should assist the surgeon in this demanding task. The task of preventing complications should start before the day of surgery, preferably during the preoperative office visit. Long-term nutritional deficits should be addressed and treated. Continuing advances in parenteral hyperalimentation (both in and out of the hospital) may help to minimize wound healing problems related to a poor nutritional state. Patients who are at high risk for urinary tract complications, either from retention or recurrent bacteriuria, should be examined and treated definitively before any surgical procedure. Further advances in the study of urodynamics, as well as improved antibiotic specificities, may minimize perioperative urologic complications.

New advances in combined or low-dose prophylaxis for deep venous thrombosis may provide safer anticoagulation without the inconvenience and cost of frequent laboratory monitoring. More effective treatment for patients with life-threatening pulmonary emboli may follow the introduction of advanced second- and third-generation thrombolytic agents. It is anticipated that additional prospective multicenter studies will attempt to verify the effectiveness of newer agents that might be associated with a lower complication rate.

Although refractory skin ulceration is a postoperative complication to be avoided, when it does occur topical growth factors may prove to a helpful adjunct. Application of recent advances in microsurgery may expand the indications for free tissue flaps to cover areas of chronic breakdown.

Annotated Bibliography

Keywords

Decubitus ulcer; Dextran; Heparin; Impedance plethysmography; Nutrition; Prostate gland; Pulmonary embolism; Pulmonary function; Sepsis; Stress; Thromboembolism; Tourniquet; Ultrasonography; Urinary tract infection; Venography; Warfarin

Nutrition

Adams S, Dellinger EP, Wertz MJ, et al: Enteral versus parenteral nutritional support following laparotomy for trauma: A randomized prospective trial. *J Trauma* 1986; 26:882–891.
　This study compared total parenteral nutrition with enteral nutrition by jejunostomy in patients with multiple injuries. Nutritional support began on the first postoperative day. The results suggested that early jejunostomy feeding is safe and efficacious in patients with multiple injuries who undergo laparotomy.

Border JR, Hassett J, LaDuca J, et al: The gut origin septic states in blunt multiple trauma (ISS = 40) in the ICU. *Ann Surg* 1987;206:427–448.
　This study included 66 patients with blunt multiple trauma. A septic state was more likely to develop in patients who had not received enteral nutrition for more than ten days. This suggests that a lack of enteral feeding produces atrophy of the gut mucosa and endotoxin transmission through the gut, creating a systemic septic state.

Cortes V, Nelson LE: Errors in estimating energy expenditure in critically ill surgical patients. *Arch Surg* 1989;124:287–290.
　Measured energy expenditure was compared with predictions of basal energy expenditure and calculated energy expenditure in 31 critically ill surgical patients. The measured energy expenditure was significantly greater than the basal energy expenditure. The authors recommend indirect calorimetry, measuring oxygen comsumption and carbon dioxide production, to assess energy expenditure more accurately and to optimize nutritional support.

Kay SP, Moreland JR, Schmitter E: Nutritional status and wound healing in lower extremity amputations. *Clin Orthop* 1987;217:253–256.
　The effect of nutritional status was studied in 41 consecutive patients who underwent lower-extremity amputation. The amputations healed in 15 of 16 patients with normal nutritional parameters. Eleven of 25 malnourished patients sustained either systemic or local postoperative complications. The authors recommend that patients admitted for lower-extremity amputation have elective surgery postponed if routine laboratory tests suggest malnutrition. Patients requiring surgery on an emergency basis should receive supplemental nutritional support perioperatively.

Moore EE, Jones TN: Benefits of immediate jejunostomy feeding after major abdominal trauma: A prospective, randomized study. *J Trauma* 1986;26:874–881.
　Seventy-five consecutive patients undergoing emergency laparotomy were randomly assigned to a control group who received no supplemental nutrition for the first five days or to a group given enteral nutrition through needle catheter jejunostomies. Elemental nutrition was given 18 hours postoperatively. The group given enteral nutrition had a markedly improved nitrogen balance and a lower mortality from sepsis.

Smith TK: Prevention of complications in orthopaedic surgery secondary to nutritional depletion. *Clin Orthop* 1987;222:91–97.

　Protein and calorie malnutrition has an adverse effect on wound healing, immunity, and fracture healing, and can ultimately lead to multiorgan failure in the highly stressed patient. Fifty percent of medical and surgical patients exhibited findings of malnutrition in a large urban teaching hospital survey. Wheareas the normal adult requires approximately 147 J of energy per kilogram of body weight per day, a patient with multiple fractures may need 252 to 294 J/day. An increase in body temperature of 1 degree increases the resting energy requirement 7% to 8%.

Thromboembolism

Consensus Conference: Prevention of venous thrombosis and pulmonary embolism. *JAMA* 1986;256:744–749.
　Evaluation of relevant trials in thromboembolism prevention, with recommended guidelines for orthopaedic surgery.

Froehlich JA, Dorfman GS, Cronan JJ, et al: Compression ultrasonography for the detection of deep venous thrombosis in patients who have a fracture of the hip. *J Bone Joint Surg* 1989;71A:249–256.
　Compression ultrasonography was demonstrated to have a sensitivity of 100% and specificity of 97% in the detection of above-calf deep venous thrombosis after fracture of the hip.

Hull R, Carter C, Raskob G, et al: Intermittent pneumatic leg compression for preventing venous thrombosis following total hip replacement. *Chest* 1987;92(suppl): 105S.
　Intermittent pneumatic compression effectively reduced the incidence of deep venous thrombosis after elective hip surgery.

Hull R, Hirsh J, Jay R, et al: Different intensities of oral anticoagulant therapy in the treatment of proximal-vein thrombosis. *N Engl J Med* 1982;307:1676–1681.
　A less intense warfarin regimen was associated wih a low frequency of recurrent venous thromboembolism and a reduced risk of hemorrhage.

Kessler CM: Anticoagulation and thrombolytic therapy: Practical considerations. *Chest* 1989;95:245–256.
　A thorough discussion of thrombolytic agents as well as the pharmacology of anticogulants.

Lagerstedt CI, Olsson CG, Fagher BO, et al: Need for long-term anticoagulant treatment in symptomatic calf-vein thrombosis. *Lancet* 1985;2:515–517.
　Extended warfarin anticoagulation (three months) was found to decrease the recurrence rate of deep venous thrombosis from 68% to 4%. Without warfarin, proximal extension of the thrombus was seen in 18% of patients and one pulmonary embolism was noted.

Lynch AF, Bourne RB, Rorabeck CH, et al: Deep-vein thrombosis and continuous passive motion after total knee arthroplasty. *J Bone J Surg* 1988;70A:11–14.
　Forty percent of patients undergoing total knee arthroplasty had calf-vein thrombosis whether continuous passive motion was used or not.

Paiement GD, Beisaw N, Lotke PA, et al: Advances in the prevention of venous thromboembolic disease after hip and knee surgery. *Orthop Rev* 1989;18(suppl):1–20.
　An extensive review and bibliography addressing this subject in a comprehensive manner.

Paiement G, Bell D, Weissinger SJ, et al: New advances in the prevention, diagnosis and cost effectiveness of venous thromboembolic disease in patients with total hip replacement. *Hip* 1986;14:94–119.

Intermittent pneumatic compression was found to be comparable to warfarin for the prophylaxis of deep venous thrombosis after elective hip surgery.

Paiement G, Weissinger SJ, Waltman AC, et al: Surveillance of deep vein thrombosis in asymptomatic total hip replacement patients: Impedance phlebography and fibrinogen scanning versus roentgenographic phlebography *Am J Surg* 1988;155:400–404.

Impedance plethysmography was compared with venography and demonstrated to have low sensitivity in detecting thrombi of the lower extremity.

Stulberg BN, Insall JN, Williams GW, et al: Deep-vein thrombosis following total knee replacement: Analysis of six hundred and thirty-eight arthroplasties. *J Bone Joint Surg* 1984;66A:194–201.

A retrospective review of 638 total knee replacements with emphasis on the incidences of deep venous thrombosis and pulmonary embolism and risk factors for thromboembolism.

Urinary Tract Infections

Carpiniello VL, Cendron M, Altman HG, et al: Treatment of urinary complications after total joint replacement in elderly females. *Urology* 1988;32:186–188.

A prospective, randomized study of 77 female patients undergoing total joint replacement demonstrated that short-term indwelling catheterization was associated with lower rates of urinary retention and urinary tract infection than intermittent catheterization.

Jinnah RH, Amstutz HC, Tooke SM, et al: The UCLA Charnley experience: A long-term follow-up study using survival analysis. *Clin Orthop* 1986;211:164–172.

Of 149 patients undergoing total hip arthroplasty, 32% developed urinary tract infections and one developed apparent seeding of the joint.

Michelson JD, Lotke PA, Steinberg ME: Urinary-bladder management after total joint replacement surgery. *N Eng J Med* 1988;319:321–326.

A prospective, randomized study of 100 patients undergoing total joint replacement demonstrated that short-term indwelling catheterization was associated with lower rates of urinary retention and bladder overdistention, without increasing the rate of urinary tract infection.

Redfern TR, Machin DG, Parsons KG, et al: Urinary retention in men after total hip arthroplasty. *J Bone Joint Surg* 1986;68A:1435–1438.

A prospective study of 64 patients undergoing total hip replacement demonstrated that decreased peak urinary flow rate was statistically associated with an increased risk of the development of perioperative urinary retention.

Ritter MA, Fechtman RW: Urinary tract sequelae: Possible influence on joint infections following total joint replacement. *Orthopedics* 1987;10:467–469.

Of a series of 277 patients undergoing total joint replacement, 35 (12.6%) had urinary tract infections, with three developing joint infections not related to the primary urinary tract infection organisms.

Schaeffer J: Catheter-associated bacteriuria. *Urol Clin North Am* 1986;13:735–747.

A comprehensive discussion of the etiology and clinical implications of catheter-associated bacteriuria.

Skin Ulcers

Allman RM, Walker JM, Hart MK, et al: Air-fluidized beds or conventional therapy for pressure sores: A randomized trial. *Ann Intern Med* 1987;107:641–648.

Air-fluidized beds are more effective than conventional therapy, particularly for large pressure sores.

Lim R, Sirett R, Conine TA, et al: Clinical trial of foam cushions in the prevention of decubitus ulcers in elderly patients. *J Rehabil Res Dev* 1988;25:19–26.

The difference between slab form and the customized contoured form of foam cushions in the prevention of decubitus ulcers is discussed.

Maklebust J: Pressure ulcers: Etiology and prevention. *Nurs Clin North Am* 1987;22:359–377.

A summary of causes and modes of prevention of pressure ulcers is presented.

The Use of Tourniquets

Hargens AR, McClure AG, Skyhar MJ, et al: Local compression patterns beneath pneumatic tourniquets aspplied to arms and thighs of human cadaver. *J Orthop Res* 1987;2:247–252.

This study documented stratification of tissue pressures with increased depth under cuff. The highest pressures were in the subcutaneous region and the lowest were near the bone. This confirmed that a wider cuff produces ischemia at a lower pressure.

Heppenstall RB, Scott R, Sapega: A comparative sudy of the tolerance of skeletal muscle in ischemia: Tourniquet application compared with acute compartment syndrome. *J Bone Joint Surg* 1986;68A:820–828,.

The authors used magnetic resonance imaging to study metabolic changes in tourniquet-induced ischemia. After three hours of compression, the cellular energy system reversed completely within 15 minutes of reperfusion.

McLaren AC Rorabeck CH: The pressure distribution under tourniquets. *J Bone Joint Surg* 1985;67A:433–438.

Pressures vary with the width of the tourniquet and the depth of the tissues beneath the tourniquet. The Esmarch tourniquet is associated with dangerous peak pressures.

Moore MR, Garfin SR, Hargens AR: Wide tourniquets eliminate blood flow at low inflation pressures. *J Hand Surg* 1987;12A:1006–1011.

Wide cuffs consistently stop blood flow at systolic pressure levels; higher pressures are required with narrower cuff.

Neimkin RJ, Smith RJ: Double tourniquet with linked mercury manometers for hand surgery. *J Hand Surg* 1983;8:938–941.

Double tourniquet technique afforded up to 3½ hours of tourniquet time in upper extremity surgery. Transient paresthesia was associated with more than two hours of tourniquet use.

Sapega AA, Heppenstall RB, Chance B, et al: Optimizing tourniquet application and release times in extremity surgery: A biochemical and ultrastructural study. *J Bone Joint Surg* 1985;67A:303–314.

Magnetic resonance imaging demonstrates that 90 minutes of tourniquet use followed by five minutes of reperfusion permits another 90-minute period of tourniquet use without permanent deleterious effect.

Van Roekel HE, Thurston AJ: Tourniquet pressure: The effect of limb circumference and systolic pressure. *J Hand Surg* 1985;10B:142–144.

A formula is derived to relate the required pressure to the systolic pressure and limb circumference.

10
Musculoskeletal Neoplasms

The essentials of evaluation and treatment of the most common neoplasms of bone and soft tissue were presented in *Orthopaedic Knowledge Update 2* and are still considered current. This chapter extends that basic information, emphasizing newer developments in the staging of musculoskeletal neoplasms, the use of magnetic resonance imaging in the diagnosis and treatment of sarcoma, and methods of pathologically assessing soft-tissue sarcomas. The treatment of chondrosarcoma, giant cell tumor of bone, malignant fibrous histiocytoma, chordoma, and metastatic disease has not changed substantially in the last few years, whereas the use of adjuvant chemotherapy in osteosarcoma has continued to evolve, as have methods of limb salvage in patients with this neoplasm.

Advances in sarcoma histology and treatment are being made on many fronts. Determination of DNA ploidy (as a marker of prognosis), prediction of drug sensitivity, advances in molecular biology, improvements in allograft transplantation, and the biomechanics of prosthetic implants are areas of current research.

Staging Systems for Malignant Tumors of the Musculoskeletal System

Staging of malignant tumors of the musculoskeletal system is necessary to determine the prognosis. Among the various prognostic factors that have been identified and used to define tumor stages are its location and relative size, the presence or absence of regional or distant metastases, and the histologic grade of the tumor. Although these factors are common to many staging systems, the relative significance assigned to them varies from system to system.

Tumor Grade

The grade of a tumor is a measure of its aggressiveness or tendency to metastasize. The assignment of grade is always based on histologic features; however, for bone tumors clinical and radiologic data may also be included in the determination of biologic aggressiveness. Because lesions with cellular atypia, frequent mitoses, extensive necrosis, significant vascularity, and small amounts of immature matrix seem to be aggressive in their behavior, these histologic features are used in the assignment of grade. Clinical symptoms such as pain, as well as radiographic manifestations such as soft-tissue extension of a bone neoplasm or involvement of bone by a soft-tissue neoplasm, are also used in staging tumors.

When histologic criteria alone are used, even expert pathologists can find it difficult to agree about the tumor grade. In addition, the number of grades needed is controversial. Enneking defined only two grades, which he based on histologic, clinical, and radiologic criteria, whereas most other staging systems include four grades

based solely on histologic criteria. Although there may be disagreement as to the number of grades and the way in which they should be assigned, it is clear that the grade should be a major factor in any staging system, and that it should assist in predicting the risk of distant metastases.

Other Factors in Staging of Tumors

The location and the size of a tumor relative to the anatomic region that it occupies may directly influence the prognosis. The risk of local recurrence and distant metastases is greater for large tumors than for small ones. In addition, anatomic structures such as cortical bone, articular surfaces, joint capsules, and major fascial septae appear to be relative barriers to local tumor spread. For purposes of staging and to aid in surgical planning, tumors (regardless of size) are grouped as either intracompartmental or extracompartmental. Intracompartmental tumors are bordered in all dimensions by natural barriers to extension. Extracompartmental tumors arise in an extracompartmental location or extend beyond natural barriers because of growth or iatrogenic contamination. An extracompartmental location can reflect the tumor's invasiveness or a delay in diagnosis. For example, an intramedullary chondrosarcoma that has not violated the cortex of the bone is considered to be intracompartmental, in contrast to a similarly placed lesion that has penetrated the cortex with a soft-tissue mass extending into the adjacent muscle. The latter reflects the aggressiveness of the lesion and is considered to be extracompartmental. Because of the likelihood of satellite nodules and tumor cells within the pseudocapsule of the lesion, an extracompartmental

Table 1. Surgical sites*

Intracompartmental	Extracompartmental
Intraosseus	Soft-tissue extension
Intra-articular	Soft-tissue extension
Superficial to deep fascia	Deep fascial extension
Paraosseus	Intraosseus or extrafascial
Intrafascial compartments	Extrafascial planes or spaces
Ray of hand or foot	Mid and hind foot
Posterior calf	Popliteal space
Anterolateral leg	Groin-femoral triangle
Anterior thigh	Intrapelvic
Medial thigh	Mid-hand
Posterior thigh	Antecubital fossae
Buttocks	Axilla
Volar forearm	Periclavicular
Dorsal forearm	Paraspinal
Anterior arm	Head and neck
Posterior arm	
Periscapular	

*Reproduced with permission from Enneking WF, Spanier SS, Goodman MA: A system for the surgical staging of musculoskeletal sarcoma. *Clin Orthop* 1980;153:106–120.

STAGE	G	T	N	M
IA	1	1	0	0
IB	1	2	0	0
IIA	2	1	0	0
IIB	2	2	0	0
IIIA	3-4	1	0	0
IIIB	3-4	2	0	0
IVA	1-4	1-2	1	0
IVB	1-4	1-2	0-1	1

Characteristics

Histological Grade (G)

G_1 Well differentiated
G_2 Moderately well differentiated
$G_{3,4}$ Poorly differentiated; undifferentiated

Primary Tumor (T)

T_1 Tumor 5cm or less in greatest dimension
T_2 Tumor more than 5cm in greatest dimension

Regional Lymph Nodes (N)

N_0 No regional lymph node metastases
N_1 Regional lymph node metastases

Distant Metastases (M)

M_0 No distant metastases
M_1 Distant metastases

Figure 1

The American Joint Commission's staging protocol for soft-tissue sarcomas. (Adapted with permission from American Joint Commission on Cancer: Soft tissues, in Beahrs OH, Myers MH (eds): *Manual for Staging of Cancer*, ed 3. Philadelphia, JB Lippincott, 1988, pp 127–131.)

STAGE	GRADE	SITE	METASTASES
IA	G_1	T_1	M_0
IB	G_1	T_2	M_0
IIA	G_2	T_1	M_0
IIB	G_2	T_2	M_0
IIIA	G_1-G_2	T_1	M_1
IIIB	G_1-G_2	T_2	M_1

Characteristics

Grade (G)

G_1 Low
G_2 High

Site (T)

T_1 Intracompartmental
T_2 Extracompartmental

Metastases (M)

M_0 No regional or distant metastases
M_1 Regional or distant metastases present

Figure 2

The Enneking system for staging of soft-tissue sarcomas and sarcomas of bone. (Adapted with permission from Enneking WF, Spanier SS, Goodman MA: A system for the surgical staging of musculoskeletal sarcoma. *Clin Orthop* 1980;153:106–120.)

lesion adjacent to a major neurovascular structure is less likely to be resectable than an intracompartmental one at the same distance. The various surgical compartments are listed in Table 1.

The primary factors determining the extent of the surgical margins to be used are the specific compartment or compartments involved and the proximity of the tumor to vital neurovascular and osseous structures. In general, intracompartmental tumors are smaller than extracompartmental tumors, allowing wider surgical margins and thus a greater probability of local control.

A soft-tissue sarcoma can be subcutaneous or deep to the superficial fascia. Approximately 25% of soft-tissue sarcomas in adults are subcutaneous. Subcutaneous sarcomas are generally smaller than deep sarcomas.

Obviously, the tumor's location has an effect on the technical aspects of local control, whereas size may or may not be a significant technical factor. Thus, location is a vital factor in the surgeon's effort to achieve local control.

Regional or distant metastases are the most important prognostic variables in any staging system. Although musculoskeletal neoplasms seldom metastasize to regional lymph nodes, distant metastases are present in approximately 10% of cases at the time of diagnosis, despite the absence of regional lymph node involvement. It is known that both regional and distant metastases confer a poor prognosis. In soft-tissue sarcomas, the probability of distant metastases increases with the size of the tumor.

At present, there are three recognized staging systems for sarcomas of soft tissue and two for sarcomas of bone. All these systems include the same variables in determining the tumor's stage but differ in the assignment of relative prognostic significance and the method of organizing them into a practical and meaningful schema. Although a biopsy is necessary for determining histologic grade, important information about the stage of a tumor can be obtained preoperatively with various imaging techniques. The tumor's size, location, and proximity to vital neurovascular structures can be determined by means of radiography, scintigraphy, computed tomography, and magnetic resonance imaging. Regional and distant metastases can be detected by chest radiography, computed tomography of the lungs, and bone scintigraphy. The recommended staging procedures for both bone and soft-tissue sarcomas include conventional radiography of the involved limb and lung, technetium Tc 99m phosphonate bone scintigraphy, magnetic resonance imaging of the limb, computed tomography of the lungs, and, for bone sarcomas, computed tomography of the involved limb.

Staging of Soft-Tissue Sarcomas in Adults

For soft-tissue sarcomas in adults, the three staging systems presently used are those developed by the American Joint Commission on Cancer, by Enneking, and by Hajdu.

The revised system of the American Joint Commission on Cancer is based on the T, N, M system and the histologic grade, G (Fig. 1). T refers to tumor size, N to nodal metastases, and M to distant metastases. There are progressive stages, with stages I, II, and III defined by histologic grade. Stage IV depends on the presence of either regional lymph node metastases (stage IVA) or distant me-

STAGE	SIZE (cm)	SITE	GRADE
0	<5	S	L
IA	<5	S	H
IB	<5	D	L
IC	>5	S	L
IIA	<5	D	H
IIB	>5	S	H
IIC	>5	D	L
III	>5	D	H

Characteristics

Site (S)

| S | Superficial to fascia (subcutaneous) |
| D | Deep to fascia |

Grade (G)

| L | Low |
| H | High |

Figure 3

Hajdu's system for staging of soft-tissue sarcomas. (Reproduced with permission from Hajdu SI: *Pathology of Soft Tissue Tumors.* Philadelphia, Lea & Febiger, 1979, pp 35–47.)

STAGE	GRADE	PRIMARY TUMOR	REGIONAL NODES	DISTANT METASTASES
IA	G_1-G_2	T_1	N_0	M_0
IB	G_1-G_2	T_2	N_0	M_0
IIA	G_3-G_4	T_1	N_0	M_0
IIB	G_3-G_4	T_2	N_0	M_0
III	Not defined			
IVA	Any G	Any T	N_1	M_0
IVB	Any G	Any T	Any N	M_1

Characteristics

Primary Tumor (T)

T_1	Tumor confined within the cortex
T_2	Tumor extended beyond the cortex
NOTE:	Juxtacortical (parosteal) sarcomas should be considered separately

Regional Lymph Nodes (N)

| N_0 | No regional lymph node metastases |
| N_1 | Regional lymph node metastases |

Distant Metastases (M)

| M_0 | No distant metastases |
| M_1 | Distant metastases |

Histological Grade (G)

G_1	Well differentiated
G_2	Moderately differentiated
G_3	Poorly differentiated
G_4	Undifferentiated

| NOTE: | Ewing's sarcoma and malignant lymphoma are defined as G_4 |

Figure 4

The American Joint Commission's staging protocol for sarcomas of bone. (Adapted with permission from American Joint Commission on Cancer: Bone, in Beahrs OH, Myers MH (eds): *Manual for Staging of Cancer*, ed 3. Philadelphia, JB Lippincott, 1988, pp 123–126.)

tastases (stage IVB). Tumor size is an important factor in this system. Stages I to III are subdivided into T_1 (greatest dimension less than 5 cm) and T_2 (greatest dimension more than 5 cm).

An alternative system developed by Enneking applies to both primary bone and primary soft-tissue sarcomas (Fig. 2). In this system, there are three major stages defined by surgical grade (G), surgical site (T), and the presence or absence of metastases (M). The surgical grade is determined mainly by histologic criteria; however, clinical and radiographic data are used in the ultimate assignment of grade. The clinical and radiographic information is more important for bone than for soft-tissue sarcomas. The surgical grade is either low (G1: less than 25% risk of metastases) or high (G2: more than 25% risk of metastases). The surgical site (T) is further subdivided into intracompartmental (A) and extracompartmental (B) categories. A tumor is assigned to stage III if there are metastases to regional lymph nodes, or if distant metastases are present (MI).

The third system, used only for staging of soft-tissue sarcomas, is that developed by Hajdu (Fig. 3).

The important prognostic variables of grade, location, size, depth, and metastases are incorporated, either directly or indirectly, in all three staging systems for soft-tissue sarcomas. Although grade is very important for the prognosis, it is difficult to devise a four-stage system acceptable to most expert pathologists. The American Joint Commission gives no detailed guidelines for the four-stage system. Both the American Joint Commission system and the Hajdu system place considerable emphasis on the size of the tumor. Although size may influence the prognosis, the proximity of a tumor to vital neurovascular structures and its size relative to the compartment involved are of more practical significance with regard to surgical margins. By using the concept of anatomic compartments, the Enne-

king system addresses the anatomic site from a surgeon's perspective more than do the other systems. The Enneking system does not allow a separate designation for superficial tumors, which are usually small, and size is only an indirect variable. Hajdu has incorporated depth as a prognostic variable in his staging system.

In all three staging systems for adult soft-tissue sarcomas, the histologic grade and the presence or absence of metastases are the most important prognostic variables. The size, depth, and anatomic site of each tumor are important, but how they should be weighted in the staging system is yet to be determined.

Staging of Sarcomas of Bone

The first staging system for sarcomas of bone was that described by Enneking (Fig. 2). This system is identical to the system used for soft-tissue sarcomas except that intracompartmental bone tumors are those confined within the cortex or periosteum (T_1), and extracompartmental bone tumors are those that extend into the soft tissues (T_2). A parosteal tumor that does not extend into the underlying cortex is also designated as T_1.

The system described by the American Joint Commission for the staging of malignant tumors of bone has not yet been completed (Fig. 4). It uses the T, N, M, G classification with T referring to the extent of the tumor (confined to or extending beyond the cortex of bone), N to nodal metastases, M to distant metastases, and G to his-

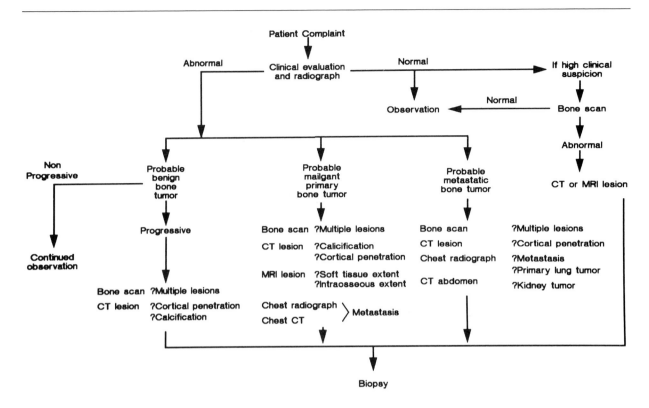

Algorithm 1

Diagnostic strategy for a bone tumor.

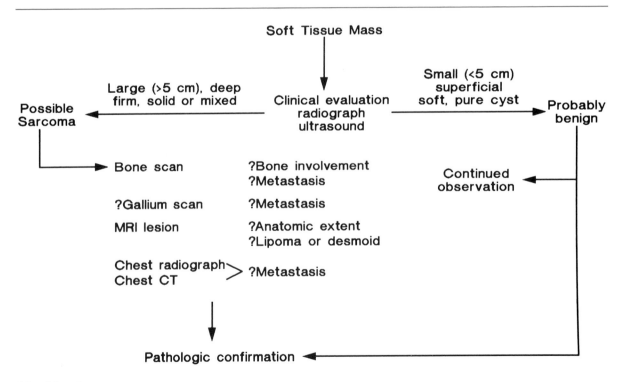

Algorithm 2

Diagnostic strategy for a soft-tissue mass.

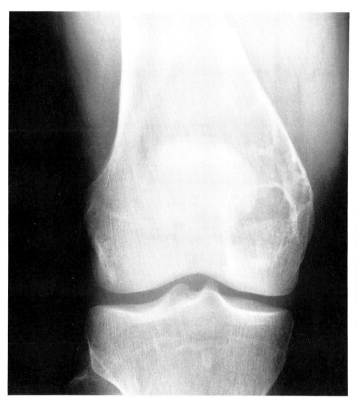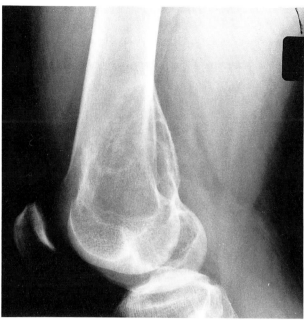

Figure 5

Typical giant cell tumor of the right distal femur in a 34-year-old man. Plain radiographs show an eccentric, moderately well-defined destructive lesion in the metaphysis and epiphysis of the distal femur without apparent penetration of the cortex or mineralization in the lesion.

tologic grade. Of the four progressive stages, I and II are defined by histologic grade and modified by cortical involvement (T_1, confined within the cortex; T_2, extending beyond the cortex). Stage III is still undefined. Stage IV is categorized by the presence or absence of nodal metastases (A) or distant metastases (B).

A careful comparison of the American Joint Commission system to the Enneking system makes it apparent that the differences are minor. The anatomic site (T) is essentially identical in the two systems. The only significant differences are that the American Joint Commission designates but has not yet defined a stage III, and considers nodal and distant metastases separately. The American Joint Commission system designates four grades on the basis of histologic features, but from a practical standpoint only two grades exist. From a surgeon's perspective, it seems that only two histologic grades are needed, and that clinical and radiographic criteria should be considered in staging sarcomas of bone.

Algorithms 1 and 2 illustrate suggested diagnostic strategies for bone and soft-tissue tumors.

Biopsy of Musculoskeletal Lesions

Biopsy is the crucial procedure that must be performed at the end of the diagnostic and staging phases for musculoskeletal lesions. The lesion should be staged before biopsy to enhance clinical, radiographic, and pathologic correlations, to facilitate immediate surgery on the basis of

frozen-section analysis, and because imaging specificity diminishes after biopsy.

There are some basic rules of biopsy placement. To tailor treatment appropriately, the surgeon must know the probable diagnosis and the clinical stage of the lesion.

The biopsy specimen must be excised en bloc if the tumor is malignant and limb salvage or amputation is contemplated. The surgeon performing the biopsy should be familiar with the available surgical alternatives for each anatomic location and diagnosis.

During the biopsy, one should not make transverse incisions or expose or dissect important neurovascular structures. The biopsy should traverse only one compartment, usually a muscle that can be sacrificed if a second procedure for malignancy is necessary.

Biopsy placement is particularly important in an open biopsy, which produces a larger hematoma and has a greater likelihood of infection, and pathologic fracture. An open biopsy should be performed in an operating room. After making a small longitudinal incision, the surgeon should take a small sample of the periphery of the tumor, which is the most representative portion. If there is soft-tissue extension, the bone should not be sampled. An excisional biopsy of small, superficial soft-tissue tumors or small, benign bone tumors may be judicious. If bone must be violated, a circular hole or oblong window should be fashioned to lessen the likelihood of pathologic fracture. If the tumor is a sarcoma, a pathologic fracture usually causes the loss of the limb. If a tourniquet is used, it should be released and hemostasis obtained before closure. The su-

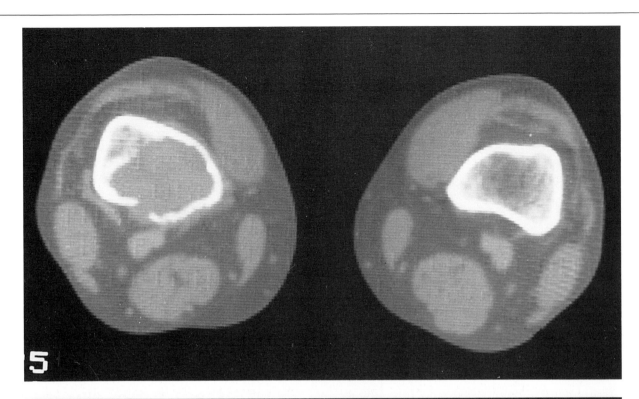

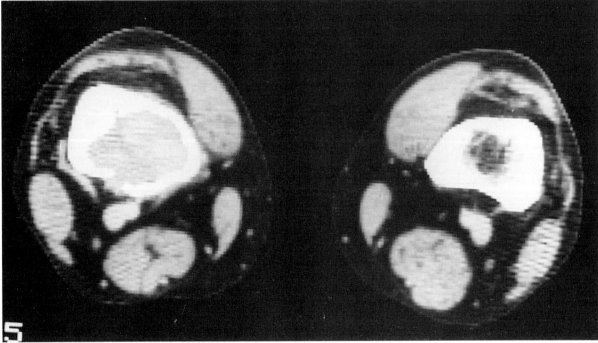

Figure 6

Computed tomograms of giant cell tumor shown in Figure 5. **Top**, "Bone windows" show penetration of the posterior cortex by the tumor. **Bottom**, "Soft-tissue windows" confirm the posterior cortical penetration and show no ossification with the tumor.

tures and any drains should be placed close to the edge of the incision. The tumor tissue should always undergo immediate frozen-section analysis to confirm the diagnosis. If the clinical and radiographic diagnosis is confirmed by frozen-section analysis, the surgeon can often continue with the definitive procedure. In such cases, the surgeon must close the wound with an adhesive seal, redrape and

reprepare the surgical area, and change instruments and surgical attire. These precautions also apply when obtaining an autogenous bone graft for a benign tumor. Recently, the use of DNA ploidy measurements, as determined by flow cytometry, has proven to be of prognostic value in many types of cancer. The technique, which involves computer analysis of fluorescent signals from cell nuclei stained

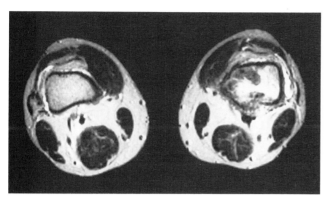

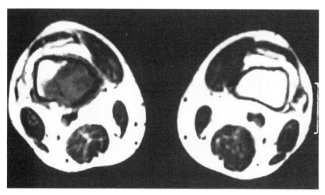

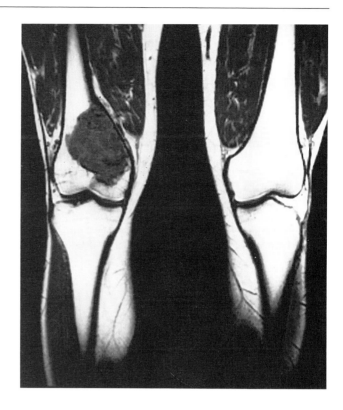

Figure 7

Magnetic resonance images of giant cell tumor shown in Figures 5 and 6. **Top left**, Axial T$_1$-weighted images show replacement of the marrow by a low-signal lesion but do not demonstrate the posterior cortical penetration as well as computed tomography does. **Bottom left**, Axial T$_2$-weighted images show a mixed-signal lesion corresponding to the anatomic area shown on the T$_1$-weighted images, but do not demonstrate cortical penetration. **Right**, Coronal T$_1$-weighted image shows excellent contrast between the low-signal tumor and the high-signal bone marrow.

with a DNA dye, yields an estimation of the number of cells in the various stages of the cell cycle. Tumors with higher DNA synthetic activity and those with aberrant concentrations of cellular DNA (termed DNA aneuploidy) are more likely to be of higher grade and to be more biologically aggressive than tumors with a cell cycle activity similar to that of normal resting cells. Several studies of bone and soft-tissue sarcomas have demostrated correlations between DNA ploidy and histologic grade and biologic behavior. Many centers are now using the technique as an adjunct to pathologic grading.

A closed biopsy yields a smaller sample. It may be performed in a radiology suite. Younger patients may require anesthesia. The accuracy of closed biopsy is greatest in homogeneous tumors, in infections, and in cases in which the diagnosis has been made radiographically. A closed biopsy is less accurate than open biopsy in primary bone tumors and in cases in which the diagnosis has not been made radiographically. Diagnosis in this instance requires expert and experienced pathologists and radiologists. A closed biopsy is preferred for tumors of the spine and pelvis and when the expected diagnosis is metastasis, infection, or round cell tumors. The surgeon who will perform the definitive procedure should perform the biopsy as well.

Magnetic Resonance Imaging of Musculoskeletal Tumors

In the past three to five years, a great deal of experience has been acquired with magnetic resonance imaging, so

that it is now possible to compare this method of imaging musculoskeletal neoplasms with computed tomography. One should bear in mind, however, that neither magnetic resonance imaging nor computed tomography provides diagnostic images of bone tumors as good as those obtained with plain radiographs.

Comparison of Magnetic Resonance Imaging and Computed Tomography

Some investigations have compared the efficacy of magnetic resonance imaging with that of computed tomography for bone and soft-tissue tumors.

For benign (Figs. 5 to 7) or malignant (Figs. 8 to 16) tumors of bone, magnetic resonance imaging is superior to computed tomography for visualization or detection of (1) extraosseous extension (Figs. 15 and 16), (2) intraosseous extension of the tumor (Figs. 7, *right*, 12, and 16), (3) joint involvement, (4) skip metastases, and (5) epiphyseal extension (Fig. 16). Also, in the presence of nonferromagnetic metal, the images do not become degraded as much as do those of computed tomography. On the other hand, computed tomography, because it shows mineralization, is superior to magnetic resonance imaging for visualizing or detecting (1) subtle cortical destruction (Figs. 6, *bottom*, and 11, *top*), (2) subtle fracture, and (3) calcification or ossification (Figs. 9, *top* and *center*, and 14). Calcification and ossification are often of diagnostic importance in the detection of punctate calcifications in car-

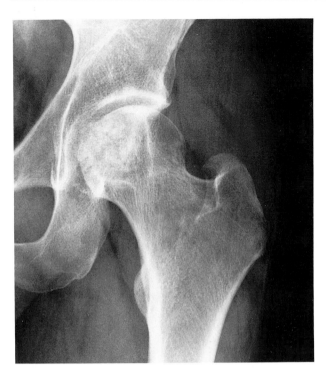
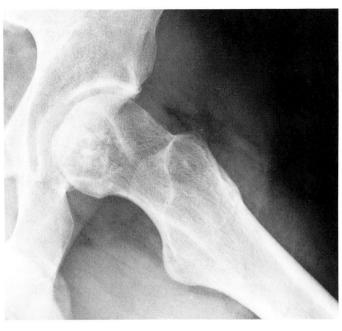

Figure 8

A clear-cell chondrosarcoma of the left femoral head in a 28-year-old man. Plain radiographs show a well-circumscribed lesion adjacent to the articular cartilage in the femoral head, with punctate mineralization within the lesion.

tilage lesions or of a thin rim of reactive bone surrounding an aneurysmal bone cyst. Some of the advantages of computed tomography also become apparent when a tomogram is compared with a plain radiograph (Figs. 8 and 13).

For soft-tissue masses (Figs. 17 and 18) and bone tumors with soft-tissue extension (Figs. 13 to 16), magnetic resonance imaging, because of its inherent superior image contrast, is preferable to computed tomography for delineation of such masses from muscle, vessels, nerves, fat, bone, and joints (Figs. 15 and 18). There is now little or no need for angiography to delineate vascular anatomy. Magnetic resonance imaging does not show mineralization in these masses, nor does it indicate cortical disruption by a bone tumor or by an extensive soft-tissue mass. However, it is superior to computed tomography in showing the relationship of a soft-tissue mass to the cortex of a bone. In all studies of soft-tissue tumors, magnetic resonance imaging is equal or superior to computed tomography in image quality, detection of the tumor, and clarity of boundaries.

In summary, because of its superb image quality, magnetic resonance imaging is excellent for delineating any soft-tissue extension of bone tumors, and it appears to be more useful than computed tomography for imaging of malignant bone tumors when anatomic delineation is of prime importance. Computed tomography still appears to be the equal of magnetic resonance imaging in demonstrating benign bone tumors and malignant bone tumors that are entirely intraosseous. For soft-tissue tumors, magnetic resonance imaging is superior to computed tomography in almost all respects and should replace computed tomography as the method of choice when information on the anatomy of a mass is desired. In future investigations,

magnetic resonance imaging technology may be used for specific diagnoses and for the prediction and definition of the response to chemotherapy and radiation therapy.

General Characteristics of Magnetic Resonance Imaging of Tumors

Two pulse sequences are necessary for tumor imaging: T_1-weighted images and T_2-weighted images. T_1-weighted images are better for showing normal anatomy; however, most tumors have the same low signal intensity as muscle, making it difficult to detect any soft-tissue extension of a bone tumor or a soft-tissue mass. On the other hand, on T_2-weighted images, the normal anatomy is somewhat degraded, but most soft-tissue masses have a high signal intensity compared with that of muscle, providing a remarkable contrast with respect to surrounding structures. Thus, in general, most musculoskeletal tumors have a low signal intensity (that is, they appear dark) on T_1-weighted images and a high signal intensity (that is, they appear light) on T_2-weighted images.

Another useful characteristic of magnetic resonance imaging is the ability to display longitudinal (coronal and sagittal) images in addition to axial images. Axial images are preferable for illustrating the relationship of a tumor to neurovascular and other soft-tissue structures. However, longitudinal imaging allows direct visualization of the medullary extent of a bone tumor and shows any invasion of joints by a musculoskeletal tumor.

Local Tumor Characteristics

Most tumors do not have any specific diagnostic characteristics on magnetic resonance imaging. However, there

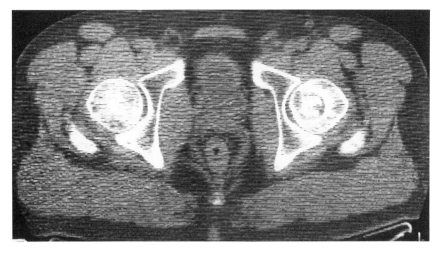

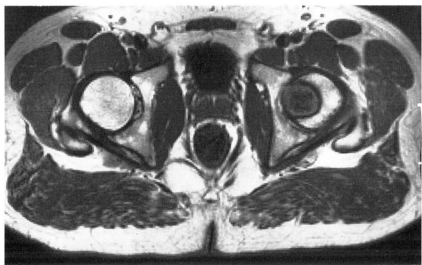

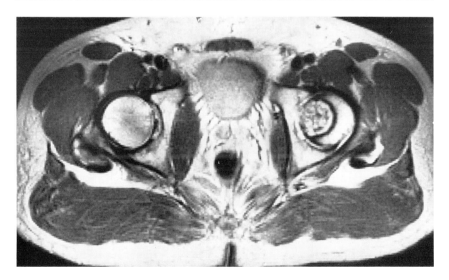

Figure 9

Same clear-cell chondrosarcoma shown in Figure 8. Computed tomogram (**top**) shows a well-demarcated lesion within the femoral head. The lesion is subarticular and exhibits marked mineralization. Axial T_1-weighted (**center**) and T_2-weighted (**bottom**) magnetic resonance images also show a well-circumscribed lesion but not the intralesional mineralization or the medial cortex of the femoral head adjacent to the lesion.

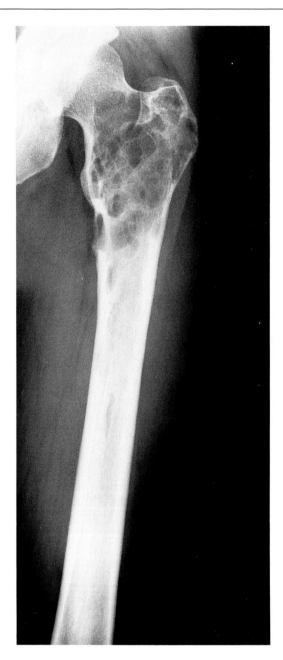

Figure 10

Extensive chondrosarcoma of the left proximal femur in a 30-year-old man. Plain radiograph shows a destructive lesion in the femoral neck and the intertrochanteric and subtrochanteric areas. Intralesional mineralization is not apparent, but the cortex seems to be violated in the subtrochanteric area. In addition, the lesion appears to extend along the diaphysis.

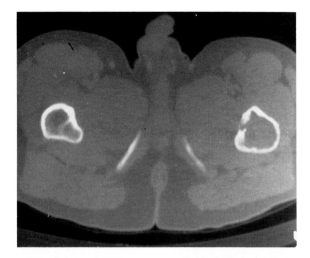

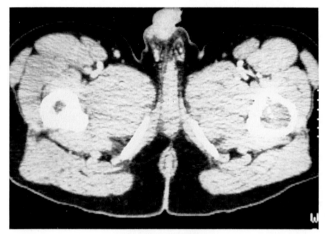

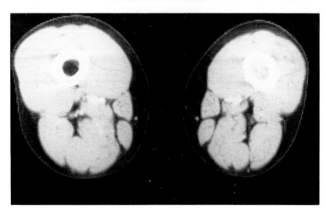

Figure 11

Computed tomograms of chondrosarcoma shown in Figure 10. **Top,** "Bone windows" confirm the cortical penetration in the subtrochanteric area. **Center,** "Soft-tissue windows" demonstrate mineralization in the subtrochanteric area, calling attention to the probable diagnosis of chondrosarcoma. **Bottom,** Tomogram of the distal diaphysis still shows bone marrow replacement by the lesion.

are some exceptions. Lipomas have high signal intensities on both T_1- and T_2-weighted images, whereas lesions that have a very high collagen content, such as those in aggressive fibromatosis or surgical scars, have low signal intensities on both T_1- and T_2-weighted images. Ossification and calcification are not visualized on magnetic resonance images. If a biopsy was performed more than six weeks before imaging, there is likely to be an abnormal low signal on both T_1- and T_2-weighted images, whereas if the biopsy was performed less than six weeks before the examination,

imaging will not differentiate residual tumor from the hematoma that follows the surgical procedure. Magnetic resonance imaging has also been shown to be unequaled in detecting local recurrences after surgical procedures. After surgery, abnormal low signal intensities on T_1- and T_2-

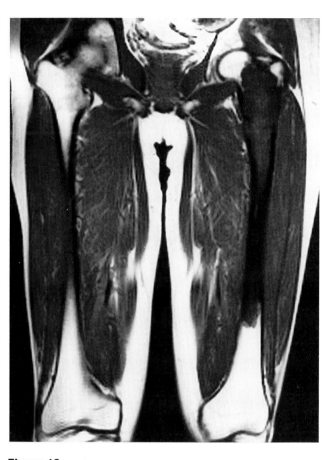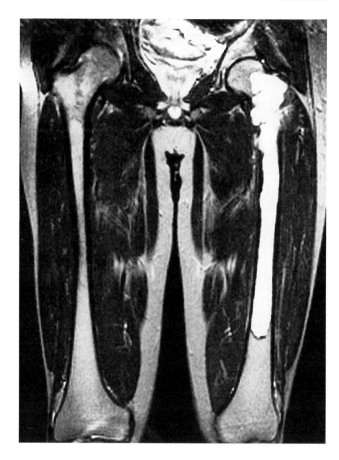

Figure 12

Magnetic resonance images of chondrosarcoma shown in Figures 10 and 11. Both T$_1$-weighted (**left**) and T$_2$-weighted (**right**) coronal images clearly show the intramedullary extent of the lesion from the femoral neck to the distal diaphysis.

weighted magnetic resonance images are not likely to represent tumor, but abnormal high signal intensities on T$_2$-weighted images may indicate a local recurrence. If a patient has undergone only radiation therapy and no surgery, a high signal intensity on T$_2$-weighted images is not diagnostic. The ability to detect a local recurrence on magnetic resonance images after a combination of surgery and radiation therapy has not been investigated adequately.

Recent hemorrhages, as well as hematomas and tumor necrosis, appear as areas of high signal intensity on both T$_1$- and T$_2$-weighted images. Similarly, heterogeneity of tumor images suggests necrosis and hemorrhage, which are characteristic of malignancy. Perineoplastic edema, which has a high signal intensity on T$_2$-weighted images, accompanies many malignant masses, but also surrounds inflammatory masses and some benign masses such as hemangiomas. Sharp margins can be visualized in both benign and malignant masses. Therefore, there are no generally reliable criteria for the diagnosis of malignant or benign bone or soft-tissue tumors by magnetic resonance imaging.

Magnetic resonance imaging is excellent for evaluating the intraosseous extent of a bone tumor and for detecting any extraosseous extensions through the cortex. However, because it does not "visualize" the cortex, subtle endosteal or periosteal erosion is not detected. For soft-tissue tumors and for the soft-tissue extension of bone tumors, magnetic resonance imaging is a superior method of delineating the lesion from the surrounding soft tissues.

Chemotherapy for Osteosarcoma

Adjuvant Chemotherapy

The rationale for adjuvant (postoperative) chemotherapy for patients with high-grade osteosarcoma was derived from the observation that about 80% of patients with no other known clinical disease died of metastases despite ablative surgery. It was assumed that these patients had subclinical pulmonary metastases at the time of surgery; therefore, it was proposed that cytotoxic agents would be most effective if administered before such metastases were detected clinically. The initial reports were optimistic but flawed by short follow-ups and the inclusion of variants of osteosarcoma that have favorable prognoses. Longer-term reports, however, substantiated an apparent favorable prognosis, with about 50% of patients alive and disease-free at five years.

However, in the late 1970s doubts about the efficacy of adjuvant chemotherapy were expressed by some investigators. They found similar 15-year survival rates when they compared patients treated with surgery and adjuvant chemotherapy with patients treated by surgery alone. The apparent improvement in the survival rate of patients treated with surgery alone may have been attributable in part to improved clinical staging by scintigraphy and computed tomography, earlier diagnosis, and the increased use of thoracotomy for lung metastases. These studies also cast

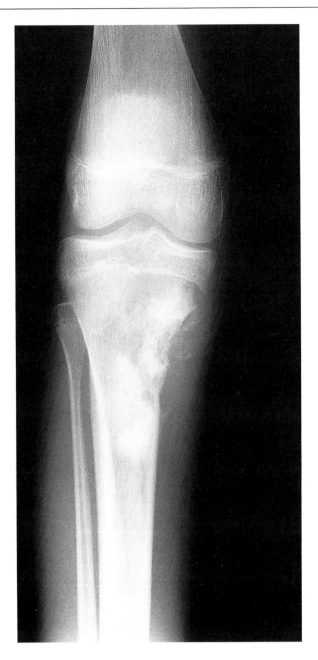 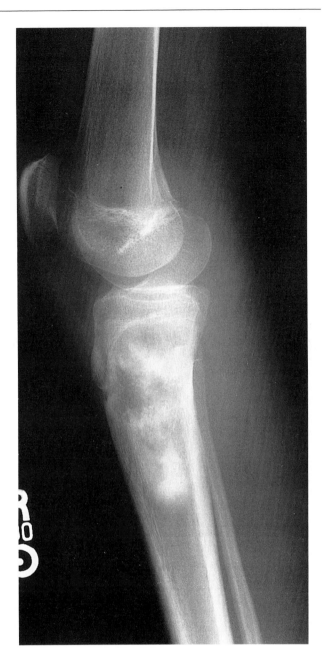

Figure 13

Osteosarcoma of the proximal right tibia in a 16-year-old boy. Plain radiographs show an ill-defined lesion in the metaphysis of the proximal tibia, extending medially into the soft tissues, with ossification within the lesion.

doubt on the validity of using historical controls for whom a 20% five-year disease-free survival rate after surgery alone was shown. Therefore, at the beginning of this decade, a demand arose for contemporary, randomized studies on the efficacy of adjuvant chemotherapy.

In a multi-institutional study and a single-institutional study, randomized, controlled trials were conducted in an effort to determine the role of adjuvant chemotherapy in improving the probability of disease-free survival of patients with nonmetastatic high-grade osteosarcoma of the limbs. Both studies confirmed that adjuvant chemotherapy had a significant positive impact on disease-free survival. The drugs found to be most effective for osteosarcoma were doxorubicin, high-dose methotrexate with leucovorin res-

cue, cis-platinum, and possibly ifosfamide. In these studies, the control groups had a disease-free survival rate of only about 20%, confirming the validity of the historical observations of the previous decade.

Neoadjuvant Chemotherapy

At the same time, some investigators were using chemotherapy both before (neoadjuvant chemotherapy) and after the surgical removal of the primary tumor. The projected disease-free survival rates of 70% to 80% were even higher than those obtained with adjuvant chemotherapy alone. After surgery, the excised specimen was graded pathologically for tumor necrosis, and the postoperative chemo-

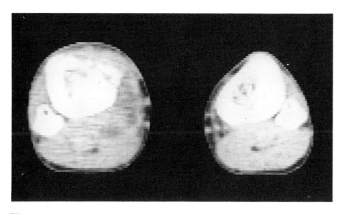
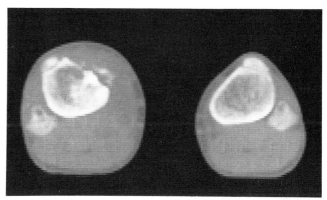

Figure 14

Computed tomograms of the osteosarcoma shown in Figure 13 demonstrate a destructive lesion with soft-tissue ossification. The soft-tissue mass is, however, poorly defined.

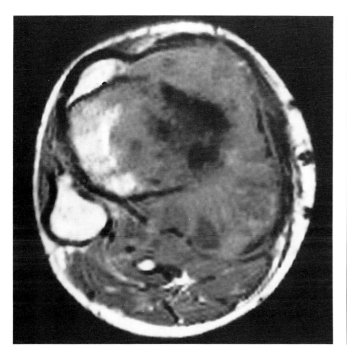
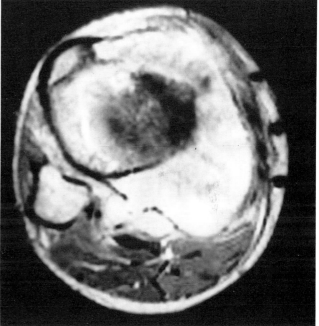

Figure 15

Magnetic resonance images of the osteosarcoma shown in Figures 13 and 14. Axial T_1-weighted (**left**) and T_2-weighted (**right**) images demonstrate the soft-tissue mass and its relationship to the neurovascular structures much better than does computed tomography. Note the diffuse high-signal edema about the lateral tibia on the T_2-weighted image.

therapy regimen was based on the histologic response of the tumor to drugs. "Responders" underwent a regimen similar to that used before surgery, and "nonresponders" underwent an alternate program. The adjustment of chemotherapy regimens on the basis of tumor response to neoadjuvant chemotherapy is called "tailored therapy."

There are several possible justifications for the use of neoadjuvant chemotherapy for patients with osteosarcoma. The most important is the commencement of systemic treatment without delay so that micrometastases, which have rapid doubling times, do not enlarge, or so that spontaneous mutations that may be drug-resistant do not occur while the patient is recovering from the surgery. Neoadjuvant chemotherapy also facilitates limb-salvage

surgery. With effective therapy, perineoplastic vascularity and edema almost always resolve, making diagnostic imaging and surgery more accurate. During the period of neoadjuvant chemotherapy, the surgeon has time for careful planning of a limb-salvage procedure and for ordering custom-made devices, implants, or allografts. Also, it appears that chemotherapy allows closer surgical margins than were previously considered advisable. A third justification for neoadjuvant chemotherapy is that it may be possible to measure the effectiveness of a given type of regimen against the primary or metastatic tumor in vivo, allowing different risk groups to be identified and an appropriate postoperative chemotherapeutic regimen (that is, tailored therapy) to be designed. Some studies have con-

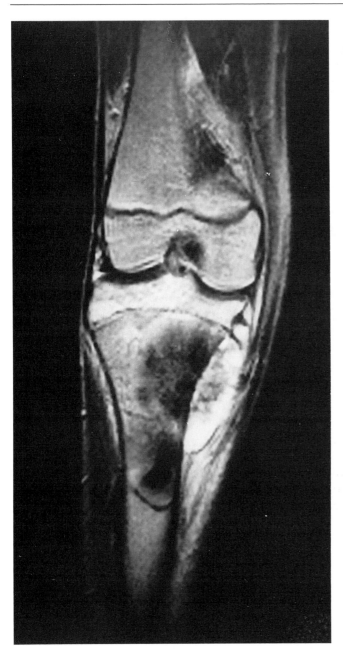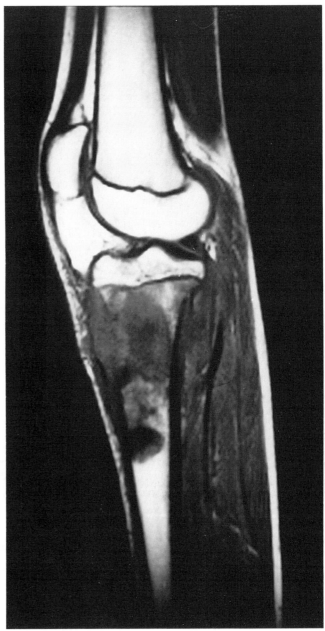

Figure 16

Magnetic resonance images of the osteosarcoma shown in Figures 13 to 15. Sagittal T$_1$-weighted (**left**) and T$_2$-weighted (**right**) images show the soft-tissue and intraosseous extent of the sarcoma. The epiphysis does not appear to be involved.

firmed that patients who respond well to neoadjuvant chemotherapy have a better probability of disease-free survival than do those who respond poorly. However, it is not known whether good responders do well because of or despite neoadjuvant chemotherapy, that is, whether the administration of neoadjuvant chemotherapy merely identifies patients with a good prognosis. In addition, it has not been established that switching therapy improves the disease-free survival of nonresponders.

A secondary advantage of neoadjuvant chemotherapy is that the entire treatment program requires the close collaboration of many specialists, enhancing the coordination of care and compliance by the patient. The patient, there-

fore, is likely to be treated by a team of experienced physicians, providing an opportunity for full discussion of the treatment plan by everyone concerned before therapy is instituted. During neoadjuvant chemotherapy, patients and their families have time to adjust psychologically to the disease and to discuss the proposed surgery; this allows the patients to make the adjustments necessary for postoperative rehabilitation.

Neoadjuvant chemotherapy for osteosarcoma appears to compare favorably with standard adjuvant chemotherapy with respect to survival. Neoadjuvant chemotherapeutic agents for osteosarcoma can be administered by intravenous or intra-arterial routes. Intravenous neoadjuvant

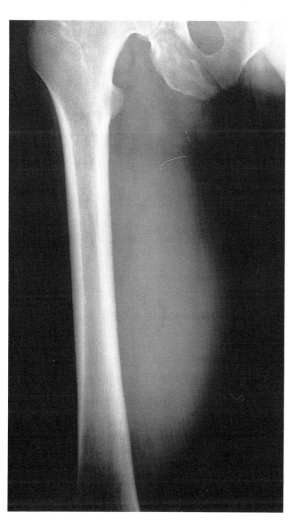
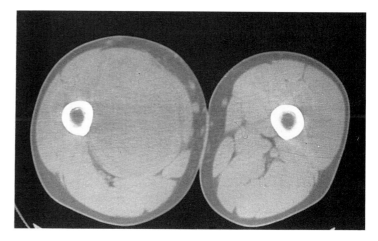
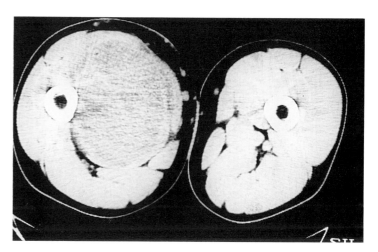

Figure 17

A large myxoid liposarcoma of the thigh in a 26-year-old man. **Left**, Plain radiograph shows a large medial water-density mass and a normal femur. **Top right** and **bottom right**, Computed tomograms of the thigh show an ill-defined soft-tissue mass in the medial quadriceps muscle.

chemotherapy may result in better rates of survival, whereas intra-arterial neoadjuvant chemotherapy may have advantages for potential candidates for limb-salvage procedures. Intra-arterial chemotherapy requires longer periods of hospitalization and expert interventional radiology. The extent of tumor necrosis induced by intra-arterial chemotherapy may not be as sensitive a prognostic indicator as is the extent of necrosis after intravenous chemotherapy.

Chemotherapy in conjunction with surgery is presently the standard treatment for conventional high-grade osteosarcoma. Most centers are now administering neoadjuvant chemotherapy and, except in a few instances, are using intravenous rather than intra-arterial routes. The efficacy of tailored chemotherapy regimens has not yet been proved, and why responders to chemotherapy have a good prognosis is unknown.

Limb Salvage in the Treatment of Sarcomas of Bone

For sarcomas of bone, surgical resection remains a required procedure. In the past, surgeons commonly performed am-

putations to attain this goal. In the last decade, however, interest in limb-salvage surgery has increased, and limb-salvage procedures have become an attractive alternative to amputation. Better diagnostic imaging methods, advances in adjunctive therapy, and innovative techniques for reconstruction of limbs have all increased the interest in limb preservation. If limb salvage is to be considered for a patient with a sarcoma of bone, it is obvious that (1) the oncologic result should not be compromised significantly and (2) the reconstruction should result in an extremity that functions better than it would after amputation.

Recently, it has been shown that there is no significant decrease in the rate of long-term survival when limb salvage instead of amputation is used for local control of osteosarcoma of the distal femur. Earlier diagnosis, adjunctive chemotherapy, surgical resection of pulmonary metastases, and better imaging techniques probably all play a role in the increased rate of survival. The technique of resection, with a wide margin and with planning by preoperative imaging, has become standardized and varies only with the site of the tumor. In addition, the prognosis

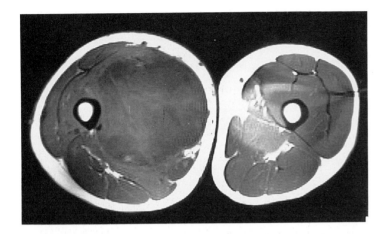

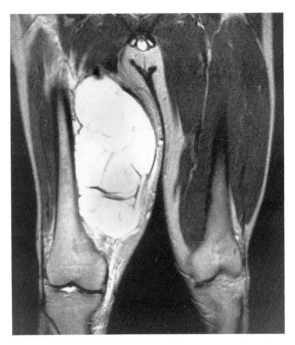

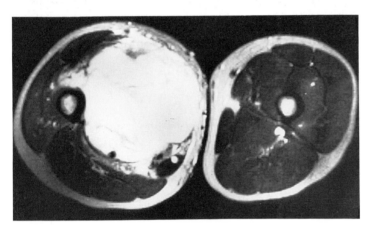

Figure 18

Magnetic resonance images of the myxoid liposarcoma shown in Figure 17. Axial T_1-weighted (**top left**) and T_2-weighted (**bottom left**) images show a large mass adjacent to the femur and encasing the superficial femoral artery. These images provide anatomic detail much superior to that of the computed tomograms. On the T_2-weighted image, note the diffuse, high-signal edema around the tumor, about the anterior femur, and posterior and medial to the superficial femoral artery. A coronal T_2-weighted image (**right**) shows a large high-signal mass adjacent to the femur.

for local control, based on the location, type, and size of the tumor, can be determined accurately. At present, there are many reconstructive techniques for various tumor locations; however, which technique is the "best" is unknown and remains a challenge for the future.

Indications and Preoperative Evaluation

If limb salvage is to be an attractive alternative to ablative surgery for a sarcoma of bone, the tumor must be in an anatomic location that allows for complete resection with wide surgical margins. For some tumors, such as osteosarcoma and Ewing's sarcoma, it is probably advisable for the patient to undergo neoadjuvant chemotherapy. After resection, it should be possible to carry out a reconstruction to provide limb function superior to the function obtained with a prosthetic device. If the extraosseous soft-tissue component of the lesion involves neurovascular structures vital to limb function, or if a wide surgical margin cannot be achieved and the remaining limb will not be functional after reconstruction, limb salvage surgery is contraindicated (Fig. 19).

Relative contraindications to limb-salvage surgery include a pathologic fracture and, possibly, skeletal imma-

turity. A pathologic fracture may spread the tumor through the fracture hematoma, beyond normal anatomic barriers, and make it extremely difficult for the surgeon to perform an appropriately wide resection. The presence of regional or distant metastases confers a poor prognosis. However, with currently available chemotherapy regimens and with resection of pulmonary metastases, it is possible for patients with distant metastases to undergo limb salvage and to expect reasonably good long-term survival rates. If a tumor in the lower extremity can be resected with a wide margin, without sacrifice of growth plates, skeletal immaturity is not a contraindication to limb salvage; however, if growth plates must be sacrificed, the resultant limb-length inequality imposes a possible contraindication for limb salvage. Recently, rotationplasty and the use of an expanding metallic prosthesis after limb-salvage surgery have been considered as alternatives to amputation in skeletally immature individuals. Thus, the ideal candidate for limb-salvage surgery is a skeletally mature individual who has an intraosseous tumor with little or no soft-tissue extension, and no pathologic fracture.

Before limb-salvage surgery for local control of a sarcoma of bone, various imaging techniques are employed to evaluate the extent of local disease and the presence or

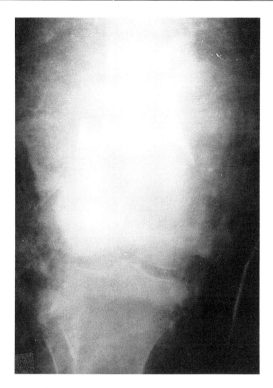

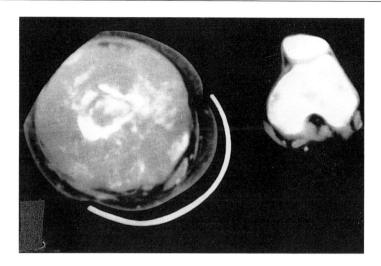

Figure 19

Osteosarcoma of the right distal femur with a pathologic fracture. **Left**, Anteroposterior radiographs show that the lesion is heavily ossified with an extensive soft-tissue mass. **Right**, Computed tomogram through the distal femur demonstrates the destructive lesion with cortical fracture and extensive soft-tissue mass. The femoral vessels and sciatic nerve cannot be distinguished; they are encased in the soft-tissue mass.

Intercalary   Intraarticular   Extraarticular

Figure 20

The three basic types of osseous resections for sarcomas of bone.

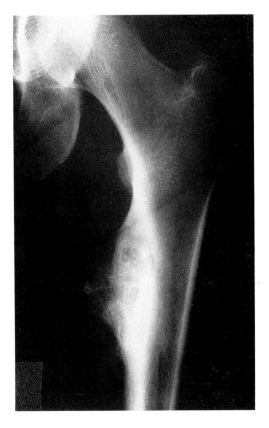 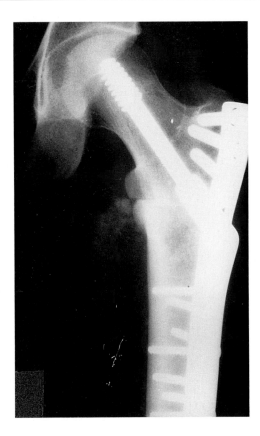 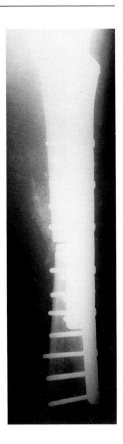

Figure 21

Periosteal mesenchymal chondrosarcoma. **Left**, Anteroposterior radiograph of the proximal femur. **Center** and **right**, Radiographs of the femur after resection and whole-segment allograft replacement with multiple plates and screws and autogenous junctional bone grafting.

absence of distant metastases. Imaging is routinely used before biopsy and then repeated after the completion of neoadjuvant chemotherapy, before the definitive resection and reconstruction. Routine imaging procedures include conventional radiography of the involved limb, chest radiography, technetium bone scintigraphy, computed tomography of the involved limb and chest, and magnetic resonance imaging of the limb. Plain radiographs are helpful in the formulation of the initial differential diagnosis and in showing the general location of the tumor. Technetium bone scintigraphy is used to detect skeletal metastases and "skip" lesions. The extent of local disease and the adjacent anatomic structures are defined by both computed tomography and magnetic resonance imaging of the involved limb. The matrix of the tumor and the fine structural anatomic details of cortical bone are best demonstrated by computed tomography, whereas the sagittal and frontal images provided by magnetic resonance imaging are most useful in showing the intraosseous proximal and distal extent of the tumor. Axial magnetic resonance images are the best means of defining local anatomy and soft-tissue extension of a bone sarcoma. Chest radiographs may detect pulmonary metastases, but computed tomography of the chest is more sensitive in detecting such metastases.

Surgical Technique and Reconstructive Alternatives

In most cases, limb salvage requires that the bone tumor, along with a surrounding cuff of normal tissue, be surgically resected en bloc. Infrequently, the sarcoma involves an expendable bone (that is, the fibula or clavicle), and all that is necessary is the resection of this bone. More commonly, reconstruction of both osseous and soft tissues is required. In most cases, a large weightbearing joint is sacrificed and must be reconstructed.

Usually, an incisional biopsy is performed before the definitive resection. Because the biopsy tract is likely to be contaminated with tumor cells, it should be excised en bloc with a margin of normal tissue, in such a way that the biopsy tract remains in continuity with the resected surgical specimen.

Skin incisions are planned so that they allow access to major neurovascular structures and include the biopsy tract. After skin flaps are created, the neurovascular structures are isolated and carefully dissected away from the region to be excised. The remaining dissection is carried out through normal tissue well beyond the reactive zone of the tumor.

Although preoperative imaging may assist the surgeon, the optimal size of the soft-tissue cuff and its distance from the tumor are generally unknown. The size of the soft-tissue cuff should be increased over any area where extraosseous tumor is present. After the soft-tissue dissection, the level of osseous resection proximal and distal to the tumor must be selected on the basis of calculations from the computed tomograph or magnetic resonance image, by means of a known landmark such as a joint.

Three basic types of osseous resection are used: inter-

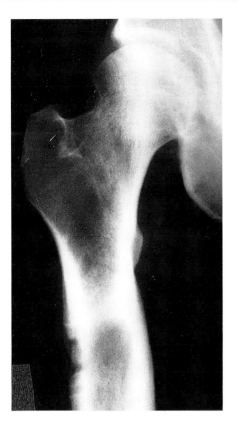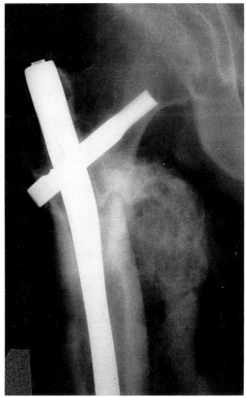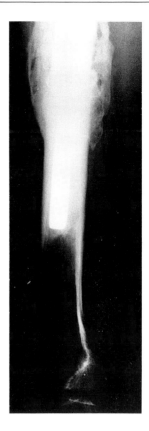

Figure 22

Chondrosarcoma. **Left**, Anteroposterior radiograph of the proximal femur shows involvement of the proximal femoral diaphysis. **Center** and **right**, Radiographs of the femur after resection and reconstruction with the resected segment, which has been autoclaved and fixed with a Zickel intramedullary nail with the addition of autogenous cancellous bone grafts.

calary (between joints), intra-articular (involving one side of a joint), and extra-articular (involving both sides of a joint) (Fig. 20).

For most diaphyseal lesions, an intercalary resection is performed by creation of an osteotomy above and below the tumor. In this procedure, both the proximal and the distal areas of the joint are spared. Most tumors involve the metaphysis, however, and occasionally some invade the joint. For a metaphyseal tumor, an osteotomy is created in the diaphysis proximal or distal to the joint, depending on the location of the tumor. The surgeon then performs either an intra-articular or an extra-articular resection. The acceptable margin of osseous tissue is unknown; a 4-cm margin of normal osseous tissue included in the specimen is considered adequate. When a tumor has invaded a joint, an extra-articular resection is necessary; however, for a tumor in a metaphysis, an intra-articular resection is all that is necessary in most cases. After the osteotomy, the specimen is dissected circumferentially with the soft-tissue cuff, and an intercalary, intra-articular, or extra-articular resection completed. Frozen sections can be obtained from the remaining soft-tissue and bone marrow margins to confirm that the margin is free of tumor cells.

Many options and techniques are available for the reconstruction of a large osseous deficit after resection of a sarcoma of bone. Whether the extremity is weightbearing, whether a joint must be sacrificed, and the size of the resection all have implications for the reconstructive options available. It is relatively simple to reconstruct the skeletal defect after an intercalary resection. Options include (1) a custom segmental metallic device with a porous ingrowth surface, which is bone-grafted with either autogenous or allograft cancellous bone; (2) a matched whole-segment allograft cylinder fixed either with plates and screws or with an intermedullary rod (Fig. 21); and (3) reimplantation of an autoclaved autogenous segment of bone (Fig. 22). This option involves removal of soft tissues from the specimen, autoclaving to eradicate the sarcomatous area, and then reimplanting the resected segment. This procedure is reported to be indicated for small, low-grade chondrosarcomas without extensive bone destruction.

Lesions that involve the metaphysis require not only replacement of a segment of bone but also reconstruction or arthrodesis of the involved joint. When an intra-articular resection is performed, the options for reconstruction include (1) a custom-made segmental total-joint replacement (Fig. 23); (2) a whole-segment osteoarticular allograft (Fig. 24); (3) an arthrodesis in which a bone graft (either autogenous or a whole-segment allograft) is used (Figs. 25 and 26) or a custom segmental metal device with an ingrowth surface and bone grafting is applied; (4) a composite consisting of an allograft and a conventional or custom total joint replacement (Figs. 27 to 29); (5) an autoclaved autogenous segment used as a composite with a total joint replacement, also indicated only for a small, low-grade chondrosarcoma; and (6) if the patient is skeletally immature, rotationplasty (Fig. 30) or an expanding prosthesis (Fig. 31). When an extra-articular resection is necessary,

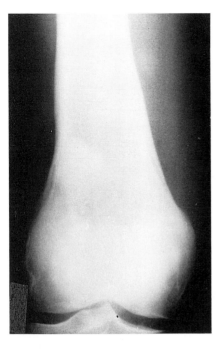
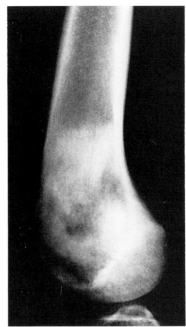
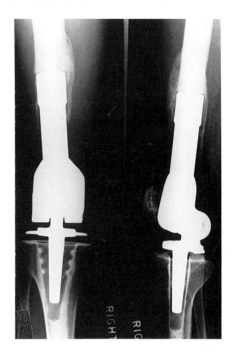

Figure 23

Osteosarcoma. **Left** and **center**, Anteroposterior and lateral radiographs of the right distal femur. **Right**, Anteroposterior and lateral radiographs after resection and replacement with a custom segmental total knee replacement. Extramedullary fixation by porous ingrowth is determined best on the medial and lateral cortex, which received an autogenous graft.

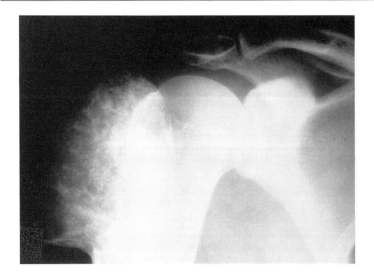
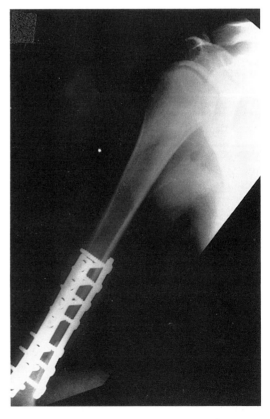

Figure 24

Large exophytic chondrosarcoma secondary to enchondromatosis (Ollier's disease). **Left**, Anteroposterior radiograph of the proximal humerus. **Right**, Radiograph of the humerus after resection and reconstruction with an osteoarticular allograft.

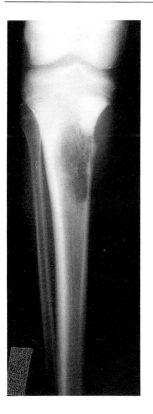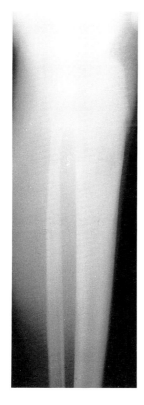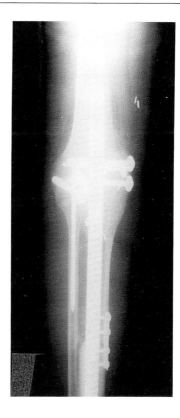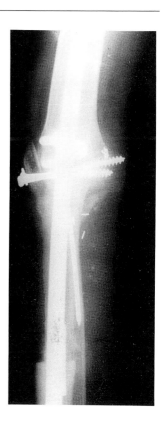

Figure 25

Osteosarcoma. **Left** and **left center**, Anteroposterior and lateral radiographs of the right proximal tibia. **Right center** and **right**, Anteroposterior and lateral radiographs after resection and reconstruction by arthrodesis with local autogenous bone grafting and an intramedullary rod for fixation. The patella was fixed as a bone graft with 6.5-mm AO cancellous screws; a small plate provides rotational control at the distal junction.

the practical options for reconstruction include an arthrodesis for the hip, knee, or shoulder (Fig. 32).

At present, the best technique for reconstruction, the best material for bridging of gaps or reconstruction of joints, and the type of bone graft or the method of fixation of either large segments of bone or prosthetic devices all remain controversial. Variables such as location of the tumor, the patient's preference, and the surgeon's experience play a role in the decision as to which reconstruction technique is used for a particular sarcoma of bone. Intercalary reconstructions are technically easier to perform and are probably more durable. If a joint is involved, an arthrodesis is the most durable type of reconstruction, provided that the patient is willing to accept decreased function.

The use of large-segment allografts for reconstruction in limb-salvage procedures has become increasingly popular. Allografts can be used as intercalary cylinders, to bridge a large gap when an arthrodesis is performed, or to serve as an osteoarticular replacement. When an osteoarticular replacement is required, an allograft can be used with or without a surface replacement total joint. The advantages of allografts include the absence of donor site morbidity, the ability to provide an accurately sized and shaped graft to fit the defect that has been created, and the ability to attach various muscle tendon units and ligaments. Disadvantages include limited availability, prolonged healing times, the potential transfer of disease, the possibility of rejection, and the occurrence of stress fractures. In addition, infection rates of 10% to 15% have been reported.

In some situations osseous reconstruction must be fol-

lowed by reconstruction of soft tissues. If joint function has been preserved, it may be necessary to reattach important muscle-tendon complexes or to do muscle transfers. When whole-segment allografts are used, the attachment of muscle-tendon complexes functions better than is the case when a joint has been replaced totally by metallic devices. The second stage of soft-tissue reconstruction involves covering of the skeletal reconstruction. Local muscle transposition flaps with or without split-thickness skin grafts should be used whenever there is any doubt about skin viability. The medial or lateral gastrocnemius flap has been used successfully after surgery for tumors around the knee and tibia.

Results of Limb Salvage

For limb-salvage surgery to be successful, the oncologic result must not be compromised, and the ultimate reconstruction should provide greater function than is achieved with an appropriate level of ablation. In addition, the patient and the surgeon must be willing to accept a high complication rate and the possibility of several secondary surgical procedures, both early and delayed. Factors such as long operating times, lengthy anesthesia, extensive blood loss, and technically difficult reconstructions all increase the number of complications compared with amputation. Early complication rates for limb-salvage surgery have been estimated to be between 20% and 35%. As many as one third of limb-salvage patients have early complications that require one or more additional surgical procedures.

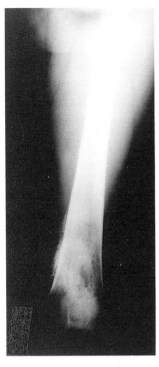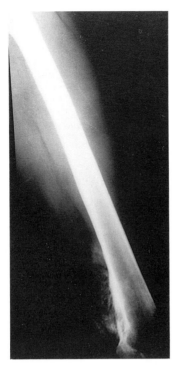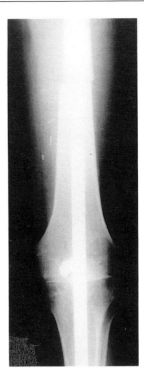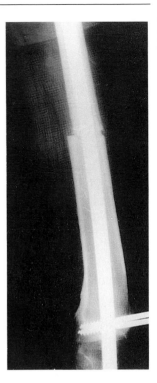

Figure 26

Parosteal osteosarcoma. **Left** and **left center**, Anteroposterior and lateral radiographs of the left distal femur. **Right center** and **right**, Anteroposterior and lateral radiographs after resection and reconstruction by arthrodesis with a whole-segment allograft and intramedullary rod fixation. The patella was fixed with two 6.5-mm AO spongiosis screws.

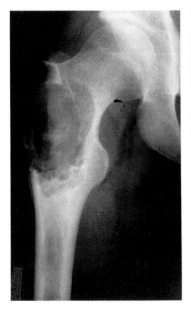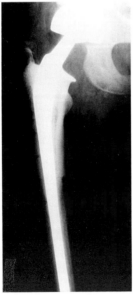

Figure 27

Chondrosarcoma. **Left**, Anteroposterior radiograph of the proximal femur. **Right**, Anteroposterior radiograph after resection and reconstruction with hemiarthroplasty using an allograft-prosthesis composite.

In addition, a number of patients may later have to undergo amputation because of a complication or a local recurrence.

When limb salvage instead of amputation is considered for sarcomas of the extremity, the following variables must be evaluated: (1) the oncologic result (survival), (2) the expected function of the involved extremity, (3) the psychosocial benefit for the patient, and (4) the possibility of early and delayed morbidity.

Long-term survival rates for patients with osteosarcoma treated by either limb salvage or amputation vary between 40% and 70% at five years. For osteosarcoma of the distal femur, there appears to be no difference between limb salvage and amputation with regard to the survival rate, provided that the limb salvage is performed by experienced surgeons using wide margins and provided that the patient receives adjunctive chemotherapy. The local recurrence rate for osteosarcoma in patients who underwent limb-salvage surgery is 5% to 10%. In some cases, this reflects the aggressiveness of the tumor and is not a result of the limb salvage. Amputation would eliminate local recurrences, but many patients would still die of disseminated disease. Therefore, there appears to be no statistically significant difference in survival rates for limb-salvage procedures and amputation for sarcomas of bone.

Because of the diversity of tumor locations and the types of reconstruction employed, it is difficult to evaluate limb function after limb-salvage surgery. Weightbearing in the lower extremity and fine motor function in the upper extremity should be used in the comparisons. There is no doubt that a resection of the proximal humerus with any type of reconstruction provides better function than does

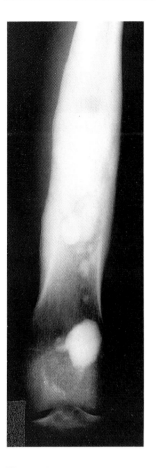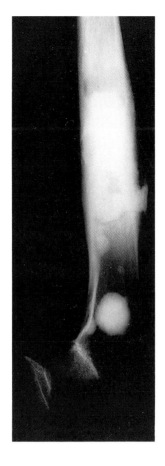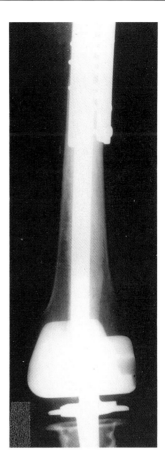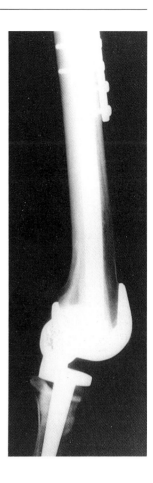

Figure 28
Osteosarcoma with a digital "skip." **Left** and **left center**, Anteroposterior and lateral radiographs of the left distal femur. **Right center** and **right**, Anteroposterior and lateral radiographs after resection and reconstruction wih a custom, prosthesis-allograft composite, rotating-hinge, total knee replacement.

a forequarter amputation. In addition, reconstructions for sarcomas in the proximal femur or for local pelvic resections provide function superior to that after hemipelvectomy. For sarcomas involving the tibia and foot, however, amputation generally provides better function than can be achieved with comparative limb-salvage procedures.

In a recent study in which oxygen consumption was used as a means of judging function after limb salvage or amputation, patients with a resection and total joint replacement of the knee for osteosarcoma of the distal femur or proximal tibia were found to expend less energy during gait than did patients with an above-the-knee amputation. In addition, it has been shown that young patients with rotationplasty maintain walking speeds comparable to those of normal children. In general, function after surgery for tumors about the knee probably is better with limb salvage than with amputation, and the reconstructions which yield the greatest function are mobile knee replacements of some type.

In most cases, patients, their families, and physicians consider it best from a psychosocial standpoint to avoid amputation in the treatment of sarcomas of bone. However, two recent publications showed no benefit of limb salvage over amputation with respect to the patients' quality of life or psychosocial adaptation. Although these studies were done on patients with sarcomas of the lower extremity only, it seems that a patient with no previous psychological disorder will adjust well after surgery regardless of whether it is limb salvage or amputation.

The morbidity associated with limb-salvage surgery may be significant. Early complication rates may be as high as 30%. Perioperative complications include fracture, cortical penetration by intramedullary devices, cement extrusion, skin necrosis, infection, arterial or venous occlusion, neuropraxia, and dislocation. Most of these early complications seem to be related to technical problems involving soft tissues. With greater experience and, ultimately, a shortened operating time, less blood loss, less soft-tissue trauma, and fewer technical complications, this high overall complication rate should decrease. The use of prophylactic muscle transposition flaps has helped eliminate the skin necrosis that often leads to deep infection.

The delayed complications of limb-salvage surgery are related primarily to problems with the durability of the chosen reconstruction and to local recurrences. Problems such as joint dysfunction (weakness and decreased range of motion), nonunions of osseous junctions, stress fractures of large-segment bone grafts or metallic implants, failure of fixation of prosthetic devices, and bone graft atrophy are possible after these reconstructions. Although the local recurrence rate may continue to decrease with better preoperative staging techniques and greater expertise with the

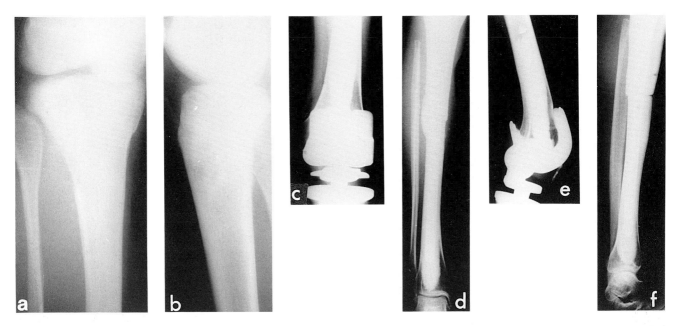

Figure 29

Osteosarcoma. **a** and **b**, Anteroposterior and lateral radiographs of the proximal tibia. **c** to **f**, Anteroposterior and lateral radiographs of the proximal tibia and distal femur after resection and reconstruction with a custom, prosthesis-allograft composite, rotating-hinge, total knee replacement.

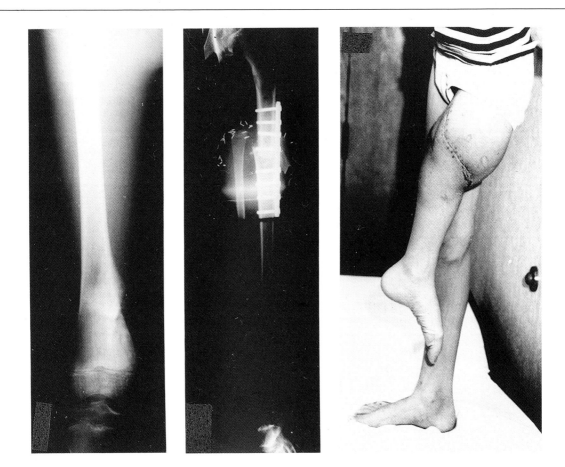

Figure 30

Osteosarcoma. **Left**, Anterior radiograph of the distal femur. **Center**, Anteroposterior radiograph after resection and reconstruction by rotationplasty. **Right**, In rotationplasty, the ankle is used as a functional knee joint.

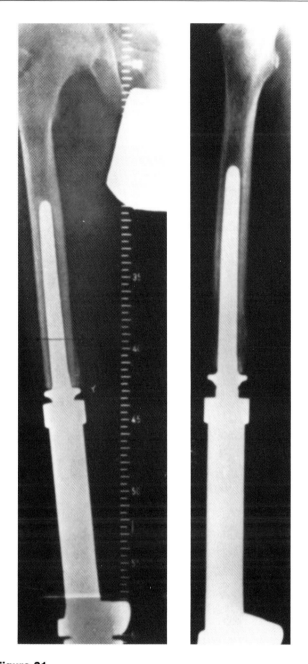

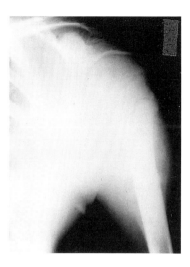

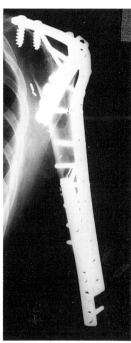

Figure 32

Osteosarcoma. **Left,** Anteroposterior radiograph of the left proximal humerus. **Right,** Anteroposterior radiograph after resection and reconstruction by an arthrodesis with a whole-segment allograft.

Figure 31

Expanding total knee replacement. **Left,** Anteroposterior radiograph of the right femur after resection of the distal portion and reconstruction. **Right,** Anteroposterior radiographs shows that the prosthesis has been lengthened by approximately 1 cm.

techniques of resection, the delayed complications of these skeletal reconstructions probably will increase as the survival time of the patients increases. At present, the optimal technique for any given tumor location is not yet known.

Advances in the Diagnosis and Treatment of Soft-Tissue Sarcomas in Adults

Immunohistochemistry of Soft-Tissue Tumors

Soft-tissue tumors are a heterogeneous group of tumors of widely varying histologic appearance. Difficulties are often encountered in the differential diagnosis, especially in the case of high-grade pleomorphic sarcomas. During the past five years, several immunologic markers for soft-tissue tumors have been identified, and antibodies have been prepared against them. The use of immunofluorescence techniques on frozen tissue is impractical because insufficient tissue is available and because morphologic detail is poor. Conversely, many antigenic sites are destroyed by the fixation and embedding procedures used in the preparation of paraffin-embedded specimens. Sections of formalin-fixed, paraffin-embedded tissues are used most frequently for the immunohistochemical detection of antigens in normal tissues and in tumors.

Three general markers are helpful in showing whether a tumor is a sarcoma, carcinoma, or lymphoma. Leukocyte common antigen is very specific and is restricted to the surface of cells of leukocyte lineage. This antigen is exceedingly helpful in distinguishing a lymphoma from a sarcoma or carcinoma. Cytokeratins are found in tumors of epithelial origin, but can be found in some sarcomas, such as synovial and epithelioid sarcomas. On the other hand, the intermediate filament vimentin is found in most mesenchymal tumors and in some carcinomas. Other antigens that are common only in soft-tissue tumors are desmin (skeletal and smooth-muscle tumors), factor VIII-associated antigen (benign and malignant vascular tumors), and S-100 protein (benign nerve sheath tumors, granular cell tumors, clear cell sarcomas, melanoma, and some malignant nerve tumors). Some of these antigens are also found in certain primary bone tumors. Algorithm 3 illustrates a schema for the use of these markers for soft-tissue tumors.

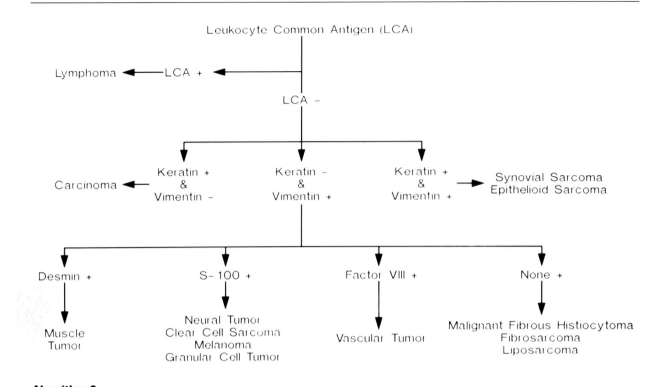

Algorithm 3
Schema for use of antigen markers in soft-tissue tumors.

Combined Surgery and Radiation Therapy

If the soft-tissue sarcoma is small, of low grade, and in a well-defined anatomic compartment or subcutaneous site, an adequate surgical margin can be achieved without amputation or radiation therapy, with preservation of excellent limb function. However, about one half of soft-tissue sarcomas in adults are in a deep extracompartmental location or are large intracompartmental tumors adjacent to major neurovascular or osseous structures. In these instances, the only traditional surgical therapy that provides adequate margins is an amputation. If amputation is to be avoided, adjuvant radiation therapy is necessary. Studies on the use of radiation therapy and conservative surgery in the 1980s have yielded results comparable to those of traditional surgery, that is, local recurrence rates were about 15% to 20%.

Radiation therapy has traditionally been administered after limited excision of a soft-tissue sarcoma in adults to kill the remaining microscopic areas of tumor adjacent to the surgical resection. The subclinical extensions of the tumor into the adjacent, grossly normal-appearing tissues are destroyed by moderate doses of radiation, making surgical removal of larger amounts of apparently normal tissue unnecessary. In the past decade, some reports on preoperative radiation therapy given alone or in combination with intra-arterial doxorubicin, a drug that acts as a radiation-therapy sensitizer, have been published. The proponents of preoperative radiation therapy contend that radiation kills or inactivates most of the tumor cells, thus decreasing the likelihood of intraoperative seeding or autotransplantation of the tumor. Also, irradiated cells shed into the circulation are less likely to establish distant metastases. Furthermore, if radiation is administered before definitive surgery, the volume to be treated is smaller. If radiation is administered after the surgical procedure, the radiation field must include all the areas that were manipulated at the time of surgery. These considerations are especially important when a large tumor is adjacent to a nonexpendable bone or a major neurovascular structure. In such instances, a conservative resection would probably cause contamination of the large surgical field. Preoperative radiation therapy could cause a large tumor to shrink, and the peripheral necrosis produced may allow the surgeon to resect the tumor without local seeding.

Preoperative radiation therapy, in particular, may lead to considerable morbidity because of difficult problems with the surgical wound. Dehiscence of the wound and severe fibrosis are especially troublesome when radiation therapy is combined with intra-arterial or intravenous doxorubicin. Preoperative radiation therapy demands meticulous technique by experienced radiation oncologists and surgeons so that morbidity is minimized.

At present, most patients with subcutaneous sarcomas or deep, small or moderate-sized sarcomas in well-defined compartments can undergo traditional surgery with wide or radical margins, with excellent preservation of function and without the need for adjuvant radiation therapy. Marginal resections combined with postoperative radiation therapy appear to be indicated for soft-tissue sarcomas for which wide or radical margins cannot be obtained without amputation. When the sarcoma is large and is located adjacent to a nonexpendable bone or a major neurovascular structure, preoperative radiation therapy may be indicated.

Adjuvant Chemotherapy for Adult Patients

High-grade soft-tissue sarcomas in adults have a moderate propensity to disseminate systemically. Approximately

60% of soft-tissue sarcomas occur in the extremities, and approximately 60% of these are cured by local management consisting of surgery or surgery combined with radiation. Regimens that include doxorubicin have been shown to have antitumor activity in patients with metastatic soft-tissue sarcomas. In the past few years, many investigations of adjuvant chemotherapy in high-grade soft-tissue sarcomas have yielded conflicting results. Differences in the primary site, histologic grading, chemotherapy regimens, and the time of initiation of the regimen make direct comparisons difficult.

Presently, no study supports the effectiveness of adjuvant chemotherapy in increasing long-term survival for sarcomas of soft tissue. The technical issues involved in achieving local control of sarcomas in the head, neck, trunk, viscera, and retroperitoneum make direct comparisons of these patients with patients who have limb sarcomas inadvisable. In future studies, histologic grading and histogenesis must be rigorously controlled. The designation of a tumor as a grade II tumor is often a compromise and is ambiguous. Nevertheless, some studies have included grade II tumors, obscuring the conclusions. In these studies, the chemotherapy regimens differed both in composition and in timing. Many regimens were applied only after conservative surgery and radiation therapy had been completed, often two to three months after the diagnosis. This can hardly be called adjuvant therapy because the patients received no systemic therapy during a significant period.

Possibly because of the drawbacks cited above and because of the small numbers of patients included in different randomized treatment plans, most studies on adjuvant chemotherapy do not show any significant gain in overall survival rates. However, a few investigators did find an increase in disease-free survival; that is, there appeared to be a significant delay in the appearance of metastases. In addition, there seems to be a trend toward a decreased local recurrence rate in those patients who undergo adjuvant chemotherapy.

Presently, there appears to be support for a national protocol in which large (more than 5 cm), high-grade (grade III) soft-tissue sarcomas in the limbs would be studied in a prospective randomized fashion. At present, however, no convincing evidence exists that adjuvant chemotherapy for adult soft-tissue sarcomas offers any benefits sufficient to offset the toxicity of the regimens.

Ewing's Sarcoma

The principles of diagnosis and treatment of this round cell sarcoma appeared in *Orthopaedic Knowledge Update*

2. Newer chemotherapeutic drugs, such as ifosamide and VP-16, appear to be effective, and several nonrandomized retrospective studies have indicated that surgical resection of the primary tumor may improve disease-free survival and decrease local recurrence. A prospective, randomized study is needed to directly compare irradiation and surgery in achieving local control of this tumor.

Trends

As we reach the last decade of the 20th century, advances in technical and biologic knowledge will continue to improve the outcomes for patients with sarcoma. It is difficult to foresee another spectacular breakthrough in tumor imaging such as magnetic resonance imaging. However, magnetic resonance technology will be refined in such a way that specific diagnoses and other biologic characteristics can be ascertained before biopsy and treatment.

New and more effective chemotherapeutic agents and biologic treatments will be found for sarcomas. More importantly, further investigation into the basic biologic characteristics of normal cells and of sarcomas by means of DNA and RNA probes will help us to understand chromosomal and oncogenic abnormalities at the molecular level.

Staging systems for bone and soft-tissue sarcomas will become more refined and reproducible. Treatment variables and patient characteristics will be integrated into staging systems that at present focus only on tumor characteristics.

More effective diagnostic methods involving monoclonal antibodies will reduce variability in the diagnosis, and will allow more succinct, reproducible clinical studies and assignment of patients to prognostic groups.

Improved techniques of radiation therapy should allow multimodality treatment with decreased morbidity. More studies of limb salvage that address limb function and psychosocial issues will be performed, so that surgeons can make more appropriate surgical decisions. Data on the advantages and disadvantages of prosthetic or allograft replacement of segmental defects after tumor resection will become available for each anatomic site and for similar diagnoses and stages, and thus appropriate comparisons will be feasible.

Lastly, more refined randomized and stratified studies of systemic and surgical treatments will be performed, allowing physicians to improve treatment strategies and outcomes for patients with sarcomas.

Annotated Bibliography

Keywords

Bone tumor; Chemotherapy; Computed tomography; Ewing's sarcoma; Limb-salvage surgery; Magnetic resonance imaging; Neoplasm staging; Osteosarcoma; Radiation therapy; Sarcoma; Scintigraphy; Soft-tissue tumor

Staging Systems for Malignant Tumors of the Musculoskeletal System

American Joint Commission on Cancer: Bone and soft tissues, in Beahrs OH, Myers MH (eds): *Manual for Staging of Cancer*, ed 3. Philadelphia, JB Lippincott, 1988, pp 123–131.

This manual outlines the staging systems of the American Joint Commission on Cancer for musculoskeletal neoplasms. Specifically, four stages with various subdivisions based on prognostic variables are listed for both bone and soft-tissue sarcomas.

Enneking WF, Spanier SS, Goodman MA: A system for the surgical staging of musculoskeletal sarcoma. *Clin Orthop* 1980;153:106–120.

The authors outline their system for the surgical staging of musculoskeletal sarcomas. They discuss the manner in which this system can be linked to the surgical strategy and to the management of such tumors of both bone and soft tissue, with prognostic correlation.

Finn HA, Simon MA, Martin WB, et al: Scintigraphy with gallium-67 citrate in staging of soft-tissue sarcomas of the extremity. *J Bone Joint Surg* 1987; 69A:886–891.

This retrospective study is a review of the utility of gallium citrate Ga 67 scintigraphy as a staging tool in the preoperative evaluation of a soft-tissue sarcoma of the extremity. Routine use of ^{67}Ga scintigraphy is recommended in the staging of soft-tissue sarcomas, particularly for detection of nonpulmonary metastases that would not be detected by other staging studies.

Biopsy of Musculoskeletal Lesions

Heare TC, Enneking WF, Heare MJ: Staging techniques and biopsy of bone tumors. *Orthop Clin North Am* 1989;20:273.

Principles of staging, biopsy, and formulating a treatment plan are discussed in this recent update by an experienced group of oncologic surgeons.

Matsuno T, Gebhardt MC, Schiller AL, et al: The use of flow cytometry as a diagnostic aid in the management of soft-tissue tumors. *J Bone Joint Surg* 1988;70A:751–759.

The authors compared histologic grading with DNA ploidy determinations by flow cytometry in 146 soft-tissue tumors. Flow cytometry appears to be a powerful research tool that in time may become a valuable adjunct to traditional assessment of the biologic aggressiveness of soft-tissue tumors.

Simon MA: Biopsy of musculoskeletal tumors. *J Bone Joint Surg* 1982;64A:1253–1257.

This is a review of current concepts concerning prebiopsy strategy, biopsy placement, closed and open biopsy techniques, and the utilization of tourniquets, frozen-section analysis, and immediate surgery.

Magnetic Resonance Imaging of Musculoskeletal Tumors

Beltran J, Simon DC, Katz W, et al: Increased MR signal intensity in skeletal muscle adjacent to malignant tumors: Pathologic correlation and clinical relevance. *Radiology* 1987;162:251–255.

In many cases of malignancy, inflammation, infection, or hematoma, increased signal intensity on T_2-weighted images is seen adjacent to the process, and biopsy of these areas reveals only edema. If the patient has not had a biopsy or radiation therapy and the mass is not inflammatory, this finding usually indicates malignancy. Alternatively, it may be difficult to determine the true anatomic extent of a sarcoma because of this phenomenon.

Pettersson H, Gillespy T III, Hamlin DJ, et al: Primary musculoskeletal tumors: Examination with MR imaging compared with conventional modalities. *Radiology* 1987;164:237–241.

For tumors confined to bone, magnetic resonance imaging was found to be equal to computed tomography for evaluation of the intraosseous extent, but inferior to computed tomography and plain radiographs for evaluation of calcification, ossification, cortical penetration, and endosteal or periosteal reaction. However, for soft-tissue tumors and bone tumors with extraosseous extension, magnetic resonance imaging was superior to all other modalities with regard to image contrast and delineation of the relationship of the tumor to muscle, vessels, fat, joints, and bones.

Sundaram M, McGuire MH, Schajowicz F: Soft-tissue masses: Histologic basis for decreased signal (short T2) on T2-weighted MR images. *AJR* 1987;148:1247–1250.

Soft-tissue masses usually have a low signal intensity on T_1-weighted images and a high signal intensity on T_2-weighted images. In seven cases in which the tumor had low signal intensity on both T_1- and T_2-weighted images, the tumors had high collagen content and low cellularity (for example, in fibromatosis).

Vanel D, Lacombe MJ, Couanet D, et al: Musculoskeletal tumors: Follow-up with MR imaging after treatment with surgery and radiation therapy. *Radiology* 1987;164:243–245.

If a high signal intensity is seen on T_2-weighted images after a patient has undergone surgery for a neoplasm, the patient is likely to have recurrent tumor. If only low signal intensity is found, it is probably caused by changes resulting from surgery. If the patient has undergone radiation therapy or if the surgery was recent, the value of magnetic resonance imaging for detection of residual tumor is limited.

Chemotherapy for Osteosarcoma

Goorin AM, Abelson HT, Frei E III: Osteosarcoma: Fifteen years later. *N Engl J Med* 1985;313:1637–1643.

An excellent review of the biology, natural history, evolution of treatment (drug and surgical), and current status of osteosarcoma.

Link MP, Goorin AM, Miser AW, et al: The effect of adjuvant chemotherapy on relapse-free survival in patients with osteosarcoma of the extremity. *N Engl J Med* 1986;314:1600–1606.

A randomized, controlled trial of intense multiagent adjuvant chemotherapy showed a significant difference in relapse-free survival between the adjuvant-chemotherapy group (66%) and a control group (17%). The natural course of the disease after surgery alone did not improve over that of the previous decade.

Simon MA, Nachman J: The clinical utility of preoperative therapy for sarcomas. *J Bone Joint Surg* 1986;68A:1458–1463.

The rationale for utilizing chemotherapy before definitive surgery (neoadjuvant chemotherapy) for osteosarcoma is reviewed. The three main advantages are treatment of micrometastases as soon as possible, facilitation of limb-salvage surgery, and identification of high-risk or low-risk groups by assessment of the histologic response of the tumor to chemotherapy.

Winkler K, Beron G, Delling G, et al: Neoadjuvant chemotherapy of osteosarcomas: Results of a randomized cooperative trial (COSS-82) with salvage chemotherapy based on histological tumor response. *J Clin Oncol* 1988;6:329–337.

After demonstrating previously that histologic assessment of tumor necrosis was predictive of disease-free survival after neoadjuvant chemotherapy in osteosarcoma, the authors undertook this study to determine whether less toxic chemotherapy could be administered preoperatively to some patients. The response rate in the control group (doxorubicin, cisplatin, methotrexate) was superior to that of the experimental group (methotrexate, bleomycin-cyclophosphamide-dactinomycin) (60% vs 26%; P <.001), suggesting that aggressive chemotherapy should be administered early in the course of treatment. Attempts with less toxic therapy are likely to be unsuccessful.

Limb Salvage in the Treatment of Sarcomas of Bone

Bos G, Sim F, Pritchard D, et al: Prosthetic replacement of the proximal humerus. *Clin Orthop* 1987;224:178–191.

The authors retrospectively reviewed 18 patients who underwent prosthetic proximal humeral replacement for either benign or malignant lesions. A high rate of complications and early failures was reported. The authors suggest that this procedure may be used as a first stage before an allograft arthrodesis, so that the effects on the allograft are avoided when a malignant tumor is treated with chemotherapy.

Lewis MM: The use of an expandable and adjustable prosthesis in the treatment of childhood malignant bone tumors of the extremity. *Cancer* 1986;57:499–502.

The author discusses the technique of using an expandable and adjustable prosthesis in treating malignant bone tumors in skeletally immature individuals. Six case reports are included. This procedure is an alternative to amputation in patients who meet the adult criteria for limb-sparing surgery and may be preferable to amputation for selected individuals.

Lord CF, Gebhardt MC, Tomford WW, et al: Infection in bone allografts: Incidence, nature, and treatment. *J Bone Joint Surg* 1988;70A:369–376.

This is a retrospective review of 283 patients who underwent massive allografts for aggressive benign tumors or sarcomas of bone or soft tissue. Postoperative infection occurred in 33 of these patients (11.7%). The risk of infection was not related to age, type of graft, anatomic site of the lesion, or the stage of the tumor. Gram-positive organisms were the most common cause of infection. In 27 of the 33 patients (82%), infection resulted in either amputation or removal of the graft.

Mankin HJ, Gebhardt MC, Tomford WW: The use of frozen cadaveric allografts in the management of patients with bone tumors of the extremities. *Orthop Clin North Am* 1987;18:275–289.

The limb was preserved and function restored in more than 70% of the 314 frozen osteoarticular and intercalary cadaveric allografts implanted since 1971 (primarily in patients with aggressive malignant tumors of bone). The procedure is, however, arduous and sometimes produces complications. The key to success is a high-quality procurement and banking program.

Murray MP, Jacobs PA, Gore DR, et al: Functional performance after tibial rotationplasty. *J Bone Joint Surg* 1985;67A:392–399.

In two children who underwent tibial rotationplasty for osteosarcoma of the distal end of the femur, muscle strength, joint motion, gait parameters, and electromyographic activity of the ankle and knee during walking, running, and stairclimbing were reviewed. Despite some abnormalities in gait, both children walked at speeds that were comparable to those of normal children. The functional results suggest that rotationplasty is a worthwhile alternative to an above-the-knee amputation for an osteosarcoma of the distal femur in skeletally immature individuals.

Office of Medical Applications of Research, National Institutes of Health, Consensus Conference: Limb-sparing treatment of adult soft-tissue sarcomas and osteosarcomas. *JAMA* 1985;254:1791–1794.

This is a summary of the National Institutes of Health 1984 consensus conference on limb-sparing treatment of soft-tissue sarcomas and osteosarcomas in adults. Limb salvage was reported to be feasible and appropriate for a significant proportion of high-grade extremity sarcomas. Optimal therapeutic strategies are described.

Sim FH, Beauchamp CP, Chao EY: Reconstruction of musculoskeletal defects about the knee for tumor. *Clin Orthop* 1987;221:188–201.

The authors studied 79 patients from 1970 to 1987 who underwent reconstruction of the knee after en bloc resection of a primary bone tumor. Results of reconstruction with custom total knee replacements, arthrodesis, and osteoarticular allograft were compared.

Simon MA: Current concepts review: Limb salvage for osteosarcoma. *J Bone Joint Surg* 1988;70A:307–310.

The results of limb salvage in the treatment of osteosarcoma should be evaluated on the basis of survival, immediate and delayed morbidity, limb function, and psychosocial benefits. These are the four factors by which limb salvage should be compared with amputations.

Simon MA, Aschliman M, Thomas N, et al: Limb-salvage treatment versus amputation for osteosarcoma of the distal end of the femur. *J Bone Joint Surg* 1986;68A:1331–1337.

A retrospective multi-institutional study of 227 patients with osteosarcoma of the distal end of the femur compared the rates of local recurrence, metastases, and survival. When compared with above-knee amputation or hip disarticulation, limb-salvage procedures for osteosarcoma of the distal end of the femur did not shorten the disease-free interval or compromise long-term survival.

Smith WS, Struhl S: Replantation of an autoclaved autogenous segment of bone for treatment of chondrosarcoma: Long-term follow-up. *J Bone Joint Surg* 1988;70A:70–75.

The authors review seven patients who had low-grade chondrosarcomas of the proximal part of the humerus or femur and who were treated by resection, autoclaving of the excised segment, and reinsertion of the segment with supplementary fresh autogenous grafting. In follow-up studies over 14 to 24 years, serial roentgenograms documented a continuing process of healing and remodeling, with no fractures, resorption, infection, or loss of function.

Springfield DS, Schmidt R, Graham-Pole J, et al: Surgical treatment for osteosarcoma. *J Bone Joint Surg* 1988;70A:1124–1130.

The authors review 53 patients whose high-grade osteosarcomas were treated by limb salvage or amputation. They suggest that a wide surgical margin and adjuvant chemotherapy are adequate for control of primary osteosarcoma, and that, if such a wide margin can be obtained by limb salvage, amputation is not required.

Advances in the Diagnosis and Treatment of Soft-Tissue Sarcomas in Adults

Chang AE, Kinsella T, Glatstein E, et al: Adjuvant chemotherapy for patients with high-grade soft-tissue sarcomas of the extremity. *J Clin Oncol* 1988;6:1491–1500.

A randomized trial of adjuvant chemotherapy in the treatment of patients with high-grade extremity sarcomas showed a significant improvement in disease-free survival, but only a trend toward improved overall survival. The effect of a reduced dose of doxorubicin was found to be comparable to that of a high-dose regimen.

Elias AD, Antman KH: Adjuvant chemotherapy for soft-tissue sarcoma: A critical appraisal. *Semin Surg Oncol* 1988;4:59–65.

The role of adjuvant chemotherapy in the treatment of adult soft-tissue sarcomas has yet to be determined. At this time, its use in this group of tumors should be considered investigational.

Gherlinzoni F, Bacci G, Picci P, et al: A randomized trial for the treatment of high-grade soft-tissue sarcomas of the extremities: Preliminary observations. *J Clin Oncol* 1986;4:552–558.

A preliminary report on a randomized trial of doxorubicin for soft-tissue sarcomas in adults showed a significant increase in the disease-free survival rate of patients who received chemotherapy over that of patients who were only observed postoperatively.

Roholl PJM, De Jong ASH, Ramaekers FCS: Application of markers in the diagnosis of soft tissue tumours. *Histopathology* 1985;9:1019–1035.

The application of immunohistochemical markers, which are useful for the diagnosis of soft-tissue tumors on paraffin sections, is reviewed.

Ewing's Sarcoma

Sailer S, Harmon DC, Mankin HJ, et al: Ewing's sarcoma: Surgical resection as a prognostic factor. *Int J Radiat Oncol Biol Phys* 1988;15:43–52.

In this retrospective study, 46 cases of Ewing's sarcoma were assessed for prognostic factors. Overall actuarial survival and local control rates were 0.52 ± 0.08 and 0.78 ± 0.07, respectively, at five years. Twelve patients had surgical resection of the tumor (with or without radiation therapy) as part of the treatment, and their five-year actuarial survival was 0.92 ± 0.08 compared with 0.37 ± 0.09 for the patients receiving radiation to the primary tumor and no surgical resection ($P = .02$ by Cox multivariate analysis). Tumor size, site, and stage were also of prognostic significance.

Wilkins RM, Prichard DJ, Burgert ED Jr, et al: Ewing's sarcoma of bone: Experience with 140 patients. *Cancer* 1986;58:2551–2555.

In this retrospective study of 140 patients with Ewing's sarcoma treated between 1969 and 1982, the presence of metastatic disease at diagnosis, an increased erythrocyte sedimentation rate, and pelvic location of the tumor were poor prognostic indicators. Patients who underwent complete excision of the primary tumor had a better survival rate (54% at five years) than those who did not (34%).

11

Infection

During the 1980s, orthopaedists and infectious disease specialists confronted new and more widespread clinical entities (toxic shock and acquired immune deficiency syndromes and Lyme disease) and problems with resistant organisms, including methicillin-resistant *Staphylococcus aureus* and methicillin-resistant coagulase-negative staphylococci. Prevention of infection was facilitated by the refinement of accurate staging systems for open fractures, the identification of operating-room environmental factors (especially important in total joint replacement), and the more routine use of perioperative antibiotics. Early and more accurate differential diagnosis of infection was enhanced by technetium, gallium, indium-labeled leukocyte, and magnetic resonance imaging studies. Basic science research and work with animal models have defined the way in which antibiotics penetrate bone. New families of antibiotics, second- and third-generation cephalosporins, and more cost-effective antibiotic delivery systems were evaluated clinically. Arthroscopy was used for drainage and debridement of pyarthroses. New emphasis was placed on the nutritional status of the host. The emphasis on accurate and thorough debridement remained a constant, reaffirmed by work characterizing polysaccharide biofilms on implanted materials.

Antibiotics

Approval of new antibiotics, such as ciprofloxacin, by the Food and Drug Administration and continuing work on local medication delivery systems, such as osmotic pumps, antibiotic-impregnated beads, and home administration of intravenous antibiotics, are facilitating shorter hospitalizations and decreasing the cost of care for many patients.

Ciprofloxacin

Ciprofloxacin is the first fluoroquinolone antibiotic with systemic activity to be marketed in the United States. Ciprofloxacin, administered orally, is bacteriocidal against most gram-negative aerobic bacilli, including *Pseudomonas aeruginosa*. Activity against gram-positive organisms is more variable, but many strains of methicillin-susceptible and methicillin-resistant *S aureus* and coagulase-negative staphylococci as well as enterococci are inhibited by drug concentrations normally achieved in vivo. Activity against anaerobic bacteria is poor. Ciprofloxacin requires only twice-daily oral administration because its serum half-life is four to five hours. Investigators have reported osteomyelitis arrest rates of 63% to 100% with ciprofloxacin.

The fluoroquinolones are developmental analogues of the original quinolone, nalidixic acid. Nalidixic acid had limited effectiveness because organisms rapidly developed resistance, and therapeutic concentrations could only be produced in the urine. In contrast, the fluoroquinolones have more complete gastrointestinal absorption, a broader antimicrobial spectrum, a lower incidence of resistance, and fewer adverse effects. These drugs inhibit bacterial cell protein synthesis and DNA replication by preventing bacterial DNA-gyrase from introducing into DNA the negative superhelical twists necessary for transcription and reproduction.

Oral therapy offers major advantages over intravenous treatment, particularly in elderly patients and in intravenous drug abusers with poor venous access. Patients with internally fixed fractures and concomitant infection can be treated orally, at home, for prolonged periods. In this setting, the clinical signs of infection have been suppressed in some patients, thus allowing bone union before hardware removal.

Ciprofloxacin has two significant drug interactions. The coadministration of magnesium- or aluminum-containing antacids can decrease its absorption by sixfold to tenfold. Thus, patients receiving long-term antacid therapy are not good candidates for oral ciprofloxacin. Ciprofloxacin has the potential to increase theophylline serum concentrations more than twofold when the drugs are coadministered. Patients receiving both drugs should have theophylline serum concentrations monitored closely.

Several cautions are worth noting. Antibiotic susceptibility should be confirmed before therapy is begun. All anaerobic organisms should be considered resistant to ciprofloxacin. When infections caused by anaerobic and susceptible aerobic organisms are encountered, metronidazole may be combined with ciprofloxacin. Although the development of resistance during treatment with ciprofloxacin is infrequent, drainage from wounds and debrided tissue should be cultured periodically to monitor for changes in flora and sensitivity. Compliance is essential to the success of oral antibiotic therapy. Candidates for outpatient management of osteomyelitis should be carefully selected because prolonged self-medication is difficult to maintain once the symptoms have resolved. Ciprofloxacin is not recommended for children because joint cartilage erosion has been documented in young experimental animals receiving the drug.

Antibiotic-Impregnated Beads

Local delivery of antibiotics to the site of infection has been facilitated by placing appropriate antibiotics in polymethylmethacrylate (PMMA) beads and by infusion from implantable pumps.

A multicenter FDA trial is underway to evaluate the safety and efficacy of local implantation of gentamicin-impregnated PMMA beads in the treatment of osteomyelitis. Each commercially prepared bead with a 7-mm diameter contains 7.5 mg of gentamicin sulfate (equivalent to 4.5 mg of gentamicin base). The beads are threaded on multifilament surgical wire.

Gentamicin is released from the beads by diffusion. Local gentamicin concentrations of 200 to 300 μg/ml have been recorded along with a concomitant serum concentration of 0.5 μg/ml. The amount of antibiotic released is proportional to the surface area of the cement, the concentration of the antibiotic in the cement, and the amount of fluid around the cement (Fig. 1).

Gentamicin is active against infections caused by a wide variety of pathogenic gram-negative (and gram-positive) bacteria, including *Escherichia coli* and *Klebsiella*, *Enterobacter*, and *Pseudomonas* sp. Microorganisms such as streptococci and some *Proteus* spp, which have minimum inhibitory concentrations higher than the maximum serum gentamicin level (4 μg/ml) attained after conventional intravenous administration, are destroyed by the substantially higher concentrations achieved by local application. Local treatment with gentamicin-impregnated beads is not appropriate for osteomyelitis caused by anaerobic organisms or enterococci.

Insertion of antibiotic-impregnated PMMA beads is not a substitute for adequate surgical debridement. The goal is to remove all infected necrotic bone, scar, and foreign material. Careful wound closure with either local tissue or liquid-impermeable synthetics is required to maintain the high local concentration of the antibiotic.

To date there have been no published reports of ototoxicity, nephrotoxicity, or allergic reactions after implantation of as many as 540 beads in a single patient.

Osmotic Pumps

Totally implantable osmotic pumps are used to deliver antibiotics locally in patients with chronic osteomyelitis. The pump consists of two chambers separated by a flexible metal bellows. One chamber is the drug reservoir, and the other contains the charging fluid in a completely sealed environment. The vapor pressure of the charging fluid exerts a constant pressure on the bellows, forcing the drug from the reservoir through an outlet filter and flow restrictor into a catheter for delivery to the selected body site. When the pump is refilled, the increasing volume within the bellows drug chamber exerts pressure on the charging fluid, causing the fluid vapor to condense to its liquid state, thereby storing energy for the next pumping cycle. The pump functions by maintaining a precise drug flow for a specified period of time.

In patients with chronic infection, the pump is generally implanted at the time of initial debridement. An identical pump has been used for several years to deliver drugs for the treatment of cancer and for the relief of pain. More than 17,000 such pumps have been implanted. Systemic perioperative antibiotics are used to lessen the chance of

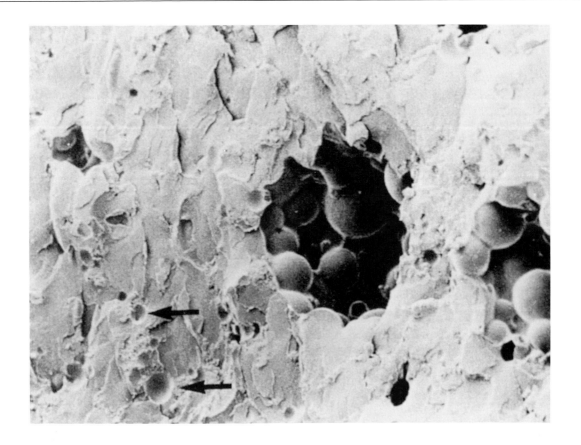

Figure 1

After three months of implantation in a sheep, the outer surface of the antibiotic-impregnated cement (0.5 g of gentamicin per packet of cement) shows visible cracks (arrows). (Reproduced with permission from Baker AS, Greenham LW: Release of gentamicin from acrylic bone cement: Elution and diffusion studies. *J Bone Joint Surg* 1988;70A:1551–1557.)

pump-pocket infection. The pump is implanted into a subcutaneous pocket fashioned in the abdominal wall, and the catheters are tunneled to the site of infection.

Amikacin, a semisynthetic derivative of kanamycin, with the broadest range of antimicrobial therapy of the aminoglycosides, is the antibiotic used most frequently with the implantable pump. Amikacin has been shown to maintain its stability in the pump. Unlike other aminoglycosides, it resists destruction by bacterial enzymes (except acetyl transferase and adenylating enzyme). Like other aminoglycosides, it inhibits protein synthesis in the bacterial cell and is bacteriocidal. Studies have shown that amikacin is active in vitro and in vivo against a wide variety of gram-positive and gram-negative organisms.

Contraindications to pump use include psychological intolerance of such a device, a body size not large enough to accommodate the size and weight of the pump, allergic reaction to amikacin, and marked changes in altitude such as might be experienced by frequent travelers.

Home Administration of Intravenous Antibiotics

Intravenous antibiotics can be delivered through either peripheral or central modes of access. Catheters that provide central access, however, require surgical placement in the operating room. The advantage for most patients is the ability to continue appropriate antibiotic therapy while at home with their families. Most insurance carriers recognize the cost-effectiveness of this home treatment program.

Patients must be monitored for signs of toxicity such as leukopenia and, depending on the antibiotic chosen, appropriate peak and trough levels must be maintained.

Microbiology

Staphylococci continue to be the most frequent cause of postoperative and posttraumatic musculoskeletal infections. Coagulase-negative staphylococci account for more than 50% of infections involving prosthetic valves, intravenous catheter tips, and sternal wounds in some hospitals. Increasingly, these organisms are resistant to methicillin.

Anaerobic organisms are more prevalent in the wounds of compromised hosts: elderly patients, those undergoing multiple revision surgery, patients with diabetes, and those whose conditions involve retained foreign bodies, necrotic tissue, or dead space. Optimal antibiotic treatment depends on prompt, accurate isolation of the organism and determination of its antibiotic sensitivity patterns.

Antibiotic resistance is increasing. Plasmids, packages of genetic material transferred from one bacterial cell to another by conjugation, transmit antibiotic resistance information. Resistance can be conferred by the production of an enzyme such as penicillinase, by an alteration in the cell-wall protein-binding site so that the antibiotic cannot attach, or by a change in the cell wall that precludes antibiotic penetration.

Lyme Disease

Lyme disease is caused by the spirochete *Borellia burgdorferi* carried by the deer tick, *Ixodes dammini*. Stage I Lyme disease becomes evident three to 30 days after the bite, with erythema chronicum migrans—an expanding red ring with central clearing and intermittent attacks of swelling in one or more large joints. Stage II Lyme disease involves neurologic sequelae (frequently Bell's palsy) and cardiac abnormalities. Stage III Lyme disease involves arthritis. The knee is most frequently affected. The erythrocyte sedimentation rate is elevated in 90% of patients. ELISA testing for Lyme disease is both sensitive and specific. Treatment is phenoxymethyl penicillin (50 mg/kg of body weight per day) or tetracycline (30 mg/kg per day) for four weeks. If a patient fails to respond to this treatment regimen, penicillin G (20 million units per day for ten days) is administered intravenously.

Bacterial Resistance in the Presence of Foreign Material

Direct examination of tissue and biomaterials from infections related to prostheses, internal fixation devices, and percutaneous sutures has shown bacteria enveloped by extracellular material that on scanning electron microscopy appears to be a fibrous extracellular matrix. This exopolysaccharide glycocalix protects the bacteria from host defense factors and accounts, in part, for their persistence and resistance to treatment. Because of the adherent growth of the organisms, accurate microbiologic sampling is difficult. Analysis of joint fluids, swabs of excised tissue, and prosthetic surface frequently yields only one species of organism from what is actually a polymicrobial population. In these instances, suppression of clinical infection can be accomplished, but a long-term cure requires surgical removal of the hardware and glycocalix.

Allograft Infection

The first report of infection complicating massive bone allograft revealed an 11.7% infection rate in 283 patients. Gram-positive organisms predominated. *Staphylococcus epidermidis* accounted for 36% of the infections. Six of the 33 patients had a single gram-negative type of organism, and nine had mixed flora. Of the first 33 infections treated, 27 failed to resolve without significant limb compromise involving either resection of the graft or amputation.

Thirteen patients had skin sloughing, six underwent additional operations for nonunion or fracture, two had massive hematomas, and one each had a urinary tract infection, a dental extraction, and decubitus. Salvage rates have improved in the last few years because of aggressive treatment of infection by removal of the graft, improved soft-tissue coverage by techniques such as gastrocnemius flaps, use of a spacer or external fixator to maintain limb length, administration of intravenous and oral antibiotics, and subsequent reimplantation of a second allograft.

Osteomyelitis

The timing of soft-tissue transfer procedures in type III open fractures, the effectiveness of magnetic resonance imaging as a diagnostic tool defining the extent of bone infection, the classification system for osteomyelitis, and the role of adjunctive hyperbaric oxygen therapy remain controversial.

Prevention of osteomyelitis in patients with type III open fractures remains challenging. There may be a significant benefit from aggressive early soft-tissue management. When free flap transfer was accomplished within 72 hours of injury, the flap failure rate was 0.75% and the infection rate was 1.5% (Table 1).

Indium-labeled leukocyte scintigraphy and magnetic res-

Table 1. Microsurgical reconstruction with free flap transfers*

Time From Injury to Surgery	Flap Failure (%)	Infection Rate (%)	Time to Bone Healing (mos)
< 72 hours	0.75	1.5	6.8
72 hours to 3 months	12.0	17.5	12.3
> 3 months	9.5	6.0	29.0

*Modified from Godina M: Early microsurgical reconstruction of complex trauma of the extremities. *Plast Reconstr Surg* 1986;78:285–292.

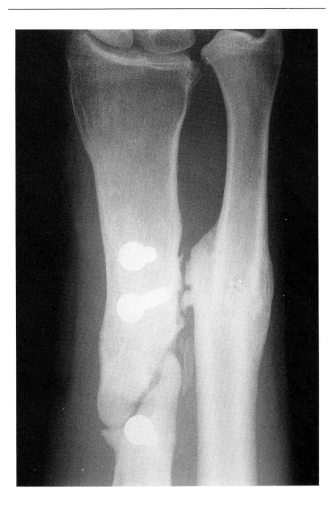

onance imaging have made it possible to diagnose subclinical osteomyelitis and its extent within the medullary canal. Indium-labeled leukocyte scintigraphy is more accurate than plain technetium or sequential technetium-gallium imaging in suspected low-grade infection of a longbone or chronic musculoskeletal infection (Figs. 2 to 4). Sequential technetium-gallium imaging is still preferred if the focus involves the vertebral column because indium is not useful in the spine.

Magnetic resonance imaging is superior to ^{111}In-labeled leukocyte scintigraphy in defining the extent of infection. A magnetic resonance image is considered to be consistent with active osteomyelitis when an area of abnormal marrow showing low signal intensity on T_1-weighted sequences corresponds to an increased signal intensity on the T_2-weighted image. Abnormal marrow caused by posttraumatic and postsurgical fibrosis and scarring is defined by a low marrow signal on T_1-weighted images with no evident increase in signal on T_2-weighted images. Cellulitis is defined by diffuse areas of intermediate signal in the soft tissues on T_1-weighted images with similar soft-tissue areas displaying increased signal on T_2-weighted images.

Soft-tissue abscesses are revealed as focal areas of intermediate signal intensity on T_1-weighted images with high signal intensity on T_2-weighted images. The extent of intramedullary and extramedullary disease seen on magnetic resonance images correlated directly with that seen on serial sectioning of amputated extremities. Magnetic resonance imaging is not able to differentiate clearly between areas of abnormal marrow resulting from chronic inactive osteomyelitis and marrow previously disrupted by trauma or surgery that has healed with fibrosis. Nonferromagnetic internal fixation devices located within the study area do not interfere significantly with image interpretation.

Comparison of published treatment results in osteomyelitis has been made more difficult by the lack of a uniform, widely accepted clinical staging system. Clearly, all patients with osteomyelitis are not identical. Table 2 summarizes some classification systems.

Debridement remains the key to adequate long-term eradication of chronic infection (Figs. 5 and 6). Controversy still surrounds the effectiveness and appropriateness of hyperbaric oxygen therapy in patients with chronic osteomyelitis.

Whether hyperbaric oxygen is more helpful in this context in revascularization of a chronic wound or in improving leukocyte function has yet to be determined. Perhaps only a class B host (Table 2), whose infection cannot be entirely removed, is a candidate for hyperbaric oxygenation. Hyperbaric oxygenation has been shown to be effective in radiation osteonecrosis and chronic osteomyelitis of the mandible.

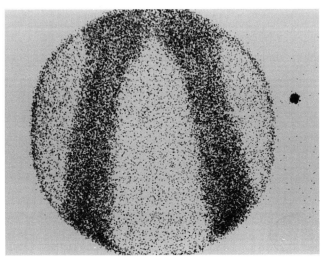

Figure 2

Nonunion of the right radius in a 28-year-old man. **Top**, There was no clinical or roentgenographic evidence of infection 44 months after closed fracture and 28 months after the last of four surgical interventions. **Bottom**, ^{111}In-labeled leukocyte scan of the forearms showed no localization of labeled cell. Culture of a bone biopsy specimen showed no growth. (Reproduced with permission from Esterhai JL, Goll SR, McCarthy KIE, et al: Indium-111 leukocyte scintigraphic detection of subclinical osteomyelitis complicating delayed and nonunion long bone fractures: A prospective study. *J Orthop Res* 1987;5:1–6.)

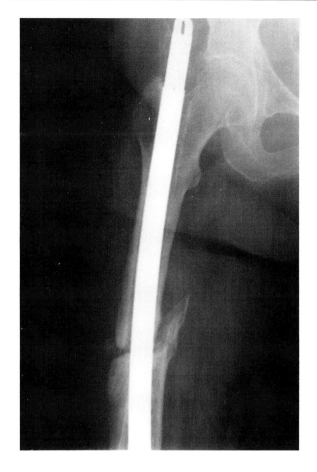

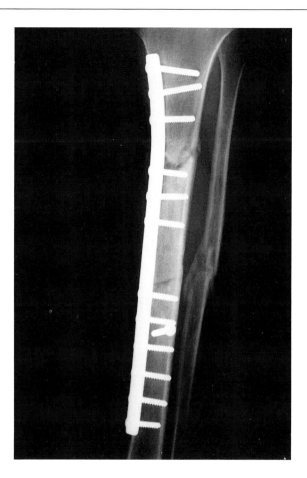

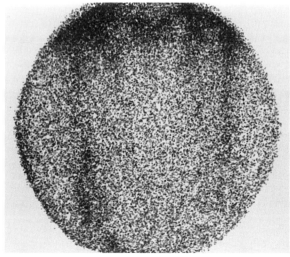

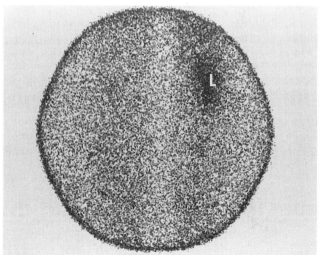

Figure 3

Nonunion of the right femur in a 61-year-old woman. **Top**, There was no clinical or roentgenographic evidence of infection 36 months after open fracture and five months after the last of five surgical interventions. **Bottom**, ¹¹¹In-labeled leukocyte scan of both thighs showed increased localization of leukocytes at the site of the nonunion. Culture of a bone biopsy specimen grew *Staphylococcus epidermidis*. (Reproduced with permission from Esterhai JL, Goll SR, McCarthy KIE, et al: Indium-111 leukocyte scintigraphic detection of subclinical osteomyelitis complicating delayed and nonunion long bone fractures: A prospective study. *J Orthop Res* 1987;5:1–6.)

Figure 4

Nonunion of the left tibia in a 20-year-old man. **Top**, There was no clinical or roentgenographic evidence of infection five months after open reduction and internal fixation of this open segmental fracture. **Bottom**, ¹¹¹In-labeled leukocyte scan of both lower legs shows intense localization of leukocytes (L) at the proximal fracture site. Culture of a bone biopsy specimen from the fracture site grew *Staphylococcus aureus* and *Pseudomonas aeruginosa*. (Reproduced with permission from Esterhai JL, Goll SR, McCarthy KIE, et al: Indium-111 leukocyte scintigraphic detection of subclinical osteomyelitis complicating delayed and nonunion long bone fractures: A prospective study. *J Orthop Res* 1987;5:1–6.)

Table 2. Osteomyelitis classification systems

System	Basis of System	Classification
Waldvogel	Etiology and region involved	Type 1: Hematogenous Type 2: Contiguous focus Type 3: Associated with major vessel disease
Kelly	Etiology and region involved	Type 1: Chronic hematogenous Type 2: Associated with fracture union Type 3: Associated with fracture nonunion Type 4: Posttraumatic or postoperative Type 5: Vertebral Type 6: Small bones of skull, face, hand, foot
Ger	Wound characteristics	Type 1: Single sinus Type 2: Chronic superficial ulcers Type 3: Multiple sinuses Type 4: Multiple skin-lined sinuses
Weiland	Extent of infection	Type I: Exposed bone with soft-tissue infection Type II: Circumferential, cortical, and endosteal infection Type III: Cortical and endosteal infection with segmental bone loss
Gordon	Severity of underlying bone damage	Type A: Tibial defect and nonunion without significant segmental loss Type B: Tibial defect > 3 cm, fibula intact Type C: Tibial defect > 3 cm, fibula fractured
University of Texas	Location of infection modified by immune system of host	Type I: Intramedullary Type II: Superficial Type III: Local Type IV: Diffuse, with segmental bone loss
		Modifications: A, Normal immune system and adequate soft-tissue envelope. B, Local or systemic compromise or both. C, Requires immunosuppressive therapy or would be made worse by aggressive treatment.

Total Joint Arthroplasty

The combination of perioperative antibiotics, laminar-air-flow operating rooms, and body-exhaust systems reduces the incidence of deep wound sepsis after total hip replacement. The single most effective variable is appropriate perioperative antibiotics. The overall incidence of sepsis after standard primary procedures was as low as 0.38% in one series. Late infection is more likely to occur after procedures that involve major bone grafting (4%).

Using antibiotic-impregnated cement is appropriate in revision surgery for patients with known previous infections, but it has not been studied sufficiently to justify routine use for ordinary prophylaxis. The similarity of success rates, the dissimilarity of protocols, and the lack of comparative studies make it difficult to determine whether the combination of antibiotic-impregnated cement and systemic antibiotics is more advantageous than either used separately. However, in patients with infected total joint arthroplasties, the potential benefits of antibiotic-impregnated cement are likely to outweigh the risks.

Cements vary in their ability to release antibiotic. Studies of tensile strength and fatigue testing have revealed that 0.5 g of gentamicin powder per 40 g of cement did not significantly change the strength of the cement. The magnitude of the changes equaled that attributable to voids in the cement.

Continued, unexplained elevation of the Westergren erythrocyte sedimentation rate remains the single most reliable clinical indication of infection after total hip arthroplasty. Of patients with proven infection, 84% had an elevated erythrocyte sedimentation rate. Erythrocytes normally repel each other because of their negative surface charge. Positively charged fibrinogen and α-, β-, and γ-globulins lead to aggregation of erythrocytes into rouleaux. The weight of the combined cells increases relative to their surface area, and the rate of fall of the cells through the plasma increases. Although the erythrocyte sedimentation rate routinely returns to normal within one month of an acute fracture, it may remain elevated for as much as one year after routine total hip arthroplasty. A rate that remains greater than 40 mm/hr after one year suggests that the patient has an infection until proven otherwise.

There is no completely reliable study that differentiates a loose, painful prosthesis from one that is also infected. Scintigraphy with ^{111}In-labeled leukocytes produces both false-positive and false-negative findings; further, the findings must be interpreted against the normal reticuloendothelial background and in conjunction with the clinical situation to avoid overreading. Indium-labeled leukocytes can accumulate in patients with osteosarcoma, pigmented villonodular synovitis, eosinophilic granuloma, Paget's disease, osteolytic carcinoma of the breast, and lymphoma with pathologic fracture. In a patient with a painful prosthesis, the initial history, physical examination, plain roentgenographs, and laboratory studies should be followed by a technetium scan. If the technetium scan is negative, infection is unlikely. If the technetium reveals increased localized uptake, an indium study should be performed. If the indium scan shows no increase in uptake, infection is unlikely.

The incidence of infection in a recently reported large series (821 cases) of total knee arthroplasties was 1.71%. Five of the 14 infections were hematogenous with an identifiable source, and one was suspected of having a hematogenous origin. Three of these followed urinary tract infections, one occurred in a patient with bacterial endocarditis, and one occurred after a routine dental cleaning. Ultimate salvage of a total knee arthroplasty, once infected, was only 31% without device removal and subsequent reimplantation. Only four of the infected prostheses were salvaged. In each of these patients, treatment was initiated within one week of the diagnosis of sepsis and the components were found to be solidly fixed at surgery. Two of the remaining knees received successful exchange prostheses.

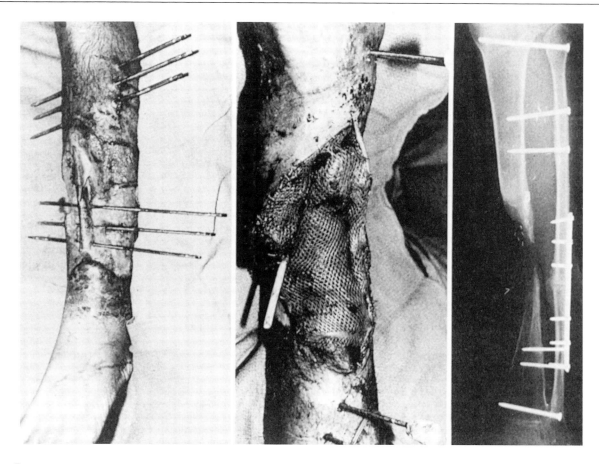

Figure 5

Chronic infection. **Left**, The infected wound, with purulent drainage; 15 cm of the tibia is exposed. **Center**, After extensive debridement, latissimus dorsi transplantation, and split-thickness skin grafting. **Right**, Radiograph of the segmental tibial defect just before tibiofibular synostosis. (Reproduced with permission from Gordon L, Chiu EJ: Treatment of infected non-unions and segmental defects of the tibia with staged microvascular muscle transplantation and bone-grafting. *J Bone Joint Surg* 1988;70A:377–386.)

An infection at the site of an arthroplasty should be treated aggressively. Salvage is possible if the infection is detected early, the components are well fixed, and the organism is sensitive to antibiotics.

Threats to Healthcare Workers From Human Immunodeficiency Virus and Hepatitis B

Use of universal precautions and hepatitis B vaccine will help decrease the risk of life-threatening infections in healthcare workers.

Acquired Immune Deficiency Syndrome (AIDS)

Orthopaedic surgeons are at increased risk for human immunodeficiency virus (HIV) infection because of their extensive involvement with trauma patients and the greater likelihood of skin penetration because of the sharpness of skeletal fragments and orthopaedic surgical instruments.

It is now estimated that 1 to 1.5 million individuals are infected with HIV, and that 54,000 new cases of AIDS per year will occur in the United States by 1991. The spectrum of disease extends from asymptomatic HIV-infected patients carrying the virus to those with AIDS. Of individuals positive for HIV, 5% to 7% per year progress to AIDS. If

the current trends continue, one half of those who are infected today will die within the next ten years.

There are several special high-risk groups: homosexual men, especially those who engage in high-risk sexual activities, intravenous drug users, particularly those who share paraphernalia, patients who have received HIV-contaminated transfusions, and the heterosexual partners of these individuals. Among hemophiliacs, 90% of those with type A disease and 55% of those with type B disease are HIV-positive.

In 1983, the Centers for Disease Control began a prospective study of the risk of HIV infection in healthcare workers, primarily nurses who had needle-stick exposures to HIV-infected blood. Of 917 workers who completed at least six months of follow-up after their exposure, four were HIV-positive. Of these four cases, three were documented seroconversions linked to the exposure. Thus, the risk in this group is approximately 0.3% after a parenteral exposure to HIV-infected blood.

Because of the concern that repeated exposures might produce a cumulative risk far exceeding this 0.3% risk per individual needle-stick, a study of 1,300 dentists practicing in New York City was conducted. The seroprevalence rate in this population was less than 0.1%. In contrast, 21% of the dentists who had not received hepatitis B vaccine tested positive for hepatitis B antibody. Thus, it appears that the

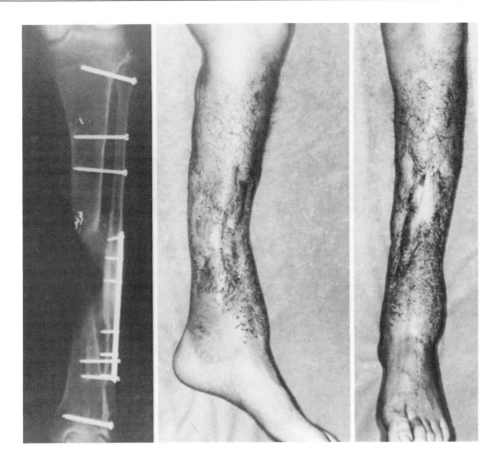

Figure 6
Same tibial defect shown in Figure 5. **Left**, Anteroposterior radiograph made 20 months after proximal and distal tibiofibular synostoses shows solid osseous union. **Center** and **right**, Sixty-two months after latissimus dorsi transplantation, the leg is fully healed. (Reproduced with permission from Gordon L, Chiu EJ: Treatment of infected non-unions and segmental defects of the tibia with staged microvascular muscle transplantation and bone-grafting. *J Bone Joint Surg* 1988;70A:377–386.)

risk of HIV transmission to healthcare workers is relatively low even after needle-stick exposure. To reduce this risk even further, the Centers for Disease Control recommend that the blood and body fluids of all patients be considered potentially infectious. This is the only reliable way to protect healthcare workers, not only against HIV but also against all other blood-borne diseases.

All physicians performing invasive procedures should reevaluate their techniques to see if any procedures could be modified or new instruments developed to reduce the risk of exposure.

Universal precautions, as recommended by the Centers for Disease Control, include the following:

1. All healthcare workers should routinely use appropriate barrier precautions to prevent skin and mucous membrane exposure when contact with blood or other body fluids of any patient is anticipated.

2. Hands and other skin surfaces should be washed immediately after gloves are removed.

3. All healthcare workers should take precautions to prevent injuries caused by needles, scalpels, and other sharp instruments or devices.

4. Although saliva has not been implicated in HIV transmission, to minimize the need for emergency mouth-to-mouth resuscitation, bags or other ventilation devices should be available in areas in which the need for resuscitation is predictable.

5. Healthcare workers who have exudative lesions or weeping dermatitis should refrain from all direct patient care.

6. Pregnant healthcare workers should be especially familiar with and strictly adhere to precautions to minimize the risk of HIV transmission.

In the operating room, appropriate protection includes impermeable gowns, leg and foot wear to the knee, and protective devices against conjunctival contamination (goggles or a faceshield). Surgeons who are at risk for possible HIV contamination must convince their hospital administrators that it is their responsibility to provide the protective equipment required.

The Centers for Disease Control further recommend that if a healthcare worker has a parenteral or mucous membrane exposure to blood or other body fluids or has a cutaneous exposure involving large amounts of blood or prolonged contact with blood, the source patient should be informed of the incident and tested for serologic evidence of HIV infection after consent is obtained.

Policies must be developed in regard to testing source patients in situations in which consent cannot be obtained. Pending federal legislation, physicians and hospital administrations must follow the laws of their individual states concerning testing. HIV testing can be performed without the patient's written consent in only a few states.

If the source patient is positive for HIV antibody or refuses the test, the healthcare worker should be counseled regarding the risk of HIV infection and examined clinically and serologically for evidence of HIV infection. The worker should be advised to report and seek medical evaluation for any acute febrile illness that occurs within 12 weeks of the exposure, since this may represent a febrile reaction to viral infection. Seronegative healthcare workers should be retested six weeks after exposure and periodically thereafter (12 weeks and six months after exposure) to determine whether transmission has occurred. Seroconversion occurs within six months in 95% of individuals who become infected. In addition, if the exposure consists of direct inoculation, through a needle-stick or into an open cut or abrasion, of blood from a person known to be infected with HIV, treatment with zidovudine (AZT), started immediately and continued for four to six weeks, should be considered. This prophylactic use is, however, controversial.

No further follow-up is necessary if the source patient is seronegative unless the source patient is at high risk for HIV infection. In this case, subsequent specimens may be obtained from the healthcare worker and, with consent, from the source patient for antibody testing. If the source patient cannot be identified, decisions regarding appropriate follow-up should be made on an individual basis.

Hospitals are establishing multidisciplinary HIV evaluation and management teams composed of representatives from internal medicine, nursing, social service, and nutrition for outpatient management and inpatient consultation. The goal is to provide AIDS patients with the most efficient and up-to-date outpatient care so that the frequency and duration of their hospitalizations are minimized.

Hepatitis

The term "viral hepatitis" is commonly used for clinically similar diseases that are etiologically and epidemiologically distinct. Two of these, hepatitis A (formerly called infectious hepatitis), and hepatitis B (formerly called serum hepatitis) have been recognized as separate entities since the early 1940s. The third, currently known as non-A, non-B hepatitis, is probably caused by at least two different agents and remains a diagnosis of exclusion. It is an important form of acute viral hepatitis in adults, and currently accounts for most posttransfusion hepatitis in the United States.

Although approximately 21,500 cases of hepatitis A, 24,300 cases of hepatitis B, and 3,500 cases of non-A, non-B hepatitis were reported in the United States in 1983, the actual number of hepatitis cases is thought to be several times higher than the reported number.

Immune globulins used in medical practice are sterile solutions of antibodies (immunoglobulins) from human plasma. They are prepared by cold ethanol fractionation of large plasma pools. Only plasma shown to be free of hepatitis B surface antigen (HBsAg) is used to prepare immunoglobulins.

Immune globulin (formerly called immune serum globulin or γ-globulin) produced in the United States contains antibodies against hepatitis A and hepatitis B. Hepatitis B immune globulin (HBIG) is an immune globulin prepared from plasma containing high titers of antibodies against hepatitis B surface antigen (anti-HBs).

Neither immune globulin nor HBIG commercially available in the United States transmits hepatitis or other viral infections. There is no evidence that HIV has been transmitted by immune globulin or HBIG.

An estimated 200,000 persons are infected with hepatitis B virus each year in the United States. Of these, 25% (50,000) become ill with jaundice, 5% (10,000) require hospitalization, and 0.1% (200) die of fulminant disease each year. Between 6% and 10% become hepatitis B carriers. The United States currently has an estimated 500,000 to 1 million carriers. Chronic active hepatitis develops in more than 25% of carriers and often produces cirrhosis. Carriers have an increased risk of developing primary liver cancer. It is estimated that 4,000 persons die of hepatitis B-related cirrhosis each year and that more than 800 die of hepatitis B-related liver cancer.

Transmission of infection by transfusion of contaminated blood has been greatly reduced since the advent of routine screening with highly sensitive tests for HBsAg.

Two types of products are available for protection against hepatitis B. Hepatitis B vaccine provides active immunization and is recommended for prophylaxis both before and after exposure. Immune globulin products provide temporary, passive protection and are indicated only in certain postexposure settings.

Two vaccines are available. Heptavax-B is a suspension of inactivated, alum-adsorbed, 22-nm surface antigen particles that have been purified from human plasma. The purification process has been shown to inactivate all classes of viruses found in human blood, including HIV.

The newer vaccine, Recombivax-HB, prepared in yeast by recombinant DNA technology, has reduced antigenicity when compared to plasma-derived HBsAg.

The vaccines are 80% to 95% effective in preventing hepatitis infection in susceptible persons. The duration of protection and need for booster doses have not been defined.

Primary vaccination consists of three intramuscular doses of vaccine with the second and third doses given one and six months after the first. The most common side effect is soreness at the injection site. One hundred episodes of severe illness, including arthralgia and Guillain-Barré syndrome, have been reported after vaccination of approximately 1 million workers. The rate of Guillain-Barré infection after vaccination apparently was no higher than expected in the general population and, thus, these temporally related illnesses were not considered to be etiologically related to the vaccine.

Immune globulin and HBIG contain different amounts of anti-HBs. HBIG has an anti-HBs titer of more than 1:100,000 by radioimmune assay.

The specific recommendations for hepatitis B prophylaxis after percutaneous exposure vary depending on whether the source is HBsAg-positive. If the healthcare worker is unvaccinated and the patient tests positive, one dose of HBIG is given immediately and hepatitis vaccination is indicated, with the first dose given within one week of exposure and the second and third doses at one and six months, respectively. A healthcare worker who has already been vaccinated should be tested for anti-HBs. If the antibody titer is inadequate, the worker should receive one dose of HBIG immediately, along with a hepatitis B vaccine booster dose.

Although several studies have attempted to assess the value of prophylaxis with immune globulin against non-A, non-B hepatitis, the results have been equivocal and no specific recommendations can be made. However, for healthcare workers with percutaneous exposure to blood from a patient with non-A, non-B hepatitis, it may be reasonable to administer immune globulin (0.06 ml/kg) as soon as possible after exposure.

No evidence of HIV seroconversion has been observed among an estimated 1 million individuals who have been vaccinated against hepatitis B with plasma-derived vaccine. As experience with the plasma-derived vaccine has increased, the unfounded fear of acquiring AIDS has gradually, although not entirely, abated. Recombinant vaccine is now readily available, is safe, and provides excellent active immunization. Those at high-risk, including ortho-paedic surgeons and operating room staff, should be vaccinated, preferably with recombinant vaccine.

Trends

The primary infectious disease challenge of the 1990s will be the prevention of infection. Those caring for trauma patients with orthopaedic injuries and for patients with severe long-bone fractures will strive to provide functional limb salvage. Imaging capabilities will allow more precise definition of the extent of injury and earlier diagnosis of infection. Soft-tissue transfer and soft-tissue substitution techniques will improve and new antibiotic delivery systems with ever-decreasing side effects will be developed. Physicians will learn to enhance host-immune competence.

Annotated Bibliography

Keywords

Acquired immune deficiency syndrome; Antibiotics; Hepatitis; Human immunodeficiency virus; Immunology; Infection; Osteomyelitis; Septic arthritis; Total joint arthroplasty

Antibiotics

Baker AS, Greenham LW: Release of gentamicin from acrylic bone cement: Elution and diffusion studies. *J Bone Joint Surg* 1988;70A:1551–1557.
Release of antibiotic from bone cement occurs from the surface and through a network of cracks and voids in the cement matrix. The cracks may have occurred through local stress and shrinkage at the time of polymerization. The bubble-like voids were probably the result of air introduced during mixing or vaporization of monomer during polymerization. The intact PMMA matrix was impermeable to gentamicin.

Greenberg RN, Kennedy DJ, Reilly PM, et al: Treatment of bone, joint, and soft-tissue infections with oral ciprofloxacin. *Antimicrob Agents Chemother* 1987;31:151–155.
The authors report excellent success in suppressing osteomyelitis with twice-daily oral administration of ciprofloxacin.

Perry CR, Ritterbusch JK, Rice SH, et al: Antibiotics delivered by an implantable drug pump: A new application for treating osteomyelitis. *Am J Med* 1986;80(suppl 6B):222–227.
Thirteen patients with chronic osteomyelitis were treated with debridement and amikacin administered by implantable pump. Serum concentration of amikacin ranged from 2.5 to 8.2 μg/ml; the wound drainage concentration ranged from 55 to more than 5,000 μg/ml. Infection was arrested in 12 of the 13 patients.

Walenkamp GH, Vree TB, van Rens TJ: Gentamicin-PMMA beads: Pharmacokinetic and nephrotoxicological study. *Clin Orthop* 1986;205:171–183.
Treatment of osteomyelitis with gentamicin-PMMA beads produced a gentamicin serum concentration of 0.03 to 0.4 μg/ml. Gentamicin was released slowly during the entire treatment.

Watt B, Brown FV: Is ciprofloxacin active against clinically important anaerobes? *J Antimicrob Chemother* 1986;17:605–613.
The authors caution against using ciprofloxacin alone in mixed anaerobic-aerobic infections.

Microbiology

Culp RW, Eichenfield AH, Davidson RS, et al: Goldsmith DP: Lyme arthritis in children: An orthopaedic perspective. *J Bone Joint Surg* 1987;69A:96–99.
The knee was involved in 41 of 43 patients with Lyme disease. Immunofluorescent serology is both sensitive and specific. Oligoarticular manifestations resemble those of pauciarticular juvenile rheumatoid arthritis.

Gristina AG, Dobbins JJ, Giammara B, et al: Biomaterial-centered sepsis and the total artificial heart: Microbial adhesion vs tissue integration. *JAMA* 1988;259:870–874.
Bacteria in their natural habitats and in biomaterial-centered infections and osteomyelitis have a common survival mode based on adhesive colonization of the substrate within and protected by the biofilm. Prevention of infection may require changing the surfaces of biomaterials by preintegration with human tissue cells to preclude bacterial adherence.

Johnson KD, Johnston DW: Orthopedic experience with methicillin-resistant *Staphylococcus aureus* during a hospital epidemic. *Clin Orthop* 1986;212:281–288.
Of 508 patients with positive cultures for methicillin-resistant *Staphylococcus aureus* infections, 38 had been hospitalized for orthopaedic procedures. Because vancomycin is the antibiotic of choice in such cases, its cost increased 300%. Thus, it is important to interrupt the transmission of such infections within and among hospitals.

Lord CF, Gebhardt MC, Tomford WW, et al: Infection in bone allografts: Incidence, nature, and treatment. *J Bone Joint Surg* 1988;70A:369–376.
Of 283 patients treated with massive bone allografts, 11.7% developed infections. Twenty-seven of 32 infected allografts

were lost. Aggressive treatment involving removal of the infected allograft, maintaining limb length, intravenous and oral antibiotic therapy, and reimplantation led to improved salvage and good to excellent results.

Osteomyelitis

Esterhai JL Jr, Pisarello J, Brighton CT, et al: Adjunctive hyperbaric oxygen therapy in the treatment of chronic refractory osteomyelitis. *J Trauma* 1987;27:763–768.

Hyperbaric oxygen therapy (100% oxygen at 2 atm, with six two-hour dives per week) had no effect on length of hospitalization, rapidity of wound repair, initial clinical outcome, or recurrence of infection after an average follow-up of 41 months.

Godina M: Early microsurgical reconstruction of complex trauma of the extremities. *Plast Reconstr Surg* 1986;78:285–292.

The author compared early and late microvascular soft-tissue transfer in patients with open fractures and severe soft-tissue loss. In patients receiving a flap within 72 hours of injury, the flap failure rate was 0.75%, the infection rate was 1.5%, and the time to bone healing was 6.8 months. In contrast, in patients who underwent microvascular soft-tissue transfer between 72 hours and three months, the flap failure rate was 12%, the infection rate was 17.5%, and the time to healing was 12.3 months.

Gordon L, Chiu EJ: Treatment of infected non-unions and segmental defects of the tibia with staged microvascular muscle transplantation and bone-grafting. *J Bone Joint Surg* 1988;70A:377–386.

Fourteen patients with infected nonunion or infected fracture of the tibia with segmental defect were treated with debridement and microvascular muscle transfer. Infection was arrested in 12 of the 14 (86%). One patient had a persistent nonunion. Eleven patients achieved full weightbearing with or without an orthosis after an average follow-up of 3.9 years.

Markel KD, Brown ML, Dewanjee MK, et al: Comparison of indium-labeled-leukocyte imaging with sequential technetium-gallium scanning in the diagnosis of low-grade musculoskeletal sepsis. *J Bone Joint Surg* 1985;67A:465–476.

The authors studied the pathologic and microbiologic findings in 30 patients with axial and appendicular skeletal infections and prosthetic infections. Indium imaging had an overall sensitivity of 83%, a specificity of 86%, and an accuracy of 83%. Indium imaging was more accurate than the technetium-gallium scans and was also easier to interpret.

Marx RE, Johnson RP, Kline SN: Prevention of osteoradionecrosis: A randomized prospective clinical trial of hyperbaric oxygen versus penicillin. *J Am Dent Assoc* 1985;111:49–54.

A prospective randomized trial comparing hyperbaric oxygen and systemic antibiotics in the prevention of osteoradionecrosis in a high-risk population who required tooth removal from irradiated mandibles showed an incidence of osteoradionecrosis of 5.4% in the oxygen-treated group and an incidence of 29.9% in the antibiotic-treated group (P = .005). Hyperbaric oxygen should be considered a prophylactic measure when postirradiation dental care involving trauma to tissue is necessary.

Sheftel TG, Mader JT, Pennick JJ, et al: Methicillin-resistant *Staphylococcus aureus* osteomyelitis. *Clin Orthop* 1985;198:231–239.

This staging system describes not only the extent of the infection but also the capability of the host to mount an effective response. Examples of systemic host compromise include malnutrition, immune deficiency, chronic hypoxia, malignancy, diabetes, extremes of age, and renal and liver failure. Local host compromise includes chronic lymph edema, venostasis, major vessel disease compromise, arteritis, extensive scarring, and radiation fibrosis.

Tang JSH, Gold RH, Bassett LW, et al: Musculoskeletal infection of the extremities: Evaluation with MR imaging. *Radiology* 1988;166:205–209.

Magnetic resonance imaging detects musculoskeletal infections with greater sensitivity than radionuclide studies and can distinguish soft-tissue infection with periosteal inflammation from osteomyelitis with intramedullary involvement.

Unger E, Moldofsky P, Gatenby R, et al: Diagnosis of osteomyelitis by MR imaging. *AJR* 1988;150:605–610.

Magnetic resonance imaging delineates the extent of infection within the medullary canal.

Total Joint Arthroplasty

Covey DC, Albright JA: Clinical significance of the erythrocyte sedimentation rate in orthopaedic surgery. *J Bone Joint Surg* 1987;69A:148–151.

The value of the erythrocyte sedimentation rate is its ability to ascertain the progression of or improvement in disease in response to therapy. Of all laboratory tests, continued elevation of erythrocyte sedimentation rate is the most reliable single indicator of infection after total hip replacement.

Grogan TJ, Dorey F, Rollins J, et al: Deep sepsis following total knee arthroplasty: Ten-year experience at the University of California at Los Angeles Medical Center. *J Bone Joint Surg* 1986;68A:226–234.

The infection rate in 821 total knee arthroplasties was 1.71%. Eight of the 14 infections were attributable to wound healing problems and six were secondary to hematogenous spread. Pain was the chief complaint.

MacMillan M, Petty W, Hendeles L: Effect of irrigation and tourniquet application on aminoglycoside antibiotic concentrations in bone. *J Orthop Res* 1988;6:311–316.

The use of vigorous irrigation in bone preparation had a deleterious effect on the local presence of systemically administered antibiotics. This effect is compounded when the surgical site is isolated by use of a tourniquet. The authors recommend either application of antibiotic-containing irrigants or antibiotic-laden polymethylmethacrylate.

Maderazo EG, Judson S, Pasternak H: Late infections of total joint prostheses: A review and recommendations for prevention. *Clin Orthop* 1988;229:131–142.

The incidence of late infection after total joint replacement is 0.6%. The three most common origins of infection are skin and soft tissue (46%), dental tissue (15%), and the urinary tract (13%). There are no prospective studies comparing antibiotic prophylactic regimens against hematogenous infection of total joint prostheses. The authors recommend oral cephalosporins or cafazolin for dental (with gum bleeding), head, neck, oral, chest, upper gastrointestinal tract, and female genital tract procedures with clindamycin, erythromycin, or vancomycin as alternatives. Patients undergoing high-risk biliary tract surgery with common duct stones, obstruction, or acute cholecystitis should receive cafazolin or aminoglycoside as well as vancomycin. Patients undergoing colon and rectal surgery should receive cefoxitin or aminoglycoside plus clindamycin.

Schutzer SF, Harris WH: Deep-wound infection after total hip replacement under contemporary aseptic conditions. *J Bone Joint Surg* 1988;70A:724–727.

The results of 659 total hip arthroplasties in 575 patients were analyzed with regard to postoperative infection. Patients whose operations included major bone grafting were at increased risk for late hematogenous sepsis. Of the total of six cases of late infection, five had an identifiable source of infection that was extrinsic to the wound.

Trippel SB: Antibiotic-impregnated cement in total joint arthroplasty. *J Bone Joint Surg* 1986;68A:1297–1302.

Antibiotic-impregnated cement is indicated in total joint arthroplasty for patients with established infection for whom reimplantation is planned because excisional arthroplasty is not an acceptable alternative.

Wukich DK, Abreu SH, Callaghan JJ, et al: Diagnosis of infection by preoperative scintigraphy with indium-labeled white blood cells. *J Bone Joint Surg* 1987;69A:1353–1360.

Indium-labeled leukocyte scintigraphy produced no false-negative but ten false-positive results in 24 patients with painful prostheses. In 26 patients with questionable osteomyelitis, there was one false-negative and eight false-positive results. The authors emphasize the importance of clinical correlation in interpreting scintigraphic information.

Threats to Healthcare Workers From Human Immunodeficiency Virus and Hepatitis B

AAOS Task Force on AIDS and Orthopaedic Surgery: *Recommendations for the Prevention of Human Immunodeficiency Virus (HIV) Transmission in the Practice of Orthopaedic Surgery.* Park Ridge, American Academy of Orthopaedic Surgeons, 1989.

The three major sections of this document deal with (1) the orthopaedic surgeon's occupational risk of contracting HIV, (2) epidemiologic and scientific data about AIDS and HIV, and (3) specific recommendations regarding orthopaedic practice and procedures.

Centers for Disease Control, Immunization Practices Advisory Committee: Recommendations for protection against viral hepatitis. *Ann Intern Med* 1985;103:391–402.

Updates all previous recommendations on the use of immune globulins and vaccines.

Imagawa DT, Moon HL, Wolensky SM, et al: HIV type I infection in homosexual men who remain seronegative for prolonged periods. *N Engl J Med* 1989;320:1458–1462.

Infection with the human immunodeficiency virus type I (HIV-I) as demonstrated by viral cultures has been described in some patients before antibodies to the virus can be detected. The virus was isolated in blood samples of 31 of 133 homosexual men at high risk for infection. Twenty-seven of these patients (87%) remained seronegative for as long as 36 months after the positive culture. The authors concluded that HIV infection in patients at high risk may occur at least 35 months before antibodies to HIV-I can be detected. Such a prolonged period of latency may be more common than previously thought. The degree of infectiousness during such periods is unknown.

12
Blood and Blood Components

In the last three years there has been a rapid expansion of scientific and clinical investigations in the areas of blood safety and transfusion practices. These areas are particularly relevant to orthopaedic surgeons, since many of their procedures routinely require considerable amounts of blood and blood products.

Transfusion in a Changing Environment

Blood banking is in a period of significant change as a result of several concurrent factors. Technical advances in transfusion medicine (such as the development of plastic blood containers and of apheresis instruments) have made available blood component therapy, in which transfusion of packed erythrocytes, plasma, platelets, cryoprecipitate, and/or clotting factor concentrate has replaced transfusion of units of whole blood. This allows more effective use of blood units donated by the 5% of the population constituting the anonymous, volunteer blood donors who fill our transfusion needs; one blood donor can now potentially supply blood components for many blood-transfusion recipients. It has become increasingly evident, however, that the education of physicians has not kept pace with these technological advances. For example, the use of fresh-frozen plasma has increased tenfold nationally during the last decade, a period in which no new indications for plasma transfusion emerged. Similarly, transfusion of platelet concentrates has increased markedly, so that unit requirements for this product now exceed those for packed erythrocytes; platelets now require platelet pheresis of additional blood donors. Although some of this can be attributed to the transfusion support given to increasingly complex cases in cancer medicine, transplantation, trauma, and the intensive care setting, one inescapable conclusion is that many patients are receiving combinations of erythrocytes, plasma, platelets, and/or cryoprecipitate as modified whole-blood equivalents but at a cost of exposure to many more blood donors for each patient.

In 1985, the acquired immune deficiency syndrome (AIDS) was identified as a disease transmissible by several routes, including the transfusion of blood and blood products. More than 2,200 AIDS cases attributable to blood transfusion had been reported by Jan 2, 1989 (Table 1). Although AIDS brought blood safety issues to the attention of the public, the medical community had long been aware that, despite efforts to make the blood supply as safe as possible, blood transfusion carries a risk. Because these risks must be discussed by the physician and the patient, the American Association of Blood Banks has recommended that informed consent be obtained and documented before an elective or anticipated blood transfusion. The elements of informed consent for homologous blood transfusions are explanations of the relative risks and benefits of a blood transfusion, presentation of alternatives to the patient, an opportunity for the patient to ask questions, and, finally, the giving of consent.

The alternatives to be discussed include the following:

(1) No transfusion—This is an alternative for a patient who refuses a transfusion because of religious beliefs. One possibility is the reevaluation of the postoperative "transfusion-trigger hematocrit" for all patients. This issue was addressed at a National Institutes of Health consensus conference, which may explain the stable or decreased level of erythrocyte transfusions during the last three years. Another possibility is the use of pharmacologic agents to eliminate or reduce the need for homologous blood transfusions, such as desmopressin and the experimental agent recombinant human erythropoietin.

(2) Autologous blood transfusion—This transfusion practice has been available for decades and was formerly used primarily in patients with rare blood types and in patients with significant alloimmunity. Because of increased public concern about blood safety, the practice of predepositing autologous blood before elective surgery has increased significantly. This is a good transfusion practice and has been widely endorsed.

(3) Designated (from a donor known to the recipient) blood transfusion—This transfusion practice is increasingly requested by patients as an alternative to homologous blood, and several state legislatures now mandate that this be offered as an alternative in elective transfusions. This transfusion practice, unlike autologous blood transfusion, is controversial—no evidence to date indicates that designated blood is safer than homologous blood; indeed, designated blood may be less safe. Homologous and designated blood products undergo testing before transfusion, but confidential donor screening also contributes to blood safety. The blood donor is given information identifying high-risk categories of those who should not donate blood (Outline 1); high-risk donors can withdraw from participation or identify themselves, confidentially, by checking a box indicating that the blood they donate should be used for research purposes only. This screening mechanism is not possible in designated blood donation because the blood donor is known to the transfusion recipient. The donation, moreover, may not be truly voluntary. Further, designated blood donation may have a potentially adverse effect on the community blood supply, since individuals who "save" their donations for the unexpected transfusion needs of their families and friends may be less inclined to become community blood donors.

This final point is important because there is growing concern about the adequacy of the national blood inventory. Although blood transfusion needs have increased 100% during the last decade, blood collections have increased only about 30%. There are several reasons for this. The conversion of many manufacturing jobs to service-

Table 1. Transfusion-associated AIDS cases in the United States*

| Year of Diagnosis | All AIDS Cases | Transfusion-Associated AIDS Cases | | | |
| | | Adults | Children | Total | |
				No.	%
Before 1981	75	0	0	0	0.0
1981	265	0	0	0	0.0
1982	1,008	8	4	12	1.2
1983	2,798	36	10	46	1.6
1984	5,603	83	9	92	1.6
1985	9,737	196	22	218	2.2
1986	13,434	232	14	336	2.5
1987	21,355	629	45	774	3.7
1988†	32,311	862	67	929	2.9
Total	82,764	2,044‡	169‡	2,213	2.7

*Information provided by Dr. John Ward, Centers for Disease Control
†Cases diagnosed and reported as of Jan 2, 1989.
‡Excludes cases of HIV infection associated with hemophilia.

related jobs means that donors no longer have access to blood-mobiles during working hours, and must travel to fixed-site donation facilities. Additionally, individuals in high-risk groups or whose tests for non-A, non-B hepatitis (4% to 8% of all blood donors) are positive are no longer accepted as donors. Finally, the false belief, held by 20% to 30% of the population of the United States, that AIDS can be acquired by donating blood has further reduced the pool of blood donors.

The continuing challenge in transfusion medicine will be to preserve the nation's blood resources at the same time that issues of blood safety, blood donor source, and transfusion practice are addressed.

Administration of Blood Products and Its Risks

Febrile reactions to leukocyte contamination of blood products and febrile or urticarial reactions to plasma proteins occur in approximately 5% of all transfusions. These are associated with some morbidity but almost never with mortality. Of the 4 million patients who receive transfusions each year, approximately 35 to 50 die during or as a direct result of the transfusion (one per 100,000 or approximately the same mortality rate as that for induction of general anesthesia). Nearly one half of these deaths are caused by ABO incompatibility resulting from administrative errors; one third are caused by microbially contaminated blood, both bacterial and viral; and the rest have diverse causes. In one six-year review of 116,273 transfusions, 2,293 recipients (5.42%) had transfusion reactions. Of these, 1,046 (45.6%) were classified as allergic, 997 (43.5%) as febrile, and 227 (9.9%) as hemolytic.

Outline 1. Individuals who should not be homologous blood donors

Any male who had a sexual relationship with another male after 1977
Any person who has ever taken illegal drugs intravenously
Any person who came to the United States from Haiti, Burundi, Rwanda, Tanzania, Uganda, or Zaire after 1977
Any person who has AIDS or one of the signs or symptoms of AIDS
Any person who has tested positive for HIV antibody
Any person who received clotting factor since 1977
Any sexual partner of any individual listed above
Any person (male or female) who was a prostitute after 1977
Any person who has been the sexual partner of a prostitute (male or female) within the last six months

Allergic reactions characteristically occur toward the end of the transfusion of erythrocytes. Rectal temperature rarely rises above 38.5 C to 39.4 C; shaking chills, pruritis, erythema, and hives occur in 60% to 90% of such reactions, whereas laryngeal edema and bronchospasm occur in less than 1%. Allergic reactions are most common in patients who have had allergic reactions previously (a subsequent risk of 50% to 60%) and patients with atopy, hay fever, or asthma. Pretreatment of such individuals with diphenhydramine HCl (50 mg), acetaminophen, and hydrocortisone (100 mg) can be helpful in diminishing such reactions. It is rarely, if ever, necessary to stop a transfusion when pruritis or urticaria indicate an allergic reaction, because this type of reaction is innocuous and will subside spontaneously within two to six hours.

Febrile transfusion reactions are most often a response to transfusion of leukocytes in donor blood containing antigens to which the recipient has leukocyte antibody; 50% to 80% of recipients who experience febrile transfusion reactions have demonstrable leukoagglutinins. The symptoms are primarily chills and fever, without pruritis, urticaria, or pain. Characteristically, 300 ml or more of blood is required to cause this entity, just as in allergic reactions, although fever may be noted after 50- to 100-ml infusions. Treatment of febrile reactions is essentially supportive and similar to that of allergic reactions. Washed (leukocyte-poor) erythrocytes can be given to such patients to prevent the febrile response; leukocyte-removal filters are also suitable, removing more than 90% of the leukocytes with 87% erythrocyte recovery.

Hemolytic transfusion reactions occur with very small amounts (30 to 40 ml) of transfused erythrocytes; 36% of such reactions result in clinical symptoms that include (in descending order of frequency) chills, fever, tachycardia, chest tightness, flank pain, and dyspnea. Nausea, bloody urine, and shock occur infrequently (7% to 8%). Pain along the infusion site can also be a symptom. In one series, the mortality rate in serious, symptomatic hemolytic transfusion reactions was 40%. Clinical management of a symptomatic, hemolytic transfusion reaction should include the following: (1) stopping the transfusion; (2) sending blood and urine samples for laboratory studies (culture, complete blood cell count, serologic evaluations, and plasma and urine free hemoglobin determination); (3) administration of fluids and mannitol and diuretic therapy to maintain an adequate renal glomerular filtration flow rate; (4) administration of 500 mg of hydrocortisone; and (5) using pressors to maintain blood pressure, if needed.

A delayed hemolytic transfusion reaction is diagnosed in approximately one case per 4,000 erythrocyte units transfused, although it is probably more common when transfusions are frequent. In 37 such cases in one series, 13 patients were asymptomatic and discovered by serologic evaluation only when a second transfusion was ordered. The 24 symptomatic patients had anemia, chills, and fever (12 patients) or anemia and jaundice (12 patients); "anemia" was secondary to increased clearance of the transfused erythrocytes, failure of the transfusion to "take," and presumably was also present in the 13 asymptomatic patients for whom a second blood transfusion was ordered. Serologic evaluation of all 37 patients revealed that 30 patients had one antibody and seven patients had more than one antibody responsible for the delayed transfusion reaction.

Diseases Transmitted by Transfusion

Non-A, Non-B Hepatitis

Posttransfusion hepatitis, particularly non-A, non-B hepatitis, is far more common than transfusion-associated AIDS. It is predicted that in the current era of AIDS screening and donor deferral, transfusion-associated AIDS may develop in 50 to 100 individuals each year, a risk similar to the risk of dying of a fatal hemolytic transfusion reaction. At the same time, a conservative estimate of a 1% to 4% incidence indicates that non-A, non-B hepatitis will develop in 30,000 to 120,000 people each year and that cirrhosis and/or hepatoma will develop in 5% of these individuals. The current incidence of transfusion-associated non-A, non-B hepatitis is unknown and can only be inferred from previous prospective studies. In the late 1970s, the incidence of posttransfusion hepatitis ranged between 7% and 12%; 90% to 95% of these cases were attributed by exclusion to non-A, non-B hepatitis. No large prospective studies of non-A, non-B hepatitis have been conducted in the United States since 1980. Estimates for the incidence of this disease ranged between 3% and 8% before the advent of surrogate testing in November 1986 for the non-A, non-B hepatitis agent but have decreased to about 50% of that rate (1% to 4%) since that time. Surrogate testing is testing of blood donors for increased levels of alanine aminotransferase enzyme and for the presence of antibody to hepatitis B core antigen. Previous studies have shown that the 4% to 8% of blood donors who test positive for either of these surrogate markers account for 60% (30% each) of posttransfusion non-A, non-B hepatitis; on the basis of these studies, surrogate testing has been instituted to screen blood products and thereby reduce postransfusion non-A, non-B hepatitis by an anticipated 50%.

The clinical significance of non-A, non-B hepatitis has been increasingly recognized. Because 75% of such cases are anicteric, it was previously thought to represent a benign disease. Prospective surveillance studies have now established that 40% of patients with non-A, non-B hepatitis demonstrate chronically increased levels of liver transaminase. Of these, 40% show evidence of chronic active hepatitis and 20% of cirrhosis. In one study, five of 20 patients with cirrhosis died of liver-related disease. Another large collaborative study suggested that cirrhosis de-

velops in 22% of hemophiliacs; the vast majority of cases are related to non-A, non-B hepatitis. Thus, prospective studies have shown that the consequences of transfusion-induced non-A, non-B hepatitis include chronic active hepatitis, cirrhosis, and liver-related death.

Hepatitis B

Serologic and chemical markers indicate that acute hepatitis B virus (HBV) infection is of relatively long duration, persisting for weeks to months. Ten percent of such infections result in a chronic carrier state with hepatitis B surface antigen (HBsAg) positivity. Infectivity by HBV inoculum from blood from these individuals has been correlated with the serologic marker for hepatitis B e antigen (HBeAg). Fewer than 10% of HBsAg-positive normal volunteer blood donors are estimated to be infectious, compared with 60% to 70% of dialysis patients and homosexual men. Hepatitis B is observed among a small proportion (less than 1%) of transfusion recipients given blood that was HBsAg-negative by current third-generation tests. Such individuals would not ordinarily be considered to be infectious; HBV transmission probably occurs under these circumstances because of the hepatitis B inoculum given with the large volume of transfused blood.

Human Immunodeficiency Virus Infection

Of the 82,764 cases of AIDS diagnosed and reported in the United States as of Jan 2, 1989, a total of 2,213 (2.9%) were classified as transfusion-associated cases on the basis of a history of blood transfusion after 1977 and no other identifiable risk factor for human immunodeficiency virus (HIV) infection (Table 1). Although pediatric (less than 13 years of age) AIDS patients make up only 1% of all reported cases, they account for approximately 7% of all transfusion-associated cases. More than two thirds of the patients with transfusion-associated AIDS are known to have died; the mean period of time between transfusion and diagnosis of AIDS for adults is three years (range, one to seven years). The distribution of transfusion-associated cases by state of residence does not differ markedly from that of all cases of AIDS, except for New York, where the distribution is 15.9% for transfusion-related AIDS and 29.3% for all cases. The risk of receiving a seropositive unit when HIV antibody screening began in 1985 was approximately 0.04%; estimates of additional transfusion-related AIDS cases that may develop from blood transfused before HIV testing range from 10,000 to 15,000.

A total of 856 cases of AIDS have been identified as associated with clotting factor concentrate; of these, 83 cases occurred in children (Table 2). Ninety percent are in patients with classic hemophilia (factor VIII deficiency) given transfusions of factor VIII concentrate, and most of the remaining cases are in patients with Christmas disease (factor IX deficiency) given transfusions of factor IX concentrate, in which commercial lots are derived from 10,000 to 30,000 donors. The estimated annual incidence of AIDS in persons with classic hemophilia in the United States was approximately 1.1% for calendar year 1986. Serologic surveys have shown that 74% of persons with classic hemophilia and 39% of persons with Christmas disease have antibody to HIV. Seroprevalence is related to the volume of clotting factor concentrate used. The risk of new HIV infection since the introduction of treated (by solvent, heat, or monoclonal antibody) preparations from plasma

Table 2. AIDS cases associated with clotting factor deficiency in the United States*

Year of Diagnosis	All AIDS Cases	AIDS Cases Associated With Clotting Factor Deficiency			
		Adults	Children	Total	
				No.	% of All Cases
Before 1981	75	0	0	0	0.0
1981	265	2	0	2	0.0
1982	1,008	6	1	7	0.7
1983	2,798	13	2	15	0.5
1984	5,603	48	3	51	0.9
1985	9,737	100	7	107	1.1
1986	13,434	124	14	138	1.0
1987	21,355	219	22	241	1.0
1988†	32,311	299	38	337	1.4
Total	82,764	773	83	856	1.3

*Information provided by Dr. John Ward, Centers for Disease Control.
†Cases diagnosed and reported as of Jan 2, 1989.

screened for HIV antibody has decreased markedly. Widespread commercial availability of a recombinant monoclonal factor VIII product will further reduce the risk of transfusion-acquired AIDS in this population of patients.

Two mechanisms to ensure blood safety are currently in place. Donor deferral from blood donation for high-risk individuals has been in place since 1983 (Outline 1). The overall prevalence of HIV antibody positivity in blood donors decreased from 0.04% in 1985 to 0.015% in 1987. However, the prevalence of HIV positivity remains at 0.06% for first-time male donors, indicating that further screening approaches must be developed for this population. The second mechanism ensuring blood safety is the enzyme-linked immunosorbent assay (ELISA) for the antibody to HIV. Although the sensitivity and specificity of this test is more than 99%, the test is not directed at the detection of the HIV agent itself, so that seronegative donors who are infected with HIV can be missed. Seven such cases have been reported. Estimations of the risks of now acquiring AIDS from 1 unit of blood transfusion range from 1 per 20,000 units to 1 per 1 million units, and the risk varies geographically (Table 3).

Cytomegalovirus Infection

The most common viral agent transmitted via blood transfusion is cytomegalovirus (CMV). Blood is not routinely tested for this agent because CMV infection is endemic in the United States and its prevalence is age-dependent; approximately 20% of blood donors have been infected by CMV by 20 years of age; this increases to approximately 70% by 70 years of age. The virus is harbored in leukocytes and can be transmitted years after clinical infection. Posttransfusion CMV infection is not a significant clinical problem in the immunocompetent transfusion recipient, although in the early years of open heart surgery, when exposure to many blood donors was routine, a "postperfusion syndrome" of fever, jaundice, and hepatosplenomegaly was recognized as caused by CMV blood transmission and infection. Current indications for CMV-negative blood products are not well-defined, but include transplantation of bone marrow in CMV-negative patients, transplants from CMV-negative donors, blood transfusions in CMV-negative women who are pregnant, treatment of premature neonates (less than 30 weeks of gestational age and/or suffering from intrauterine growth retardation and birthweight of less than 1,200 g) born to CMV-negative mothers, and treatment of AIDS patients who are CMV-negative.

Human T-Cell Lymphotropic Virus Type I Infection

Other newly identified human retroviruses are also potential candidates for transfusion-transmitted infections. Human T-cell lymphotropic virus type I (HTLV-I) infection has been associated with adult T-cell leukemia in Japan (more than 300 cases), tropical spastic paraparesis (as many as 75% of cases) in the Caribbean, and myelopathy

Table 3. Risk of HIV transmission by blood transfusion*

No. of Units Transfused	Baseline	Pessimistic Estimates	Very Pessimistic Estimates	Very Optimistic Estimates
1.0	1 in 99,000	1 in 33,000	1 in 20,000	1 in 1,133,000
2.0	1 in 50,000	1 in 17,000	1 in 10,000	1 in 556,000
2.9†	1 in 34,000	1 in 11,000	1 in 7,000	1 in 391,000
5.0	1 in 20,000	1 in 7,000	1 in 4,000	1 in 227,000
10.0	1 in 10,000	1 in 3,000	1 in 2,000	1 in 113,000
20.0	1 in 5,000	1 in 2,000	1 in 1,000	1 in 57,000
30.0	1 in 3,000	1 in 1,000	1 in 1,000	1 in 38,000

*Reproduced with permission from *Confronting AIDS.* Washington, DC, National Academy Press, 1986.
†Approximately the average number of units transfused (units of blood transfused per year divided by the number of patients receiving tarnsfusions per year).

in Japan (more than 85 cases). The prevalence of HTLV-I seropositivity in the United States is very low (approximately 0.025% of donor pools tested) but blood donor screening for antibody to HTLV-I was implemented in January 1989 because of these disease associations.

Immunosuppression From Erythrocyte Transfusions

The immunosuppressive effect of blood transfusion was first noted in renal transplantation. Preoperative blood transfusions were observed to increase substantially (by as much as 20%) the survival of cadaveric renal transplants. This salutary effect has been lessened, if not abolished, by the postoperative use of cyclosporin to prevent renal graft rejection. Blood transfusions have also been associated with an increased incidence of metastasis from cancer when the blood transfusions are given at the time of surgical removal of the primary tumor and also with an increased risk of death from metastases in patients given transfusions. All of the 30 clinical studies reported have been retrospective, nonrandomized studies subjected to careful multivariate analysis; on balance, these studies certainly support the need for further work in this area.

Benefits of Blood Transfusion

Oxygen Transport

Tissue oxygen delivery, as the primary function of hemoglobin, is preserved during significant reductions in erythrocyte volume by a complex series of interactions, but most notably by enhanced cardiac output; thus, there are significant compensatory mechanisms for anemia in patients with normal cardiopulmonary reserves. Because of the new appreciation of the risks of blood products, the "transfusion-trigger" for perioperative erythrocyte transfusion is being reexamined. A hemoglobin level of 100 g/L (10 g/dl) is often used in decision-making; survey studies indicate that more than 50% of surgeons would order a preoperative transfusion for an asymptomatic individual whose hemoglobin level is less than 100 g/L (10 g/dl). Many anesthesiologists also regard this hemoglobin level as a transfusion indication per se. However, experience with renal transplant patients during the last 25 years has stimulated interest in reevaluating preoperative hemoglobin requirements. A prospective study of 282 patients with preoperative hemoglobin levels of less than 100 g/L (10 g/dl) indicated that many patients can undergo anesthesia and surgery safely with hemoglobin levels as low as 80 g/L (8 g/dl). In another study of 15 Jehovah's Witnesses, all of whom had preoperative hemoglobin levels of less than 70 g/L (7 g/dl), there were no deaths from anemia. Surgical studies monitoring mixed venous Po_2 and the oxygen extraction ratio suggest that such measures may be useful in making "transfusion-trigger" decisions for individual patients.

Wound Healing

There is a widely recognized rule of thumb that states that wound healing suffers when the hemoglobin level is below about 80 g/L (8 g/dl). This belief arose decades ago as a result of several uncontrolled retrospective clinical studies of wound dehiscence. Experimental animal studies do indicate that nutritional anemia (iron deficiency) is detrimental to wound healing, but poor wound healing persists when the anemia is corrected with erythrocytes. Similarly, poor wound healing associated with blood-loss anemia can be corrected when blood volume is enhanced without changing the hemoglobin level. Subsequently, many studies have shown that normovolemic anemia is irrelevant to wound healing in experimental animals until the hematocrit level decreases to 0.15 (15%) or lower.

Special Considerations in Blood and Blood Component Therapy

Massive Transfusion

Nearly all studies of platelet hemostasis in patients receiving massive transfusions have shown a strong tendency for dilutional thrombocytopenia to develop. This thrombocytopenia is directly related to the number of transfusions received and is a consequence of the loss of blood that contains viable platelets and its replacement with blood and/or other fluids containing either nonviable or no platelets. However, the likelihood of thrombocytopenia developing in any given patient is related to many other factors governing the circulating platelet count. Patients undergoing massive transfusions in whom diffuse clinical bleeding (that is, more than that normally associated with the surgical procedure) begins are potental candidates for platelet transfusions. Such patients ordinarily have either a platelet count of less than 100×10^9/L or a prolonged bleeding time. In these patients there is usually bleeding from venipuncture sites, mucous membranes, and other areas besides the surgical or trauma site. A prospective, randomized, double-blind clinical trial showed that prophylactic platelet transfusions in patients receiving massive transfusions did not affect blood requirements or clinical outcome. Therefore, the arbitrary infusion of platelets after some fixed level of transfusion is inappropriate.

When platelet transfusion is deemed appropriate, 1 unit of platelet concentrate containing at least 55×10^9 platelets would be expected to increase the circulating platelet count by about 10×10^9/L in the average 75-kg man. Thus, transfusion of 4 to 8 pooled platelet concentrates should raise the count by 40 to 80×10^9/L and should provide adequate hemostasis (shown by a reduction in bleeding time and control of hemorrhagic manifestations). Ordinarily a single transfusion should be sufficient. However, in many cases complications reduce the survival of transfused platelets. Thus, posttransfusion platelet counts and bleeding manifestations should be carefully monitored to determine if additional transfusions are required.

Similarly, fresh-frozen plasma should not be given prophylactically to patients with massive bleeding who do not have significantly (at least 150% of that of controls) abnormal coagulation tests. It is also inappropriate to use plasma or albumin for blood volume expansion or for support in resuscitation or trauma; crystalloid infusion (Ringer's lactate) has been shown to be equivalent to colloid infusion in these circumstances.

Replacement of Clotting Factors by Plasma or Its Derivatives

Fresh-frozen plasma contains 1 unit/ml activity of all clotting factors except for factor VIII, which is temperature-labile and has 85% (0.85 μ/ml) activity. Schedule and dose replacement of any clotting factor depend on the desired level and its half-life. Dose calculation is a function of plasma volume, which is approximately 40 ml/kg of body weight; for example, to provide 100% factor IX coverage in a 70-kg patient with Christmas disease undergoing minor surgery requires 11 units of plasma initially (100% × 40 ml/kg × 70 kg = 2,800 units of factor IX) and 50% replacement every six hours for the first day and daily thereafter. For higher (200%) levels in patients undergoing major surgery and who have hereditary hemorrhagic disorders and limited cardiopulmonary reserves and for whom large infusion volumes are poorly tolerated, commercial clotting factor concentrates may be necessary. The disadvantages of these concentrates include exposure to many donors (as many as 20,000 donors contribute to a given commercial lot) and the risk of thrombosis from the activated clotting factors in the concentrate. In classic hemophilia or von Willebrand's disease, cryoprecipitate may be given; each bag is derived from one blood donor and contains fibrinogen (300 mg), factor VIII (80 to 100 units), and factor XIII (fibrin-stabilizing factor). In this case, 2,800 units of factor VIII can be supplied by 3,800 ml of plasma, or 35 bags of cryoprecipitate, with 50% replacement every 12 hours thereafter. The advantage of cryoprecipitate over plasma is one of volume; the advantage of cryoprecipitate over commercial factor VIII concentrate is exposure to fewer donors and a lower risk of thrombosis.

Cryoprecipitate can also be used as a source of fibrinogen in consumptive coagulopathies associated with hypofibrinogenemia. Each bag of cryoprecipitate contains approximately 300 mg of fibrinogen; patient plasma volume = 60 ml of blood/kg × (1−hematocrit) so that in a patient with a hematocrit reading of 0.30 (30%) and approximately 42 ml of plasma/kg, the number of bags of cryoprecipitate required for a therapeutic increment of 100 mg/dl of fibrinogen is approximately 1 bag of cryoprecipitate per 6 kg of body weight.

In response to the overuse of fresh-frozen plasma and its attendant risks and questionable benefits, certain guidelines for the use of fresh-frozen plasma should be followed. It may be used to correct multiple coagulation factor deficiency under the following conditions: oral anticoagulant overdose, massive transfusion, plasmapheresis, liver disease, and disseminated intravascular coagulation. Fresh-frozen plasma may be considered (but is not mandatory) in a patient who is bleeding abnormally (bleeding not controlled by sutures or cautery), whose prothrombin time or partial thromboplastin time is less than 40% of normal, and whose platelet count is more than 50×10^9/L.

The dose of fresh-frozen plasma used should be adequate to replace coagulation factors. For example, an adult with liver disease usually requires 3 to 9 units (approximately 15 ml/kg) of fresh-frozen plasma to shorten the prothrombin time significantly. One or 2 units does little to correct the deficiency. Fresh-frozen plasma should be administered rapidly at the time of bleeding or within an hour of the anticipated bleeding. Its maximal effect declines two to four hours after transfusion. For correction of a warfarin overdose, vitamin K is the primary treatment. Fresh-frozen plasma should be given only when the bleeding is life-threatening and the eight- to 12-hour waiting period for vitamin K to take effect is too long. For monitoring purposes, prothrombin time and/or partial thromboplastin time should be determined immediately before and immediately after the transfusion of fresh-frozen plasma.

Alternatives to Homologous Blood Transfusion

Autologous Blood Predeposit

Patients scheduled for elective orthopaedic surgery are particularly well-suited for enrollment in an autologous blood predeposit program, since the need for perioperative transfusion is significant. Further, most cases can be scheduled as long as 42 days in advance, the maximum period for prestoring liquid-packed erythrocytes. One unit of autologous blood can be procured from the patient every 72 hours until 72 hours before surgery, as long as the hematocrit reading is at least 0.34 (34%); iron supplementation is routine. Thus, 2 to 4 units of autologous blood can easily be procured. The amount of autologous blood predonated may, however, be limited because of functional iron deficiency, the endogenous erythropoietin response to serial phlebotomy, or both. Recent studies indicate that not all autologous blood donors have an adequate erythropoietin response; this has implications for subsequent homologous blood exposure (Table 4): 43% of such patients receive homologous blood compared with less than 13% of patients who successfully predeposit the requested amount of autologous blood.

Successful predeposit of autologous blood depends on the amount requested. In one study (Table 4), 110 of 117 patients (94%) asked to predeposit 3 units or less of autologous blood were able to do so; only 35 of 58 patients (61%) asked to predeposit 4 or more units were able to do so. Further studies designed to maximize such predeposits must include the use of recombinant erythropoietin.

Autologous blood predeposit programs at hospitals with active orthopaedic surgical services have seen a tenfold increase in activity during the last three years. The percentage of participation by eligible orthopaedic patients has increased from less than 5% to more than 50% in many programs. Although this approach is still underutilized, its safety and efficacy should make it a standard practice.

Frozen autologous blood predeposit is also an option for patients anticipating future blood needs. Because blood stored in this manner is not always suitable for emergency needs (because of logistical and transport considerations over long distances) and because liquid blood storage is more cost-effective for elective, anticipated transfusion needs, this option continues to be most appropriate for patients who have alloantibodies or who have rare erythrocyte antigens.

Autologous Blood Salvage and Reinfusion

Autologous blood salvage and reinfusion, either intraoperatively or postoperatively, complements the predeposit approach. Blood salvaged intraoperatively from a sterile field is most commonly reinfused after processing through a cell-saver via centrifugation and washing, either in the operating suite or the blood bank. Processing has the advantage of removing activated products of coagulation and the heparin anticoagulant used in the collection system. Use of the cell-saver in Harrington rod spinal fusions was shown to reduce the homologous blood transfusion needed from 5.1 ± 2.7 units to 2.0 ± 1.5 units. Further, 50% of patients who underwent intraoperative autologous blood salvage avoided homologous blood transfusion, compared with 4.2% of the patients who did not. In another study, intraoperative autologous blood salvage and reinfusion significantly reduced the amount of banked

Table 4. Consequences of understoring autologous blood*

Success of Patients	No. of Patients	Patients Subsequently Exposed to Homologous Blood	
		No.	%
Requested amount donated	145	19	13.1
≤ 3 units requested	110	16	14.5
≥ 4 units requested	35	3	8.6
Requested amount not donated	30	13	43.3
≤ 3 units requested	7	4	57.1
≥ 4 units requested	23	9	39.1

*Reproduced with pemission from Goodnough LT: Autologous blood donation, letter. *JAMA* 1988;259:2405.

homologous blood required in total hip replacements and spinal fusions. A third study of 25 children undergoing spinal surgery showed that reinfusion of 10,000 ml of salvaged autologous blood (hematocrit reading, 0.55 [55%]), along with 7,300 ml of autologous blood procured by preoperative phlebotomy, eliminated the need for homologous blood.

The impact of induced hypotension on homologous blood requirements has also been studied. In one such investigation of patients undergoing spinal fusion procedures, induced hypotension did not reduce homologous blood requirements.

Acute Preoperative Hemodilution

Acute preoperative hemodilution is a third method of autologous blood transfusion. This has been demonstrated to be a safe and effective means of reducing homologous blood needs during surgery. This maneuver consists of an isovolemic exchange of whole blood with crystalloid and/or colloid (hydroxyethyl starch) solutions after induction of general anesthesia and before surgery. Two to 6 units of autologous blood can be procured with hemodilution of the preoperative hematocrit reading to 0.22 to 0.25 (22% to 25%). This can be done manually or by automation. Blood replacement starts at intraoperative hematocrit readings of 0.20 to 0.22 (20% to 22%), transfusing "last blood out" as "first blood in." This maneuver has two advantages: fresh autologous whole blood is available for the patient in the operating room and surgical erythrocyte loss is less (by as much as 50%) in the anemic patient. This practice has been shown to be both safe and effective in a variety of operations, including orthopaedic (adults and children) and gynecologic procedures and open heart surgery. One study of 12 pediatric patients undergoing spine surgery demonstrated both the safety and the efficacy of this procedure.

Pharmacologic Interventions

The increasing use of pharmacologic agents has also provided an alternative to homologous blood transfusion, particularly in combination with autologous blood interventions. Desmopressin is a synthetic analogue of an antidiuretic hormone (vasopressin) that has no clinically significant vasomotor effects. This drug has been shown to increase plasma activity levels of antihemophilic factor (factor VIII) and von Willebrand factor. Thus, desmopressin can be used to treat patients with mild hemophilia, carriers of hemophilia with low factor VIII concentrations, and patients with von Willebrand's disease. When given by slow intravenous injection in a dose of 0.3 μg/kg of

body weight, factor VIII activity increases threefold to fivefold and in von Willebrand's disease the bleeding time is shortened or even made normal. Because of its antidiuretic effect, excessive free water administration should be avoided. Desmopressin also reduces surgical blood loss and homologous blood transfusion requirements in patients without clotting factor deficiencies who undergo open heart surgery (correcting the qualitative platelet defect secondary to ex vivo corporeal circulation) and in patients with normal platelet function who undergo Harrington rod spinal fusion surgery. Finally, desmopressin improves or corrects the prolonged bleeding times in patients with acquired platelet defects such as those caused by uremia, cirrhosis, and aspirin ingestion; these patients may benefit from desmopressin therapy in the perioperative period.

Fibrin glue has been used in a wide variety of surgical procedures. Although fibrin glue is not a pharmacologic agent, this preparation is readily derived from aliquots of the patient's own (autologous) plasma before elective surgery. Fibrin glue has been shown to be useful in otologic (middle ear) surgery and various thoracic procedures; ongoing studies will help define its role in orthopaedic surgery.

Recombinant Erythropoietin

This experimental drug has broad potential applications in transfusion medicine, in both surgical and nonsurgical settings. Data from clinical trials have shown the relative safety and efficacy of this drug in patients with renal failure. A study in anesthetized baboons subjected to acute blood loss demonstrated the ability of this drug to stimulate erythropoiesis postoperatively. Finally, studies in patients predepositing autologous blood have shown an absence of endogenous erythropoietin response during the phlebotomy interval. Clinical investigations are underway to study the usefulness of this drug as a perisurgical adjuvant therapy in vascular surgery and as a means of facilitating autologous blood predeposit before elective orthopaedic surgery.

Erythrocyte Substitutes

Perfluorochemical emulsion (Fluosol-DA) is a synthetic oxygen carrier studied for use in acutely anemic patients who refuse blood transfusions. The data in this select group of patients indicated that this preparation is unnecessary in moderate anemia (mean hemoglobin level >70 g/L [7 g/dl]) and ineffective in severe anemia (hemoglobin level <35 g/L [3.5 g/dl]). Its efficacy is limited by the percentage of the drug that can be solubilized, by its oxygen-carrying capacity, and by biologic half-life. More recent research has been done on human and bovine hemoglobin polymers in an effort to develop erythrocyte substitutes that address these limitations.

Trends

Blood banking went through a period of rapid change in the 1980s. This process will continue to evolve in the 1990s. Areas that will undergo further development include (1) mechanisms of informed consent for anticipated blood transfusions; (2) autologous blood transfusion and designated blood transfusion as alternatives to homologous blood transfusion; (3) the "transfusion-trigger" hematocrit; (4) pharmacologic interventions to reduce blood transfusion needs; (5) synthetic blood substitutes, such as hemoglobin polymers; and (6) processes for inactivating viral agents.

Because of this intense scrutiny of issues of blood safety, we have been able to reaffirm that the blood supply is as safe as ever but that blood should be transfused only when necessary.

Annotated Bibliography

Keywords

Acquired immune deficiency syndrome; Blood transfusion; Cytomegalovirus; Hemophilia; Hepatitis; HTLV-I; Human immunodeficiency virus; Immunology

Transfusion in a Changing Environment

Kruskall MS, Umlas J: Acquired immunodeficiency syndrome and directed blood donations: A dilemma for American medicine. *Arch Surg* 1988;123:23–25.
  Reviews why directed blood donation is a controversial practice.

Toy PTCY, Strauss RG, Stehling LC, et al: Predeposited autologous blood for elective surgery: A national multicenter study. *N Engl J Med* 1987;316:517–520.
  Demonstrates that autologous blood donation is an underutilized practice.

Administration of Blood Products and Its Risks

Baker RJ, Moinichen SL, Nyhus LM: Transfusion reaction: A reappraisal of surgical incidence and significance. *Ann Surg* 1969;169:684–693.
  This six-year review of 116,000 transfusions showed that 5% produced reactions.

Blumberg N, Heal JM: Transfusion and host defenses against cancer recurrence and infection. *Transfusion* 1989;29:236–245.
  In this review article, the authors provide evidence that homologous blood is immunologically suppressive.

Moore SB, Taswell HF, Pineda AA, et al: Delayed hemolytic transfusion reactions: Evidence of the need for an improved pretransfusion compatibility test. *Am J Clin Pathol* 1980;74:94–97.
  Although the documented incidence of transfusion reaction was one in 4,000, the authors found that such reactions occurred far more often.

Diseases Transmitted by Transfusion

Aledort LM, Levine PH, Hilgartner M, et al: A study of liver biopsies and liver disease among hemophiliacs. *Blood* 1985;66:367–372.
  The authors report that cirrhosis develops in 22% of hemophiliacs.

Hardy AM, Allen JR, Morgan WM, et al: The incidence rate of acquired immunodeficiency syndrome in selected populations. *JAMA* 1985;253:215–220.
  Reviews the epidemiology of AIDS.

Myhre BA: Fatalities from blood transfusion. *JAMA* 1980;244:1333–1335.
  Approximately 35 to 50 deaths result from blood incompatibility in the United States each year.

Benefits of Blood Transfusion

Gould SA, Rosen AL, Sehgal LR, et al: Fluosol-DA as a red-cell substitute in acute anemia. *N Engl J Med* 1986;314:1653–1656.
  Fluosol-DA did not reduce the mortality in severely anemic patients (those with hematocrit readings ≤0.12 [12%]).

Stehling LC, Ellison N, Faust RJ, et al: A survey of transfusion practices among anesthesiologists. *Vox Sang* 1987;52:60–62.
  Most anesthesiologists regard a hemoglobin level of 100 g/L (10 g/dl) or less as an indication for transfusion.

Special Considerations in Blood and Blood Component Therapy

Counts RB, Haisch C, Simon TL, et al: Hemostasis in massively transfused trauma patients. *Ann Surg* 1979;190:91–99.
  The authors found that prophylactic plasma transfusion is not necessary in such cases.

Reed RL II, Ciavarella D, Heimbach DM, et al: Prophylactic platelet administration during massive transfusion: A prospective, randomized, double-blind clinical study. *Ann Surg* 1986;203:40–48.
  The authors found that prophylactic platelet transfusion is not necessary in such cases.

Virgilio RW, Rice CL, Smith DE, et al: Crystalloid vs. colloid resuscitation: Is one better? A randomized clinical study. *Surgery* 1979;85:129–139.
  The authors found that crystalloid is equivalent to colloid.

Alternatives to Homologous Blood Transfusion

Eschbach JW, Egrie JC, Downing MR, et al: Correction of the anemia of end-stage renal disease with recombinant human erythropoietin: Results of a combined phase I and II clinical trial. *N Engl J Med* 1987;316:73–78.

Recombinant erythropoietin was efficacious in 100% of cases.

Goodnough LT: Autologous blood donation, letter. *JAMA* 1988;259:2405.

Surgeons can accurately predict how many units of autologous blood must be predeposited to avoid exposure to homologous blood.

Goodnough LT: Directed blood procurement does not benefit patients who are already enrolled in an autologous blood predeposit program. *Am J Clin Pathol*, in press.

A controversial transfusion practice (directed donation) should not replace a good transfusion practice (autologous donation).

Goodnough LT, Wasman J, Corlucci K, et al: Limitations to donating adequate autologous blood prior to elective orthopedic surgery. *Arch Surg* 1989;124:494–496.

Of patients unable to predeposit the requested amount of autologous blood, 40% receive homologous blood.

Kafer ER, Isley MR, Hansen T, et al: Automated acute normovolemic hemodilution reduces blood transfusion requirements for spinal fusion. *Anesth Analg* 1986;65:S76.

Acute preoperative hemodilution reduces homologous blood needs.

Kobrinsky NL, Letts RM, Patel LR, et al: 1-Desamino-8-D-arginine vasopressin (desmopressin) decreases operative blood loss in patients having Harrington rod spinal fusion surgery: A randomized, double-blinded, controlled trial. *Ann Intern Med* 1987;107:446–450.

Desmopressin may reduce blood loss and transfusion needs during such surgery.

Kruger LM, Colbert JM: Intraoperative autologous transfusion in children undergoing spinal surgery. *J Pediatr Orthop* 1985;5:330–332.

Intraoperative salvage and reinfusion effectively reduces the need for homologous blood transfusion.

Lennon RL, Hosking MP, Gray JR, et al: The effects of intraoperative blood salvage and induced hypotension on transfusion requirements during spinal surgical procedures. *Mayo Clin Proc* 1987;62:1090–1094.

Induced hypotension did not reduce homologous blood needs.

Mann M, Sacks HJ, Goldfinger D: Safety of autologous blood donation prior to elective surgery for a variety of potentially 'high-risk' patients. *Transfusion* 1983;23:229–232.

The authors found autologous blood donation to be a safe procedure.

Silvergleid AJ: Safety and effectiveness of predeposit autologous transfusions in preteen and adolescent children. *JAMA* 1987;257:3403–3404.

Autologous blood donation is safe and effective in children.

Wasman J, Goodnough LT: Autologous blood donation for elective surgery: Effect on physician transfusion behavior. *JAMA* 1987;258:3135–3137.

Surgeons tolerate lower hematocrit readings in patients receiving autologous blood than in matched controls.

Trends

Gould SA, Sehgal LR, Rosen AL, et al: Polyhemoglobin: An improved red blood cell substitute. *Surg Forum* 1985;36:30–31.

Soluble hemoglobin has a longer half-life and can carry more oxygen than Fluosol-DA.

13
Bone Grafts

There are many approaches to reconstructing or replacing deficits of the skeleton, including the use of synthetic materials, biologic tissues, and combinations of these. These options have greatly expanded the scope of clinical disorders that can be treated, but also underscore the fact that no single type of implant or graft is ideally suited for all circumstances. Studies in the past several years have provided increased knowledge of the biology, immunology, and biomechanics of bone grafts and a better definition of the relationship between the graft and its host environment. This information serves as the basis for choosing the most appropriate approach to reconstruction in selected cases, in terms of both graft type and surgical techniques.

Bone grafts are generally classified according to their tissue composition (cortical, cancellous), anatomic considerations (site of origin, size, shape), nature of blood supply (nonvascularized, revascularized), preservation method (fresh, frozen, freeze-dried), additional chemical or physical manipulations or exposures (demineralization, irradiation), and the degree of genetic disparity between donor and recipient (Table 1). Changes in any of these factors can influence the physiologic or structural properties of the graft; this, in turn, may affect its clinical efficacy in specific circumstances.

Although there is some rationale for designating viable osseous tissues as "grafts" and nonviable biologic preparations as "implants" (transplanted vs implanted), common usage has tended to lump both categories together—as "grafts"—with the appropriate descriptive adjectives appended: fresh revascularized segmental fibular autograft, freeze-dried irradiated cancellous wafer allograft, frozen distal femoral osteochondral allograft, and the like.

Biology

Our understanding of bone graft incorporation has not changed significantly. Incorporation represents a predictable sequence of events, reflecting a partnership between graft-derived and host-derived factors. After implantation, grafts become enveloped in a hematoma. Unless the blood supply is immediately reestablished by vascular reanastomosis, most cellular elements die within a few days and incite an inflammatory response. The host-tissue reaction is transformed into a fibrovascular stroma over the next one to three weeks. Blood vessels as well as host cells dedicated to bone resorption and new bone formation converge at the graft. Because of its more open structure, cancellous tissue permits more rapid permeation of blood vessels than does cortical bone. In cortical bone the vascular response must find, traverse, and widen preexisting Volkmann and haversian canals to reestablish the blood flow.

The initial host cell activity within bone grafts is resorptive and is mediated by osteoclasts derived from circulating monocytes of hematopoietic origin (Figs. 1 to 3). Osteoblasts, also arising from bone marrow precursors, subsequently elaborate osteoid on bony surfaces that were previous sites of resorption. This suggests the expression of humoral signals or exposure of protein messengers at points of previous osteoclastic activity. The repair and remodeling observed during graft incorporation is analogous to intact bone homeostasis and presumably relies on a cascade of systemic factors and locally derived signals, including bone morphogenetic protein. This molecule has been partially isolated and demonstrated to be in the 17- to 18-kd range.

The host contributes all blood vessels and most, if not all, the cells required to incorporate a bone graft. The graft itself serves as a scaffold or template on which the vascular and cellular response occurs. This passive role is termed "osteoconduction" and contrasts with the active phenomenon of "osteoinduction" whereby the graft matrix and perhaps residual cells provide signals to the host that are responsible for recruiting the required cellular activity.

Variations in the sequence and intensity of these cellular events occur when autologous tissues are compared with allogeneic alternatives, when autografts are immediately revascularized, and when allografts are pretreated before implantation.

Autografts

Nonvascularized Grafts

Fresh, nonvascularized autogenous bone grafts continue to be the standard to which other osteogenic alternatives are compared. Segmental grafts evaluated in long-bone deficits in several canine models have demonstrated graft resorption as well as osteoconductive and osteoinductive properties. As in normal fracture repair, the addition of electrical stimulation does not influence the end point of repair as judged histologically or biomechanically. When grafts were used to supplement calcar stock in dogs undergoing total joint replacement, 30% to 50% of the graft was involved in new bone formation by three months and 50% to 80% of the mass demonstrated the presence of fluorochrome markers of osteogenesis six months after the graft procedure.

Revascularized Grafts

Autografts transferred on a vascular pedicle or immediately reanastomosed to a blood supply do not undergo cell necrosis and do not require the lengthy repair process characteristic of conventional graft incorporation. Indeed, these grafts remain viable and heal at the host osteosyn-

Table 1. Advantages and disadvantages of available materials used for reconstruction of bone defects

Materials	Advantages	Disadvantages
Autografts		
Fresh	Optimal biologic behavior; no transfer of disease; histocompatible; best choice when donor site morbidity is acceptable and supply is sufficient	Limited availability; donor site morbidity
Revascularized	Little dependence on host bed; rapid healing	Limited availability of donor sites; technically difficult; sacrifice of normal structures
Allograft implants		
Fresh	No preservation required; articular cartilage viable; well suited to joint resurfacing alone	Most intense immune response; need and availability may not coincide; little time to test for sterility or disease
Frozen	Simple; permits cartilage cryopreservation; decreased immunogenicity; no change in biomechanical properties; well suited to massive osteoarticular and segmental deficits	Requires careful screening of donors; expensive over the long-term; cannot be sterilized secondarily; transit over long distances requires freezing temperature to be maintained; cartilage viability is limited
Freeze-dried	Can be stored indefinitely at room temperature; easy to transport; can be recovered clean and sterilized secondarily; compatible with demineralization; well suited to intercalary segmental loss or cystic defects	Storage and preservation techniques expensive and complicated; biomechanical changes; lengthy and perhaps less reliable incorporation; incompatible with cartilage cryopreservation
Demineralized	Potent osteoinducer; easy to contour; well suited to cystic defects and small or irregular bony gaps for supplementing stable fusions	Little intrinsic strength; complex processing; radiolucent
Synthetics		
Tricalcium phosphate	Restores volume; osteoconductive	No bonding to bone; unpredictable resorption; lengthy incorporation
Hydroxyapatite ceramic	Bonds to bone; restores volume	Brittle
Polymethylmethacrylate (PMMA)	Immediate strength; conforms to defect	Particulate wear debris; barrier to bone regeneration
Nonresorbable polymers (Teflon, foams, polyethylene)	Biocompatible in bulk form	May provoke inflammatory reaction in particulate form
Resorbable synthetics (polyglycolic acid, polylactic acid)	Osteoconductive; vehicle for additives	Unpredictable resorption
Bioactive silicate	Bonds to bone	Brittle

thesis sites by events analogous to fracture repair. To date, noninvasive attempts to monitor and study this repair process in canine models have been unsuccessful. In particular, technetium bone scans are a reliable indicator of blood flow to the graft only during the first postoperative week. Plain radiographs, although a crude measure of the biologic characteristics of the graft, remain the standard noninvasive measure of bone graft incorporation. However, magnetic resonance imaging is likely to provide new and useful information in the future.

Autoclaved Grafts

An autoclaved autograft in a rabbit ulnar defect was unable to bridge the deficit unless supplemented with demineralized bone matrix, whether the additional graft material was autogenous or allogeneic. In contrast, the use of autoclaved autogenous segments in humans, after resection of skeletal tumors, has been associated with clinical success in a few centers.

Allografts

Fresh Grafts

Nonvascularized fresh allogeneic bone in canine models uniformly behaves in a manner biologically inferior to autografts. In addition to cellular necrosis, allografts elicit a host immune response manifested histologically as an in-

flammatory exudate, slower new bone formation, and less apparent osteoinduction. In animals, if fresh allografts are reanastomosed to a blood supply and immunosuppression is withheld, the extent and speed of biologic failure parallels the degree of histocompatibility differences. This same pattern holds true for nonvascularized allografts in animals, but has not been confirmed to occur in a similar fashion in human recipients of bone allografts.

In a rat knee-joint model, fresh revascularized allografts transferred against a strong histocompatibility mismatch demonstrated rapid cell death. The initial immunologic response probably targeted the vascular endothelial cells of donor origin, causing disruption of the blood supply. Graft osteogenic cells are probably a secondary target of the immune response. Indeed, if the histocompatibility differences are minor, the intensity of the cellular response is lessened and more gradual in its evolution. The blood vessels remain patent and the earliest cell necrosis occurs in osteoblasts, with osteoclast death occurring later. Physeal chondrocytes appear to survive transplantation across weak histocompatibility barriers.

Preserved Grafts

Most bone allografts used clinically are subjected to some form of preservation technique, most commonly deep-freezing, freeze-drying, demineralization, or combinations of these approaches. In almost all animal models, the histologic sequence of events associated with allograft incor-

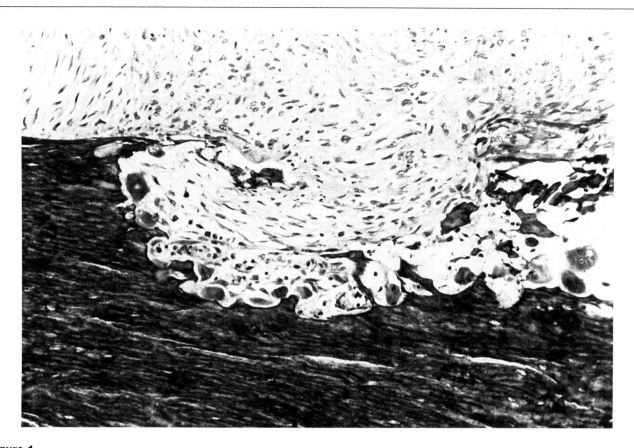

Figure 1
The graft (cortical bone) is engulfed in a fibrovascular response, from which osteoclasts arise and vigorously resorb preexisting bone at the periphery of the transplant.

poration is identical to that in fresh autografts, but preserved allografts take longer to repair and do so less completely than autogenous grafts. A recent evaluation of freeze-dried allografts in a segmental defect in dogs showed no histologic, histomorphometric, or biomechanical differences between fresh and frozen allografts, nor was there any improvement in these factors when recipients of the preserved grafts were given azathioprine for immunosuppression. Conversely, frozen allografts induced new bone formation within the medullary canal of dogs undergoing noncemented hip arthroplasty.

Allogeneic demineralized bone matrix has been shown to be osteoinductive in subcutaneous sites in rats as well as in segmental long-bone defects in rats and rabbits. Similarly, autolyzed antigen-extracted allogeneic bone has been effective in repairing segmental deficits in rabbit ulnas. It has not, however, been as useful in canine cranial defects, perhaps reflecting differences in the skull as a recipient site rather than inadequacies of this processed bone.

Synthetic Bone Substitutes

Two synthetic preparations of particular interest as graft substitutes are hydroxyapatite and tricalcium phosphate. Both materials can be found or manufactured with pore sizes from 50 to 600 μ and have been evaluated in animal models, usually canine or rabbit, either as single materials, mixed together, or supplemented with autograft or other sources of bone morphogenetic protein. Hydroxyapatite and tricalcium phosphate in cancellous skeletal sites are invaded by blood vessels and osteogenic cell populations. Tricalcium phosphate is biodegradable and replaced by new bone, whereas hydroxyapatite is nonbiodegradable but serves as an effective osteoconductive material. Neither hydroxyapatite or tricalcium phosphate is significantly inductive nor are their activities substantially enhanced by a pulsed electromagnetic field. These materials appear suitable for filling cystic defects, where the intrinsic mechanical strength of the graft is unimportant.

Influence of Drugs and Irradiation

Many drugs, including chemotherapeutic agents and nonsteroidal anti-inflammatories, negatively influence new bone formation in the intact skeleton and, to some degree, the repair associated with fractures. Similar findings exist for irradiation. Although these effects have not yet been studied in bone grafts, it is reasonable to assume that they also occur in bone graft incorporation. Preliminary data suggest an increased incidence of nonunions in human recipients of osteochondral allografts simultaneously treated with chemotherapy. It has also been demonstrated that physical barriers placed between the graft and its host bed, such as polymethylmethacrylate, also interfere with bone graft incorporation.

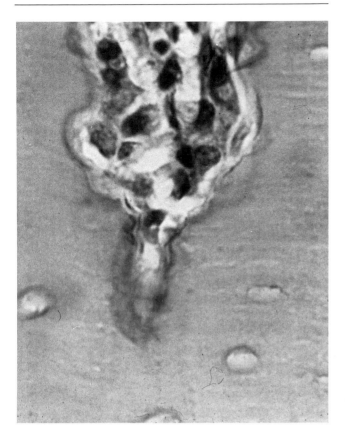

Figure 2

The resorptive response is conducted through former Volkmann's and harversian canals into the "dead" graft (characterized by empty lacunae). Osteoclasts widen these channels, by resorbing matrix, before deposition of new bone.

Immunology

No bone graft issue is more perplexing than the relationship of allograft immunogenicity to the biology of incorporation. Many investigators have demonstrated in several animal models that allografts evoke immune responses against cell surface histocompatibility antigens and that these responses can be diminished by deep-freezing or freeze-drying the graft before implementation. Similarly, the response can be moderated by more closely matching donors and recipients, as shown in rats and dogs. Invasive and noninvasive tests in these animal models also strongly suggested that there are adverse biologic consequences related to these immunologic responses, and that these consequences are manifested as less reliable incorporation.

To date, however, these correlations between graft immunogenicity and biology observed in animal models have not been demonstrated in humans. There are suggestions that the worst clinical failures, few in number, reflect immune "rejection" and some early indications that sensitization to class II major histocompatibility antigens after transplantation is protective while presensitization to class I histocompatibility antigens before surgery is detrimental to graft biology. Since most (about 75%) human recipients of massive frozen osteochondral allografts have satisfactory clinical results and since noninvasive techniques provide only a crude measure of graft biology, the clinical

significance of immune reactions against bone allografts has not been established and the need to match allograft donors and recipients by factors other than size or mechanical fit cannot yet be substantiated.

Clinical Applications

Autografts

In cases in which there is good soft-tissue coverage and no infection, fresh autogenous bone graft is usually used to graft skeletal defects and is the method most likely to succeed biologically or by clinical criteria. There are many reports describing the successful use of cancellous and corticocancellous autografts, usually iliac crest in origin, in the treatment of nonunions of long bones and the femoral neck. Satisfactory results can also be anticipated if infected nonunions are extensively debrided, the missing soft tissue replaced with free muscle transfer, and the bone graft then applied to the deficit. Conventional fresh autografts have also been used effectively to replace inadequate bone stock of the acetabulum or femur during total hip arthroplasty, to decrease the incidence of trochanteric nonunions, to supplement the glenoid at the time of total shoulder arthroplasty, to repair segmental defects of long bones, to augment bone stock in spinal fusion, and in the arthrodesis of joints such as the subtalar articulation.

Revascularized Grafts Revascularized autografts of fibula or iliac crest restore segmental defects associated with local compromise of soft tissue or bone, including infection, congenital pseudarthrosis of the tibia, and ununited fractures of the femoral neck. They are particularly well suited to lengthy deficits in long bones. These grafts are associated with relatively rapid repair (four months in the upper extremity and eight to nine months in the lower extremity) and can be expected to hypertrophy over time. There is evidence, however, that the fibular donor site is a source of prolonged muscle weakness and gait disturbance, so these findings must be balanced against the potential advantages of this approach.

Allografts

Allografts, particularly deep-frozen and freeze-dried grafts, continue to be used with predictable success in a number of clinical circumstances. Massive frozen osteochondral allografts are associated with satisfactory results in 75% to 85% of cases after limb-sparing tumor resections. Massive allografts have been used with increasing frequency to replace inadequate bone stock in the proximal femur at the time of revision total joint replacement or in the proximal tibia or distal femur during arthroplasty of the knee. Prostheses are generally cemented directly into allografts, with long stems extending beyond the osteosynthesis site. Care must be taken to prevent polymethylmethacrylate from becoming interposed between the allograft and the host side of the bony junction, or nonunion and failure of the construct will eventually occur.

Preserved allografts have also been used successfully in spinal fusions, with nonunion rates comparable to those of autografts in several series.

Infection remains a particularly devastating complication of allografts because more than 80% of infected grafts are associated with clinical failure. Infection rates, reported

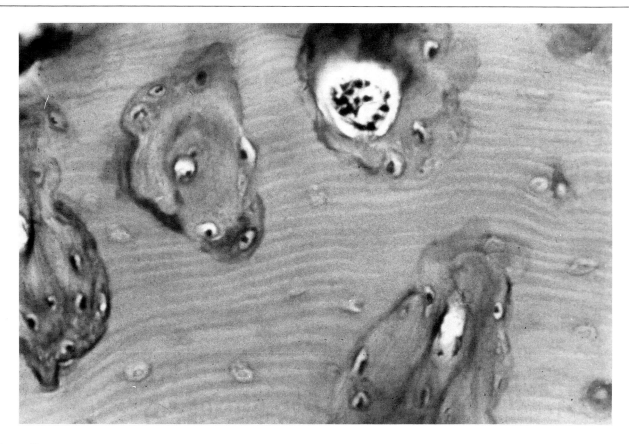

Figure 3
The resorption sites are then filled in by osteoblastic activity of host origin. This produces, in cross section, the appearance of viable osteons within a background of nonviable interstitial bone (representing unremodeled graft). The net result is a physiologically and biomechanically satisfactory composite.

to be as high as 10% to 12%, undoubtedly reflect several unique features of the procedure in which these massive implants are utilized. Generally, allograft reconstruction follows another operation to remove a bony malignancy, including a generous cuff of soft tissue; these patients often receive chemotherapy or irradiation after the procedure, and there is some reason to believe that immunologic responses to allografts may also contribute to the incidence of infection. It is reasonable, especially with low-grade virulent gram-positive organisms, to remove the infected graft, vigorously debride the host bed, reimplant another allograft, and treat the patient with appropriate antibiotics. This approach was successful in nine of 11 patients in one recent study.

Alternative Approaches

There is evidence suggesting that autoclaved autografts can provide a satisfactory osteoconductive matrix in patients undergoing limb-sparing tumor resections and reimplantation of the autoclaved segment. This observation is contrary to data obtained from animal models, but provides a useful clinical alternative. Recently, investigators used human bone morphogenetic protein to treat nonunions and segmental deficits. The rate of clinical success was high, but such studies are difficult to control and evaluate. Nonetheless, this represents an area of intense interest for the future.

Bone Banking

The clinical use of bone and cartilage allografts depends on banking techniques that ensure safe and viable tissues that are available in a timely fashion.

Consent Laws

Bone transplantation is only one part of the national program to recover potentially useful organs and tissues and make them available to the patients who need them most. It is currently possible to transplant kidneys, hearts, heart-lung units, livers, pancreas, corneas, skin, reproductive tissues, bone marrow, and blood in addition to bone and cartilage, and to do so with reasonable success. None of these organs or tissues, however, is available in sufficient numbers to respond to current or projected needs. One effort to enhance the supply has resulted in modification of the consent process. Most states now have "required request" or "routine inquiry" statutes. Although the individual (or next-of-kin) retains the right to decide whether or not to participate as an organ or tissue donor, healthcare institutions are required to identify potential donors and ask for the donation rather than wait for the donor to volunteer. This approach has not yet substantially increased the number of donors, but the rate of tissue donation has increased.

Donor Selection

The American Association of Tissue Banks has produced standards for the banking of musculoskeletal tissues that are widely used in the United States and elsewhere. Donors are selected by review of the medical history and appropriate laboratory tests to exclude individuals harboring significant and potentially transmissible diseases (infection, malignancy, hepatitis, venereal disease, AIDS) and those with disorders affecting the biomechanical or biologic properties of bone (collagen disorders, metabolic bone disease) or providing an opportunity to transfer toxic substances (poisons, radioactivity). Protecting the recipient from inadvertent transfer of disease is of paramount importance, and serologic tests are available to screen potential donors for hepatitis, venereal disease, and AIDS. It is imperative these tests be used and that the medical record be scrutinized.

HIV Testing

In one reported case, a bone allograft served as a vector for transmission of the human immunodeficiency virus (HIV), resulting in the death of the recipient. This occurred before adequate screening tests were available, but makes clear the need to minimize the spread of potentially harmful disease through organ or tissue transplants. Current recommendations by the American Association of Tissue Banks, which are supported by the Centers for Disease Control, include a careful medical history and the use of serologic tests for HIV antibodies obtained at the time of tissue donation. To eliminate the "window" during which infection may be present but there are no detectable antibodies, living donors should be tested again three to six months after the first test. When reliable tests for the HIV virus itself (an antigen test) become available, retesting will no longer be necessary.

Banking Methods

Grafts can be removed in a sterile environment using standard operating-room techniques, and the tissues maintained in sterile packages, usually deep-frozen. Alternatively, tissues recovered in a clean but nonsterile fashion can be subjected to secondary methods of eliminating contamination, including exposure to ethylene oxide, high-dose irradiation (in the range of 10 to 30×10^3 Gy), or strong acids (such as hydrochloric acid). These secondarily sterilized grafts are usually freeze-dried for long-term preservation. The AAA technique combines antigen extraction with chloroform methanol, demineralization, and sterilization with hydrochloric acid followed by lyophilization.

The advantages of deep-freezing (usually −70 to −80 C) include retention of biomechanical properties, relatively low costs, easy storage, and the opportunity to cryopreserve cartilage (with glycerol or dimethyl sulfoxide). Freeze-drying permits storage for indefinite periods at room temperature in evacuated containers, but there is some loss of structural integrity (although this may be unimportant unless the grafts are used as weightbearing segments). Demineralization appears to enhance osteoinduction, but these grafts have little intrinsic mechanical strength.

Trends

The applications of autogenous and allogeneic bone grafts have increased substantially in many areas. In the early 1970s, 100,000 to 200,000 bone grafts were used annually in the United States, with a smaller number representing allografts. Some estimates for the 1990s approach 1 million surgical procedures each year involving the application of bone graft material, and both the number and the percentage of allogeneic grafts are increasing. This reflects more indications, improved banking methods that ensure safety and efficacy, and recognition of the morbidity associated with autogenous graft sites.

Annotated Bibliography

Keywords

Allograft; Autograft; Bone banking; Bone graft; Hydroxyapatite; Immunology; Radiation therapy; Tricalcium phosphate

Biology

Friedlaender GE: Bone grafts: The basic science rationale for clinical applications. *J Bone Joint Surg* 1987;69A: 786–790.
  This is a concise summary of cellular events characteristic of bone graft incorporation, stressing the relationship between graft and host-derived contributions and their clinical implications.

Friedlaender GE (ed): Bone grafting. *Orthop Clin North Am* 1987, vol 18, No. 2.
  A wide spectrum of contributions discusses the biology, immunology, biomechanics, banking, and clinical applications of bone allografts.

Goldberg VM, Stevenson S: Natural history of autografts and allografts. *Clin Orthop* 1987;225:7–16.
  This is a comprehensive review of the investigators' experience with fresh autografts and fresh, frozen, and freeze-dried allografts in a canine model. Autografts are superior to allogeneic tissues in terms of biology, but the qualitative patterns of successful repair also occur in allografts.

Autografts

Bargar WL, Paul HA, Merritt K, et al: The calcar bone graft. *Clin Orthop* 1986;202:269–277.
  Iliac crest autografts used as calcar supplements in a canine total hip model demonstrated 20% to 50% uptake of fluorochromes at three months and 50% to 80% at six months. All grafts were incorporated without substantial resorption.

Köhler P, Kreicbergs A: Incorporation of autoclaved autogeneic bone supplemented with allogeneic demineralized bone matrix: An experimental study in the rabbit. *Clin Orthop* 1987;218:247–258.

Seven of seven ulnar deficits in rabbits healed with autoclaved autograft and demineralized allogeneic bone matrix, but five of seven went on to nonunion when autoclaved autograft was used alone.

Lindsey RW, Grobman J, Leggon RE, et al: Effects of bone graft and electrical stimulation on the strength of healing bony defects in dogs. *Clin Orthop* 1987;222:275–280.

Pulsed electromagnetic fields caused no difference in the biomechanical strength of canine long-bone defects autografted and evaluated after eight weeks.

Oklund SA, Prolo DJ, Gutierrez RV, et al: Quantitative comparisons of healing in cranial fresh autografts, frozen autografts and processed autografts, and allografts in canine skull defects. *Clin Orthop* 1986;205:269–291.

Fresh autografts were superior to frozen autografts and demineralized autograft or allograft. In the canine skull, none of the grafts demonstrated osteoinduction.

Shaffer JW, Field GA, Wilber RG, et al: Experimental vascularized bone grafts: Histopathologic correlations with postoperative bone scan. The risk of false-positive results. *J Orthop Res* 1987;5:311–319.

Technetium bone scans were valid predictors of graft perfusion in revascularized canine ulnas only during the first postoperative week.

Allografts

Burchardt H, Glowczewskie F, Miller G: Freeze-dried segmental fibular allografts in azathioprine-treated dogs. *Clin Orthop* 1987;218:259–267.

Radiography, tetracycline labeling, biomechanics, and histologic studies were used to evaluate canine grafts. Fresh autografts fared best, and all allografts, regardless of preservation or use of immunosuppression, were similar and fared worse than autografts.

Gepstein R, Weiss RE, Saba K, et al: Bridging large defects in bone by demineralized bone matrix in the form of a powder: A radiographic, histological, and radioisotope-uptake study in rats. *J Bone Joint Surg* 1987;69A:984–992.

The authors describe the osteoinductive nature of demineralized bone matrix in filling radial defects in rats.

Gotfried Y, Yaremchuk MJ, Randolph MA, et al: Histological characteristics of acute rejection in vascularized allografts of bone. *J Bone Joint Surg* 1987;69A:410–425.

The authors describe patterns of cellular necrosis associated with strong and weak histocompatibility differences in a rat knee model. Strong differences cause rapid "rejection," whereas more closely matched grafts demonstrated early osteoblastic cell death and later effects in osteoclasts.

Janovec M, Dvorak K: Autolyzed antigen-extracted allogeneic bone for bridging segmented diaphyseal bone defects in rabbits. *Clin Orthop* 1988;229:249–256.

The authors describe the efficacy of this processed bone in rabbit ulnar defects.

McDonald DJ, Fitzgerald RH Jr, Chao EY: The enhancement of fixation of a porous-coated femoral component by autograft and allograft in the dog. *J Bone Joint Surg* 1988;70A:728–737.

Both autograft and allograft induced new bone formation and achieved the pull-out strength of noncemented femoral components in dogs.

Synthetic Bone Substitutes

Bucholz RW, Carlton A, Holmes R: Interporous hydroxyapatite as a bone graft substitute in tibial plateau fractures. *Clin Orthop* 1989;240:53–62.

There were no radiographically detectable differences in treating tibial plateau fractures with interporous hydroxyapatite compared with bone autograft.

Eggli PS, Müller W, Schenk RK: Porous hydroxyapatite and tricalcium phosphate cylinders with two different pore size ranges implanted in the cancellous bone of rabbits: A comparative histomorphometric and histologic study of bony ingrowth and implant substitution. *Clin Orthop* 1988;232:127–138.

Tricalcium phosphate is biodegradable and hydroxyapatite is not. Both preparations are associated with more rapid newbone formation when the pore size is reduced, and resorption is mediated by osteoclasts and, probably, macrophages.

Holmes RE, Bucholz RW, Mooney V: Porous hydroxyapatite as a bone graft substitute in diaphyseal defects: A histometric study. *J Orthop Res* 1987;5:114–121.

The authors describe bony ingrowth of a hydroxyapatite preparation without implant resorption in the canine radius.

Moore DC, Chapman MW, Manske D: The evaluation of a biphasic calcium phosphate ceramic for use in grafting long-bone diaphyseal defects. *J Orthop Res* 1987;5:356–365.

A sintered hydroxyapatite and tricalcium phosphate preparation, evaluated in 2.5-cm diaphyseal defects in dogs, was not osteoinductive and was much more effective when mixed with cancellous autografts at the time of implantation.

Influence of Drugs and Irradiation

Friedlaender GE: The influence of various physical modalities and drugs on bone regeneration and ingrowth, in Fitzgerald RH Jr (ed): *Non-Cemented Total Hip Arthroplasty.* New York, Raven Press, 1987, pp 135–141.

The author reviews adverse influence of drugs, such as chemotherapeutic agents and nonsteroidal anti-inflammatory agents, on intact bone and fracture repair in rats using histomorphometry and biomechanical testing in torsion.

Immunology

Czitrom AA, Langer F, McKee N, et al: Bone and cartilage allotransplantation: A review of 14 years of research and clinical studies. *Clin Orthop* 1986;208:141–145.

Using radiation-reconstituted chimerae, the authors determined that the probable source of bone graft immunogenicity is myeloid cells of the granulocytic lineage. They also confirmed that freezing and freeze-drying reduce immunogenicity.

Horowitz MC, Friedlaender GE: Immunologic aspects of bone transplantation: A rationale for future studies. *Orthop Clin North Am* 1987;18:227–233.

The authors hypothesize that bone rejects in an immunologic fashion, similar to soft tissue, but uniquely modified by its mineralized nature. Immunologic considerations are reviewed.

Muscolo DL, Caletti E, Schajowicz F, et al: Tissue-typing in human massive allografts of frozen bone. *J Bone Joint Surg* 1987;69A:583–595.

Although the two worst clinical failures in a group of 26 patients were the most poorly matched immunologically, there was otherwise no clear correlation between genetic disparity and massive frozen allograft incorporation.

Stevenson S: The immune response to osteochondral allografts in dogs. *J Bone Joint Surg* 1987;69A:573–582.

Results of fresh and frozen proximal radial grafts in DLA-matched and DLA-mismatched beagles, followed clinically and by immunologic assays, suggested that histocompatibility matching in dogs is important.

Clinical Applications

Autografts

Aberg M, Rydholm A, Holmberg J, et al: Reconstruction with a free vascularized fibular graft for malignant bone tumor. *Acta Orthop Scand* 1988;59:430–437.

Vascularized fibula is particularly useful when graft site or recipient has been compromised by the use of irradiation or chemotherapy.

Blick SS, Brumback RJ, Lakatos R, et al: Early prophylactic bone grafting of high-energy tibial fractures. *Clin Orthop* 1989;240:21–41.

The rate of union in fractures, mostly grade III, treated by debridement of posterolateral autografts two weeks after wound closure was 96%.

Gordon L, Chiu EJ: Treatment of infected non-unions and segmental defects of the tibia with staged microvascular muscle transplantation and bone-grafting. *J Bone Joint Surg* 1988;70A:377–386.

The authors stress the importance of well-vascularized soft tissue in the support of bony repair.

Harrington KD, Johnston JO, Kaufer HN, et al: Limb salvage and prosthetic joint reconstruction for low-grade and selected high-grade sarcomas of bone after wide resection and replacement by autoclaved autogeneic grafts. *Clin Orthop* 1986;211:180–214.

In 42 patients treated with autoclaved segments of autogenous tumor-bearing bone, there were two local recurrences, five nonunions, and no fatigue fractures, resulting in a satisfactory overall outcome.

Hirst P, Esser M, Murphy JC, et al: Bone grafting for protrusio acetabuli during total hip replacement: A review of the Wrightington method in 61 hips. *J Bone Joint Surg* 1987;69B:229–233.

The authors' experience with femoral head autografts for protrusio acetabuli was satisfactory, but they caution against placing bone cement between host bed and graft.

Johnson EE, Marder RA: Open intramedullary nailing and bone-grafting for non-union of tibial diaphyseal fracture. *J Bone Joint Surg* 1987;69A:375–380.

The authors stress the importance of adequate debridement, internal fixation, and autografting to produce a high rate of union.

Johnson EE, Urist MR, Finerman GAM: Repair of segmental defects of the tibia with cancellous bone grafts augmented with human bone morphogenetic protein: A preliminary report. *Clin Orthop* 1988;236:249–257.

All six 3- to 17-cm traumatic tibial defects united after autografts supplemented with human bone morphogenetic protein.

Salibian AH, Anzel SH, Salyer WA: Transfer of vascularized grafts of iliac bone to the extremities. *J Bone Joint Surg* 1987;69A:1319–1327.

The authors used revascularized segments of iliac crest and adjacent soft tissue to reconstruct upper- and lower-extremity defects.

Youdas JW, Wood MB, Cahalan TD, et al: A quantitative analysis of donor site morbidity after vascularized fibula transfer. *J Orthop Res* 1988;6:621–629.

The authors found that all 11 donors of fibular material had prolonged postoperative muscle weakness. This morbidity must be balanced against the advantages of a revascularized graft.

Allografts

Gitelis S, Heligman D, Quill G, et al: The use of large allografts for tumor reconstruction and salvage of the failed total hip arthroplasty. *Clin Orthop* 1988;231:62–70.

The authors achieved 86% good or excellent results using massive frozen bone allografts for limb-sparing tumor reconstruction and revision total joint arthroplasty.

Jofe MH, Gebhardt MC, Tomford WW, et al: Reconstruction for defects of the proximal part of the femur using allograft arthroplasty. *J Bone Joint Surg* 1988;70A:507–516.

Results were good or excellent in 80% of 44 patients with allografts and proximal femoral implants. Despite complications of fractures and injection, this approach is a satisfactory alternative for these reconstructive challenges.

Lord CF, Gebhardt MC, Tomford WW, et al: Infection in bone allografts: Incidence, nature, and treatment. *J Bone Joint Surg* 1988;70A:369–376.

The infection rate in 283 patients with massive frozen allografts was 11.7%, reflecting the extensive nature of the surgical procedure. Most infections lead to failure of the allograft, but vigorous debridement and antibiotics have allowed successful reimplantation of a second allograft.

McCarthy RE, Peek RD, Morrissy RT, et al: Allograft bone in spinal fusion for paralytic scoliosis. *J Bone Joint Surg* 1986;68A:370–375.

Clinical experience, in terms of pseudarthrosis, with frozen femoral head allografts was equal to or better than experience with autografts.

Oakeshott RD, Morgan DAF, Zukor DJ, et al: Revision total hip arthroplasty with osseous allograft reconstruction: A clinical and roentgenographic analysis. *Clin Orthop* 1987;225:37–61.

Results were satisfactory in 85% of 72 patients receiving 112 frozen allografts during revision total hip reconstruction.

Trancik TM, Stulberg BN, Wilde AH, et al: Allograft reconstruction of the acetabulum during revision total hip arthroplasty: Clinical, radiographic, and scintigraphic assessment of the results. *J Bone Joint Surg* 1986;68A:527–533.

Frozen femoral head allografts used to reconstruct the acetabulum were well incorporated.

Bone Banking

Buck BE, Malinin TI, Brown MD: Bone transplantation and human immunodeficiency virus: An estimate of risk of acquired immunodeficiency syndrome (AIDS). *Clin Orthop* 1989;240:129–136.

The authors estimate the approximate risks of acquiring AIDS from bone grafts on the basis of the accuracy of available screening approaches.

Centers for Disease Control: Transmission of HIV

through bone transplantation: Case report and public health recommendations. *MMWR* 1988;37:597–599.

Documents a case of HIV transmission through bone graft vector and provides recommendations to minimize this fatal occurrence in the future.

Friedlaender GE: Bone banking: In support of reconstructive surgery of the hip. *Clin Orthop* 1987;225:17–21.

The author, stressing safety and efficacy, describes methods of donor selection, tissue recovery, and preservation and storage of allografts used in conjunction with total hip arthroplasty.

Tomford WW, Ploetz JE, Mankin HJ: Bone allografts of femoral heads: Procurement and storage. *J Bone Joint Surg* 1986;68A:534–537.

The authors described their approach to banking femoral heads in frozen form, which is especially suited to the needs of community hospitals.

14
Soft-Tissue Implants

Although soft-tissue implants can be used at many anatomic sites, the area most often involved is the knee, particularly the anterior cruciate ligament (ACL).

Implants can be divided into three categories: autografts, allografts, and synthetics.

The ACL is known to be a primary stabilizer of the knee. ACL-deficient knees can eventually become unstable, leading to joint degeneration and disability. As a result, surgeons have attempted its primary surgical repair as well as reconstruction to preserve knee joint stability and mechanics.

Autogenous tissues have traditionally been used to reconstruct the ACL and recent advances have improved the clinical outcome. Many centers report successful short-term results in 80% to 90% of patients treated with bone-patellar tendon-bone autografts or semitendinosus grafts (with or without the gracilis tendon). However, concern about donor site morbidity has led to the use of allografts and synthetics as ACL replacements.

ACL replacement by allografts and synthetics is still in its infancy and should be considered experimental. Data concerning allograft and synthetic replacement are preliminary, and long-term follow-up is necessary to determine the safety and efficacy of these procedures.

Allografts

Among the different human allograft tissues used as ACL replacements are bone-patellar tendon-bone units, fascia lata, the Achilles tendon, the tibialis anterior tendon, and groups of flexor tendons.

When compared with autograft tissues, allografts offer the advantage of a potentially unlimited supply of tissues in various shapes and sizes, without resultant donor site morbidity. However, allografts are not without potential problems. Immune response and the possibility of transmission of infectious agents are concerns.

Immunology

Cells, matrix, and collagen are thought to have immunogenic potential. Cell surface antigens are the main source of immunogens.

Preservation techniques can alter the immunogenic capabilities of allografts. Fresh allografts are strongly immunogenic, deep-frozen allografts have a diminished response, and freeze-dried tissue has the least capability of inducing an immunogenic response. Those preservation techniques that diminish the immunogenicity of allografts also affect the mechanical strength of these implants.

Retrieval

Retrieval first involves the screening of potential donors. Donor selection criteria have been established by the American Association of Tissue Banks (Outline 1). These criteria were instituted to minimize the risk of transmission of infectious or neoplastic processes.

Retrieval may be done in a sterile manner or in a clean nonsterile manner.

In sterile retrieval, tissue must be removed within 12 hours of cessation of cardiopulmonary function (24 hours if the body is stored at 4 C). Because sterile retrieval requires a sterile surgical technique, secondary sterilization of the tissue is not needed. Tissue retrieved in this manner can, therefore, be preserved by either lyophilization or deep freezing. In clean nonsterile retrieval, tissue can be removed 24 hours after death. Because a sterile surgical technique is not required, secondary sterilization of the tissue is needed. The two presently available secondary sterilization techniques are chemical sterilization with ethylene oxide and irradiation.

Secondary Sterilization Either γ-rays or electron beam radiation can be used. A dose of 15 to 25 $\times$ 10^3 Gy is recommended to ensure that the tissue is not altered biomechanically. However, some spore-forming viruses can survive this treatment.

Gas sterilization involves exposure of the tissue to ethylene oxide, followed by aeration to allow dissipation of residual ethylene oxide and/or its breakdown products of ethylene glycol and ethylene chlorhydrin. Some adverse effects are suspected and may be responsible for adverse clinical results. Approximately 50% of 35 patients who underwent ACL replacement with ethylene oxide-treated bone-patellar tendon-bone allografts were satisfied with the procedure after two years. There were five complete failures; these were thought to result from ethylene oxide residues. In another study, a persistent chronic effusion developed in seven of 109 patients (6.4%). Graft removal led to resolution of the process. Ethylene chlorhydrin, a by-product of ethylene oxide, was found in the synovium and allograft of one patient.

Ethylene oxide-treated allografts currently are not rec-

Outline 1. American Association of Tissue Banks guidelines for donor exclusion

Infection or sepsis by history, physical examination, and laboratory testing
Positive blood culture
History of intravenous drug abuse
History of neoplasm other than basal cell carcinoma of the skin, carcinoma in situ of the uterus, or intracranial neoplasm
History of hepatitis, syphilis, slow virus, infection, AIDS, ARC, or high risk for AIDS or ARC
History of autoimmune diseases
Positive serologic tests
Toxic substance in potentially toxic amounts in the tissues to be collected
Evidence of serious illness of unknown cause

ommended for use in ACL reconstruction until a better understanding of allograft processing and preservation is achieved.

Preservation

Sterilely retrieved tissue can be deep-frozen or lyophilized (freeze-dried). Deep-frozen tissue kept at –70 C or below can be stored for as long as five years. Lyophilized tissue can be stored at room temperature for five years. Nonsterilely retrieved tissue can be secondarily sterilized with irradiation or ethylene oxide.

Biologic and Biomechanical Properties Incorporation of allograft tissue is similar to that seen with autografts. In the animal model, allograft tissues act as free grafts and undergo the processes of necrosis, revascularization, and cellular proliferation.

Allograft tissue can possess different biomechanical properties depending on tissue type and preservation, processing, and storage techniques.

Deep-frozen patellar tendon allografts have a greater ultimate strength than Achilles tendon or fascia lata. A comparison of fresh-frozen and freeze-dried specimens showed no statistically significant difference in strength, although ultimate strength was slightly decreased in the freeze-dried group.

Biomechanical testing of fresh-frozen, freeze-dried, freeze-dried ethylene oxide-treated, and freeze-dried irradiated bone-patellar tendon-bone units, fascia lata, and Achilles tendon showed that ultimate strength was significantly reduced in the freeze-dried irradiated allografts. Fresh-frozen allografts had the greatest ultimate strength.

A recent study examining the order of irradiation and lyophilization on the strength of patellar tendon allografts revealed that allografts that were lyophilized and then irradiated were significantly weaker than grafts that were irradiated before lyophilization. A dose of 20×10^3 Gy of γ-irradiation does not significantly alter the initial material properties of deep-frozen bone-patellar tendon-bone allografts, but a dose of 30×10^3 Gy significantly reduces maximum stress and strain energy density to maximum stress.

Clinical Results

In one reported series, 106 patients underwent intra-articular ACL reconstruction wih fresh-frozen allografts of a mixed variety, including Achilles tendon, the tibialis and/or peroneus tendons, or thick flexor tendons. Grafts were implanted through a medial parapatellar arthrotomy. Two thirds of the patients also underwent an extra-articular procedure. After a minimum follow-up of three years (average, 57 months), 80 patients underwent further testing. Sixteen also underwent follow-up arthroscopy. Results were excellent or good in 75 patients and unsatisfactory in five. Three of the five failures were graft failures. Knee stability was restored in 90% of the patients (both those who had undergone extra-articular procedures and those who had not). Arthroscopically, the grafts resembled normal ACLs.

Synthetic Ligaments

Synthetic ligaments for use in ACL replacement offer many advantages over autograft and allograft tissues. Unlike autografts and allografts, which are weak postoperatively un-

til revascularization and reorganization are complete, synthetics have no initial weakness. As a result, synthetic ligament replacements do not require postoperative protection, facilitating rehabilitation and allowing a quicker return to activity.

In addition, synthetics obviate the need to harvest autogenous tissues, thus avoiding donor site morbidity. As an alternative to allograft tissue, synthetics offer the advantages of increased availability, lack of immune response, and no risk of transmitting infection.

Although synthetic ligament use is widespread and many different synthetics are available elsewhere, this is not true in the United States. Three synthetic ligaments have been approved by the FDA for use in the United States—the Gore-Tex ligament, the Stryker Dacron ligament prosthesis, and the Kennedy ligament augmentation device (Table 1).

A true prosthesis does not require autogenous tissue for support, has enough strength to provide immediate stability, and does not rely on intra-articular healing to augment its strength. The Gore-Tex and Stryker Dacron ligaments are examples.

Augmentation devices act as mechanical supports, reinforcing autogenous tissue and thereby increasing the initial strength of the autograft. However, augmentation devices must permit load-sharing with the graft tissue so that stress shielding does not occur. The Kennedy device is an example.

Only these three synthetic ligaments are sold in the United States because all ligaments must be approved by the FDA. Manufacturers or "sponsors" must meet many criteria before a ligament is approved for use.

Biologic and Biomechanical Properties

Table 2 summarizes a study of fixation strength and bone ingrowth in a canine model. It is important to remember, however, that the devices were implanted in dogs rather than in humans, that they were unstressed, and that they were not fixed with screws or staples as is done in humans. Moreover, although the comparison showed the Kennedy device to be significantly weaker than the Gore-Tex and Stryker ligaments, the Kennedy device is an augmentation device and not a true prosthesis. Its function is only temporary and biologic fixation is not required.

Abrasion testing is an important component of mechanical testing. Because all synthetic ligaments are subject to wear and abrasion, what effect, if any, the wear particles may have on the surrounding knee environment must be determined.

A study of the biochemical effects of synthetic ligament wear particles on a lapine synovial cell culture, as well as the histologic effects of wear particles injected into rabbit knees, showed that wear particles from all the synthetic ligaments tested increased the levels of neutral proteinases (collagenase and gelatinase) and chondrocyte activation factor (shown to be interleukin-1) in vitro. In vivo results showed wear particle accumulation throughout the synovial and subsynovial tissues, with the highest concentrations located in the retrotibial and retrofemoral synovial fields. Wear particles in the synovium were visible by polarized light microscopy. A foreign-body response was also noted in the form of mild to moderate synovial hypertrophy.

Although effusion and chronic synovitis are complica-

Table 1. Prosthetic ligaments available in the United States

Device	Material	Approved by the FDA	Indications
Gore-Tex	Polytetrafluorethylene	1986	Previous failed intra-articular reconstructions
Kennedy	Polypropylene	1987	Augmentation of autogenous tissue used in the Marshall-MacIntosh procedure for ACL reconstruction
Stryker	Dacron polyester	1989	Previous failed intra-articular reconstructions

Table 2. Fixation strength and bone ingrowth in synthesis

Device	Maximum Pull-Out Strength (N)	Bone Ingrowth
Gore-Tex	438.1 ± 131.9	Marked ingrowth of trabecular bone into interstices of prosthesis
Kennedy	78.4 ± 47.9	No evidence of ingrowth; fibrous tissue interface between the prosthesis and remodeled trabecular bone
Stryker	445.7 ± 151.0	Marked trabecular ingrowth into the periphery of the prosthesis; no ingrowth into central-core Dacron tapes

tions associated with ACL replacement, their cause is poorly understood. In one study of Dacron ACL replacements, abrasion synovitis was noted in more than 20% of the cases. In other studies, some synovial biopsy specimens from patients with chronic sterile effusions after ACL replacement with a synthetic ligament have contained wear debris. No positive correlations could be made, however. Further research is necessary to determine the effects of particulate debris in humans as well as to determine if any relationship exists between wear debris and sterile effusion.

Clinical Results

Comparing various synthetic materials is difficult because of the many variables involved. These include the patient's age, degree of injury, associated injuries, any previous surgery, and rehabilitation and the type and technique of surgery used to implant the synthetic.

The Gore-Tex Ligament The Gore-Tex ligament is a true prosthesis composed of expanded polytetrafluoroethylene. It is constructed as a three-bundle braid with eyelets at each end for fixation. Bicortically placed screws are used for immediate fixation.

In October 1986, the FDA approved commercial distribution for use in patients with previously failed intra-articular reconstructions. A considerable amount of clinical data is now available. More than 8,000 Gore-Tex ligaments have been implanted worldwide and more than 1,100 in the United States. After more than three years of follow-up (average, 40 months), knee stability was evaluated in approximately 120 of 187 patients in the original clinical study. Overall, 84% of the patients reported improvement. Complications included failure in 11 cases, instability requiring surgical intervention in 12 cases, infection in five cases, and effusions in nine cases.

In a similar study of 39 patients with a minimum of two years of follow-up, KT 1000 testing showed an average displacement of about 2 mm when 20 lb of force was anteriorly directed on the tibia. Complications included graft failure, instability, sterile effusion, need for screw removal, and infection (Table 3).

In another series, 97 patients with an average follow-up of 52 months (range, 18 to 75 months) were tested both subjectively and objectively. The replacements were considered successful (objective and subjective improvement)

Table 3. Complications with 39 Gore-Tex ligaments

Complications	No.	%
Graft failure	4	10.2
Infection	1	2.5
Instability	3	7.6
Screw removal	3	7.6
Sterile infusions	9	23.1

in 45%, pseudosuccessful (objective failure but subjective improvement) in 13%, and failures (both objective and subjective failure) in 42%.

After two to six years of follow-up, 99 Gore-Tex ACL reconstructions were evaluated objectively and subjectively, including physical examination, KT-1000 arthrometer measurements, and radiographs. More than one third of patients said the knee seemed to loosen with time and 41% noted swelling of the knee. Nonetheless, 86% considered their knees were improved. The Lachman test was at least slightly positive in 68% of cases; the pivot shift test was negative in 36%, mild in 50%, and moderate in 14%. Arthrometry revealed a side-to-side difference of more than 5 mm at maximum load in 52% of cases. The prosthesis had to be removed in 10% of cases.

The Stryker Dacron Ligament Prosthesis The Stryker ligament is a true prosthesis composed of a central core of four high-strength Dacron tapes that provide its inherent strength. The central core is enveloped by a Dacron velour sleeve that allows fibrous ingrowth.

In 84 patients whose knees were symptomatically unstable and in whom primary repair of the ACL or autogenous reconstruction had failed, complications included graft failure in 3.6%, septic arthritis in 3.6%, synovitis in 2.4%, and extra-articular infections in 1.2%. However, in most of this group, the Stryker ligament was used to augment autogenous tissues rather than functioning as the sole replacement. Follow-up ranged from three to 24 months (average, 23 months).

In another series of 61 patients, a two-tunnel surgical technique was used for ACL replacement. Complications included rupture in nine cases and synovial fistula in one case. The minimum follow-up was five years.

The Kennedy Ligament Augmentation Device The Kennedy

device was designed to augment autogenous tissues in reconstruction of the ACL. It is composed of polypropylene yarn braided in a flat diamond form.

Augmentation devices should increase the initial strength of the biologic graft and protect the biologic graft from elongation and disruption during necrosis, revascularization, and cell proliferation. As the graft matures, the augmentation device should share the applied forces wih the remodeling tissue to enhance the remodeling process and avoid stress-shielding. Load-sharing can be accomplished in one of three ways:

(1) The first technique is to fix the device at both ends. Once the graft has undergone remodeling, the device is released at one end to allow stresses to pass through the newly revascularized tissue.

(2) In the second method, the biologic graft is coupled to an augmentation device with biodegradable properties. This allows the prosthesis to be fixed at both ends. With time, the augmentation device slowly undergoes biodegradation, allowing a gradual transference of stresses to the biologic graft.

(3) The currently used technique is to couple the biologic graft and the augmentation device with sutures; the augmentation device is then fixed at one end only. Because the composite is only as strong as the weakest component, failure resulting from inadequate suture fixation remains a concern.

Clinically, the Kennedy device is usually used in combination with the Marshall-MacIntosh ACL reconstruction procedure. This involves the autogenous central third of the patellar tendon and the central two thirds of the quadriceps tendon. The FDA approved the device for this use in May 1987.

Ninety percent of patients who participated in one prospective multicenter study reported subjective improvement after two years. Complications included breakage in 3%, superficial infection in 3%, deep infection in 1%, patellar tendon rupture in 3%, and joint effusion in 13%.

In a retrospective study, 43 patients underwent autogenous intra-articular ACL reconstruction without augmentation and 48 patients underwent the procedure with augmentation by the Kennedy device. Mean follow-up was 64 and 50 months, respectively. Objective measurements indicated that the augmented procedure produced much better results.

Other Synthetic Ligaments Synthetic ligaments not approved by the FDA include the Xenograft tendon and the carbon and Leeds-Keio ligaments.

In the early 1980s clinical trials of the bovine Xenograft tendon began in Europe. The Xenograft tendon was treated with glutaraldehyde, which was supposed to have a dual function—sterilizing the graft and, by cross-linking collagen, protecting it from in vitro enzymatic attack. It functioned as a true prosthesis. The clinical results were mixed, and failure and synovitis were common. In 1987, the FDA voted against granting premarketing approval.

The carbon ligament was designed to function as a biodegradable scaffold, allowing host tissue ingrowth while providing the initial strength needed to stabilize the joint.

Scaffolds may be used with or without autogenous tissues. Potential problems with biodegradable scaffolds are twofold. As host tissue matures, a biodegradable scaffold should allow a gradual transference of stress to the host tissue. If the degradation is too rapid, the host tissue may be exposed to stresses that are too great, resulting in failure. If the tissue biodegrades too slowly, however, the host tissue is subject to stress shielding.

Clinical results with the carbon ligament were mixed. Problems included abrasion and partial fragmentation of the carbon fibers and concern about the nature of the tissue ingrowth. In 1986, the FDA unanimously disapproved the carbon ligament because of concern about the long-term effects of particles released from the device.

The Leeds-Keio ligament is made of pure polyester in an open-weave design. The Leeds-Keio ligament has enough initial strength (2,000 N) to act as a prosthesis, but it was designed to function as a permanent scaffold. Therefore, it can stabilize the joint while allowing host tissue ingrowth. This ingrowth further increases the strength of the implant. Whether the fibrous tissue ingrowth possesses structural ligamentous properties is still unknown. Clinical results with the Leeds-Keio ligament are encouraging. As of yet, the FDA has neither approved nor disapproved it.

Trends

Using meniscal allografts to replace severely damaged or absent menisci has received recent attention. Meniscal transplantation is still new and experimental, but much research on various surgical, preservation, and storage techniques is being done.

In a canine model, cryopreserved meniscal allografts healed to the host tissue with minimal articular cartilage changes beneath the transplanted meniscus. The investigators concluded that meniscal allografts appear to be suitable replacements for menisci in the canine model.

An important issue is the effect of preservation and storage on cell viability and the mechanical properties of the tissue. Dimethyl sulfoxide cryopreservation did not significantly alter the tensile properties of canine meniscal tissue after one week of storage.

The histologic characteristics of the meniscal tissue were apparently unaffected by the cryopreservation technique, although metabolic activity was reduced. Biosynthetic activity was approximately 50% of normal, and autoradiographic examination revealed that approximately 10% of the cells were metabolically active after two weeks of storage. As storage time increased, activity decreased.

Although few orthopaedic surgeons have attempted meniscal transplantation in humans and no large series is available as yet, meniscal transplantation may one day be an option for the patient with severely damaged, absent, or unrepairable menisci.

The search for knowledge about and clinical applications of soft-tissue implantation in other anatomic areas, including the posterior cruciate ligament and the intervertebral disk, continues. Much effort is needed so that one day ideal replacement materials, whether synthetic, autograft, allograft, or a combination of these, will be available.

Annotated Bibliography

Keywords

Allograft; Anterior cruciate ligament; Grafting; Immunology; Meniscus; Synthetic ligament

Allografts

Retrieval

Jackson DW, Simon TM, Windler G: Intra-articular reactions following reconstruction of the anterior cruciate ligament with ethylene oxide sterilized bone-patellar tendon-bone allografts. Presented at the meeting of the American Orthopaedic Society for Sports Medicine, Las Vegas, Feb 12, 1989.

Freeze-dried bone-patellar tendon-bone allografts sterilized with ethylene oxide were used as ACL replacements in 109 patients. Three years later, 6.4% of the patients had developed a persistent intra-articular reaction characterized by persistent synovial effusion with collagenous particulates and cellular inflammatory responses. The reaction ceased on removal of the allograft. Ethylene chlorhydrin (an ethylene oxide residue) was detected by gas chromatography within the allograft and synovium of one patient. The authors recommended that these grafts not be used in ACL reconstruction.

Roberts TS, Drez DJ Jr, McCarthy W, et al: Anterior cruciate reconstruction using freeze-dried, ethylene oxide sterilized bone-patellar tendon bone allografts: Two year results in 35 patients. Presented at the 56th Annual Meeting of the American Academy of Orthopaedic Surgeons, Las Vegas, Feb 13, 1989.

The authors studied 35 patients who underwent ACL reconstructive surgery with freeze-dried bone-patellar tendon-bone allografts sterilized with ethylene oxide. Results after two years were poor, with only one half considered satisfactory and five considered failures. The poor results were attributed to ethylene oxide residues, and the authors recommended that grafts sterilized with ethylene oxide not be used in ACL reconstruction.

Technical Manual for Tissue Banking. McLean, Virginia, American Association of Tissue Banks, 1987.

This manual describes methods of acquisition, retrieval, processing, preservation, storage, quality control, and distribution of transplantable tissues.

Preservation

Arnoczky SP, Warren RF, Ashlock MA: Replacement of the anterior cruciate ligament using a patellar tendon allograft: An experimental study. *J Bone Joint Surg* 1986;68A:376–385.

Fresh and deep-frozen bone-patellar tendon-bone allografts were compared in a canine model. The deep-frozen allografts underwent necrosis, revascularization, and cellular proliferation similar to those seen in autogenous tissues. The grafts were completely revascularized by six months; at one year the graft resembled a normal ACL. The fresh allografts incited a marked inflammatory and rejection response.

Butler DL, Noyes FR, Walz KA, et al: Biomechanics of human knee ligament allograft treatment. *Trans Orthop Res Soc* 1987;12:128.

The authors showed that modulus and maximum stress of irradiated freeze-dried fascia lata were significantly less than those of fresh-frozen, freeze-dried, or ethylene oxide-treated freeze-dried fascia lata. However, each of the grafts was obtained from a different donor. In a study of specimens obtained from two donors, both freeze-dried ethylene oxide-treated bone-patellar tendon units and fascia lata had significantly decreased modulus and maximus stress when compared with fresh-frozen tissues. No significant reductions were noted in the fresh-frozen irradiated group, perhaps because the irradiation dose was only 19.5×10^3 Gy.

Curtis RJ, Delee JC, Drez DJ Jr: Reconstruction of the anterior cruciate ligament with freeze dried fascia lata allografts in dogs: A preliminary report. *Am J Sports Med* 1985;13:408–414.

The canine ACL was reconstructed with freeze-dried fascia lata by means of the two-tunnel and over-the-top techniques combined with extra-articular back-up. Histologically, the allografts underwent necrosis; this was followed by revascularization and fibrous ingrowth. Biomechanically, the allografts initially were stronger than the contralateral control ACL, but by 12 weeks the allografts possessed only 19% of the strength of the contralateral ACLs. By 24 weeks, however, the allografts possessed 67% of the strength of the contralateral ACLs.

Gibbons MJ, Butler DL, Grood ES, et al: Dose dependent effects of gamma irradiation on the material properties of frozen bone-patellar tendon-bone allografts. *Trans Orthop Res Soc* 1989;14:513.

Using graft bone-patellar tendon-bone grafts, the authors demonstrated that a 20×10^3 Gy dose does not significantly alter the initial material properties of the tissue. However, a 30×10^3 Gy dose significantly reduces maximum stress and strain energy density to maximum stress.

Haut RC, Powlison AC: Order of irradiation and lyophilization on the strength of patellar tendon allografts. *Trans Orthop Res Soc* 1989;14:514.

A comparison of fresh-frozen, fresh-frozen irradiated $(20 \times 10^3$ Gy), irradiated then freeze-dried, and freeze-dried then irradiated bone-patellar tendon-bone grafts showed that fresh-frozen irradiated grafts had a 25% decrease in strength whereas the irradiated then freeze-dried grafts had approximately a 35% decrease in strength. However, the freeze-dried then irradiated grafts had a 75% decrease in strength. The authors concluded that irradiation has a deleterious effect on dry tissue.

Nikolaou PK, Seaber AV, Glisson RR, et al: Anterior cruciate ligament allograft transplantation: Long-term function, histology, revascularization, and operative technique. *Am J Sports Med* 1986;14:348–360.

The authors studied both allografts and autografts for ACL replacement. In the autograft group, revascularization was seen by week 8; by week 24 the microangiographic appearance was normal. Histologically, the graft underwent necrosis, revascularization, and then remodeling; by 24 weeks the graft appeared histologically normal. Biomechanically, the graft possessed 87.3% of control strength at 36 weeks. Similar results were found with allograft ACL, but the time course was longer. Control values for strength to failure for the ACLs tested were extremely low when compared with those in other studies.

Paulos LE, France EP, Rosenberg TD, et al: Comparative material properties of allograft tissues for ligament replacement: Effects of type, age, sterilization and preservation. *Trans Orthop Res Soc* 1987;12:129.

This study showed that there was no statistical difference in strength between fresh-frozen and freeze-dried allografts, although a trend to slightly decreased ultimate stress was noted in the freeze-dried group. Radiation sterilization significantly reduced the ultimate stress of specimens tested. Age-related changes were similar in the deep-frozen and the freeze-dried grafts. Deep-frozen bone-patellar tendon-bone grafts possessed the greatest ultimate stress value.

Spire B, Dormont D, Barre-Sinoussi F, et al: Inactivation of lymphadenopathy-associated virus by heat, gamma rays and ultraviolet light. *Lancet* 1985;1:188–189.

The authors reported on the effects of heat, γ-irradiation, and ultraviolet light on HIV. They concluded that the virus was inactivated by heating to 56 C for 30 minutes. In addition, HIV was not inactivated by ultraviolet radiation in doses much greater than those usually employed under laminar flow hoods. The authors also concluded that the virus was not infectious after exposure to 2.5×10^3 Gy of γ-irradiation.

Clinical Results

Shino K, Inoue M, Horibe S, et al: Reconstruction of the anterior cruciate ligament using allogenic tendon: Long-term follow-up. Presented at the meeting of the American Orthopaedic Society for Sports Medicine, Las Vegas, Feb 12, 1989.

The authors reported on 106 patients who underwent ACL reconstruction with deep-frozen allogeneic tendons (Achilles, tibialis, peroneus, or thick flexor tendons). Two thirds of all patients received extra-articular augmentations as well. Of the 80 patients examined after a follow-up of more than three years, 75 had satisfactory results and five had unsatisfactory results. Physical examinations and instrumented knee testing showed good stability in 90%, including those with the extra-articular augmentations. In 16 patients, arthroscopy after 36 months or more showed the graft to be well vascularized and viable.

Shino K, Kimura T, Hirose H, et al: Reconstruction of the anterior cruciate ligament by allogeneic tendon graft: An operation for chronic ligamentous insufficiency. *J Bone Joint Surg* 1986;68B:739–746.

Using a variety of deep-frozen allogeneic tendons (Achilles, tibialis anterior, and flexor tendons), the authors reconstructed the ACL in 83 patients, 31 of whom were examined after a minimum follow-up of two years. In some patients extra-articular repairs were also done. Thirty patients returned to sporting activities. The pivot shift sign was negative in 29 patients and slightly to mildly positive in two patients. Differences in stability (measured with knee testing apparatus) were not statistically significant between normal and reconstructed knees. No deep infections or signs of rejection were noted. Two patients had superficial wound infections and one patient required reoperation for release of adhesions.

Synthetic Ligaments

Biologic and Biomechanical Properties

Arnoczky SP, Torzilli PA, Warren RF, et al: Biologic fixation of ligament prostheses and augmentations: An evaluation of bone ingrowth in the dog. *Am J Sports Med* 1988;16:106–112.

Xenograft, Gore-Tex, and Stryker ligaments and one Kennedy ligament augmentation device were compared with respect to biologic fixation. The devices were placed unstressed in corticocancellous bone of the proximal femur and humerus of dogs. Biomechanically, only the Kennedy device had significantly weaker pullout strength than the other materials. With the Stryker, Xenograft, and Gore-Tex ligaments, trabecular bone was seen surrounding and growing into the prosthetic devices. The extent of ingrowth was related to the configuration of the synthetic material. No evidence of bone ingrowth was seen with the Kennedy device. Unlike the Stryker, Xenograft, and Gore-Tex ligaments, the Kennedy device is an augmentation device rather than a true prosthesis and, therefore, should

not be expected to have the same biologic and fixation properties as a true prosthesis.

Klein W, Jensen K: Arthritis in artificial ACL ligaments. Presented at the Sixth Congress of the International Society of the Knee, Rome, May 1989.

The authors reported their experience with a Dacron ACL replacement. In a series of 59 patients, more than 20% experienced an abrasion synovitis that in many cases resembled septic arthritis or a low-grade chronic infection. The patients were treated by arthroscopic means, including prosthesis removal and synovectomy. Early results were satisfying but the long-term results are still unknown.

Olson EJ, Kang JD, Fu FH, et al: The biochemical and histological effects of artificial ligament wear particles: In vitro and in vivo studies. *Am J Sports Med* 1988;16:558–570.

The effects of wear particles from ligament substitutes and augmentation devices (Gore-Tex, Stryker, Versigraft Carbon, Xenograft, Leeds Keio, and human patellar tendon and the Kennedy device) were studied both biochemically and histologically in a rabbit model. All ligaments increased the levels of enzyme (neutral proteinases) production by rabbit synoviocytes. In vivo, a foreign-body response to the wear particles was noted. The authors suggest a hypothetical model to explain the effects of wear particles in the knee.

Clinical Results

Arnoczky SP, Cuzzell JZ, McDevitt CA, et al: Meniscal replacement using a cryopreserved allograft: An experimental study in the dog. *Trans Orthop Res Soc* 1984;9:220.

Meniscal transplantation of cryopreserved menisci in a canine model was assessed. The allografts became reattached to the capsular tissues by fibrous connective tissue and were revascularized throughout the peripheral margin. The authors also noted that articular cartilage changes beneath the meniscus were minimal five months postoperatively.

Arnoczky SP, McDevitt CA, Schmidt MB, et al: The effect of cryopreservation on canine menisci: A biochemical, morphologic, and biomechanical evaluation. *J Orthop Res* 1988;6:1–12.

Menisci were cryopreserved and then stored in liquid nitrogen for various periods (0 to 12 weeks). Short-term storage did not affect the meniscal tissue biomechanically or histologically. Biosynthetic activity was decreased to 53% of normal immediately after storage and to 50% after two weeks of storage. The activity then steadily declined to 17% at 12 weeks. Similarly, autoradiographic examination of the tissue revealed that only 10% of meniscal cells were metabolically active immediately after storage. Activity decreased to less than 3% at 12 weeks.

Baratz ME, Rehak DC, Fu FH, et al: Peripheral tears of the meniscus: The effect of open versus arthroscopic repair on intraarticular contact stresses in the human knee. *Am J Sports Med* 1988;16:1–6.

The authors used pressure-sensitive film to show that the biomechanical properties of the meniscus are altered when a meniscal tear is created. Specifically, the contact area was decreased and the contact stresses were increased at the cartilage-cartilage interface. The tears were then repaired either in an open fashion or arthroscopically. After repair, the contact stresses and the contact area were measured and found not to differ significantly from those of the normal meniscus. Also, the open and arthroscopic techniques were equally successful, with neither technique offering a distinct advantage in terms of return of biomechanical properties.

Daniel D, Van Kampen CL: Synthetic augmentation of

biologic anterior cruciate ligament substitution, in Friedman MJ, Ferkel RD (eds): *Prosthetic Ligament Reconstruction of the Knee.* Philadelphia, WB Saunders, 1988, pp 65–70.

Various methods of biologic augmentation in ACL replacement surgery are described. Mechanically coupling the augmentation device and autogenous tissue and securing the augmentation device to the bone at only one end is the technique most often used. The authors used the basic spring theory to examine forces in the autogenous tissue-augmentation composite.

Daniel D, Woodward WP, Loose G, et al: The Marshall/MacIntosh anterior cruciate ligament reconstruction with the Kennedy ligament augmentation device: Report of the United States Clinical Trial, in Friedman MJ, Ferkel RD (eds): *Prosthetic Ligament Reconstruction of the Knee.* Philadelphia, WB Saunders, 1988, pp 71–78.

The authors present two-year follow-up results for 148 of 157 patients who received the Kennedy ligament augmentation device as part of a prospective multicenter study. Augmented grafts were compared with nonaugmented grafts from another study. The clinical results were good in both groups.

Indelicato PA, Pascale MS, Huegel MO: Early experience with the GORE-TEX polytetrafluoroethylene anterior cruciate ligament prosthesis. *Am J Sports Med* 1989;17:55–62.

Thirty-nine patients were prospectively studied after ACL replacement with the Gore-Tex ligament. The minimum follow-up was two years. Results were satisfactory in 34 patients but four had a complete rupture of the prosthesis. More than 80% had Lachman, anterior drawer, and pivot shift scores of 0 to 1. Complications included effusion, graft failure, and infection.

Lukianov AV, Gillquist J, Grana WA, et al: An anterior cruciate ligament (ACL) evaluation format for assessment of artificial or autologous anterior cruciate reconstruction results. *Clin Orthop* 1987;218:167–180.

The evaluation format is broken into three major categories: (1) history and surgery, (2) initial evaluation and follow-up, and (3) complications. Part 1 has five sections: patient information, history of the injury, previous surgery, surgery performed, and postoperative course. Part 2 has six sections: Lysholm knee function scoring scale, Tegner activity scale, physical examination (including Lachman and pivot shift testing), complications, supplementary data, and Tegner activity level scale definitions. Part 3 describes complications.

Nordt WE, Terry GC: Report on the Gore-Tex prosthetic ligament for use in ACL and PCL reconstruction. Presented at the meeting of the American Orthopaedic Society for Sports Medicine, Traverse City, June 1989.

The authors used the Gore-Tex ligament in 114 patients (134 procedures) for replacement of the ACL, PCL, or both. After an average of 51 months, 104 patients were available for follow-up. The patients were tested both objectively and subjectively, and the outcomes were classified as (1) successful, objectively and subjectively, (2) pseudosuccessful, objective failure

but subjective improvement, and (3) failed, objectively and subjectively. Overall, 41% were successes, 16% were pseudosuccesses, and 43% were failures. ACL substitution only was successful in 45%, pseudosuccessful in 13%, and failed in 42%. PCL substitution only was successful in 17%, pseudosuccessful in 30%, and failed in 53%.

Roth JH, Kennedy JC, Lockstadt H, et al: Polypropylene braid augmented and nonaugmented intraarticular anterior cruciate ligament reconstruction. *Am J Sports Med* 1985;13:321–336.

This retrospective study compared nonaugmented autogenous reconstruction of the ACL with the modified Marshall-MacIntosh procedure to augmented autogenous reconstruction with the Kennedy ligament augmentation device. Mean follow-up for the 38 nonaugmented procedures was 64 months and that for the 45 augmented procedures was 50 months. On Lachman, pivot shift, and anterior drawer testing, the augmented grafts were significantly better than the nonaugmented grafts. On KT 1000, Cybex isokinetic strength analysis, and one-leg hop for distance, there was no statistically significant difference between the two groups. The authors concluded that the augmentation procedure is safe and improves the efficacy of the intra-articular autograft reconstruction.

van Steensel CJ, Schreuder O, van den Bosch BF, et al: Failure of anterior cruciate-ligament reconstruction using tendon xenograft. *J Bone Joint Surg* 1987;69A:860–864.

Forty patients who underwent ACL reconstruction with the Xenograft tendon were divided into two groups. Group 1 consisted of the first 30 patients who received grafts that had been rinsed according to the manufacturers' recommendations; group 2 consisted of the next ten patients who had received grafts that had been rinsed for a much longer period (72 hours). The rinse period was increased because synovitis developed postoperatively in many patients. Synovitis developed in six patients in group 1 but in no patients in group 2. Five of the grafts had to be removed. A total of 22 patients (17 patients in group 1 and five in group 2) had ruptured grafts.

Wills PP, Collins MR: Intraarticular Gore-Tex anterior cruciate ligament reconstruction: 2–6 year follow-up. Presented at the meeting of the American Orthopaedic Society for Sports Medicine, Traverse City, June 1989.

A series of 99 Gore-Tex ACL reconstructions was examined two to six years later by an independent surgeon and a trained technician. Of the patients, 91% had returned to athletics and 86% rated their knees as improved. More than one third said their knees had loosened as time passed. The Lachman test was rated at least slightly positive in 68%. Pivot shift was negative in 36%, mild in 50%, and moderate in 14%. Arthrometry showed an average side-to-side difference of 5.9 mm at maximum manual load; 52% of the patients had a side-to-side difference of more than 5 mm at maximum load. The prosthesis had to be removed or replaced in 10% of patients during the study period. The authors concluded that the Gore-Tex prosthetic ACL reconstruction is a reasonable alternative after failed intra-articular autograft.

15

Prostheses: Materials, Design, and Strategies for Implant Fixation

The performance of prostheses depends on the properties of the materials used, the design of the device, and the method of fixation (that is, attachment to the musculoskeletal system). Material properties consist of mechanical characteristics such as strength and modulus of elasticity, tribologic features including wear, resistance to degradation (for example, corrosion), and "biocompatibility." Design considerations encompass the size, shape, and configuration of the device. Strategies for fixation include the use of bone cement, interference (friction) fit (either "line-to-line" fit or press-fit), bone adaptation to irregular surface features (macrointerlock), bone ingrowth into a porous coating (microinterlock or "biologic fixation"), and/or "direct bone bonding" (for example, bone formation on the surface of hydroxyapatite coatings). *Orthopaedic Knowledge Update I* described the chemical composition and mechanical properties of the materials used in the fabrication of prostheses. The corresponding chapter in *Orthopaedic Knowledge Update 2* focused on issues related to implant fixation. By the end of the 1980s, long-term follow-up evaluations have made it possible to define problems with prostheses more clearly.

Contemporary designs and cement techniques have now extended the anticipated lifetime of total knee and hip replacements to 15 years (Fig. 1). Problems such as infection and stem breakage that occurred early in the development of total hip replacement have for the most part been solved. Primary contemporary concerns are those that have become apparent with the extended longevity of joint replacements: wear of the bearing surfaces and loss of bone stock as a result of the osteolytic response to particulate wear debris and to stress-shielding effects. In ad-

dition, the long-term biologic and clinical sequelae of metal ion release, particularly in uncemented devices in young individuals, remain unknown.

The foremost issue associated with the design of uncemented prosthetic components is achieving initial mechanical stability. A consensus is developing that such stability requires filling of the medullary canal proximally, with or without distal filling. Advances in the design of canal-filling femoral stems have come about because of algorithms for computer-designed devices, modular off-the-shelf prostheses, and methods of designing custom devices.

Although improvements in cement techniques have extended the durability of fixation, the limited fatigue life of this substance continues to focus attention on uncemented strategies for fixation in the younger patient. Questions about the amount, location, and functional importance of bone ingrowth into porous coatings have not all been answered. These concerns have prompted consideration of other strategies such as nonporous canal-filling titanium devices for "osseointegration" and hydroxyapatite coatings for "bone bonding."

Materials

The chemical composition and properties of biomaterials used for prostheses were discussed in *Orthopaedic Knowledge Updates I* and *2*. New methods for treating these materials have improved their performance. Progress has been made in two new classes of biomaterials, carbon-fiber-reinforced polymer composites and calcium phosphates, for orthopaedic applications.

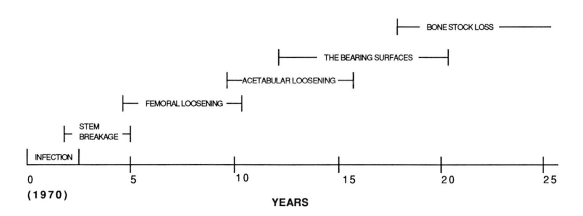

Figure 1

As each major problem affecting the longevity of total hip replacements was solved, other, more long-term problems appeared. (Reproduced with permission from Poss R, Brick GW, Wright RJ, et al: The effects of modern cementing techniques on the longevity of total hip arthroplasty. *Orthop Clin North Am* 1988;19:591–598.)

Metals

The introduction of high-strength "supermetals" almost eliminated concerns about femoral-stem breakage. Questions that remain relate to the biologic response to ions released from metallic implants. In addition, with the ever-increasing number of larger-diameter femoral stems has come the awareness of bone loss caused by stress-shielding effects related to the stiffness of metallic devices, particularly cobalt-chromium alloys. The issues of ion release and stress-shielding have contributed to increased interest in titanium alloy (6% aluminum and 4% vanadium) for the fabrication of hip and knee replacements. However, this has brought to light the low wear-resistance of this metal.

Metal Ion Release Investigations in humans and in animal models reveal increased levels of metal ions in subjects with joint replacement prostheses and other types of implants. Results are often variable with respect to the concentration of specific metal ions in certain tissues and fluids. One recent investigation of 14 patients undergoing conventional cemented cobalt-chromium hip replacement showed postoperative increases in serum (Fig. 2) and urinary chromium levels. However, an attempt to determine the valency of chromium from the concentration of metal ion in blood clots was not successful. This experiment was based on the fact that erythrocytes display a unidirectional uptake of chromium with a valency of +6 while effectively excluding chromium with a valency of +3. This distinction is important because the former is much more biologically active than the latter.

Cellular Response to Metal *Orthopaedic Knowledge Update I* outlined several test procedures employed for the evaluation of the "biocompatibility" of metals, discussing issues related to the "systemic response of metal sensitivity" and the local response of tumorigenicity. It was noted that neither of these biologic responses had yet been related to clinical implant failure of a prosthesis. Unfortunately, knowledge about the biologic and clinical sequelae of metal ion release has not significantly advanced during the past several years. However, a few recent studies of the synovial cell response to metal particles and ions have generated information that could form the basis of future clinical insights. Recent investigations have shown that laboratory-prepared particulate cobalt-chromium particles induced rapid proliferation of macrophages and focal degeneration of synovial tissues in rats when injected intra-articularly, in much the same way as happens in the articular tissues around loose total joint prostheses in human subjects. Another study showed that cobalt ions added to synovial cells in culture increase levels of collagenase (Fig. 3) and prostaglandin E_2. It has been suggested that these findings may be relevant to aseptic loosening of joint prostheses in that metal ions could activate synovial cells in the joint capsule and "pseudomembrane" at the implant-bone interface to produce agents that promote osteolysis.

Most work on metal ion release has focused on cobalt-chromium alloys. Recently, research addressing similar issues for titanium alloy has been initiated. Histologic studies of pigmented tissues surrounding titanium implants has generally shown considerably fewer macrophages and mul-

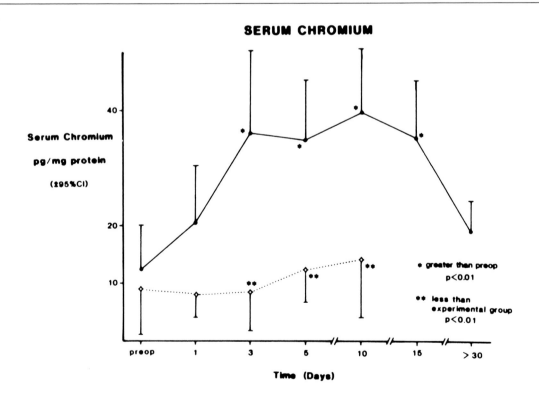

Figure 2
Patients undergoing total hip arthroplasty showed a significant postoperative increase in serum chromium concentration. The solid line shows the mean values for 14 patients who received conventional cemented cobalt-chromium hip prostheses; the broken line shows the mean values for seven control patients who underwent orthopaedic procedures other than implantation. (Reproduced with permission from Bartolozzi A, Black J: Chromium concentrations in serum, blood clot and urine from patients following total hip arthroplasty. *Biomaterials* 1985;6:2–8.)

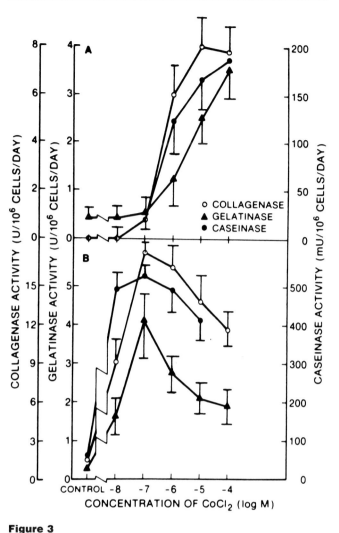

Figure 3
Effect of CoCl₂ on the production of neutral proteinases by synovial cells in vitro. **A,** Values for human cells. **B,** Values for rabbit cells. (Reproduced with permission from Ferguson GM, Watanabe S, Georgescu HI, et al: The synovial production of collagenase and chondrocyte activating factors in response to cobalt. *J Orthop Res* 1988;6:525–530.)

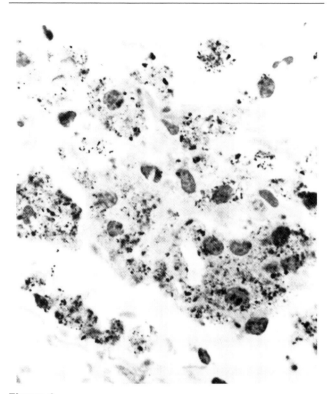

Figure 4
Photomicrograph showing titanium alloy metallic debris within histiocytes. (Reproduced with permission from Agins HJ, Alcock NW, Bansal M, et al: Metallic wear in failed titanium-alloy total hip replacements. *J Bone Joint Surg* 1988;70A:347–356.)

tinucleated foreign-body giant cells than found around cobalt-chromium particles and polymeric particulate debris. However, a recent study of titanium alloy particulate debris generated by the abrasion of a femoral stem against bone cement provided histologic evidence of a histiocytic response to the metallic particles (Fig. 4). This histiocytic response, along with an associated lymphoplasmacytic reaction, indicates that understanding of the biologic response to titanium alloy particles remains incomplete.

Neoplasms The use of uncemented, porous-coated metallic stems (with large surface areas) in younger patients continues to raise concern about the long-term clinical consequences of metal ion release. In the years 1986 through 1989, there were four reported cases of tumors at the sites of total joint replacement prostheses (Table 1). The differences in tumor types, times to appearance, and types of prostheses confound attempts to associate the neoplasms with the implant materials, released particles, and ions.

In a recent epidemiologic investigation, more than 1,300 patients with total joint replacements were monitored to determine the incidence of remote-site tumors. The incidences of tumors of the lymphatic and hematopoietic systems were found to be significantly greater than expected in the decade after arthroplasty while incidences of cancer of the breast, colon, and rectum were significantly less than expected. The investigators acknowledged that although the association might result, in part, from an effect of the prosthetic implants, other mechanisms, particularly drug therapy, require consideration.

Wear of Titanium Alloy Although titanium alloy has the advantages of a lower modulus of elasticity and favorable "biocompatibility," it has a relatively low resistance to abrasion. Titanium's poor wear-resistance has caused concern about its use as a femoral head and condylar surface. This has led to the introduction of modularity in femoral-stem designs that allows cobalt-chromium heads on titanium stems. In many total knee replacement designs, titanium femoral components have been replaced by cobalt-chromium components.

The need to improve the wear-resistance of titanium alloy, particularly to allow its continued use in knee replacements, has led to the implementation of the new surface-treatment technique of "ion implantation." In this method, ions of a specific element (for example, nitrogen) are "implanted" into the surface of titanium alloy by exposing the prosthesis to the appropriate ion beam excited by high voltage (Fig. 5). Previous investigations for nonmedical applications have shown that the wear-resist-

Table 1. Tumors at sites of orthopaedic prostheses reported from 1986 to 1989

Tumor Type	Prosthesis*	Time From Surgery to Appearance of Tumor
Malignant fibrous histiocytoma	Cemented hip (Weber-Huggler II)	10 years
Osteosarcoma	Cemented hip (Charnley-Muller)	10 years
Epithelioid sarcoma (possibly malignant histiocytoma or fibrosarcoma)†	Cemented knee	4½ years
Soft-tissue sarcoma	Uncemented hip (ceramic-ceramic articulation)	1¼ years

*All metallic components were fabricated from cobalt-chromium alloy.
†An enchondroma or bone infarct had been found on preoperative radiographs of the distal femur.

ance of titanium alloy is greatly enhanced by ion implantation. A recent study tested the improved wear-resistance of ion-implanted commercially pure titanium articulating against polyethylene in a hip joint simulator. Despite the titanium's improved wear-resistance, these articulations still generated more polymeric wear than cobalt-chromium-polyethylene combinations. This difference was attributed to the inferior surface polish on the titanium specimens. This and another investigation showed that a benefit of ion implantation is a reduction in wear-accelerated titanium alloy corrosion, reflected in decreased ion release. An important unanswered question relates to the durability of the ion-implanted metallic surface.

The articulating surface of titanium implants is not the only potential source of titanium wear debris. It has been shown that the abrasion of bone cement against titanium femoral stems can lead to the generation of large quantities of titanium wear debris. It has been proposed that the less stiff titanium femoral stems place a cement sheath at greater risk for fracture because of the known increase in stress on the cement (when compared with cobalt-chromium components). Once fractured, the sheath can abrade the titanium surface.

Polymers

Polymethylmethacrylate and ultrahigh-molecular-weight polyethylene remain the important polymers in joint re-

placement. Although the last few years have not produced solutions to all the problems of these two polymers, important advances have been made that should allow for improved performance.

Properties of Polyethylene Ultrahigh-molecular-weight polyethylene continues to play the dominant role in the fabrication of "low-friction" total joint replacements. Unfortunately, polyethylene wear debris is often found in the tissues at revision surgery. Particles of this polymer, particularly those less than 0.5 to 10 μ in size, have been associated with an osteolytic response (Fig. 6) often determined to be the cause of failure (loosening). A consensus appears to be developing that it is this wear and the biologic sequelae of both polyethylene and polymethylmethacrylate particle debris that currently limit the life of total joint replacements. Analyses of polyethylene components retrieved at revision surgery and finite-element stress analyses have begun to reveal the wear mechanisms responsible for component failure. In addition to surface features consistent with abrasive wear, the polyethylene components often display delamination (Figs. 7 and 8) that appears to be initiated by subsurface intergranular defects (Fig. 9) and propagated by excessive fatigue stresses beneath the contact zone. One study confirmed that the design variables affecting the amount of damage are component thickness and the conformity of the articulating surfaces. Surface

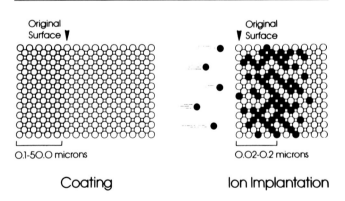

0.1-50.0 microns   0.02-0.2 microns

Coating   ### Ion Implantation

Figure 5

Schema comparing conventional coating and ion implantation processes. Because the implanted ions are intermingled with the substrate, the ion-implanted layers are less likely to detach the way a conventional coat might. However, it is not known whether the ion-implanted layers will eventually wear away. (Reproduced with permission from Solnick-Legg H, Legg K: Ion beam and plasma technology for improved biocompatible surfaces. *Mater Res Soc Bull* 1989, pp 27–30.)

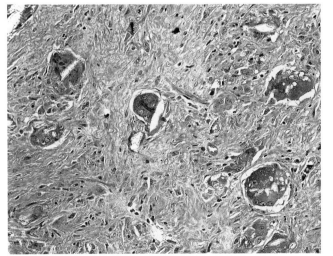

Figure 6

Histologic micrograph showing macrophages and giant cells engulfing polymeric particulate debris.

damage is more severe in thin (less than 4 to 6 mm) components and in components with relatively flat tibial articulating surfaces. This investigation also found that surface damage is expected to be more extreme in carbon-fiber-reinforced polyethylene components than in components made from plain polyethylene. This latter determination is based on finite-element stress analysis that showed that higher-modulus carbon-fiber-reinforced polyethylene increased stress 35% to 40% over plain polyethylene (Fig. 10). These elevated stresses can produce subsurface fatigue damage that can ultimately lead to delamination. Related studies using a "fracture mechanics" approach showed that carbon-fiber-reinforced material has a lower crack-resistance than unreinforced polyethylene, making it more susceptible to fatigue failure. The predicted poor performance of carbon-fiber-reinforced polyethylene has been confirmed by the common finding of large amounts of carbon debris at revision surgery.

Examination of retrieved acetabular sockets has suggested that a considerable amount of particulate debris could result from abrasion of a loose acetabular component against the acrylic cement and surrounding bone. It has been proposed that this condition is initiated by polyethylene wear debris from the articulating surface infiltrating the cement-bone junction. The ability of polyethylene particles to infiltrate the implant-bone interface, particularly when it is fibrous, has been demonstrated in a recent animal investigation. These results could also explain why such particles are found at distant sites around femoral stems.

A confounding aspect of the breakdown of polyethylene is its unpredictable postimplantation time course. There is a suggestion that the degradative processes in polyethylene are nonlinear, explaining its increased wear rate approximately ten years after implantation. Although the cause of the degradative process is unknown, it may be related, in part, to the oxidation of polyethylene. Associated with this degradation are increases in density and modulus of elasticity. These changes could make the polyethylene component more susceptible to fatigue damage and wear.

Many investigations in animals and in tissue recovered from revision surgery have revealed a histiocytic response to polyethylene particles as well as to polymethylmethacrylate. It has been shown that this macrophage response can lead to bone resorption, thereby potentiating the loosening process (Fig. 11). Although some investigators suggest that polyethylene particles may elicit a more "virulent" reaction than cement particles, there is no experimental evidence that directly compares the responses. Recent studies have addressed the response of cells to biomaterial surfaces. One recent investigation has shown that tissue-culture medium conditioned by macrophages exposed to orthopaedic biomaterials has bone-resorption activity in vitro. Greater bone-resorption activity was present in medium conditioned with macrophages on hydrophilic and rough surfaces than on hydrophobic and smooth surfaces. High-density polyethylene elicited approximately 20% more bone resorption than polymethylmethacrylate. The clinical importance of these findings is not yet clear.

In an attempt to improve the mechanical properties of polyethylene, a method has been implemented to change the way in which the polyethylene molecule is folded. By reducing the number of folds in each molecular chain that constitutes the ultrahigh-molecular-weight polyethylene component, it is possible to alter the mechanical proper-

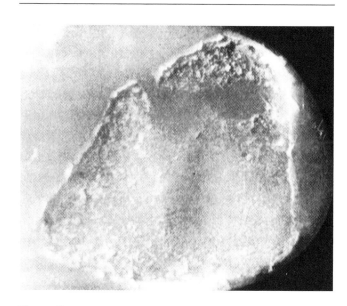

Figure 7

A large area of delamination on the articulating surface of a polyethylene tibial component that had been implanted for seven years. (Reproduced with permission from Wright TM, Bartel DL: The problem of surface damage in polyethylene total knee components. *Clin Orthop* 1986;205:67–74.)

ties. The "enhanced" polyethylene displays higher creep resistance and greater resistance to oxidation than does medical-grade polyethylene. Moreover, there is a reduction in the coefficient of friction and an improvement in other properties that may contribute to less wear. However, there is an increase in the modulus of elasticity that could lead to higher contact stress. Additional laboratory investigations and human trials are required to characterize fully the performance of this "enhanced" polyethylene.

Composites Potential problems related to metal ion release and the relatively high modulus of elasticity of metallic substances continue to spur investigational work focused on the development of high-strength polymeric materials for the fabrication of total joint replacements. This investigative work has generally focused on polymer composites reinforced with carbon fiber. The term "composites" is used to describe a material formed by the combination of two or more substances in such a way that the benefits of each substance can be better used to meet a specific application. For example, high-strength, high-modulus carbon fibers can be combined with brittle, low-strength, ductile polymers to produce composite femoral stems comparable in strength to titanium devices but with one half the stiffness (and one quarter the stiffness of cobalt-chromium prostheses). Another composite being developed is a carbon-carbon combination. Carbon-fiber-reinforced carbon materials are produced by heating (carbonizing) carbon-fiber-reinforced polymer composites. It has been suggested that these carbon-carbon materials have greater chemical stability and higher static and fatigue strength than carbon-polymer substances. Moreover, it has been suggested that soluble compounds are less likely to be released from the carbon-carbon material. However, all of these putative advantages require additional experimental validation.

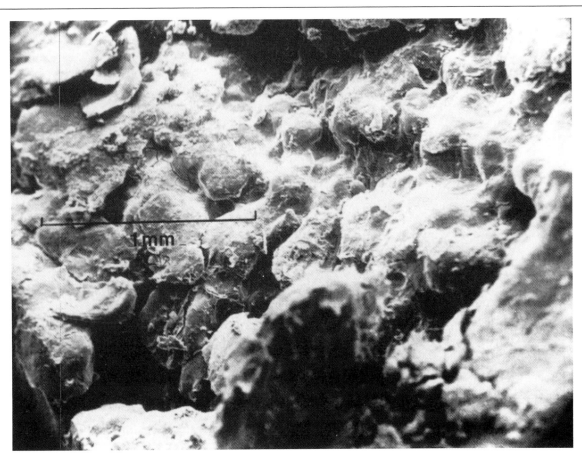

Figure 8

Scanning electron micrograph of exposed delamination surfaces through an area of heavy intergranular cracking. (Reproduced with permission from Landy M, Walker PS: Wear of ultra-high-molecular-weight polyethylene components of 90 retrieved knee prostheses. *J Arthrop* 1988, suppl, pp S73–S85.)

The benefits of more flexible composite stems have been suggested by mathematical models of the proximal femur with the femoral component. These finite-element analyses demonstrate that the stresses in the proximal cortical bone with the conventional cobalt-chromium femoral stem are less than one half the magnitude of the stresses in the intact femur. However, if the material properties of the carbon-composite material are substituted for those of cobalt-chromium alloy, these stresses are increased to approximately 75% of the stresses in the intact femur. In other words, the degree of stress protection can be reduced from approximately 50% to 25% by the use of a carbon-fiber-reinforced material, without otherwise modifying the component design.

The fabrication of a composite prosthesis requires technology very different from that employed for the fabrication of metallic devices. To obtain the greatest component strength, continuous (rather than "chopped") carbon fibers are employed in the polymeric matrix (Tables 2 and 3). Bonding of the polymer to the carbon fiber is essential to achieve the highest strength. In practice, thin layers, or plies, of carbon fibers are impregnated with the matrix polymer. Plates of the desired thickness are produced by compression-molding a stack of the plies (Fig. 12). The mechanical properties of the resulting plate depend on ply orientation and stacking sequence (Table 4). One goal is

to achieve a lower modulus without unacceptable compromise of strength. Achieving the desired mechanical properties is a complex problem because of the many variables: carbon-fiber and polymer-matrix mechanical properties, volume fraction of fiber in the composite, and ply orientation and stacking sequence. The resultant prosthesis can be machined from the plates to its final shape. An alternative method of fabrication is to compression-mold precut plies into the shape of the device.

Many of the laboratory and animal investigations of carbon-fiber-reinforced polymers have used polysulfone as the matrix material. However, recent laboratory studies have suggested that another polymer, polyetheretherketone, may also be suitable for the fabrication of composites. To date there have been no animal investigations directly comparing the bone remodeling around composite femoral stems with metallic devices of identical design employed as controls. Previous canine studies compared the cortical bone remodeling around the prosthetic device with the untreated contralateral cortex. Although the results of laboratory and animal studies have been encouraging, considerably more investigative work needs to be performed before such composite systems can be considered for the fabrication of prostheses.

One concern in considering the use of composite materials for the fabrication of femoral stems is whether to

SURFACE

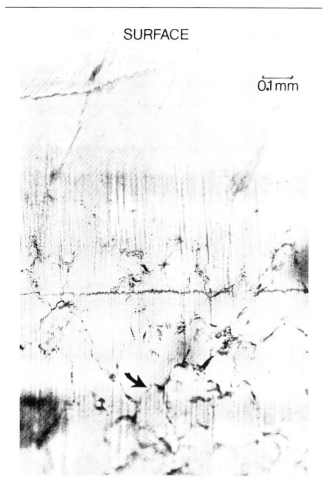

Figure 9

High-power view of a subsurface crack (arrow) developing along planes of intergranular cracking. (Reproduced with permission from Landy M, Walker PS: Wear of ultra-high-molecular-weight polyethylene components of 90 retrieved knee prostheses. *J Arthrop* 1988, suppl, pp S73–S85.)

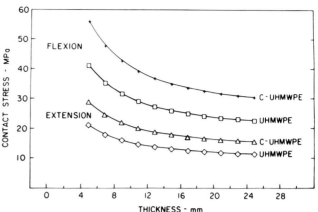

Figure 10

Variations in the maximum compressive contact stresses on the surface of the tibial components with varying thicknesses of the layer of polyethylene. The elasticity solution was used to compute the stresses for a load of 1,500 N for layers of plain and carbon-fiber reinforced polyethylene when the knee was in extension and when it was in flexion. The higher contact stresses that occur with thinner (4 to 6 mm) layers can promote failure that might appear as delamination. (Reproduced with permission from Bartel DL, Bicknell DL, Wright TM: The effect of conformity, thickness, and material on stresses in ultra-high molecular weight components for total joint replacement. *J Bone Joint Surg* 1986;68A:1041–1051.)

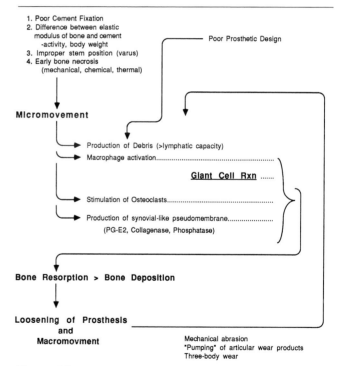

Figure 11

Pathogenesis of loosening and foreign-body giant cell reaction. (Reproduced with permission from Maguire JK Jr, Coscia NF, Lynch MH: Foreign body reaction to polymeric debris following total hip arthroplasty. *Clin Orthop* 1987;216:213–223.)

coat them with a substance that can serve as an attachment vehicle to surrounding bone. Because of the relatively low abrasion-resistance of the carbon and polymeric elements, there is concern that abrasion with surrounding bone could lead to large amounts of particulate wear debris if they were used in a "press-fit" mode. This matter is complicated by the fact that these substances do not lend themselves to being coated with porous materials or ceramics.

There are several potential disadvantages of carbon-polymer and carbon-carbon materials for the fabrication of prostheses. These substances generally display poor impact-resistance. Therefore, extreme care must be exercised during the implantation procedure so as to guard against sharp blows delivered to the device. The radiolucency of these materials may prove to be a disadvantage in post-operative radiographic evaluation of device performance. This property also prevents certain radiologic procedures from being employed for quality control during their manufacture. Other nondestructive tests for quality control of these devices have not yet been used on a large-scale basis. Finally, manufacturing difficulties may add significantly to the cost of the composite prosthesis.

Ceramics

Orthopaedic Knowledge Update I presented information about the use of ceramic materials for the fabrication of components for total joint replacements, particularly the

Table 2. Properties of two types of fibers commonly used in composites*

| Property | Carbon PAN-Based Fiber | | Polyamide Fiber |
	Type I	Type II	
Diameter (μ)	7.0 to 9.7	7.6 to 8.6	11.9
Young's modulus (10^3 MPa)	390	250	125
Modulus perpendicular to fiber axis (10^3 MPa)	12	20	No data
Tensile strength (10^3 MPa)	2.2	2.7	2.8 to 3.6

*Reproduced with permission from Skinner HB: Composite technology for total hip arthroplasty. *Clin Orthop* 1988; 235:224–236.

Table 3. Properties of composite matrix materials*

Properties	Polysulfone	Polyetheretherketone	Ultrahigh-Molecular-Weight Polyethylene
Density (g/cc)	1.25	1.32	No data
Tensile strength yield (MPa)	70.3	92	20
Compressive strength yield (MPa)	96	118	14.7
Tensile modulus (GPa)	2.48	3.6	0.602
Elongation (%)	50 to 100	50	No data
Flexural strength (MPa)	106	170	13.3
Poissons's ratio	0.37	0.42	No data
Fatigue endurance limit (MPa)	6.9	70	15.8

*Reproduced with permission from Skinner HB: Composite technology for total hip arthroplasty. *Clin Orthop* 1988;235:224–236.

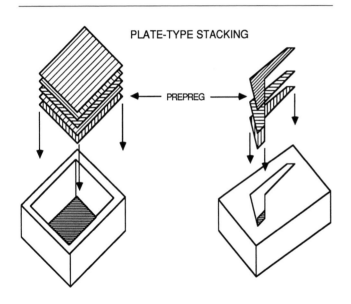

PLATE-TYPE STACKING

PREPREG

Figure 12

Plies of continuous carbon fibers impregnated with polymer are stacked and compression-molded to form plates out of which prostheses can be machined. In an alternative method, precut plies are stacked so as to produce devices in final form.

femoral head for articulation with polyethylene acetabular cups. Little has been added to our knowledge regarding this class of ceramics for orthopaedic applications since then.

A class of materials referred to as "bioactive ceramics" was also reviewed in *Orthopaedic Knowledge Update 2*. This term is generally used to describe the calcium-containing substances that undergo a surface reaction that facilitates "bone bonding." The substance previously referred to as Bioglass has not appeared in the orthopaedic literature in the last several years, perhaps because of the difficulty in adapting it for use as a coating because of its limited mechanical properties. However, another group of bioactive substances, the calcium phosphates, have undergone intense recent investigation.

Calcium Phosphates In recent years calcium phosphate ceramics have been studied as bone-substitute materials and as coatings for total joint replacements. In part, the rationale underlying this work is based on the fact that bone matrix contains a calcium phosphate that resembles the mineral, hydroxyapatite (bone mineral is actually calcium-deficient carbonate apatite). This and other calcium phosphate minerals were initially produced by heat-treating (sintering) to fabricate ceramics of higher strength. Calcium phosphate products fabricated to date include dense- and porous-block and particulate forms of hydroxyapatite and another mineral form, tricalcium phosphate (also referred to as whitlockite). Hydroxyapatite is relatively insoluble, and is, therefore, often referred to as "permanent." Tricalcium phosphate is relatively soluble and is referred to as "resorbable." This terminology is unfortunate because it implies that tricalcium phosphate is broken down by the cell-mediated process that occurs in bone resorption. However, such has not been found to be the case. Rather, the degradation of tricalcium phosphate appears to be a combination of physicochemical dissolution and fragmentation. One new substance undergoing investigation is a blend of these two mineral forms, hydroxyapatite-tricalcium phosphate (HA-TCP).

Many animal studies have demonstrated that bone matrix is deposited directly on the surface of calcium phosphate implants (Fig. 13). The strength of attachment is considerably greater than expected from simple adaptation of bone to surface irregularities (that is, connection as well as contact occurs). Examination of the fracture surface generally reveals failure through the bone or ceramic substance, but not through the interface. Recent studies suggest that soon after implantation "biologic apatites" are deposited on the surface of the synthetic calcium phosphate

Table 4. Elastic moduli of a carbon fiber-polyetheretherketone composite*†

Lay-up Orientations (%)	Longitudinal Elastic Modulus (GPa)	Transverse Elastic Modulus (GPa)	Safety Factor‡
0	134.0	8.9	14.5
0/90	7.2	7.2	5.0
0/45	72.9	11.9	7.4
45/−45	14.4	14.4	10.4
30/−30	20.7	3.9	8.2
90	8.9	134.0	0.62

*Reproduced with permission from Skinner HB: Composite technology for total hip arthroplasty. *Clin Orthop* 1988;235:224–236.

†Composite composed of 24 layers, each 0.05 cm thick, under a tensile stress similar to that expected in an implanted total hip femoral stem.

‡Ratio of failure strain to calculated strain for lamina closest to failure in tension. (Thermal effects could reduce the indicated value by as much as half.)

implant. This layer of biologic apatite may facilitate later protein adsorption and cell adhesion. To date, the orthopaedic applications of these bone-substitute materials has been investigational, including the filling of bony defects such as iliac crest bone-graft donor sites, and in tumors, cysts, and fractures. One recent animal investigation used HA-TCP as grout around an uncemented, porous-coated femoral stem in a canine revision model. It was found that when an interference fit was not obtained, the HA-TCP did not produce additional bone ingrowth or mechanical stability.

Calcium phosphate coatings on joint replacements (for example, on femoral stems and actabular cups) are applied by a plasma-spraying technique (Fig. 14). Particles of hydroxyapatite or other calcium phosphate are introduced into a flame that directs the particles for deposition onto the metallic prosthetic component. Coatings 50 to 200 μ thick are fabricated in this way. There are several questions about these coatings. It is known that the high temperature of the flame used in the coating process can alter the composition and structure of the hydroxyapatite powder. Analysis of coatings produced in this way showed significant percentages of tricalcium phosphate and "unknown" substances. A related matter concerns the solubility of these surfaces. Recent studies suggest that the dissolution rate may be several micrometers per year. One recent canine study indicated that coatings that were relatively stable under unloaded conditions in vitro were partially degraded and, in some instances, detached from the metal stems by two years.

Animal investigations have shown that bone bonds directly to the hydroxyapatite coating (Fig. 15). Studies comparing the strength of attachment of bone to hydroxyapatite-coated and uncoated porous specimens repeatedly show much higher bond strengths for the hydroxyapatite-coated specimens. However, the bond strength is only increased for the first several weeks postoperatively. After six weeks, the bond strengths are generally comparable. Other recent animal investigations have shown the benefits of hydroxyapatite coatings on specimens that are separated from their bone bed by a gap, and for implants in osteopenic bone. In each of these conditions, hydroxyapatite-coated porous implants displayed more bone ingrowth and higher attachment strengths than uncoated controls.

Clinical trials of hydroxyapatite-coated stems are in progress. Both fully coated and partially coated designs are undergoing investigation. To date, clinical and radiographic follow-up data are favorable. The radiolucent zone

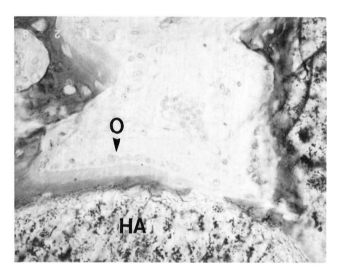

Figure 13

Histologic study showed bone deposition directly on the surface of the synthetic hydroxyapatite (HA) ten days after implantation in rabbit bone. O, osteoblasts.

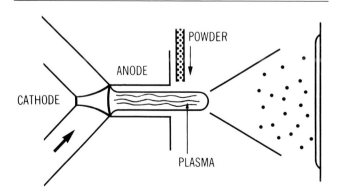

Figure 14

Schema of the plasma-spraying procedure. (Reproduced with permission from de Groot K, Geesink R, Kein CPAT, et al: Plasma sprayed coatings of hydroxyapatite. *J Biomater Res* 1987;21:1375–1381.)

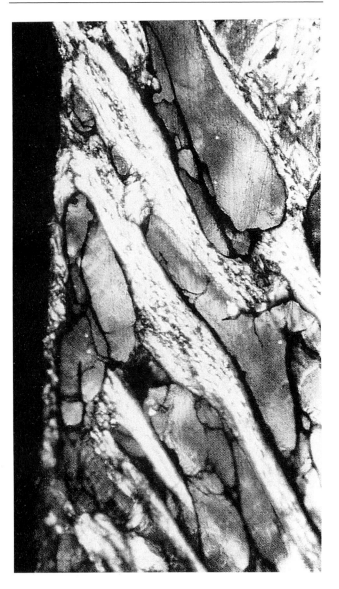

Figure 15

A thin "plate" of bone on the surface of a hydroxyapatite-coated titanium femoral stem three weeks after implantation in a dog (x 100). (Reproduced with permission from Geesink RGT, de Groot K, Klein CPAT: Chemical implant fixation using hydroxyl-apatite coatings. *Clin Orthop* 1987;225:147–170.)

(bordered by a sclerotic line) often seen around nonporous devices was not found around hydroxyapatite-coated prostheses. Histologic examination of retrieved devices showed a "shell" of trabecular bone, approximately 100 μ thick, on the surface of the hydroxyapatite coating, suggesting bone bonding.

It is clear that more extensive laboratory, animal, and clinical investigations are needed before hydroxyapatite-coated devices can be approved for widespread use in humans.

Design Considerations

Just as advances in cement technique have led to a significant improvement in the clinical behavior of cemented devices, so too have advances in design led to better performance of uncemented femoral stems. Initial mechanical stability is essential; there is now a consensus that attachment vehicles such as porous coatings cannot serve as a primary means of stabilization for femoral stems in the absence of initial stable fixation. Recent investigations have shown that such coatings may contribute to stability, preventing micromotion, over longer periods.

As the diameter of femoral stems has become larger in attempts to fill the canal, the stiffness of the device has increased significantly. The bending stiffness of femoral stems is the product of the modulus of elasticity multiplied by the cross-section moment of inertia. Because the moment of inertia increases (to the fourth power) with the diameter of the stem, a small increase in diameter leads to a large increase in bending stiffness. Because the modulus of titanium alloy is approximately one half that of cobalt-chromium alloy, titanium has been used in the fabrication of femoral stems to reduce bending stiffness.

Femoral Stems

The general conclusion that can be drawn from clinical reports of uncemented stems is that the results improve with the degree of fit achieved at surgery, indicating that immediate stable fixation achieved by filling the medullary canal, especially, proximally, is of paramount importance. During the last few years, strategies implemented for "canal-filling" include computer design of femoral components, modular prostheses, custom-designed prostheses employing computed tomographic data, and intraoperative molding of the prepared canal for the immediate on-site fabrication of custom stems.

Algorithm for Computer Design One recent approach is based on the proposition that a stem shape that closely resembles the endosteal anatomy of the femur, particularly in the proximal region, can achieve intimate contact and stability and approximate the load-transfer patterns of the normal femur. The fit achieved with such an "anatomic" design, with the emphasis on maximum fit in certain priority areas of contact, could result in maximal load transfer to cortical bone and resist not only axial and bending loads but also the important torsional loads. A stem that completely filled the medullary canal (for example, an exact replica of the canal) is not considered a practical design objective because such a prosthesis could not actually be implanted or removed.

An algorithm was developed for designing a stem that would provide an optimal fit into the "average" femoral canal. The percentage of the canal filled by the resulting "anatomic" design was compared with that filled by a conventional symmetric prosthesis (Fig. 16). The results showed that more of the canal was filled by the anatomic device and that the anatomic device was in relatively close contact (within 1 mm) with the endosteal cortex in the identified "priority" regions of the femur. Other studies in cadaveric bone showed that these collarless, uncemented devices without porous coatings led to higher surface strains in the proximal femur than are produced with cemented implants. These strains are hoop strains that are larger than those occurring in the normal femur. The long-term consequence of these higher hoop strains have yet to be determined.

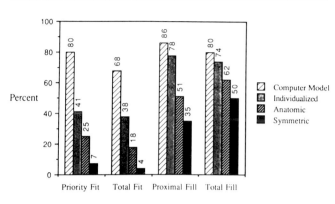

Figure 16

Fit and fill results of different stems fitted in bone sections. (Reproduced with permission from Poss R, Walker P, Spector M, et al: Strategies for improving fixation of femoral components in total hip arthroplasty. *Clin Orthop* 1988;235:181–194.)

Modularity The concept of modularity was first introduced when cobalt-chromium alloy (and later aluminum oxide ceramic) balls were used with titanium femoral stems. This concept was extended to include sleeves to fit over the proximal portion of the stems to enhance proximal canal filling and caps to be fitted onto the distal end of the stem to fill the canal at the isthmus. The latter approach was used to achieve distal fixation without uniformly increasing the diameter of the stem and its bending stiffness.

A potential problem related to the implementation of modular prostheses fabricated from titanium alloy (and perhaps other metal alloys) is the fretting wear that can result from the relative motion between mated parts under cyclic loading. A laboratory study of one particular design with a modular collar and neck revealed considerable wear at the junction of the components. This finding emphasizes the need for comprehensive laboratory testing (under cyclic load conditions in an aqueous environment) before such devices are used clinically.

Custom Design Joint replacement protheses, particularly femoral stems, can be fabricated in such a way that they are customized to the individual patient. Initially this concept was implemented in the fabrication of revision prostheses for situations that could not be treated effectively with off-the-shelf devices. The design of such custom prostheses is based on reconstructed images of the patient's femur by computed tomography. There is a question about the cost-effectiveness of this approach for generalized use in primary arthroplasty.

Another method of preparing customized stems for primary and revision arthroplasty involves the fabrication of intraoperative molds of the femoral canal (after surgical preparation), and the on-site production of a titanium alloy stem for immediate implantation. In this approach, a thin elastomeric "balloon" filled with an impression material is inserted into the prepared medullary canal to produce an accurate model of the cavity. A laser scan of the canal model is coupled to a milling machine that cuts a replica of the model into a block of titanium alloy. The finished stem is cleaned, passivated, sterilized, and returned to the operating room within about 90 minutes. It should be emphasized that, to date, the routine use of custom implants is supported only by theoretic data. There is considerable

question as to whether this approach will prove to be cost-effective.

Flexible Stems Proximal bone loss around stiff femoral stems (Fig. 17) is a potentially serious problem. Approximately 20% of 301 cobalt-chromium alloy devices that were fully or partially (two thirds) porous-coated showed bone resorption proximal to the distal border of the coating, as did 28% of 232 stems more than 13.5 mm in diameter (Table 5). In contrast, the incidence of significant bone loss was only 5.6% in stems 12 mm or less in diameter. It is not known whether nonporous (that is, not bonded) prostheses of comparable size would have elicited as much bone loss. Finite-element stress analyses of bonded and unbonded stems have not proven whether bonding is a first-order or second-order influence on the stress-shielding effects that lead to bone resorption.

Even though titanium alloy has one half the elastic modulus of cobalt-chromium alloy, titanium alloy femoral stems with diameters of more than approximately 16 mm can significantly reduce stresses in surrounding bone. Recent animal investigations have shown that partially or

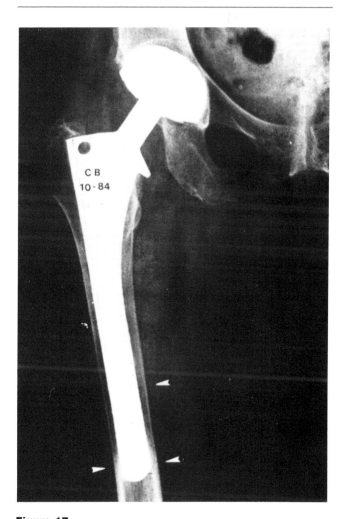

Figure 17

Radiograph shows bone loss caused by stress-shielding around a relatively stiff fully porous-coated cobalt-chromium femoral stem. (Reproduced with permission from Engh CA, Bobyn JD: *Biological Fixation in Total Hip Arthroplasty.* Thorofare, Slack, 1985.)

Table 5. Overall effect of stem size on second- or third-degree bone resorption*

Stem Size (mm)	No. of Cases	Combined Incidence (%)
9.0	7	0
10.5	129	2
12.0	43	16
13.5	66	27
15.0	10	25
16.5	51	35
18.0 or more	15	29

*Reproduced with permission from Engh CA, Bobyn JD: The influence of stem size and extent of porous coating on femoral bone resorption after primary cementless hip arthroplasty. *Clin Orthop* 1988;231:7–28.

fully porous-coated stems produced as much as 20% cortical bone loss after six months. These findings prompted attempts to develop materials with a lower modulus of elasticity. The European experience has been with a polymeric (polyacetal) stem, referred to as the "isoelastic" prosthesis. This uncemented prosthesis, which has only a thin metal spine, is press-fit into the canal. Surface irregularities provide for "macrointerlock." After two years, the first 400 patients treated at one center had no stem fractures. The revision rate of 1% and clinical performance encouraged the investigators to continue the trial.

Another approach is to develop designs with lower cross-section moments of inertia. Laboratory investigations and clinical trials in Europe have shown that metallic stems with distal longitudinal splits are significantly more flexible than conventional prostheses. Clinical follow-up studies of this device have yet to appear.

Strategies for Implant Fixation

Contemporary cement techniques have significantly improved the longevity of cemented total hip and knee replacement prostheses. Because cement has a limited fatigue life, alternative cementless methods of fixation are generally employed in younger patients and, in many instances, in revision arthroplasty. Although good early results have been obtained for many types of uncemented implants, unfavorable outcomes have also been reported. No one uncemented method of fixation stands out as being clearly superior to the others. Moreover, the interpretation of results obtained from animal and human trials continues to be confounded by variables other than just the method of fixation. For example, radiographic findings such as subsidence, loosening, or resorption by surrounding bone are influenced not only by the nature of the fixation but also by the inherent mechanical stability of the component design, its stiffness, the enduring quality of the host bone, and polyethylene wear debris.

Bone Cement

Techniques implemented in recent years to improve the performance of bone cement include modifications in the methods of preparing the bony site for implantation of cement and changes in the way bone cement is prepared and delivered to the surgical site. In preparing the implant site, care must be taken to remove bone and blood debris. Modifications in the preparation and handling of cement include the use of vacuum and/or centrifugation during preparation, and specially designed syringes for the delivery of cement under enough pressure to ensure sufficient intrusion of cement into surrounding bone interstices.

Recent investigations have shown that the mechanical properties of cement, in particular its fatigue performance, can be improved through preparative methods that reduce the voids in the substance and through the use of cements of higher average molecular weights. These advances have resulted from the implementation of the engineering approach called "fracture mechanics." Fracture is related to two events, crack initiation and crack growth. In many substances, a fracture is the result of the formation of surface cracks that, once formed, quickly proceed throughout the substance (that is, rapid crack growth). In other materials or situations, fracture is controlled by the rate of crack growth rather than the initiation of microcracks in the substance. Experimental methods can determine if the fracture of a particular substance is controlled by crack initiation or by crack growth.

It has been proposed that it is the voids that form during the mixing of cement that serve as multiple sites of crack initiation. The hypothesis is that reducing the number of voids (cracks) will decrease the likelihood of fracture. Investigation has shown that the fatigue strength of cement does increase in cement mixed under vacuum and by centrifugation to reduce the number of voids even in the presence of surface irregularities. This work has led to the implementation of these methods for cement preparation in the operating room. However, other investigators have assumed that microcracks will always be present in the cement sheath as it is cured in vivo because of the (desired) irregular topography resulting from the intrusion of cement into the surrounding bone interstices. This approach incriminates crack growth, rather than crack initiation, as the mechanism controlling the resistance of bone cement to fracture (that is, its fatigue strength). It was shown that bone cements with higher average molecular weights were more resistant to crack growth.

Unfortunately, it appears that little recent progress has been made in developing improved bone cement substances.

Biologic Fixation: Bone Ingrowth Into Porous Coatings

The biologic fixation achieved by bone ingrowth into porous coatings continues to be implemented as an alternative to cementing prosthetic devices. However, questions remain as to the contribution of this bone ingrowth to the stability of the device. It is accepted that inherent mechanical stability of the prosthesis is a prerequisite for bone ingrowth. The porous coating may contribute less to the ultimate load-carrying capacity of the device than to limiting the relative micromotion between the stem and surrounding bone.

Biologic fixation can be considered a two-stage process consisting of the initial bone ingrowth and the subsequent stress-induced adaptive remodeling (Fig. 18). Surgical trauma associated with implementation of the device initiates the wound-healing of bone "regeneration." As bone forms within the surgical defect (that is, the bed produced to accept the prosthesis), it also forms within the pores of the device. If this bone regeneration is impaired by factors (such as micromotion) that destroy the stromal elements of regeneration, a "repair" process results. The end result of tissue repair is scar (that is, fibrous ingrowth). As the bone regeneration (bone ingrowth) process subsides, stress-

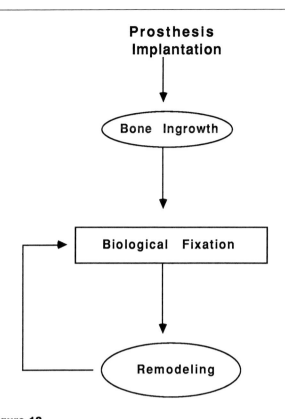

Figure 18

Diagram depicting the influence of bone ingrowth and remodeling on biologic fixation.

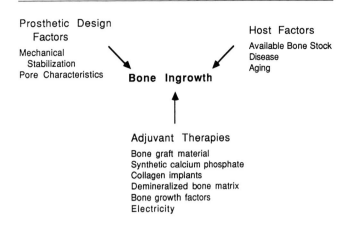

Figure 19

Factors affecting bone ingrowth.

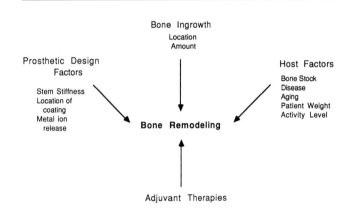

Figure 20

Factors affecting bone remodeling.

induced bone remodeling begins. Many factors influence bone ingrowth and bone remodeling during biologic fixation (Figs. 19 and 20).

Many patients in whom porous-coated devices are implanted may require postoperative treatment with certain procedures and drugs that could adversely influence bone ingrowth. For example, agents used to prevent heterotopic ossification can inhibit the bone ingrowth process. Animal models have revealed that γ-radiation, sodium etidronate, and nonsteroidal anti-inflammtory drugs such as indomethacin inhibit bone ingrowth, as reflected by the reduced amount of bone in the pores of the specimens and the lower attachment strength. Anticancer drugs such as cis-platinum also inhibit bone ingrowth. In general, it is to be expected that agents that have an adverse influence on bone regeneration will inhibit bone ingrowth during biologic fixation.

Many investigators have attempted to identify treatments and agents that accelerate the bone ingrowth process. These agents include autogenous and allogeneic bone-graft particles, synthetic calcium phosphate particles and coatings, demineralized bone matrix and partially purified bone morphogenic protein, collagen, and bone growth factors. It has been proposed that these agents facilitate the bone ingrowth process by serving as a grouting medium to enhance stabilization and/or to accelerate the cellular or extracellular processes constituting bone regeneration. To date, animal studies have shown that some agents can increase the amount of bone ingrowth and the strength of attachment within the first few weeks after implantation but no agents increase bone ingrowth and strength of attachment after six to eight weeks, perhaps because the ul-

timate strength of attachment of a porous-coated device is controlled by the mechanical properties of the surrounding bone. There is no indication that agents used to accelerate the bone ingrowth process have a long-term influence on the bone density around these implants.

Electrical stimulation has also been investigated to augment porous-coated devices. Although initial studies using direct-current stimulation found a marginal increase in the amounts of bone ingrowth and interfacial shear strength within a few weeks postoperatively in animals, later studies using pulsed electromagnetic fields showed no effect. The efficacy of electricity in enhancing biologic fixation remains in question.

Porous coatings currently undergoing widespread clinical use are fabricated by sintering cobalt-chromium alloy and titanium alloy microspheres and commercially pure titanium fibers and by plasma-spraying titanium. For porous materials with pore sizes large enough to accommodate the elements of bone (that is, cells, capillaries, and matrix), no clear benefit of one type of material over another has been shown. Previously, it had been proposed that porous polymeric coatings might offer advantages over porous metallic materials by virtue of the absence of metal ion release and their low modulus of elasticity. The relatively high incidence of failure (revision) and the finding of fragmentation of the coating and detachment from the metallic substrate suggest that the current forms of these porous polymeric materials have insufficient strength.

Press-Fit Prostheses and Osseointegration

Favorable clinical results have been obtained with uncemented, nonporous devices for which an "interference" or "friction" fit is obtained at the time of implantation. These devices have smooth or irregular surfaces and are generally referred to as "press-fit" prostheses.

Bone can be found in close apposition to the surface of a metallic device, in some cases with no interposed fibrous tissue. The term osseointegration has been accepted as a convenient means of describing a sitation in which no fibrous issue is observed between bone and a metallic surface by light microscopy. There are no data that demonstrate that prostheses perform any better clinically after osseointegration.

Hydroxyapatite Coatings

Although there is some question about the degree to which bone bonds to metallic implants, studies have indicated that osseous tissue can bond to certain "biologically active glasses" and calcium phosphates. Evidence for bone attachment to these substances generally has come from biomechanical tests in which implants were pushed or pulled out of bone. The interfacial shear strength is considerably higher than that found with uncoated control materials, often titanium alloy. Because of their limited strength, the biologically active glasses have not yet been introduced into clinical practice as bone-substitute materials or as coatings for prostheses.

Synthetic calcium phosphates in the mineral form of hydroxyapatite and tricalcium phosphate are being used clinically for certain oral and maxillofacial applications as bone-substitute materials. They are only now undergoing investigation for orthopaedic applications. Hydroxyapatite coatings produced by plasma-spraying are now being clinically investigated as coatings for femoral stems. Important unresolved issues relate to the solubility and mechanical properties of these coatings. In particular, there is some concern as to whether they will remain bonded to the metallic substrate under cyclic loading in an aqueous environment in vivo.

The advantage of hydroxyapatite coatings over other methods of biologic fixation may be in the rate at which the stem is "incorporated" into the host bone. It is possible that these stems become more rapidly stabilized after implantation. However, direct evidence of this more rapid stabilization is only now emerging from some investigations.

Mechanisms of Implant Failure

Loosening, Micromotion, and Subsidence

Implant loosening has been related to several factors: (1) the mechanical overload failure of supporting cancellous bone, (2) fracture and fragmentation of bone cement with a subsequent osteolytic response, (3) osteolytic response related to polyethylene wear debris, and (4) loss of supportive bone mass because of stress-shielding affects. A related issue that has attracted attention in recent years is the relative micromotion that occurs between implant and bone under applied loading. To date, the effect of micromotion has been considered in relation to the adverse effects on bone ingrowth, and its contribution to pain. Another related issue is permanent migration (subsidence that can occur with some prosthetic components).

The degree of relative motion that can occur between the prosthetic surface and surrounding tissue is now being investigated. This motion (measured in μ) can represent both slippage of the device in the tissue bed and elastic and plastic deformation of the interfacial tissue and surrounding bone. Slippage is of particular importance because it represents subsidence or migration of the device, and may potentiate biologic responses that lead to loosening of the prosthesis and pain. Investigations of certain designs of knee and hip replacements in animals and human cadavers have shown that micromotion of 100 μ or more can occur. This magnitude of relative movement of a porous coating in surrounding bone could impair the bone regeneration response that leads to bone ingrowth. Micomotion may also influence the formation and exacerbation of the "pseudomembrane" that has been found around loose cemented and uncemented prostheses.

A few years ago a new method of analysis was employed to evaluate the migration of total knee replacements in radiographs. The method, roentgen stereophotogrammetry, involves insertion of tantalum markers into the polyethylene tibial component and into the proximal tibia at the time of surgery. This provides distinct points of identification on radiographs. In one study, migration of 0.19 to 1.2 mm was found for cemented and uncemented devices of several designs after four years. Some prostheses continued to migrate throughout the period of the investigation, which was five years. In addition to migration, all prostheses showed reversible displacement, with the maximum deflection ranging from 0.2 to 1.0 mm. The clinical consequences of this migration have yet to be determined. In another study, femurs implanted with cemented stems have been retrieved from human subjects after varying implantation times. The stems and femurs were instrumented so the relative motion could be measured when the stem was loaded under physiologic conditions. In some cases the untreated contralateral femur was implanted with a device so it could act as a control, providing information about the type of micromotion expected immediately after implantation. Results of these investigations showed that cementing the stem led to immediate and lasting stability with little micromotion (approximately 40 μ being recorded). In a similar study of uncemented, porous-coated devices in dogs, acute implantation (modeling the immediate postoperative situation) displayed significantly more micromotion (as much as 150 μ). However, six months after implantation, presumably after bone ingrowth had occurred, the degree of relative motion was reduced to the level found with bone cement.

Retrieval Analysis

To obtain direct evidence of the bone ingrowth into porous-coated prostheses, histologic studies were performed on devices obtained at revision surgery. These analyses generally revealed little ingrowth of bone into the porous-coated prostheses. However, in most of these early studies, revision of the implant was required because of loosening. Therefore, it was difficult to make definitive statements regarding the extent of bone ingrowth into specific devices only on the basis of these retrieved specimens.

In recent years increasing numbers of devices have had to be revised for problems other than loosening (for example, malposition). In addition, cadaveric specimens have become available for analysis. Histologic investigations of these devices have revealed that bone does grow into a variety of total hip and knee replacement devices although, as is almost universlly reported, a minority of the available surface is ingrown with bone.

A recent analysis of femurs retrieved from patients who underwent successful total hip replacement (follow-up was as long as 17 years in some cases) revealed several important findings: (1) The marked stress-shielding in the proximal femur induced by implantation of a cemented stem persists to a large degree and is not compensated for by "adaptive remodeling." (2) Histologic examination revealed a benign and enduring interface between trabecular bone and cement. (3) The authors suggested that the initial site of fixation failure is at the prosthesis-cement interface.

Trends

Twenty-two years after the widespread implementation of total joint replacement in the United States, ten-year success rates of more than 90% have been reported for cemented total hip and knee replacement prostheses. Problems such as infection and stem breakage, which appeared to be major problems soon after the introduction of total joint replacements, are now uncommon. Current concerns are problems that become manifest after ten to 15 years of implantation: metal ion release, wear and mechanical degradation of polyethylene, and bone loss caused by stress-shielding. Because of concerns about the long-term mechanical properties of bone cement, strategies for cementless fixation in younger patients continue to be pursued.

It is of some interest that the materials currently used in the fabrication of joint replacement prostheses are essentially those that were available when the procedure was first developed in the 1960s. Improvements in performance have come through (1) prosthetic design modifications, (2) changes in the way bone cement is handled intraoperatively, and (3) more judicious selection of and experience with prostheses. The solution to these longer-term problems of joint arthroplasty may come through the introduction of new materials: "modified" polyethylene, carbon-fiber-reinforced polymer composites, and calcium phosphate coatings. One of the more important goals for

the 1990s is learning about the performance of these substances. Because none of these materials has been widely used for nonmedical applications, orthopaedic investigators will need to generate fundamental information about the composition, structure, and properties of the materials as well as their behavior in orthopaedic applications.

During the 1990s the magnitude of certain problems associated with metallic devices must be better assessed. It is known that metal ions are released from cobalt-chromium alloy implants, but the biologic implications of their accumulation with time are unknown. It is known that bone loss in the proximal femur is associated with rigid metallic stems, but it is not known whether such bone loss will remain nonsymptomatic and of no significant clinical consequence. It is known that there is a nonlinear degeneration of polyethylene components, with increasing wear found after ten years, but it is not known whether current polyethylene components, and those to be fabricated with "enhanced" polyethylene, will suddenly fail after ten to 15 years.

Other unsettled issues that must be clarified in coming years relate to the necessity of coatings serving as attachment vehicles for joint replacement prostheses. A prerequisite for success is a prosthetic design with inherent mechanical stability, but it may be necessary to have some type of "bonding" of the prosthesis to surrounding bone to limit the micromotion that promotes loosening. A related issue concerns which surface coatings may be indicated for certain patients. The location and extent of bone ingrowth continue to vary. Studies are needed to determine whether limited regions of bone ingrowth significantly contribute to the stability of the prosthesis. The hydroxyapatite coating appears promising, but whether these coatings will remain bonded to the metallic substrates over time and whether these ceramic particles contribute to loosening and osteolysis must be determined.

Investigations of the tissue surrounding loose prostheses have revealed their cellular constituents and biochemical activity. This tissue has certain characteristics in common with inflamed synovium. Pehaps a drug will be found that slows the progression of the pseudomembrane around a loose device, extending the time before revision is required. A better understanding of how the implant-bone interface forms and remodels could provide some indication of the value of locally delivered "bone growth factors" as adjuvants to enhance the process of osseointegration and bone bonding.

Even limited success in achieving the goals of this agenda for the 1990s would mean significant improvements in the performance of total joint arthroplasty.

Annotated Bibliography

Keywords

Bone cement; Bone ingrowth; Calcium phosphate ceramics; Ceramics; Cobalt-chromium alloy; Hydroxyapatite; Neoplasms; Polyethylene; Polymers; Prosthesis; Titanium alloy

Materials

Metals

Agins HJ, Alcock NW, Bansal M, et al: Metallic wear in failed titanium-alloy total hip replacements. *J Bone Joint Surg* 1988;70A:347–356.

Tissues from failed titanium alloy total hip prostheses displayed intense histiocytic and plasma-cell reactions in the pseudocapsular tissue, with copious metallic staining of the lining cells. Eight of these hips were cemented; one was implanted with no cement. Titanium, aluminum, and vanadium were found in the tissues. The concentrations of the three elements in the soft tissues were similar to those in the metal of the prostheses.

Bartolozzi A, Black J: Chromium concentrations in serum, blood clot and urine from patients following total hip arthroplasty. *Biomaterials* 1987;6:2–8.

Blood and urine specimens from 14 patients with cement cobalt-chromium alloy hip replacement prostheses revealed a significant postoperative increase in serum chromium content in comparison with seven control patients. It was not possible to determine if the chromium ions had a valency of +3 or +6.

Betts F, Hansraj KK, Bansa M, et al: Metal release from cobalt-chrome prostheses: Analysis of tissues from revision total hip replacements. Presented at the 15th Annual Meeting of the Society for Biomaterials, Lake Buena Vista, Florida, 1989.

Tissue samples taken from the joint capsule and cement-bone interface from human subjects contained various degrees of metal. Relative concentrations of the ions generally reflected the alloy composition, indicating that most of the metal was present in the form of metal particles.

Buchanan RA, Rigney ED Jr: Ion implantation of surgical TI-6Al-4V for improved resistance to wear-accelerated corrosion. *J Biomed Mater Res* 1987;21:355–366.

Nitrogen ion implantation of titanium alloy significantly improved the resistance to wear-accelerated corrosion in saline and serum solutions.

Ferguson GM, Watanabe S, Georgescu HI, et al: The synovial production of collagenase and chondrocyte activating factors in response to cobalt. *J Orthop Res* 1988; 6:525–530.

Addition of cobalt ions in the form of cobalt fluoride solutions to media containing lapine or human synovial cells stimulated their production of neutral proteinases and collagenase. Production of prostaglandin E_2 by lapine cells was enhanced 30% to 40% by cobalt solutions that slightly depressed the production of prostaglandin E_2 by human cells. Lapine synovial cells stimulated by $CoCl_2$ also produced a substance that provoked the synthesis of collagenase, gelatinase, caseinase, and prostaglandin E_2 by monolayers of articular chondrocytes.

Gillespie WJ, Frampton CMA, Henderson RJ, et al: The incidence of cancer following total hip replacement. *J Bone Joint Surg* 1988;70B:539–542.

The incidence of tumors at remote sites after total hip replacement in 1,358 individuals was studied. In the decade following implantation, the incidence of tumors of the lymphatic and hematopoietic systems was significantly greater than expected and that of cancer of the breast, colon, and rectum was significantly less than expected.

Haag M, Adler CP: Malignant fibrous histiocytoma in association with hip replacement. *J Bone Joint Surg* 1989; 71B:701.

A malignant fibrous histiocytoma was found at the site of a cemented Weber-Huggler type II hip replacement prosthesis, the stem of which was fabricated from a metal alloy containing chromium, nickel, and cobalt. The tumor was found at reoperation, ten years after implantation. The authors noted that in recent years malignant fibrous histiocytoma, formerly a rare tumor, has been reported much more frequently, particularly as a soft-tissue tumor of the lower limbs in older men.

Howie DW, Vernon-Roberts B: The synovial response

to intra-articular cobalt-chrome wear particles. *Clin Orthop* 1988;232:244–254.

Cobalt-chromium alloy particulate wear debris injected into rat knee joints induced rapid proliferation of macrophages and focal degeneration of synovial tissues similar to the response seen in the tissues around loose total joint prostheses in humans. Initially, there was ulceration of the synovium and necrosis of macrophages at the site of large concentrations of particles in the subsynovium. Particles were endocytosed by macrophages. The decreasing number of particles and macrophages in the synovial tissue with time supports the concept that joints possess the ability to dispose of wear particles.

Martin A, Bauer TW, Manley MT, et al: Osteosarcoma at the site of total hip replacement. *J Bone Joint Surg* 1988;70A:1561–1567.

Osteosarcoma was found at the site of a cemented Charnley-Muller hip replacement prosthesis made of cast cobalt-chromium alloy. The tumor was found ten years after implantation. Higher concentrations of cobalt and chromium were found in the tumor than in control samples. Increased nickel was also found in one of the samples from the tumor. The authors review previous findings of tumors at the sites of orthopaedic prostheses and internal fixation devices.

Rostlund T, Albrektsson B, Albrektsson T, et al: Wear of ion-implanted pure titanium against UHMWPE. *Biomaterials* 1989;10:176–181.

Ion implantation of nitrogen into commercially pure titanium femoral heads led to an improvement in the wear properties. Ion implantation reduced the release rate of metal from the head and significantly reduced the wear of the polyethylene acetabular cups against which the titanium balls articulated. However, the mean polymer wear rate with titanium specimens (ion-implanted or not) was 36% higher than that with cobalt-chromium alloy heads. This difference was attributed to differences in surface finish. There was evidence to indicate that the ion-implanted layer on the titanium specimens gradually rubbed off the contact zones.

Ryu RK, Bovill EG Jr, Skinner HB, et al: Soft tissue sarcoma associated with aluminum oxide ceramic total hip arthroplasty: A case report. *Clin Orthop* 1987;216: 207–212.

An aggressive soft-tissue sarcoma was detected 15 months after implantation of a total hip replacement prosthesis consisting of a cobalt-chromium alloy stem with a ceramic ball and ceramic cup (implanted without cement).

Visuri T, Koskenvuo M: Cancer risk after McKee-Farrar total hip replacement. *Acta Orthop Scand* 1989;60(suppl 231):25.

The cancer incidence in 443 patients implanted with McKee-Farrar total hip replacement prostheses, operated on between 1967 and 1973, was monitored to the end of 1981. Although the risk of total cancer incidence did not increase, the risk for leukemias and lymphomas increased, while the risk for breast cancer decreased. This study was performed in Finland.

Weber PC: Epithelioid sarcoma in association with total knee replacement: A case report. *J Bone Joint Surg* 1986;68B:824–826.

In this case report, an epithelioid sarcoma was found at the site of a cobalt-chromium alloy total knee replacement prosthesis 44 months after implantation.

Polymers

Bartel DL, Bicknell VL, Wright TM: The effect of conformity, thickness, and material on stresses in ultra-high molecular weight components for total joint replacement. *J Bone Joint Surg* 1986;68A:1041–1051.

Stress analysis showed that contact stresses in the polyethylene component of total knee replacement prostheses can exceed the yield strength of the material for certain designs. The contact stress was increased by decreasing the thickness of the polyethylene component and by use of less conforming geometry. Results showed that polyethylene should be more than 8 to 10 mm thick when possible, and designs with conforming articulating surfaces employed if possible. Stresses were lower in acetabular components articulating with femoral heads 28 mm in diameter than in those articulating with femoral heads 22 mm in diameter. The use of carbon-fiber-inforced polyethylene resulted in stresses that were higher by as much as 40%.

Christel P, Meunier A, Leclercq S: Development of a carbon-carbon hip prosthesis. *J Biomed Mater Res* 1987; 21:191–218.

The method of preparing carbon-fiber-reinforced carbon composites is described, as are the composition, structure, and mechanical properties of the substance. Bone was found apposed to nonweightbearing implants of the carbon-carbon-material. Mechanical studies displayed the favorable performance of carbon-carbon femoral stems tested in the laboratory.

Connelly GM, Rimnac CM, Wright TM, et al: Fatigue crack propagation behavior of ultrahigh molecular weight polyethylene. *J Orthop Res* 1984;2:119–125.

The fatigue crack propagation resistance of carbon-fiber-reinforced polyethylene was found to be significantly worse than that of conventional nonreinforced polyethylene. This result, which was attributed to poor bonding between the carbon fibers and the polyethylene matrix and the ductile nature of the matrix, contraindicated the use of the carbon-fiber-reinforced polyethylene material for the fabrication of components for total joint replacement prostheses.

Eyerer P: Property changes of UHMW polyethylene during implantation: First hints for the development of an alternative polyethylene. *Adv Biomater*, 1987, pp 62–68.

New, retrieved, and shelf-stored polyethylene acetabular cups were analyzed for the presence of insoluble constituents, density, and chemical composition. The percentage of soluble constituents increased with implantation time, especially near the inner and outer surface of the cup. This was attributed to oxidative molecular degradation. The density of the polyethylene substance also changed with implantation time, and varied with location in the cup. These results showed that different aging processes occurred in vivo and in vitro.

Howie DW, Vernon-Roberts B, Oakeshott R, et al: A rat model of resorption of bone at the cement-bone interface in the presence of polyethylene wear particles. *J Bone Joint Surg* 1988;70A:257–263.

Injection of polyethylene particles into the knee joint of rats induced resorption of bone and the formation of a membrane at the interface of a nonweightbearing plug of bone cement implanted through the knee joint into the distal part of the femur. Polyethylene particles were found infiltrating the fibrous tissue around the acrylic plug.

Landy MM, Walker PS: Wear of ultra-high-molecular-weight polyethylene components of 90 retrieved knee prostheses. *J Arthrop*, 1988, suppl, pp S73–S85.

This analysis of polyethylene components retrieved from 90 total knee replacement prostheses, with implantation times as long as ten years, revealed abrasion of the polyethylene from cement or bone, and delamination of the polyethylene surface. This delamination appeared to be initiated by intergranular material defects, and propagated by the excessive subsurface stresses beneath the contact zone.

Magee FP, Weinstein AM, Longo JA, et al: A canine

composite femoral stem: An in vivo study. *Clin Orthop* 1988;235:237–252.

Carbon-fiber-reinforced polysulfone-composite femoral stems were evaluated radiographically, by computed tomography, and by postmortem histologic study. Radiography and computed tomography showed that the cortical dimensions of the operated on limb remained unchanged when compared with the control femur, indicating the absence of proximal bone loss that might be the result of stress-shielding effects. A radiodense shell of bone formed around the stem immediately after implantation, and reached its maximum thickness at six to eight months. Bone and fibrous tissue were histologically observed around the prosthesis.

Maguire JK Jr, Coscia MF, Lynch MH: Foreign body reaction to polymeric debris following total hip arthroplasty. *Clin Orthop* 1987;216:2113–223.

Tissue obtained from the cement-bone interface of two failed total hip replacements was evaluated histologically. Polyethylene and polymethylmethacrylate particulate debris was associated with macrophages and multinucleated foreign-body giant cells.

Murray DW, Rae T, Rushton N: The influence of the surface energy and roughness of implants on bone resorption. *J Bone Joint Surg* 1989;71B:632–637.

This cell culture investigation found that macrophages released increased amounts of mediators that stimulate bone resorption when adherent to foreign surfaces. The greatest bone-resorption activity and prostaglandin E_2 release was found when the cells were cultured on rough hydrophilic surfaces and the least when they were cultured on smooth hydrophobic surfaces. Smooth hydrophilic and rough hydrophobic surfaces were in between, with the former stimulating slightly more, although the differences were not significant. With surfaces of the same surface energy, rough topography stimulated more resorptive activity than the smooth surface. Generally, more resorptive activity was found with hydrophilic than with hydrophobic surfaces. In these experiments it was found that polyethylene yielded 20% more bone resorption activity than polymethylmethacrylate.

Skinner HB: Composite technology for total hip arthroplasty. *Clin Orthop* 1988;235:224–236.

This article reviewed materials that might be employed in the fabrication of carbon-fiber-reinforced polymer-composite total hip replacement prostheses. The mechanical properties of the nonreinforced and reinforced polysulfone and polyetheretherketone depended on carbon-fiber orientation and the sequence in which oriented laminates of composite sheets were stacked before molding. Potential problems related to testing of the mechanical properties of composites and the relatively low abrasion-resistance of composites are noted.

Wright TM, Bartel DL: The problem of surface damage in polyethylene to total knee components. *Clin Orthop* 1986;205:67–74.

This analysis of retrieved polyethylene components from total knee replacement prostheses found that the amount and severity of polyethylene damage increased significantly with patient weight and implantation time. The authors identified seven modes of surface damage.

Wroblewski BM, Lunch M, Atkinson JR, et al: External wear of the polethylene socket in cemented total hip arthroplasty. *J Bone Joint Surg* 1987;69B:61–63.

Nineteen of 59 cemented polyethylene acetabular cups removed at revision surgery displayed areas of wear between the outside of the socket and the acetabular bone. This was associated with lack of acrylic cement in those areas and also related to the depth of the wear on the articulating surface of the socket. These results suggest that poloyethylene particulate debris and the associated osteolytic response at the bone-cement junction are secondary to socket loosening and abrasion of the cup against the bone of the acetabulum, rather than to particles migrating from the metal-polyethylene interface.

Ceramics

Fitzgerald RH, Chao EYS, McDonald DJ, et al: A comparison of autografts, allografts, and tricalcium phosphate hydroxyapatite crystals in Fitzgerald R Jr (ed): *Non-Cemented Total Hip Arthroplasty*. New York, Raven Press, 1988, pp 159–174.

A synthetic calcium phosphate "bone-substitute material" made of tricalcium phosphate and hydroxyapatite was employed to fill a gap, purposely produced surgically, between the porous coating of a canine femoral stem and surrounding bone. In this application the bone-substitute material had no more bone ingrowth or strength of attachment than did unfilled gaps.

Design Considerations

Engh CA, Bobyn JD: The influence of stem size and extent of porous coating on femoral bone resorption after primary cementless hip arthroplasty. *Clin Orthop* 1988; 231:7–28.

The influence of stem size and extent of porous coating on femoral bone resorption was examined in 411 cases of primary cementless hip arthroplasty. Pronounced resorption occurred in all cases. The use of larger-diameter stems increased the occurrence of marked bone resorption. Stems with diameters of 13.5 mm or more had five times the incidence of pronounced resorption than stems 12 mm or less in diameter. Stems with two-thirds and full porous coatings showed a twofold to fourfold increase in the incidence of pronounced bone resorption. The clinical findings agreed with theoretic calculations of the degree of stress-shielding to be expected as a result of the bending stiffness of the device.

Poss R, Robertson DD, Walker PS, et al: Anatomic stem design for press-fit and cemented application, in Fitzgerald R Jr (ed): *Non-Cemented Total Hip Arthroplasty*. New York, Raven Press, 1988, pp 343–363.

An algorithm that allows computer design of canal-filling femoral stems for press-fit application is described. These anatomic devices filled the canal better than a conventional symmetric design. Related studies showed that the hoop strains produced by insertion of the noncemented press-fit stems are higher than normal, and higher than those occurring with cemented implants. Micromotion and rotation of the press-fit stems, wedged into place, were found to be very small (less than 50 μ).

Poss R, Walker PS, Spector M, et al: Strategies for improving fixation of femoral components in total hip arthroplasty. *Clin Orthop* 1988;235:181–194.

Prosthetic design features, including strategies for cementless fixation of femoral components, are reviewed.

Sumner DR, Turner TM: The effects of femoral component design features on femoral remodeling, in Fitzgerald R Jr (ed): *Non-Cemented Total Hip Arthroplasty*. New York, Raven Press, 1988.

The amount of bone loss in the cortex of dogs implanted with titanium stems with differing extents of porous coating was determined. The area of the cortex at selected transverse sections of the operated on femur was compared with the cortical area at corresponding levels in the unoperated limb. Fully coated devices led to approximately 35% loss in cortical bone area in transverse sections taken at the midstem region. Results obtained with fiber-metal, beaded, and plasma-sprayed porous coatings were comparable. Less bone loss was found around partially coated devices.

Strategies for Implant Fixation

Davies JP, O'Connor DO, Burke DW, et al: The effect of centrifugation on the fatigue life of bone cement in the presence of surface irregularities. *Clin Orthop* 1988; 229:156–161.

The fatigue life of bone-cement test specimens with both smooth and irregular surfaces is significantly increased with centrifugation. Specimens that were composites of bone cement and trabecular bone also displayed increased fatigue life after being centrifuged. These data support the concept that reduction of porosity of bone cement by centrifugation may extend the duration of fixation of the components in cemented total joint replacements.

Goodman SB, Fornasier VL, Kei J: The effects of bulk vrs. particulate polymethylmethacrylate on bone. *Clin Orthop* 1988;232:255–262.

Bulk and particulate forms of polymethylmethacrylate were implanted into the proximal tibias of rabbits. Histologically, bulk forms of bone cement were surrounded by a thin, fibrous tissue membrane. Particulate polymethylmethacrylate stimulated a much thicker, florid, foreign-body reaction composed of histiocytes and giant cells. The foreign-body response to particulate acrylic cement was similar to that seen in failed cemented total joint replacement prostheses in humans.

Rimnac CM, Wright TM, McGill DL: The effect of centrifugation on the fracture properties of acrylic bone cements. *J Bone Joint Surg* 1986;68A:281–287.

In this study, centrifugation did not alter the static or cyclic fatigue properties of bone cement. Tests of fracture toughness and fatigue-crack propagation of centrifuged specimens of commercial cements (with and without antibiotic additions) demonstrated no significant difference from control values. Among the cements tested, the one with the highest molecular weight displayed the highest fracture toughness when tested with and without the addition of antibiotics. These results indicated that centrifugation of bone cement does not improve the cement's resistance to fracture in the presence of surface imperfections, such as those found at the bone-cement interface.

Biological Fixation: Bone Ingrowth Into Porous Coatings

Barth E, Roenningen H, Solheim LF, et al: Influence of cis-platinum on bone ingrowth into porous fiber titanium: Mechanical and biochemical correlations. Presented at the 12th Annual Meeting of the Society for Biomaterials, 1986.

Cis-platinum in therapeutic doses reduced the interfacial strength and inhibited bone ingrowth in fiber-titanium implants in rats for a period of ten weeks or less after completion of medication. This agent resulted in a reduced level of mineralization of ingrown bone for seven weeks after the completion of treatment.

Berry JL, Geiger JM, Moran JM, et al: Use of tricalcium phosphate or electrical stimulation to enhance the bone-porous implant interface. *J Biomed Mater Res* 1986;20: 65–77.

This study found no enhancement of the interfacial strength or amount of bone ingrowth into porous metallic specimens impregnated with tricalcium phosphate powder or treated with electrical stimulation, when compared with untreated controls in this canine study one, two, three, four, five, and ten weeks after implantation.

Cook SD, Thomas KA, Kay JF, et al: Hydroxyapatite-coated porous titanium for use as an orthopaedic biologic attachment system. *Clin Orthop* 1988;230:303–312.

Hydroxyapatite-coated porous titanium implants placed transcortically in the femurs of dogs did not display a higher attachment strength than uncoated porous controls. Histologic and microradiographic sections yielded similar qualitative results in the amount of bone grown into each system. However, histologically, differences were noted at the ingrown bone-porous material interface between the two implant types. The hydroxyapatite coating supported mineralization directly onto its surfaces, and a thin osseous layer was found lining all hydroxyapatite-coated surfaces. An extremely thin fibrous layer was observed separating the uncoated titanium particle surface from ingrown bone. There was not extensive direct apposition or lining of the ingrown bone to the uncoated porous titanium particle surfaces.

Haddad RJ Jr, Cook SD, Thomas KA: Biological fixation of porous-coated implants. *J Bone Joint Surg* 1987; 69A:1459–1466.

This article reviews the development of porous-coated implant devices and outlines the design parameters for the ingrowth of tissue. Clinical results with several different total hip and knee replacement systems are represented.

Keller JC, Trancik TM, Young FA, et al: Effects of indomethacin on bone ingrowth. *J Orthop Res* 1989;7:28–34.

The percentage of bone ingrowth in porous specimens implanted in rabbits treated with indomethacin was found to be less than the percentage of bone ingrowth in untreated control animals.

Magee FP, Longo JA, Hedley AK: The effect of age on the interface strength between porous coated implants and bone. Presented at the 15th Annual Meeting of the Society for Biomaterials, Lake Buena Vista, Florida, 1989.

The interfacial shear strength of porous metallic test specimens implanted into diaphyseal region of the femurs of old dogs was less than in young animals 40 days after implantation.

Martin RB, Paul HA, Bargar WL, et al: Effects of estrogen deficiency on the growth of tissue into porous titanium implants. *J Bone Joint Surg* 1988;70A:540–547.

The push-out strength of porous metallic test specimens from ovariectomized dogs was 31% less than in the control animals. Ovariectomy caused no difference in the amount of ingrowth of bone but resulted in a significant increase in the amount of fibrous connective tissue within the porous specimen. The presence of this fibrous tissue appeared to have an important effect on bone-implant fixation. In the control dogs, strength correlated positively with ingrowth of bone and negatively with ingrowth of fibrous tissue; in the ovariectomized dogs, strength correlated positively with ingrowth of fibrous tissue and not at all with ingrowth of bone. The results of this study suggest that the fixation of porous-surfaced implants may be reduced in postmenopausal or ovariectomized women.

McDonald DJ, Fitzgerald RH Jr, Chao EYS: The enhancement of fixation of a porous-coated femoral component by autograft and allograft in the dog. *J Bone Joint Surg* 1988;70A:728–737.

Revision total hip arthroplasty without cement was performed in dogs to compare the abilities of autologous grafts and allografts to enhance histologic ingrowth of bone and biomechanical strength. At 17 weeks porous-coated titanium femoral stems inserted at the time of the revision with autograft and allograft displayed greater amounts of bone ingrowth histologically than nongrafted specimens. Push-out testing showed greater ultimate shear strength proximally than distally in the grafted specimens, and at the proximal level there was a significant difference between the autograft group and the untreated controls.

Rivero DP, Fox J, Skipor AK, et al: Calcium phosphate-coated porous titanium implants for enhanced skeletal fixation. *J Biomed Mater Res* 1988;22:191–201.

Four weeks after implantation, the mean shear strength of skeletal fixation of calcium phosphate-coated fiber-metal implants in dogs was 24% greater than for paired controls. No difference in strength of fixation between treated and control implants was present at other periods. No significant increase of the volume of bone ingrowth was established for treated implants compared with paired controls at any time.

Rivero DP, Skipor AK, Singh M, et al: Effect of disodium etidronate (EHDP) on bone ingrowth in a porous material. *Clin Orthop* 1987;215:279–286.

The mean shear strength of fixation of porous metallic test specimen implanted in dogs treated with disodium etidronate was reduced by 76% compared with the controls. There was an inhibition of mineralization of the tissue in the pores of the animals treated with disodium etidronate. These findings suggest that cementless skeletal fixation of porous-coated implants by bone ingrowth may be delayed or prevented by the administration of disodium etidronate.

Spector M: Current concepts of bone ingrowth and remodeling, in Fitzgerald R Jr (ed): *Non-Cemented Total Hip Arthroplasty*. New York, Raven Press, 1988.

Factors influencing the bone ingrowth and remodeling stages of biologic fixation are reviewed. Individual factors contributed in different ways to ingrowth and remodeling. As large-diameter femoral stems are required to fill larger canals to provide the initial mechanical stability required for bone ingrowth, the high stiffness (fourth power of the diameter) can lead to adverse adaptive remodeling (that is, bone loss from stress-shielding).

Press-Fit Prostheses and Osseointegration

Poss R, Robertson DD, Walker PS, et al: Anatomic stem design for press-fit and cemented application, in Fitzgerald R Jr (ed): *Non-Cemented Total Hip Arthroplasty*. New York, Raven Press, 1988.

The design rationale employed for the development of a press-fit femoral stem is reviewed.

Hydroxyapatite Coatings

Geesink RG, de Groot K, Klein CP: Chemical implant fixation using hydroxyl-apatite coatings: The development of a human total hip prosthesis for chemical fixation to bone using hydroxyl-apatite coatings on titanium substrates. *Clin Orthop* 1987;225:147–170.

A bone-bonding shear strength of 64 MPa was measured for plasma-sprayed apatite coatings on titanium substrates implanted into dogs. Histologic sections confirmed the close bonding between the coating and living bone. In a canine total hip arthroplasty study, the hydroxyapatite-coated implants proved superior to uncoated controls with respect to radiographic and histologic appearance. Uncoated prostheses were surrounded by fibrous tissue and were easily extracted from the femur at any time. The hydroxyapatite-coated implants were rigidly fixed within three weeks with bone formation up to the implant surface. Bony defects as large as 2 mm in depth were filled with bone within six weeks.

Mechanisms of Implant Failure

Loosening, Micromotion, and Subsidence

Maloney WJ, Jasty M, Burke DW, et al: Biomechanical and histological investigations of cemented total hip replacements: A study of autopsy retrieved femurs after in vivo cycling. *Clin Orthop*, 1989;249:129–140.

Eleven whole cadaveric femurs were retrieved at autopsy from patients who had previously undergone cemented total hip arthroplasty. Implant duration ranged from two weeks to 210 months. Clinically and radiographically the implants were stable. The stability offered by cement in these well-fixed prostheses was remarkable, with the maximum axial micromotion being 40 μ. The strain gauge and photoelastic strain coating studies revealed that marked stress-shielding persists in the proximal medial femoral cortex long after a cemented femoral component is inserted. Even 17 years after surgery, the strain in the calcar region did not normalize.

Maloney WJ, O'Connor DO, Zalenski EB, et al: Stress shielding and micromotion in cemented total hip replacement after up to seventeen years of in vivo service in humans. Presented at the 15th Annual Meeting of the Society for Biomaterials, Lake Buena Vista, Florida, 1989.

Eight whole femurs with cemented femoral components were retrieved from human subjects two weeks to 210 months after surgery. In all specimens, axial micromotion was less than 30 μ in both coronal and stair-climbing loading. With one exception, transverse micromotion was less than 45 μ with coronal loading. In contrast, transverse micromotion as high as 155 μ was measured during stair-climbing. Marked reduction in the axial compressive strains in the femoral cortex were found in the calcar region compared with the distal strains medially.

Ryd L: Micromotion in knee arthroplasty: A roentgen stereophotogrammetric analysis of tibial component fixation. *Acta Orthop Scand* 1986;220(suppl):1–80.

Roentgen stereophotogrammetric analysis of migration of total knee replacement components was evaluated and found to have an accuracy ten times better than that of conventional radiography. Two types of micromotion of the tibial component were studied—migration, that is, gradual motion over time, and inducible displacement, that is, instant motion and response to external forces. Of the 96 knee replacements, which used four different types of fixation, 89 were clinically successful. Follow-up ranged from two to five years. Migration occurred in all prostheses, with a mean maximum deflection of approximately 1 mm after four years. The major part of the migration occurred during the first year, after which most components did not migrate further. All prostheses showed reversible inducible displacement, the maximum deflection ranging from 0.2 to 1.0 mm.

Zalenski E, Jasty M, O'Connor DO, et al: Micromotion of porous-surfaced, cementless prostheses following six months of in vivo bone ingrowth in a canine model. *Trans Orthop Res Soc* 1989;14:377.

An average axial micromotion of 11.7 μ was measured immediately after implantation of femoral stems in canine femurs. More motion was apparent in the rotational direction, with a mean bone-implant displacement of 24.2 μ. The micromotion of the prostheses after six months of bone ingrowth was less than the initial micromotion. The axial micromotion of the six-month implant was 3.4 u, with the rotational micromotion being 8.13 μ.

Retrieval Analysis

Caviglia HA, Sumner DR, Jacobs JJ, et al: A quantitative assessment of bone ingrowth in femoral THR components retrieved from human patients. *Trans Orthop Res Soc* 1989;14:580.

The histologic investigation of porous-coated femoral stems retrieved from human subjects included ten devices removed for reasons unrelated to fixation. In eight of these ten, bone ingrowth was found in at least 20% of the porous surface. The other two had bone ingrowth in at least 5% of the porous surface. The mean extent of bone ingrowth was 4.2% (range, 12.2% to 95.7%) and the volume fraction of bone ingrowth was 16.1% (range, 4.3% to 65.0%). The most bone ingrowth was observed in the medial porous surface, followed by the posterior and anterior surfaces at proximal middle and distal levels. Three of ten prostheses that had been in place for less than ten weeks displayed woven bone. Components in place for longer periods contained lamellar bone ingrowth.

Collier JP, Mayor MD, Chae JC, et al: Macroscopic and microscopic evidence of prosthetic fixation with porous-coated materials. *Clin Orthop* 1988;235:173–180.

A series of 162 uncemented porous-coated hip prostheses underwent detailed macroscopic and histologic examination. Twenty-eight of the 104 femoral hip components displayed some regions of bone ingrowth and 16% of the acetabular components showed evidence of bone in the pores of the coating. In no case was more than 50% of the surface of the cup ingrown by bone. Prostheses retrieved for pain showed a somewhat higher incidence of bone ingrowth (seven of 21) than those retrieved for all other reasons (21 of 85), indicating that bone ingrowth alone is not sufficient to guarantee relief from pain. In general, femoral components were more likely to display bone ingrowth along the lateral quadrant of their porous coating. The incidence of bone ingrowth of femoral components was nearly twice that of acetabular devices. The pore size, geometry, and porous-coating composition did not appear to influence the appearance of bone in fibrous tissue ingrowth.

Cook SD, Thomas KA, Haddad Jr RJ: Histologic analysis of retrieved human porous-coated total joint components. *Clin Orthop* 1988;234:90–101.

Sixty-two cementless total knee components and 28 cementless total hip prostheses retrieved from human subjects underwent histologic evaluation for the presence of bone ingrowth. In approximately one third of the components, no bone ingrowth or apposition was observed. No component had more than 10% of the available porous material ingrown with bone. In all components, the majority of the porous coating contained fibrous tissue that in some cases displayed an orientation indicating evidence of load-transmission capability. The presence and magnitude of bone ingrowth did not correlate with the degree of clinical pain relief or the radiographic appearance of the implant.

Goldring SR, Jasty M, Roelke M, et al: Biological factors that influence the development of a bone-cement membrane, in Fitzgerald R Jr (ed): *Non-Cemented Total Hip Arthroplasty.* New York, Raven Press, 1988.

Prostaglandin E_2 levels and bone resorbing activity of tissues surrounding loose and rigidly fixed total joint replacement components were determined. There was a significant elevation in prostaglandin E_2 levels of the pseudomembrane around the loose prostheses in comparison with the rigidly fixed components.

Goldring SR, Jasty M, Roelke MS, et al: Formation of a synovial-like membrane at the bone-like cement interface: Its role in bone resorption and implant loosening after total hip replacement. *Arthritis Rheum* 1986;29:836–842.

Histologic evaluation of tissue surrounding the loosened components after joint replacements revealed the presence of a lining resembling synovium adjacent to the cement. The tissue was heavily infiltrated with particulate cement as well as polyethylene associated with a foreign body-type giant cell reaction. That this tissue response may be responsible for the bone lysis associated with loosening was suggested by the demonstration of high prostaglandin E_2 levels and enhanced bone-resorbing activity in the tissue-culture medium of fragments from this membrane.

Sumner DR, Jasty M, Turner TM, et al: Bone ingrowth in porous-coated cementless acetabular components retrieved from human patients. *Trans Orthop Res Soc* 1987;12:509.

Nineteen cementless acetabular cups, removed for reasons other than loosening, underwent histologic investigation for bone ingrowth. Implants that had been in place for less than two months contained thin trabeculae and some haversian systems. At later times, mature trabeculae and haversian bone were observed. The ingrown bone occasionally penetrated the entire depth of the coating and in some regions nearly 100% of the available pore space was filled by bone. Bone ingrowth seemed to occur preferentially in the vicinity of some of the screw holes. The area of the fiber-metal pad occupied by bone ingrowth varied from 0% to 80%. Some bone ingrowth was found in 17 of 18 cases in which the implant had been in place for more than one week.

Sumner DR, Jacobs JJ, Turner TM, et al: Quantitative study of bone ingrowth in tibial components retrieved from human subjects. Presented at the 15th Annual Meeting of the Society for Biomaterials, Lake Buena Vista, Florida, 1989.

Fifteen noncemented porous-coated tibial components of one design were retrieved from human subjects for histologic evaluation of bone ingrowth. The mean extent of bone ingrowth (that is, the percentage of surface area of porous coating ingrown with bone) was 25.1% with a range of 2.9% to 44.1%. There was more bone anteriorly than posteriorly (32% vs 16%) but no difference in the mediolateral distribution of bone ingrowth. In eight of these components all four fixation pegs had bone ingrowth; in the remaining two components, three of the four pegs had bone ingrowth.

16
Microsurgery

In the 1980s microsurgery matured as an independent discipline. Microsurgery is now practiced at most surgical centers as well as at many community-based hospitals.

Although the techniques of nerve and vascular repair have changed little in the past decade, basic research has significantly improved our knowledge of both neural and vascular pathophysiology. The old controversy about "epineurial vs perineurial suture" has been replaced by a more general debate over the roles of mechanical and humoral factors in the control of peripheral nerve regeneration. Similarly, the pathophysiology of vascular injury and repair is better understood and can now be manipulated pharmacologically. As the "discovery" phase of free tissue transfer winds down, emphasis has shifted from the description of new donor sites to reevaluation and refinement of those already in use; in many instances this has involved "upgrading" a flap from composite to fasciocutaneous, or from fasciocutaneous to fascial. The clinical applications of free tissue transfer have also evolved substantially. An accelerated timetable for reconstruction after major trauma has significantly reduced morbidity. Burn resurfacing and limb salvage are now possible in carefully selected patients not previously thought to be candidates for microsurgery.

Peripheral Nerve

Recent efforts to improve the results of end-to-end nerve repair have focused on fascicular matching. Electrical or histochemical techniques are used to identify and selectively reunite sensory or motor fascicles in proximal and distal stumps. The most significant clinical findings are in patients who have undergone electrical fascicular identification. Light general anesthesia or Bier block anesthesia is used for initial dissection and exposure of nerve ends. The anesthetic is then terminated, and fascicles of the proximal stump are individually stimulated. Sensory fascicles are identified and mapped by the anatomic area in which the patient reports sensation; motor fascicles are identified by the lack of sensory response. General anesthesia is then induced. In acute cases, the motor fascicles in the distal stump are identified by stimulation and observation of muscle contraction. If the lesion is chronic, distal motor fascicles can be identified only by retrograde dissection from peripheral motor branches. In a series of 18 patients treated with this technique, six of seven undergoing ulnar nerve suture regained 80% of their intrinsic motor power, and seven of 11 undergoing median nerve suture regained 75% of opposition strength. The results of this small series were sufficiently promising to warrant further investigation.

Histochemical detection of the enzyme acetylcholinesterase is a well-established technique for identification of motor fascicles. Full-thickness biopsy specimens are re-moved from proximal and distal stumps, immersed in fixative, and sectioned transversely. These sections are then reacted to demonstrate acetylcholinesterase within myelinated motor axons. However, long reaction times mandate two operations: the first for biopsy, and the second, a day later, for nerve repair. This cumbersome procedure is rarely used. Recently developed histochemical procedures permit more rapid fascicular identification, and thus have potential clinical application. Modifications of the acetylcholinesterase technique omit tissue fixation (reaction is done on frozen sections) and require only one hour. Other enzymes have also been found to differentiate sensory from motor axons. Among these is carbonic anhydrase, found principally in myelinated sensory axons. It can be detected on rapidly fixed tissue sections in 90 minutes. Clinical trials of both techniques must be undertaken before they can be recommended for routine use.

The nerve gap is currently managed by joining proximal and distal stumps with autologous nerve grafts. Alternative experimental techniques include using tissue expanders to eliminate the gap, providing nerve grafts with an immediate vascular supply, or bridging the gap with an empty tube or basement membrane scaffold. In one recent report, tissue expansion was used to overcome a 3.5-cm median nerve gap. Conduction was not disturbed when expander pressure was less than 40 mm Hg. Wire markers placed in the epineurium showed significant creep of proximal nerve onto the expander. Immediate microsurgical graft revascularization, discussed in *Orthopaedic Knowledge Update 2*, has potential advantages over routine grafting, but its clinical superiority has not been demonstrated.

Mechanical and humoral influences on axon regeneration have yet to be modified in such a way as to improve the results of end-to-end clinical nerve repair. However, both have been used in efforts to overcome nerve gaps. In one study of primates, tropic (directional) and/or trophic (nutritive) influences from the distal stump guided regenerating axons across the gap. Axons within the distal stump were reduced in caliber and conduction velocity and amplitude after grafting. Mechanical guidance of regenerating axons was used to bridge digital nerve gaps in a small clinical series. Sensation was regained in seven of eight cases. A trial of grafting larger mixed nerves is underway and should more clearly define indications for this technique.

Microvascular Surgery

Experimental Techniques

Three new techniques of microvascular repair have recently undergone experimental trials (Table 1). A mechanical coupling device (Fig. 1) achieves anastomosis by plac-

Table 1. Experimental microsurgical techniques

Technique	Advantages	Disadvantages
Mechanical coupling device	Rapid (3 to 5 min); 98% patency; continuous endothelial contact; easily matches different vessel diameters	Requires excess vessel length; medial atrophy at repair site; permanent implant around vessel
Thermic sleeve	Rapid (30 to 60 sec, after intussusception); simple, no special equipment needed; 100% arterial patency	Initial stenosis at ends of overlap; requires excess vessel length; 78% venous patency
Carbon dioxide laser	Rapid endothelialization; 95% arterial patency	Initially fragile repair; 10% false aneurysm rate; expensive; saves little time

ing proximal and distal vessel ends through separate rings, everting the vessel ends by impaling them on small pins on the anastomotic surface of the ring, and then joining the rings together. The thermic sleeve technique involves intussusception of the proximal stump into the distal stump and "spot welding" the edges of the distal stump to the sides of the proximal stump with a bipolar cautery. In the laser-assisted repair technique, three stay sutures are placed in the artery and the intervening spaces are spot welded with the carbon dioxide laser. None of these techniques is in widespread clinical use. The thermic sleeve technique is easy and cost-effective but constricts the luminal area. The mechanical coupling device may have clinical applications, especially if resorbable ring pins can be fabricated. The carbon dioxide laser technique is costly and offers few advantages over conventional sutures.

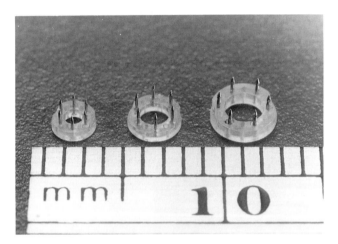
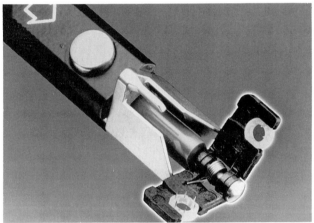
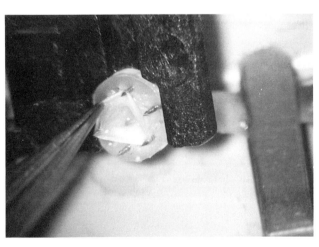
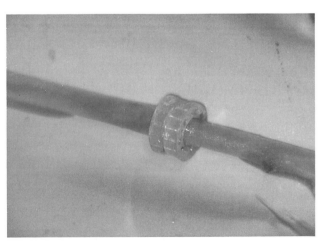

Figure 1

The mechanical coupling device. **Top left,** Anastomatic rings. Pins for vessel fixation alternate with holes that accept the pins on the opposing ring. Luminal diameters of 1, 1.5, and 2 mm are available. **Top right,** The rings are premounted on two spring-loaded "wings," which are held open by a reusable applicator. **Bottom left,** The end of the vessel is pulled through one of the rings with jewelers' forceps. The wall of the vessel is then everted 90 degrees and hooked onto the ring pins. **Bottom right,** When both ends of the vessel are mounted, the ring-holding wings are brought together to join the two rings and the completed anastomosis is ejected automatically.

Pharmacologic Manipulation

In further experimental work, patency of arterial repair was improved by pharmacologic manipulation of vasospasm and thrombosis. Control arterial repairs performed in a rat-tail model of epinephrine-induced vasospasm had a patency rate of only 45%. Topical application of 20% lidocaine, which acts on the membrane of both nerve and smooth muscle, improved patency to 60%; topical thorazine, which blocks formation of the calcium-calmodulin complex, inhibiting muscle contraction, improved patency to 95%. Although only thorazine produced a statistically significant difference in this study, both agents were more effective than 2% lidocaine in preliminary clinical trials. Similarly dramatic results were obtained with systemic heparin treatment in a thrombogenic model. Control arterial patency one week after inversion grafting of rabbit femoral arteries (turning the grafted arterial segment inside out) was only 19%. A 72% heparin infusion improved patency to 67%. Heparin, which in microsurgery is now used principally to "salvage" impending failures, may thus have a wider role in maintaining arterial patency. However, both topical and systemic techniques of thrombosis prophylaxis must be tested in controlled clinical trials before they are recommended for general use.

In extreme clinical situations, a free tissue transfer may be salvaged with streptokinase. This enzyme converts plasminogen to plasmin, which degrades fibrin clots as well as fibrinogen and other proteins. In recently reported cases, streptokinase was infused directly into free latissimus dorsi and fibular transfers after repeated clotting of arterial and venous anastomoses, respectively. This technique should only be used as a last resort because of the potentially severe complications of hypersensitivity reaction, fever, and hemorrhage.

Digital Ischemia

Digital ischemia requires a thorough history, physical examination, and laboratory evaluation to identify underlying vascular disease, connective tissue or clotting disorders, or proximal embolic sources. Conservative treatment involves cessation of smoking, job modification to avoid exposure to cold or vibration, and pharmacologic manipulation with vasodilators, ganglionic blocking agents, calcium channel blockers, or steroids when appropriate. If conservative treatment fails, pulse volume recordings should be obtained. Cold stress by immersion in water at 12 C normally produces a transient decrease in digital perfusion, with a return to normal within five minutes (Fig. 2). Patients who do not return to normal within this time (Fig. 3) should have the test repeated after lidocaine digital block, which produces a pharmacologic digital sympathectomy. Those in whom digital perfusion is significantly improved (Fig. 4) are candidates for surgical digital sympathectomy. In this procedure the neurovascular bundles are exposed from the distal palm to the proximal interphalangeal joint, the digital nerve branches to the artery (usually four) are removed, and the adventitia is stripped from the artery. Results are best in young patients with vasculitis or primary vasospastic disease, and worst in those with connective tissue disorders such as scleroderma.

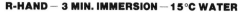

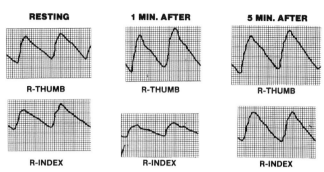

Figure 2

Pulse volume recordings from the thumb and index fingers show the normal response to cold stress and recovery. (Reproduced with permission from Wilgis EFS: Digital sympathectomy for vascular insufficiency. *Hand Clin* 1985;1:361–367.)

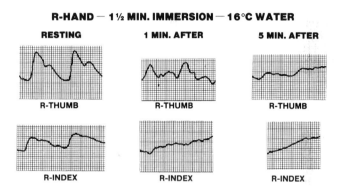

Figure 3

These pulse volume recordings demonstrate an abnormal response to cold stress, with poor recovery of waveforms. (Reproduced with permission from Wilgis EFS: Digital sympathectomy for vascular insufficiency. *Hand Clin* 1985;1:361–367.)

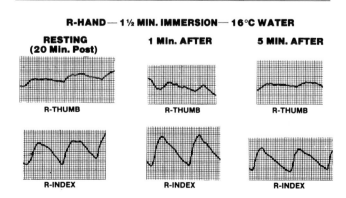

Figure 4

In this patient with vasospastic disease, the pulse volume recordings shows the effect of a 2% lidocaine block on the response to cold stress. There is no adverse response in the blocked index finger but the response in the unblocked thumb continues to be poor. (Reproduced with permission from Wilgis EFS: Digital sympathectomy for vascular insufficiency. *Hand Clin* 1985;1:361–367.)

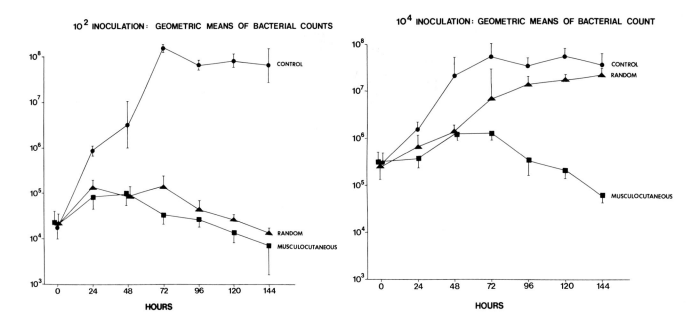

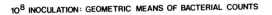

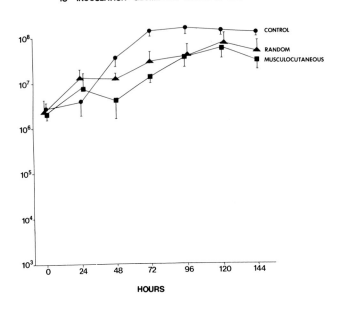

Figure 5

Mean bacterial counts after closure in minimally contaminated **(top left)**, moderately contaminated **(top right)**, and heavily contaminated **(bottom)** wounds. Minimally contaminated wounds were successfully treated with either random-pattern cutaneous or myocutaneous flaps, whereas only myocutaneous flaps were successful in moderately contaminated wounds. The random-pattern cutaneous flaps failed to control bacterial proliferation and the flaps were lost. Neither type of flap was successful in heavily contaminated wounds. (Reproduced with permission from Murphy RC, Robson MC, Heggers JP, et al: The effect of microbial contamination on musculocutaneous and random flaps. *J Surg Res* 1986;41:75–80.)

Free Tissue Transfer

Physiology

Recent experimental work has clarified the role of muscle flaps in infection control and bone revascularization. Related investigations of the vascular response to tissue expansion have led to the free microvascular transfer of expanded tissue. Muscle flaps have been used increasingly to provide coverage of contaminated wounds that could not

be covered with traditional, random-pattern flaps. Bacterial proliferation, potentiated by a marginal blood supply, has been shown to play a major role in cutaneous flap necrosis. Previous research has shown that myocutaneous flaps provide both greater oxygen tension to distal portions of the flap and increased resistance to direct bacterial innoculation than do cutaneous flaps. Myocutaneous flaps also decrease bacterial counts.

In one recent study, rats were given 10% full-thickness

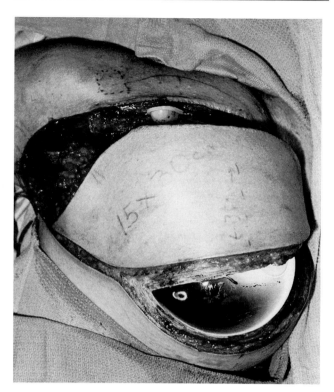

Figure 7

The partially elevated scapular flap, measuring 15 × 30 cm, showing
the expander (inferior flap margin) and the filler valve (superior
margin) still in place. (Reproduced with permission from Leighton
WD, Russell RC, Feller AM, et al: Experimental pretransfer expansion
of free-flap donor sites: II. Physiology, histology, and clinical
correlation. *Plast Reconstr Surg* 1988;82:76–87.)

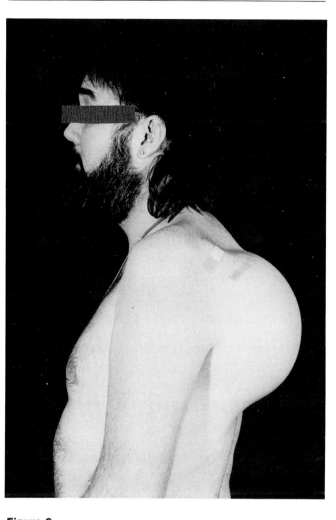

Figure 6

Tissue expander enlarged with 1,565 ml of normal saline beneath a
left scapular fasciocutaneous flap. (Reproduced with permission from
Leighton WD, Russell RC, Feller AM, et al: Experimental pretransfer
expansion of free-flap donor sites: II. Physiology, histology, and
clinical correlation. *Plast Reconstr Surg* 1988;82:76–87.)

scald burns that were inoculated with varying concentrations of *Pseudomonas aeruginosa*. Five days later the
wounds were covered with flaps (either random-pattern
cutaneous flaps or myocutaneous flaps) or left uncovered
(controls). All wounds with minimal contamination (10^4
organisms per gram) at the time of flap coverage healed.
Bacterial counts 120 hours after coverage with both cutaneous and myocutaneous flaps were significantly less
than those in controls (Fig. 5, *top left*). With moderate
contamination (10^5/g), bacterial counts at 120 hours were
significantly less in myocutaneous flaps than they were in
controls or cutaneous flaps (Fig. 5, *top right*); these wounds
healed, whereas the others dehisced. After heavy contamination (10^6/g) neither flap prevented bacterial proliferation and flap loss (Fig. 5, *bottom*).

It is not known whether the blood supply and infection
resistance of myocutaneous flaps, which are superior to
those of other flaps, can specifically benefit the process of
bone healing in the treatment of osteomyelitis. One of the
first steps in this process is bone revascularization. A recent
experimental study measured differences between revas-

cularization by muscle and skin. Isolated bone segments
were placed beneath pig myocutaneous or cutaneous flaps.
Four weeks later, measurable blood flow was found in ten
of 11 bone segments covered with muscle but in only three
of 17 covered with skin. Blood flow was increased in both
myocutaneous and cutaneous flaps, suggesting that factors
other than blood flow alone may have been responsible for
the significant difference between the two experimental
groups. However, the experiments do suggest that the beneficial role of muscle coverage in chronic osteomyelitis may
reflect promotion of bony healing in addition to control of
bacterial flora.

Tissue vascularity also plays a significant role in the free
transfer of previously expanded flaps. An experimental
study analyzed changes in the vascularity and histologic
characteristics of expanded pig buttock (cutaneous) and
latissimus dorsi (myocutaneous) free flaps. Arterial inflow
to both flaps was significantly greater than that of control,
unexpanded flaps. Angiography demonstrated proliferation of blood vessels within all expanded flaps. In addition,
expanded cutaneous flaps were characterized by neovascular branches originating in the pedicle and spreading to
enter the base of the flap. Histologically, there was thinning
of all soft-tissue layers beneath the skin, with mild dermal
thinning and no changes in the epidermis. These findings
were then applied to a clinical case (Figs. 6 and 7). A fasciocutaneous scapular flap was expanded and successfully
transferred to cover an anterior tibial defect. This new tech-

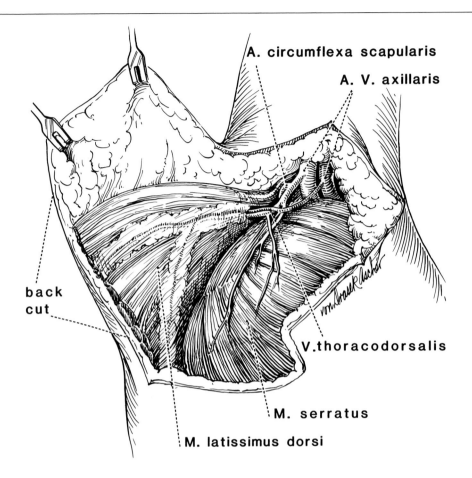

A. circumflexa scapularis

A. V. axillaris

back cut

V. thoracodorsalis

M. serratus

M. latissimus dorsi

Figure 8

Dissection of the tailored latissimus dorsi flap. Once the distal margin of the flap has been reached (as marked on the skin), a back-cut is made across the skin and muscle, permitting the muscle to be displaced posteromedially to expose the vessels of the axilla and the branches of the thoracodorsal artery and vein. (Reproduced with permission from Godina M: Early microsurgical reconstruction of complex trauma of the extremities. *Plast Reconstr Surg* 1986;78:285–292.)

nique has significant potential for modifying the size and thickness of known flaps and may also facilitate the primary closure of donor sites.

Timing of Reconstruction

When free tissue transfers are available, early radical debridement is now possible even in the largest wounds. This combined technique has decreased rates of infection and improved bone healing without increasing flap mortality. There are several advantages to obtaining wound closure within 72 hours of injury. Vessels adjacent to the wound have not yet become fibrotic, there is no granulation tissue with attendant superficial infection, and desiccation and progressive necrosis of exposed bone and tendon have not yet occurred. Further, the surgeon need not deal with poorly perfused scar, colonized or infected areas of infected tissue, or pockets within the wound. The technique of wound care includes early skeletal fixation, using external fixators if necessary. Debridement in a bloodless field under tourniquet control avoids blood loss and allows better visualization of questionable tissue. The tourniquet is then released and remaining tissues are examined for viability. Partially traumatized nerve and vessels with blood flow are preserved. When free tissue transfer is performed, an end-to-side approach to undamaged vessels is preferred.

A series of 134 patients with severe trauma to an extremity underwent free flap coverage within 72 hours of injury. Flap failure occurred in 0.75% and infection in 1.5%. These results were significantly better than those obtained by the same surgeon in other patients who underwent coverage more than 72 hours after injury. In another series, 22 consecutive patients underwent sequential debridement before their wounds were covered (average time to coverage was 17 days). Flap failure occurred in 9% and infection in 14%, results far better than the expected 50% incidence of flap loss and infection.

Expanded Indications

Increasing confidence in free tissue transfer has resulted in exploration of applications previously thought to be beyond the scope of microsurgery. Recent clinical series have evaluated the role of free tissue transfer in the coverage of fourth-degree burns and in the salvage of limbs with severe peripheral vascular disease.

Burns Single-stage debridement and reconstruction of limited areas of fourth-degree burns permit early wound closure, early return to mobility, decreased hospitalization time, and possible salvage of limbs that might otherwise be lost. A series of 70 free tissue transfers was performed

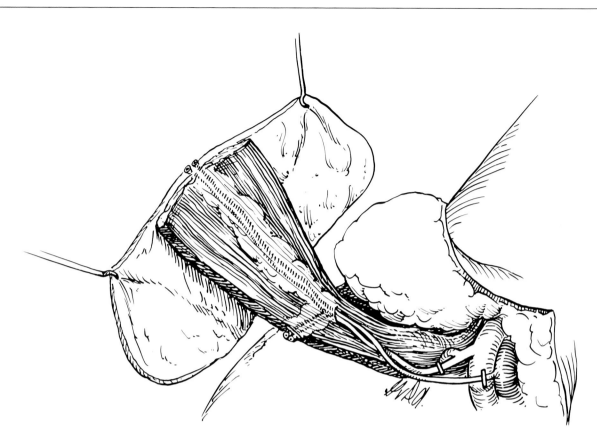

Figure 9

The proximal incision through the skin is made, and the thoracodorsal artery is dissected off the muscle as far distally as possible. At this point, the muscle is again transected, leaving the bulky portion near the insertion in the donor site. (Reproduced with permission from Godina M: Early microsurgical reconstruction of complex trauma of the extremities. *Plast Reconstr Surg* 1986;78:285–292.)

in patients with total burn areas of 1% to 15% of the body surface (mean, 3.2%). Flap survival was 100% when healed wounds were reconstructed, but only 80% when recent burns were treated. Great care must be taken in planning free flap coverage of recent burns. Preoperative angiography should be considered if there is any question of damage to recipient vessels. Recipient vessels must be well beyond the margins of burn; in recent electrical burns, however, it may be impossible to determine these margins.

Peripheral Vascular Disease Severe peripheral vascular disease has traditionally precluded the use of free tissue transfer for lower extremity salvage, reflecting the misconception that diabetic foot problems are caused by small-vessel disease. In a recent clinical series, ten microsurgical free tissue transfers were performed in diabetics with severe peripheral vascular disease; indications were osteomyelitis in two cases and neurotrophic ulcers in eight cases. Endarterectomy was performed on the recipient artery at the time of surgery and flaps were taken from the upper trunk to minimize atherosclerosis within the donor vessels. In this series there were no anastomotic flap failures, but one leg was amputated because of sepsis. In carefully selected patients, free tissue transfer may thus permit limb salvage in diabetic patients with severe peripheral vascular disease. This technique may be especially useful in a patient whose other leg has already been amputated.

Individual Flaps

Recent emphasis has been on the refinement of known donor sites rather than on the creation of new ones. Anatomic knowledge of donor areas has been improved, with the focus on the vascular relationships between skin and underlying fascia. Techniques of flap elevation and donor site closure have been stressed.

Latissimus Dorsi Flap The latissimus dorsi free flap is the mainstay of reconstructive microsurgery. Its desirable qualities include a large, reliable pedicle, an acceptable donor site, and the large volume of tissue available for transfer. Because transfer of excessive bulk may lead to poor contour, a limited portion of the muscle with overlying skin should be used (Figs. 8 and 9). Properly done, this produces a flap of precisely tailored volume with a long pedicle, minimizing the need for a vein graft.

Fibular Bone Graft The free vascularized fibular bone graft can also be tailored to produce two parallel struts, increasing the potential usefulness of this valuable reconstructive tool (Fig. 10). The proximal strut maintains both the periosteal and the endosteal blood supply, while the distal strut survives on the periosteal blood supply alone. This technique has been applied successfully in three patients with segmental defects of the distal femur and in one with adjacent defects in the radius and ulna.

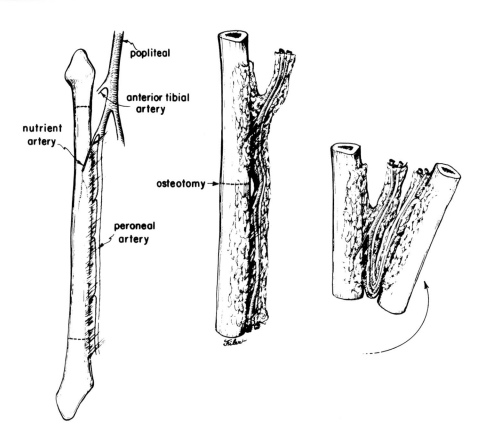

Figure 10

The blood supply to the fibular shift is provided by the peroneal artery (**left**). A lateral osteotomy, performed distal to the entry of the nutrient artery, preserves a cuff of muscle that contains the artery (**center**). The two segments of bone can then be doubled up, preserving the periosteal blood supply to the distal segment (**right**).

Temporoparietal Flap The temporoparietal free flap is ideal when a skin graft is preferable to a bulky flap but the recipient bed is not adequate for skin grafting. The flap, described as a microvascular transfer of a recipient bed, is based on the superficial temporal artery. It can be skin grafted on either side, and it may retain the gliding function of the donor site. This characteristic may prove to be useful for tendon coverage. The flap can also be tailored along vessel arborizations to conform to irregular surfaces. The donor site lies within the hair-bearing area and is usually inconspicuous. Overall, this is an ideal flap for covering limited areas, particularly when gliding function is desired. However, damage to the adjacent facial nerve is a potentially disastrous consequence.

Dorsalis Pedis Flap The dorsalis pedis artery free flap has had limited clinical acceptance, largely because of donor site complications and the perception that its vascular supply is unreliable. Several studies found that the connection between the dorsalis pedis and first dorsal metatarsal arteries was lacking, making the flap unsuitable for transfer, in 10% to 20% of cases. However, recently described techniques of flap evaluation and donor site closure have minimized both vascular and donor site problems. The flap is based on the vascular axis of the dorsalis pedis and the first dorsal metatarsal. Significant wound problems oc-

curred only when bone was taken with the flap. Others, however, have reported that the vascular anatomy may preclude raising the flap. The dorsalis pedis artery may not communicate with the first dorsal metatarsal artery or may not even exist. A thorough preoperative vascular examination is therefore mandatory.

Back Tissue Flaps The tissues of the upper back provide a variety of overlapping free tissue donor sites. Recent studies of the blood supply to the dorsal thoracic fascia have led to the clinical use of the fascia, both as a fascial free flap and as an extension of myocutaneous flaps. The circumflex scapular artery was found to lie within the dorsal thoracic fascia rather than within the subcutaneous tissue. Scapular and parascapular flaps are, therefore, fasciocutaneous flaps, and the dorsal thoracic fascia itself can be transferred as a free flap. The circumflex scapular artery was also found to communicate with myocutaneous perforators of the trapezius and latissimus dorsi. Thus, dorsal thoracic fascia can also be used to extend the myocutaneous latissimus dorsi flap.

Trends

The microsurgical landscape of the human body has been well described in more than two decades of anatomic exploration. Further progress in microsurgery is thus likely to reflect the development of techniques and the physiologic manipulation of basic processes to enhance nerve regeneration, improve patency of vascular repair, reduce ischemic tissue damage, and even create new tissues for microsurgical transfer. Techniques of fascicular identification and matching may find clinical use in the treatment of acute, sharp nerve divisions without tissue loss. However, many nerve injuries are complicated by tissue loss and thus are not candidates for this approach. To improve results in these cases, the ability of regenerating axons to make appropriate distal connections must be enhanced. Initial experiments suggest that electrical stimulation of axon regeneration may serve this function, as well as speeding axon regeneration. An ingenious alternative currently being tested involves placement of a porous microchip at the repair site to redirect impulses from the proximal stump to appropriate axons in the distal stump.

In microvascular surgery, the quest for a simple, rapid, reliable technique of vascular repair is still in its infancy. Improvements in the mechanical coupling device, with absorbable rings for smaller vessels, may help in the evolution of such a technique. Physiologic manipulation of microsurgical results should become increasingly possible as our knowledge of microvascular physiology improves. Research within related disciplines on thrombolysis and tissue preservation should be particularly helpful. Tissue plasminogen activator, currently used to reduce coronary thrombosis, might also be useful in protecting microvascular repairs. Similarly, free radical scavengers, used to minimize ischemic tissue damage, could have a similar role in replantation and free tissue transfer. Advances may even come from novel applications of existing technology. The capsule that forms around a tissue expander beneath an axial flap is well vascularized and could perhaps be transferred as a free flap based on the axial vessels. Free flaps could thus be tailored for specific applications without sacrificing important donor tissues.

Annotated Bibliography

Keywords

Bone graft; Burns; Cutaneous flap; Grafting; Myocutaneous flap; Peripheral nerve; Peripheral vascular disease

Peripheral Nerve

Carson KA, Terzis JK: Carbonic anhydrase histochemistry: A potential diagnostic method for peripheral nerve repair. *Clin Plast Surg* 1985;12:227–232.
Carbonic anhydrase is an enzyme found predominantly within the sensory axons of peripheral nerve. A technique is presented for rapid demonstration of the enzyme to aid fascicular matching in clinical nerve repair.

Dellon AL, Mackinnon SE: An alternative to the classical nerve graft for the management of the short nerve gap. *Plast Reconstr Surg* 1988;82:849–856.
Primate ulnar nerve axons regenerated across a 3-cm gap enclosed within a polyglycolic acid tube. Mean fiber diameters and axonal conduction velocities and amplitudes were reduced after both tube and sural nerve graft techniques.

Gaul JS: Electrical fascicle identification as an adjunct to nerve repair. *Hand Clin* 1986;2:709–722.
Median and ulnar nerve fascicles were identified and matched by electrical stimulation in awake patients. In a series of 18 patients treated with this technique, six of seven undergoing ulnar nerve suture regained 80% of their intrinsic motor power, while seven of 11 undergoing median nerve suture regained 75% of opposition strength.

Manders EK, Saggers GC, Diaz-Alonso P, et al: Elongation of peripheral nerve and viscera containing smooth muscle. *Clin Plast Surg* 1987;14:551–562.
A tissue expander was used beneath the proximal stump of an injured median nerve to overcome a 3.5-cm gap.

Norris RW, Glasby MA, Gattuso JM, et al: Peripheral nerve repair in humans using muscle autografts: A new technique. *J Bone Joint Surg* 1988;70B:530–533.
Digital nerve gaps of 1.5 to 2.5 mm were bridged with autologous muscle basement membrane in eight patients. Seven regained sensibility to MRC grade 3+, although sensory examinations were performed without blocking the uninjured digital nerve.

Yunshao H, Shizhen Z: Acetylcholinesterase: A histochemical identification of motor and sensory fascicles in human peripheral nerve and its use during operation. *Plast Reconstr Surg* 1988;82:125–132.
A rapid modification of the Karnovsky and Roots method of demonstrating acetylcholinesterase is described. This technique can now be used for clinical fascicular identification in a single surgical procedure.

Microvascular Surgery

Experimental Techniques

Berggren A, Ostrup LT, Lidman D: Mechanical anastomosis of small arteries and veins with the unilink apparatus: A histologic and scanning electron microscopic study. *Plast Reconstr Surg* 1987;80:274–283.
The unilink apparatus is a miniaturized version of the ring pin instrument devices by Nakayama. A 98% patency rate was obtained for rabbit arteries and veins with a ring measuring 1.5 mm in diameter.

Duarte A, Valauri FA, Buncke HJ: Microvascular thermic sleeve anastomosis: A sutureless technique. *J Reconstr Microsurg* 1987;4:53–60.
This rapid technique of microvascular anastomosis combines intussusception of the proximal stump within the distal stump and "spot welding" the two together with biopolar cautery. Patency rates were 100% for arteries and 78% for veins.

Travers V, Kanaujia RR, Ochi M, et al: Microvascular anastomosis using carbon dioxide (CO_2) laser: Evaluation by SEM after corrosion cast. *J Reconstr Microsurg* 1987;4:61–67.
An arterial patency rate of 95% was obtained by placing

three stay sutures in the rat femoral artery and sealing the opposed ends with a carbon dioxide laser.

Pharmacologic Stimulation

Geter RK, Winters RR, Puckett CL: Resolution of experimental microvascular spasm and improvement in anastomotic patency by direct topical agent application. *Plast Reconstr Surg* 1986;77:105–115.

Impairment of experimental anastomotic patency by epinephrine-induced vasospasm is minimized by topical application of thorazine.

Greenberg BM, Masem M, May JW Jr: Therapeutic value of intravenous heparin in microvascular surgery: An experimental vascular thrombosis study. *Plast Reconstr Surg* 1988;82:463–472.

Prophylactic heparin infusion significantly diminished the incidence of thrombosis in an arterial inversion graft model. Scanning electron microscopy showed fewer aggregate platelets and less fibrin deposition in the heparin-treated grafts.

Lipton HA, Jupiter JB: Streptokinase salvage of a free-tissue transfer: Case report and review of the literature. *Plast Reconstr Surg* 1987;79:977–981.

A composite transfer of fibula, peroneal and soleus muscle, and skin to the forearm was jeopardized by repeated venous thromboses beginning 40 hours after the transfer. Streptokinase (10,000 units) infusion through the arterial system of the flap every ten minutes for one hour restored and maintained good blood flow.

Digital Ischemia

Wilgis EFS: Digital sympathectomy for vascular insufficiency. *Hand Clin* 1985;1:361–367.

Patients with digital ischemia who do not respond to conservative treatment are given a cold stress test. Those showing a vasospastic response to cold that is significantly diminished by lidocaine digital block are candidates for surgical digital sympathectomy.

Free Tissue Transfer

Physiology

Fisher J, Wood MB: Experimental comparison of bone revascularization by musculocutaneous and cutaneous flaps. *Plast Reconstr Surg* 1987;79:81–90.

A radioactive microsphere technique was used to demonstrate that isolated bone segments had significant blood flow four weeks after coverage with a muscle flap but not after coverage with a cutaneous flap.

Leighton WD, Russell RC, Feller AM, et al: Experimental pretransfer expansion of free-flap donor sites: II. Physiology, histology, and clinical correlation. *Plast Reconstr Surg* 1988;82:76–87.

Expansion of cutaneous and myocutaneous flaps in the pig resulted in neovascular proliferation and increased axial blood flow to the flaps. All tissues beneath the skin were thinned, with changes most prominent over the center of the expander. A successful clinical transfer of an expanded flap is presented.

Murphy RC, Robson MC, Heggers JP, et al: The effect of microbial contamination on musculocutaneous and random flaps. *J Surg Res* 1986;41:75–80.

In the moderately contaminated wound (10^5 bacteria per gram of tissue) myocutaneous flaps can decrease bacterial counts and obtain wound closure when random cutaneous flaps cannot.

Timing of Reconstruction

Godina M: Early microsurgical reconstruction of complex trauma of the extremities. *Plast Reconstr Surg* 1986;78:285–292.

Free flap coverage of extremity wounds within 72 hours resulted in decreased flap failure and infection rates and diminished bone healing times when compared with cases in which coverage was obtained after 72 hours. Radical debridement of devitalized tissues is the essential part of this techique.

Yaremchuk MJ, Brumback RJ, Manson PN, et al: Acute and definitive management of traumatic osteocutaneous defects of the lower extremity. *Plast Reconstr Surg* 1987;80:1–14.

Twenty-two consecutive high-energy lower extremity injuries (Gustilo type IIIb) were serially debrided and covered by predominately free tissue transfer an average of 17 days after injury. The early infection rate was 14%, there were no long-term infections, and only two flaps were lost.

Expanded Indications

Colen LB: Limb salvage in the patient with severe peripheral vascular disease: The role of microsurgical free-tissue transfer. *Plast Reconstr Surg* 1987;79:389–395.

Microsurgical free tissue transfer may allow limb salvage in carefully selected diabetics with peripheral vascular disease. The technique is particularly valuable in patients who have undergone amputation of the other leg.

Shen TY, Sun YH, Cao DX, et al: The use of free flaps in burn patients: Experiences with 70 flaps in 65 patients. *Plast Reconstr Surg* 1988;81:352–357.

Fourth-degree burn wounds of limited size can be successfully covered with microvascular free tissue transfers. Extreme caution should be exercised in attempting to cover electrical burns in which the recipient vessels may be damaged over considerable distances.

Individual Flaps

Brent B, Upton J, Acland RD, et al: Experience with the temporoparietal fascial free flap. *Plast Reconstr Surg* 1985;76:177–188.

The temporoparietal fascial free flap is an ideal source of ultrathin tissue coverage with minimal donor site morbidity.
Godina M: The tailored latissimus dorsi free flap. *Plast Reconstr Surg* 1987;80:304–306.

A technique of tailored, partial transfer of the latissimus dorsi muscle permits exact matching of flap and recipient site, eliminating the excess bulk often seen with this flap.

Jones NF, Swartz WM, Mears DC, et al: The "double barrel" free vascularized fibular bone graft. *Plast Reconstr Surg* 1988;81:378–385.

The fibular shaft is bisected transversely, preserving the peroneal blood supply to the distal half. This creates two vascularized struts that can be placed parallel to one another to provide increased mechanical stability.

Kim PS, Gottlieb JR, Harris GD, et al: The dorsal thoracic fascia: Anatomic significance with clinical applications in reconstructive microsurgery. *Plast Reconstr Surg* 1987;79:72–80.

The circumflex scapular artery lies within the dorsal thoracic fascia and communicates with the myocutaneous perforators of the latissimus dorsi. The dorsal thoracic fascia can be transferred as a free flap or used to extend the latissimus dorsi myocutaneous flap.

Lister G, Scheker L: Emergency free flaps to the upper extremity. *J Hand Surg* 1988;13A:22–28.

Thirty-one emergency free flaps were applied to the upper exremities with a 93.5% success rate and only one infecion. Patients in whom radical debridement would destroy a chance of meaningful function are not candidates for this approach.

Petry JJ, French TS, Wortham KA: The effect of the "patency test" on arterial endothelial surface. *Plast Reconstr Surg* 1986;77:960–964.

The "milking patency test" produces significant endothelial damage and should be avoided.

Zuker RM, Manktelow RT: The dorsalis pedis free flap: Technique of elevation, foot closure, and flap application. *Plast Reconstr Surg* 1986;77:93–104.

The dorsalis pedis free flap has had limited acceptance because of its unreliable vascularity and frequent donor site morbidity. The authors describe meticulous techniques of flap elevation and foot closure that have resulted in 45 successful dorsalis pedis transfers.

17
Pain

During the last two decades there have been rapid and dramatic advances in our understanding of the neuroanatomy and neuropharmacology of the pain sensory system. This has been translated into practical benefits for the care of acute postoperative pain as well as the more chronic painful afflictions.

Definitions

The International Association for the Study of Pain defines pain as "an unpleasant sensory and emotional experience associated with actual or potential tissue damage, or described in terms of such damage." At its most basic level, pain is both a physical phenomenon (presence of discrete neural pathways) and a psychological or emotional experience ("It hurts."). Teleologically, pain serves the useful function of prevention of tissue damage. Pain is actually a homeostatic mechanism. It is only in the postoperative setting or when pain becomes chronic that it serves no useful function.

"Acute" pain implies the presence of actual tissue damage or the potential for tissue damage unless the noxious stimulus is removed. Acute pain also signifies the presence of an intact, properly functioning nervous system. There is autonomic hyperactivity—hypertension, tachycardia, sweating and vasoconstriction, and the like. The pain is only temporary.

"Chronic" pain implies the absence of a threat of tissue damage. Yet, the patient describes sensations in terms of acute damage ("pain" and "suffering"). There is no autonomic hyperactivity. The normal transmission pathways become altered or develop spontaneous activity. Pain becomes chronic when it persists or progresses beyond three or, for some investigators, six months.

Neural Pathways for Pain Sensation

The Pain Sensory System

Between the site of tissue damage and the perception of pain is a series of complex electrochemical events. Four physiologic processes are involved: transduction, transmission, modulation, and perception (Fig. 1).

Transduction is the process whereby noxious stimuli cause electrical activity at sensory nerve endings. Transmission refers to the propagation of impulses throughout the sensory system. There are three neural components to the transmission system: (1) the primary sensory afferent neurons carrying information to the spinal cord; (2) a series of ascending relay neurons between the spinal cord, brain stem, and thalamus; and (3) the thalamocortical projections.

Modulation refers to the process controlling the amount of afferent activity transmitted from the periphery to the central nervous system. Through distinct neural pathways containing norepinephrine, serotonin, and endogenous opioids, transmission is selectively inhibited and facilitated at the level of the dorsal horn of the spinal cord. (Pain is also modulated at the level of the brain stem and thalamus.) Unfortunately, the process whereby neural impulses produce a subjective, emotional experience such as pain is totally obscure.

Transduction The ability of tissues to elicit pain when noxious stimuli are applied depends on their innervation by nociceptors. Nociceptors are primary afferent neurons whose peripheral terminals respond selectively to noxious stimuli. These nociceptors subserve the physiologic process of transduction whereby energy (chemical, thermal, or mechanical) at the site of the noxious stimulus is encoded into a train of neural impulses.

All nociceptors are directly sensitive to thermal and mechanical stimuli. Repetition of the stimulus increasingly sensitizes many nociceptors. Sensitization of nociceptor activity is accomplished by the release of chemical mediators. These compounds may leak out of damaged cells whose membrane integrity has been compromised (potassium, histamine, acetylcholine, serotonin, adenosine triphosphate). They also may be enzymatically synthesized locally (bradykinin, prostaglandins, leukotrienes). Nociceptors themselves may release substances that enhance transduction. The exact composition of these substances is as yet undetermined, but a likely constituent is substance P, an 11-amino acid polypeptide. Neurons containing substance P are found in a variety of pain-sensitive tissues. Substance P is a potent direct vasodilator. It also indirectly causes histamine release from mast cells. Through release of substance P and similar mediators at their distal terminals, nociceptors not only signal tissue damage, but play a direct role in the inflammatory mechanisms enhancing transduction.

Transmission Information regarding tissue damage is transmitted via peripheral nerves. Peripheral nerves serve a variety of functions (sensory, motor, autonomic) reflected in the composition of their constituent axons (Table 1). Individual axons may be distinguished on the basis of myelination and diameter. The most numerous axonal types composing a peripheral nerve are A-α, A-δ, and C fibers, with lesser numbers of A-β and A-γ fibers.

The large-diameter A-α fibers are myelinated and conduct at speeds greater than 100 m/sec. A-α and A-β fibers subserve fine somatosensory discrimination.

The most numerous axonal type within a peripheral nerve is the C fiber. C fibers are small in diameter and slowly conducting. Although most C fibers are primary afferents with their cell bodies located in the dorsal root

219

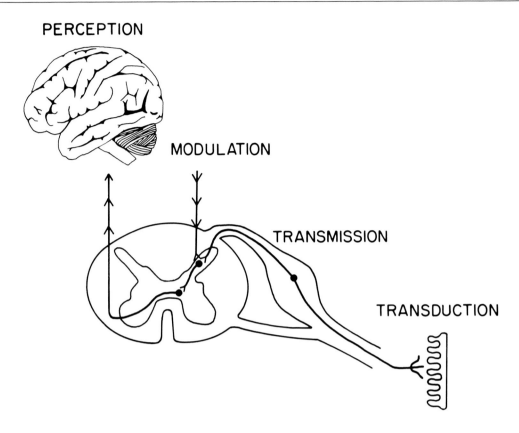

PERCEPTION

MODULATION

TRANSMISSION

TRANSDUCTION

Figure 1

The four physiologic processes of the pain sensory system.

ganglion, 20% are sympathetic postganglionic efferents with cell bodies located in the ganglia of the sympathetic chain. Sensory fibers responsive to noxious stimuli are almost always of the A-δ and C fiber types. These smaller-diameter fibers carry signals from nociceptors to the spinal cord.

Pathways Within the Central Nervous System As the nociceptive A-δ and C fibers approach the dorsal horn, they take a ventrolateral position within the dorsal root. The large myelinated A-α and A-β fibers continue medially and enter the dorsal columns. Collaterals of A-α fibers synapse throughout the dorsal horn and are important in diminishing nociceptive transmission. The smaller A-δ and C fibers ascend or descend in Lissauer's tract for a short distance before entering the spinal gray matter.

The gray matter of the spinal cord has a laminar cytoarchitectural organization. Lamina I (marginal layer) lies juxtaposed to the dorsal columns and Lissauer's tract (Fig. 2). It has a reticular appearance because of numerous nerve bundles coursing through it. Lamina II has a gelatinous appearance, for which reason it is called the substantia gelatinosa. Laminae I, II, and V are the synaptic termination for primary sensory afferent neurons.

Knowledge of the neurotransmitters synthesized in the dorsal root ganglia of primary sensory afferents and responsible for the excitation of spinal neurons is incomplete (Fig. 2). Cytochemical studies implicate a number of peptides, amino acids, catechols, and indoleamines. For example, substance P, somatostatin, and vasoactive intes-

tinal peptide are found in discrete populations of cells within the dorsal root ganglion. With transection of the dorsal root, dorsal horn concentrations of all the peptides decrease precipitously, suggesting that they are normally synthesized within the dorsal root ganglion cell bodies and transported to the spinal cord via axoplasmic flow.

Substance P is present in high concentrations in laminae I and II, somatostatin primarily in lamina II, and vasoactive intestinal peptide in lamina I. Other possible neurotransmitters are listed in Figure 2.

From laminae I, II, and V and various interneuronal laminar connections, projecting axons coalesce into the spinothalamic tract located in the anterolateral quadrant of the spinal cord. Spinothalamic tract neurons segregate into medial and lateral divisions as they approach the thalamus and terminate in their respective thalamic areas. Spinothalamic tract neurons projecting to the lateral thalamus are largely derived from laminae I, II, and V. Neurons from the lateral thalamus project strictly to the somatosensory cortex. In contrast, those neurons projecting to the medial thalamus are derived from deeper laminae (VI, VII, and VIII). These neurons have many synaptic connections with the reticular formation of the brain stem. Axons projecting from this reticular formation (spinoreticular pathway) are interspersed with the medially projecting spinothalamic tract neurons and share many similar anatomic and physiologic properties. From the medial thalamus, neurons project widely to the basal ganglia, the prefrontal and motor cortex, and the somatosensory and visual cortical areas.

The functional specialization of the medial and lateral

Table 1. Classification of peripheral nerves

Fiber Type*	Myelination	Location	Physiologic Function
A-α	Yes	Afferents and efferents to muscles and joints	Motor, proprioception
A-β	Yes	Afferents and efferents to muscles and joints	Motor, proprioception
A-γ	Yes	Efferents to muscle spindles	Muscle tone
A-δ	Yes	Sensory afferents	Pain, temperature, touch
B	Yes	Preganglionic sympathetic	Autonomic
C (80%)	No	Sensory afferents	Pain, temperature, touch
C (20%)	No	Postganglionic sympathetic	Autonomic

*Fibers are listed in order from largest (A-α) to smallest (C).

spinothalamic pathways can be suggested by phylogenetic argument. All vertebrates possess a spinoreticular pathway. In lower vertebrates possessing a spinothalamic tract, the tract projects to the medial thalamus. Being phylogenetically more primitive, it is referred to as the paleospinothalamic tract. As the projections from the medial thalamus are widespread with a large projection to the frontal lobe, the medial thalamic pathway (paleospinothalamic tract) may be more involved with nonspecific arousal or the affective-motivational aspects of pain. With increased encephalization in higher vertebrates, the lateral spinothalamic pathway appears (neospinothalamic tract). As its projections are restricted to the somatosensory cortex, the lateral thalamic pathway may subserve the sensory-discriminative (somatotopic localization) aspects of pain.

Modulation Insightful clinical observers argued that descending systems exist to modulate pain. Recently, pathways that modulate afferent activity at the level of the dorsal horn have been traced in anatomic and physiologic detail. Stimulation of cells in the periaqueductal gray matter, dorsolateral tegmentum of the pons, and rostroventral medulla increases activity within a descending neural pathway called the dorsolateral funiculus. The terminals of axons in the dorsolateral funiculus are concentrated in laminae I, II, and V—the same laminae that contain the terminals of primary sensory afferents and the cell bodies of the spinothalamic tract. Cell bodies residing in the dorsolateral pontine tegmentum contain norepinephrine, while those in the rostroventral medulla contain serotonin. Electrical stimulation of these anatomic sites produces analgesia and inhibition of nociceptive dorsal horn neurons.

Endogenous Opioids An endogenous opioid system also contributes to descending modulation. All endogenous opioids contain the amino acid sequence tyrosine-glycine-glycine-phenylalanine and are formed by cleavage from larger precursor molecules. Endogenous opioids can be grouped by their derivation from three precursor molecules: proenkephalin A, pro-opiomelanocortin, and prodynorphin (proenkephalin B).

Both met-enkephalin and leu-enkephalin are derived from proenkephalin A. Enkephalins are found in the gastrointestinal tract, sympathetic nervous system, and adrenal medulla. They are also found in high concentration in anatomic areas important for nociception (or antinociception)—the periaqueductal gray matter, the rostroventral medulla, and laminae I, II, V, and X. The enkephalins show the characteristic pharmacologic properties of the opioid family of compounds—reversal by naloxone and cross-tolerance to morphine. Enkephalins are weak analgesics whose potency can be augmented by inhibition of their degradative enzymes.

β-Endorphin is derived from pro-opiomelanocortin. Adrenocorticotropic hormone is also derived by cleavage from pro-opiomelanocortin and is formed on a one-to-one molar basis with β-endorphin, perhaps suggesting an as yet undefined neuroendocrine function for β-endorphin. β-Endorphin is the most potent of the endogenous opioids and is found in the hypothalamus, periaqueductal gray matter, and locus ceruleus.

Prodynorphin gives rise to dynorphin and α-neoendorphin. Despite having an anatomic localization similar to that of the enkephalins, the dynorphins are not potent analgesics.

Microinjection of opioids into discrete anatomic areas of the central nervous system that contain endogenous opioids can produce intense analgesia in animals. This analgesia can be reversed by subsequent local injection of naloxone. These and other animal studies indicate that systemic or perispinal (intrathecal, epidural) administration of narcotics produces analgesia by mimicking the action of endogenous opioids.

Multiple Opiate Receptors The various pharmacologic properties of the opioids—production of analgesia, respiratory depression, gastrointestinal motility, and the like—are a function of their affinities for various receptor types. These opiate receptors have discrete anatomic locations as well as prototypic ligands as determined by binding studies (Table 2).

Opiate analgesia is mediated through a complex interaction with μ-, δ-, and κ-receptors. There are two μ-receptor subtypes. The μ_1-receptor is primarily concerned with analgesia and the μ_2-receptor is involved with the physiologic processes of gastric motility and respiration. The highest concentrations of μ_1-receptors are found above the level of the spinal cord. The δ- and κ-opiate receptors are responsible for spinal analgesia. Interestingly, the opioids presently used for intrathecal or epidural administration are typically μ_1-agonists, and are therefore not the most efficacious for perispinal administration. Thus, narcotic analgesia is not a simple "lock-and-key" mechanism at the receptor site, but the result of complex interactions at various receptors throughout discrete areas of the central nervous system.

The Gate Control Theory of Pain

The gate control theory of pain, as originally developed by Melzack and Wall, attributes transmission through the dor-

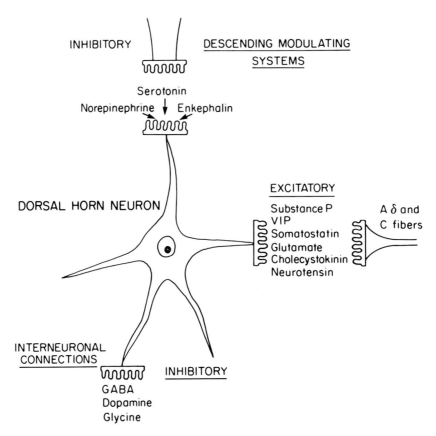

Figure 2

A number of peptides, catecholamines, and indoleamines are implicated as neurotransmitters at the dorsal horn.

sal horn to the interplay between myelinated and unmyelinated inputs (Fig. 3). This interaction was thought to occur at two sites: inhibitory interneurons within lamina II (substantia gelatinosa) and dorsal horn transmission neurons (T cells). It was hypothesized that both myelinated and unmyelinated primary afferents directly excited T cells and that the lamina II interneurons presynaptically inhibited afferent input to T cells by inhibition of transmitter release from both m yelinated and unmyelinated primary afferents. The myelinated afferents, it was suggested, directly excited lamina II neurons, thus inhibiting input to T cells, while the unmyelinated sensory afferents inhibited the inhibitory substantia gelatinosa neurons, thereby increasing T cell activity.

The gate control theory remains just that—a theory. The T cell itself has never been anatomically or functionally identified. Nonetheless, the gate control hypothesis succeeds as a global "image" for pain. It fails only in the attribution of specific interactions to particular loci. The elucidation of descending antinociceptive systems and the neurotransmitters involved makes the concept of the dorsal horn as the focal point (gate) for integration and modulation of nociception quite valid.

Thus, the neural pathways for pain sensation are not mere cables ("labeled lines") in the complex circuitry of the central nervous system. Pain sensation is a dynamic, fluid process capable of modification and modulation at several levels with particular, highly specific agents. It is this key concept that offers a promise of major break-

throughs in the management of painful afflictions within the next several decades.

Postoperative Pain Relief

Knowledge of the neural mechanisms of pain sensation establishes a rational approach for the treatment of postoperative pain by manipulation of the physiologic processes involved: transduction, transmission, and modulation. Thus, the concept of "balanced analgesia" (combining analgesic modalities) is becoming established on more firm physiologic grounds.

Transduction

Transduction as a nociceptive process has been heretofore largely ignored with respect to analgesic intervention. Release of chemical mediators at the peripheral terminals of nociceptors can enhance transduction. There has been a flurry of recent research in analgesics that can reduce sensitization after peripheral injury.

Prostaglandins have long been known as important nociceptive chemical mediators. Although marketed in Europe, intravenous cyclo-oxygenase inhibitors have not been available in the United States. An intravenous nonsteroidal anti-inflammatory medication with potency similar to that of the opioids is currently undergoing trials.

Capsaicin, a substance P antagonist, has been used in the treatment of post-herpetic neuralgia and holds promise

Table 2. Opiate receptor classification

Receptor	Prototypic Drug	Proposed Actions
μ_1	Most endogenous, naturally occurring or synthetic opioids	Supraspinal analgesia
μ_2	Morphine	Respiratory depression, cardiovascular effects
δ	Enkaphalins	Spinal analgesia
κ	Ketocyclazocine and dynorphin	Spinal analgesia, sedation
ϵ	β-Endorphin	Hormone?
σ	N-allynormetazocine	Psychotomimetic effects

in the treatment of other maladies. Long-acting local anesthetics can be directly applied to wounds via subcutaneous catheters or instilled into joints after arthroscopic procedures.

Transmission

Neural blockade is classically accomplished with local anesthetics. Local anesthetics inhibit axonal transmission by binding to sodium ionic channels. Via the epidural or, less frequently, the intrathecal routes, they can provide excellent postoperative analgesia. Their use as single agents requires fairly high concentrations with the attendant risk of motor blockade and cardiovascular instability. Continuous catheter techniques with dilute concentrations of local anesthetic in combination with opioids can provide analgesia for prolonged periods without cardiovascular instability and motor blockade.

Modulation

The perispinal application of opioids to the neuraxis (epidural or intrathecal routes) can provide intense analgesia without autonomic or motor blockade. Unlike systemic opioids, even small doses are effective because they act directly at the dorsal horn.

When administered epidurally, opioids diffuse to the area of the dorsal root ganglion where the dura is the thinnest. The degree of lipophilicity of an opioid determines its diffusion across the dura, and, therefore, the onset and duration of its effects. Lipophilic drugs such as fentanyl and sufentanil easily diffuse through the dura to the receptors at the dorsal horn. However, their lipophilicity also allows easy diffusion to venous drainage systems, eventually reducing their concentration. Thus, lipophilic agents have a quick onset but short duration of action. Morphine, however, is more hydrophilic because of its hydroxyl groups and crosses the dura less readily. Its maximum cerebrospinal fluid concentration occurs 90 minutes after epidural injection. Onset of analgesia is, therefore, delayed. Similarly, morphine's duration of action is prolonged (sometimes as much as 24 hours) because its hydrophilicity does not permit reuptake into veins. This permits rostral migration of morphine via passive cerebrospinal fluid flow.

The enhanced water solubility of morphine that permits rostral spread in the cerebrospinal fluid is responsible for the rare delayed respiratory depression seen with perispinal morphine. The peak incidence of respiratory depression usually occurs six to ten hours after administration, but may occur as late as 20 to 24 hours after administration. This necessitates careful monitoring of all patients who receive perispinal morphine. The respiratory depression seen with lipophilic agents occurs within the first one or two hours after administration. Factors predisposing to respiratory depression with perispinal opioids include (1) advanced age, (2) the use of hydrophilic agents (morphine), (3) high doses, (4) thoracic administration, and (5) the coincident administration of opioids by other routes.

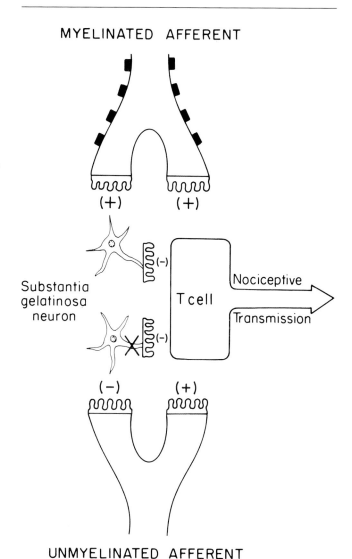

MYELINATED AFFERENT

UNMYELINATED AFFERENT

Figure 3

The gate theory of pain as originally proposed by Melzack and Wall.

Concomitant intravenous infusion of naloxone (5 μg/kg/hr) inhibits the respiratory depression caused by perispinal morphine without affecting analgesia. Coincident administration of naloxone with lipophilic agents opposes their analgesic effect. Naloxone can also be used to treat the other side effects of perispinal opioids—nausea, vomiting, urinary retention, and pruritis.

Epidural clonidine, an α_2-agonist, has been used in experimental models as an effective analgesic. There is a high concentration of α_2-receptors in the superficial layers of the dorsal horn, and the descending noradrenergic modulation to the cord is mediated through these receptors. Therefore, clonidine holds promise as another analgesic that can be directly applied to the neuraxis.

The efficacy of transcutaneous electrical nerve stimulation is based on the gate control hypothesis whereby pain relief is achieved through selective stimulation of large-diameter myelinated primary afferents. There is no associated pain as A-δ and C fibers have high electrical thresholds and remain unactivated. Because transcutaneous electrical nerve stimulation is associated with a specific sensation induced by simulation of large-diameter myelinated afferents, it is difficult to design a placebo-controlled study. However, the technique is completely innocuous and noninvasive and is of great benefit to some patients.

Chronic Neuropathic Pain

There are several mechanisms that can give rise to painful nervous system dysfunction: (1) deafferentation, (2) loss of segmental inhibition by destruction of large-diameter myelinated fibers, (3) ectopic impulse generation in primary sensory afferents, (4) "vicious cycles" between the sympathetic nervous system and the somatosensory system, and (5) lesions of the central nervous system. The neuropathic pain syndromes of particular import to the orthopaedist are neuromas (mechanism 3) and reflex sympathetic dystrophy (mechanism 4).

Neuromas

After injury, a peripheral nerve axon forms sprouts that grow toward the transected distal portion. These sprouts are for the most part small and unmyelinated. Depending on whether or not the connective tissue sheath is intact, the axons either continue to grow and reach the distal structure or they end blindly in a tangled mat called a neuroma. The area of sprouting becomes sensitive to mechanical stimulation (the basis of Tinel's sign). Regenerating axons also develop spontaneous activity at the site of sprouting as well as near the cell body in the dorsal root ganglion.

Neuromas are responsive to anticonvulsant medications, such as phenytoin and carbamazepine, that reduce discharge rates from sites of ectopic impulse generation. Repeated injections of a local anesthetic-steroid mixture also reduce pain through inhibition of sodium channel conductance and membrane stabilization, respectively.

Reflex Sympathetic Dystrophy and Causalgia

Reflex sympathetic dystrophy is a pain syndrome caused by traumatic injury to a nerve and sustained by efferent activity arising from sympathetic fibers. The nomenclature regarding reflex sympathetic dystrophy has been confusing because of the names that each individual medical specialty attributed to it. When a known injury occurs to a major nerve trunk, it is called causalgia. When the predisposing injury is unknown, or there is no clear major nerve involvement, or there is need for a more general term, it is called reflex sympathetic dystrophy.

The precipitating factors for reflex sympathetic dystrophy are myriad and sometimes lead to confusion regarding diagnosis. Precipitating factors of most import to the orthopaedist include soft-tissue injury, arthritis, fasciitis, tendinitis, bursitis, venous or arterial thrombosis, fractures, sprains, dislocations, surgical procedures, and imobilization with a cast or splint.

The diagnosis of reflex sympathetic dystrophy is made clinically. Patients describe a "burning" quality to their pain. Allodynia (pain to soft touch) and hyperpathia (an exaggerated and prolonged response to a painful stimulus) are typically present. Normal cutaneous sensation is preserved.

The symptoms may begin gradually, days to weeks after the initial injury, or they begin immediately. The temporal progression of reflex sympathetic dystrophy occurs in three stages. The "acute" stage is manifested by descriptions of "burning" pain with hyperpathia and allodynia. The affected part is usually edematous with vasomotor instability. There is accelerated hair and nail growth.

During the "dystrophic" phase, the affected area becomes cool, cyanotic, and indurated. Hair and nail growth are affected. Roentgenography shows diffuse osteopenia.

During the "atrophic" phase, irreversible tissue damage becomes manifest. The pain spreads proximally. The skin is shiny and appears almost "sclerodermatous."

A "vicious" neural cycle initiates and perpetuates reflex sympathetic dystrophy by activation or sensitization of primary afferent nociceptors in the skin. The "efferent limb" causing this activation or sensitization appears to begin with activation of sympathetic preganglionic neurons in the intermediolateral gray matter (Fig. 4). Although most patients with reflex sympathetic dystrophy show no electrophysiologic evidence of clinical nerve damage, propagation of activity in the "afferent limb" may result from

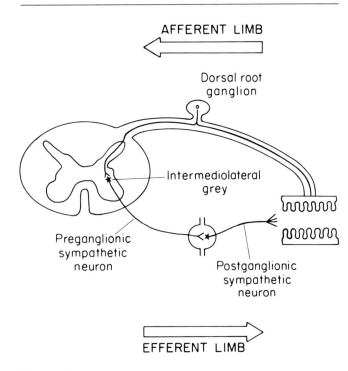

Figure 4

The "vicious" cycle of reflex sympathetic dystrophy.

enhanced nociceptor activity in response to norepinephrine or to the formation of ephapses. Ephapses are artificial electrical junctions formed by regenerating sprouts of nociceptive primary afferents and sympathetic efferents. Afferent activity activates sympathetic preganglionic neurons in the intermediolateral gray matter; these neurons in turn synapse within the sympathetic ganglia. The postganglionic sympathetic neuron releases norepinephrine at its peripheral terminals, sensitizing primary afferent nociceptors and establishing the cycle.

The treatment for reflex sympathetic dystrophy is early intervention with sympathetic blockade (stellate ganglion block or lumbar paravertebral sympathetic ganglion block, depending on the extremity involved, or Bier block using reserpine, guanethidine, bretylium, or corticosteroid along with local anesthetic). Of particular note is the fact that pain relief outlasts the duration of action of the local anesthetic. With repeated blockade, pain relief becomes progressively longer, becoming permanent in many cases.

Other treatments include physical therapy, transcutaneous electrical nerve stimulation, corticosteroids, and phenoxybenzamine. Physical therapy alone has been shown to be beneficial and should form an integral part of any care plan. Although some authorities argue as to whether transcutaneous electrical nerve stimulation can affect sympathetic tone, it is worth considering as a treatment modality because of its extreme safety. Both oral prednisone and phenoxybenzamine can achieve good remission of reflex sympathetic dystrophy, although some patients require retreatment.

The sooner reflex sympathetic dystrophy is diagnosed and treated, the better the ultimate prognosis. Once reflex sympathetic dystrophy enters the "dystrophic" phase, it becomes progressively more refractory to treatment.

Trends

Much has been learned about the neurobiology of pain within the last decade. With this foundation, the future management of acute and chronic pain will bear little resemblance to present clinical practice. Revolutionary pharmacologic and physiologic modulators will be introduced in the next decade.

Annotated Bibliography

Keywords

Endogenous opioids; Endorphin; Nerve fibers, Neural transmission; Pain; Reflex sympathetic dystrophy

Neural Pathways for Pain Sensation

The Pain Sensory System

Fields HL: *Pain.* New York, McGraw-Hill, 1987, p 354.
 A clear, concise, and comprehensible description of the neuroanatomy, physiology, and pathology of the pain sensory system. It is the best primary text available.

Transduction

Price DD, Dubner R: Neurons that subserve the sensory-discriminative aspects of pain. *Pain* 1977;3:307–338.
 The neuronal types involved in the transduction and transmission of sensory-discriminative nociceptive information are reviewed.

Raja SN, Meyer RA, Campbell JN: Peripheral mechanisms of somatic pain. *Anesthesiology* 1988;68:571–590.
 Cutaneous, muscular, and joint nociceptor types and the biochemical mechanisms of their sensitization are reviewed.

Transmission

Torebjörk HE, Hallin RG: Perceptual changes accompanying controlled preferential blocking of A and C fibre responses in intact human skin nerves. *Exp Brain Res* 1973;16:321–332.
 A noninvasive method was used to stimulate and record neural activity in unanesthetized human skin, demonstrating that A-α and C fibers are responsible for nociception.

Pathways Within the Central Nervous System

Cervero F, Iggo A: The substantia gelatinosa of the spinal cord: A critical review. *Brain* 1980;103:717–772.
 The neuroanatomy and neurophysiology of Rexed's lamina II are extensively reviewed.

Jessell TM, Jahr CE: Fast and slow excitatory transmitters at primary afferent synapses in the dorsal horn of the spinal cord, in Fields HL, et al (eds): *Advances in Pain Research and Therapy.* New York, Raven Press, 1985, vol 9.
 There are fast and slow components to excitation of spinal neurons by nociceptive input. Substance P is implicated as a "slow" excitatory neurotransmitter while glutamate, aspartate, and adenosine triphosphate may be "fast" excitatory neurotransmitters.

Kevetter GA, Willis WD: Collateralization in the spinothalamic tract: New methodology to support or deny phylogenetic theories. *Brain Res Rev* 1984;7:1–14.
 Components of the spinothalamic tract system are reviewed. The presence of collateralization is discussed with regard to theories of the phylogenetic development of pathways.

Otsuka M, Konishi S, Yanagisawa M, et al: Role of substance P as a sensory transmitter in spinal cord and sympathetic ganglia. *Ciba Found Symp* 1982;91:13–34.
 The role of substance P at the primary sensory afferent spinal synapse is discussed.

Rexed B: The cytoarchitectonic organization of the spinal cord in the cat. *J Comp Neurol* 1952;96:415–495.
 The laminar organization of the spinal cord was first completely described by Rexed in this classic article.

Modulation

Duggan AW: Pharmacology of descending control systems. *Philos Trans R Soc London [B]* 1985;308:375–391.

The role of serotonin, norepinephrine, and opioid peptides in supraspinal and segmental inhibition of afferent dorsal horn input is reviewed in the rat and cat models.

Yaksh TL, Reddy SV: Studies in the primate on the analgetic effects associated with intrathecal actions of opiates, alpha-adrenergic agonists and baclofen. *Anesthesiology* 1981;54:451–467.

Powerful analgesia can be produced by selectively activating opiate, adrenergic, and baclofenergic receptor systems in the spinal cord.

Endogenous Opiates

Grevert P, Albert LH, Goldstein A: Partial antagonism of placebo analgesia by naloxone. *Pain* 1983;16:129–143.

This double-masked study suggests that endogenous opiates may be involved in the production of placebo-induced analgesia.

Palkovits M: Distribution of neuropeptides in the central nervous system: A review of biochemical mapping studies. *Prog Neurobiol* 1984;23:151–189.

The somatotopic distributions of the individual endogenous opioids are extensively reviewed.

Ruda MA: Opiates and pain pathways: Demonstration of enkephalin synapses on dorsal horn projection neurons. *Science* 1982;215:1523–1525.

Using immunocytochemistry and horseradish peroxidase, axonal endings containing enkephalin immunoreactivity were found to make direct contact with the soma and dendrites of dorsal horn spinothalamic tract neurons. This suggests that a major site of enkephalin-mediated antinociception is at the spinothalamic tract projection neurons themselves.

Yaksh TL, Noueihed R: The physiology and pharmacology of spinal opiates. *Annu Rev Pharmacol Toxicol* 1985;25:433–462.

The endogenous opioids are extensively reviewed in this definitive work.

Multiple Opiate Receptors

Fang FG, Fields HL, Lee NM: Action at the mu receptor is sufficient to explain the supraspinal analgesic effect of opiates. *J Pharmacol Exp Ther* 1986;238:1039–1044.

Although μ- and δ-selective ligands produced analgesia, μ-receptor activity was shown to be responsible for supraspinal analgesia in the mouse model.

Pasternak GW: Multiple morphine and enkephalin receptors and the relief of pain. *JAMA* 1988;259:1362–1367.

Opiate receptor subtypes and their pharmacologic activities are clearly and concisely reviewed.

The Gate Control Theory of Pain

Melzack R, Wall PD: Pain mechanisms: A new theory. *Science* 1965;150:971–979.

The gate control theory was first discussed in this classic article.

Postoperative Pain Relief

Transduction

Cashman JN, Jones RM, Foster JM, et al: Comparison of infusions of morphine and lysine acetyl salicylate for the relief of pain after surgery. *Br J Anaesth* 1985;57:255–258.

The analgesic effects of constant infusions of morphine or lysine acetyl salicylate were compared in patients undergoing herniorrhaphy. Lysine acetyl salicylate offered as much analgesia as morphine with significantly less drowsiness, nausea, and vomiting.

O'Hara DA, Fragen RJ, Kinzer M, et al: Ketorolac tromethamine as compared with morphine sulfate for treatment of postoperative pain. *Clin Pharmacol Ther* 1987;41:556–561.

Ketorolac tromethamine is a nonopioid investigational drug that inhibits prostaglandin synthesis and has analgesic, anti-inflammatory, and antipyretic properties. Given intramuscularly in this study, it was as analgesic as morphine with significantly fewer side effects.

Watson CP, Evans RJ, Watt VR: Post-herpetic neuralgia and topical capsaicin. *Pain* 1988;33:333–340.

Topical 0.025% capsaicin was used to treat post-herpetic neuralgia in this nonrandomized, noncontrolled study. It appears to be a useful modality worthy of a double-masked, controlled trial.

Modulation

Camporesi EM, Nielsen CH, Bromage PR, et al: Ventilatory CO_2 sensitivity after intravenous and epidural morphine in volunteers. *Anesth Analg* 1983;62:633–640.

Significant respiratory depression was noted with epidural morphine as compared with intravenous morphine. Significant depression was seen as early as three hours after injection and continued for 24 hours, highlighting the need for adequate monitoring.

Cousins MJ, Mather LE: Intrathecal and epidural administration of opioids. *Anesthesiology* 1984;61:276–310.

This is the definitive review of clinical perispinal analgesia with opioids.

Gueneron JP, Ecoffey C, Carli P, Benhamou D, Gross JB: Effect of naloxone infusion on analgesia and respiratory depression after epidural fentanyl. *Anesth Analg* 1988;67:35–38.

Low-dose intravenous infusion of naloxone (5 μg/kg/hr) antagonized the analgesia from a 200-μg epidural injection of fentanyl, but not the respiratory depression. High-dose intravenous infusion of naloxone (10 μg/kg/hr) significantly decreased the quality of analgesia, but also antagonized repiratory depression.

Rawal N, Schött U, Dahlström B, et al: Influence of naloxone infusion on analgesia and respiratory depression following epidural morphine. *Anesthesiology* 1986;64:194–201.

Low-dose naloxone infusion (5 μg/kg/hr) prevented respiratory depression after epidural injection of 4 mg of morphine without affecting analgesia.

Schulze S, Roikjaer O, Hasselstrøm L, et al: Epidural bupivacaine and morphine plus systemic indomethacin eliminates pain but not systemic response and convalescence after cholecystectomy. *Surgery* 1988;103:321–327.

Use of epidural bupivacaine (affects transmission), epidural morphine (affects modulation), and systemic indomethacin (affects transduction) completely ablated postoperative pain, providing the strongest evidence to date on the validity of the concept of "balanced analgesia."

Chronic Neuropathic Pain

Schwartzman RJ, McLellan TL: Reflex sympathetic dystrophy: A review. *Arch Neurol* 1987;44:555–561.

The clinical presentation and pathophysiology of reflex sympathetic dystrophy are extensively reviewed.

18
Spinal Cord Monitoring

Spinal cord monitoring is used in the diagnosis of spinal conditions and in spinal surgery. Significant neurologic complications are associated with spinal surgery in 0.5% to 1.5% of cases (the rate varies with the type of case and the instrumentation used), indicating the importance of monitoring cord function during surgery. Current methods make this feasible but much progress is still needed before electronic monitoring systems will become standard. For now, the intraoperative "wake-up" test remains the most widely used means of monitoring cord function during surgery.

Monitoring Techniques

Neuroanatomy

Spinal cord monitoring is based on the transmission of impulses up and down the spinal cord. The tracts involved depend on the stimulus sites used. The traditional cross-sectional representation of cord pathways is the accepted configuration in analyzing spinal cord function as depicted by spinal cord monitoring. Because there are a significant number of tracts in the cord, different types of monitoring have been developed for studying different regions of the cord.

The most widely used tracts are the posterior columns, which carry most of the impulses generated by stimulation of a mixed peripheral nerve such as the median nerve or the posterior tibial nerve. The limitations of this anatomic arrangement led to the development of other methods using tracts located in other parts of the cord, particularly the anterior areas. Research delineating which pathways are used under various stimuli generally supports the established anatomic model of the spinal cord.

Although the posterior columns are the main transport for stimuli generated by somatosensory evoked potentials, major spinal cord damage in other tracts of the cord is also reflected in the function of the posterior columns. Careful monitoring will detect all major cord injuries. Nonetheless, because the anterior spinal artery is a vital, easily damaged structure, investigators have tried to find other, more sensitive techniques through the stimulation of motor pathways. These approaches are not yet in general clinical use.

Each of the different techniques needed for effective monitoring of the entire cord has different characteristics and different advantages and disadvantages. For example, stimulating a peripheral nerve and recording its expression over the appropriate cerebral cortex uses tracts that pass through a number of higher centers and synapses. This creates a wide variety of responses and a very weak signal.

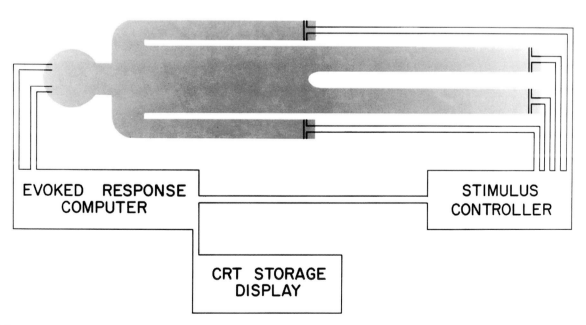

Figure 1

Schema depicting the variety of stimulus and recording sites available for evoked potential monitoring. The computer generates the stimulus, coordinates the stimulus and recording sequence, records the evoked response, and analyzes, displays, and stores the data.

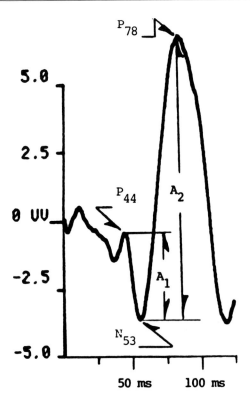

Figure 2

This is a typical intraoperative recording generated from 64 stimulations of the posterior nerve at a rate of 1.2 Hz and averaging the responses with a bandwidth of 0.3 to 100 Hz. Primary peak latencies are denoted by both their polarity (positive or negative) and their time of occurrence in milliseconds after stimulus. In this example, the peaks are denoted P44, N53, and P79. Peak-to-peak amplitudes are measured as absolute differences of successive peaks (A1 and A2), which are respectively 3.25 and 10.5 μV.

Interpretation is, therefore, more complex, but the information derived is greater than that obtained with a simple system. Also, this approach is noninvasive and can be done in a variety of settings, making it versatile.

Thus, neuroanatomy dictates the configuration of any system of monitoring. The location of the motor centers and tracts makes the development of stimulus sites so difficult that transcranial magnetic impulses are now being studied as a way of producing motor impulses. Adding to the complexity of the task, the central and peripheral nervous systems respond to a variety of different stimulus characteristics and transmit with a variety of velocities and frequencies. Changes in stimulus and recording criteria can seriously affect the data generated and the effectiveness of any given approach.

System Analysis

Basic Methods Somatosensory cortical evoked potentials (SCEPs) were first used in a clinical setting in 1959. The technique consisted of repetitively stimulating a mixed peripheral nerve and recording on an oscilloscope the signals generated by the cortical sensory center serving that stimulated nerve. Electroencephalographic recordings were timed to correspond with the onset of the peripheral nerve stimulus. The individual electroencephalographic sweeps

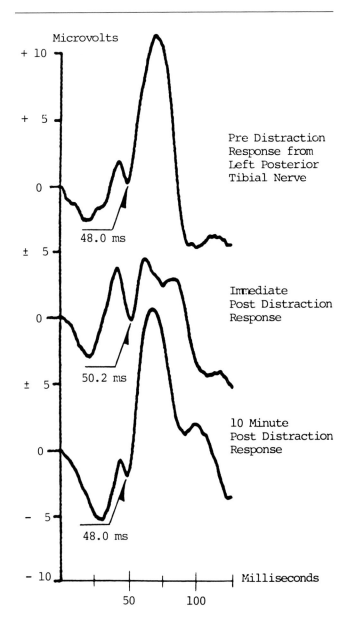

Figure 3

A series of intraoperative SCEP recordings in a patient with idiopathic scoliosis undergoing spinal instrumentation. The predistraction recording from stimulation of the left posterior tibial nerve is within normal limits. The immediate postdistraction recording shows an increase in primary peak latency and a decrease in overall recording amplitude. However, this change returned to baseline in less than 15 minutes and later recordings were interpreted as showing the patient to be neurologically intact, which was the case. System parameters were the same as in Figure 2.

generated by the stimulus were summed by having a camera positioned in front of the oscilloscope with the lens open so that each recording was superimposed on the sweeps preceding it. This method of summing responses produced distinct, polyphasic wave patterns. Although these recordings were imprecise, they were the forerunners of present-day recordings.

In the technique used today, a computer applies a stimulus in a repetitive fashion, simultaneously triggering the recording system. Signals are picked up by electrodes

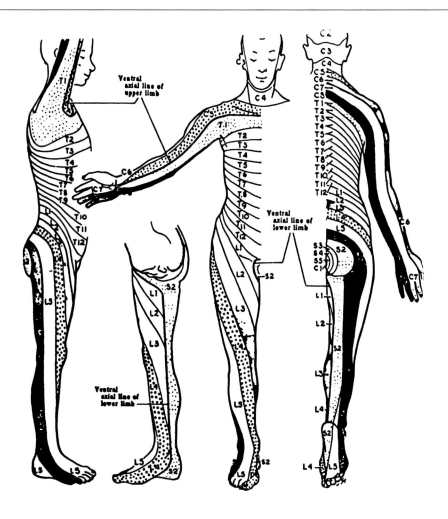

Figure 4

This is the standard dermatomal mapping diagram used to determine electrode placement sites. The obliquity of the dermatomal axes can be seen. Electrodes are placed within a given dermatome so that they are close to easily identifiable anatomic sites such as the tibial tuberosity and not directly over a point of motor insertion.

placed over the appropriate contralateral area of the scalp or near the segment of the central nervous system transmitting the signals (Fig. 1). Individual responses generated by individual stimuli are then electronically summed to average out background noise and enhance the signal-to-noise ratio. If the system is working well, it generates a clean, reproducible recording that can be analyzed and interpreted (Fig. 2).

Data Analysis Recordings are made before the surgical procedure and at critical times during it (for example, when corrective distraction is applied). The preoperative recordings serve as a control, indicating the initial status of the central nervous system. During surgery, recordings obtained after the induction of anesthesia serve as the best baseline. The patient's intraoperative physiologic status must, therefore, be kept as stable as possible so that any change in the recordings cannot be attributed to alterations in the patient's internal physiologic or biochemical environment.

The most common measurements used to interpret the recordings are latency and amplitude (Fig. 2). Latency measures the time in milliseconds between the onset of a stimulus and the point at which a peak of the waveform generated occurs. There are a number of components to the response, but those occurring in the first 50 to 60 ms reflect transmissions from the spinal cord and higher centers. The peaks receive designations such as "P38" or "N54" that indicate their polarity (positive or negative) and their time of arrival (38 or 54 ms). Upward deflection is by convention positive. Peaks occurring before 15 ms or after 100 ms have meaning but are not used in routine analysis.

Amplitude is measured in microvolts and represents the voltage differential between one peak and the next peak in the sequence. As an example, the "peak-to-peak" amplitude of "N54" is the differential between "P38" and "N54." This can range from 1 to 5 μV or more.

Changes in either the latency or the amplitude occur naturally, but if environmental conditions are stable and the changes exceed certain guidelines, there is an increasing likelihood that signal transmission is being compromised. Current guidelines are that an increase in the latency of more than 10% or a decrease of 50% or more in peak-to-

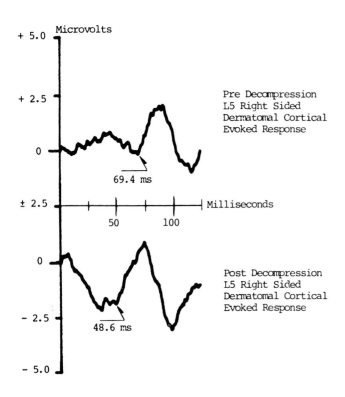

+ 5.0   Microvolts

+ 2.5

0

Pre Decompression
L5 Right Sided
Dermatomal Cortical
Evoked Response

69.4 ms

± 2.5 ─── Milliseconds
50   100

0

Post Decompression
L5 Right Sided
Dermatomal Cortical
Evoked Response

- 2.5

48.6 ms

- 5.0

Figure 5

These recordings were taken from a case in which dermatomal mapping was used during a lumbar decompression. The predecompression recording from the right L-5 dermatome shows increased latency, indicating involvement of the L-5 root. The postdecompression recording shows marked improvement in the latency. This correlated with postoperative relief of radiculopathy. System parameters for these recordings were a stimulus rate of 0.8 Hz, a summation of 64 responses, and a recording bandwidth of 0.3 to 100 Hz.

peak amplitude is cause for concern. If these changes persist for more than 15 to 20 minutes, the cause of these changes must be determined and appropriate action taken.

Although there are isolated reports of false-negative findings (that is, the recordings were satisfactory but the patient suffered a major neurologic loss), such cases are very rare. On occasion, the changes seen are borderline and difficult to correlate with clinical findings. In 60% to 70% of such cases, there are no neurologic sequelae. In the rest, the sequelae are, for the most part, transient mild parasthesias that resolve before the patient leaves the hospital.

The Database Surgeons and institutions must establish their own databases with their own equipment. A great many variables can affect the recordings and, therefore, databases are likely to vary. The database also depends on the development of a controlled protocol that establishes the parameters and variables of the system. In addition, those responsible for the system must be well trained because presently available commercial systems are quite complex.

Terminology

Although many different terms have been used to describe the various types of spinal cord monitoring, one proposed system is based on the various combinations of stimulating and recording conditions that can be used. Accordingly, the formula used to "build" spinal cord monitoring descriptors is stimulus site plus recording site plus evoked potentials. Thus, the initial letters of somatosensory, cortical, and evoked potential equals SCEP. SSEP, then, represents somatosensory spinal evoked potential. In some currently used exceptions (such as MEP and DEP, which indicate motor evoked potential and dermatomal evoked potential, the recording site part of the nomenclature is omitted because further clinical development of these systems is needed.

Evoked Potential Monitoring Systems

Over the years, several electronic monitoring systems have evolved. SCEP monitoring is the most widely used electronic system in North America and SSEP monitoring is almost the only system used in Japan and is widely used in Europe. The advantages of SCEP monitoring are its noninvasiveness and its versatility; its disadvantages are its small signal and its sensitivity to anesthetics and changes in physiologic variables. SSEP monitoring produces larger signals and is insensitive to anesthetic agents, but is relatively invasive and has limited diagnostic use. Both systems monitor only the sensory components, although both are highly accurate and reliable. Other systems being developed stimulate the motor tracts and record distally or stimulate a sensory dermatome and record proximally.

Nonelectronic Monitoring Methods

The Wake-Up Test This test was first used in adult patients with severe scoliosis who were wakened in the operating room to confirm distal motor function after spinal instrumentation. This method is safe when done properly and is the current "gold standard" for monitoring in cases in which intraoperative neurologic damage is a risk. The test is conducted by the anesthesiologist, who must lighten the anesthesia to a level at which the patient can respond to verbal commands to move the hands. Next, foot and ankle motions are requested. The responsible surgeon must observe the patient's feet for motion and decide whether neural competency is present. The advantages of this approach are its relative simplicity and its low cost. Its limitations are that the results can be difficult to evaluate (particularly if the patient has a preexisting neurologic deficit), it measures neuologic status at only one moment in time, and it addresses only the motor tracts. The wake-up test can be used as the only monitoring test or in conjunction with electronic monitoring.

The Ankle Clonus Test The ankle clonus test is an alternative, nonelectronic, intraoperative approach to monitoring. The patient's ankle reflexes are monitored during the induction of anesthesia and the findings compared with those when the patient is partially awakened intraoperatively after spinal manipulation. As in the "wake-up" test, visual interpretation can be difficult, but users of this approach report that it is a reliable test of neurologic integrity. This test is not widely used and has the same general advantages and disadvantages as the wake-up test.

Clinical Applications

Intraoperative Uses

Spine surgery with a recognizable risk of neurologic damage requires spinal cord monitoring. Examples include correction of spinal deformity through application of forces, management of unstable spines, vertebral osteotomies, decompression for tumors, and epidural or intradural procedures in the region of the spinal cord. Electronic monitoring systems are now developed to the point that they are preferred in more complex, higher-risk cases because of their sensitivity, reproducible results, and versatility. These systems are more demanding, complex, and expensive, but the information derived from them can be significantly more useful. Figure 3 is a set of intraoperative SCEP recordings taken during spinal instrumentation for scoliosis. The recordings made shortly after the application of distraction showed changes in amplitude and latency; these resolved within 15 minutes. Because the recordings returned rapidly to a normal range, the interpretation was that the patient was neurologically intact. The patient awoke with no deficits.

There are still many questions about the effectiveness of these systems in detecting neurologic complications. Data vary from study to study in format and completeness, but several statements can be made regarding the general sensitivity and specificity of electronic monitoring. The number of false-negatives (cases in which the recordings were well within normal ranges but the patient awoke with new neural deficits) is very small. Conversely, false-positives (cases in which significant changes occurred intraoperatively but no neurologic deficits were noted postoperatively) are reported in 5% to 25% of cases. True-positives and true-negatives are reported in 1% and 60% of cases, respectively. Thus, the sensitivity of electronic monitoring is high because of the low false-negative rate but specificity levels are more modest because of the higher incidence of false-positives. However, these specificity levels are considered acceptable because the consequences of false-positives are much less grave than those of false-negatives. Much of the current developmental work in monitoring addresses the issue of improved correlation between changes in evoked potential recordings and changes in clinical function.

The wake-up and ankle clonus tests are appropriate in lower-risk cases such as correction of idiopathic adolescent scoliosis in a teenager. Although procedures using the anterior approach to the spine are generally low-risk, monitoring is considered desirable, particularly if instrumentation or peridural procedures are utilized.

Spinal cord monitoring is also helpful in the surgical treatment of cervical and lumbar spine diseases, such as spondylosis and spinal stenosis, in which extensive dissection and decompression are needed. In such cases, electronic systems can serve both protective and diagnostic functions by providing feedback about neural conduction during decompression in the form of improving or deteriorating recordings. The ability of these systems to provide selective diagnostic information about specific root function is improving. When this approach is used, the preoperative recordings provide not only control data but also information about the specific location or level of the abnormality.

Monitoring has also been used in cases of spinal trauma, particularly when instability and/or neurologic deficits are present. In such cases, the wake-up test provides limited information and electronic monitoring is preferred. Preoperative baseline records are essential and monitoring right-left differences, frequent repetitions, and comparing the findings with those for the unaffected extremities are valuable. Although spinal cord monitoring has correlated well with recovery in incomplete injuries, it has not been predictive in cases of complete cord injury.

Other orthopaedic uses for evoked potential monitoring are now being identified. Among these is the monitoring of sciatic nerve function during hip surgery, particularly revision cases in which the incidence of sciatic nerve palsy is significant. Modified and simplified SCEP or SSEP systems are being used. Recent reports have shown altered recordings in more than 50% of total hip replacements. These findings improved when traction was removed and no postoperative palsies were reported. Evoked potentials have proven helpful in brachial plexus injury and can be helpful in determining the location and extent of lesions.

Trends

The use of spinal cord monitoring to aid in diagnosis is perhaps one of the most promising areas of growth. There are increasing reports of the use of a DEP system to define the specific nerves involved in lumbar radicular pain. When specific dermatomal testing montages are selected, information can be gained about the status of transmission along a specific root. This approach can be used to obtain data from as low as S-4 proximally to the upper cervical area. In the lumbar area, root monitoring can be done as far caudally as S-5 by stimulating the anal nerve and S-3 and S-4 through the pudendal nerve. Above that, the specific nerve dermatome (Fig. 4) is stimulated with electrodes placed along the central dermatomal axis approximately 4 to 6 cm apart with the cathode proximal. Stimulation levels are set to give sensation but no motor response. Recordings can be made from the spinal areas intraoperatively, but cortical electrodes placed over the appropriate contralateral cortex are diagnostically useful because individual roots can be assessed to determine specific deficits and correlate them with other clinical and diagnostic findings. This can be helpful when data are conflicting or vague. This also provides a baseline for monitoring the effects of corrective decompressive surgery. Figure 5 shows a series of DEP recordings taken during lumbar decompression for radiculopathy. The unilateral involvement of the L-5 root can be seen in the predecompression recordings; improvement is apparent after the decompression. Postoperatively, the patient had significantly improved radiculopathy.

Similar root level diagnostic testing can be done in the cervical area via either the dermatomal approach or the more invasive method of inserting an extradural stimulating electrode in the lower cervical spine and passage proximally. Spinal-spinal or spinal-cortical evoked potentials are recorded for each cervical level in which the presence or absence of local root dysfunction can be determined. This method is not widely used in North America but is widely used in Japan, where this technique was developed.

Annotated Bibliography

Keywords

Ankle clonus test; Central nervous system; Evoked potentials; Peripheral nervous system; Spinal cord; Wake-up test

Monitoring Techniques

Brown RH, Nash CL Jr, Berilla JA, et al: Cortical evoked potential monitoring: A system for intraoperative monitoring of spinal cord function. *Spine* 1984;9:256–261.

The authors review their series of more than 300 cases monitored intraoperatively with SCEPs. They describe the system and its technical and physiologic limitations and problems. In four cases changes in the recordings led to changes in the surgical technique, resulting in normal postoperative neural status. No false-negatives or false-positives occurred.

Grundy BL: Intraoperative monitoring of sensory-evoked potentials. *Anesthesiology* 1983;58:72–87.

The author reviews the rationale for and methods of sensory monitoring, including the important anesthetic aspects of this approach.

Nuwer MR, Dawson E: Intraoperative evoked potential monitoring of the spinal cord: Enhanced stability of cortical recordings. *Electroencephalogr Clin Neurophysiol* 1984;59:318–327.

The authors studied 115 patients with various spinal abnormalities by means of SCEPs. They studied stimulus frequency and intensity, scalp recording sites and configuration, filter settings, and anesthesia. All affected recording amplitude.

Peterson DO, Drummond JC, Todd MM: Effects of halothane, enflurane, isoflurane, and nitrous oxide on somatosensory evoked potentials in humans. *Anesthesiology* 1986;65:35–40.

Median nerve SCEP recordings were studied in 21 healthy subjects under a variety of anesthetic agents. Recordings were done while the anesthetics were gradually increased. All agents decreased amplitude and increased latency. These changes were most pronounced with enflurane and least pronounced with halothane. The addition of nitrous oxide increased these effects.

Salzman SK, Beckman AL, Marks HG, et al: Effects of halothane on intraoperative scalp-recorded somatosensory evoked potentials to posterior tibial nerve stimulation in man. *Electroencephalogr Clin Neurophysiol* 1986;65:36–45.

The authors studied a series of 116 patients undergoing spinal surgery with halothane anesthesia in concentrations from 0.25% to 2.0%. They achieved recordings in 91% of these cases; when a continuous 0.5% concentration was used, monitoring was achieved in 96% of cases. Amplitude decrease and latency increase were the most noted changes with halothane. The peak occurring at 30 ms appeared most resistant to degradation.

Clinical Applications

Aminoff MJ, Goodin DS, Barbaro NM, et al: Dermatomal somatosensory evoked potentials in unilateral lumbosacral radiculopathy. *Ann Neurol* 1985;17:171–176.

The authors compared SCEPs with DEPs in the detection of L-5 and S-1 involvement in 19 cases. All the SCEP recordings were normal and five of 19 DEP recordings were considered accurate. In ten cases, the DEP information was misleading. In three cases the SCEP and DEP recordings and radiologic tests were normal while the electromyographic findings were abnormal. The authors question the ultimate utility of evoked potential techniques in the evaluation of patients with suspected radiculopathies.

Ben-David B: Spinal cord monitoring. *Orthop Clin North Am* 1988;19:427–448.

This article reviews the use of spinal cord monitoring in surgery including both the wake-up test and the various electrophysiologic methods. The various methods are compared and the advantages and disadvantages of each are presented.

Bieber E, Tolo V, Uematsu S: Spinal cord monitoring during posterior spinal instrumentation and fusion. *Clin Orthop* 1988;229:121–124.

SCEP monitoring was used in 257 patients undergoing posterior scoliosis fusion with instrumentation. Intraoperatively, six (2%) had significant increases in latency or loss of recordings within 15 to 20 minutes. All cases resolved after intraoperative removal of the instrumentation. All but one of these patients tolerated reinsertion of instrumentation at reduced force. The others underwent in situ fusion and none had postoperative deficits.

Blight AR: Motor evoked potentials in CNS trauma. *Cent Nerv Syst Trauma* 1986;3:207–214.

The author reviews the current state of MEP monitoring, including stimulus and recording options. He concluded that MEP monitoring complements somatosensory evoked potentials and that they have their own set of limitations and constraints in data extraction and interpretation.

Bradshaw K, Webb JK, Fraser AM: Clinical evaluation of spinal cord monitoring in scoliosis surgery. *Spine* 1984;9:636–643.

Forty patients were monitored intraoperatively with SCEP and the wake-up test. The results of the SCEP and wake-up tests were in full agreement. There were no false-positive or false-negative SCEP recordings. Two cases of transient neurologic deficits are described in detail, both of which the monitoring detected early. The technique is described as clinically valuable.

Chabot R, York DH, Watts C, et al: Somatosensory evoked potentials evaluated in normal subjects and spinal cord-injured patients. *J Neurosurg* 1985;63:544–551.

The authors studied 24 normal subjects and 34 patients with spinal cord trauma. SCEP recordings showed differences in peak latency, interpeak latency, and amplitude between persons with normal neurologic findings and those with deficits. They did not distinguish among the different types or degrees of neurologic deficit.

Cohen BA, Huizenga BA: Dermatomal monitoring for surgical correction of spondylolisthesis: A case report. *Spine* 1988;13:1125–1128.

The authors use this case report to describe in detail their use of DEP monitoring in more than 50 cases. There were no false-negatives. This method provided increased sensitivity with an amplitude reduction of 20% and a latency increase of 4% being significant.

Dinner DS, Lüders H, Lesser RP, et al: Intraoperative spinal somatosensory evoked potential monitoring. *J Neurosurg* 1986;65:807–814.

The authors studied a series of 220 spinal cases by means of peripheral nerve (tibial and median) stimulation and a variety of rostral recording sites, including epidural, subcortical, and scalp sites. There was postoperative neurologic deterioration in seven cases; three of these had significant intraoperative changes. An additional four patients showed substantial changes in the monitoring but had no postoperative neurologic changes. The authors calculated the false-negative rate of their multimodality monitoring approach to be 1.87%.

Herron LD, Trippi AC, Gonyeau M: Intraoperative use of dermatomal somatosensory-evoked potentials in lumbar stenosis surgery. *Spine* 1987;12:379–383.

The use of DSEPs was evaluated in 30 cases involving the L-4, L-5, and S-1 dermatomes. In six cases of unilateral and 24 cases of bilateral abnormality, latency increased an average of 9 ms compared with 3.4 ms in the undecompressed side. The average reduction in latency was 9.9 ms in patients with good results, 8.2 ms in patients with fair results, and 6.0 ms in patients with poor results. Although these differences were not statistically significant, the authors state that DSEPs were helpful, particularly in cases in which there was primary root involvement or level selection was difficult.

Keim HA, Hajdu M, Gonzalez EG, et al: Somatosensory evoked potentials as an aid in the diagnosis and intra-operative management of spinal stenosis. *Spine* 1985;10:338–344.

The authors used SCEPs to examine 20 patients with lumbar spinal stenosis. They also studied 11 of the 20 intraoperatively. In patients with symptomatic lower extremities, the posterior tibial nerve was abnormal in 95%, the peroneal nerve in 90%, the sural nerve in 60%, and the saphenous nerve in 12%. They concluded that SCEPs were more sensitive than other electro-diagnostic modalities and that they were helpful in identifying additional levels and adequate intraoperative decompression.

Kubota S, Nagashima C, Ohmori S: Segmental spinal somatosensory evoked potentials in cervical myelopa-thies due to spondylosis, ossification of the posterior longitudinal ligament and developmental cervical steno-sis. *Neuro-Orthop* 1988;5:25–35.

SSEPs were used in 35 cases to study three different patho-logic conditions. Cord vulnerability was noted to be variable with ossification of the posterior longitudinal ligament being the most significant factor. Stenosis was the least significant. This finding correlated in general with anteroposterior diameter although other factors were involved.

Lesser RP, Raudzens P, Lüders H, et al: Postoperative neurological deficits may occur despite unchanged intra-operative somatosensory evoked potentials. *Ann Neurol* 1986;19:22–25.

Six patients demonstrated postoperative neurologic deficits despite unchanged somatosensory evoked potentials during in-traoperative monitoring. The authors cite various reasons for this, including mishaps in unmonitored areas of the cord. They indicate that monitoring is still valuable, but that the physician should be aware of its possible limitations.

Levy WJ: Transcranial stimulation of the motor cortex to produce motor-evoked potentials. *Med Instrum* 1987;21:248–254.

The author describes experiments in cats in which the motor cortex was stimulated by electrodes placed on the skull and the roof of the hard palate and the responses recorded epidurally in the mid-thoracic area. This produced stimulation of the pyram-idal tracts, creating high-quality recordings superior to the so-matosensory recordings. This approach, although demanding, may be valuable for use in humans.

Lueders H, Gurd A, Hahn J, et al: A new technique for intraoperative monitoring of spinal cord function: Multi-channel recording of spinal cord and subcortical evoked potentials. *Spine* 1982;7:110–115.

The authors describe a system of monitoring in which multi-ple recording sites were used to measure peripheral nerve stim-uli. Forty surgical patients were studied with simultaneous recordings taken from below the surgical site, the interspinous ligament rostral to the site, the subcortical scalp, and cortical scalp areas. The authors concluded that the interspinous liga-ment recordings were the most useful; the subcortical responses were also helpful. They believed that the SCEP recordings were too variable to be of help and discontinued using them. One case of intraoperative changes is described.

Machida M, Asai T, Sato K, et al: New approach for diagnosis in herniated lumbosacral disc: Dermatomal somatosensory evoked potentials (DSSEPs). *Spine* 1986;11:380–384.

The authors studied 50 normal subjects and 40 patients undergoing lumbar disk surgery. DEPs were abnormal in 34 of 40 patients with herniated disks confirmed at surgery. Myelog-raphy produced eight false-positive or false-negative findings. The authors concluded that DEPs were a valuable, noninvasive diagnostic tool.

Machida M, Weinstein SL, Yamada T, et al: Dissocia-tion of muscle action potentials and spinal somatosen-sory evoked potentials after ischemic damage of spinal cord. *Spine* 1988;13:1119–1124.

The authors report their experience with MEP and SSEP monitoring in 30 patients undergoing spinal instrumentation. The motor system was stimulated through electrodes placed through the ligamentum flavum rostral to the surgical area and the compound muscle action potentials (CMAPs) were re-corded distally. In three cases changes were seen in the CMAPs but not in the SSEPs during derotation. They also studied ten dogs and noted similar dissociate responses with ligation of the thoracolumbar aorta or intercostal arteries. They recommended CMAP monitoring in derotation procedures.

Machida M, Weinstein SL, Yamada T, et al: Spinal cord monitoring: Electrophysiological measures of sensory and motor function during spinal surgery. *Spine* 1985;10:407–413.

The authors studied both afferent and efferent pathways while monitoring spinal cord function intraoperatively. Periph-eral nerve and spinal cord stimulus sites were used along with scalp, epidural, and muscle recording sites. Distal spinal cord stimulation and proximal cortical recording produced the best efferent responses, although the others were also effective. Prox-imal spinal cord stimulation and distal muscle recording was thought to be a useful adjunct.

Machleder HI, Moll F, Nuwer M, et al: Somatosensory evoked potentials in the assessment of thoracic outlet compression syndrome. *J Vasc Surg* 1987;6:177–184.

Of 80 patients with thoracic outlet compression syndrome, 74% had abnormal findings on the affected side, shown by de-creased amplitude and increased latencies. Changes in the re-cordings were correlated with changes in symptoms in 92% of the 47 patients for whom both preoperative and postoperative recordings were available.

More RC, Nuwer MR, Dawson EG: Cortical evoked potential monitoring during spinal surgery: Sensitivity, specificity, reliability, and criteria for alarm. *J Spinal Disorders* 1988;1:75–80.

SCEPs were used to monitor 158 patients undergoing correc-tive surgery for spinal deformity. Of these patients, 88% had stable recordings while 3% with preexisting neurologic deficits had unstable recordings. Eight patients had transient decreases in amplitude of more than 40% and one had partial paraplegia postoperatively. In no case was the hardware removed.

Mostegl A, Bauer R, Eichenauer M: Intraoperative

somatosensory potential monitoring: A clinical analysis of 127 surgical procedures. *Spine* 1988;13:396–400.

The authors present 127 cases in which SCEPs were used to monitor spinal surgery. They report brief decreases in the 73 patients undergoing posterior instrumentation and no significant changes in the 46 anterior cases despite ligation of vessels in 38 cases. True-positives were noted in six cases. The authors advocate using SCEPs supplemented with the wake-up test.

Nash CL Jr, Brown RH: Current concepts review: Spinal cord monitoring. *J Bone Joint Surg* 1989;71A:627–630.

The authors update the Current Concepts Review of 1983.

Owen JH, Laschinger J, Bridwell K, et al: Sensitivity and specificity of somatosensory and neurogenic-motor evoked potentials in animals and humans. *Spine* 1988;13:1111–1118.

The authors studied 55 animals by applying compression, ischemia, or distraction while recording SCEPs, SSEPs, and NMEPs. Reliable NMEP recordings were generated in more than 90% of animals. Both SCEPs and SSEPs were less sensitive. Comparative studies done in 111 patients resulted in 90% reliable recording of NMEPs and no postoperative neurologic deficits. The authors recommend the clinical use of NMEPs, SEPs, and the wake-up test as needed for patients undergoing osteotomy or instrumentation.

Perlik S, Fisher MA, Patel DV, et al: On the usefulness of somatosensory evoked responses for the evaluation of lower back pain. *Arch Neurol* 1986;43:907–913.

The authors compared electrodiagnostic and computed tomographic data for 30 patients with low back pain and unilateral radiculopathy. Of 27 patients with positive computed tomographic findings, 15 had positive myelographic findings and 21 had positive SCEPs. The authors concluded that SCEPs were helpful, particularly when sensorimotor or reflex signs were absent.

Rodriquez AA, Kanis L, Rodriquez AA, et al: Somatosensory evoked potentials from dermatomal stimulation as an indicator of L5 and S1 radiculopathy. *Arch Phys Med Rehabil* 1987;68:366–368.

The authors studied 50 patients with electromyography and dermatomal mapping and compared the results with those of myelography and/or computed tomography. The specificity of electromyography and DEPs were similar although the DEPs were not as sensitive or accurate. The two tests produced 27% false-negative and 9% false-positive results. The authors concluded that DEPs were not helpful in diagnosing radiculopathy.

Roy EP III, Gutmann L, Riggs JE, et al: Intraoperative somatosensory evoked potential monitoring in scoliosis. *Clin Orthop* 1988;229:94–98.

Sixty-three patients with scoliosis undergoing spinal surgery were studied. Monitoring was done with SSEP techniques; more than 85% of the patients had no changes in the recordings or neurologic status. False-positive findings occurred in 11% who had significant changes in the intraoperative recordings but no postoperative neurologic changes. Decreases in body temperature were thought to play a role in altering intraoperative records in these cases. One patient had both monitoring and postoperative sensory changes while one patient had a false-negative result (postoperative motor changes without intraoperative monitoring changes).

Ryan TP, Britt RH: Spinal and cortical somatosensory evoked potential monitoring during corrective spinal surgery with 108 patients. *Spine* 1986;11:352–361.

The authors note that cortical recording monitoring was successful in 107 of 108 patients. All 33 cases in which spinal epidural recordings were used were successful. The authors concluded that caudal and rostral epidural, subcortical, and cortical electrode sites were the most reliable for maximum patient safety.

Satomi K, Okuma T, Kenmotsu K, et al: Level diagnosis of cervical myelopathy using evoked spinal cord potentials. *Spine* 1988;13:1217–1224.

The authors studied 65 patients by means of median nerve and distal spinal cord stimulus sites and recording posteriorly over the ligamentum flavum from C-1 to T-1 in posterior cases and the intervertebral disk spaces in anterior cases. Using this approach and grading the responses obtained at each level, they were able to identify the primary lesion areas in 94.7% of posterior and 74.1% of anterior cases.

Szalay EA, Carollo JJ, Roach JW: Sensitivity of spinal cord monitoring to intraoperative events. *J Pediatr Orthop* 1986;6:437–441.

This study reviews 50 patients monitored with SCEPs. Waveform changes were correlated with intraoperative events; 22 of the 50 had stable recordings, 14 had technically poor recordings, 12 had false-positive recordings, and two had true-positive recordings. The authors concluded that SCEPs were sensitive but not necessarily specific.

Whittle IR, Johnston IH, Besser M: Recording of spinal somatosensory evoked potentials for intraoperative spinal cord monitoring. *J Neurosurg* 1986;64:601–612.

The authors report their experience with 26 patients undergoing intradural and extradural procedures. Monitoring with SSEPs provided good recordings in patients with and without neural deficits. Loss of waveform occurred with profound hypotension, longitudinal distraction, dorsal myotomy, and removal of intradural tumors. The SSEPs were considered useful in extradural surgery but had limitations with intradural cases.

19
Anesthesia for Orthopaedic Surgery

During the past two decades there has been a marked increase in the use of regional anesthesia in orthopaedic surgery as new local anesthetic drugs and new techniques have been introduced. Laboratory and clinical studies have clearly defined the physiologic and toxic effects of local anesthetic drugs, as well as the effects of regional anesthesia on various organ systems. The role of anesthesia in modifying perioperative morbidity and mortality has also been studied extensively. For example, studies have shown that the endocrine and metabolic changes occurring during surgery ("surgical stress") are inhibited by continuous epidural anesthesia. It has also been shown that regional (spinal and epidural) anesthesia decreases intraoperative blood loss during hip surgery. Further, the incidences of deep venous thrombosis and pulmonary embolism are significantly decreased by regional anesthesia. These findings suggest that, at least in orthopaedic surgery, regional anesthesia has a number of advantages over general anesthesia.

General Considerations

Preoperative Evaluation

The preoperative visit elicits relevant information such as the patient's present state of health, medical history, and previous reactions to anesthetic agents. This information allows the anesthesiologist to choose a particular technique on the basis of many factors, including the patient's age and physical state, the type and duration of the surgery planned, and the surgeon's needs.

Currently, about one in four patients admitted for surgery is more than 65 years old and approximately one in ten is more than 75 years old. Physiologic function decreases and significant illness with multiple organ system involvement is common in the geriatric population. Morbidity and mortality rates in the elderly appear to be related to medical problems present before surgery. Thus, a careful preoperative assessment is particularly important in the older patient.

Perioperative Medication

Perioperative medication depends on the patient's age and physical status and the surgical procedure planned. Preoperative medication is intended to allay anxiety and produce sedation without compromising cardiovascular or respiratory function. Preoperative sedation should be kept to a minimum in the elderly. The benzodiazepines produce sedation and amnesia. The use of opioids is recommended for major surgical procedures, especially when general anesthesia is used.

It is essential to obtain a drug history when assessing a patient preoperatively. Patients with cardiovascular disease, for example, may be taking many types of drugs, including antihypertensives, diuretics, antiarrhythmics, and cardiac glycosides. With the exception of diuretics, the patient should continue to take these medications until the time of surgery. This ensures good control of the underlying process for which patients are being treated. Other classes of drugs require careful consideration when preparing a patient for surgery and anesthesia; among these are insulin, steroids, psychotropic drugs, and the like.

Positioning

Careful positioning of the patient is of utmost importance. Patients with rheumatoid arthritis often have limited neck motion secondary to cervical spine involvement. Limitation of motion may be present in other joints as well. These patients require gentle positioning, especially when they are under general anesthesia. With a regional anesthesia technique, the patient can participate in the positioning. Extra padding is required for protection of particularly vulnerable parts, such as the ulnar and peroneal nerves. Avoiding pressure or stretching of the brachial plexus is important. The eyes must be protected by taping them closed and padding (especially when the patient is in the prone position) to prevent corneal abrasion.

Muscle and ligamentous relaxation during anesthesia may result in backache. The potential for backache increases with longer surgery and is not affected by the choice of anesthesia.

Regional Anesthesia

Regional anesthesia appears to offer a number of advantages over general anesthesia. This is especially true in orthopaedic surgery. The advantages of regional anesthesia may include a more rapid postoperative recovery, reduced intraoperative blood loss, and decreased incidences of deep venous thrombosis and pulmonary embolism. In addition, regional anesthesia can be prolonged into the postoperative period to provide analgesia.

Regional anesthesia appropriate for orthopaedic surgery includes central neural blockades (spinal and epidural blocks) and peripheral nerve blocks.

The main indication for a central neural block is surgery involving the lower extremities. Most data comparing the effects of regional anesthesia with those of general anesthesia are from patients undergoing hip surgery. This includes total hip replacement and surgery for fractured hip.

Blood Loss After Total Hip Replacement

Hip surgery is often associated with substantial blood loss. Both epidural anesthesia and subarachnoid block (spinal anesthesia) reduce blood loss. Some studies have reported reductions in blood loss of 50% or more.

In one study comparing general and spinal anesthesia in terms of blood loss in 234 total hip replacements, the mean blood loss for patients given general anesthesia was 1,088 ml, which was significantly more than the blood loss for patients given spinal anesthesia (594 ml). There was no correlation between intraoperative blood loss and blood pressure except when systolic blood pressure was maintained at or above 150 mm Hg. Thus, factors other than a decrease in blood pressure must be responsible for the decreased blood loss observed during regional anesthesia. Controlled ventilation during general anesthesia results in increased intrathoracic pressure. This in turn results in decreased venous return and increased peripheral venous pressure. This increased venous pressure may have been partially responsible for the increased bleeding in patients given general anesthesia. There was also a higher incidence of postoperative complications (pulmonary embolus, phlebitis, confusion, and local complications) with general anesthesia. Blood replacement needs were also significantly lower in the patients given spinal anesthesia.

Other investigators also reported significantly less blood loss after total hip replacement under epidural anesthesia than under general anesthesia (743 ml vs 1,168 ml in one study and 1,001 ml vs 1,504 ml in another). Blood transfusion was required in 70% of patients who received general anesthesia but in only 10% of patients during spinal block. One group, in two different studies, reported 28% and 39% decreases in blood loss in patients undergoing total hip replacement under epidural anesthesia. Postoperative blood loss was also significantly lower and fewer blood transfusions were needed in patients given epidural anesthesia. Significantly decreased postoperative blood loss was not reported in all studies, however. Some investigators found no differences between anesthetic techniques. The effects of regional anesthesia on blood loss after surgery for fractures of the hip are less consistent, perhaps because these procedures are associated with less blood loss than total hip replacement.

The mechanisms of diminished bleeding with regional anesthesia are probably multifactorial. Spontaneous respiration without an increase in intrathoracic pressure and a concomitant increase in venous return are important factors. Another significant factor is the lower blood pressure usually obtained with central neural blockade. This relative hypotensive anesthesia may also decrease intraoperative blood loss during hip replacement.

Deep Venous Thrombosis

Thromboembolism is a frequent complication after major surgery. The development of deep venous thrombosis can be predicted by the nature and number of risk factors present. For a young, healthy patient undergoing minor surgery, the incidence of deep venous thrombosis is approximately 2% and that of pulmonary embolism is about 0.002%. However, when risk factors such as age, congestive heart failure, malignancy, trauma, and orthopaedic or other major surgery are added, the incidence of deep venous thrombosis increases markedly. Patients undergoing hip surgery are at high risk for the development of deep venous thrombosis. Pulmonary embolism is probably the major cause of death after elective total hip replacement and it is one of the main causes for the high mortality associated with fracture of the femoral neck.

There is now evidence to suggest that the type of anesthetic technique, and regional anesthesia in particular, may decrease the incidences of deep venous thrombosis and pulmonary embolism in patients undergoing elective total hip replacement or surgery for fractured hip.

The method employed to detect deep venous thrombosis is important. A purely clinical assessment is inaccurate. Deep venous thrombosis will be present in 50% or fewer of patients with calf tenderness after surgery; most patients in whom deep venous thrombosis is diagnosed by more sensitive methods have no physical signs. At present, venography is the most sensitive method for determining the presence of deep venous thrombosis.

Spinal anesthesia is associated with a lower incidence of deep venous thrombosis than general anesthesia (29% vs 53% in one study of hip replacement and 40% vs 76.2% in a study of femoral neck fractures).

One study of 60 patients compared the incidences of thromboembolism and pulmonary embolism after total hip replacement under epidural and general anesthesia. All drugs with antiplatelet activity, such as acetylsalicylic acid and nonsteroidal anti-inflammatory drugs, were discontinued seven days before surgery and for 11 days after surgery. The patients underwent venography and perfusion lung scans two weeks before and two weeks after surgery. Thirty patients received general anesthesia (fentanyl, nitrous oxide-oxygen) and 30 patients received epidural anesthesia (0.5% bupivacaine with epinephrine). The group given epidural anesthesia received intermittent doses of epidural bupivacaine for postoperative analgesia for the first 24 hours after surgery. Parenteral narcotics were used for postoperative analgesia after general anesthesia. The overall incidence of deep venous thrombosis was 40% in the epidural group and 77% in the group given general anesthesia. When the location of the thrombosis was evaluated, the incidence of deep venous thrombosis in the popliteal and femoral veins was also significantly lower after epidural anesthesia (13% vs 67%). The frequency of pulmonary embolism, as assessed by perfusion lung scan, was 10% after epidural anesthesia and 33% after general anesthesia. Thus, epidural anesthesia appears to offer advantages over general anesthesia with respect to deep venous thrombosis formation in patients undergoing total hip replacement (Fig. 1).

Possible explanations for this beneficial effect of regional anesthesia have been proposed. Both spinal anesthesia and epidural anesthesia are associated with a reduction of blood viscosity, partially as a result of hemodilution and partially because of increased erythrocyte deformability. Arterial inflow, the venous emptying rate, and venous capacity are greater in patients given epidural anesthesia than in those given general anesthesia. The rheologic improvement seen with epidural anesthesia was more pronounced at the end of surgery and in the period immediately after surgery. This hyperkinetic limb blood flow may protect against "stasis" and thrombus formation. General anesthesia may create a predisposition to deep venous thrombosis by producing stasis in deep veins of the lower limb and substantially reducing blood flow in the lower limb.

Postoperative fibrinolytic activity is decreased in all patients regardless of the type of anesthesia employed. However, the degree of inhibition of fibrinolytic activity is lower after epidural anesthesia. This improved fibrinolytic activity may play a role in the decreased incidence of deep venous thrombosis after epidural anesthesia.

Local anesthetics themselves inhibit platelet adhesion,

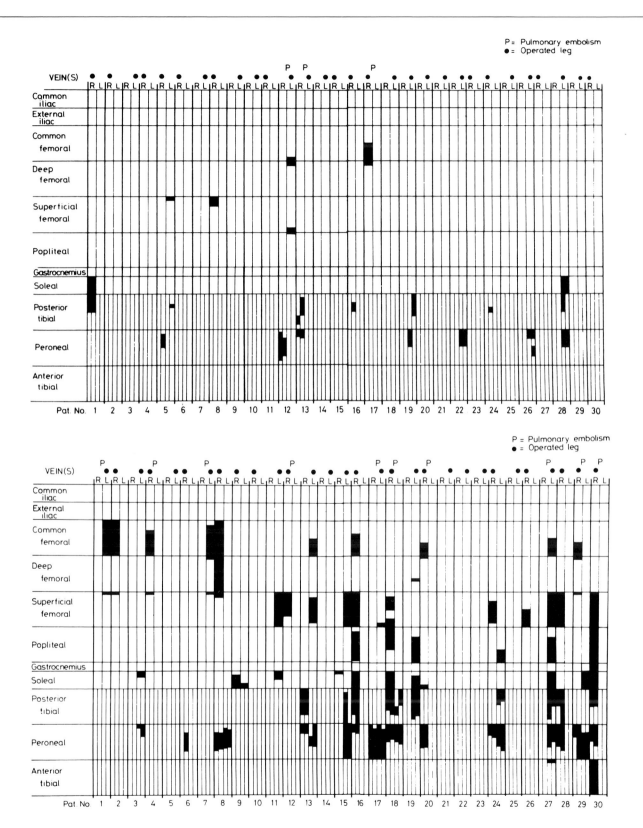

Figure 1

Sites, extents, and distributions of deep venous thrombosis and pulmonary embolism in patients given continuous epidural anesthesia (**top**) and general anesthesia (**bottom**). (Reproduced with permission from Modig J, Borg T, Karlström G, et al: Thromboembolism after total hip replacement: Role of epidural and general anesthesia. *Anesth Analg* 1983;62:174–180.)

aggregation, and release and leukocyte migration and aggregation. This was first shown with lidocaine, indicating that lidocaine may have an antithrombotic effect. More recently, investigators using bupivacaine for epidural anesthesia demonstrated a significant inhibitory effect on platelet aggregation in patients given epidural anesthesia. They concluded that the possible thromboprophylactic effects of epidural anesthesia and analgesia with bupivacaine may result from an inhibitory effect on platelet aggregation as well as increased blood flow in the lower limb.

It has been suggested that the frequency of thromboembolism after hip arthroplasty increases when surgery is associated with a large blood loss. One study examined the effects of hypotensive anesthesia on the incidence of thromboembolism. The authors studied four groups of patients. One group was given hypotensive anesthesia with sodium nitroprusside and dextran-70 for thromboprophylaxis. The second group was also given sodium nitroprusside but received a combination of dihydroergotamine mesylate and heparin for prophylaxis. The third group was given normotensive anesthesia with halothane and dextran-70 for prophylaxis. The fourth group was also given halothane anesthesia but received dihydroergotamine mesylate and heparin for prophylaxis. Hypotensive anesthesia reduced surgical blood loss and the number of blood transfusions. Deep venous thrombosis occurred in 48% of the patients. Anesthesia type made no difference in the incidences of deep venous thrombosis and pulmonary embolism. Thus, blood loss and blood transfusions are probably of minor importance in deep venous thrombosis after hip arthroplasty.

Deliberate Hypotension

Controlled or deliberate hypotension during general anesthesia has been employed for different surgical procedures for a number of years. Since it was first described by Cushing in 1917, the use of deliberate hypotension for surgery has been extensively studied, and today is a widely accepted technique. When properly used, deliberate hypotensive anesthesia is safe; it decreases blood loss and the need for blood transfusions. Further, the technique provides a relatively bloodless field, facilitating surgery and shortening the surgical procedure. The popularity of hypotensive anesthesia has fluctuated, especially for procedures other than cerebral aneurysm surgery. Current concerns about the possible transmission of infectious disease with blood replacement have increased interest in the technique of deliberate hypotension.

Blood pressure is decreased by the use of a variety of drugs. Deep anesthesia with an inhalation anesthetic (halothane, enflurane, isoflurane) has been used. However, more frequently, blood pressure is decreased by direct arterial or venous dilators, by ganglionic blocking drugs, α-adrenergic blockers, combined α- and β-adrenergic blockers, and calcium channel blockers. With the decrease in peripheral resistance and/or decrease in cardiac output, there is a proportional decrease in perfusion pressure. Adequate tissue blood flow persists over a wide range of subnormal blood pressures. Fine adjustments may be needed to achieve the desired pressure. These can be made by optimizing the patient's body position, alteration of airway pressure, control of heart rate, or by the use of vasoactive drugs that complement the effect of the primary hypotensive agent.

In orthopaedic surgery the main occasions for the use of deliberate hypotension are total hip replacement and back surgery for scoliosis.

Total Hip Replacement

Deliberate hypotension has been extensively used during total hip replacement. The significant decreases in blood loss and blood transfusions have been well documented.

Recent discussions of the use of hypotensive anesthesia for total hip replacement have compared different drugs used to produce hypotension. Sodium nitroprusside is the most widely used hypotensive agent because of its rapid onset, relatively consistent effect, and short half-life. Further, blood flow to vital organs is maintained at a perfusion pressure of 50 mm Hg. Potential side effects include cyanide and thiocynate toxicity, rebound hypertension, tachycardia, coagulation abnormalities, increased pulmonary shunting, and hypothyroidism.

Several other drugs have been studied in an attempt to find the ideal hypotensive agent. A comparison of diltiazem (a calcium channel blocker) and sodium nitroprusside in total hip replacement showed that diltiazem produced a weak and inconsistent decrease in blood pressure. It may produce moderate hypotension without tachycardia but the modulation of blood pressure is unpredictable. In this study, the dose of diltiazem had to be increased considerably to obtain the desired blood pressure. This increase in dose led to a significant depression in atrioventricular conduction. In addition, the hypotension produced by diltiazem lasted for approximately 30 to 60 minutes after discontinuation of the drug. It was concluded that blood pressure is difficult to control with diltiazem, and that the added depression of atrioventricular conduction is undesirable.

In a comparison of isoflurane (an inhalation anesthetic) to sodium nitroprusside for total hip replacement, the decrease in mean arterial pressure, the perioperative blood replacement needs, and postoperative hematocrit levels were the same with both drugs. However, isoflurane decreased systemic vascular resistance and oxygen consumption without changing cardiac index or pulmonary shunting. Thus, it was concluded that isoflurane is a good alternative to sodium nitroprusside. It is easy to use, efficient in producing a level of moderate hypotension, and decreases blood loss in total hip arthroplasty.

Although the advantages and safety of hypotensive anesthesia are well established, there is still concern about potential organ damage from hypoperfusion. The brain, for example, is particularly vulnerable to ischemia. One recent study investigated the effects of hypotensive anesthesia on cerebral blood flow and metabolism in patients undergoing total hip replacement. The patients ranged in age from 52 to 82 years. Deliberate hypotension was induced by sodium nitroprusside infusion. Mean arterial pressure was reduced to a mean of 52.1 mm Hg. Heart rate remained unchanged. There were no significant changes in cerebral blood flow or cerebral metabolic rate during hypotension or after blood pressure had returned to normal. No changes were observed in the serum levels of lactate and glucose. There was an expected decrease in cerebral vascular resistance. Cerebral blood flow is autoregulated within a wide range of perfusion pressures. If mean arterial pressure is below the lower limit of autoregulation, cerebral blood flow falls. In this study, cerebral blood flow remained unchanged, indicating that autoregulation was preserved.

One study compared the hemodynamic changes occurring with the use of acrylic cement during hypotensive and normotensive anesthesia. Considerable evidence exists concerning changes in blood pressure and cardiac output after the introduction of cement during hip arthroplasty. Three different drugs were used to induce hypotension—trimethaphan, nitroglycerine, and sodium nitroprusside. The induction and maintenance of anesthesia and fluid replacement was the same in all groups. There was a moderate decrease in mean arterial pressure after the insertion of cement into the acetabulum in the normotensive and the trimethaphan groups (11% and 8%, respectively). In contrast, the insertion of cement into the femoral canal significantly reduced mean arterial pressure in the normotensive and trimethaphan groups. Stroke volume and cardiac output were also moderately decreased in those two groups. However, the insertion of cement in the two groups treated with sodium nitroprusside and nitroglycerine caused no significant changes in any of the hemodynamic factors studied. Heart rate was unchanged in all groups.

The changes in mean arterial pressure and cardiac output observed in the normotensive group of patients indicate that the monomer is a potent vasodilator. The investigators concluded that sodium nitroprusside and nitroglycerine are preferable to trimethaphan for induction of hypotension during hip arthroplasty.

Spinal Fusion

Spinal fusion to correct scoliosis may be associated with substantial blood loss. Preoperative autologous blood harvesting is recommended to minimize or eliminate the use of banked blood. In addition, several techniques have been recommended in an attempt to decrease blood loss (for example, subcutaneous infiltration of saline with epinephrine 1:500,000 before incision). Careful positioning of the patient to avoid abdominal compression and to prevent venous engorgement is essential. Using a cell saver is recommended to reduce the need of transfusion. Normovolemic hemodilution to a hematocrit level of 0.24 to 0.26 (24% to 26%) and reinfusion of the harvested blood at the end of surgery decrease the need for homologous transfusions.

Induced hypotension during general anesthesia decreases blood loss significantly. In normotensive patients, hypotension can be induced to a mean arterial pressure of 60 mm Hg. Although different drugs have been utilized to induce hypotension, sodium nitroprusside and nitroglycerine are the most commonly used hypotensive agents.

The hypotensive effects of these two drugs have been studied in children and adolescents undergoing surgery for scoliosis. Nitroglycerine failed to produce rapid, predictable, and sustained decreases in blood pressure even at high doses. Sodium nitroprusside, however, produced rapid and reliable hypotension in all patients, including children in whom nitroglycerine was not effective.

The most recent study on the use of hypotensive anesthesia for scoliosis surgery reported the effects of moderate hypotension on blood loss, the need for transfusion, and the length of surgery in patients undergoing spinal fusion and Harrington rod instrumentation. Enflurane was employed to produce moderate hypotension. Blood pressure

was reduced and maintained at 20 to 30 mm Hg below the preoperative systolic pressure. This moderate hypotension was maintained from the time of incision to the beginning of closure.

The result was a reduction in blood loss of approximately 40%. The need for transfusion was reduced by nearly 45%, whereas the operating time was only shortened by 10%. Hemoglobin and hematocrit values in the postoperative period showed no statistically significant differences between normotensive and hypotensive anesthesia. Further, there were no complications related to the anesthetic technique.

To decrease the morbidity that may be associated with hypotensive anesthesia in scoliosis surgery (cord ischemia and subsequent neurologic deficit), a thorough preoperative evaluation and adequate intraoperative monitoring are essential.

Cervical Osteotomy

Flexion deformity of the cervical spine in ankylosing spondylitis is a chronic process during which the spinal cord adapts to the anatomic distortion. This process often progresses to extreme degrees of flexion deformity. Neurologic function, however, remains intact. Severe flexion deformity of the cervical spine may also be associated with rheumatoid arthritis. Surgical correction with extension of the neck is often required. This procedure is associated with difficult airway management and possible damage to the spinal cord (Figs. 2 and 3).

Until recently, surgical correction of flexion deformity was done with the use of local anesthesia supplemented with incremental doses of intravenous narcotics and sedatives and, occasionally, inhalation of nitrous oxide. This technique maintains the airway and minimizes the dangers of airway obstruction. It also allows continuous intraoperative assessment of neurologic function in an awake patient.

This surgical procedure can be safely performed with the patient under general anesthesia. A flexible fiberoptic bronchoscope allows the patient's trachea to be intubated with minimal discomfort and minimal or no trauma to the airway. Fiberoptic intubation in an awake patient requires adequate topical anesthesia applied to the nasopharynx, larynx, and trachea. Intravenous sedation should be used with caution. With experience, safe intubation of the trachea can be accomplished in awake patients capable of maintaining their own airways.

Neurologic function can easily be evaluated with somatosensory evoked potential monitoring. Cortical evoked potentials are obtained after stimulation of a peripheral nerve. These potentials can be affected by anesthetic gases, and low body temperature. They are independent of Pco_2 until the value decreases to less than 25 mm Hg. Somatosensory evoked potentials yield information about nerve conduction velocity along the peripheral sensory nerves and the sensory tracts of the central nervous system. Monitoring of somatosensory evoked potentials may help minimize the risk of neurologic injury during surgery on the spine.

Local Anesthesia for Arthroscopy

Local infiltration anesthesia is commonly used by surgeons for minor superficial procedures or to supplement an in-

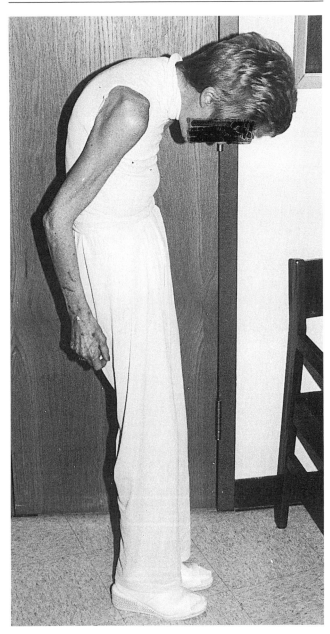

Figure 2
Patient with ankylosing spondylitis who subsequently underwent cervical osteotomy for correction of flexion deformity.

adequate regional block. Although most arthroscopic examinations of the knee and most surgical arthroscopic procedures are performed with the patient under general or regional anesthesia, an increasing number of these procedures are done on an outpatient basis with the patient receiving local anesthesia.

Recently, several reports of arthroscopy under local anesthesia have have been published. Various local anesthetic drugs (lidocaine, prilocaine, bupivacaine) have been employed with good results. In addition to infiltration of the area for arthroscopy, local anesthetic solutions are used for continuous irrigation or for intra-articular injection before insertion of the arthroscope.

Several benefits (such as avoidance of complications that may occur after general or regional anesthesia) have been attributed to the use of local anesthesia for arthroscopic procedures. This type of anesthesia has also been found to be safe, reliable, and inexpensive. Difficulties that may be encountered are bleeding and lack of relaxation. The judicious use of intravenous sedation with a short-acting narcotic such as fentanyl and a benzodiazepine such as midazolam is recommended to decrease discomfort and provide relaxation.

Intra-articular Bupivacaine

Intra-articular bupivacaine has been used to produce local anesthesia for arthroscopic procedures and to provide analgesia after such procedures. Bupivacaine has been used in concentrations of 0.25%, 0.5%, and 0.75%. The volume varies between 20 and 40 ml. Systemic absorption of bupivacaine after intra-articular injection results in detectable blood levels of the drug as early as five minutes after injection. A study comparing the effects of intra-articular injection of 20 ml of 0.25%, 0.5%, and 0.75% bupivacaine assessed the efficacy and acceptability of the procedure as well as the venous serum bupivacaine levels. The procedure was well accepted by both patients and surgeons. There were no significant differences among the different concentrations of bupivacaine in terms of the patient's comfort or surgical condition. However, serum levels of bupivacaine were consistently higher when the 0.75% solution was used. The maximum concentration occurred at 30 minutes with all concentrations studied and serum levels started to decline slowly at approximately 60 minutes. In this study, one patient who received 0.75% bupivacaine had a maximum concentration of 1.06 μg/ml.

Toxic reactions to bupivacaine rarely occur at plasma levels below 3 to 4 μg/ml. Central nervous system toxicity generally occurs at lower plasma levels of local anesthetic than does myocardial toxicity. However, bupivacaine exhibits a high degree of myocardial toxicity and the plasma levels at which central nervous system manifestations and cardiac toxicity occur are very close. Although 3 to 4 μg/ml is considered to be the toxic plasma level, a case of central nervous system toxicity with seizure was reported in a patient with a plasma level of 1 μg/ml. Thus, 0.25% or at most 0.5% concentrations of bupivacaine should be used for this procedure. A study of pharmacokinetics of intra-articular bupivacaine for arthroscopy, using 20 ml of 0.25% bupivacaine, found that the maximum concentration (0.48 ± 0.20 μg/ml) occurred at 43 ± 23 minutes. The elimination half-life was 189 ± 84 minutes. This maximum concentration was safe and well below the lowest level associated with clinical toxicity.

Malignant Hyperthermia

Malignant hyperthermia is a hypermetabolic disorder of skeletal muscle. Although it has been described as a heritable syndrome, and a heritable component is present in many cases, this is not invariably apparent from a patient's family history. Malignant hyperthermia is inherited in an autosomal dominant fashion and has been described as multifactorial, as having multiple penetrance, and as having a multigene origin. Malignant hyperthermia can be triggered by exposure to certain anesthetic drugs. Classically, malignant hyperthermia consists of increased body temperature, skeletal muscle rigidity, and acidosis but there is great variability in its clinical presentation.

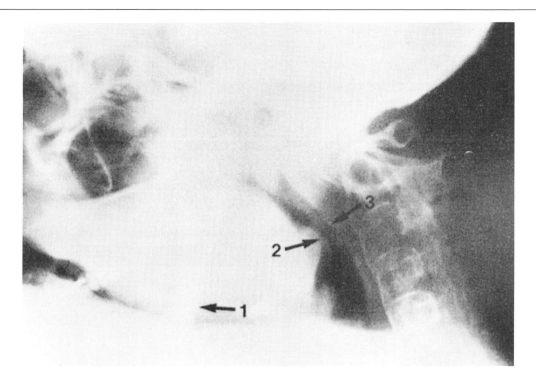

Figure 3

Lateral roentgenogram of the upper cervical spine of patient with flexion deformity secondary to rheumatoid arthritis. It shows a narrow anteroposterior dimension of the hypopharynx at the level of the epiglottis. 1, mandible; 2, epiglottis; 3, posterior pharynx. (Reproduced with permission from Ovassapian A, Land P, Schafer MF, et al: Anesthetic management for surgical corrections of severe flexion deformity of the cervical spine. *Anesthesiology* 1983;58:370–372.)

The classic initial signs are tachycardia and tachypnea. These result from sympathetic stimulation secondary to hypermetabolism and hypercarbia. An increase in blood pressure follows; this may be associated with ventricular arrhythmias. Muscle rigidity or increased muscle tone may then appear. Blood desaturation in the surgical field becomes apparent, and body temperature may increase 1 C to 2 C every five minutes. Other associated signs are molting of the skin, sweating, and cyanosis. Arterial blood gases show hypercarbia, oxygen desaturation, and respiratory and metabolic acidosis. Hyperkalemia, hypercalcemia, and myoglobinuria are also present. Renal failure secondary to myoglobinuria and disseminated intravascular coagulation can result.

Most commonly, the first manifestations occur in the operating room shortly after induction of or on emergence from anesthesia. However, malignant hyperthermia can occur any time intraoperatively, in the recovery room, or in the early postoperative period.

Malignant hyperthermia has been associated with a high mortality rate, especially before dantrolene sodium was accepted by the FDA in 1979 for its treatment. Early diagnosis and prompt therapy are mandatory. Death will result if the syndrome is not treated promptly.

Malignant Hyperthermia in Association With Other Syndromes

Some diseases or syndromes have been associated with malignant hyperthermia (Outline 1). It is assumed that an individual with one of these diseases or syndromes is predisposed to malignant hyperthermia and will develop ma-

Outline 1. Diseases reported to be associated with malignant hyperthermia*

Almost certainly related
  Central core diseases
Possibly related
  Duchenne's muscular dystrophy
  King-Denborough syndrome
  Other myopathies, such as:
    Becker's muscular dystrophy
    Fukuyama-type congenital muscular dystrophy
    Mitochondrial myopathy
    Myotonia congenita
    Periodic paralysis
    Sarcoplasmic reticulum adenosine triphosphatase deficiency syndrome
Apparently coincidental
  Neuroleptic malignant syndrome
  Sudden infant death syndrome
  Other diseases, such as:
    Glycogen storage disease
    Lymphomas
    Osteogenesis imperfecta

*Adapted from Brownell AKW: Malignant hyperthermia: Relationship to other diseases. *Br J Anaesth* 1988;60:303–308.

lignant hyperthermia if exposed to a triggering agent. The relationship between malignant hyperthermia and other syndromes can be categorized as one of "significant association" and "associations that seem only to be a chance occurrence."

Duchenne's Muscular Dystrophy This progressive disease results in severe disability at a very early age, with death occurring in early adulthood. These patients may require multiple orthopaedic procedures. Several complications with unusual presentations, which may mimic or actually be malignant hyperthermia, have been reported. These complications more commonly follow anesthetics with triggering agents, such as halothane and succinylcholine. Among them are ventricular arrhythmias associated with hyperkalemia, acidosis, and, occasionally, increased temperature and myoglobinuria.

In a recent retrospective study of complications asssociated with Duchenne's muscular dystrophy in patients undergoing surgery, 18 of 65 general anesthetics were associated with minor or more serious complications. Of the 18 complications, ten were associated with an increase in heart rate and body temperature. Thus, patients with Duchenne's muscular dystrophy should be considered at risk for developing malignant hyperthermia during general anesthesia.

Trends

Advances in orthopaedic surgery have been paralleled by concomitant advances in anesthesia. New anesthetic techniques, sophisticated monitoring, and the well-documented benefits of various anesthetic modes for orthopaedic surgery assure improved outcomes.

General anesthesia continues to be the most commonly used type of anesthesia, and certain surgical procedures require the use of general anesthesia. However, the morbidity associated with certain types of surgery can be altered by the anesthetic technique. An example of this is the use of hypotensive anesthesia for scoliosis surgery. Hypotensive anesthesia significantly decreases blood loss without increasing morbidity. The decreased blood loss leads to a decrease in blood transfusion requirements; this in turn lessens the possibility of complications such as transmission of viral diseases.

There is sufficient evidence to suggest that regional anesthesia offers significant advantages over general anesthesia in many types of orthopaedic procedures. The benefits of regional anesthesia include decreased blood loss after hip arthroplasty and decreased incidences of deep venous thrombosis and pulmonary embolism.

Finally, among the technical advances related to anesthesia are the management of difficult airways with the aid of fiberoptic bronchoscopy and monitoring of spinal cord function with somatosensory evoked potentials during spinal surgery. Techniques for monitoring motor tracts have been developed (electrical transosseal cortical stimulation and magnetic stimulation of the motor cortex). These techniques have been extensively investigated and are just beginning to be applied for clinical monitoring. Although still considered experimental, these techniques will probably be adopted as effective clinical tools.

Annotated Bibliography

Keywords

Anesthesia; Ankylosing spondylitis; Arthroscopy; Hypotension; Malignant hyperthermia; Osteotomy; Pulmonary embolism; Spinal fusion; Surgery; Thrombosis; Total hip replacement

General Considerations

Martin JT: Complications associated with patient positioning. *Anesth Analg* 1988;67(suppl 4S):1–6.

Potential complications associated with patient positioning are reviewed. Complications are not rare but most are preventable. The importance of the team approach to careful positioning in order to avoid potential injury is emphasized.

Regional Anesthesia

McKenzie PJ, Loach AB: Local anaesthesia for orthopaedic surgery. *Br J Anaesth* 1986;58:779–789.

A general review of the use of local anesthetics and regional anesthesia for orthopaedic surgery and the possible advantages of regional anesthesia. It includes a discussion of peripheral nerve blocks for surgery of the extremities.

Blood Loss After Total Hip Replacement

Keith I: Anaesthesia and blood loss in total hip replacement. *Anaesthesia* 1977;32:444–450.

The author examines the effects of three anesthetic techniques on blood loss. Blood loss was significantly reduced in patients who received epidural anesthesia compared with those who received general anesthesia with controlled ventilation. General anesthesia with spontaneous ventilation resulted in a greater blood loss than epidural anesthesia. However, the difference was not statistically significant. Postoperative blood loss was not related to anesthetic technique.

Sculco TP, Ranawat C: The use of spinal anesthesia for total hip-replacement arthroplasty. *J Bone Joint Surg* 1975;57A:173–177.

The authors report a significant reduction in intraoperative and postoperative blood loss as well as in the amount of blood transfused after total hip replacement with the patient under spinal anesthesia. The reduced blood loss was not related to hypotension.

Deep Venous Thrombosis

Henry CP, Odoom JA, ten Cate H, et al: Effects of extradural bupivacaine on the haemostatic system. *Br J Anaesth* 1986;58:301–305.

Epidural analgesia with 0.5% bupivacaine produced an inhibitory effect on platelet aggregation and platelet release. The inhibition of platelet aggregation may play a role in decreasing the incidence of deep venous thrombosis in patients given epidural anesthesia.

McKenzie PJ, Wishart HY, Smith G: Long-term outcome after repair of fractured neck of femur: Comparison of subarachnoid and general anaesthesia. *Br J Anaesth* 1984;56:581–585.

Patients undergoing surgery for femoral neck fracture demonstrated a significantly lower incidence of deep venous thrombosis after spinal anesthesia (40%) compared with patients given general anesthesia (76.2%) for the same surgical procedure.

Modig J, Borg T, Karlström G, et al: Thromboembolism after total hip replacement: Role of epidural and general anesthesia. *Anesth Analg* 1983;62:174–180.

Deep venous thrombosis occurred in 40% of patients given continuous epidural anesthesia and in 77% of those given general anesthesia. The incidence of popliteal and femoral vein deep venous thrombosis was also significantly lower after epidural anesthesia (13% vs 67%), as was the incidence of pulmonary embolism (10% vs 33%). Blood loss and blood requirements were significantly reduced by epidural anesthesia. Thus, epidural anesthesia is apparently beneficial in patients undergoing total hip replacement.

Thorburn J, Louden JR, Vallance R: Spinal and general anaesthesia in total hip replacement: Frequency of deep vein thrombosis. *Br J Anaesth* 1980;52:1117–1121.

Deep venous thrombosis after total hip replacement occurred in 29% of patients given spinal anesthesia but in 53% of those given general anesthesia. In addition, blood loss was reduced by 50% in the spinal anesthesia group. Spinal anesthesia apparently offers significant advantages over general anesthesia in this setting.

Deliberate Hypotension

Total Hip Replacement

Bernard JM, Pinaud M, Carteau S, et al: Hypotensive actions of diltiazem and nitroprusside compared during fentanyl anaesthesia for total hip arthroplasty. *Can J Anaesth* 1986;33:308–314.

The hypotensive effects of diltiazem and nitroprusside were studied in patients undergoing total hip replacement. Diltiazem induced and maintained moderate hypotension with an associated decrease in cardiac output. The significantly lower heart rate was probably a result of depression of atrioventricular conduction. Hypotension persisted for approximately 30 minutes after surgery ended. Arterial pressure was difficult to control with diltiazem.

Bernard JM, Pinaud M, Ganansia MF, et al: Systemic haemodynamic and metabolic effects of deliberate hypotension with isoflurane anaesthesia or sodium nitroprusside during total hip arthroplasty. *Can J Anaesth* 1987; 34:135–140.

In a study comparing isoflurane with sodium nitroprusside as a hypotensive agent in total hip replacement, the mean arterial pressure was decreased to 50% of the awake level by both drugs. The perioperative blood replacement and hematocrit levels were similar in both groups. Isoflurane appears to be an alternative to sodium nitroprusside for inducing hypotension.

Bünemann L, Jensen K, Thomsen L, et al: Cerebral blood flow and metabolism during controlled hypotension with sodium-nitroprusside and general anaesthesia for total hip replacement a.m. Charnley. *Acta Anaesthesiol Scand* 1987;31:487–490.

Cerebral blood flow and cerebral metabolic rate of oxygen were studied during hypotensive anesthesia, induced by sodium nitroprusside, in patients undergoing total hip replacement. Cerebral blood flow was unchanged during hypotension, indicating either that cerebral autoregulation was preserved or that the decreased cerebral vascular resistance caused by sodium nitroprusside helped preserve cerebral blood flow. There were no changes in cerebral metabolic rate of oxygen or lactate and glucose serum levels. There were no complications attributable to the hypotensive anesthesia technique.

Fredin H, Gustafson C, Rosberg B: Hypotensive anes-

thesia, thromboprophylaxis and postoperative thromboembolism in total hip arthroplasty. *Acta Anaesthesiol Scand* 1984;28:503–507.

The influence of hypotensive and normotensive anesthesia in combination with thromboprophylaxis on blood loss, deep venous thrombosis, and pulmonary embolism after total hip replacement was investigated. Hypotensive anesthesia reduced surgical bleeding. The incidences of deep venous thrombosis and pulmonary embolism were the same for normotensive and hypotensive patients. It appears that blood loss and blood replacement, which have been linked to the frequency of deep venous thrombosis, are probably of minor importance in causing deep venous thrombosis after hip surgery.

Vazeery AK, Skeie S, Anda O: Changes in cardiac output and systemic arterial pressure after insertion of acrylic cement during trimetaphan, sodium nitroprusside and glyceryl trinitrate-induced hypotension: A comparison with changes during normotension. *Br J Anaesth* 1983;55:783–790.

Normotensive patients showed a moderate decrease in mean arterial pressure after insertion of cement into the acetabulum, and a significantly greater decrease in mean arterial pressure after the insertion of cement into the femur. The cardiac index and cardiac output also decreased. Although these hemodynamic changes did not occur in hypotensive patients given sodium nitroprusside or nitroglycerine, mean arterial pressure decreased with monomer insertion in hypotensive patients given trimetaphan. It appears that sodium nitroprusside and nitroglycerine are better hypotensive agents in total hip replacement.

Spinal Fusion for Scoliosis

Patel NJ, Patel BS, Paskin S, et al: Induced moderate hypotensive anesthesia for spinal fusion and Harrington-rod instrumentation. *J Bone Joint Surg* 1985;67A:1384–1387.

Moderate hypotensive anesthesia was induced with enflurane supplemented by fentanyl. Blood loss, blood transfusion requirements, and surgical time were all significantly reduced. There were no complications attributable to anesthetic technique. Moderate hypotension may offer benefits for scoliosis surgery, without increasing morbidity.

Yaster M, Simmons RS, Tolo VT, et al: A comparison of nitroglycerine and nitroprusside for inducing hypotension in children: A double-blind study. *Anesthesiology* 1986;65:175–179.

Deliberate hypotension was defined as a mean arterial pressure below 55 mm Hg. Nitroglycerine failed to reduce mean arterial pressure to desired levels. Sodium nitroprusside consistently decreased mean arterial pressure even in patients who did not respond to nitroglycerine. Heart rate was decreased by both drugs. Cardiac output increased with sodium nitroprusside; Pao_2 increased and the alveolar-arterial oxygen diffusion gradient decreased with both drugs. Sodium nitroprusside appears to be the agent of choice for reliable and sustained induction of hypotension in children and adolescents.

Cervical Osteotomy

Ovassapian A, Land P, Schafer MF, et al: Anesthetic management for surgical corrections of severe flexion deformity of the cervical spine. *Anesthesiology* 1983;58: 370–372.

Severe flexion deformity of the cervical spine associated with rheumatoid arthritis was surgically corrected with the patient under general anesthesia. Somatosensory evoked potentials were monitored. Surgical correction of the most severe cervical flexion deformity can be accomplished with the patient under general anesthesia, careful management of the airway, and the use of somatosensory evoked potential monitoring.

Local Anesthesia for Arthroscopy

Besser MI, Stahl S: Arthroscopic surgery performed under local anesthesia as an outpatient procedure. *Arch Orthop Trauma Surg* 1986;105:296–297.

The authors present 875 patients who underwent arthroscopy under local anesthesia; 523 underwent arthroscopic surgery. The patients were discharged within one hour of completion of surgery. This technique of anesthesia is reported to be safe and reliable. It decreases morbidity and lowers hospital and patient costs as well.

Gerber H, Censier K, Gächter A, et al: Intra-articular absorption of bupivacaine during arthroscopy: Comparison of 0.25%, 0.5% and 0.75% solution, abstract. *Anesthesiology* 1985;63:A217.

Venous serum levels of bupivacaine after intra-articular injection were studied. The comfort of the patients and the surgeon's acceptance of the techniques were evaluated. Comfort was adequate at all three concentrations. The procedure was fully accepted by patients and surgeons. Slow absorption, with peak levels still present at 45 minutes, was reported. The concentrations of bupivacaine should not exceed 0.5%. Patients should not be discharged for at least one hour after injection.

Katz JA, Kaeding C, Hill J, et al: The pharmacokinetics of bupivacaine when injected intra-articularly following knee arthroscopy. *Reg Anesth*, 1988, suppl 13, pp 15–51.

The injection of 100 mg of bupivacaine into the knee joint results in safe peak plasma concentration within the first hour of tourniquet release. Peak concentrations can be minimized by increasing the time from injection to tourniquet release.

Kirkeby OJ, Aase S: Knee arthroscopy and arthrotomy under local anesthesia. *Acta Orthop Scand* 1987;58:133–134.

Local infiltration of lidocaine combined with intra-articular injection of the same local anesthetic was used. Only one patient found the procedure very painful. There were no complications. The authors concluded that this is a safe and practical technique for diagnostic arthroscopy and arthroscopic surgery.

Malignant Hyperthermia

Larsen U, Juhl B, Sorensen O, et al: Complications during anaesthesia in patients with Duchenne's muscular dystrophy (a retrospective study). *Can J Anaesth* 1989; 36:418–422.

This report examines the complications encountered in 44 patients with Duchenne's muscular dystrophy who underwent 84 surgical procedures. Sixty-five general anesthetics were administered, 18 of which were associated with complications. In ten cases these included tachycardia and increased body temperature. These ten patients had received an anesthetic that included halothane and/or succinylcholine.

20
Congenital Abnormalities

Isolated congenital malformations, such as clubfoot or hip dislocation, are discussed elsewhere in this volume. The concern here is with congenital abnormalities that affect much of the skeleton, the connective tissue, or the muscles. The causes of these syndromes are just beginning to be understood and may involve genetic factors, fetal environmental factors, or both. Often the specific local deformity becomes less important when the entire array of abnormalities is considered.

Skeletal Dysplasias

A skeletal dysplasia is a generalized developmental disorder that affects both bone and cartilage. Although each individual disorder is rare, the skeletal dysplasias when taken together affect a substantial number of patients. Most, if not all, appear to involve simple mendelian inheritance, either autosomal dominant or autosomal recessive. Various classifications have been offered but the standard remains *The International Nomenclature of Constitutional Disorders of Bone*, based on a symposium held in Paris in 1976. Nevertheless, many patients with skeletal dysplasia fail to fit into any of the groups classified in this volume. Ultimately, a better understanding of the biochemical factors involved should produce a more logical classification. For the present, however, most skeletal dysplasias are known by the region of the bone affected roentgenographically (epiphyses, metaphyses, and the like). Early diagnosis assists in planning for the child's social as well as orthopaedic needs and permits accurate genetic counseling. In some conditions, a diagnosis can be made prenatally by amniocentesis or ultrasonographic measurement of disproportionately short femurs.

Multiple Epiphyseal Dysplasia

This is one of the most common bone dysplasias and is characterized by short stature and irregular epiphyses. In many cases, height at maturity may be only 152 cm. The irregular epiphyseal growth usually, but not always, involves the joints symmetrically. There is a wide range of involvement (Fig. 1). The ossification centers appear late, and are often fragmented and irregular. There is minor vertebral involvement. The femoral capital epiphyses are always affected, with the femoral heads eventually becoming flattened. Precocious arthritis is the rule. The child characteristically has a waddling, painful gait with a stiff hip; understandably, Legg-Calvé-Perthes disease is often the initial (incorrect) diagnosis. Multiple epiphyseal dysplasia is almost always inherited as an autosomal dominant condition.

Spondyloepiphyseal Dysplasia

The several varieties of spondyloepiphyseal dysplasia are usually distinguished by the severity of dwarfing and the magnitude of coxa vara. Autosomal dominance is the usual mode of transmission, but the very severe cases are sporadic. Spondyloepiphyseal dysplasia congenita is the most severe form; it is characterized by dwarfism with a profoundly disproportionate short trunk and gross disorganization of the upper end of the femur. Lumbar lordosis with a protuberant abdomen and thoracic kyphosis with pectus carinatum are usual. Because of the associated atlantoaxial instability, myelopathy develops in many patients. The ossification of the femoral capital epiphyses is delayed, often not appearing until the child is 5 years old. Coxa vara develops early, often with discontinuity of the femoral necks. This combination of absent ossification, high-riding femurs, and limited hip abduction gives the false impression of congenitally dislocated hips. Arthrograms demonstrate that the femoral head is within the acetabulum. Arthrography is, therefore, recommended in the planning of appropriate surgical procedures. The gait is waddling, hip motion is progressively lost, and precocious arthritis ensues. As yet, there is no consensus regarding the management of the hip. Genu valgum and rigid clubfeet occur regularly.

Metaphyseal Chondrodysplasia

There are several eponymic forms of chondrodysplasia, all of which affect the metaphyses, especially the upper end of the femur with secondary coxa vara. The initial features include a waddling gait, lumbar lordosis, genu varum, and short stature. The classic roentgenographic features of expanded metaphyses with irregular cupped physeal plates resemble rickets, and serum calcium and phosphorus levels should be measured to exclude that diagnosis (Fig. 2). The epiphyses themselves are spared, so precocious arthritis is not a feature. Metaphyseal chondrodysplasias are usually diagnosed not at birth, but during the child's second or third year. The roentgenographic changes in the metaphyses disappear after physeal closure. Most metaphyseal chondrodysplasias are inherited as autosomal dominant disorders.

Achondroplasia

Although this is an autosomal dominant disorder, nearly all cases are new mutations. This is the most common type of short-limbed dwarfism, with a prevalence of between 0.5 and 1.5 per 10,000 births. The characteristic short limbs, bulging forehead, and depressed nasal bridge seen at birth are characteristic of achondroplasia. The trunk is of almost normal length, but the extremities are short; the proximal segment is more severely affected than the distal segment (rhisomelia). At maturity the average height is 130

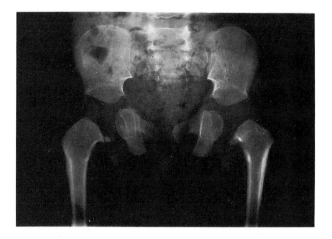

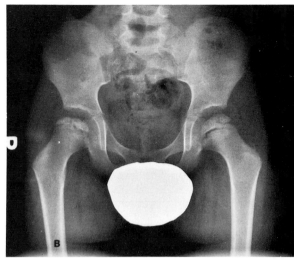

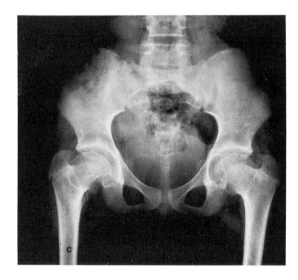

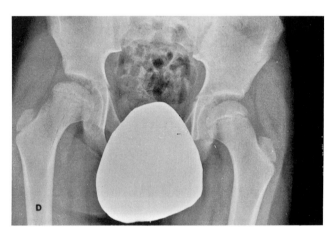

Figure 1

The spectrum of multiple epiphyseal dysplasia. **Top left,** Failure of ossification of the femoral heads in this 22-month-old girl could be mistaken for hip dysplasia with or without osteonecrosis. **Top right,** Bilateral irregular ossification of the femoral heads in this boy at the age of 4 years 4 months could be mistaken for Legg-Calvé-Perthes disease. **Bottom left,** In this 11-year-old girl, the flattened and enlarged femoral heads with coxa vara and short femoral necks represent a more severe expression of multiple epiphyseal dysplasia. **Bottom right,** The same patient shown at top right at the age of 9 years 7 months. The femoral heads have lost height and the multiple epiphyseal dysplasia has a milder appearance.

cm for men and 125 cm for women. The underlying cause of achondroplasia is not known; no biochemical abnormalities have been detected. It is presumed that the growth disturbance results from abnormal enchondral ossification.

Infants and young children with this condition are hypotonic and walking is often delayed until the age of 3 years. Intelligence is normal. Respiratory problems are common in children because of the constricted thoracic cage and bony encroachment of the upper airways. Some 3% of the children have undetected hydrocephalus. The bulging forehead often invalidates head circumference measurements, and the delay in developmental milestones and hypotonia may further confuse the issue. If coexisting hydrocephalus is suspected, a computed tomographic scan of the head is recommended.

Thoracolumbar kyphosis is usual in infancy, and characteristically resolves spontaneously as the child begins to walk. A wedged vertebra at the thoracolumbar junction

may cause the kyphosis to persist or progress; this is a rare but potentially serious problem. The pathognomonic roentgenographic features of the spine include short pedicles and progressive narrowing of the interpedicular distances from L-1 to L-5 (Fig. 3). This spinal stenosis produces substantial disability in as many as 20% of adults with achondroplasia. Spinal claudication, impotence, and progressive neurologic deficit may begin as early as the third or fourth decade of life. Paralysis is most likely if the thoracolumbar kyphosis has persisted. Evaluation by magnetic resonance imaging or computed tomography is preferred to myelography. Extensive decompressive laminectomy is indicated, but care must be taken to assess any kyphosis.

The craniocervical junction is abnormal in patients with achondroplasia. The foramen magnum is small and misshapen; this can lead to compression of the medulla or upper cervical spine. The prevalence of this complication

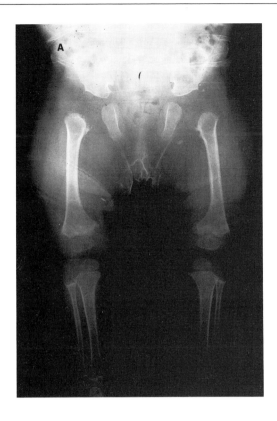
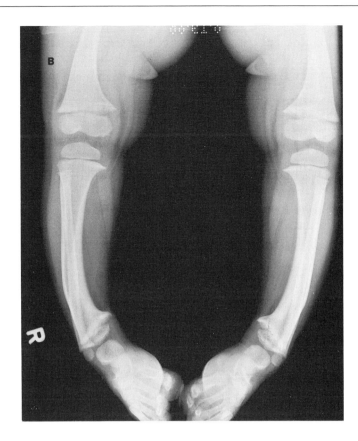

Figure 2

Metaphyseal chondroplasia and rickets. **Left**, Radiograph of an 18-month-old girl with metaphyseal chondroplasia shows expanded metaphyses, irregular physes, and normal epiphyses. **Right**, Radiograph of a 23-month-old girl with hypophosphatemic (vitamin D-resistant) rickets. The irregular and cupped epiphyses and bowlegs are also characteristic of metaphyseal chondroplasia and may cause the two conditions to be confused.

is not known, but the condition has been shown to cause sleep apnea and respiratory dysfunction as well as long-tract signs. Computed tomography accurately evaluates the anatomy and may identify patients who are at greater risk for respiratory or neurologic complications. Suboccipital surgical decompression has been beneficial.

Several clinical and roentgenographic features have no clinical significance but serve only to confirm the diagnosis. These include the trident hand, in which the long and ring fingers deviate from each other, the subluxated radial head with limited elbow extension, and the pelvic shape of flat acetabula and small sciatic notches. Precocious arthritis and hip disability are not features of achondroplasia (Fig. 3).

The distal femoral metaphysis is flared and the somewhat chevron-shaped distal femoral epiphysis is recessed into it. The fibula is disproportionately long when compared with the tibia. Nevertheless, the precise cause of the bowlegs in achondroplasia is not clear. The long fibula may force the foot into varus. Bracing for genu varum is ineffective, with the orthosis simply opening the joint medially because of ligamentous laxity. The orthosis restricts motion, and thereby interferes with the activities of daily living. In some cases, osteotomy of both the tibia and the fibula to restore plumb-line alignment is indicated. Patellofemoral mechanics must be maintained or restored.

The advent of sophisticated rigid but dynamic axial fixation systems (such as the Ilizarov system) and the de-

velopment of techniques for controlled symmetric distraction of the physeal plate (chondrodiastasis) or the lengthening of long bones by callus distraction (callotasis) have been applied to patients with achondroplasia. Surgery before the age of 10 years is not advocated. The lower limb is lengthened by about 30% (7.5 cm each in the femur and the tibia); time to healing is about ten months. There is a high incidence of complications with these techniques (20% to 40%) and the patient remains unbalanced because the arms are relatively short unless humeral lengthening is also undertaken. The application of these limb-lengthening techniques has been justified by cosmetic, psychological, and functional rationales, but it remains controversial inasmuch as the major medical problem affecting patients with achondroplasia is not height but the associated spinal, neurologic, and pulmonary dysfunction.

Diastrophic Dysplasia

This short-limbed dwarfism is far less common than achondroplasia but produces striking orthopaedic deformity. There is a rigid clubfoot that is resistant to surgical techniques, an abducted "hitchhiker's" thumb, and anterior hip flexion deformities. The axial skeleton is malformed and malaligned with a short, sharp, rigidly angular kyphosis in the upper thoracic spine, cervical kyphosis, odontoid hypoplasia, scoliosis, and prominent pectus carinatum. This autosomal recessive disorder produces a pri-

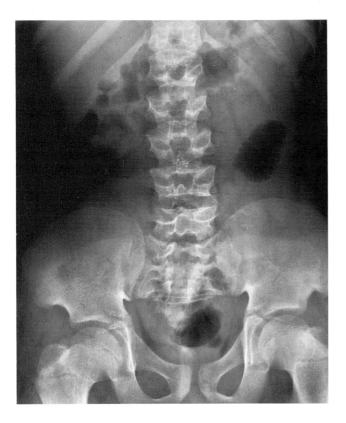

Figure 3
Radiograph of the pelvis and lumbar spine of a 10-year-old girl with achondroplasia. The diagnostic features include progressive narrowing of the interpedicular interval from L-1 to L-5, flared iliac wings, short femoral necks, and no evidence of precocious hip arthritis.

mary cartilage abnormality that is indirectly demonstrated by a misshapen ear with hemorrhage in the pinna, the so-called cauliflower ear. Cardiorespiratory problems are frequent.

The Storage Diseases

These include the mucopolysaccharidoses and the mucolipidoses. The mucopolysaccharidoses are diagnosed by the presence of mucopolysaccharides in the urine. They show strikingly similar roentgenographic and clinical features, and are clinically separated by the severity of the findings and the particular complex sugar present in the urine (for example, heparan sulfate, keratan sulfate). Biochemical analysis of polysaccharide metabolism in fibroblast cultures has established heterogeneity within several of the primary mucopolysaccharidoses. Different eponymic diseases are caused by the same enzyme defect, and several enzyme defects can cause the same eponymic disease. The specific enzyme deficiencies for ten mucopolysaccharidoses have now been elucidated (Table 1).

All affected patients have somewhat thickened and coarse facial features, short stature, and stiff joints, especially in the hands. Typical roentgenographic findings include oval vertebral bodies, often beaked anteriorly, and a characteristic pelvis with wide flat ilia, large capacious

Table 1. The mucopolysaccharidoses

Type	Syndrome	Biochemical Defect
I	Hurler; Scheie	α-L-Iduronidase
II	Hunter	Sulfoid uronate sulfatase
IIIA	Sanfilippo A	Heparan N-sulfatase
IIIB	Sanfilippo B	N-Acetyl-α-D-glucosaminidase
IIIC	Sanfilippo C	Acetyl CoA: α-glucosaminide-N-acetyltransferase
IIID	Sanfilippo D	N-Acetyl-α-D-glucosaminide-β-sulfatase
IVA	Morquio A	N-Acetylgalactosamine-6-sulfatase
IVB	Morquio B	β-Galactosidase
VI	Maroteaux-Lamy	Arylsulfatase B
VII	Sly	β-Glucuronidase

acetabula with unossified femoral head cartilage, and apparent coxa valga.

The roentgenographic and clinical features become more apparent as the child gets older, and these storage diseases can be quite difficult to diagnose at birth. All are inherited as autosomal recessive disorders except mucopolysaccharidosis II (Hunter's syndrome), which is X-linked. Mucopolysaccharidoses I and IV are the most common.

Mucopolysaccharidosis I Mucopolysaccharidosis I (Hurler's syndrome, Scheie's syndrome) is not clinically diagnosable at birth. As the mucopolysaccharide accumulates in the tissues, coarse facial gargoyle features and hepatosplenomegaly gradually develop during the first few months of life, becoming obvious by the age of 18 months. Mental retardation, short stature with a disproportionately short trunk, thoracolumbar kyphosis, and corneal opacities become increasingly apparent with age. It is a progressive disease warranting only symptomatic treatment because death from cardiopulmonary complications is usual by the age of 10 to 15 years.

Mucopolysaccharidosis IV Children with mucopolysaccharidosis IV (Morquio's syndrome), on the other hand, have normal intelligence and survival well into adult life is usual. Short stature is apparent by the age of 3 years and thereafter rapidly progresses to a short-trunk disproportionate dwarfism with a prominent pectus carinatum. The extensive array of orthopaedic deformities includes odontoid hypoplasia and atlantoaxial instability, often leading to myelopathy; platyspondyly and thoracolumbar kyphosis, also leading to myelopathy; and severe genu valgum accentuated by profound ligamentous laxity.

Mucolipidoses The mucolipidoses are a group of storage diseases with many phenotypic and skeletal features similar to those of the mucopolysaccharidoses, including coarse facial features, thoracic cage deformity, and stiff joints. There is no excessive mucopolysaccharide in the urine, but tissue culture analysis demonstrates peculiar intracellular inclusions in the fibroblasts. Specific enzyme defects have been found for two of the four mucolipidoses.

Multiple Hereditary Exostosis

Multiple hereditary exostosis is one of the most common skeletal dysplasias. It is an autosomal dominant disorder that has a wide spectrum of involvement from very mild to very severe. This variation occurs in affected members of the same family. Intelligence is normal. Stature is unaffected in those mildly affected, but more than 75% of patients are below the mean height for their age. In addition to the limbs being short in general, side-to-side differences occur, making leg-length discrepancies very common. Further, disproportionate growth between the radius and ulna and between the tibia and fibula leads to various angular malformations and disturbances in joint mechanics. Cartilage-capped exostoses (osteochondromas) arise from the metaphyseal region, pointing away from the epiphysis; as the child grows, they appear to move down the diaphysis. These bony lumps are usually noted during early childhood, but may be detected at birth. They increase in size and number as the child grows, ceasing growth at skeletal maturity. The flat bones of the pelvis and scapulas are not spared, nor are the posterior elements of the vertebrae.

Particularly troublesome sequelae include peroneal nerve compression, diastasis of the ankle, and genu valgum, which can be managed by asymmetric stapling. Diminished pronation-supination and progressive ulnar deviation of the hand caused by shortening of the ulna are common problems in the forearm.

Chondrosarcoma is the most serious complication and, although its incidence is difficult to determine, probably occurs in less than 2% of affected individuals more than 20 years old. A change in the size of an exostosis or the onset of pain in an affected adult should be evaluated. Monitoring patients by means of annual technetium bone scans has been recommended.

Enchondromatosis

Enchondromatosis (Ollier's disease) is a rare nongenetic disorder characterized by unossified cartilage in the metaphyses and the diaphyses. Roentgenographically these may be no more than streaking in the proximal femur or the iliac wings, but there may also be large masses of cartilage at the ends of a long bone. Involvement is markedly asymmetric and often entirely unilateral. The affected limb is short, bone deformity may be severe, and pathologic fractures are always a risk. The spine is usually spared. The lesions continue to enlarge during growth, but stop enlarging at the time of puberty. The incidence of malignant degeneration is about 25% by the age of 40 years. However, the risk is far greater if hemangiomas are present (Maffucci's syndrome). The chondrosarcomas that develop in patients with enchondromatosis tend to be low-grade and can be managed effectively with current surgical techniques.

Maffucci's Syndrome

This skeletal dysplasia consists of multiple enchondromas and hemangiomas. The vascular malformations are subcutaneous cavernous hemangiomas, and produce little disability. The enchondromas are located throughout the skeleton, but there is a predilection for the small bones of the hands and feet. They tend to be distributed asymmetrically, producing angular deformity and limb-length discrepancy. For the adult patient with Maffucci's syndrome, sarcomatous transformation of the enchondroma is almost a certainty. Serial technetium bone scans are a valuable way to monitor such patients. The chondrosarcomas tend to be of low-grade malignancy. There is also a predilection for the development of nonskeletal malignancies, especially in the abdominal viscera and central nervous system; most of these prove to be fatal. Such nonskeletal malig-

nancies often develop at the same time or within a few years of the secondary chondrosarcomas. Thus, periodic surveillance of the brain and abdomen for undetected malignant lesions is indicated. This rare syndrome has no genetic basis.

Connective Tissue Disorders

Marfan's Syndrome

Marfan's syndrome is defined solely by its clinical features and its mode of inheritance. No laboratory test is available to confirm the clinical impression. The diagnosis is made when the patient meets at least two, and preferably more, of the major diagnostic criteria: (1) a positive family history; (2) cardiac disease, usually dilation of the ascending aorta or mitral valve prolapse; (3) dislocation of the ocular lens; (4) a variety of musculoskeletal abnomalities, including a characteristic body habitus (dolichomelia), arachnodactyly, pectus excavatum, scoliosis, and ligamentous laxity.

Marfan's syndrome is an autosomal dominant disorder, but fully a quarter of the patients have no family history of the condition and represent new mutations.

Early diagnosis of cardiac lesions is accomplished by echocardiography. Newer medical and cardiovascular surgical techniques are prolonging life expectancy, which previously was the early 40s. Contact sports, weight-lifting, and other isometric exercises have traditionally been prohibited, but there is no evidence that restricting sports is of any benefit.

Patients with Marfan's syndrome are characteristically more than 182 cm tall, and the slenderness of their limbs exaggerates their height. However, both clinical and radiographic measurements of the marfanoid habitus overlap with those of the normal population, and no one calculation is more specific than another.

The ligaments are lax and the joints are hypermobile; chronic and recurrent subluxations of the patella, the shoulder, the sternoclavicular joint, and the thumb metacarpophalangeal joint are common. Pes planovalgus, genu valgum, and genu recurvatum are additional manifestations of this generalized disorder of connective tissue. It follows, therefore, that the results of soft-tissue surgery to correct joint instability are often disappointing. Therapy designed to improve muscle strength and relieve symptoms is a sound initial program.

Although most patients with Marfan's syndrome have some distortion of spinal alignment, scoliosis is significant enough to require treatment in only 20%. The chest has a diminished anteroposterior diameter and a lack of the normal thoracic kyphosis produces a characteristic flat-back appearance. Scoliosis often develops before the age of 9 years and may worsen rapidly. The curves respond poorly to orthoses, in part because of the accompanying thoracic lordosis. Pseudarthroses often complicate spinal fusion. Progesterone and estrogen therapy to induce premature puberty in girls (as a means of controlling both height and curve progression) has not been successful. High-grade symptomatic spondylolisthesis occurs in patients with Marfan's syndrome.

Dural ectasia and anterior meningocele may be present and are thought to result from the transmission of normal cerebrospinal fluid pulsations through dura composed of weakened and defective collagen.

An unexplained high incidence of protrusio acetabuli occurs in young patients with Marfan's syndrome. It may be progressive, symptomatic, and accompanied by chondrolysis. The long narrow foot, with a disproportionately long great toe, makes fitting shoes a problem, and the valgus hindfoot may need to be controlled by an orthosis or arthrodesis.

The specific biochemical errors that account for the pathologic changes in Marfan's syndrome are unknown. Studies have suggested, however, that there is an aberration in the structure of collagen, and defective side-chain cross-linking has been implicated.

Homocystinuria

The clinical resemblance of homocystinuria to Marfan's syndrome often results in a misdiagnosis. Homocystinuria, which is inherited as an autosomal recessive disorder, is an inborn error of methionine metabolism, characterized by a deficiency of the enzyme cystathionine synthase. The abnormally high concentration of homocystine in the blood is reflected in the urine, where it can be detected by the cyanide-nitroprusside test. However, this test may give a false-negative result in some homocystinuric patients, and a quantitative serum amino acid analysis, therefore, is indicated in patients for whom there is a high index of suspicion. Homocystinuria shares certain phenotypic features with Marfan's syndrome. The patients are taller than average and have long, thin limbs. However, instead of the ligamentous laxity and hypermobility present in Marfan's syndrome, patients with homocystinuria have joint stiffness, and finger contractures are common. Pes cavus is almost always present. One third of patients have scoliosis and progressive kyphosis is not uncommon. Genu valgum is often severe enough to justify osteotomy, but recurrence is common. Osteoporosis is a distinctive feature and leads to vertebral flattening with end-plate indentation. The skeleton is spared in infancy, but by the end of the first decade the osteoporosis, vertebral collapse, and elongation of the long bones have evolved. The ocular lens dislocates, but, in contrast to Marfan's syndrome, it luxates downward and toward the nasal side.

An important and devastating feature of homocystinuria is the propensity for spontaneous thrombotic episodes. Thrombi may occur in medium-sized arteries and veins, producing widespread occlusive phenomena, including thrombophlebitis, claudication, pulmonary embolism, and renal artery thrombosis. The propensity for such thrombosis is enhanced by general anesthesia, by surgery, and by contrast studies that involve manipulation of the arteries and veins.

The toxic effects of homocystine on the nervous system produce mental retardation, seizures, and disturbed behavior.

Homocystinuria is treatable. Patients treated with pyridoxine from infancy develop a normal skeleton. The toxic level of homocystine in the system can be reduced by oral administration of pyridoxine hydrochloride (vitamin B_6), the coenzyme for cystathionine synthase, and by a methionine-restricted diet (one that substitutes vegetables for animal and dairy protein).

Multiple Endocrine Neoplasia Type 2b

This is a rare genetic disorder, but its phenotypic similarity to Marfan's syndrome and a high incidence of slipped capital femoral epiphysis make it of some orthopaedic significance. The first symptoms of this syndrome affect the musculoskeletal system and include tall stature, scoliosis, slipped capital femoral epiphyses, and cavus feet. The tongue is bumpy and the lips thickened because of ganglioneuromatosis in this area. The major cause of mortality is the endocrine tumors—medullary thyroid carcinoma and pheochromocytoma. Prompt recognition of this syndrome permits treatment of a thyroid cancer before metastasis, and of a pheochromocytoma before a hypertensive crisis.

Ehlers-Danlos Syndrome

Ehlers-Danlos syndrome is a heterogeneous group of disorders characterized by abnormality of the skin, the joint ligaments, and other connective tissue. The spectrum is highly variable; those mildly affected show no more than a slight deviation from normal and those severely affected have a life-threatening disease. The various forms of Ehlers-Danlos syndrome are separated on the basis of their clinical features, their pattern of inheritance, and by specific biochemical abnormalities (Table 2). The expanding classification of the Ehlers-Danlos syndrome now includes 11 distinct types. However, as many as one half of all patients who have clear manifestations of this syndrome cannot easily be fitted into the present schema, and specific biochemical defects have been found in only a few instances.

The cutaneous manifestations include hyperextensible skin. Although it is not lax, it can be stretched over an unusually large range. It has a soft, velvety texture. It is fragile, and healing results in shiny scars that have been likened to cigarette paper or papyrus. There is a tendency for wounds to dehisce. Some children have been mistakenly thought to be victims of child abuse.

Connective tissues supporting the blood vessels can also be affected, with the development of varicose veins and aneurysms. In patients with type IV, shear forces from normal activity may produce a catastrophic rupture of large and medium-size arteries. Similarly, the supporting structures of the colon, bladder, and uterus are weakened; diverticula develop and occasionally a hollow viscus ruptures spontaneously. Spontaneous pneumothorax and mitral valve prolapse also occur.

The joints are hypermobile; in many cases they are unstable as well. Dislocations may be acute, chronic, or repetitive. Chronic effusions and arthralgias are common. Symptomatic shoulder instability is usually multidirectional. Patellar dislocation and subluxation are present in almost all cases. Dislocations along the thumb ray (interphalangeal, metacarpophalangeal, and carpometacarpal joints) are particularly disabling. Muscle strengthening is the best initial therapy. The benefits of ligament surgery are only temporary. Arthrodesis of the trapeziometacarpal joint has been helpful.

Osteogenesis Imperfecta

This group of disorders is characterized by fragility of bone, but there is a wide variation in severity. In its most severe form the child is either stillborn with multiple fractures, or dies in the early neonatal period. In the mildest form it may be detected only when osteoporosis develops in adults with no history of repetitive fractures. Various classifications have been offered, but the most popular one (Table 3) incorporates the time and frequency of fractures,

Table 2. Ehlers-Danlos syndrome

Type	Inheritance	Biochemistry	Major Clinical Features		
			Skin	**Joints**	**Other**
I Gravis	Autosomal dominant	Unknown	Fragile; hyperextensible; easily bruised	Laxity with dislocation	Scoliosis; varicose veins; hernia; premature birth
II Mitis	Autosomal dominant	Unknown	Moderately hyperextensible; mild bruising	Moderate laxity in hands and feet; no dislocations	——
III Benign hypermobile	Autosomal dominant	Unknown	Normal	Severe laxity; frequent dislocations	——
IV Ecchymotic	Autosomal dominant or autosomal recessive	Decreased type III collagen synthesis and/or secretion	Thin; severe bruising; deep tissues very friable	Laxity only in hands and fingers; occasional dislocations	Aneurysms; spontaneous artery rupture; rupture of uterus and colon; early vascular death
V X-linked	X-linked recessive	Deficiency of peptidyl lysine oxidase (?)	Strikingly hyperextensible; mild fragility and bruising	Minimal laxity; no dislocations	——
VI Ocular-scoliotic	Autosomal recessive	Deficiency of peptidyl lysine hydroxylase	Moderately hyperextensible; moderate fragility and bruising	Moderate laxity with dislocations	Severe scoliosis; ocular fragility; congenital clubfeet; "floppy baby"
VII Arthrochalasis multiplex congenita	Autosomal dominant and autosomal recessive	Deficiency of procollagen n-protease; resistant terminal cleavage site in procollagen 2	Moderate fragility and hyperextensibility	Severe laxity; frequent dislocations; bilateral congenital dislocated hips	Scoliosis; short stature; abnormal facies
VIII Periodontosis	Autosomal dominant	Protease-sensitive collagen (?)	Mild hyperextensibility; severe fragility	Moderate laxity, especially fingers; no dislocations	Periodontal disease with tooth loss
IX Occipital horns	X-linked recessive	Deficiency of peptidyl lysine oxidase and abnormal copper metabolism	More lax than hyperextensible	Hands and feet lax but elbows stiff	Widespread skeletal dysplasia; occipital bony exostoses; congenitally dislocated radial heads; urinary tract dysplasia
X Platelet dysfunction	Autosomal recessive	Abnormal fibronectin	Moderately hyperextensible; easily bruised	Laxity in hands and feet; no dislocations	Defect in platelet aggregation
XI Familial joint laxity	Autosomal dominant	Unknown	Normal	Severe laxity; frequent dislocations; patellar subluxation; congenital dislocated hip	——

the color of the sclera, and the genetic factors; unfortunately, it does not always allow the diagnosis to be established in a newborn. Because the outcome cannot be precisely predicted, management of this disorder is entirely clinical. Osteogenesis imperfecta often includes many of the features of other connective tissue disorders. The ligaments are lax, the skin is often thin and distensible, and bruising occurs easily. Poor scar formation is present in some.

The skeleton is exceedingly fragile. Acute fractures generally heal promptly with normal-appearing callus, but remodeling into mature lamellar bone does not occur, making the limb again susceptible to fracture. Nonunions occur in almost 20% of patients, and are more common than

Table 3. Classification of osteogenesis imperfecta

Type	Inheritance	Sclera	Clinical Features
I	Autosomal dominant	Blue	Fractures during childhood; hearing loss; subgroups with and without opalescent teeth; most common type
II	Autosomal recessive	Blue	Lethal in perinatal period; crumpled long bones; flattened vertebrae; very rare
III	Autosomal recessive	White	Birth fractures and progressive deformity; markedly short stature; subgroups with and without opalescent teeth; spinal deformity and costovertebral anomalies
IV	Autosomal dominant	White	Skeletal fragility; no hearing loss; moderate growth failure; may have opalescent teeth

once thought. All fractures in patients with osteogenesis imperfecta must be properly splinted and braced. A vigorous hyperplastic callus is occasionally seen and rare, malignant degenerations of this hyperplastic callus have been reported. Multiple microscopic fractures occur on the tension side of the long bones, leading to rather marked deformity. Multiple realignment osteotomies using telescoping intramedullary rods are recommended to maintain functional alignment in both the upper and lower extremities. It is best to realign all the bones simultaneously. Weightbearing using supportive braces should begin as soon as possible. Innovative brace designs, such as vacuum pants orthoses, have been developed in an attempt to achieve comfortable standing, reduce the number of fractures, and possibly improve bone density. Fractures usually cease at puberty.

Prognosis for ambulation is guarded. Most of those born with multiple fractures and those who survive the respiratory complications of the neonatal period will be wheelchair-dependent. Most patients whose fractures do not begin until after ambulation starts will, however, remain ambulatory.

Other signs of abnormal collagen are present in only some patients with osteogenesis imperfecta; these include blue scleras and abnormal dentin that gives the teeth an opalescent appearance and a propensity for decay. A floppy mitral valve may also be detected. All patients with osteogenesis imperfecta should undergo regular audiologic examinations.

The presence of blue scleras, wormian bones in the skull, opalescent teeth, and a characteristic small triangular face helps distinguish children with osteogenesis imperfecta from battered children, a differentiation that can be a challenge in the emergency room.

Severe scoliosis is present in one half of the patients. Bracing is ineffective because of the plasticity of the chest wall. Posterior spinal instrumentation has worked successfully, although augmentation with methylmethacrylate has occasionally been required. Even in those without scoliosis, osteoporosis and multiple vertebral compression fractures lead to symptomatic back deformity.

Ultrastructural and biochemical analysis of the skeleton and fibroblast cultures have shown that heterogeneity is far more extensive than is suggested by clinical classifications. The basic biochemical abnormality appears to be in the processing of procollagen to type I collagen. There is no evidence that systemic medication has had any beneficial effect. Calcium, phosphorus, magnesium, vitamin C, vitamin D, parathormone, fluoride calcitonin, and diphosphonate have all been tried but to no avail.

Arthrogryposis Multiplex Congenita and Arthrogryposis Syndromes

Children with arthrogryposis have deformed, fusiform limbs, smooth creaseless skin, rigid joints, and a variety of congenital malformations including clubfeet, dislocated knees, and dislocated hips. However, more than 100 syndromes whose main features include congenital contractures have been called arthrogryposis. Multiple causative factors have been uncovered, including aberration of the fetal environment, infectious agents, drugs, maternal illness, and physical insults. All act either directly or indirectly on the motor system of the fetus to cause immobilization of the limbs. The most frequent pathologic finding is a reduction in the number of anterior horn cells in the spinal cord. The risk of arthrogryposis recurring in a family ranges from zero in those disorders resulting from a teratogen or an unfavorable intrauterine environment to as high as 50% for those syndromes resulting from an autosomal dominant gene.

Arthrogryposis Multiplex Congenita (Amyoplasia)

Classic arthrogryposis multiplex congenita is now commonly called amyoplasia. Amyoplasia has consistent features that enable it to be differentiated from the myriad of other similar syndromes. These include (1) characteristic limb position, which is symmetric, and includes adducted internally rotated shoulders, extended elbows, and flexed wrists, hyperflexed abducted hips, and clubfeet, (2) essentially normal facies, with no significant dysmorphic features, (3) a lack of visceral malformations, (4) normal intelligence, and (5) no family history of arthrogryposis.

Amyoplasia is not a genetic disorder. There is, curiously, an increased incidence of one of a pair of identical twins having amyoplasia.

Roentgenographic changes in the joints are adaptive; all are secondary to the failure of motion and the fixed joint position. Scoliosis, which occurs in one third of patients, takes the form of a C-shaped curve. Congenital scoliosis is very rare. There are no diagnostic laboratory tests. Electromyographic and nerve conduction studies yield inconsistent findings. Muscle biopsy specimens from patients less than 4 months old are difficult to interpret. Specimens from patients more than 4 months old may show both neuropathic and myopathic changes. Thus, the diagnosis of amyoplasia remains a clinical one.

The combination of a breech presentation and stiff malpositioned limbs makes delivery difficult and fractures common. Despite the relative frequency of this disorder, little is known about its natural history or the functional status of adults. Nearly one in four children will be unable to walk, and an even larger number will, at maturity, remain partially or completely dependent on others.

The goals of treatment are alignment and stability of the lower limb to permit ambulation and mobility of the upper limb for self-care skills. Initial treatment begins in the newborn nursery with active physical therapy, and then splinting to maintain what has been gained by exercise. Surgery to release inelastic periarticular structures is best done early, before adaptive changes in the skeleton.

There is agreement regarding the importance of reducing a unilateral congenital dislocated hip, but management of bilateral dislocation remains controversial. Because gait is not compromised and motion, although limited, remains, most orthopaedic surgeons do not favor reduction.

Knee flexion deformity beyond 30 degrees precludes both bracing and ambulation. Hamstring and posterior capsule release, followed by prolonged bracing to delay recurrence, gives satisfactory results, but an extension osteotomy of the distal femur is, nevertheless, often needed toward the end of growth. The clubfoot in arthrogryposis resists all nonsurgical techniques, has a high incidence of surgical complications, and has a very high recurrence rate after surgery. Early posterior, medial, lateral, and plantar soft-tissue release, combining capsulotomies and tendon excision, has been successful in some cases. Talectomy has been a satisfactory salvage procedure, but is gaining favor as a primary procedure. The upper extremity must be considered as a whole, and the two arms must be considered together. The goals of treatment are to allow self-help skills, such as toileting and feeding, and mobility skills, such as pushing out of a chair and using crutches. The neuromuscular scoliosis of arthrogryposis responds poorly to nonsurgical measures.

Larsen's Syndrome

This genetic disorder (usually autosomal dominant, but autosomal recessive cases have also been described) is characterized by multiple congenital dislocations of the large joints. There is a unique pattern, with bilateral anterior dislocation of the tibia on the femur, bilateral dislocated hips, bilateral elbow dislocation, and bilateral clubfeet. The most consistent finding is bilateral congenital dislocation in the knee. Dislocation of the knee is rare; therefore, whenever it is encountered, Larsen's syndrome must be considered. The facial features are characterized by a flattened appearance with a prominent forehead. The ligaments are lax, and stable joint reductions are difficult to achieve by either surgical or nonsurgical means. Abnormal segmentation of the cervical vertebrae causes remarkable malalignment with a severe cervical kyphosis that may lead to quadriplegia. A more idiopathic type of scoliosis is present in the thoracic and lumbar spine.

Distal Arthrogryposis Syndrome

In distal arthrogryposis syndromes, the congenital contractures predominantly affect the distal portion of the limb (hands and feet) and, on occasion, the face. They are a heterogeneous group that, in general, are inherited in an autosomal dominant pattern. The hand and foot deformities respond better to treatment than do similar deformities in amyoplasia. The diagnosis is confirmed if the hands have an ulnar deviation of the fingers at the metacarpophalangeal joint, flexion contractures at the metacarpophalangeal and proximal interphalangeal joints, a deeply cupped palm, and a flexed adducted thumb with motion limited by a thick web extending from the palm to the proximal phalanx. The various patterns of clubfoot deformity include, on occasion, congenital vertical talus. The Freeman-Sheldon or whistling face syndrome is one of the distal arthrogryposes and is so termed because of the deeply set eyes, bulging fleshy cheeks, and extremely small mouth with pursed lips. The hand and foot deformities, however, are typical of those found in all distal arthrogryposis syndromes.

Multiple Pterygium Syndrome

This syndrome is characterized by cutaneous webs across the flexor aspects of the limbs. When fully manifest, the multiple pterygium syndrome includes webs across every flexion crease, including the lateral neck, the popliteal space, the axillae, the antecubital, interdigital, and intercrural regions, and chin to sternum. When the webs are not as well developed, this syndrome is easily confused with amyoplasia. One means of differentiating them, however, is that 80% of patients with pterygium syndrome have congenital vertical tali, and more than 50% have significant congenital scoliosis with multiple areas of defective segmentation. Lordoscoliosis with substantial trunk shortening is common. If surgery to release the popliteal web is undertaken, it is best accomplished early, before secondary deformity of the knee joint occurs. The leading edge of the web contains a thick fibrous band running from ischium to the os calcis; just beneath it, a veil of muscle fibers hides the sciatic nerve. Multiple pterygium syndrome is an autosomal recessive disorder.

Neurocutaneous and Vascular Syndromes

Neurofibromatosis

Neurofibromatosis (von Recklinghausen's disease) is one of the most common genetic disorders in humans, occurring in one per 3,000 newborns. It is an autosomal dominant disorder that affects both sexes equally. Many patients appear normal at birth because the full manifestations of neurofibromatosis may not be present until after puberty. Some 40% of patients have a major orthopaedic problem. The severity of the disease varies, and there is a wide range of expression, which makes early diagnosis difficult. Café-au-lait spots, although usually present at birth, may take up to a year to appear. Thereafter their number and size increase; thus, an emphasis on number, size, or shape is inappropriate during the first decade of life. Neurofibromas begin to appear by the age of 10 years and increase in number during puberty. They are composed of benign Schwann cells and fibrous connective tissue and may occur anywhere on the body. They may be sessile or peduncular on the skin or may develop along the path of a peripheral nerve or nerve roots. They rarely cause any neurologic deficit. The so-called plexiform neurofibroma, on the other hand, is usually present at birth and may be diagnosed by a dark-brown pigmentation of the overlying skin. The skin may hang in pendulous folds. Plexiform neurofibromas may lead to limb overgrowth and gigantism, they may infiltrate the neuraxis, or they may grotesquely disfigure the face. They are highly vascular, and surgical extirpation is either impractical or impossible.

Scoliosis is frequent and may be the initial complaint. Curves are either of the dystrophic or the idiopathic type. The dystrophic curve is short and sharp, with widening of the neural foramina, erosion of the pedicles, distortion of the vertebral bodies, and thinning of the ribs. It is relentlessly progressive and may prove refractory to brace treatment. Only prompt surgical fusion leads to good results. The idiopathic type of curve behaves like an idiopathic scoliosis and can be managed accordingly.

Pseudarthrosis of a long bone may accompany neurofibromatosis. The bone is usually the tibia, but may be the ulna, femur, clavicle, radius, or humerus. The relationship between congenital pseudarthrosis and neurofibromatosis is well documented, but the precise mechanism remains obscure because surgical specimens typically fail to show neurofibromas at the pseudarthrosis site. The prognosis for establishing union remains guarded, and the technique offering the best chance for success is still a matter of opinion. Free vascularized grafts are generating considerable interest.

Limb overgrowth, partial gigantism, and macrodactyly have a relationship with plexiform neurofibromas, but the precise pathologic mechanism has not been completely explained. Overgrowth is not symmetric or uniform, as in idiopathic hemihypertrophy; the dermis and the subcutaneous tissues become disproportionately hypertrophic while the skeleton is affected more erratically.

Erosive defects and cystic changes in the skeletons of children with neurofibromatosis roentgenographically can resemble a number of benign—and occasionally malignant—conditions.

Children with neurofibromatosis are short, with large heads. Often they experience precocious puberty. Almost one half have an intellectual handicap.

Proteus Syndrome

The signs of Proteus syndrome overlap with those of other overgrowth conditions, such as idiopathic hemihypertrophy, Klippel-Trenaunay syndrome, Maffucci's syndrome, and—most importantly—neurofibromatosis. Indeed, it has been suggested that John Merrick (the Elephant Man) had Proteus syndrome. The bizarre array of abnormalities seen in Proteus syndrome include partial gigantism of the hands or feet or both, macrodactyly, thickening and deep furrowing of the skin on the palms of the hands and soles of the feet, cutaneous hemangioma, pigmented nevi, subcutaneous lipoma, varicosities, macrocephaly, and cranial hyperostosis. Scoliosis and genu valgum are common. The progressive nature of the deformities is striking, and can lead to grotesque overgrowth, facial disfigurement, angular malformations, and severe scoliosis. Surgical intervention is helpful, but there is nonetheless a high rate of recurring deformity.

Klippel-Trenaunay Syndrome

It is well known that vascular malformations can contribute to overgrowth, and that the overgrowth may be severe. The most frequently encountered vascular malformation syndrome is that described by Klippel and Trenaunay. This syndrome was originally thought to be a triad of cutaneous hemangioma, varicose veins, and limb hypertrophy. However, deep arteriovenous malformations are the major cause of disability. The cutaneous hemangiomas are of the port-wine variety. Varicose veins are a consistent finding; a tortuous and dilated vein on the lateral border of the leg is typical. However, the arteriovenous malformations can range from a functionally insignificant microscopic fistula to one that has a substantial hemodynamic effect. Abnormalities in the lymphatics may also occur. Hemangiomas in the developing limb may significantly interfere with morphogenesis, leading to congenital amputations. Overgrowth may be limited to part or all of the limb and affects both the soft tissue and the skeleton. Management depends on a thorough evaluation and understanding of the vascular abnormality. Surgical excision of the arteriovenous malformation is rarely successful; often the most practical approach to the severely hypertrophied part is amputation.

Chromosomal Syndromes

Down's Syndrome

With an incidence of one per 660 births, Down's syndrome is the most common chromosomal abnormality in humans. Its frequency increases with maternal age. Cytogenetic studies reveal that 95% of cases are the result of trisomy 21; mosaics account for 2%, and translocations involving the 21st chromosome account for the remainder.

The degree of mental impairment varies within rather wide limits, and performance always seems better than formal intelligence testing would indicate. Congenital heart disease is present in 50% of the patients; major congenital abnormalities in the gastrointestinal tract are common and a frequent cause of death in early infancy. Leukemia is present in about 1% of patients with Down's syndrome. Seizures increase with age. Endocrine dysfunction, such as hypothyroidism and juvenile-onset diabetes mellitus, is frequent, and a susceptibility to infection persists through life. There is premature aging, with patients always looking older than their chronologic age, and a progressive dementia closely resembling Alzheimer's disease ensues. Nevertheless, the use of antibiotics, improved heart surgery, and the rearing of most children with Down's syndrome at home has greatly increased life expectancy.

Despite our knowledge that the cause of Down's syndrome is the extra genetic information on the 21st chromosome, nothing is known yet of the basic underlying biochemical mechanisms. Children with Down's syndrome exhibit a generalized growth retardation, with a mean height of 154 cm in men and 145 cm in women. They have disproportionately short legs. On the average, the onset of independent ambulation is delayed to between the second and third year. The gait is broad-based, with side-to-side waddling and outwardly turned feet. Ligamentous laxity and hypotonia are a consistent finding in young children with Down's syndrome. Although ligamentous laxity tends to decrease with age, it plays an important role in many of the orthopaedic abnormalities encountered. Orthopaedic problems are second only to heart disease as a cause of morbidity in this syndrome.

Some 15% of children with Down's syndrome show roentgenographic evidence of an increased atlanto-dens interval of 5 mm or more. However, the significance of this finding is not clear. At least 85% of patients with atlanto-dens intervals of 5 mm or more have no neurologic signs or symptoms. Data are lacking to support the notion that C1-C2 instability predisposes to progressive subluxation and myelopathy. Those who develop signs of myelopathy usually do so before the age of 10 years; the myelopathy is chronic and insidious. Girls, for unknown reasons, are more susceptible. The variety of symptoms and signs of C1-C2 instability and the difficulty of communicating with these patients often delay diagnosis. Thus, it is recommended that all patients with Down's syndrome undergo roentgenographic evaluation of the cervical spine. This is best performed after the child has begun walking and after there is sufficient ossification of the vertebrae to allow for accurate measurements (usually when the child is 3 to 4 years old). Whether or not a single roentgenographic examination is sufficient and whether or not C1-C2 instability can later develop in children with no initial instability are controversial issues. Controlled long-term longitudinal studies are lacking. Children with increased atlanto-dens intervals but no evidence of myelopathy have been advised to avoid sports that require stressful weight-bearing on the head, such as gymnastics, tumbling, and diving. Restricting all sports is not justified. Indeed, because so many patients with catastrophic C1-C2 subluxation or dislocation have readily detectable physical signs for several weeks, a physical examination with careful attention to neurologic signs may well be better than a radiographic examination for screening children who plan to participate in the Special Olympics or other activities. Children with an increased atlanto-dens interval and myelopathy require cervical spine fusion.

Abnormalities in the configuration of the odontoid are also present; these include hypoplasia and ossicle terminale. When present in conjunction with an atlanto-dens dislocation, it is a warning that the C1-C2 subluxation is irreducible and that prolonged attempts at reduction may worsen neurologic function. The radiographic anatomy of some odontoid ossicles is more consistent with avulsions, implicating a traumatic rather than a developmental cause.

Cervical spine screening of persons with Down's syndrome has disclosed that anomalies exist not only at the C1-C2 articulation but throughout the cervical spine. They include hypoplasia of the posterior arch of C-1, which can make attempts to achieve C1-C2 fusions difficult, posterior subluxation of the occiput on C-1 when the neck is extended, spondylolysis of midcervical vertebrae, and precocious arthritis of the cervical spine, especially at C-4 through C-6.

One half of patients with Down's syndrome have a scoliotic curve of the idiopathic type, with the apex at the midthoracic region. Congenital scoliosis is uncommon. Progression is more likely to occur in female institutionalized patients. Management of the spinal deformity by orthosis or with surgery is appropriate. Lumbar spondylolysis and spondylolisthesis are common.

The radiographic appearance of the hip in a newborn with Down's syndrome suggests stability. The femoral head is well covered and the acetabulum is ossified laterally, so that a high center-edge angle is seen. Clinically, however, the hip is hypermobile, although stable. The problems of hip instability begin some time during the first decade, and may affect as many as one in 20 persons with Down's syndrome (Fig. 4). In some there is an acute dislocation, in others a habitual dislocation with spontaneous reduction, and in still others a chronic subluxation with acetabular dysplasia. This progressive loss of hip stability and acetabular dysplasia may continue even after skeletal maturity. Treatment depends on the age of the patient, the status of the dislocation, and the configuration of the acetabulum. In children, the status of the redundant hip capsule, the acetabulum, and the proximal femur must all be taken into consideration. Overall, results have been satisfactory. In adults, reconstructive surgery, including total joint replacement, has been successful but the long-term results are not known.

Slipped capital femoral epiphysis, a regular occurrence in patients with Down's syndrome, has a high frequency of acute slips, chondrolysis, and osteonecrosis.

Most knee problems are related to ligamentous instability and the patella. About one third of patients have subluxation and as many as 10% have frank dislocation. Ligamentous laxity is responsible for the disrupted patellofemoral mechanics. Nevertheless, most patients are ambulatory and have little obvious disability. Surgical correction of a subluxating patella in Down's syndrome is best approached with extreme caution because of recurring dislocations postoperatively, symptomatic chondromalacia, and loss of knee motion.

The planovalgus configuration of the foot, although a characteristic feature of Down's syndrome, is usually asymptomatic, requiring neither orthopaedic appliances nor surgical intervention. Metatarsal primus varus, common in childhood, often persists and leads to symptomatic hallux valgus. There is a curious, and as yet unexplained, association of juvenile rheumatoid arthritis with Down's syndrome.

Turner's Syndrome

Turner's syndrome occurs in females with a single X chromosome (XO). Some cases, however, are mosaic (XO/XX), and others result from a deletion of part of the X chromosome. Short stature, sexual infantilism, web neck, and cubitus valgus are the diagnostic features. The ovaries are replaced by streaks of stromal tissue. The low hairline and web neck are suggestive of Klippel-Feil syndrome, but roentgenography shows no vertebral abnormalities and no cervical spine disability ensues. Growth retardation is a cardinal feature; if untreated, women will be only 137 to 142 cm tall. Idiopathic scoliosis is common, and may begin early in childhood. The delay in skeletal maturation allows an extended period of time for curve progression.

The current treatment for growth retardation and sexual infantilism consists of combinations of estrogen, growth hormone, and androgens, and may cause a rapid progression of the scoliosis. Cubitus valgus occurs in 80% of patients, but remains asymptomatic with full rotation of the forearm and full flexion and extension of the elbow. Genu valgum is common. A prominence on the proximal tibia is present but requires no treatment. There is relative shortening of the fourth and occasionally the fifth metacarpal and, in some instances, the corresponding metatarsal. Clinically, this creates a depressed knuckle and a short toe, and serves as a good clue to the diagnosis of Turner's syndrome in a young girl who has scoliosis and small stature.

Noonan's Syndrome

Because the phenotype of Noonan's syndrome—short stature, web neck, and cubitus valgus—is identical to that of Turner's syndrome, this condition has been called male Turner's syndrome. Noonan's syndrome, however, occurs in males who have a normal XY genotype and also in girls who have a normal XX genotype. Some 40% of patients with Noonan's syndrome have scoliosis and a distinctive chest wall deformity consisting of pectus carinatum superiorly and pectus excavatum inferiorly. Other characteristics include a degree of mental retardation and right-sided congenital heart defects. It has been said that children with Noonan's syndrome are at risk for developing malignant hyperthermia at the time of surgery. These reports may represent confusion of Noonan's syndrome with King-Denborough syndrome, a rare myopathic arthrogryposis that shares some phenotypic features with Noonan's

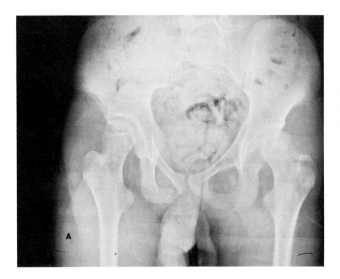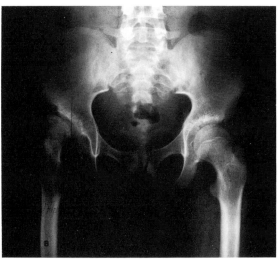

Figure 4

Down's syndrome with acetabular dysplasia and hip subluxation. **Left**, Radiograph of a 15-year-old boy with asymptomatic bilateral acetabular dysplasia and progressive subluxation. **Right**, Radiograph of a 9-year-old girl with unilateral acetabular dysplasia and symptomatic subluxation.

syndrome. In any case, surgery on children with Noonan's syndrome, as well as those with myopathies and arthrogryposis, requires precautions against malignant hyperthermia.

Prader-Willi Syndrome

Prader-Willi syndrome is one of the most common syndromes seen in dysmorphology clinics, occurring once in every 5,000 live births. Because of the metamorphosis from a hypotonic, floppy infant with feeding problems to an intellectually impaired, incredibly obese adult, diagnosis was once difficult. Identification of the syndrome was based entirely on the changing physical findings. However, high-resolution banding of chromosomes has now revealed that the Prader-Willi syndrome is a result of a specific deletion of part of the long arm of chromosome 15. Congenital dislocated hips are common, occurring in almost 10% of cases. Developmental milestones are considerably delayed, but all patients eventually walk.

After the first birthday, the apparent disinterest in food is changed to a preoccupation with it. There is relentless weight gain, so that it is not unusual for a 6-year-old patient to weigh 67.8 kg. The fat is unevenly distributed about the trunk, lower abdomen, buttocks, and thighs, and spares the neck, face, and limbs. The child appears insatiable and effortlessly consumes large amounts of food and unappetizing items discarded by others. Behavior modification in controlled environments has sometimes been helpful. Despite the increased weight, there is little increase in height, and only a few patients reach 152 cm. The small hands and feet are diagnostic features of this syndrome. The patients are mentally retarded, but the magnitude of the deficiency is variable, ranging from moderate to just borderline. The mental impairment seems to parallel the magnitude of obesity. Children have hypoplastic genitalia that may not be apparent until they get older.

The major orthopaedic problem in children with Prader-Willi syndrome is a deviation of spinal alignment, with scoliosis reported in 50% to 90%. The curves are of juvenile onset. Structural vertebral malformations are uncommon. Obesity makes clinical diagnosis difficult, and routine roentgenograms are recommended. It is difficult to fit an orthosis properly because of the trunk shape, and compliance is poor. Many curves progress more than 45 degrees, to the point at which surgery is indicated; however, the morbid effects of obesity, including hypoventilation and diminished cardiac reserve, substantially increase the risks of anesthesia.

Disturbed Fetal Environment

The developing fetus is susceptible to alterations in and invasions of its environment by viruses, bacteria, chemicals, and drugs.

Fetal AIDS

The causative agent of the acquired immune deficiency syndrome (AIDS) is the human immunodeficiency virus (HIV), a retrovirus that can be transmitted across the placenta to the child in utero. The incubation period of clinically expressed pediatric AIDS is 18 to 27 months, and the serologic response to HIV in children is weaker and often false-negative. With the current fear of AIDS transmission in the operating room, it may be worthwhile to try and recognize the characteristic dysmorphic cranial and facial features in the newborn infected with HIV. A prominent box-like forehead, wide-spaced eyes, growth failure, and a small head are diagnostic clues.

Fetal Alcohol Syndrome

There is a distinct pattern of malformations in the children of alcoholic mothers, but lesser manifestations can occur, and there is substantial disagreement regarding the dangers of moderate alcohol use during pregnancy. Epidemiologic studies have established a clear association between maternal alcohol use and fetal damage, but the precise biochemical mechanism for teratogenesis is unknown. The affected child has disturbances in growth, in central nervous system function, in facial appearance, and in the normal morphogenesis of the skeleton. The children are small at birth and remain below normal in both height and weight. Evidences of brain damage include mental retardation, delayed motor milestones, and hypotonia or hypertonia; many cases are misdisagnosed as cerebral palsy. A dysmorphic face is characteristic. Fifty percent of children with fetal alcohol syndrome have orthopaedic problems. There is a generalized restriction of joint movement at birth, with particular stiffness of the elbows and the metacarpophalangeal and interphalangeal joints. Ten percent have hip dislocation. Fusion of the cervical vertebrae, similar to that in Klippel-Feil syndrome, thoracic hemivertebrae, congenital scoliosis, and myelodysplasia may all occur. Bone fusions of the upper extremity are a unique feature of fetal alcohol syndrome and include proximal radioulnar synostosis and carpal bone fusions.

Intrauterine Exposure to Therapeutic Drugs

Intrauterine exposure to hydantoin can result in hypoplasia of the fingernails, abnormal distal phalanges, absent distal interphalangeal crease, and, in more severe instances, a partial or total absence of the fingers. Exposure to warfarin during pregnancy may result in a newborn with stippled epiphyses, stippled vertebrae, and a clinical pattern resembling that of chondrodysplasia calcificans punctata (Conradi's disease).

Miscellaneous Syndromes

Rett's Syndrome

Rett's syndrome was originally described some two decades ago, but was not widely recognized until recently. It is now being diagnosed with regularity. It is a progressive dysfunction of the brain that occurs only in girls. Initially it may be mistaken for cerebral palsy, mental retardation, or autism. At birth, the girls appear to be healthy and remain so until 6 to 12 months old. Then, there is a rather sharp curtailment of motor and intellectual development, followed by a progressive loss of motor and cognitive skills, inappropriate social interaction, and an inability to communicate. They exhibit a rather striking movement disorder of the hands, in which there are stereotypic hand motions ranging from simple to highly complicated. Handwashing, hand-wringing, hand-to-mouth, and hand-clapping dominates almost the entire waking time. Despite these complex stereotypic movements, the girls cannot perform even the most elementary purposeful hand functions such as grasp, feeding, or playing with toys. Abnormal chewing and tongue thrusting are frequent, and feeding is a slow and laborious process. Except for the hands, there is a loss of spontaneous body motion; this and the inability to communicate suggest autism.

Spasticity and increased tone develop by the end of the first decade, and patients then exhibit all the associated complications of spastic cerebral palsy: elbow and knee contractures, ankle equinus, and spastic hip dislocation. In those who were able to walk, ambulation is lost after a period of unsteadiness or ataxia. Seizures develop, as well as a disorder of respiration with hyperventilation and breath-holding spells. The hands and feet exhibit an annoying vasomotor instability. Scoliosis is present in 80%

of patients and is usually a C-shaped curve. It is progressive despite bracing. Air-swallowing, seizures that respond poorly to medication, and spasticity make bracing nearly impossible. The life span of girls with Rett's syndrome seems unaffected, and thus aggressive treatment of the scoliosis appears to be justified. Early spinal fusions by methods that avoid postoperative immobilization are recommended. Other therapeutic modalities for dealing with spasticity, including physical and occupational therapy, bracing, and orthopaedic surgery have been tried with variable benefits. The cause of this condition has not been elucidated, although it is thought to be a disturbance in the X chromosome.

Hemihypertrophy

Leg-length discrepancy and body asymmetry may be the result of acquired disorders such as trauma or osteomyelitis, chronic inflammatory disease such as juvenile rheumatoid arthritis, or neurologic diseases such as polio or cerebral palsy. Overgrowth may be secondary to a vascular malformation or neurofibromatosis. In addition, certain syndromes whose causes are unknown have body asymmetry as a feature. Two such examples are Beckwith-Wiedemann syndrome, in which a large child has macroglossia, omphalocele, enlarged abdominal viscera, and asymmetric overgrowth, and Russell-Silver syndrome, in which a short child has a small, triangular face, genitourinary malformations, and one limb smaller than the other. Even after all these syndromes are considered, the most likely diagnosis for a child with body asymmetry is idiopathic hemihypertrophy.

In this condition exactly one half of the body is enlarged. One arm, one leg, one half of the trunk, and one half of the face are enlarged. One of each pair of visceral organs is enlarged. The hypertrophy may be more prominent in just one limb (usually the leg). The skeleton is enlarged in both length and width, as are all the soft tissues. The asymmetry is evident at birth, and the enlarged limb always grows faster than the other. There is no catch-up phenomenon, and skeletal maturity is attained at the same time on both sides, although the centers of ossification may be different in size. The leg-length discrepancy increases in a linear fashion. If the difference approaches 2.5 cm by the age of 4 years, a major discrepancy can be expected at maturity. Longitudinal measurements are needed, with epiphysiodesis of the distal femur and/or proximal tibia remaining the treatment of choice. There is no effective way to reduce the girth of the limb, which is often an important cosmetic issue. Scoliosis is usually a consequence of the leg-length discrepancy. Structural renal malformations are common. There is a measurable risk, about 5%, that an intra-abdominal malignant tumor will develop; the most common is Wilms' nephroblastoma.

Congenital Constriction Band Syndrome

The cardinal feature of this syndrome is the presence of anular constricting grooves in the digits and limbs, and occasionally across the face and around the trunk. The distribution is random, with no two cases of constriction band syndrome looking exactly alike. The constriction bands are present at birth and no new ones develop. The bands are distributed asymmetrically around the fingers and toes, and the distal end of the limb is more likely to be affected, with the central fingers and medial two toes the most susceptible. The consequences of these constriction bands can vary from a shallow cutaneous crease to a deep gutter down to and involving the bone. The most severe manifestation is a transverse amputation. The amputation behaves as an acquired amputation with troublesome appositional overgrowth, a situation quite distinct from congenital amputations resulting from failure of formation. A diagnostic syndactyly is present. In this fenestrated acrosyndactyly, the fingertips are connected by soft tissue, the proximal interdigital spaces are preserved, and the digits lie above and below each other rather than in the same plane. One third of patients have a clubfoot. In most instances there is an anular constriction band in the supramalleolar region or proximally in the calf. Proximal bands in general are more likely to have an associated

neurologic deficit, and this must be borne in mind when clubfoot treatment is undertaken. A significant leg-length discrepancy exceeding 2.5 cm occurs in 20% of patients. Orthopaedic surgeons should recognize that neonatal mortality is occasionally associated with congenital constriction band syndrome. One third of the patients are products of premature births. Cleft lip and oblique facial clefts may be present, some leading to grotesque disfigurement. Asymmetric encephaloceles are yet another complication.

The syndrome has an incidence of one per 5,000 births. It is nongenetic and its cause is thought to be fibrous strands from a damaged amnion and chorion that wrap around already developed limbs, leading to grooves, indentations, and amputations. This condition was once termed Streeter's dysplasia.

Annotated Bibliography

Keywords

Achondroplasia; Arthrogryposis; Congenital constriction band syndrome; Down's syndrome; Ehlers-Danlos syndrome; Enchondromatosis; Homocystinuria; Marfan's syndrome; Mucolipidoses; Mucopolysaccharidoses; Neurofibromatosis; Osteogenesis imperfecta; Prader-Willi syndrome; Rett's syndrome; Skeletal dysplasias

General Considerations

Goldberg MJ: *The Dysmorphic Child: An Orthopedic Perspective.* New York, Raven Press, 1987.
The musculoskeletal and significant nonorthopaedic aspects of the most frequently encountered syndromes are presented with an emphasis on the differential diagnosis of children who have similar orthopaedic deformities.

McKusick VA: *Mendelian Inheritance in Man,* ed 7. Baltimore, Johns Hopkins University Press, 1986.
A catalog of autosomal-dominant, autosomal-recessive, and X-linked phenotypes with the essential basic clinical information, detailed biochemistry, and up-to-date bibliography.

Skeletal Dysplasias

Aldegheri R, Trivella G, Renzi-Brivio L, et al: Lengthening of the lower limbs in achondroplastic patients: A comparative study of four techniques. *J Bone Joint Surg* 1988;70B:69–73.
The results of limb lengthening in 61 patients with achondroplasia and 11 with hypochondroplasia are presented with details of length achieved, healing time, and complications. Chondrodiastasis, callotasis, and osteotomy are compared.

McKusik VA, Scott CI: A nomenclature for constitutional disorders of bone. *J Bone Joint Surg* 1971;53A:978–986.
Now nearly two decades old, this classification for skeletal dysplasias seems to be withstanding the test of time.

Reid CS, Pyeritz RE, Kopits SE, et al: Cervicomedullary compression in young patients with achondroplasia: Value of comprehensive neurologic and respiratory evaluation. *J Pediatr* 1987;110:522–530.
A study of 26 young patients with achondroplasia showed

that 85% had respiratory abnormalities. Although most resulted from primary problems of the pulmonary system, in nine patients cervicomedullary cord compression was a factor.

Schwartz HS, Zimmerman NB, Simon MA, et al: The malignant potential of enchondromatosis. *J Bone Joint Surg* 1987;69A:269–274.
An analysis of the types of malignant skeletal and nonskeletal tumors in 37 patients with enchondromatosis and seven with Maffucci's syndrome, and a calculation of life survival rates.

Wynne-Davies R, Gormley J: The prevalence of skeletal dysplasias: An estimate of their minimum frequency and the number of patients requiring orthopaedic care. *J Bone Joint Surg* 1985;67B:133–137.
An estimation that during the period from 1950 to 1979 there were 10,000 individuals with skeletal dysplasias in Britain, of whom 6,000 required substantial orthopaedic care. The types and extent of handicap are detailed.

Connective Tissue Disorders

Boers GH, Polder TW, Cruysberg JR, et al: Homocystinuria versus Marfan's syndrome: The therapeutic relevance of the differential diagnosis. *Neth J Med* 1984,27:206–212.
A lucid discussion of the biochemistry of these conditions and the rationale for treatment, along with excellent photographs.

Byers PH, Holbrook KA: Molecular basis of clinical heterogeneity in the Ehlers-Danlos syndrome. *Ann NY Acad Sci* 1985;460:298–310.
Because advances in the understanding of the molecular basis of the clinical features of Ehlers-Danlos syndrome have been slow, this review remains valuable in understanding the biochemical and genetic aspects of ten of the 11 types of Ehlers-Danlos syndrome.

Gamble JG, Rinsky LA, Strudwick J, et al: Non-union of fractures in children who have osteogenesis imperfecta. *J Bone Joint Surg* 1988;70A:439–443.
Ten of 52 patients with osteogenesis imperfecta had 12 nonunions. All had functional disability as a result; union was achieved in eight of the nine who underwent surgery.

Arthrogryposis Multiplex Congenita and Arthrogryposis Syndromes

Dias LS, Stern LS: Talectomy in the treatment of resistant talipes equinovarus deformity in myelomeningocele and arthrogryposis. *J Pediatr Orthop* 1987;7:39–41.

Fourteen patients with spina bifida and four with arthrogryposis underwent talectomy after failed posteromedial release. Effective hindfoot correction was achieved but 25% required further surgery to correct forefoot adduction deformity.

Green AD, Fixsen JA, Lloyd-Roberts GC: Talectomy for arthrogryposis multiplex congenita. *J Bone Joint Surg* 1984;66B:697–699.

After an average of 11 years of follow-up, 24 of 34 feet with rigid clubfoot treated by talectomy were considered satisfactory. Talectomy as either a primary procedure or after other operations has failed.

Staheli LT, Chew DE, Elliott JS, et al: Management of hip dislocations in children with arthrogryposis. *J Pediatr Orthop* 1987;7:681–1685.

The medial approach was used to reduce dislocated hips in children with arthrogryposis. Stability was achieved, acetabular development was satisfactory, and range of motion was better than in those treated by anterolateral incision or closed reduction. Osteonecrosis occurred in one of 13 cases.

Neurocutaneous and Vascular Syndromes

Clark RD, Donnai D, Rogers J, et al: Proteus syndrome: An expanded phenotype. *Am J Med Genet* 1987;27:99–117.

Eleven cases of this syndrome illustrate the magnitude and the worsening of the physical findings, including the orthopaedic aspects of macrodactyly, gigantism, scoliosis, and exostosis.

Crawford AH Jr, Bagamery N: Osseous manifestations of neurofibromatosis in childhood. *J Pediatr Orthop* 1986;6:72–88.

A detailed review of the skeletal manifestations of neurofibromatosis in 116 children diagnosed before the age of 12 years and followed up for an average of five years. This report also includes the cutaneous and neoplastic aspects of this disorder.

Tibbles JA, Cohen MM Jr: The Proteus syndrome: The Elephant Man diagnosed. *Br Med J* 1986;293:683–685.

This is an interesting historical argument. Because the Elephant Man became so well-known, patients and parents of children with neurofibromatosis may be unnecessarily anxious.

Chromosomal Syndromes

Allanson JE: Noonan syndrome. *J Med Genet* 1987;24:9–13.

An extensive bibliography accompanies this overview of Noonan's syndrome; the references to the cases of malignant hyperthermia are of particular value.

Cassidy SB: Prader-Willi Syndrome. *Curr Probl Pediatr* 1984;14:1–55.

A monograph covering all aspects of this syndrome from historical notes to the cytogenetics of chromosome 15, as well as management of orthopaedic and nonorthopaedic manifestations.

Davidson RG: Atlantoaxial instability in individuals with Down syndrome: A fresh look at the evidence. *Pediatrics* 1988;81:857–865.

A review of the case histories of 31 persons with Down's syndrome in whom atlantoaxial dislocation later developed concludes that routine roentgenographic screening unnecessarily restricts sports participation, and does not prevent these neurologic catastrophes.

Dugdale TW, Renshaw TS: Instability of the patellofemoral joint in Down syndrome. *J Bone Joint Surg* 1986;68A:405–413.

An evaluation of 210 institutionalized persons with Down's syndrome and 151 persons in the community reveals that less than 10% had dislocated or dislocatable patellas and that only three were unable to walk because of patellofemoral instability.

French HG, Burke SW, Roberts JM, et al: Upper cervical ossicles in Down syndrome. *J Pediatr Orthop* 1987;7:69–71.

Serial radiographs and radiographic anatomy in six young adults with Down's syndrome suggest that the ossicles at C-2 represent an avulsion of the dens rather than a developmental ossiculum terminale.

Pueschel SM, Scola FH: Atlantoaxial instability in individuals with Down syndrome: Epidemiologic, radiographic, and clinical studies. *Pediatrics* 1987;80:555–560.

Fifty-nine of 404 (14.6%) persons with Down's syndrome had C1-C2 instability. Of these, 53 were asymptomatic and six required fusion for myelopathy. There were no clinical or roentgenographic changes in 95 patients followed up longitudinally.

Disturbed Fetal Environment

Ernhart CB, Sokol RJ, Martier S, et al: Alcohol teratogenicity in the human: A detailed assessment of specificity, critical period, and threshold. *Am J Obstet Gynecol* 1987;156:33–39.

A detailed prospective study of 359 neonates revealed that the critical period for alcohol teratogenicity is around the time of conception, and that certain anomalies, but not all, occur in a dose-response manner.

Marion RW, Wiznia AA, Hutcheon RG, et al: Fetal AIDS syndrome score: Correlation between severity of dysmorphism and age at diagnosis of immunodeficiency. *Am J Dis Child* 1987;141:429–431.

Characteristic dysmorphic facial features were evaluated in 37 children born with HIV infection and were found to have been helpful in establishing the diagnosis before clinical AIDS developed.

Miscellaneous Syndromes

Askins G, Ger E: Congenital constriction band syndrome. *J Pediatr Orthop* 1988;8:461–466.

A retrospective review of 55 affected patients detailing the more common findings of syndactyly and amputations, but also those less frequently recognized, such as neurogenic clubfoot and leg-length discrepancy.

Naidu S, Murphy M, Moser HW, et al: Rett syndrome: Natural history in 70 cases. *Am J Med Genet* 1986;24(suppl 1):61–72.

A review of all aspects of this syndrome in 70 females 2½ to 34 years old, with emphasis on the time of appearance and severity of each characteristic. This is but one of 40 articles in this supplement volume devoted to Rett's syndrome.

21

Neuromusculoskeletal Disorders and Gait

Human gait consists of a series of limb-segment rotational movements that produce stable forward propulsion at a constant speed in an energy-conserving manner. Forces produced by muscles interacting with the body's gravitational and inertial properties result in joint-angle changes. The needs for support and propulsion vary with the phase of the gait cycle (for example, weight acceptance, single stance, swing). Muscular forces and the resulting limb positions and angular changes of the joints vary throughout the cycle. The sum of these movements is the stride length produced and, in association with the number of steps taken per minute (cadence), the overall velocity. (These latter features constitute a measure of overall performance.) All these parameters of gait—timing of muscle activity, joint angle changes, and time-distance features (for example, step length, phase times, cadence, and velocity)—are reproducible from cycle to cycle and person to person and are normally controlled by the central nervous system. The normal gait pattern was described in *Orthopaedic Knowledge Updates I* and *2*. Diseases or injuries to joints, ligaments, bones, or muscles produce a pattern that is abnormal, but still controlled by a normal central nervous system. Gait dysfunction caused by such disorders appears to be governed by a set of rules of compensation. These compensatory mechanisms may result in loss of energy efficiency and increased joint forces and muscle effort so that walking can be maintained. Diseases affecting the nervous system may or may not allow normal compensatory reactions and, in association with spasticity or weakness, can produce a walking pattern that is not readily identified by standard clinical methods.

The evaluation of gait is now being refined by objective, quantifiable methods using electronic and computer hardware and software. Recent advances permit "instant" gait analysis, making clinical use of the gait laboratory feasible. These systems can measure a variety of gait characteristics.

Instrumentation Systems

The function of a gait-analysis laboratory is to quantitate and assess an individual patient's walking performance. It can measure gait events, ground-reaction forces, kinematics (movement of the body and its segments in three dimensions), electromyographic activity, and, in some cases, oxygen consumption. Computer equipment is required to process the data and allow visual checks of the functioning of the system. Moments around joints and deforming forces can be calculated from the measured variables. The type of information produced and the nature of the recently introduced measuring systems fall into three categories: movement analyses, dynamic electromyographic analyses, and foot-floor reaction forces and pressures. Like any other laboratory test, gait-analysis testing yields only information; the tests themselves do not provide an interpretation of the data. This is left to the clinician, usually an orthopaedist, a physical therapist, or a kinesiologist-engineer.

Automated Motion Analysis

To provide an accurate measurement of human movement, motion-analysis systems must (1) visualize and accurately record all movements desired, (2) identify and quantify where in space each area of interest exists at every instant in the gait cycle, and (3) calculate parameters of interest to clinicians, that is, joint angles, velocity, stance times, and the like. At least five systems are commercially available. All use videotape cameras, specialized electronic hardware, and computers.

Dynamic Electromyographic Measurements

During any functional movement, including walking, a particular muscle is activated only for a given period of time. No muscle is activated for more than 30% to 40% of the entire gait cycle. Comparing the value of an activated muscle with its unactivated value yields a better understanding of a given disorder. This has been most valuable in determining treatments for neuromuscular disorders, such as cerebral palsy, head trauma, or stroke. In such cases, knowing the timing of muscles helps determine which muscles should be lengthened, transferred, or left alone.

Dynamic electromyographic recording shows when a particular muscle is activated and the muscle's inherent properties that are activated. The magnitude does not represent the absolute force of the muscle and cannot be used alone to compare a muscle's force from one testing session to another or between subjects. Comparing the relative magnitude of the electromyographic activity during gait with a maximal voluntary contracture of the muscle during the same session provides useful clinical information. Timing can be used to compare a subject's performance with normal values and to determine whether the muscle maintains the same phase of activity from condition to condition and from subject to subject.

The electromyographic signal recorded is the sum of many motor units and muscle fibers being activated. During activation, the magnitude and the frequency of the signal change. The number of muscle fibers and motor units recorded varies with the method of sampling. In one method, electrical (bipolar) wires no larger than a human hair are inserted into the muscle. If the sampling site is properly selected, the few motor units tested by this method accurately represent the entire muscle. A second method uses surface electrodes that represent more motor units and more muscle fibers.

Studies have shown that three strides of electromyographic data per subject provide information as reliable as that obtained from 12 strides. Electromyographic examination of eight muscles about the ankle at three walking velocities (free, fast, slow) and during manual muscle testing demonstrated that the intensity of muscle action during walking was related to the manual muscle test grades. Walking at the normal free velocity required grade 3 (fair) muscle action. During slow gait, the muscle functioned at grade 2 (poor) level. Fast walking necessitated muscle action midway between fair and normal, interpreted as good (grade 4).

Foot-Floor Force and Pressure Recordings

The change in ground-reaction forces (in direction, magnitude, and area of contact) during the stance phase of walking is one of the most relevant factors in the assessment of human gait. Body weight and inertial forces are only effective in moving the body forward and providing stability if they are resisted by the ground. Measurement of ground-reaction forces via platforms embedded in the ground provides an understanding of these forces. Force platforms do not provide information regarding the areas of contact or pressure distribution of the foot on the ground. Harris mats provide an inexpensive qualitative "snapshot" of all the areas of contact of the foot with the ground during the entire stance phase. Miniature shoe-borne (inserts) load cells or in-ground fixed "pedaborographic" devices provide a quantitative means of identifying the foot's vertical forces and the area of their distribution at each instant in the stance phase.

The normal foot-floor pattern in children, young adults, and elderly people varies from person to person but shows a considerable step-to-step consistency and symmetry of the forces from both feet for a given subject. The force pattern in abnormal gait secondary to disorders of the foot also shows marked repeatability.

Walking aids are necessary to support, restrain, and/or propel the locomotion of a person with a functional deficit. For which purpose the aid is used varies with the nature and magnitude of the gait disorder. Force platforms have demonstrated variability in aid loading and between ipsilateral and contralateral support among subjects with total hip replacement. In contrast, symmetric sagittal-plane restraining and propelling aid loadings predominated in subjects with fractures. Aid impulses directed laterally were greater than the combined impulses directed anteriorly and posteriorly in some hemiplegic subjects during three-point gait. This suggests that more accurate assessment of crutch supports are needed if such devices are to be used properly to assist gait in neuromusculoskeletal disorders.

Measuring the external moments about the hip, knee, or ankle joints requires the synchronization of the force platform data to motion data and further calculations. For amputees, this information for normal and prosthetic limbs allows adjustments to be made immediately to the hydraulic mechanism so that optimal function of prosthetic equipment can be determined objectively.

Recent Findings by Instrumented Gait Analysis

Arthritis

Patients with juvenile rheumatoid arthritis walk with significantly decreased velocity, cadence, and stride length. Although most of these patients have knee involvement,

hip extension at the end of single-limb stance, ankle plantar flexion during weight release, and an anterior pelvic tilt are the most significant motion abnormalities noted; all are significantly increased throughout the gait cycle. However, no significant differences in step width, in the percentage of time spent in each phase of the gait cycle, or in knee-joint excursion have been noted.

A better understanding of the characteristics of joint loading, stress distribution, and the biologic response of bone to stress may improve an implant's function and longevity. A comparison of a cemented and a noncemented total hip replacement showed that the gait variables providing the best objective evidence of a change in the patient's ambulatory status and correlating best with the clinical impression of gait function were all measurements of weightbearing capacity and not of joint motions. Maximal vertical force and average velocity were the only gait variables that distinguished between the two total hip replacements, although step rate, single-limb support, and weight acceptance showed a similar trend.

The variations in individual and composite muscular anatomy can be recorded noninvasively by computed tomography. In 18 normal hips in which the abductor muscles were mapped in detail, the inclination of the axis of the abductor muscle ranged from 17 to 26 degrees (standard deviation, 2.9 degrees) in the frontal plane and from −12 to 14 degrees (standard deviation, 4.2 degrees) in the sagittal plane. Patterns associated with trauma, arthritis, and the like can differ from normal.

A simplified three-dimensional model of the hip, incorporating straight lines of muscle action between attachment sites, simulates a variety of hip configurations during simple hip motions in three principal anatomic planes. The three contributions of a muscle (flexion-extension, abduction-adduction, and internal-external rotation) tending to rotate the thigh segment relative to the pelvis can be identified. With such a model, muscles can be classified by their action or turning effect at, for example, 0, 40, and 90 degrees of hip flexion. Certain muscles exhibit significant changes in their action during these simple motions, emphasizing the importance of hip position to muscle function. A muscle that produces primarily a flexion moment may also produce secondary abduction and tertiary internal rotation moments. The functions of muscles crossing the hip and knee joints can also be computed by the changing relative positions of joint centers and muscle origins and insertions during a gait cycle. The amount of force necessary to produce a given moment about a joint depends on the limb's position. In addition, muscle function changes significantly with limb position.

In patients tested by gait evaluation before undergoing high tibial osteotomy and then one year and about three years after surgery, the moment tending to adduct the knee joint during walking preoperatively was predictive of postoperative clinical results. The patients could be divided into high adduction-moment and low adduction-moment groups on the basis of the magnitude of the knee's adduction moment. The adduction moment was reduced in both groups after surgery, but the average postoperative adduction moments in the low adduction-moment group were still significantly lower than those in the high adduction-moment group. The two groups were indistinguishable on the basis of preoperative knee score, initial varus deformity, immediate postoperative correction, age, and weight. However, after an average follow-up of 3.2 years, patients with low preoperative adduction moments had substantially better clinical results than did patients with high adduction moments. A significant recurrence of varus deformity was noted in the high adduction-moment group.

After total knee replacement, even asymptomatic patients with excellent clinical results may have an abnormality of gait consisting of shorter-than-normal stride length, reduced mid-stance knee flexion, and abnormal patterns of external flexion-extension moment of the knee. Differences in gait resulting from the designs of the prostheses can be identified during the more stressful activity of stair-climbing. Some evidence suggests that, two years or more after surgery, the less constrained cruciate-retaining designs produce a more normal gait during stair-climbing than do the more constrained cruciate-sacrificing designs.

In elderly subjects, gait speed and step length are significantly greater on carpeted surfaces than on vinyl surfaces.

Cerebral Palsy

The gait of spastic children shows abnormal values for time-distance parameters (velocity, stride length, cadence). Recent evidence suggests that these parameters change with age as they do in normal children; although gait velocity and stride length values are lower than normal, they do increase with age, with stride length increasing and stride frequency (cadence) decreasing as they do normally. Stance and swing times, when normalized with regard to stride duration, show no change with age, again as happens normally. Studies have indicated that the metabolic energy level and heart rate of children with spastic cerebral palsy may be abnormally increased during walking. The higher metabolic cost may be attributable, at least in part, to poor patterns of exchange between the potential and kinetic energy types of the head, arms, and trunk segment, to very low levels of kinetic energy that preclude exchange, or to both.

Abnormal timing of muscle activity in the lower extremity is a hallmark of the gait of children with cerebral palsy. Gait electromyograms, however, cannot differentiate idiopathic toe-walking from spastic cerebral palsy. Idiopathic toe-walkers studied by gait electromyography showed muscle timing abnormalities similar to those in children with cerebral palsy and equinus deformities. Available data (family history, male predominance, and learning disabilities) suggest that idiopathic toe-walking is a true and separate entity.

Stance-phase stability and swing-phase clearance, prerequisites for normal ambulation, are often lost in the gait of children with cerebral palsy. A major emphasis in the management of the crouch gait of children with cerebral palsy has been the correction of the excessively flexed knee and hip in stance. Less attention has been paid to swing clearance. Lengthening of the hamstrings improves stance-phase knee extension but may not greatly alter swing-phase knee flexion. Because it was once assumed that the rectus femoris was active when the flexed hip was in stance, its proximal release was recommended. However, this often resulted in a stiff-legged gait with poor swing initiation. Dynamic electromyographic records of children with cerebral palsy have now demonstrated that the rectus femoris is more often active in the swing phase, when it also acts as a knee extensor. Recent reports suggest that transferring the rectus femoris distally to either the medial or the lateral hamstrings in such cases improves swing-phase knee flexion and toe clearance. Because hamstring activity contributes to the crouch gait by increasing knee flexion at the end of swing and for part or all of stance, a lengthening procedure combined with a rectus femoris transfer may be indicated in some patients. This combined procedure produced better swing-phase knee flexion and less residual knee flexion in stance than did hamstring lengthening alone. Poor outcomes seemed to be associated with either foot rotation in excess of 8 degrees internally or externally or postoperative knee flexion in stance.

The defect of knee flexion in stance may contribute to excessive length of the patellar tendon. It has been suggested that this excess is caused by the long-term stretching effect on the rectus femoris when the hamstrings are chronically active in stance. Excessive length can be identified by greater passive extension than active extension of the knee and a high position of the patella on lateral radiographs. Surgical treatment in such cases consists of shortening the patellar tendon and, when necessary, combining this with lengthening of the hamstrings. Satisfactory results with this procedure after an average follow-up of four years were recently reported.

The phasic activity of the long-toe flexors has been thought to contribute to hindfoot deformity in children with cerebral palsy. Although gross abnormalities in the phasic timing of the flexor hallucis longus and flexor digitorum longus have been observed, wire electrode dynamic electromyography failed to implicate these muscles. Unless toe curling is clinically evident and symptomatic, electromyography of the long-toe flexors is apparently unnecessary.

Paraplegia

Functional electrical stimulation has been studied as a technique for supporting gait in paraplegic patients with traumatic lesions of the upper motor neurons. It is useful in cases in which the involved area is between the T-4 and T-12 levels. Functional electrical stimulation can be used to activate viable muscles. Functional electrical stimulation in such cases takes advantage of both the intact spinal cord caudad to the level of the functional transection and existing spinal reflexes. Recent reports have shown that stimulation can lead to clinical improvement within one to three years, although these cases are still limited in number. Also, the treatment programs used different stimulation patterns, different frequencies and magnitudes of voltage, and different periods of stimulation. The application of the stimulus (through the skin or directly to the nerve or muscle) and whether orthotic devices were used also varied from study to study.

A simple way for functional electrical stimulation to assist standing is tetanic stimulation of the quadriceps muscle to lock the knee joints. The hip joints are in hyperextension and the ankle joints remain free. The upper limbs are used for balancing. This posture requires minimal corrective forces exerted by the hands. It is not a very stable position because some forward-backward sway is permitted and the knees can jackknife when the knee-bending moment exceeds the moment generated by the quadriceps muscle. Fatiguing of the quadriceps is also a problem. Standing time is short, from several minutes to an hour, depending on the condition of the patient's muscles.

Cyclical functional electrical stimulation fatigues muscle considerably less. Combining this principle with the activation of different muscles at different times prolongs standing time by a factor of two to five, allowing some patients to stand for as long as five hours at a time (an achievement comparable to normal). Co-contraction of two or three muscles further expands the range of suitable patients and improves standing by increasing the permissible range of body sway.

With foot- or hand-switch activation, accurate sequencing of functional electrical stimulation pulses can enable paraplegics not only to stand but to walk. This is called open-loop control; the sequencing pattern of the gait cycle is fixed. A common pattern combines surface stimulation of the quadriceps and gluteus maximus muscles with stimulation of the hip, knee, and ankle flexors alternately for each leg. A portable microprocessor-controlled stimulator that automatically activates muscles through percutaneous intramuscular wire electrodes is a more sophisticated functional electrical stimulation approach. A basic open-loop pattern of stimulation is adapted for each individual. The subject initiates each step with a hand-operated switch. Each individual can choose a pattern of stimulation not only for walking but for exercising, sitting, and ascending or descending stairs. Subjects using this protocol have progressed to using a walker or axillary crutches.

Typically, walking velocity is slow. About 80% of the subject's body weight can be supported by the feet. Preliminary results indicate that functional electrical stimulation uses little energy when the subject is seated or when it is used as an orthotic device for standing, confirming its beneficial effect. However, walking by means of functional electrical stimulation requires exhaustive efforts. Functional electrical stimulation is, therefore, advisable primarily for young subjects. Despite the successful performance of many tasks, the systems are not yet adequate for unsupervised use outside a laboratory.

To minimize the number of muscles to be stimulated and provide more stance stability, several functional electrical stimulation protocols use ankle-foot orthoses as ancillary aids. The Oswestry Parawalker has enabled adult patients with complete thoracic-level paraplegia to achieve a reciprocal gait with an inherently low energy demand. To diminish the work demands on the girdle musculature of the upper limb during walking, some of these patients underwent electrical stimulation of the gluteal muscles in stance phase. This increased the stability of the adduction and also provided forward propulsion by driving the stance leg into extension. Bilateral stimulation of the quadriceps muscles facilitated standing and sitting in the orthosis.

Additional stability and reduced expenditures of energy are achievable through closed-loop control; by feeding information to the controller during the activity, the stimulation pattern can be changed. During normal gait, studies have found that compensatory reactions after gait perturbations may well be induced by peripheral signals. Electromyographic responses induced in the leg by gait perturbations seem to be evoked by group II afferents and mediated via the spinal pathway. The cerebral potential evoked by an electrical stimulus of the tibial nerve during walking seems to be of smaller amplitude and longer latency than that seen when the nerve is stimulated during quiet standing. During gait, the signals of group I afferents thus seem to be blocked at both segmental and supraspinal levels. The cerebral potentials evoked during gait most probably reflect the processing done by supraspinal motor centers to coordinate the widespread arm and trunk muscle activation necessary to reestablish body equilibrium.

Other rehabilitation techniques can be used to increase stability and propulsion. For example, when normal subjects were loaded with increasing weights (2 to 6 kg) applied around the ankles, stride length increased in relation to velocity and the duration of single support in relation to stride duration increased; swing increased and stance and double support decreased. The results contrasted in all respects to those obtained with the load carried in the hand; with ankle loading the swing phase was loaded and with hand loading stance was loaded.

Hemiplegia

In hemiplegia caused by a stroke or head injury, the time-distance parameters of gait are commonly well below normal values, even in functionally independent walkers. The stance and double-support phases of gait are prolonged. Throughout the stance phase, the gait of these patients is characterized by equinus deformity of the ankle, decreased flexion of the knee (hyperextension in the most severely involved patients), and increased flexion of the hip (this varies with the severity of the equinus deformity of the ankle and hyperextension of the knee). Lateral shift to the paralyzed side is decreased. During the swing phase, with the affected limb in less knee flexion and less dorsiflexion than normal, circumduction to achieve toe clearance is often present. Specific gait parameters that can be measured routinely (speed, cadence, independence, and appearance) seem to be the best predictors of gait performance and correlate with one another and with the clinical examination of balance, weightbearing ratio, motor control, and normalized strength of the paralyzed lower limbs. Performance goals for such patients should be based on values from impaired rather than healthy subjects and should be adjusted for the individual patient's type of injury, type of ambulation aid, and functional category.

The abnormal gait patterns of hemiplegic patients with equinovarus deformities can be further divided into three groups: type I, characterized by a compensated back-knee deformity and symmetric steps; type II, with hyperextension of the knee, increased stance flexion of the hip, steps of the unaffected limb decreased to 50% of normal, and a prolonged period of double-limb support; and type III, the most severely abnormal gait, which produces such instability that the uninvolved limb cannot advance past the affected stationary limb.

Gait analysis confirms that properly selected hemiplegic patients treated with orthotic devices or tendon surgery can significantly improve their walking performance. Ankle-foot orthoses can increase walking speed if plantar flexion is optimally adjusted; an improperly adjusted orthosis may produce an exaggerated knee-flexion moment, resulting in knee instability, or it may fail to correct the knee-extension moment and the back-knee deformity. Long-term follow-ups of adult patients with acquired spastic equinus and equinovarus deformity suggest that lengthening of the Achilles tendon, lateral transfer of part of the anterior tibial tendon, and other appropriate muscle releases at least one year after onset of the hemiplegia can correct the deformity. More than 50% of such patients achieve brace-free gait. Postoperative analyses of gait, performed at least one year after surgery, showed that the prolonged stance and double-support phases of gait can approach normal values. Patients with gait deficiencies should, therefore, undergo correction of the equinus deformity of the ankle as an initial procedure, as major dynamic derangement in gait can result from spastic equinus deformity alone. Although the surgery does not correct hip and knee deformities, gait can improve so much that additional surgery or bracing may prove unnecessary.

Short, intensive, multichannel electrical stimulation therapy is also being evaluated in hemiplegics after stroke or head injury. This technique is based on the principle of agonist facilitation and antagonist inhibition. In normal, nonparaplegic gait, functional electrical stimulation applied to the calf muscles performs in a manner similar to normal calf muscle function: in the first third of the stance phase it induces knee extension; when applied later in single-limb stance, it increases the amount of plantar flexion and knee flexion. Strengthened vastus muscle contraction can increase the amount and duration of stance-phase knee extension and interacts with functional electrical stimulation of the calf to increase the amount of heel rise in late single-limb stance. In contrast, in hemiplegic gait, functional electrical stimulation of the calf increases knee flexion and ankle plantar flexion only after opposite heel strike; a persistent lower-limb extensor synergy prevents knee flexion from occurring simultaneously with plantar flexion and a heel rise, while the hemiplegic limb is still weightbearing.

The stimulation of the soleus, quadriceps, hamstring, and gluteus maximus muscles with individually preprogrammed sequences by means of surface electrodes can gradually increase the walking distance and allow properly selected subjects to achieve independent ambulation with a crutch after as few as 14 stimulation sessions. A comparison of several months of multisite electrical stimulation of gait in hemiplegic patients with standard rehabilitation methods showed faster recovery rates in midtherapy (3.15 times in step length and 2.25 times in gait velocity) and at the end of therapy (2.14 times in step length, 1.42 times in gait velocity, and 1.63 times in kinesiologic gait analysis). The differences between the two groups, however, faded after eight months without treatment. Some kinesiologic deficits reappeared, primarily those in the more distal muscle groups. These findings indicate a need for a simpler intermittent long-term electrical stimulation program.

Muscular Dystrophy

An analysis of the sequential values for the moments developed around the knee during the walking cycle shows that the equinus gait of boys with Duchenne's muscular dystrophy is a necessary adaptation to keep the forces about proximal joints, particularly the knee, within the limits controllable by weakened muscles. These findings explain why in some patients lengthening of the Achilles tendon to correct contracture at the ankle permits only brace-assisted gait.

Functional rating scales have been developed for evaluation of upper-extremity and lower-extremity function in Duchenne's muscular dystrophy. The Vignos scale is accepted for lower-extremity function and the Brooke scale for upper-extremity function. Studies have been done to determine whether the upper extremity and the lower extremity lose strength and function in parallel in Duchenne's muscular dystrophy and other proximal limb girdle neuromuscular disorders. Recent reports suggest that a maximum of 86% of variation in upper-extremity rank could be explained purely by obtaining lower-extremity rank. The significant relationship between upper-extremity and lower-extremity strength and functional grade must be recognized when walkers are needed to assist weightbearing. Measures of lower-body function or strength can reflect upper-extremity function in drug trials in which global effects are expected. The two measurements are not, however, equivalent and cannot be used to predict specific upper-extremity functions.

Myelodysplasia

In children with myelodysplasia, the metabolic demands of swing-through ambulation with conventional bracing (hip-knee-ankle-foot orthosis) are significantly increased over those during wheelchair use. In contrast, a reciprocal-gait orthosis had a metabolic demand similar to that in wheelchair use. This suggests a more favorable prognosis for long-term functional ambulation in patients with higher-level myelodysplasia if such devices are used.

Nerve Palsy

Peroneal paralysis produces abnormalities during both the stance and the swing phases of gait. During early stance, there is a decrease in the length of the heel-strike phase and a reduction in the peak plantar-flexion moment. During mid-stance, the range of inversion-eversion increases, suggesting mediolateral instability. The second vertical force peak and the aft-shear force peak are reduced, as are the peak dorsiflexion moment and the opposite step length. These reductions are believed to result from mediolateral instability during push-off. Subjects demonstrate steppage gait during the swing phase and increased inversion just before heel strike.

Trends

The proper management of orthopaedic disorders requires an understanding of the abnormality and how the abnormality affects function. In the next decade, gait analysis will be used more widely to evaluate the latter. To date, it has been most valuable in assessing and treating neuromuscular control problems. With increasing use, gait-analysis laboratories will further refine when certain surgical procedures for stroke, head trauma, and cerebral palsy are most appropriate, under what conditions of movement they can best be used, and how such surgical procedures can be combined with newer types of braces and functional electrical stimulation to restore function. Advancements in electronic technology will allow improved assessment of a variety of sports activities, leading to better understanding of and treatment for sports-related disorders. As musculoskeletal reconstructive surgery continues to improve, gait analysis will be increasingly needed to compare the efficacy of one type of procedure with that of another in terms of functional outcome. Increasingly, the principles, techniques, and equipment used in gait analysis will also be used to assess disorders of the upper extremity and the spine.

Annotated Bibliography

Keywords

Arthritis; Cerebral palsy; Electromyography; Gait; Hemiplegia; Juvenile rheumatoid arthritis; Muscular dystrophy; Myelodysplasia; Nerve palsy

Instrumentation Systems

Arsenault AB, Winter DA, Marteniuk RG, et al: How many strides are required for the analysis of electromyographic data in gait? *Scand J Rehabil Med* 1986;18:133–135.

This study was conducted to obtain information on the number of strides needed per subject in an electromyographic study of gait. Ten strides were recorded for eight subjects, including data for the soleus, rectus femoris, biceps, vastus medialis, and tibialis anterior muscles. The authors concluded that three strides per subject provided information as reliable as that obtained from 12 strides.

Claeys R: The analysis of ground reaction forces in pathological gait secondary to disorders of the foot. *Int Orthop* 1983;7:113–119.

The normal gait pattern is characterized by a marked population variability, a considerable step-to-step consistency, and symmetry of the forces from both feet. The force pattern in pathologic gait secondary to disorders of the foot also shows a marked repeatability but is characterized by a pronounced asymmetry. A specific disorder of the foot does not necessarily result in a typical corresponding force pattern.

Opila KA, Nicol AC, Paul JP: Forces and impulses during aided gait. *Arch Phys Med Rehabil* 1987;68:715–722.

The relative contributions of limbs and aids were quantified in three patient groups: those with total hip replacements, those with tibial fractures, and those with paraplegia. Results showed (1) variability in aid loadings among the subjects with total hip replacements and between ipsilateral and contralateral sticks; (2) symmetric restraining and propelling aid loadings in those with fractures; and (3) greater aid impulses medially than anteroposteriorly in four of seven subjects performing three-point gait.

Perry J, Ireland ML, Gronley J, et al: Predictive value of manual muscle testing and gait analysis in normal ankles by dynamic electromyography. *Foot Ankle* 1986; 6:254–259.

Eight muscles about the ankle of seven normal subjects were electromyographically assessed during manual muscle testing and walking. Electromyographic activity increased as more muscle force was required during the different manual muscle test levels and at increased walking speeds. No manual test isolated activity to the specific muscle being tested. The intensity of muscle action during walking was related to the manual muscle test grades.

Shiavi R, Bugle HJ, Limbird T: Electromyographic gait assessment. *J Rehabil Res Dev* 1987;24:13–30.

The profiles of the linear envelopes of surface electromyograms of seven major muscles in adults were studied as a function of walking speed. The timing of most phases (expressed as percentage of the stride) decreased as speed increased. This suggests that the time base should be further normalized by stance and swing phases.

Recent Findings by Instrumented Gait Analysis

Arthritis

Lechner DE, McCarthy CF, Holden MK: Gait deviations in patients with juvenile rheumatoid arthritis. *Phys Ther* 1987;67:1335–1341.

Thirty children with juvenile rheumatoid arthritis and 30 healthy children were tested with a computerized gait-analysis system. In the subjects with juvenile rheumatoid arthritis, velocity, cadence, and stride length were significantly decreased. The anterior pelvic tilt of subjects with juvenile rheumatoid arthritis was significantly increased throughout the gait cycle. Hip extension at the end of single-limb stance and ankle plantar flexion during weight release were significantly decreased. There were no significant differences in step width, in the percentage of time spent in each phase of the gait cycle, or in knee-joint excursions.

Mansour JM, Preira JM: Quantitative functional anatomy of the lower limb with application to human gait. *J Biomech* 1987;20:51–58.

The functions of muscles crossing the hip and knee joints were computed on the basis of the changing relative positions of joint centers and muscle origins and insertions during one gait cycle. The function of several of the major muscles crossing the hip and knee joints was recorded for the different limb positions corresponding to normal gait. The amount of force necesary to produce a given moment about a joint depended on the limb position. In addition, muscle function changed significantly with limb position.

Willmott M: The effect of a vinyl floor surface and a carpeted floor surface upon walking in elderly hospital in-patients. *Age Ageing* 1986;15:119–120.

Fifty-eight elderly hospital patients walked along a 10-m length of carpeted corridor and a 10-m length of vinyl-tiled corridor. Gait speed and step length were significantly greater on the carpeted than on the vinyl surface.

Cerebral Palsy

Gage JR, Perry J, Hicks RR, et al: Rectus femoris transfer to improve knee function of children with cerebral palsy. *Dev Med Child Neurol* 1987;29:159–166.

Stance-phase stability and swing-phase clearance, prerequisites for normal ambulation, are often lost in the gait of children with cerebral palsy. The authors transferred the distal end of the rectus femoris in conjunction with hamstring lengthening in 37 knees, and compared the results with those for a control group of 24 knees in which only hamstring lengthening was done. In the first group, swing-phase knee flexion was improved by 16.0 ± 14.4 degrees, compared with 9.5 ± 7.5 degrees in the control group, and residual knee flexion in stance was reduced to 8.19 ± 8.1 degrees, compared with 15.1 ± 13.8 degrees in the control group.

Kalen V, Adler N, Bleck EE: Electromyography of idiopathic toe walking. *J Pediatr Orthop* 1986;6:31–33.

Eighteen idiopathic toe-walkers were evaluated by gait electromyography to define muscle-timing abnormalities. This group was compared with a matched group of normal children walking on their toes and to a group of patients with cerebral palsy and equinus deformities. Although historical data (family history, male predominance, and learning disabilities) suggested that idiopathic toe-walking is a true entity, the gait electromyograms were not diagnostic.

Norlin R, Odenrick P: Development of gait in spastic

children with cerebral palsy. *J Pediatric Orthop* 1986;6: 674–680.

The gait of 50 spastic children, 3 to 16 years old, showed abnormal values for the basal parameters of phases of the stride. Although values for gait velocity and stride length were lower than normal, they increased with age. Stance phase was longer than in normal children, the same tendency shown by double support. Most changes with age were the same as those in normal children. The prolonged stance and double support suggest deteriorated postural control, resulting in an increased need for support.

Normand X, Dubousse J: Remise en tension de l'appareil extenseur du genou dans la demarche en triple flexion chez l'enfant infirme moteur [Reinforcement of the tension of the knee extensor apparatus in triple flexion gait in children with motor disorders]. *Rev Chir Orthop* 1985;71:301–310.

Surgical reinforcement of the knee extensor mechanism improves the gait of children with cerebral palsy who walk with a crouch gait with flexion of the hips and knees. In these patients, the defect is related to excessive length of the patellar tendon. Surgical treatment combines shortening of the patellar tendon with lengthening of the hamstrings and tenotomy of the rectus femoris. In a series of 18 patients, the authors obtained 15 satisfactory results. The procedures were bilateral and the average follow-up was four years.

Olney SJ, Cosigan PA, Hedden DM: Mechanical energy patterns in gait of cerebral palsied children with hemiplegia. *Phys Ther* 1987;67:1348–1354.

The mechanical energy costs of walking were studied in ten children with cerebral palsy and hemiplegia to determine whether their values were substantially different from normal and, if so, to discover the movements responsible. A two-dimensional, sagittal-plane cinematographic analysis of the subjects' normal walking was undertaken. In most cases, the energy costs were above normal and were attributable to poor patterns of exchange between the potential and kinetic energy types of the head, arms, and trunk segment, to very low levels of kinetic energy that precluded exchange, or to both.

Perry J: Distal rectus femoris transfer. *Dev Med Child Neurol* 1987;29:153–158.

A major concern in the management of children with cerebral palsy is crouch gait with its excessively flexed knee and hip stance. Dynamic electromyographic records of 45 children with cerebral palsy demonstrated that the rectus femoris was likely to be active in swing phase, but that its release is appropriate only when electromyography confirms that the rectus is functioning in stance. Routine inclusion of a proximal rectus femoris release (without confirmation that the muscle's action was limited to stance) resulted in a stiff-legged gait.

Skinner SR, Lester DK: Gait electromyographic evaluation of the long-toe flexors in children with spastic cerebral palsy. *Clin Orthop* 1986;207:70–73.

In this prospective study, the electrical activities of the long-toe flexors in 37 children with varus or valgus hindfoot deformity were measured by wire electrode dynamic electromyography. Although gross abnormalities in the phasic timing of the flexor hallucis longus and flexor digitorum longus were observed, these muscles could not be implicated in the origin of hindfoot deformity.

Paraplegia

Braun Z, Mizrahi J, Najenson T, et al: Activation of paraplegic patients by functional electrical stimulation: Training and biomechanical evaluation. *Scand J Rehabil Med* 1985;12(suppl):93–101.

The authors describe a training method for activating the

lower-limb muscles of paraplegics by functional electrical stimulation. Four patients, who had been paralyzed for seven to 30 years, achieved a good standing position by stimulation of the quadriceps, sometimes supplemented by stimulation of the gluteus maximus or medius muscles. Gait was achieved by activation of the flexion reflex in a single stimulation and by tilting the trunk. No mechanical support was required to lock the joints. However, to maintain the equilibrium of the body, external supports (parallel bars, walkers, or Canadian crutches) were used. During treatment, gait improved because of reduced spasticity and better body stability.

Dietz V, Quintern J, Berger W: Afferent control of human stance and gait: Evidence for blocking of group I afferents during gait. *Exp Brain Res* 1985;61:153–163.

The cerebral potentials evoked by electrical stimulation of the tibial nerve during stance and in the various phases of gait of normal subjects were compared with the cerebral potentials and leg muscle electromyographic responses evoked by perturbations of stance and gait. Only in the stance condition was a smaller, shorter (40 ms) latency response seen. Thus, during gait the signals of group I afferents are blocked at both segmental and supraspinal levels. The electromyographic responses induced in the leg by gait perturbations may be evoked by group II afferents and mediated via a spinal pathway.

Eke-Okoro ST, Larsson LE, Sandlund B: Simulation of paretic gait in normal subjects by loading the ankles. *Scand J Rehabil Med* 1985;17:147–150.

Normal subjects were loaded with increasing weights (2 to 6 kg) applied around the ankles. Under these conditions, stride length increased in relation to velocity. The percentage of single-support duration increased in relation to stride duration. When loads applied to the two ankles were the same, the increase was symmetric. Consequently, there was also an increase in swing and decreases in stance and double support. The results differed in all respects from those in previous experiments during which the loads were carried in the hands.

Isakov E, Mizrahi J, Graupe D, et al: Energy cost and physiological reactions to effort during activation of paraplegics by functional electrical stimulation. *Scand J Rehabil Med* 1985;12(suppl):102–107.

In this study, the aim was to evaluate the influence on the cardiopulmonary system of muscular contractions of the paralyzed limbs in paraplegia, activated by functional electrical stimulation during treatment, and the energy cost of standing and walking while using functional electrical stimulation as an orthotic aid. After a six-month training period, the results indicated that functional electrical stimulation has a low energy cost in the sitting position and as an orthotic device for standing, confirming its beneficial effect in spastic paraplegia. However, efforts during ambulation by means of functional electrical stimulation were exhaustive and it is therefore advisable primarily for young subjects.

Marsolais EB, Kobetic R: Functional electrical stimulation for walking in paraplegia. *J Bone Joint Surg* 1987; 69A:728–733.

In paraplegic subjects who had functional transection of the spinal cord between the fourth and the 11th thoracic vertebrae, independent reciprocal walking was achieved by means of a portable microprocessor-controlled stimulator that electrically activated the muscles through percutaneous intramuscular wire electrodes.

McClelland M, Andrews BJ, Patrick JH, et al: Augmentation of the Oswestry Parawalker orthosis by means of surface electrical stimulation: Gait analysis of three patients. *Paraplegia* 1987;25:32–38.

The Oswestry Parawalker orthosis enabled 15 adults with complete thoracic-level paraplegia to achieve a reciprocal gait with an inherently low energy demand. To further diminish the work demands on the girdle musculature of the upper limb during ambulation, three of these patients underwent electrical stimulation of the gluteal muscles in stance phase. This increased the stability of the adduction and also provided forward propulsion by driving the stance leg into extension.

Hemiplegia

Dietz V, Quintern J, Berger W: Stumbling reactions in man: Release of a ballistic movement pattern. *Brain Res* 1986;362:355–357.

Four different modes of perturbation were applied during gait, either alone or in combination, to determine the extent to which compensatory reactions in the leg are released as fixed patterns or, alternatively, are generated by feedback mechanisms. Results indicate that the first agonist burst induced by a perturbation is stimulus-specific and immutable after release, and the appearance of the following burst of the triphasic pattern depends on the actual conditions. This suggests that a mechanism similar to that in ballistic hand and finger movements is operative, with the difference that the compensatory reactions after gait perturbations are induced by peripheral signals.

Holden MK, Gil KM, Magliozzi MR: Gait assessment for neurologically impaired patients: Standards for outcome assessment. *Phys Ther* 1986;66:1530–1539.

The authors compared the time-distance gait values of two groups of neurologically impaired subjects with those of healthy subjects and analyzed the influence of nine clinical characteristics. Velocity, cadence, step length, stride length, and ratio of stride length to lower-extremity length were recorded for 37 subjects with hemiplegia and 24 subjects with multiple sclerosis. Time-distance values were well below normal values, even in functionally independent subjects. Overall, the subjects with hemiparesis had lower values than the subjects with multiple sclerosis.

Maležič M, Bogataj U, Gros N, et al: Evaluation of gait with multichannel electrical stimulation. *Orthopedics* 1987;10:769–772.

Short, intensive multichannel electrical stimulation therapy was evaluated in 14 hemiplegic patients after stroke or head injury. The stimulation of the peroneal nerve and the soleus, quadriceps, hamstring, gluteus maximus, and triceps brachii muscles with individually preprogrammed sequences was applied by surface electrodes at the beginning of gait rehabilitation. The patients started walking with the support of a therapist, gradually increasing the walking distance. All achieved independent ambulation with a crutch after an average of 14 stimulation sessions.

Maležič M, Kljajic M, Acimovic-Janežič R, et al: Therapeutic effects of multisite electric stimulation of gait in motor-disabled patients. *Arch Phys Med Rehabil* 1987; 68:553–560.

Therapeutic effects in ten hemiplegic patients and one paraplegic patient treated by multisite electrical stimulation of gait were compared with effects in ten hemiplegic patients treated by standard rehabilitation methods after 2.6 months of extensive therapy. The results for the stimulated group in midtherapy indicated faster recovery rates (3.15 times in step length and 2.25 times in gait velocity) than in the control group; at the end of therapy, the stimulated group had higher improvement levels (2.11 times in step length, 1.42 times in gait velocity, and 1.63 times in kinesiologic gait analysis). The differences between the two groups faded after 8.4 months without treatment, and some kinesiologic deficits reappeared, mostly those in the more distal muscle groups. These findings indicate a need for simpler orthotic electrical stimulation after multisite therapy in several cases.

Pinzur MS, Sherman R, DiMonte-Leine P, et al: Adult-onset hemiplegia: Changes in gait after muscle-balancing procedures to correct the equinus deformity. *J Bone Joint Surg* 1986;68A:1249–1257.

Fifty-four adult patients with acquired spastic equinus and equinovarus deformity were treated with lengthening of the Achilles tendon, lateral transfer of the anterior tibial tendon, and appropriate muscle releases. Preoperatively, the stance and double-support phases of gait were prolonged. Throughout the stance phase, the gait of these patients was characterized by equinus deformity of the ankle, decreased flexion of the knee (hyperextension in the most severely involved patients), and increased flexion of the hip (which also varied with the severity of the equinus deformity of the ankle and hyperextension of the knee). After an average follow-up of 30 months (range, 24 to 62 months), the equinus deformity was corrected in all patients and 59% of them were brace-free. Postoperative analysis of gait, performed at least one year after surgery, in 27 patients, showed that the stance and double-support phases of gait (which had been prolonged before surgery) approached normal.

Muscular Dystrophy

Lord JP, Portwood MM, Fowler WM, et al: Upper vs lower extremity functional loss in neuromuscular disease. *Arch Phys Med Rehabil* 1987;68:8–9.

This study tested the hypothesis that upper-extremity and lower-extremity strength and functional losses are parallel in Duchenne's muscular dystrophy and other neuromuscular disorders. Vignos (lower extremity) grades, Brooke (upper extremity) grades, and manual muscle test scores were determined for 27 patients with Duchenne's muscular dystrophy, ten patients with fascioscapulohumeral muscular dystrophy, 24 patients with myotonic muscular dystrophy, and 29 patients with other proximal myopathies. Coefficients of determination indicated that a maximum of 86% of variation in upper-extremity rank could be explained purely by observing lower-extremity rank. Although there was a significant relationship between upper-extremity and lower-extremity strength and functional grade, these measurements were not entirely equivalent.

Khodadadeh S, McClelland MR, Patrick JH, et al: Knee moments in Duchenne muscular dystrophy. *Lancet* 1986;2:544–545.

The gait of seven boys with Duchenne's muscular dystrophy who could walk unaided and 21 normal boys was analyzed by means of a video recording technique linked to a Kistler force plate. The equinus gait of boys with Duchenne's muscular dystrophy was shown to be a necessary adaptation to keep the force about proximal joints, particularly the knee, within limits controllable by weakened muscles.

Myelodysplasia

Flandry F, Burke S, Roberts JM, et al: Functional ambulation in myelodysplasia: The effect of orthotic selection on physical and physiologic performance. *J Pediatr Orthop* 1986;6:661–665.

The metabolic demands of ambulation in a reciprocal-gait orthosis were compared with those in conventional bracing (hip-knee-ankle-foot orthosis) and wheelchair use in eight children with myelodysplasia. Heart rate was significantly increased during swing-through gait compared with that during wheelchair use (P < .01). Oxygen consumption studies showed a significant increase in swing-through gait over that in wheelchair use. These values for the reciprocal-gait orthosis approximated those for wheelchair use. These results suggested a more favorable prognosis for long-term functional ambulation in patients with higher-level myelodysplasia fitted with reciprocal-gait orthoses.

Nerve Palsy

Valencic V, Vodovnik L, Stefancic M, et al: Improved motor response due to chronic electrical stimulation of denervated tibialis anterior muscle in humans. *Muscle Nerve* 1986;9:612–617.

Nine patients with complete denervation of the tibialis anterior were admitted to a stimulation program to restore dorsiflexion of the foot. Best results were obtained with pulses 20 ms in width and with a 20-ms interval. After three weeks of training (20 minutes twice a day), dorsiflexion was increased in all patients. In some, gait was improved during the swing phase by electrical stimulation. Thus, the training program reversed the course of disuse atrophy.

22
Rehabilitation: Amputation, Prosthetics, and Orthotics

The surgeon who performs limb amputation must have a clear understanding of the entire rehabilitation process facing the amputee. The overall approach to amputation is to reconstruct rather than ablate the limb. The surgical aim is to form an ideal residual limb, in addition to removing the diseased limb segment. To achieve this rehabilitation goal, the amputation level should maximize length, the residual limb should retain maximal musculoskeletal function, and the amputee should be matched with the most appropriate prosthesis.

Amputations and Prostheses

Maximum Limb Length

Greater limb function correlates with greater limb length. This is especially true when greater length means saving an additional functional joint. The search continues for more accurate predictors of healing levels. Doppler waveform analysis, arteriography, and thallium scans have been joined by transcutaneous oxygen analysis and dermofluorometry. These newer methods measure vascular characteristics at points closer to the end-organ, thus defining healing levels more discretely. The information gained from these tests is frequently helpful, but the surgeon should be cautious about making decisions entirely on the basis of these laboratory results since inaccuracies still exist. Results of the physical examination and the laboratory measurements should contribute to the final decision.

Transcutaneous Oxygen and Fluorometric Prediction of Amputation Level

Two new techniques have been analyzed as adjuncts in determining the most distal amputation level that will heal. Both techniques can make valuable contributions to the information on which this critical decision relies, but fall short of an accurate predictor when taken alone. Ischemic limbs exhibit a continuous linear decrease in cutaneous Po_2 measurements when passing from viable into nonviable levels. Although more failures to heal occurred when amputations were attempted at tibial levels in which Po_2 was less than 20 mm Hg, no value, not even 0 mm Hg, was associated with 100% failure. Thus, Po_2 is a measure of relative risk for healing failure rather than an absolute predictor.

A somewhat better predictive measure was achieved with the use of dermofluorometry. This method allows sampling of many skin sites, producing a more detailed map of skin vascularity. The index calculated produced a distinct cutoff below which healing did not occur. It promises to be useful in situations in which Doppler pressures are least reliable, that is, in patients with peripheral vessel wall calcification.

These methods provide more accurate information about the vascularity in the limb to be amputated. Other factors that must be weighed include the extent and severity of infection, the patient's nutritional status, age, and eventual ambulatory status, and any concomitant medical problems. This decision remains complex.

Functional Residual Limb

Creating the optimal residual limb may require many reconstructive surgical techniques, combined with a knowledge of prosthetic socket design. The ideal limb is covered with durable, sensate skin, has adequate soft-tissue padding for the bony elements, and provides a broad bone end for weightbearing and/or prosthetic manipulation.

Recently several new surgical techniques have been successfully applied to limb amputation. Free vascularized soft-tissue flaps have been used to achieve bone coverage at the end of amputated limbs. Skin expansion followed by local muscle rotation has also been used to improve soft-tissue padding for prominent bone ends. These techniques should be considered for primary or revision surgery to avoid bone shortening.

In traumatic amputations, microsurgical techniques have made limb reimplantation possible. The functional outcome of a reimplanted limb must be weighed against that of a prosthesis. As experience with the eventual function of reimplanted limbs is being gained, clearer guidelines are emerging.

Prosthetic Design

Prosthetic devices continue to evolve because of new materials and new design features. Orthopaedic surgeons must have a working knowledge of the indications for each major design option. This knowledge will improve both their surgical technique and their prosthetic prescriptions. They will be asked to make recommendations regarding the utility of a specific prosthetic design for a specific patient. Clinical factors (such as residual limb characteristics, patient motivation, and other medical problems) are combined with prosthetic characteristics (such as socket design, weight, and performance) to achieve maximal function.

Narrow Mediolateral Socket

A new socket shape has been added to the traditional quadrilateral socket for the above-knee prosthesis. The narrower dimension in the mediolateral socket diameter, in combination with alignment of the femur in adduction, offers greater prosthetic control for some amputees. Studies have shown that many patients with above-knee amputations stand with the femur on the amputated side held in abduction (Fig. 1). The quadrilateral socket has been criticized because of its nonanatomic conformation and poor residual limb control of coronal plane stability. The diameter of the socket is wider in the coronal plane than in the sagittal plane (Fig. 2). The ischium is forced to rest above the socket on the posterior brim shelf (Fig. 3) and is held in this position because of a relatively narrow anteroposterior diameter. As a result, proximal thigh distortion decreases comfort during both sitting and prolonged standing (Fig. 4).

Initially referred to as the normal shape-normal alignment (NSNA) prosthesis, this new design is now more commonly known as the contoured adducted trochanteric-controlled alignment method (CAT-CAM) prosthesis. It improves socket comfort by transmitting body weight to the prosthesis through the well-padded gluteal muscle mass rather than the ischium. The socket maintains the femur in an adducted position throughout the stance phase of gait, thus improving the efficiency of the hip abductor muscles. The combination of this socket shape and alignment (Fig. 5) gives the amputee better prosthetic control by min-

imizing relative limb-socket movement, narrowing the base of support by the femoral adduction, and decreasing overall energy expenditure during walking. Indications for this design include adequate thigh segment length and good muscle-bone reattachment (myodesis).

Flexible Prosthetic Sockets

Investigators have combined stiff with flexible materials to produce more comfortable sockets in both upper- and lower-extremity prostheses. A strong, lightweight, stiff material is used as the skeletal framework, while a flexible material completes the walls. This combination often produces prostheses that are as strong as completely rigid designs but significantly lighter and more comfortable, particularly for patients with above-knee amputations who must bear weight through the socket while sitting and while standing.

In one group with above-knee amputations fitted with ISNY (Icelandic-Swedish-New York) flexible sockets, socket-mounted motion transducers recorded wall expan-

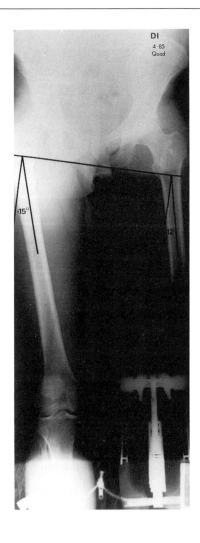
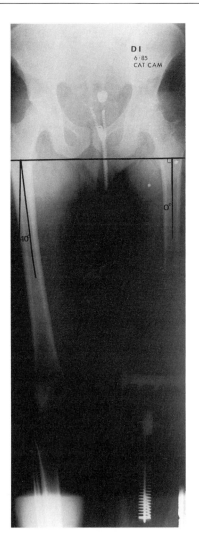

Figure 1
Stance after above-knee amputation. **Left**, The amputed femoral shaft in a quadrilateral socket is abducted 12 degrees. In contrast, the intact limb is adducted 15 degrees. **Right**, In the same patient, a CAT-CAM socket holds the amputated femur in a more normal alignment.
(Reproduced with permission from Flandry F, Besken J, Chambers RB, et al: The effect of the CAT-CAM above-knee prosthesis on functional rehabilitation. *Clin Orthop* 1989;239:249–262.)

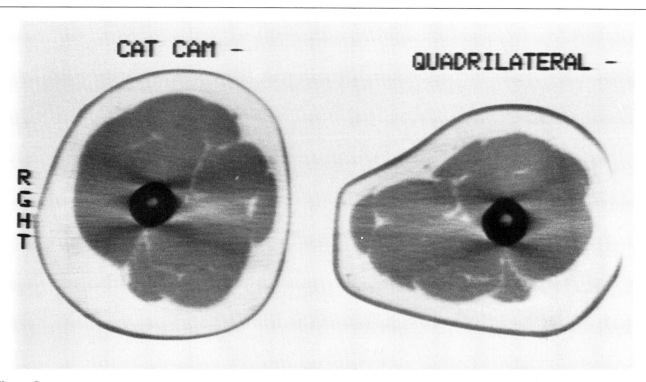

Figure 2

CAT-CAM and quadrilateral above-knee socket sleeves were fabricated to fit a normal subject. Computed tomographic scans demonstrate that the thigh musculature is more distorted by the quadrilateral socket sleeve. (Reproduced with permission from Flandry F, Besken J, Chambers RB, et al: The effect of the CAT-CAM above-knee prosthesis on functional rehabilitation. *Clin Orthop* 1989;239:249–262.)

sion synchronous with contraction of the underlying musculature during walking. This helps explain how the flexible socket improves walking comfort and suggests the possibility of improved muscular efficiency with these sockets. Gait analysis of a single subject walking with two different sockets (one with flexible walls and the other with rigid walls) on the same prosthesis showed no differences between the two socket designs. The single subject studied suggests that there may be no gait penalty for the increased socket comfort of the combined rigid-flexible socket. Additional objective data are needed to confirm these preliminary favorable findings.

Lightweight Materials

Attempts to decrease the weight of prostheses continue with a host of new materials and new fabrication techniques. The geriatric amputee with limited cardiovascular reserve but no musculoskeletal deficits (for example, joint contractures) should benefit from a prosthesis of lighter weight. Those amputees who desire to engage in sports and who are willing to forgo aesthetics may benefit from a non-anatomic limb made of the newly developed materials. The theoretic advantages of lightweight materials have yet to be confirmed by rigorous comparative studies. Anecdotal reports from amputees have praised the lighter limbs, but one must be cautious of ascribing all the benefits expressed to the lighter weight alone. In a study of 24 patients with below-knee amputations before and after conversion to an ultralightweight prosthesis, the amputees favored the lighter prosthesis but there was no measurable change in prosthetic use when wearing time and step counts were compared. Many conversion studies and amputee prefer-

ence studies are based on comparisons of old ill-fitting prostheses with new well-fitting ones. The improved fit accounts for improved amputee comfort. Further studies are needed to confirm which patient will benefit from decreased weight.

Energy-Storing Prosthetic Feet

A new generation of prosthetic feet has been introduced—energy-storing feet. These feet assist the amputee by absorbing energy during one part of the gait cycle and then releasing that energy during a later part of the cycle. This energy transfer, combined with improvements in joint motion, has led to reevaluation of how closely prostheses can simulate normal lower-limb function. Most reports have been anecdotal. Active amputees reported a greater ability to run and jump. One study of a few patients with below-knee amputations compared the SACH (solid ankle cushioned heel) foot with one of the energy-storing designs (Flex-Foot). Several gait parameters were closer to normal with the energy-storing prosthetic foot, leading to a more symmetric gait pattern. This was particularly evident for single-limb stance time, control of tibial advancement, and contralateral heel-strike forces. Although these data are preliminary, the energy-storing foot is promising.

Externally Powered Upper-Extremity Prostheses

In upper-extremity amputations, the dexterity and cosmesis of the terminal device as well as its weight, are of primary importance. Myoelectric limbs offer many of these features, along with an external power source. As miniaturization continues throughout the electronics field, myoelectric prostheses continue to improve the precise con-

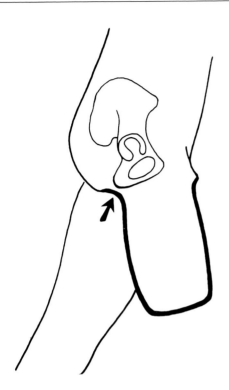

Figure 3

In the ischial weightbearing quadrilateral socket, the ischium is forced to rest on the posterior brim shelf. (Reproduced with permission from Flandry F, Besken J, Chambers RB, et al: The effect of the CAT-CAM above-knee prosthesis on functional rehabilitation. *Clin Orthop* 1989;239:249–262.)

trol of terminal devices. High repair rates, problems with the skin-electrode interface, and a lack of ruggedness have limited myoelectric prostheses to sedentary tasks only. A study of unilateral prosthesis use in adults found that body-powered prostheses were used preferentially by amputees working in jobs that required heavy lifting or handling greasy or sharp materials. Occupations in which myoelectric prostheses were used included office work, supervisory work, and jobs involving contact with the general public. Task character remains the most important factor in determining the most useful design for upper-extremity prostheses.

Single-Purpose Terminal Devices

Another way to improve upper-extremity function after amputation is to use terminal devices designed for a single task. These devices are used primarily in recreational sports and some specialized occupations. Three amputee saxophonists, for example, returned to concert-level proficiency by using special modifications to both the terminal devices and the instruments. Such custom task-related components can be rewarding. These changes are all designed to minimize the functional loss that accompanies amputation.

Orthotics and Rehabilitation

Since World War II, the application of engineering principles to the design and fabrication of orthoses has produced rapid advances.

Rationale for Orthotic Prescription

The orthotic prescription is intended to stabilize body segments and control motion. Simply defined, an orthosis is a device applied to the body to provide stability. Stabilization is achieved by externally grasping the body segment above and below the desired point requiring control. Consequently, all orthoses are force systems whether they are used to support a fracture, stabilize a joint, or correct a deformity. It logically follows that a successful orthotic fit depends on secure external attachment to the body segments.

An orthosis may exert large forces on the skin to counteract the ground-reaction force and provide stability at the ankle or knee. Although conventional metallic upright structural supports and leather cuffs with buckles remain useful, the introduction of synthetic materials during the past several decades has produced orthotic devices that provide better cosmesis, lighter weight, and closer fit. Vacuum-forming plastic shells over positive molds of the patient's limb provide a custom fit over bony prominences, distribute load more evenly, and help to avoid excessive skin pressure.

When prescribing an orthosis, the physician must carefully balance the need for joint stabilization with the amount of motion to be allowed. A joint may permit complex control by providing stability in one plane while allowing motion in another. Stops may be added to restrict the arc of permitted motion.

Different biomechanical solutions are needed for different clinical problems. For example, the treatment of choice for dropfoot resulting from peroneal nerve palsy is usually a flexible ankle-foot orthosis, made entirely of flexible plastic, that permits ankle plantar flexion after heel strike and stabilizes the limb more rapidly by placing the entire foot in contact with the ground. Conversely, equinus deformity in a stroke patient resulting from dorsiflexion weakness combined with moderate or severe plantar-flexion spasticity is usually best treated with a rigid orthosis that prevents ankle motion. This restriction helps prevent stretch-excitation (clonus) of the gastrocsoleus muscle that would impede forward progress during walking.

Gait Analysis

Although many of the advances in orthotics are the result of the introduction of new materials, a successful orthotic prescription still depends on an accurate assessment of the functional needs of the patient. When the abnormality is limited and the orthosis must control a single joint, the principles are relatively simple. When the abnormality affects the entire lower limb, as in most central nervous system disorders, considerable knowledge of the principles of biomechanics and gait analysis are required to achieve an optimal result.

Physiologic Considerations

Physiologic demand during walking is increased in most gait impairments requiring prostheses, orthoses, or crutches. The magnitude of the increase depends on how much the lower-extremity disability shifts antigravity support from the legs to the arms and shoulder girdle. Further, patients with gait impairments often have a reduced exercise capacity because of the effects of deconditioning, inactivity, or associated secondary disease. Therefore, the

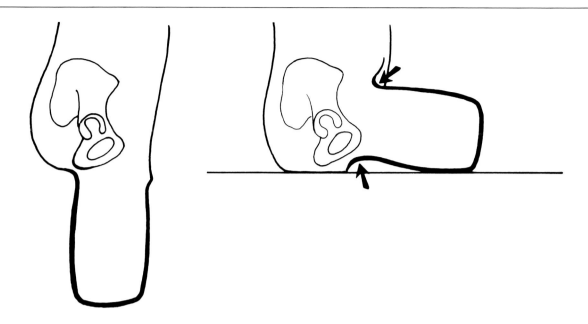

Figure 4
Proximal thigh distortion decreases comfort during sitting and prolonged standing. (Reproduced with permission from Flandry F, Besken J, Chambers RB, et al: The effect of the CAT-CAM above-knee prosthesis on functional rehabilitation. *Clin Orthop* 1989;239:249–262.)

patient's level of physical conditioning, strength, and endurance must be assessed when orthoses and upper-extremity gait-assist devices are prescribed. Failure to provide for the increased energy requirement often explains why patients with severe disabilities discontinue walking despite orthotic or prosthetic prescriptions and gait training. Physical therapy conditioning programs to increase physical work capacity are often essential.

Amputation Walking without a prosthesis and with a three-point crutch-assisted gait is associated with a high rate of oxygen consumption and a high heart rate in comparison to walking with a prosthesis and without crutches. The high physiologic demand results from the tremendous exertion required to elevate the entire body weight with each step.

Fracture Three-point gait after an injury to the lower limb that requires unilateral nonweightbearing similarly requires intense physical exertion. The energy expenditure of three-point gait was measured in patients with recent fractures. After five minutes of crutch ambulation, oxygen uptake was 32% greater than the value for normal walking, the heart rate was 53% above normal, and the respiratory quotient was markedly increased above the anaerobic threshold, indicating that the arm and shoulder-girdle muscles were working under anaerobic conditions (Table 1). These findings explain why patients with recent fractures, who are unable to bear weight on the injured limb, are severely restricted walkers. Fracture patients should be allowed full or partial weightbearing on the injured limb at the earliest possible time consistent with adequate healing to lessen physiologic stress. A therapy program to improve exercise capacity may be helpful in older patients.

Paralysis Increased energy expenditure during walking was also found in patients with spinal cord injuries who required orthoses because of paralyzed lower-limb muscles.

Paraplegics needing bilateral knee-ankle-foot orthoses to walk and who used a swing-through gait had an average rate of oxygen consumption that was 43% more than that of the patients who used wheelchairs and 38% more than required for normal walking. The average walking speed was slow in comparison with wheelchair propulsion or normal walking (Table 2). Thus, most paraplegics who require bilateral knee-ankle-foot orthoses and who use a swing-through gait prefer to use wheelchairs and discontinue walking.

Even paraplegics with musculature sufficient for a reciprocal gait pattern are limited in their ability to walk. The increase in the rate of energy expenditure beyond that required for normal walking depends directly on the extent of motor paralysis in the lower limbs and the forces exerted by the arms on crutches (Fig. 6).

Hip-Knee-Ankle-Foot Orthosis In its basic form a hip-knee-ankle-foot orthosis consists of two knee-ankle-foot orthoses linked to a rigid thoracolumbar support by a hip joint mechanism. The knee joints are locked during walking. The hip joints limit motion to flexion and extension.

Because this device does not improve intrinsic propulsive input or antigravity hip stability, two different approaches have been used to achieve hip extension. In the first, a cable mechanism is attached to the orthosis to link both lower limbs (Fig. 7). This device is called a reciprocal-gait orthosis. Active hip flexion is required. The hip in swing phase, powered by the patient's hip flexors during unrestrained hip flexion, exerts a force via the cable that extends the stance phase and stabilizes the pelvis, facilitating reciprocal gait. In one study, 24 of 41 children fitted with reciprocal-gait orthoses achieved ambulatory status.

Another investigator added functional electrical stimulation to a hip-knee-ankle-foot orthosis to provide stability and limb motion. The gluteal and quadriceps muscles were stimulated in stance, providing hip extensor stability and

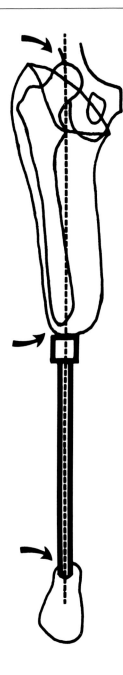

Figure 5
The CAT-CAM or normal shape-normal alignment concept uses a socket shape and a prosthesis alignment method to maintain the femur in adduction, distribute weightbearing over the gluteal muscles, and prevent movement of the limb within the socket. (Reproduced with permission from Flandry F, Besken J, Chambers RB, et al: The effect of the CAT-CAM above-knee prosthesis on functional rehabilitation. *Clin Orthop* 1989;239:249–262.)

Table 1. Energy expenditure in three-point crutch gait*

Data	Gait	
	Three-Point	Normal
Heart rate (beats/min)	153	100
Oxygen uptake rate (ml/kg·m)	15.7	11.9
Oxygen cost (ml/kg·m)	0.32	0.15
Velocity (m/min)	50	80

*Reproduced with permission from Waters RL, Campbell JM, Perry J: Energy cost of three-point crutch ambulation in fracture patients. *J Orthop Trauma* 1987;1:170–173.

fatigue, and muscle pain indicated that excessive demand and overuse of the remaining muscle fibers accounted for these symptoms. Thus, it is important to prescribe orthoses to protect weak muscles from overuse.

Many of these patients stopped using orthoses after their adolescent years because they were able to substitute for paralyzed musculature by means of altered posture or "trick maneuvers," or by using their remaining, although weakened, muscles. Newer orthotic designs encourage better patient compliance and can prevent common problems such as genu recurvatum, genu valgum, or mediolateral ankle instability. Patients should not have to wait until their problems are intractable before accepting orthotic assistance.

The Weightbearing Upper Limb

During mammalian evolution from quadrupeds to bipeds, the forelimbs evolved as dextrous prehensile devices, losing their weightbearing function. In patients with paraplegia, the upper extremities must assume the burden of mobility and weightbearing activities. Repetitive stresses are placed on the upper-extremity joints during wheelchair propulsion and transfers that exceed the customary tolerances. Pain, particularly at the shoulder, progressively increases after injury. Arthrograms of paraplegics with shoulder pain have found a high incidence of rotator cuff tears.

More than 70% of paraplegics monitored for more than ten years have symptoms and signs of carpal tunnel syndrome. Measurements of carpal tunnel pressures at rest and during loading indicate that median nerve neuropathy is probably the result of the cumulative effects of high transient carpal tunnel pressures recorded during the repetitive loading required by wheeling and transfer maneuvers.

Functional Electrical Stimulation

Functional electrical stimulation is a method of eliciting muscle contraction by electrically activating either the intact peripheral nerve or the substance of the muscle. This technique may be considered in treating central nervous system disorders such as spinal cord injury or stroke. In these conditions the anterior motor neuron and its axon are intact and, therefore, the muscle contracts in response to nerve stimulation.

In contrast, peripheral axons in lower motor neuron disorders such as polio or nerve transection are unable to conduct nerve action potentials and do not respond to stimulation. To achieve a motor response from direct muscle stimulation, a high level of stimulation is required, usually beyond the limits of pain and skin tolerance, and the

permitting knee motion. This improved performance, which was measured objectively by significantly increased walking speed and decreased work done by the arm and shoulder girdle muscles.

Orthotic Prescriptions for Patients Who Have Had Polio

Muscle pain and declining ambulatory capability are common in patients who have had polio. Electromyographic studies on such patients complaining of new weakness,

Table 2. Energy expenditure of paraplegics in walking and wheeling*

Data	Swing-Through Gait	Reciprocal Gait	Wheeling
Heart rate (beats/min)	140	131	123
Oxygen uptake rate (ml/kg·min)	16.3	13.8	11.5
Oxygen cost (ml/kg·m)	0.88	0.75	0.16
Velocity (m/min)	29	26	72

*Reproduced with permission from Waters RL, Campbell JM, Perry J: Energy cost of three-point crutch ambulation in fracture patients. *J Orthop Trauma* 1987;1:170–173.

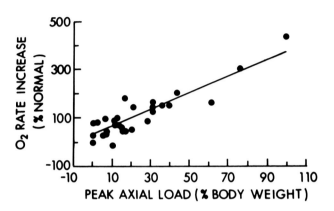

Figure 6

In patients with spinal cord injuries, the percentage by which energy expenditure is increased over normal depends on the peak axial load exerted by the arms on crutches. (Reproduced with permission from Flandry F, Besken J, Chambers RB, et al: The effect of the CAT-CAM above-knee prosthesis on functional rehabilitation. *Clin Orthop* 1989; 239:249–262.)

quality of the recruitment pattern of the motor response is comparatively poor and inadequate for functional purposes.

Despite success with surface stimulation for therapeutic purposes, the success of functional electrical stimulation has been limited. It is difficult to stimulate deep muscles and it may not be possible to obtain a discrete response in a specific individual muscle. From a clinical standpoint, patients experience problems with "gadget tolerance" and find it difficult and inconvenient to don and operate equipment with many wires, electrodes, and stimulator controls. Devices to stimulate the peroneal nerve in the swing phase to correct footdrop in stroke patients by means of skin electrodes and a footswitch triggering mechanism are commercially available.

In contrast to functional electrical stimulation, therapeutic electrical stimulation has received widespread clinical application. Therapeutic stimulation is not used for functional restoration of movement but as a therapeutic exercise for motor re-education and/or increasing muscle strength.

Lower Extremities

In 30 patients with lower-limb paralysis secondary to spinal cord injury that produced upper motor neuron paralysis, electrical stimulation enabled the legs to power a cycle ergometer. Increased strength, endurance, and bulk of stimulated muscles were noted. The subjects were able

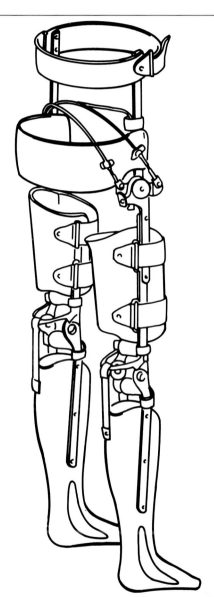

Figure 7

In a reciprocal-gait orthosis, a cable mechanism attached to two hip-knee-ankle-foot orthoses links the lower limbs. Active hip flexion, powered by the patient's hip flexors, exerts a force via the cable to extend the contralateral hip and facilitate reciprocal gait. (Reproduced with permission from Flandry F, Besken J, Chambers RB, et al: The effect of the CAT-CAM above-knee prosthesis on functional rehabilitation. *Clin Orthop* 1989;239:249–262.)

to perform more work per unit of time, indicating a training effect.

Recent investigations have focused on multichannel systems capable of restoring complex motor functions. In one study, a four-channel, computer-controlled device worn by the patient achieved a reciprocal gait with crutch assistance. The peroneal nerve was stimulated during the swing phase to elicit a flexion response; the quadriceps was stimulated during the stance phase. The patients required walkers.

Because of the limitations of surface electrodes, a percutaneous electrode system for restoring gait in paraplegics has been developed. Electrode implantation involved locating a motor point by systematic probing within a muscle. When the desired muscle contraction was obtained, the wire electrode was inserted and the needle withdrawn. A 32-channel stimulator allowed multichannel stimulation of different muscle groups. As many as 24 patterns of preprogrammed activities, such as standing and climbing stairs, can be selected from a menu stored on the stimulator. Because this system permits many different muscles to be stimulated, gait velocity and performance were superior to those achieved with surface stimulation alone. However, percutaneous electrodes were not thought to be suitable for long-term use because of the need for frequent reimplantation as a result of movement and breakage. Also, the patients still required walkers.

Surgical implantation of a peroneal nerve stimulator has been used to correct footdrop caused by hemiplegia. The surgical component consisted of a cuff electrode (wrapped around the peroneal nerve) connected to an implanted receiver. An external stimulator transmitted power to the receiver via a radiofrequency signal. A footswitch trigger activated the device in the swing phase. Some patients have used this stimulator for more than 12 years without evidence of nerve damage. Obtaining a balanced dorsiflexion response was difficult because only a single stimulation channel was available. This study indicates the potential feasibility and safety of surgically implanted nerve electrodes in humans.

Upper Extremities

Multichannel functional electrical stimulation systems have been used to restore upper-limb function in patients with C-5 and C-6 quadriplegia. The muscles stimulated for grasp-and-release are the flexors and extensors of the fingers and thumb (flexor digitorum superficialis and profundus, flexor pollicis longus, adductor pollicis, flexor pollicis brevis, abductor pollicis brevis, extensor digitorum, and extensor pollicis longus). Movement of the contralateral shoulder permits computerized control of hand and forearm musculature. Grasp patterns rather than control of individual muscles are provided because the patient cannot consciously coordinate the level of activity of each muscle while also performing a task. A static wrist-hand orthosis is used for neutral wrist stabilization in patients with C-5 quadriplegia. Although percutaneous stimulator systems are important as a means of assessing functional electrical stimulation in a reversible, minimally invasive way, percutaneous electrodes are unsuitable for prolonged use.

Trends

Amputation vs Reimplantation

Microsurgical techniques have allowed severed limbs to be successfully reattached after traumatic amputation. In such cases, the surgeon must decide whether to complete and close the amputation or to reimplant the detached part. Microsurgical techniques have been developed to anastomose ever-smaller structures, decrease the length of surgery, and delay death of the separated tissue. Information on long-term function is now becoming available. In a series of single-digit reimplantations (excluding the thumb) followed up for an average of more than four years, finger survival was high (86%), but some of the reimplanted fingers did not function well enough to warrant reattachment. Those fingers with anastomoses proximal to the insertion of the superficial flexors actually compromised overall hand function. Decisions about this surgical choice should reflect what is technically possible and what is functionally beneficial.

Follow-up and Reassessment

Continual evaluation of functional outcome must be provided to the initial decision-makers in the amputation process. The surgeon performing reconstructive amputations will continue to improve in surgical technique, patient selection, and level selection if long-term information on patient outcome is provided.

Prosthetic and Orthotic Design

In the future, attempts to find improved materials that are stronger, lighter, and more cosmetic will continue. Exotic materials such as graphite fiber and composite materials developed for the aerospace industry will achieve wider acceptance because of their lighter weight and superior strength as new fabrication techniques lower production costs. In this regard, computer-assisted designs and manufacturing technology will undoubtably play an increasing role.

At present, new socket designs for above-knee prostheses may improve prosthetic control so that elderly patients, previously thought not to be prosthetic candidates, can benefit from prosthetic use.

Functional Electrical Stimulation

The simplicity with which functional electrical stimulation systems can be operated will determine their ultimate utility. It is evident that surgically implanted systems are necessary to minimize the need for external electrodes, minimize external hardware, and achieve superior motor response.

Present work shows that it is possible to achieve electrically induced reciprocal gait with open-loop control without providing feedback about joint position. However, preliminary investigations indicate that position-sensors providing closed-loop control by means of feedback information to the computer will smooth the motion and reduce the total amount of stimulation needed.

At present, there are no available sensors suitable for long-term implantation in humans. It can be anticipated that the first generation of sensors will be mounted externally to the orthoses to provide continuous feedback about joint position. Hybrid orthoses with anterior and posterior stops may also be useful to protect insensitive joints from overstimulation and to prevent neuropathic changes. Pressure sensors on the plantar surface of the foot will permit the load distribution and the center of pressure to be calculated.

In the upper extremity, feedback about joint position, contact, force, slippage, pressure, and temperature will enhance functional electrical stimulation systems. Because quadriplegic patients who benefit from this technique are confined to wheelchairs, constraints on stimulator size and weight are not as important as they are in paraplegic patients. For this reason, development may proceed more rapidly in the upper limb than in the lower limb.

Annotated Bibliography

Keywords

Amputation; Electrical stimulation; Gait; Orthosis; Paraplegia; Polio; Prosthesis; Quadriplegia

Amputations and Prostheses

Charles D, James KB, Stein RB: Rehabilitation of musicians with upper limb amputations. *J Rehabil Res Dev* 1988;25:25–32.
Specially adapted prostheses and instruments were used for three saxophone-playing amputees. The quality of the rehabilitation was sufficient for these musicians to return to teaching and performing.

Convery P, Hughes J, Jones D, et al: A clinical evaluation of an ultralightweight polypropylene below-knee prosthesis. *Orthot Prosth* 1986;40:30–37.
Although 24 patients with below-knee amputations expressed a preference for the ultralight prosthetic limb, no conclusions could be reached regarding the effectiveness of this design because several other prosthetic changes were made at the same time.

Flandry F, Beskin J, Chambers RB, et al: The effect of the CAT-CAM above-knee prosthesis on functional rehabilitation. *Clin Orthop* 1989;239:249–262.
Five unilateral above-knee amputations in which quadrilateral sockets were used were converted to contoured adducted trochanteric-controlled alignment method (CAT-CAM) sockets to determine the effect on ambulatory function. Four of five patients had an improved gait pattern, faster walking speed, and lower physiologic energy expenditure after conversion.

Kawamura I, Kawamura J: Some biomechanical evaluations of the ISNY flexible above-knee system with quadrilateral socket. *Orthot Prosth* 1986;40:17–23.
Socket movement for a quadrilateral above-knee prosthesis was measured with transducers embedded in the socket walls of prostheses used by three amputees while walking. Wall movements temporally corresponded to the underlying muscle contractions in the residual limb.

Krebs D, Tashman S: Kinematic and kinetic comparison of the conventional and ISNY above-knee socket. *Clin Prosth Orthot* 1985;9:22–36.
Gait parameters were compared for a single patient with an above-knee amputation while walking with two prostheses, one with an ISNY socket and one with a rigid socket. Data collected and analyzed included joint position of the pelvis and both lower limbs in three dimensions, floor-reaction forces, and movement of the prosthesis in three dimensions. No significant differences between the two designs were found.

Long I: Normal shape-normal alignment (NSNA) above-knee prosthesis. *Clin Prosth Orthot* 1985;9:9–14.
A technique for fabricating and aligning this above-knee prosthesis is described.

Millstein SG, Heger H, Hunter GA: Prosthetic use in adult upper limb amputees: A comparison of the body powered and electrically powered prostheses. *Prosth Orthot Int* 1986;10:27–34.
A group of 314 patients with unilateral work-related limb amputations were examined one to 49 years after being fitted with prostheses. Results indicated complete or useful acceptance of the prosthesis in 83% of those with electrically powered limbs, 88% of those with cable-driven hooks, and 40% of those with cosmetic prostheses. In general, the cable-driven hook was preferred for precision and heavy work. The electrically powered limbs had good acceptance despite increased initial and maintenance costs. Electrically powered limbs provided better function for patients with proximal amputations.

Radocy B: Upper extremity prosthetics: Considerations and designs for sports and recreation. *Clin Prosth Orthot* 1987;11:131–153.
Sports-specific designs for upper extremity prosthetic modifications are reviewed. Twenty-four sports, from archery to wind surfing, are covered.

Sabolich J: Contoured adducted trochanteric-controlled alignment method (CAT-CAM): Introduction and basic principles. *Clin Prosth Orthot* 1985;9:15–26.
The article reviews the theoretic principles on which the CAT-CAM prosthesis is based. The advantages of this socket shape and alignment are compared with those of more traditional socket designs.

Silverman DG, Rubin SM, Reilly CA, et al: Fluorometric prediction of successful amputation level in the ischemic limb. *J Rehabil Res Dev* 1985;22:23–28.
Prediction of healing was determined by conventional methods and the results compared with those of fluorometric methods in 39 lower-extremity amputations. Results for fluorometric prediction were good, with accurate predictions in 36 of the 39 amputations. A fluorometric healing zone was proposed.

Urbaniak JR, Roth JH, Nunley JA, et al: The results of replantation after amputation of a single finger. *J Bone Joint Surg* 1985;67A:611–619.
A review of 59 consecutive single finger amputations (excluding the thumb) 53 months after reimplantation showed that finger survival was age-related, with poorer survival rates for patients less than 30 years old. Functional results were related to the anatomic location of the anastomosis, with poorer function when digits amputated proximal to the insertion of the superficial flexors were reimplanted.

Wagner P, Sienko S, Supan T, et al: Motion analysis of SACH vs Flex-Foot in moderately active below-knee amputees. *Clin Prosth Orthot* 1987;11:55–62.
Gait parameters were measured in three patients with below-knee amputations while they walked with both SACH and Flex-Foot prostheses. An additional three patients used Flex-Foot prostheses alone. The Flex-Foot provided more normal

ankle dorsiflexion (20 degrees) in later stance than did the SACH foot. The force with which the sound limb struck the floor was closer to normal with the Flex-Foot; this force was greater than normal with the SACH foot. All other gait parameters were similar.

Wyss CR, Harrington RM, Burgess EM, et al: Transcutaneous oxygen tension as a predictor of success after an amputation. *J Bone Joint Surg* 1988;70A:203–207.

Transcutaneous oxygen measurements were correlated with healing outcome in 206 lower-extremity amputations. Increased probability of failure was correlated with decreasing oxygen tension. No absolute healing zone could be identified by oxygen tension criteria.

Orthotics and Rehabilitation

Bayley JC, Cochran TP, Sledge CB: The weight-bearing shoulder: The impingement syndrome in paraplegics. *J Bone Joint Surg* 1987;69A:676–678.

Paraplegic patients have a high incidence of shoulder pain from impingement syndrome resulting from manual wheelchair use and the need for the arms to perform weightbearing activities.

Clark DR, Perry J, Lunsford TR: Case studies: Orthotic management of the adult post polio patient. *Orthot Prosth* 1986;40:43–50.

Appropriate orthoses can prevent or correct common deformities, such as genu recurvatum, genu valgum, and mediolateral ankle instability, that commonly occur in patients without orthoses who have had polio.

Gellman H, Chandler DR, Petrasek J, et al: Carpal tunnel syndrome in paraplegic patients. *J Bone Joint Surg* 1988;70A:517–519.

Paraplegic patients have a high incidence of carpal tunnel syndrome secondary to the effects of repetitive contact of the hands on the rims of wheelchairs and the high carpal tunnel pressures generated during weightbearing activities.

Gellman H, Sie I, Waters RL: Late complications of the weight-bearing upper extremity in the paraplegic patient. *Clin Orthop* 1988;233:132–135.

The incidence of pain at the upper-extremity joints progressively increases in paraplegic and quadriplegic patients confined to wheelchairs.

McCall RE, Schmidt WT: Clinical experience with the reciprocal gait orthosis in myelodysplasia. *J Pediatr Orthop* 1986;6:157–161.

Prescription of a reciprocal gait orthosis improved gait performance in 32 of 41 children with myelodysplasia.

Perry J, Barnes G, Gronley JK: The postpolio syndrome: An overuse phenomenon. *Clin Orthop* 1988;233:145–162.

Electromyographic studies in patients who have had polio show that muscle pain and diminishing ability to walk are common because of excessive demand on and overuse of remaining muscle fibers. Orthoses should be prescribed to stabilize the ankle and knee to prevent muscle overuse.

Waters RL, Campbell JM, Perry J: Energy cost of three-point crutch ambulation in fracture patients. *J Orthop Trauma* 1987;1:170–173.

Unilateral nonweightbearing crutch ambulation in otherwise healthy patients with fractures increases the rate of oxygen consumption and heart rate because of the severe exercise demand on the arms and shoulder-girdle muscles required to lift and swing the entire body forward with each step.

Waters RL, Yakura JS, Adkins R, et al: Determinants of gait performance following spinal cord injury. *Arch Phys Med Rehabil*, in press.

In adult patients with spinal cord injuries, the velocity, cadence, and increase in the rate of energy expenditure beyond the amount required for normal walking depend on the extent of lower-extremity paralysis. The peak force exerted by the upper extremities on crutches is inversely related to the extent of lower-limb paralysis.

Functional Electrical Stimulation

Keith MW, Peckham PH, Thrope GB, et al: Functional neuromuscular stimulation neuroprostheses for the tetraplegic hand. *Clin Orthop* 1988;233:25–33.

Functionally useful grasp-and-pinch was restored in quadriplegic patients by means of percutaneous intramuscular electrodes. Practical restoration of grasp-and-pinch by functional electrical stimulation will require the development of surgically implanted systems.

Kralj A, Bajd T, Turk R: Enhancement of gait restoration in spinal injured patients by functional electrical stimulation. *Clin Orthop* 1988;233:34–43.

Independent reciprocal gait was restored in paraplegic patients by a surface functional electrical stimulation system that synchronized bilateral stimulation of the peroneal nerves and the quadriceps muscles.

Marsolais EB, Kobetic R: Functional electrical stimulation for walking in paraplegia. *J Bone Joint Surg* 1987;69A:728–733.

Complex lower-limb motion, gait restoration, and stair-climbing were restored in paraplegic patients by means of a 32-channel system activating all key lower-limb muscles via percutaneous electrodes inserted into the motor point region of each muscle.

McClelland M, Andrews BJ, Patrick JH, et al: Augmentation of the Oswestry Parawalker orthosis by means of surface electrical stimulation: Gait analysis of three patients. *Paraplegia* 1987;25:32–38.

A hybrid system using functional electrical stimulation and a hip-knee-ankle-foot orthosis restored reciprocal gait after spinal cord injury.

Ragnarsson KT: Physiologic effects of functional electrical stimulation-induced exercises in spinal cord-injured individuals. *Clin Orthop* 1988;233:53–63.

Electrostimulation of centrally paralyzed muscles in paraplegic patients resulted in improved strength, muscle bulk, endurance, and exercise capacity.

Waters RL, McNeal DR, Faloon W, et al: Functional electrical stimulation of the peroneal nerve for hemiplegia: Long-term clinical follow-up. *J Bone Joint Surg* 1985;67A:792–793.

Long-term functional electrical stimulation with a surgically implanted cuff electrode wrapped around the peroneal nerve to correct footdrop has been safely used in hemiplegic patients monitored for as long as 12 years.

II
Upper Extremity

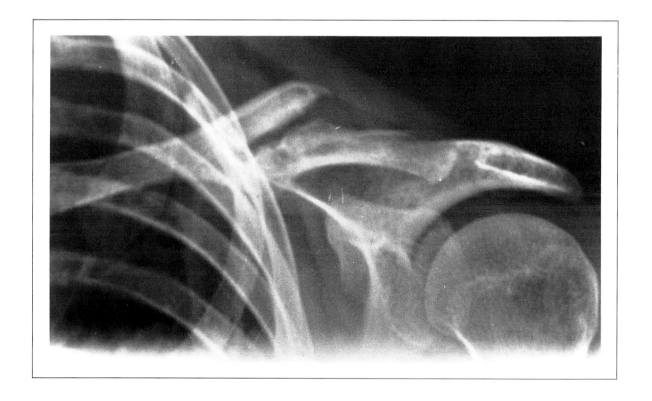

23
Upper Extremity: Pediatric Reconstruction

The first half of the 1980s was dominated by an intensified interest in the early definitive management of congenital abnormalities. With the use of magnification and microtechniques, traditional procedures (for example, syndactyly release, centralization of radial clubhand, and excision and Z-plasty of congenital constriction bands) were done earlier and new techniques (such as toe-to-hand transfer and interposition nerve grafting for brachial plexus palsy) were introduced. For the first time, reliable one-stage transfer of living tissue (microsurgical composite tissue transfer) was possible, and transplantation of human upper-extremity parts became a reality. Dramatic reports of toe-to-hand transfer for congenital anomalies, reconstruction of perinatal brachial plexus injuries by nerve grafting, and vascularized bone transfers were reported in the mid-1980s. In response, traditional and nonmicrosurgical alternatives were analyzed within the context of the effects of intervention on the natural history of the deformity, and the efficacy of these new procedures was documented. As the decade draws to a close, the new technology is being integrated into more traditional interventions, and a comfortable merger of new and traditional treatments has occurred.

Embryology

The upper limb forms from the arm bud on the lateral wall of the embryo (Wolff's crest), beginning in the third postovulatory week (days 26 to 30 of embryonic life). Extensive cell migration and multiplication occur during weeks 3 through 6; differentiation occurs during the next seven to ten days, and further refinements of tissue structure occur in the ensuing weeks. Although embryogenesis ceases in the eighth week, the hand continues to differentiate until week 13 and growth continues to birth. The hand develops from the apical ectodermal ridge. In the early hand anlage, autonomous founder cells differentiate into somatopleuric cells (tendon), angioblasts (blood vessels), neural crest (melanocytes and Schwann cells), and blood-derived cells (chondro-osteocytes). At six weeks of gestation, the hand plate has interdigital notches; by seven weeks, these have formed finger rays with separation of the fingertips and the thumb. During the eighth week, the finger separations continue and interdigital thenar and hypothenar pads begin to appear. During the ninth week, finger separation is almost complete and the thumb is rotated into an opposable position. Further differentiation continues until the 18th week of gestation (Fig. 1).

Diagnosis

In utero detection of upper-extremity malformations is possible with sonography or fetoscopy. The latter technique is quite accurate, but requires insertion of a fiberoptic fetoscope into the amniotic sac. Diagnosis by noninvasive, real-time, high-resolution ultrasonography accurately defines subtle congenital anomalies such as clinodactyly, polydactyly, and symbrachydactyly as early as 20 weeks of gestation. Ultrasonographic evaluation of fetal movement patterns and observation of extremity motion allow the early prediction of other potential congenital defects as well.

Localized Disorders

Shoulder

Sprengel's deformity, a failure of the scapula to descend normally, is the most common congenital anomaly of the shoulder. In 30% of cases an omovertebral bar consisting of bone, cartilage, or fibrocartilage connects the superior angle of the scapula to the cervical spine, and this structure must be resected to effect adequate surgical release. An accessory ossicle at the insertion of the levator scapulae has been reported and, if indeed present, may play a role analogous to that of the omovertebral bar. Resection of this ossicle alone does not reduce the deformity but such resection is necessary before additional surgical procedures can be used.

Radial Deficiencies

Radial deficiencies, defined as a total or partial absence of the preaxial (radial) portion of the upper extremity, can be divided into four types on the basis of the amount of remaining radius. In type I, the distal radius is short; in type II, the radius is hypoplastic; in type III, it is partially absent; and in type IV, it is completely absent.

In the radial clubhand, bilateral deficiencies are more frequent than unilateral deficiencies and type IV is the most common presentation (67%). Many associated anomalies are present and involve the cardiac (Holt-Oram syndrome), skeletal, hematologic, cutaneous, gastrointestinal, genitourinary, and neurologic systems, as well as the upper and lower extremities. Hematologic manifestations include Fanconi's anemia, radial platelet syndrome, and amegakaryocytosis thrombocytopenia. Almost 50% of patients with radial deficiencies (mostly type IV) have normal thumbs. In types I through III, normal thumbs are rare. They are absent in 60% of cases (Fig. 2); when present, the thumbs are often hypoplastic.

Treatment Creating a centralized but mobile and cosmetically acceptable wrist with a functional hand in the patient with a radial deficiency required a new surgical technique. To achieve centralization of the wrist over the distal ulna without excessive stiffness, extrinsic muscle units are rebalanced as necessary. Excessive curvature of the ulna, if

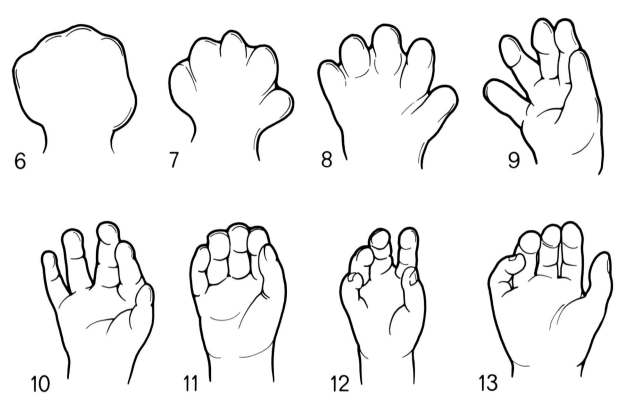

Figure 1
Hand differentiation from the sixth to 13th weeks of gestation. (Based on data from Kimura and Kitawaga.)

present, is corrected by wedge osteotomy, and the centralized wrist is kept stable by a longitudinal pin. To maintain motion, excision of carpal bone or excessive shortening of the distal ulna should be avoided. With adequate preoperative passive stretching, proper surgical technique, and postoperative brace compliance, good or satisfactory results can be expected in 80% of patients.

To provide better stabilization of a centralized wrist at the time of pollicization, the portion of the second metacarpal that would otherwise be discarded can be used to replace part of the missing radius, providing a buttress. This technique can be useful in wrists in which muscle balance is difficult to obtain. Long-term studies have shown that the wrist deformity recurs when wrist support and muscle balance are inadequate.

Hypoplastic Thumbs

Thumb hypoplasia can be classified into five grades: grade I, poor thenar musculature, small thumb; grade II, hypoplastic thenar muscles, small thumb, adducted metacarpophalangeal joint; grade III, deficient but attached metacarpal; grade IV, floating thumb; and grade V, absent thumb. There is a positive correlation between severity of thumb hypoplasia and the extent of radial involvement. Surgery should be directed at obtaining a functional thumb. In grades IV and V, pollicization is the treatment of choice, with augmentation of intrinsic motor power if necessary by opponens-plasty. Grades I through III can be managed by augmentation of intrinsic muscles, release of

any contractures, deepening of the web space, and/or bone grafting.

Ulnar Deficiencies

Ulnar deficiencies involve the postaxial (ulnar) portion of the upper extremity. These deficiencies are rare; radial deficiencies occur ten times more frequently. There is a high incidence of associated skeletal anomalies. The wrist is always ulnarly deviated but, unlike radial deficiency, there is rarely progression of deformity. Three-digit hands occur in approximately 60% of cases and fixed flexion deformity of one or more interphalangeal joints is common (67%).

Classification of ulnar deficiencies is based primarily on radiographic features of the elbow and forearm (Fig. 3). These do not necessarily correlate with prognosis and do not provide sufficient information for therapeutic decisions. A new classification based on long-term follow-up of 34 extremities has been designed to provide early prognostic information and treatment protocols.

Four subtypes of ulnar deficiency based on radiographic and clinical criteria have been proposed (Table 1). Types A and B have an abnormal elbow with fixed flexion deformity. Type A has a functional range of motion, no cubital webbing, and good function. No treatment is generally necessary for type A, although conversion to a one-bone forearm has been suggested. Follow-up of patients who underwent one-bone forearm conversion showed loss of pronation and supination but no progression of shortening and no further wrist deformity. Type B has limited range of motion, cubital webbing, and poor function. Radical

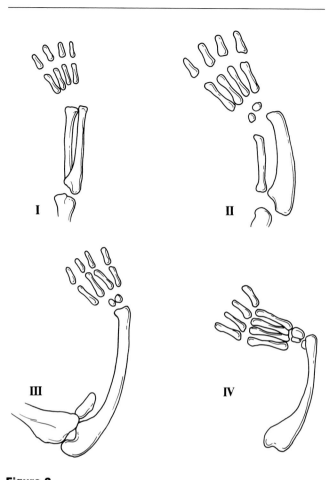

Figure 2

Classification of longitudinal deficiency of the radius. (Based on data from Bayne and Klug.)

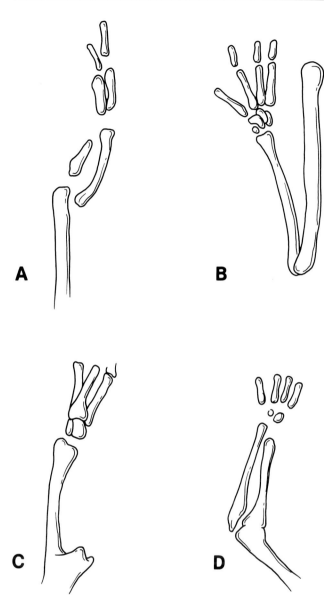

Figure 3

Classification of longitudinal deficiency of the ulna. (Based on data from Miller and associates.)

elbow release has proved to be inadequate for type B ulnar deficiencies, and, unless hand function is good, amputation and above-elbow prosthetic adaptation have been suggested, although this recommendation is not universally accepted. Types C and D have radiohumeral synostosis. Type C is characterized by the "hand-on-flank deformity"—a hyperpronated forearm, bowed radius, and flexed and rotated elbow with the hand facing posteriorly. Humeral osteotomy has been recommended to improve function. Type D has a straight radius, neutral forearm rotation, and good function, and it rarely requires intervention.

Central Deficiencies

Central defects are rare and include three general categories: type I (typical), type II (atypical), and type III, the two-, three-, or four-digit hand (Fig. 4). All types have central metacarpal deficiencies, with type III hands having the best function, although generally one, two, or three central rays are completely absent. Type I defects are often bilateral and familial, and the patient has similar foot anomalies. The central defect is V-shaped; syndactyly of the thumb-index ray is common and thumb metacarpal adduction contracture is frequent. The type II defect is the most severe manifestation and is generally unilateral, nonfamilial, and without concomitant foot involvement. The U-shaped central cleft can create a "lobster-claw" appear-

ance. In one series of 35 cleft hands, most deformities were unilateral and associated with cleft feet. In many extremities, a partial synostosis of phalanges, metacarpals, or intercarpal osseous anomalies is found at the origin of the cleft.

Treatment Type III central defects often require little intervention other than release of the syndactylized digits and maintenance of adequate digit-thumb web spaces. In the more severe types I and II, treatment must be individualized and is directed at closing the central defect and improving grasp and release.

Congenital Radioulnar Synostosis

The natural history of this deformity appears to be more benign than previously reported. In-depth analysis of un-

Table 1. Classification of ulnar deficiency*

Type	Description	
	Radiologic	Clinical
A	Dislocated radial head; bowed radius; progressive ulnar ossification	Average flexion contracture, 40 degrees; abnormal elbow motion; abnormal pronation-supination; no cubital web; good function
B	Dislocated radial head; absent ulna	Flexion contracture, > 110 degrees; average flexion, 125 degrees; poor function
C	Radiohumeral synostosis; bowed radius; delayed ulnar ossification	"Hand-on-flank" deformity; limited function because of position of the hand
D	Radiohumeral synostosis; straight radius; ulna of near-normal length	Average elbow flexion, 5 degrees; good function

*Based on data from Miller and associates.

treated patients with unilateral and bilateral involvement showed that most have few or no functional limitations and are able to perform jobs requiring extensive use of the forearm. The deformity is rare, frequently bilateral, more commonly observed in male patients, and has a multifactorial origin, exhibiting both genetic transfer and spontaneous mutations.

Four distinct radiographic patterns based upon the presence and location of the bony synostosis and the position of the radial head are now identifiable. Type I is characterized by a fibrous synostosis with a normal radial head, type II by an osseous synostosis with normal radial head, type III by an osseous synostosis with a hyperplastic and posteriorly dislocated radial head, and type IV by a short osseous synostosis and an anteriorly dislocated radial head. No functional differences have been noted among these types. Detailed functional assessment failed to demonstrate any relationship between forearm position and function in most patients; average forearm rotation was 30 degrees of pronation. Although some patients may require

osteotomy of the forearm, the natural history of this entity suggests that surgical indications should be based on documented subjective and objective limitations but not on arbitrary forearm position.

Madelung's Deformity

A wrist disorder characterized by progressive ulnar and volar angulation of the radius, Madelung's deformity, when symptomatic, has been managed by dorsal radial closing wedge osteotomy and distal ulnar resectioning or shortening. Alternative management of the distal ulna includes arthrodesis of the distal radioulnar joint and creation of a proximal pseudarthrosis of the ulna (Sauvé-Kapandji procedure).

Congenital Pseudarthrosis of the Forearm

Congenital pseudarthrosis of the forearm is extremely rare, and it is generally associated with neurofibromatosis. It may involve the radius, the ulna, or both. Pathologic stud-

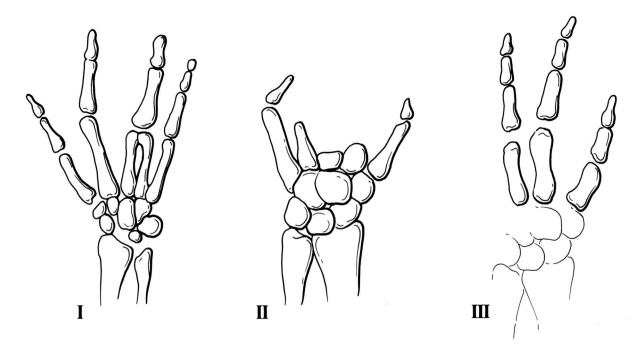

Figure 4
Types of central defects. (Based on data from Blauth and Falliner.)

ies suggest two types: The first type appears as a cystic lesion, which progresses to fracture and pseudarthrosis. This lesion may be similar in appearance and activity to fibrous dysplasia, but it does not heal after fracture or grafting. In the second, more destructive type, there is marked narrowing of the diaphysis of the radius and ulna with obliteration of the medullary canal and diaphyseal sclerosis. The periosteum is thickened and there is proliferation of fibrous tissue at the nonunion site. Failure to obtain stability or union may lead to radial head dislocation, early osteoarthritis, or both. To prevent angular deformity and its sequelae, early radical bone resection and grafting (using vascular fibula or a nonvascularized autograft) is necessary. The Ilizarov technique has been successful in obtaining union after radical resection of the pseudarthrosis.

Syndactyly

Syndactyly is one of the most common congenital deformities of the hand. Treatment depends on the type and degree of syndactyly (Outline 1) but web-space contracture after release of syndactyly appears to be a common problem. A modified zigzag incision and a large, dorsally based flap successfully maintain the web space in 95% of patients. Full-thickness skin grafts are necessary on one digit, and success has been correlated with appropriate timing of the operation (delaying surgery until the hand is larger, that is, until the child is more than 12 months old) and the experience of the surgeon.

The association of syndactyly with other congenital anomalies must be remembered and documented before surgical release of the syndactyly.

Polydactyly

Polydactyly (more than five digits per hand) remains the most common congenital hand deformity, with an incidence of one in 300 in blacks and one in 3,000 in whites. The complete or partial additional digits may be preaxial (radial) or postaxial (ulnar). Autosomal recessive and autosomal dominant patterns of inheritance have been documented. Polydactyly can be an isolated malformation or part of a generalized syndrome, and thus should be a signal for a complete diagnostic examination to exclude other significant malformations.

Preaxial polydactyly is more common in whites, is often associated with syndactyly, and is more likely to be associated with a generalized syndrome. Conversely, postaxial, ulnar-border polydactyly is more common in blacks and Orientals and can be either autosomal recessive or autosomal dominant. Although generalized syndromes can be associated with postaxial polydactyly, most patients with this deformity do not have such syndromes. In Japan, polydactyly is more commonly preaxial in the hand and postaxial in the foot.

Thumb Polydactyly Preaxial polydactyly of the thumb has been recognized as part of the range of genetic expression that can include thenar hypoplasia. Family members of affected children should be screened carefully so that appropriate genetic counseling can be provided.

In planning the surgical management of polydactyly, especially with regard to the thumb, it is important to remember that portions of the amputated digit can be used, if necessary, to enhance the reconstruction of an adjacent digit by increasing its diameter and correcting joint devia-

tion. Adjacent and collateral ligaments can be used. The amputated part can also provide a bone graft for a deviated digit.

The duplicated thumb can present a complex reconstructive problem. Simple excision of one digit may result in joint incongruity, joint instability, decreased range of motion, weak punch, and progressive angular deformity. Duplications involving a bifid proximal phalanx (Wassel type III) or a duplicated proximal phalanx (Wassel type IV) are very likely to have unsatisfactory results with simple excision. These deformities may require reconstruction of the collateral ligaments, realignment and augmentation of the long tendons, reattachment of intrinsic muscles, and correction of oblique articular surfaces by osteotomy. More distal duplications (Wassel types I and II) do well with the Bilhaut-Cloquet procedure (creation of a complex syndactyly after excision of part of each digit). The basic principles of thumb polydactyly reconstruction are (1) retaining the duplicate with the best functional and cosmetic potential; (2) using a single nail when possible; (3) aligning the digital skeleton; (4) stabilizing the joint by augmentation of collateral ligaments, joint surfaces, and appropriate alignment; and (5) balancing extrinsic and intrinsic motor power.

Macrodactyly

Macrodactyly, a rare congenital anomaly manifested by disproportionate digital enlargement, can occur as part of a generalized disorder such as neurofibromatosis or as an isolated phenomenon. "True" macrodactyly includes bone and soft-tissue enlargement and is generally preaxial (thumb, index, and long fingers). Approximately 50% of hands with macrodactyly have single-digit involvement; the second and third digits are most frequently involved; and digital nerves are almost always involved and enlarged (nerve enlargement in the lower extremity is rare). Treatment must be individualized; multiple soft-tissue and debulking procedures are often necessary. Ray resection is occasionally necessary but should be used as a last resort. The goal of treatment should be maintenance of function without sacrificing appearance. Resection of digital nerves has not been shown to be effective in diminishing digital size, and it should be avoided.

Outline 1. Classification of syndactyly (related syndromes)

Type	Description
I	Isolated (genetically distinct)
	Zygodactyly (simple cutaneous long, ring)
	Sympolydactyly (long, ring)
	Ring-little finger
	Complete hand (Haas)
	Including metacarpal synostosis
II	Poland's
III	Acrocephalosyndactyly syndromes
	Apert's
	Saethre-Chotzen's
	Waardenburg's
	Pfeiffer's
	Summitt's
IV	Acrocephalopolysyndactyly
V	Congenital band constriction syndrome (Streeter)
VI	Facial syndromes
	Orofacial
	Oculodental digital
VII	Occasional syndromes

Constriction Band Syndrome

Congenital constriction band syndrome (Streeter's dysplasia, amniotic band syndrome) is a noninherited disorder of unknown etiology. Involvement of more than one extremity is frequent and the upper extremity is involved in approximately 50% of cases. Upper-extremity malformations include the presence of constrictive bands with or without distal edema, terminal amputations of the digits, syndactyly, acrosyndactyly (fenestrated syndactyly), and amputation of the forearm or arm. Of the digits, fingers are involved more frequently than the thumb, which is protected within the palm. Correction may be by single- or two-stage Z-plasty. Recent reports have suggested that appearance is improved when the limb of the Z-plasty is kept in the mid-lateral portion of the digit.

Congenital Amputations

Congenital amputations may be secondary to amputation of a formed part (constriction band syndrome), failure of parts to form (limb-bud insult), teratogens, or a genetic defect.

Treatment must be patient-oriented and should be directed at restoring function and length. For transverse deficiencies in the arm or forearm, electrically powered upper-limb prostheses are reportedly effective. When the prostheses are provided early in life, the acceptance rate is higher and improved prosthetic function has been demonstrated.

Whether or not intervention is appropriate in more distal amputations is an area of current controversy. Therapeutic alternatives include segmental digital transposition, microsurgical composite tissue transfer, phalangeal and metacarpal distraction lengthening, nonvascularized toephalanx transfer, and vascularized osseous transfer.

Generalized Disorders

Cerebral Palsy

Recent epidemiologic data refute many of the classic concepts regarding the origin of cerebral palsy. Cerebral palsy is a manifestation of abnormal brain function and is not necessarily secondary to a fixed brain lesion that occurred in the perinatal period. Most cerebral palsy syndromes are not secondary to perinatal brain damage or asphyxia and only 10% to 15% of patients sustained perinatal damage. Rather, these data suggest as yet unidentified genetic, teratologic, and/or congenital influences.

There has been no consistent decrease in the frequency of cerebral palsy in the last two decades and approximately 300,000 to 500,000 children are now affected. A relatively small percentage of patients with cerebral palsy are considered candidates for surgical intervention in the upper extremity. The upper extremity must be considered within the context of the child's overall disability. The extremity must be evaluated in terms of function, distal weakness, proximal weakness, dexterity, and tone. Muscle tone must be assessed to determine whether it is phasic, hypertonic, or hypotonic. Appropriate balance across joints must be estimated, and whether contractures have developed must be determined. Distal power and speed correlate directly with function and must be assessed. In addition, neurophysiologic tests such as electromyography or torque generators may aid in the clinical evaluation. Recent studies

have shown that function is impaired more severely in children with left-sided hemiplegia than in those with right-sided hemiplegia and that the abnormal tone in the hemiplegic arm is increased by activities in the contralateral extremity. Further, orientation of the child's body in space may affect upper-extremity function. Testing to determine whether interventional procedures, including surgery, will be beneficial requires stable body position in an orientation that will maximize upper-extremity function.

General treatment principles were outlined in *Orthopaedic Knowledge Update 2.*

Transfers To Restore Wrist and Finger Extension Long-term follow-up of tendon transfers to the extensors of the wrist and fingers has shown that transfers of the flexor carpi ulnaris to the extensor carpi radialis brevis result in extension contractures and difficulty in finger release, but that transfers of the flexor carpi ulnaris to the extensor digitorum communis do improve finger extension and release without sacrificing the ability to grasp. Transfer of the flexor carpi ulnaris to the extensor digitorum communis is indicated when the patient has difficulty with finger and wrist extension sufficient to compromise function but a "sophisticated" cerebral palsy hand (functional intelligence, sensibility, hand placement capability, and satisfactory passive range of motion).

Arthrogryposis

Arthrogryposis is a musculoskeletal disorder characterized by generalized immobility of multiple joints. The entity may be primarily neurogenic (in which case it is often associated with other congenital abnormalities) or myopathic.

Arthrogryposis multiplex congenita has been linked with malignant hyperthermia, and agents that might trigger malignant hyperthermia should be avoided during anesthesia.

Improved upper-extremity function in children with arthrogryposis is generally limited to active and passive elbow range of motion or hand grasp and release. The results of correcting wrist flexion deformity by proximal row carpectomy are unpredictable and this procedure should be avoided. External distraction (Ilizarov technique) may prove to have a role in the management of this disorder.

Controversies

Congenital Brachial-Plexus Injury

The controversy over early (when the child is 6 to 9 months old) surgical intervention—neurolysis, microsurgical repair, or both—vs nonsurgical treatment—early motion, physical therapy, and splinting—is yet to be resolved.

The controversy continues because there is no uniform appreciation of the "true" natural history of the injury, no uniform acceptance of a functional classification for the entire upper extremity, and no adequate documentation of the effects of early surgical intervention on the natural course of the process.

The incidence of brachial-plexus birth palsy has remained relatively constant at 2 to 2.5 per 1,000 live births. Recent studies have confirmed that more than 80% of unselected neonates with upper-extremity neurologic dysfunction at birth will attain normal or near-normal function. Although it is reasonable to conclude that the

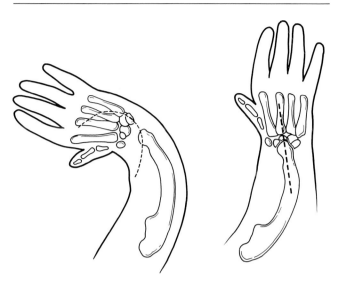

Figure 5

Technique of classic centralization including resection of carpal bones to form a slot for the distal ulna. (Based on data from Lamb.)

prognosis for brachial-plexus palsy is generally favorable, it is also reasonable to acknowledge that some children do poorly and have completely disrupted yet potentially repairable peripheral nerve injuries. Although conventional nonsurgical management is justified for most infants, this is not true in every case.

Experienced surgeons using appropriate magnification can explore an infant's brachial plexus; can assess nerve function by sensory evoked potentials, nerve action potentials, or both; and can, by neurolysis, end-to-end repair, nerve graft, or neurotization, restore appropriate functional units with acceptable and minimal morbidity. In young patients, nerve grafting or neurotization will, in

most cases, provide sensory input and motor power to the proximal shoulder and elbow. It is important to note that this motor power improves function. Further, patients operated on earlier have a uniformly better prognosis for nerve recovery.

In more than 100 reported cases undergoing surgical treatment, morbidity was minimal and functional results averaged one grade higher on the Mallet classification, which evaluates the entire extremity. In completely transected C-5 and C-6 peripheral lesions, functional biceps and shoulder motor power can be restored in most cases. Passive range of motion and splinting cannot restore function in transected nerves; therefore, the concern should not be whether early surgery is indicated, but rather how early those patients who need surgery can be identified.

The natural history of the injury suggests that: (1) patients who have biceps function before 3 months of age have an excellent prognosis for normal recovery; (2) patients who have their first evidence of biceps function between 3 months and 6 months of age will attain near-normal function; and (3) absence of biceps function by the age of 6 months correlates with "poor" functional recovery and with nerve transections that are often peripheral and therefore perhaps amenable to surgery.

Currently, most newborns who have a brachial-plexus palsy have a favorable prognosis for complete recovery. However, for those infants in whom biceps function is not clinically or electrographically present by 6 months, surgical intervention is safe and provides the possibility of improved function. With absence of biceps recovery by 6 months of age used as an indication for surgery, brachial-plexus exploration and repair of peripheral nerve injuries by nerve grafting or neurotization of a proximal avulsed trunk improves function in muscles that would otherwise remain denervated.

Radial Clubhand

There is little debate over the functional and aesthetic merits of centralization of a radially deficient hand in the pa-

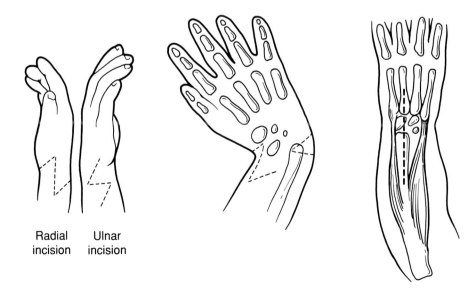

Figure 6

Technique of centralization without carpal bone excision. (Based on data from Watson and associates.)

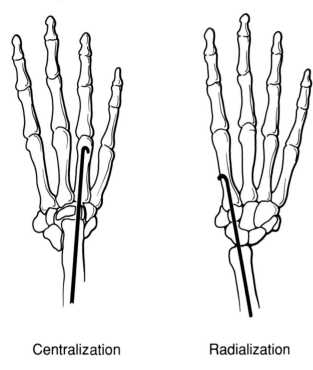

Centralization   Radialization

Figure 7

Management of radial clubhand. "Classic" centralization on the left maintains wrist position by mechanically placing the ulna into carpal bones; radialization of the ulna maintains wrist position by muscle balance, using the lever arm of the hand to maintain position.

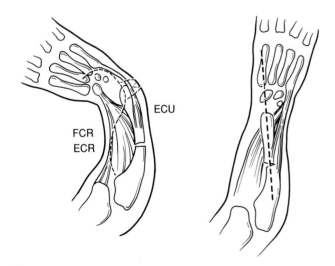

Figure 8

Technique of radialization in which the carpal bones are displaced and fixed ulnar to the long axis of the ulna and maintained by tendon transfer. (Based on data from Buck-Gramcko.)

tient with good ipsilateral elbow motion. It is also generally agreed that centralization with maintenance of wrist flexion and extension is preferable to arthrofibrosis or fusion of the wrist. Finally, it is generally agreed that patients who undergo early intervention tend to have better results than those who undergo late intervention. The best techniques to achieve these goals, however, are still subject to question.

Traditional methods of surgical correction have included isolated soft-tissue release with or without ulnar osteotomy, bone graft replacement of the radius, spike centralization of the ulna into the carpal bones, and fusion. In 1977, Lamb presented an alternative technique of centralization. Since that time, his technique of using the principle of mechanical centralization of the ulna into a slot in the carpal bones has been the standard method. From 1984 on, however, three significant modifications of Lamb's technique, also based on extensive experience, have been presented.

On the surface, these new techniques, especially when contrasted with Lamb's classic description, appear confusing. It must be remembered that Lamb's technique was based on soft-tissue release sufficient to place the undamaged head of the ulna gently into a slot in the carpal bones. Although it was not stated specifically, the gentle placement of the ulna into this slot required some balancing of the forces across the wrist. Lamb also stressed that tendon transfers were occasionally performed if there appeared to be "a strong deforming force." The basis of the technique, however, was the principle that the slot must be equal in depth to the diameter of the ulna in order to maintain the position of the ulna mechanically and thereby prevent excessive deviation of the hand (Fig. 5). Kirschner wires and splinting were used to assure maintenance of position for six to 12 months. Minor modifications involving longer periods of K-wire placement were advocated by others, and were occasionally used by Lamb. Night splinting was used for indefinite periods—often until skeletal maturity.

The three modifications of centralization have three basic tenets in common: (1) the wrist is balanced dynamically by extrinsic muscle tendon transfer and/or carpal-ulnar alignment; (2) the distal ulna is placed on and not within the carpal bones; and (3) rigid transarticular immobilization is minimized to obtain earlier motion.

The major differences from Lamb's technique involve leaving the carpal bones intact and the relatively short duration of "wrist" immobilization. In the "modified centralization" technique, soft-tissue structures, including skin, are rebalanced and an undamaged capitate and lunate are placed over the ulna with the third metacarpal in line with the ulna (Fig. 6). Z-plasties are used to achieve skin coverage, redirecting the arms of the incision ulnarly and radially.

Radialization, in contrast, overcorrects the carpus on the ulna and maintains position by muscle rebalancing with transfer of the extensor carpi radialis and the flexor carpi radialis to the ulnar side of the hand (Fig. 7). The distal ulna is aligned with the second metacarpal and fixed in that position (Fig. 8). As in "modified centralization," no carpal bones are resected, optimal timing is when the patients are young, and immobilization is short.

Both modified centralization and radialization provide improved flexion, but only marginal improvement in dorsiflexion. Overall, long-term maintenance of correction appears to be good with both techniques.

The third alternative, again a modification of centralization, utilizes carpal centralization without resection or notching. This technique includes muscle balancing by combined extensor carpi ulnaris and flexor carpi ulnaris advancement and radial release or lengthening of contracted structures. Excessive tension or ulnar bowing is

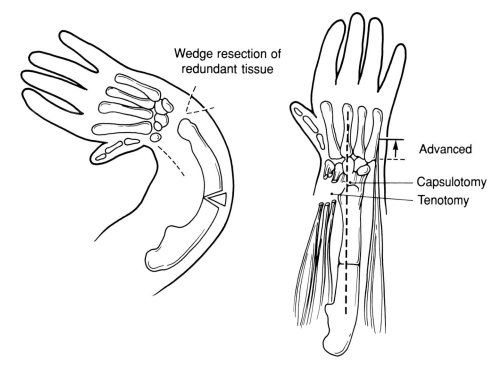

Wedge resection of
redundant tissue

Advanced

Capsulotomy
Tenotomy

Figure 9

Technique of centralization without carpal bone resection that relies on muscle balancing to maintain position after pin removal. The ulna is straightened by osteotomy if necessary. (Based on data from Bayne and Klug.)

treated by either shortening of the midshaft ulna or osteotomy to correct angulation (Fig. 9). In a long-term review of 101 radial deficiencies treated on the basis of these principles, with the goal being a stable wrist centralized on the distal ulna with maintenance of functional wrist motion, good results were obtained in 53% of patients; these included a good hand and forearm angle of less than 30 degrees and a range of motion of more than 40 degrees, with the functional range including 20 degrees of flexion and 20 degrees of extension.

Comparison of these three new techniques shows that all are capable of providing a well-centralized hand with maintenance of adequate functional wrist motion. Radialization appears to decrease the recurrence of radial deviation and is probably the most forgiving procedure because it provides a strong tendon transfer to a mechanically advantaged lever. The data for these three techniques confirm that results are predictable in patients treated by experienced surgeons. The basic principles are maintenance of a centralized mobile wrist by restoration of muscle balance without carpal resection. Results are more predictable in younger patients in whom adequate muscle transfers and rebalancing are possible.

It must be remembered, however, that the net result of hand function does not necessarily depend on wrist position. Rather, it depends on the stiffness of the digits (quite variable in radially deficient hands), the presence or absence of the thumb and/or the ability to create an acceptable pollicized digit, the range of motion of the elbow and shoulder, and the length of the forearm and humerus.

Safe and reliable techniques for lengthening the radius and/or humerus without loss of joint stability or range of motion while maintaining neurologic function have excit-

ing potential applications in extremities with radial deficiencies. Sporadic use of modifications of the Ilizarov lengthening techniques has been mentioned anecdotally and, if accurate, may revolutionize the treatment of this problem.

Congenital Absence of Digits

The treatment of congenital absence or hypoplasia of digits remains controversial. Alternatives include nonintervention, prosthetic adaptation, segmental digital transposition, distraction lengthening (phalangeal or metacarpal), microvascular composite tissue transfer, and nonmicrovascular periosteal-osseous transfer.

Congenital hand defects are different from posttraumatic deficits. Nerves, tendons, vessels, and proximal osseous structures are rarely present and when available are often abnormal, making composite tissue transfer difficult. Children are marvelously adaptable, and doing nothing is often the best therapeutic path to take. In many patients, however, appropriate intervention based on a patient-oriented approach should be considered to achieve optimal function. Realistic goals to achieve length, flexibility, power, and stability must be identified and the appropriate form of treatment employed.

Length can be obtained by transfer of toe phalanges with intact periosteum and epiphyseal plates or by distraction lengthening. In nonvascularized toe-phalanx transfer, epiphyseal plates may remain open and growth will continue. Younger children (less than 18 months) are more likely to demonstrate epiphyseal growth, but the length of bone transferred is smaller and failure to grow may result in length insufficient to improve long-term function. The presence of flexor and/or extensor tendons and adequate skin pouches also correlates with epiphyseal growth. Distraction lengthening of the metacarpal or phalanx can be performed in children of any age, although it is technically easier in older children. Further, transferred phalanges, if of sufficient size, may be lengthened at a later time. Complications of both toe-phalanx transfer and distraction lengthening are manageable. Patient cooperation is necessary for distraction lengthening, but not for phalanx transfer. Segmental digit transfer (that is, transfer of all or part of one phalanx or metacarpal to another phalanx or metacarpal) can be used to augment deficient tissue and provide stability, but growth will not occur unless an epiphysis is involved.

Microvascular transfer of the second toe can be employed. The rationale for toe transfer has been the ability to obtain length, stability, mobility, and strength—often difficult with other techniques. Unfortunately, transferred

digits generally lack mobility and have flexion contractures with an active range of motion of less than 60 degrees. The major indication is construction of a thumb when there is insufficient tissue for pollicization.

All the proposed techniques have a place in the management of congenital hand deformity. In appropriately selected young patients with skin pouches or sufficient redundant tissue with an intact tendon anlage, nonmicrovascular periosteal-osseous transfer should be considered. If this is done too early and epiphyseal growth does not occur, there may be insufficient length for function and inadequate bony structure for additional lengthening by distraction techniques. If all or part of a digit is to be amputated, segmental transfer should be considered.

Distraction lengthening is the most versatile technique for older children and adults. Vascularized toe transfer, although technologically manageable, should be reserved for the achievement of specific functional goals.

Annotated Bibliography

Keywords

Arthrogryposis; Brachial plexus; Central deficiency; Cerebral palsy; Clubhand; Congenital abnormalities; Constriction band syndrome; Embryology; Macrodactyly; Madelung's deformity; Polydactyly; Radial deficiency; Shoulder; Sprengel's deformity; Syndactyly; Ulnar deficiency

Embryology

Beatty E: Upper limb tissue differentiation in the human embryo. *Hand Clin* 1985;1:391–403.
A detailed analysis of the embryonic development of the upper limb and its relevance to the management of congenital anomalies of the upper extremity.

Kimura S, Kitagawa T: Embryological development of human palmar, plantar, and digital flexion creases. *Anat Rec* 1986;216:191–197.
Embryology of developing hand and digits.

Diagnosis

Jeanty P, Romero R, d'Alton M, et al: In utero sonographic detection of hand and foot deformities. *J Ultrasound Med* 1985;4:595–601.
Examples of early diagnosis and detection of fetal anomalies using high-resolution ultrasound.

Localized Disorders

Askins G, Ger E: Congenital constriction band syndrome. *J Pediatr Orthop* 1988;8:461–466.
A retrospective study of 55 patients outlining epidemiologic considerations.

Bayne LG: Congenital pseudarthrosis of the forearm. *Hand Clin* 1985;1:457–465.
Detailed review of this rare anomaly and a current treatment protocol.

Bayne LG, Klug MS: Long-term review of the surgical

treatment of radial deficiencies. *J Hand Surg* 1987;12A:169–179.
Review of 101 cases of radial deficiency (clubhand). Centralization and muscle balancing were employed and wrist motion was maintained. A new classification and the authors' technique are presented.

Blauth W, Falliner A: Zur Morphologie und Klassifikation von Spalthänden [Morphology and classification of cleft hands]. *Handchir Mikrochir Plast Chir* 1986;18:161–195.
Report of large series of patients with cleft hand. The authors point out the relationship of intercarpal and metacarpophalangeal synostosis as a factor in cleft formation, and present another classification.

Buck-Gramcko D: Radialization as a new treatment for radial club hand. *J Hand Surg* 1985;10A:964–968.
Overcorrection of deformity plus muscle rebalancing provides good results.

Cleary JE, Omer GE Jr: Congenital proximal radio-ulnar synostosis: Natural history and functional assessment. *J Bone Joint Surg* 1985;67A:539–545.
Thirty-six congenital synostoses (26 patients) were evaluated to determine the untreated natural history of this anomaly. The four radiographic patterns observed did not correlate with function. In contradistinction to previous studies, forearm position was not related to function in most patients, and the authors believe that surgery is rarely indicated.

Fabry G, Lammens J, Van Melkebeek J, et al: Treatment of congenital pseudarthrosis with the Ilizarov technique. *J Pediatr Orthop* 1988;8:67–70.
Union was achieved in four cases.

Kalen V, Burwell DS, Omer GE: Macrodactyly of the hands and feet. *J Pediatr Orthop* 1988;8:311–315.
Experience with seven cases, comparison with other published results, and recommendations for management.

Lamb DW: Radial club hand: A continuing study of

sixty-eight patients with one hundred and seventeen club hands. *J Bone Joint Surg* 1977;59A:1-13.
A classic article.

Lamoureux J, Verstreken L: Progressive upper limb lengthening in children: A report of two cases. *J Pediatr Orthop* 1986;6:481–485.
Treatment of cubitus varus and radial aplasia by limb lengthening.

Masada K, Tsuyuguchi Y, Kawabata H, et al: Terminal limb congenital malformations: Analysis of 523 cases. *J Pediatr Orthop* 1986;6:340–345.
Detailed evaluation of 523 cases.

Miller JK, Wenner SM, Kruger LM: Ulnar deficiency. *J Hand Surg* 1986;11A:822–829.
Experience with 34 ulnar-deficient limbs. Treatment recommendations were based on a new classification.

Nakamura J, Kanahara K, Endo Y, et al: Effective use of portions of the supernumerary digit to correct polydactyly of the thumb. *Ann Plast Surg* 1985;15:7-13.
Techniques for using portions of the deleted extra digit to augment the size, joint stability, tendon competency, and/or alignment of the remaining digit.

Sandzen SC Jr: Classification and functional management of congenital central defect of the hand. *Hand Clin* 1985;1:483–498.
A detailed review of the management of central hand defects.

Tsuge K, Watari S: New surgical procedure for correction of club hand. *J Hand Surg* 1985;10B:90–94.
Report of a new procedure replacing part of missing radius with resected second metacarpal at the time of pollicization.

Tsuyuguchi Y, Yukioka M, Kawabata H, et al: Radial ray deficiency. *J Pediatr Orthop* 1987;7:699–704.
Experience with 37 radial ray deficiencies emphasizing treatment of the hypoplastic and/or absent thumb.

Watson HK, Beebe RD, Cruz NI: A centralization procedure for radial clubhand. *J Hand Surg* 1984;9A:541–547.
Good results in 12 wrists treated by realignment and balancing.

Generalized Disorders

Hoffer MM, Lehman M, Mitani M: Long-term follow-up on tendon transfers to the extensors of the wrist and fingers in patients with cerebral palsy. *J Hand Surg* 1986;11A:836–840.
Transfer of the flexor carpi ulnaris to wrist extensors had unpredictable (often poor) results, whereas superior function was obtained in most cases by transfer of the flexor carpi ulnaris to the extensor digitorum communis tendon.

Nelson KB, Ellenberg JH: Antecedents of cerebral palsy: Multivariate analysis of risk. *N Engl J Med* 1986;315: 81–86.
Analysis of 189 children with cerebral palsy showed that asphyxia and identifiable perinatal insults did not account for most cases.

Controversies

Congenital Brachial-Plexus Injury

Gilbert A, Khouri N, Carlioz H: Exploration chirurgicale du plexus brachial dans la paralysie obstétricale: Constatations anatomiques chez 21 malades opérés. *Rev Chir Orthop* 1980;66:33–42.

Jackson ST, Hoffer MM, Parrish N: Brachial-plexus palsy in the newborn. *J Bone Joint Surg* 1988;70A:1217–1220.

Meyer RD: Treatment of adult and obstetrical brachial plexus injuries. *Orthopedics* 1986;9:899–903.

Radial Clubhand

Bayne LG, Klug MS: Long-term review of the surgical treatment of radial deficiencies. *J Hand Surg* 1987;12A: 169–179.

Buck-Gramcko D: Radialization as a new treatment for radial club hand. *J Hand Surg* 1985;10A:964–968.

Lamb DW: Radial club hand: A continuing study of sixty-eight patients with one hundred and seventeen club hands. *J Bone Joint Surg* 1977;59A:1–13.

Watson HK, Beebe RD, Cruz NI: A centralization procedure for radial clubhand. *J Hand Surg* 1984;9A:541–547.

Congenital Absence of Digits

Gilbert A: Toe transfers for congenital hand defects. *J Hand Surg* 1982;7:118–124.

Goldberg NM, Watson HK: Composite toe (phalanx and epiphysis) transfers in the reconstruction of the aphalangic hand. *J Hand Surg* 1982;7:454–459.

Lister G, Scheker L: The role of microsurgery in the reconstruction of congenital deformities of the hand. *Hand Clin* 1985;1:431–442.

Smith RJ, Gumley GJ: Metacarpal distraction lengthening. *Hand Clin* 1985;1:417–429.

24
Throwing Injuries in the Athlete

Throwing and pitching require complex adaptive mechanisms and a high level of neuromuscular coordination. Overuse injuries of the shoulder and elbow are common. A better understanding of throwing injuries and increased diagnostic capabilities have resulted in improved prevention and treatment techniques. The association of hidden shoulder subluxation and secondary rotator cuff abnormality has been recognized recently as a major cause of shoulder pain in the throwing athlete. The elbow is compromised medially by progressive distraction forces and posterolaterally by compression forces. Most throwing injuries can be effectively treated conservatively, if recognized early. Arthroscopy has aided in confirming and elucidating previously unrecognized abnormalities and plays a role in the surgical management of injuries in the upper extremity. The presence of the open epiphyseal growth plate in the adolescent athlete provides an additional site for overuse injury.

Biomechanics of Throwing

Athletic injuries to the shoulder and elbow are common. The observation that athletes often had selective weakness of specific muscles, rather than generalized muscle impairment, led investigators to question whether single-plane motion analysis could be applied to sports-specific activities. Electromyographic data demonstrated that the rapid and precise motion patterns characterizing individual sports simulate more selective muscle action, as well as specific periods of greater intensity. The concept of the separate and independent action of the deltoid and rotator cuff helped to explain the selective muscle weakness of the throwing athlete.

Although each sport has its own basic pattern, different sports also have much in common. Most overhand sports begin with a preparatory phase to position the arm. Subsequently, the arm is cocked to provide a tense, highly forceful unit ready for an accelerated release. The muscles then respond to decelerate the limb, to reduce the residual force, and to avoid injury. The baseball pitch is divided into five stages (Fig. 1): stage 1, the wind-up or preparation phase, ends when the ball leaves the gloved hand; stage 2, early cocking, shoulder abduction and external rotation that begins as the ball is released from the nondominant hand and terminates with contact of the forward foot on the ground; stage 3, late cocking phase that continues until maximum external rotation at the shoulder is obtained; stage 4, acceleration phase that starts with internal rotation of the humerus and ends with ball release; and stage 5, follow-through phase that starts with ball release and ends when all motion is complete.

Shoulder

During the baseball pitch, the deltoid is responsible for arm elevation with active forward flexion and abduction of the humerus. The supraspinatus has been thought to play an important role in humeral abduction. Its action in pitching demonstrates peak activity in the late cocking when the arm is already abducted and most susceptible to subluxation. The supraspinatus contributes to the stability of the joint by drawing the humeral head toward the glenoid. The marked greater use of the supraspinatus by amateur pitchers, compared with professionals, is an argument for preliminary conditioning. Fatigue from overuse can readily subject the amateur to shoulder injuries. As the athlete becomes proficient, efficient and economic use of the muscles takes place, preventing overuse and injury.

The infraspinatus and teres minor are responsible for external rotation and stability of the shoulder by drawing the head toward the glenoid fossa. The activity patterns are similar for both muscles, with peak activity during late cocking and follow-through, although both lag behind the supraspinatus in timing.

The subscapularis has its peak activity in late cocking when it contracts eccentrically to protect the anterior joint, which is under extreme tension. It then continues to function as an internal rotator to help carry the arm across the chest during acceleration and follow-through.

The role of the biceps at the shoulder has been controversial. The similarity of the biceps and brachialis firing patterns supports the concept that the biceps functions predominantly at the elbow rather than the shoulder. Evaluation of the long head of the biceps in shoulders with rotator cuff tears reveals significantly increased activity of the long head of the biceps during shoulder flexion and abduction.

The pectoralis major and latissimus dorsi function together as internal rotators, and eccentrically contract to protect the joint, along with the subscapularis, during late cocking. Further increase of their activity during acceleration indicates that intense internal rotation and forceful arm depression provide the primary propulsive force.

The serratus anterior controls the scapula to provide a stable glenoid. Serratus anterior activity is important for scapular protraction during late cocking. This allows the scapula to keep pace with the humerus, which is horizontally flexing and externally rotating. The relatively low level of trapezius activity provides supplementary scapular stabilization during acceleration. During follow-through, the trapezius serves to decelerate scapular protraction.

Anterior Glenohumeral Instability

Evaluation of skilled throwers with isolated anterior glenohumeral instability revealed differences from normal subjects. Mildly increased activity of the biceps during ac-

293

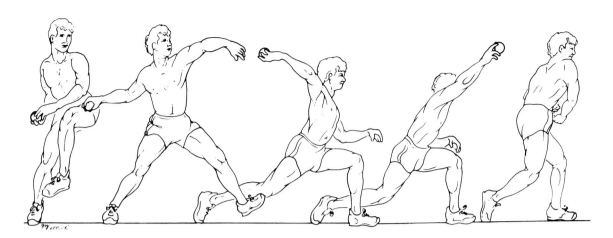

Figure 1
The five stages of pitching a baseball: wind-up, early cocking, late cocking, acceleration, and follow-through.

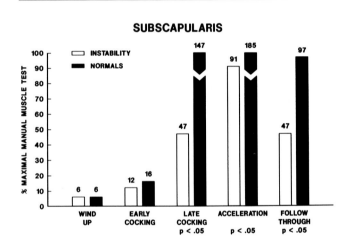

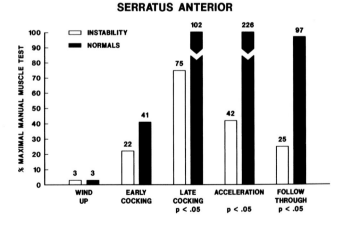

Figure 2
Activity in normal and unstable shoulders during baseball pitching. **Top**, Subscapularis. **Bottom**, Serratus anterior. (Reproduced with permission from Glousman R, Jobe F, Tibone J, et al: Dynamic electromyographic analysis of the throwing shoulder with glenohumeral instability. *J Bone Joint Surg* 1988;70A:220–226.)

celeration in those with instability could represent a compensatory mechanism to help stabilize the humeral head against the glenoid. This is consistent with the difference occurring in late cocking and acceleration, when the arm is most susceptible to subluxation.

In patients with instability, the pectoralis major, subscapularis, and latissimus dorsi all demonstrated markedly decreased activity during the pitch. Inhibition of the synergistic activity of these muscles (Fig. 2, *top*) allows persistent or accentuated external rotation. This may be a factor in producing, or maintaining, long-term anterior instability.

Decreased serratus anterior activity (Fig. 2, *bottom*) in patients with instability diminishes horizontal protraction of the scapula, which normally begins during late cocking. Early fatigue of the serratus anterior then adds to the stress on the anterior restraints. As part of a conservative or postoperative surgical rehabilitation program, the thrower with subluxation should strengthen these specific muscles.

Elbow

Analysis of the elbow revealed low to moderate activity in all muscles during all phases of the pitch. During the wind-up phase, the forearm is slightly pronated and flexed, and the wrist is extended. During early cocking, the elbow is flexed, the wrist and metacarpophalangeal joints are extended, and the forearm is slightly pronated. In late cocking, the elbow is flexed, the wrist is extended, and the forearm is pronated. During the short, explosive acceleration stage, the elbow is extended and the wrist and metacarpophalangeal joints are flexed to propel the ball forward. Follow-through is terminated by maximal pronation of the forearm, as the humerus is internally rotated and adducted across the chest. The low to moderate muscle activity seen during the pitch (Fig. 3) suggests that elbow function is more for positioning to accept the transfer of energy from the shoulder and trunk. Electromyographic analysis did not substantiate that medial elbow problems are a result of increased use of flexor muscles when a curve ball rather than a fast ball is thrown. This implies that the muscles about the elbow do not protect against overloading, especially excessive valgus loads. Monitoring of the

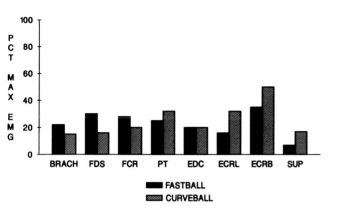

Figure 3

Muscle activity during the acceleration phase of pitching. BRACH, brachioradialis; FDS, flexor digitorum superficialis; FCR, flexor carpi radialis; PT, pronator teres; EDC, extensor digitorum communis; ECRL, extensor carpi radialis longus; ECRB, extensor carpi radialis brevis; SUP, supinator. (Reproduced with permission from Sisto DJ, Jobe FW, Moynes DR, et al: An electromyographic analysis of the elbow in pitching. *Am J Sports Med* 1987;15:260–263.)

style of delivery, and the number of innings pitched, is therefore important to decrease elbow injuries.

Conditioning of the Throwing Arm

Rehabilitation and conditioning programs have been developed on the basis of electromyographic studies of sports-specific muscle activity. These programs emphasize both general conditioning and selective exercises. Proper warm-up enhances performance while reducing the risk of injury. The warm-up should start with a cardiovascular exercise that raises body temperature and blood flow. General body stretching follows, with emphasis on the shoulder and elbow. Static stretching is continued until full range of motion is fluid. Finally, easy tossing may be started, progressing slowly until competitive speed and intensity are achieved. Emphasis has also been placed on strengthening and endurance exercises as part of a training program in the preseason and on a maintenance program during the season.

Endurance requires a high-repetition and low-load program. Special attention is given to selective rotator cuff and parascapular muscles involved in throwing (Fig. 4).

Shoulder

Rotator Cuff Injuries

The rotator cuff serves several vital roles in shoulder function, acting in concert with the glenohumeral capsule to provide stability as a dynamic restraint. The rotator cuff also acts to position the humeral head in space with depression, compression, and fixation, creating a fulcrum that permits the deltoid to function. The impact of rotator cuff impairment during athletic activity has been well documented. The combined downward displacement of the head and joint compression during arm elevation, provided by the rotator cuff, is important for humeral head stabilization. The functional arc of elevation of the shoul-

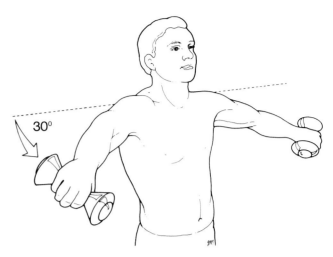

Figure 4

Selective exercise for the supraspinatus.

der is forward, not lateral, and impingement occurs predominantly against the anterior edge of the acromion and the coracoacromial ligament. Certainly, there are pathologic conditions that can lead to impingement, such as subacromial spurs and coracoid anomalies. In most young athletes, a primarily subacromial abnormality is rare, and impingement is thought to result from rotator cuff dysfunction caused by inhibition of its downward displacement force. Electromyographic studies have demonstrated the importance of the rotator cuff in throwing, and the fatigue and lack of endurance that occur without adequate training and rehabilitation.

Athletes with rotator cuff diseases usually respond to a well-managed conservative program. Inflammation is reduced with rest, nonsteroidal anti-inflammatory medications, and, occasionally, a subacromial steroid injection. Strength and endurance are improved by selective exercises for the rotator cuff, beginning with isometrics and advancing to isotonic exercises with increasing weights. Isokinetic exercises have also been used in the later stages of rehabilitation.

Surgical management of rotator cuff disease has been reserved for failures of conservative management (in the absence of a complete rotator cuff tear).

The results of open anterior acromioplasty and coracoacromial ligament resection for chronic impingement, along with repair of partial or complete rotator cuff tears, if present, have been reviewed. Pain relief was predictable, as 88% of patients were subjectively improved. However, return to competitive throwing was poor and unpredictable. Only 27% of professional and college throwers returned to their previous level.

Arthroscopy has recently been advocated for acromioplasty and coracoacromial ligament resection. Results of arthroscopic acromioplasty have been similar to those of open decompression, with decreased surgical morbidity and earlier return of function. Anatomic cadaver studies have demonstrated that arthroscopic techniques remove an adequate amount of acromial bone and that resection of the coracoacromial ligament can be accomplished. Unfortunately, it is unlikely that arthroscopic acromioplasty will improve the ultimate return of throwing athletes to

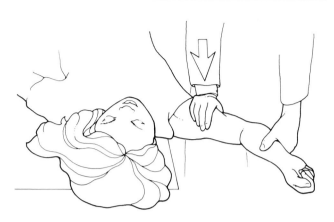

Figure 5

The relocation test. During the apprehension maneuver, posteriorly directed force on the humerus reduces the symptoms.

competitive status. The success of arthroscopic debridement of partial undersurface rotator cuff tears remains unclear. One of the major advantages of arthroscopic surgery is the ability to evaluate the glenohumeral joint for associated abnormalities. Before arthroscopic surgery, open procedures for impingement and rotator cuff disease were performed without inspection of the glenohumeral joint. Subtle lesions, such as labral tears or capsular laxity, were, therefore, sometimes undetected. Possibly some of the throwing athletes who were unable to return to play after surgery for impingement problems had unrecognized associated glenohumeral lesions.

Impingement and Associated Instability

Anterior subluxation of the glenohumeral joint has been described by many surgeons. The "dead-arm syndrome" of instability in a patient with a history of pain or weakness, without a frank dislocation, is familiar. Recently, many athletes with chronic impingement have been found to have underlying concomitant instability. In such cases, instability may be the primary problem and underlying rotator cuff tendinitis only a secondary phenomenon.

The shoulder is inherently an unstable joint. Stability is provided by the static glenohumeral ligaments and reinforced by the dynamic rotator cuff. The position of abduction and external rotation and the forces applied during throwing stress the stabilizers to physiologic limits. If injury occurs at a rate that exceeds tissue repair, overuse damage and progressive attenuation of the static restraints may result in subluxation. The lax capsule may permit abnormal excursion of the joint, resulting in fatigue and traction injury to the rotator cuff and parascapular muscles. Muscular dysfunction and fatigue may then allow the humeral head to impinge on the coracoacromial arch. Electromyography has demonstrated that selective impairment of rotator cuff and parascapular muscle activity occurs in throwing athletes with glenohumeral instability.

Most athletes with impingement and associated instability are between the ages of 16 and 35 years, and are involved in overhand activities, including throwing, tennis, volleyball, and waterpolo. In patients with instability who have been treated for impingement syndrome without treatment of the instability, the symptoms have persisted.

The history and physical examination are essential in establishing the diagnosis. Often, patients with subluxation describe pain during the overhand phase of their sport, specifically in throwing during the late cocking and acceleration phases. This differs from the nonspecific pain that progresses with repeated throwing in rotator cuff tendinitis. Pain from subluxation is usually along the posterior glenohumeral joint, and can be confused with infraspinatus tendinitis. A positive anterior apprehension sign and evidence of instability on palpation confirm the diagnosis. Usually, the anterior apprehension sign produces pain at the posterior glenohumeral joint but not a sense of impending subluxation. During the apprehension test with the arm in abduction and external rotation, a posteriorly directed force on the humerus relocates the joint and reduces the symptoms. This "relocation test" (Fig. 5) has been helpful in eliciting findings of instability in subtle cases. With concomitant rotator cuff disease, a positive impingement sign and pain with supraspinatus testing are present.

The signs of subluxation are often subtle. With secondary rotator cuff tendinitis, the impingement signs are more obvious and dramatic, obscuring the diagnosis. Therefore, in some patients, an examination under general anesthesia and an arthroscopic evaluation are necessary to confirm the diagnosis. These patients may be placed into four different groups, based on the clinical presentation and arthroscopic findings. Group 1 includes those with pure and isolated impingement findings. Group 2 includes those with impingement findings and associated instability caused by labral and capsular trauma. Group 3 includes those with impingement findings and associated instability caused by hyperelasticity, producing a lax joint. Group 4 includes those with isolated instability and no impingement findings.

Proper management and diagnosis are difficult in groups 2 and 3. The findings that correlate with anterior instability include a history of phase-specific pain and findings of apprehension. Other findings include anteroinferior labral tearing, laxity of the inferior glenohumeral ligament, posterior humeral head chondromalacia, and associated posterior labral abnormality.

Undetected instability should be ruled out in any athlete with impingement findings. If instability is diagnosed, it should be addressed primarily. Subacromial decompression is generally unsuccessful if performed when instability is present. In rare cases in which a complete rotator cuff tear exists with anterior subluxation, the rotator cuff must be repaired, but the primary instability must also be treated.

Anterior Subluxation

The primary goal when treating throwing athletes with shoulder pain is to establish the correct diagnosis. The history, physical examination, and plain radiographs may be complemented by computed tomographic arthrography. At this time, this is the radiographic procedure of choice. Its accuracy depends on the experience and interest of the examiner. Magnetic resonance imaging has been unreliable in demonstrating subtle labral-capsular and osseous lesions. Arthroscopy is the most accurate diagnostic tool for shoulder instability and has often revealed lesions missed by other radiographic procedures, including computed tomographic arthrography. Arthroscopy allows visualization of both the acromion (superior surface) and undersurface of the rotator cuff. The glenoid labrum and capsular ligaments can be visualized and palpated, not only for tears but for attenuation that often occurs in nontraumatic subluxation.

The initial treatment is a conservative program that allows most athletes to avoid reconstructive surgery. The rehabilitation consists of a four-phase program that begins with rest, to allow an inflamed and stretched capsule to recover. This can be complemented by anti-inflammatory medications. A strengthening program is then initiated for the rotator cuff and parascapular muscles, with emphasis on the internal rotators and serratus anterior. The exercises should be done in the scapular plane, avoiding extension. An endurance program is then begun. Finally, a throwing program is initiated with slow progression to competitive distance, speed, duration, and frequency.

Those for whom a rehabilitation program fails may require surgery. Many procedures have been developed to correct glenohumeral instability. The overall success of surgical stabilization in allowing the athlete to return to a competitive level has been variable. The Bristow procedure has been unsuccessful in returning athletes to competitive throwing because of loss of external rotation. Other procedures, such as the Putti-Platt or Magnussen-Stack, automatically result in loss of external rotation. Many surgeons have recommended the Bankart procedure to minimize loss of external rotation. A review of the Bankart procedure in 1978 included 30 throwing athletes, of whom ten had returned to their preinjury level. In a second review in 1981, 64% of patients with dominant arm involvement had returned to forceful throwing. The recent anterior capsulolabral reconstruction is designed to restore stability by rebuilding the capsulolabral complex that was worn away by overhand athletic activity.

The role of arthroscopic surgery in reconstruction is undefined. Results published for reconstruction of traumatic unidirectional dislocations have been variable. Arthroscopic reconstruction of nontraumatic subluxation has yielded poor results in preliminary studies.

Elbow

Injuries to the elbow are caused by valgus forces applied during the cocking and acceleration phases of throwing. Tension overload may injure the pronator-flexor muscle-tendon unit at the medial epicondyle, the ulnar nerve, and the ulnar collateral ligament. Lateral compression from valgus stress may cause osteochondral injuries to the capitellum and radial head. Forced extension injuries to the olecranon and olecranon fossa occur during the follow-through phase of throwing. Enlargement of the medial epicondyle is frequently found in conjunction with fragmentation, beaking, and occasional separation. These roentgenographic changes can be seen in both symptomatic and asymptomatic athletes. With progressive injury, bony changes develop, with reactive spurs along with loose bodies and degenerative changes. Flexion contractures of the elbow are common, occurring in more than one half of adult professional pitchers, and may be associated with a valgus deformity.

Injuries to the Medial Epicondyle

Repetitive valgus stress may create an overuse injury to the flexor-pronator muscle group and its attachment at the

medial epicondyle. In the adolescent, before fusion of the secondary ossification center, a stress fracture may occur at the epiphysis of the medial epicondyle. Findings are usually isolated to point tenderness at the medial epicondyle with loss of terminal elbow extension. Radiographic examination may reveal fragmentation and widening of the epiphyseal plate. A bone scan can be used to confirm a growth-plate injury in subtle cases. Treatment consists of rest from throwing and range-of-motion exercises. A progressive throwing program is resumed, usually at six weeks, when there is absence of pain and return of motion and strength. Complete fractures through the epiphyseal plate are usually associated with a traumatic injury such as a fall, although they can be caused by a sudden contracture of the flexor muscle group during throwing. In the presence of marked displacement or valgus instability, the fracture must be surgically stabilized.

Changes develop in the adult throwing athlete because of chronic stress at the attachment of the flexor-pronator muscle group to the medial epicondyle. Tendinitis (medial epicondylitis) responds to a conservative program except in rare cases. Symptoms consist of point tenderness at the epicondyle and occasional tenderness at the proximal flexor muscle group. Resisted palmar flexion of the wrist and fingers reproduces pain at the proximal flexor muscle and medial epicondyle. Treatment consists of rest from activities (throwing and lifting) that produce pain. Ice and nonsteroidal anti-inflammatory medications aid in the initial treatment. When symptoms persist, a cortisone injection is given adjacent to but not within the tendon. The second phase of treatment consists of a flexibility and strengthening program followed by a progressive tossing and throwing program. For those few individuals whose symptoms remain recalcitrant to conservative care, surgical debridement of granulation tissue and degenerative tendon is performed with reattachment of healthy tendon back to bleeding bone. Before surgery is considered, a well-supervised conservative program maintained for at least six months should be tried. Symptoms of ulnar neuritis or ulnar collateral ligament abnormalities must not be confused with medial epicondylitis.

Ulnar Nerve

Ulnar neuritis may be secondary to many factors, including direct trauma, recurrent subluxation, traumatic or degenerative osteophytes, progressive cubitus valgus, and developmental anomalies. In the throwing athlete, the ulnar nerve is usually injured by repeated mechanical stretching, friction, and compression secondary to the large tensile forces generated. In addition, a secondary traction neuritis may develop in an attenuated ulnar collateral ligament. Entrapment of the ulnar nerve may be caused by a thickened arcuate ligament. This may occur in conjunction with hypertrophy of the flexor musculature. In addition to pain and paresthesias at the cubital tunnel, with or without radiation, a perception of weakness or heaviness of the hand may also be noted. Findings include tenderness at the ulnar groove, positive Tinel sign, and, occasionally, abnormal ulnar nerve sensation with intrinsic atrophy and weakness of the hand. Associated conditions of medial epicondylitis and ulnar collateral ligament tendinitis or attenuation should be excluded. Results of electromyography and nerve conduction studies may be normal.

The treatment of ulnar neuritis consists of rest, ice, and

nonsteroidal anti-inflammatory agents. When conservative care fails, surgical decompression with anterior transfer of the ulnar nerve is required. Controversy exists regarding the surgical technique to be used. Recent reports have recommended a submuscular anterior transposition to protect the nerve against direct and indirect trauma.

Ulnar Collateral Ligament

The ulnar collateral ligament is composed of three bands (Fig. 6). The anterior oblique band is taut throughout the range of motion of the elbow and is considered to be the primary stabilizer. It runs from the undersurface of the medial epicondyle to a point at the medial aspect of the ulnar surface, just below the coronoid process. The posterior oblique band is taut in flexion and lax in extension. It runs from the undersurface of the medial epicondyle to the posterior medial olecranon. The transverse band is nonfunctional.

Tension with repetitive stress that exceeds the tensile strength of the ulnar collateral ligament can cause microscopic tears. Improper throwing mechanics that increase the valgus stress at the elbow may accentuate medial tension. Symptoms include medial elbow inflammation and pain accentuated during the cocking and acceleration phases of throwing. Tenderness elicited along the course of the ligament is increased on valgus stress. Treatment consists of rest, anti-inflammatory agents, and evaluation of throwing mechanics. With further repetitive overuse stress, the ligament weakens and may attenuate, causing functional instability; occasionally, it ruptures. A clinical valgus stress test demonstrates medial instability by flexing the elbow to unlock the olecranon from its fossa. Clinical evaluation may be complemented by a radiographic gravity valgus stress test.

Indications for surgical reconstruction include a motivated athlete who desires to continue throwing, failure of a conservative treatment program, and valgus instability. Occasionally, an acute tear can be repaired primarily, but most often the ligament is attenuated with degeneration and requires reconstruction. A free tendon graft (usually

palmaris longus), is placed anatomically to reconstruct the anterior oblique band of the ulnar collateral ligament (Fig. 7). The graft is placed in a figure-of-eight pattern. The ulnar nerve often has inflammation and adhesions secondary to the underlying valgus instability. Therefore, it is recommended that the nerve be decompressed and transferred anteriorly as part of the ligament reconstruction procedure. A complete rehabilitation program takes at least one year before the tendon graft has sufficient strength to stabilize the elbow for competitive throwing.

Osteochondritis Dissecans

Valgus stress during throwing creates compression at the radiocapitellar joint. Repetitive stresses may lead to osteochondral injury. Osteochondritis dissecans of the capitellum is believed to be caused by vascular insufficiency. Repeated stress from throwing has been implicated as a causative factor and certainly may contribute to progression of the disease. Osteochondrosis or Panner's disease occurs in children and consists of fragmentation of the entire capitellar ossific nucleus, with minimal residual deformity after healing. Some believe that osteochondritis dissecans represents a later stage of the same disease, with progression to loose bodies, permanent residual motion loss, and deformity of the capitellum.

Typically, the throwing athlete has lateral elbow pain, swelling, a flexion contracture, and occasional catching or locking. The lesion is usually localized to the anterolateral capitellum. Computed tomography is helping in defining the extent of the lesion and localizing loose bodies not seen on plain radiographs. The treatment of osteochondritis dissecans is dictated by the progression of the disease. If the capitellar fragment is intact, the lesion usually heals with rest. Healing is slow and all throwing activities must be stopped. Drilling and bone grafting to promote healing have been suggested, but have not been directly compared to simple rest and observation. When the lesion has become fragmented and loose bodies are present, the prognosis worsens. Most reports suggest that treatment will restore elbow function but the patient may not be able to return to vigorous overhand sports or heavy labor, especially if a congruous articulation is disrupted. Surgical treatment consists of loose-body removal. Pinning, bone grafting, or curettage to bleeding bone are somewhat controversial. Arthroscopy can aid in the evaluation of chondral lesions and in limited procedures such as loose-body removal and curettage. The best treatment is early recognition before fragmentation occurs and prolonged rest until complete healing is obtained.

Adult Osseous Injuries

Changes in the lateral compartment are often sequelae of osteochondritis dissecans or progressive wear from lateral compression during throwing. Enlargement of the capitellum and radial head occur, as well as osteophytes, chondral lesions, and occasional loose bodies. Hypertrophy of the coronoid process may contribute to motion loss. Palliative treatment consists of removal of loose bodies, debridement of osteophytes, and chondral lesions. Arthroscopic surgery allows surgical debridement with early motion and a shorter rehabilitation program.

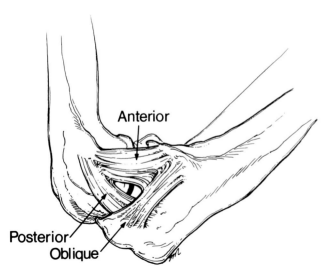

Figure 6

Anatomy of the ulnar collateral ligament.

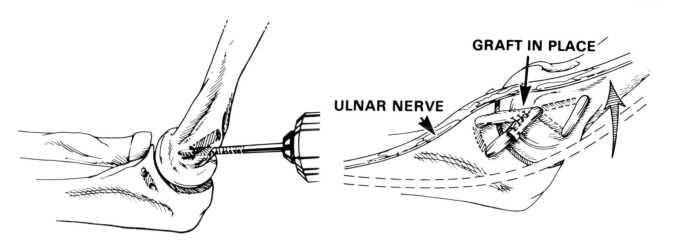

Figure 7

Ulnar collateral ligament reconstruction with a free tendon graft. (Reproduced with permission from Jobe FW, Stark H, Lombardo SJ: Reconstruction of the ulnar collateral ligament in athletes. *J Bone Joint Surg* 1986;68A:1158–1163.)

Posterior Compartment Injuries

Pathologic bony changes are frequent in the adult throwing athlete because of the forces generated during throwing (Fig. 8). Changes in the posterior compartment from extension overload and impingement of the olecranon tip against the olecranon fossa have been noted. Impingement causes osteophyte enlargement, reactive scar tissue, and loose bodies. Radiographic evaluation usually demonstrates osteophyte formation at the olecranon tip. Tomograms are helpful for illustrating loose bodies.

The symptoms include progressive posterior elbow pain, accentuated during the follow-through phase of throwing, and loss of terminal extension. Removal of loose bodies, reactive scar tissue, and impingement osteophytes relieves the pain and improves function. In selected cases, debridement, although palliative and not curative, can be accomplished arthroscopically, decreasing morbidity and allowing an earlier return to activity.

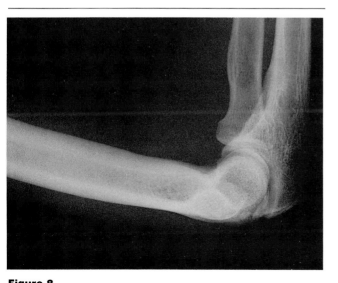

Figure 8

Pathologic changes in the throwing athlete include olecranon osteophyte and loose bodies.

Adolescent Problems

The young athlete involved in throwing sports is vulnerable to the same stresses and injuries as the adult. The open epiphyseal plate presents a unique problem. Young athletes have the desire but not the strength or endurance to meet adult standards for duration and frequency of play. The strength of the joint capsule and ligament is greater than that of an open epiphyseal plate. Forces applied to the shoulder or elbow usually stress the weakest link. It is common for an injury causing a sprained ligament in an adult to cause an epiphyseal plate fracture in an adolescent.

The term Little-League shoulder once referred to a shoulder painful from overuse. It is now recognized that the rotational stresses from throwing may cause a fatigue fracture at the physis of the proximal humerus. Symptoms often include diffuse shoulder pain with throwing. The epiphysis of the proximal humerus is tender and roentgenograms may show widening of the physis and, rarely, periosteal stripping or callus. A bone scan can confirm a physeal injury in subtle cases. Treatment consists of rest. Attention to mechanics, preseason conditioning, and avoidance of excessive throwing are the keys to prevention.

Little-League elbow initially referred to an avulsion of the ossification center of the medial epicondyle caused by pitching in the adolescent athlete. Since the initial description, at least a dozen pathologic conditions have been included and today the term refers to a nonspecific overuse injury of the elbow. The athlete usually complains of pain, which may be diffuse, swelling, decreased motion, and an occasional inability to throw. Most cases of elbow pain caused by excessive pitching can be treated successfully with rest. Repeated stress and pain that is overlooked may cause progressive and permanent injury to the joint. Degenerative changes in the lateral compartment are associated with a poor prognosis and often result in permanent loss of motion and, occasionally, pain. The key to prevention is early recognition of injury, rest, and rehabilitation.

As a response to the numerous overuse injuries from pitching, some with permanent sequelae, Little League pitching rules have been developed. The key is recognition of fatigue by a coach or trainer, counting the number of pitches, and adhering to a schedule. It is suggested that a player who pitches four or more innings should have three days of rest, with a maximum of six innings pitched in a calendar week.

Controversies

Arthroscopy has been established as an important tool in the evaluation and management of glenohumeral and elbow problems in the throwing athlete. Loose bodies can be removed, labral fragments excised, and joint laxity diagnosed. The use of arthroscopy for the treatment of shoulder instability, rotator cuff tears, and subacromial impingement has been reported, but its efficacy has not yet been firmly established. Proponents maintain that arthroscopic treatment can be as effective as open procedures and that there is less surgical morbidity and earlier return of function. This position is being comfirmed in some instances as there is increasing evidence that the treatment of subacromial impingement in the absence of an associated rotator cuff tear can be effectively managed arthroscopically. However, whether an associated smaller rotator cuff tear can be treated successfully with simple arthroscopic debridement of the torn edges is still unknown. Subtle joint instabilities can be diagnosed arthroscopically by identifying capsular laxities and associated abnormalities but arthroscopic reefing (tightening the capsule by shortening it) and stabilization of the shoulder capsule have not proven to be as effective as open procedures.

Removal of loose bodies is a universally accepted indication for arthroscopy. Critical debridement and arthroscopic removal of osteophytes continues to be assessed, with efficacy being shown to date.

The best method of surgical reconstruction in the throwing athlete with glenohumeral instability consumes much discussion time but has not been determined. Most reports emphasize an anatomic repair of a Bankart lesion and correction of inferior capsular attenuation. Recent preliminary reports emphasize the importance of an early supervised range-of-motion and rehabilitation program to enhance the athlete's ability to return to skilled throwing. Operations that do not directly correct the capsular lesion but compensate for its presence, for example, the Bristow and Putti-Platt procedures, appear to be less effective in returning the athlete to competitive throwing.

Annotated Bibliography

Keywords

Arthroscopy; Glenohumeral instability; Impingement; Osteochondritis dissecans; Rotator cuff; Sports medicine; Subluxation; Ulnar collateral ligament; Ulnar nerve

Throwing Injuries

Andrews JR: Bony injuries about the elbow in the throwing athlete, in Stauffer ES (ed): American Academy of Orthopaedic Surgeons *Instructional Course Lectures, XXXIV*. St. Louis, CV Mosby, 1985, pp 323–331.
Valgus stress during pitching is the primary cause of elbow injury. Lateral compression injuries are manifested as osteochondritis dissecans in adolescent pitchers. Medial tension injuries may require surgery. The medial collateral ligament is the primary stabilizer during valgus overload. Extension injuries occur in older athletes and surgical correction is considered palliative.

Andrews JR, Carson WG Jr, McLeod WD: Glenoid labrum tears related to the long head of the biceps. *Am J Sports Med* 1985;13:337–341.
Tears of the superior glenoid labrum were observed arthroscopically in 73 baseball pitchers. Three-dimensional high-speed cinematography of pitching and arthroscopic analysis revealed that large forces on the biceps tendon during throwing may cause tears of the superior labrum.

Andrews JR, St. Pierre RK, Carson WG Jr: Arthroscopy of the elbow. *Clin Sports Med* 1986;5:653–662.
The authors present a diagnostic and surgical arthroscopic technique for the elbow. Clinical data for 62 patients (79% involved in athletics) showed that the highest percentage of excellent and good results occurred in patients in whom mechanical disorders were corrected (removal of loose bodies and resection of impinging olecranon osteophytes).

Bennett JB, Tullos HS: Ligamentous and articular injuries in the athlete, in Morrey BF (ed): *The Elbow and Its Disorders*. Philadelphia, WB Saunders, 1985, pp 502–522.
A comprehensive review of ligamentous anatomy and acute and chronic overuse injuries to the ligaments and articular cartilage in the child and adult.

Ellman H: Athroscopic subacromial decompression: Analysis of one- to three-year results. *Arthroscopy* 1987; 3:173–181.
Anterior acromioplasty was performed by arthroscopic techniques. Of the initial 50 consecutive cases, 88% had excellent or good results. The procedure is technically demanding, and the criteria for open acromioplasty must be met. Arthroscopic subacromial decompression is generally unsuccessful if performed when the primary diagnosis is instability.

Garth WP Jr, Allman FL Jr, Armstrong WS: Occult anterior subluxations of the shoulder in noncontact sports. *Am J Sports Med* 1987;15:579–585.
Undetected shoulder subluxation can be manifested as pain in overhand athletics involving abduction and external rotation (throwing). Failure to recognize the instability and the scarcity of physical findings for subluxation often lead to an incorrect diagnosis (impingement syndrome, posterior capsular syndrome). Roentgenographic evaluation and arthroscopy are important aids in establishing the diagnosis.

Gartsman GM, Blair ME Jr, Noble PC, et al: Arthroscopic subacromial decompression: An anatomical study. *Am J Sports Med* 1988;16:48–50.
Anterior acromioplasty was performed effectively and pre-

dictably with arthroscopic instruments in cadavers. This compared favorably to conventional open osteotome acromioplasty.

Glousman R, Jobe F, Tibone J, et al: Dynamic electromyographic analysis of the throwing shoulder with glenohumeral instability. *J Bone Joint Surg* 1988;70A: 220–226.

Fifteen male athletes who were skilled in throwing and who had chronic anterior instability were found to have marked inhibition of the internal rotators (subscapularis, pectoralis major, and latissimus dorsi) and scapular protractor (serratus anterior) muscles. An association between anterior shoulder subluxation and rotator cuff function was demonstrated. The neuromuscular imbalance increases anterior laxity and is either part of the primary instability or a secondary phenomenon.

Howard FM: Controversies in nerve entrapment syndromes in the forearm and wrist. *Orthop Clin North Am* 1986;17:375–381.

In a young athlete, medial epicondylectomy may lead to weakness and altered elbow biomechanics. Decompression without transposition is reversed for limited compression within the cubital tunnel. Anterior transposition is the procedure of choice.

Ireland ML, Andrews JR: Shoulder and elbow injuries in the young athlete. *Clin Sports Med* 1988;7:473–494.

Common athletic injuries to the adolescent shoulder and elbow are described. Specific conditions are predicted on the basis of the biomechanics of the sport and age of the patient.

Jackson DW, Relman PR: Diagnosis of the painful athletic shoulder. *Techn Orthop* 1985;4:1–14.

The authors describe the functional anatomy and biomechanics of the shoulder. Emphasis is placed on the history, physical examination, and radiographic findings for the painful shoulder.

Jobe FW, Giangarra CE, Glousman RE: The anterior capsulo-labral reconstruction in skilled throwers with anterior shoulder instability. Presented at the Fifth Open Meeting of the American Shoulder and Elbow Surgeons, Las Vegas, January 1989.

In response to the increasing awareness of instability as the major underlying cause of shoulder dysfunction in the throwing athlete, the authors present a new procedure and rehabilitation program. Of 19 athletes with an average follow-up of 25 months, 15 (79%) returned to their competitive level (collegiate or professional). Four of seven pitchers (57%) and three of five professional pitchers (60%) returned to their competitive level.

Jobe FW, Glousman RE: Anterior instability in the throwing athlete. Presented at the meeting of the American Orthopaedic Society for Sports Medicine, Palm Desert, June 1988.

Recent experience has shown that rotator cuff impingement is a phenomenon secondary to underlying anterior shoulder subluxation. The diagnosis is often confused because impingement signs are obvious and instability signs are subtle. Successful treatment (usually conservative) depends on a correct diagnosis and a selective muscle rehabilitation program.

Jobe FW, Ling B: The shoulder in sports, in Post M (ed): *The Shoulder*, ed 2. Philadelphia, Lea & Febiger, 1988.

A systemic review of the anatomy, biomechanics, and pathologic conditions of the shoulder in athletics. Emphasis is placed on diagnosis and rehabilitation protocols.

Jobe FW, Nuber G: Throwing injuries of the elbow. *Clin Sports Med* 1986;5:621–636.

Repetitive upper-extremity activities such as pitching place significant strain on the elbow. Chronic stress leads to overuse

injury. Specific injuries and their treatment are discussed. Attention to conditioning, warm-up, and recognition of arm injury is stressed.

Jobe FW, Stark H, Lombardo SJ: Reconstruction of the ulnar collateral ligament in athletes. *J Bone Joint Surg* 1986;68A:1158–1163.

Reconstruction for insufficiency of the elbow ulnar collateral ligament was performed in 16 skilled throwing athletes. Ten returned to the previous level of competition (including professional baseball pitching), one returned to a lower level, and five retired from professional athletics.

Johnson LL: Open versus arthroscopic techniques for shoulder instability. Presented at the Fourth Open Meeting of the American Shoulder and Elbow Surgeons, Atlanta, February 1988.

Arthroscopic stabilization for recurrent anterior shoulder instability is technically demanding and requires strict attention to detail. Failure with redislocation occurred in 20% of the cases reviewed.

McManama GB Jr, Micheli LJ, Berry MV, et al: The surgical treatment of osteochondritis of the capitellum. *Am J Sports Med* 1985;13:11–21.

Of 14 patients treated with arthrotomy, loose-body removal, and curettage, 12 returned to competitive athletic activity without restrictions. Seven cases were associated with throwing.

McMaster WC: Anterior glenoid labrum damage: A painful lesion in swimmers. *Am J Sports Med* 1986;14: 383–387.

Swimmer's shoulder, previously thought of as impingement, has been shown by arthrography and arthroscopy to be an injury typical of overhand sports—functional instability and labral abnormality.

Matthews LS, Vetter WL, Oweida SJ, et al: Arthroscopic staple capsulorrhaphy for recurrent anterior shoulder instability. *Arthroscopy* 1988;4:106–111.

The authors review 25 consecutive arthroscopic repairs in 23 patients; 11 had documented recurrent anterior dislocations and 12 had recurrent subluxation. Excellent or good results were achieved in 67%, fair results in 8%, and poor results in 24%. Five of six with poor results underwent additional surgery. Four of six failures were in the subluxation group.

Morgan CD, Bodenstab AB: Arthroscopic Bankart suture repair: Technique and early results. *Arthroscopy* 1987;3: 111–122.

Twenty-five recurrent traumatic unidirectional anterior shoulder dislocations were stabilized arthroscopically with a transglenoid absorbable suture. A Bankart lesion was documented and repaired in all cases. All results were rated excellent.

Newberg AH: The radiographic evaluation of shoulder and elbow pain in the athlete. *Clin Sports Med* 1987;6: 785–809.

Important anatomic features of the shoulder and elbow joint and the abnormalities to which the athlete is most susceptible are discussed. Current radiographic techniques and their indications are illustrated.

Nirschl RP: Soft-tissue injuries about the elbow. *Clin Sports Med* 1986;5:637–652.

Common athletic elbow injuries, including lateral and medial tendinitis, are discussed. Conservative and surgical treatments and a rehabilitation program are illustrated.

Nottage WM, Duge WD, Fields WA: Computed arthrotomography of the glenohumeral joint to evaluate anterior instability: Correlation with arthroscopic findings. *Arthroscopy* 1987;3:273–276.

Thirty patients' arthroscopic and computed tomographic arthrographic findings were compared. Nineteen of 22 patients (86%) with proven instability had positive arthrographic findings. Findings included labral attenuation (eight cases), capsular stripping (17 cases), labral detachment (11 cases), Hill-Sachs lesion (eight cases), glenoid rim fracture (two cases), bucket-handle labral tear (one case), and hypertrophic labral lesion (one case). The overall error rate was 10% (two false-negatives and one false-positive). Eight patients had no findings of instability on either arthrography or arthroscopy.

Pappas AM, Zawacki RM, McCarthy CF: Rehabilitation of the pitching shoulder. *Am J Sports Med* 1985;13:223–235.

The kinesiology and pathomechanics of throwing are discussed and diagnostic examination procedures described. A rehabilitation and conditioning program is illustrated that emphasizes flexibility and dynamic muscular balance.

Pappas AM, Zawacki RM, Sullivan TJ: Biomechanics of baseball pitching: A preliminary report. *Am J Sports Med* 1985;13:216–222.

Fifteen professional pitchers were filmed with high-speed cinematography. Three phases of throwing were studied (cocking, acceleration, and follow-through). Arm position, phase timing, and peak shoulder velocities were recorded and analyzed.

Perry J, Glousman RE: Biomechanics of the athletic arm, in Nicholas J, Hershman E (eds): *The Upper Extremity in Sports Medicine*. St. Louis, CV Mosby, in press.

The authors describe normal and abnormal biomechanics of the upper extremity, including electromyographic analysis of the shoulder and elbow during athletic activity. Evaluation of various sports revealed that the emphasis and role of individual muscles are sport-specific. Through an understanding of normal mechanics and differences in pathologic states, a basis for training and rehabilitation is presented.

Rafii M, Minkoff J, Bonamo J, et al: Computed tomography (CT) arthrogram of shoulder instabilities in athletes. *Am J Sports Med* 1988;16:352–361.

Sixty athletes with shoulder pain were evaluated by computed tomographic arthrography. Patients with anterior glenohumeral instability all had an anteroinferior tear or detachment of the glenoid labrum, as well as violation of the insertion of the joint capsule onto the scapula. Surgical correlation obtained in 25 cases revealed the arthrographic findings to be 95% accurate.

Sisto DJ, Jobe FW, Moynes DR, et al: An electromyo-

graphic analysis of the elbow in pitching. *Am J Sports Med* 1987;15:260–263.

Eight collegiate pitchers were evaluated by electromyography to analyze the muscle-firing pattern at the elbow. Results showed low to moderate activity in all muscles during all phases of the pitch. The function of the elbow is probably positioning to accent the transfer of energy from the shoulder and trunk.

Tibone JE, Elrod B, Jobe FW, et al: Surgical treatment of tears of the rotator cuff in athletes. *J Bone Joint Surg* 1986;68A:887–891.

Forty-five athletes with partial or complete tears of the rotator cuff were treated with an anterior acromioplasty and repair of the tear. Thirty-nine (87%) were subjectively improved. However, only 25 patients (56%) returned to their former competitive level. Twelve of 29 (41%) returned to throwing and pitching. Seven of 22 (32%) returned to the same competitive level of professional or collegiate throwing and pitching.

Tibone JE, Jobe FW, Kerlan RK, et al: Shoulder impingement syndrome in athletes treated by an anterior acromioplasty. *Clin Orthop* 1985;198:134–140.

Thirty-five shoulders in which conservative treatment had failed were evaluated after anterior acromioplasty. Thirty-one (89%) were subjectively improved. However, only 15 patients (43%) returned to the preinjury level of athletics, and only four of 18 athletes involved in pitching and throwing returned to their preinjury status.

Torg JS, Balduini FC, Bonci C, et al: A modified Bristow-Helfet-May procedure for recurrent dislocation and subluxation of the shoulder: Report of two hundred and twelve cases. *J Bone Joint Surg* 1987;69A:904–913.

The Bristow procedure was performed for recurrent dislocation or subluxation of the glenohumeral joint in 212 shoulders. Eight (3.8%) redislocated and ten (4.7%) had one or more subjective episodes of subluxation. Only three of 19 athletes (16%) whose dominant arms were treated returned to their preinjury level of throwing.

Warren RF: Instability of shoulder in throwing sports, in Stauffer ES (ed): American Academy of Orthopaedic Surgeons *Instructional Course Lectures, XXXIV*. St. Louis, CV Mosby, 1985, pp 337–348.

An overview of the assessment of the unstable athletic shoulder. Conservative treatment is outlined. The Bankart procedure is used for surgical reconstruction.

Zarins B, Andrews JR, Carson WG: *Injuries to the Throwing Arm*. Philadelphia, WB Saunders, 1985.

A comprehensive review of the throwing motion and diagnostic techniques for evaluating the shoulder and elbow. Rehabilitation and conditioning protocols are described.

25

Shoulder: Trauma and Related Instability

Despite the increased use of arthroscopic surgery, open capsular repairs (Bankart type) remain the standard with which other procedures are compared in the management of recurrent traumatic anterior shoulder instability. Posterior and multidirectional instabilities are now more frequently recognized and are initially treated without surgery. The pendulum has swung toward nonsurgical management of all grade III acromioclavicular joint injuries. Treatment of three- and four-part fractures of the proximal humerus is tailored to the "personality" of the fracture and the health of the patient. Although a number of new studies on humeral shaft and clavicular nonunions have added to our understanding of these problems, the basic principles of surgical debridement of the nonunion, iliac bone graft, and stable fixation still apply.

Glenohumeral Instability

Classification

As the pathophysiology of instability has been better defined, the language of instability has become more complex. No longer can "recurrent dislocator" be accepted as a complete diagnosis. Four components determine the instability group that applies to each patient: frequency, etiology, direction, and degree (Outline 1). Most patients who undergo surgical treatment have recurrent traumatic anterior dislocations. Although somewhat cumbersome, a classification scheme such as this accurately defines the instability groups and will be helpful in the evaluation of future studies.

Radiologic Evaluation

For an initial dislocation or with any trauma to the shoulder, a trauma series must be obtained. The trauma series consists of anteroposterior, transcapular lateral (Y-view), and axillary views. These three views clearly delineate the abnormality. The axillary view is the most effective method of determining the position of the humeral head relative to the glenoid fossa.

For recurrent instability, a separate series of three radiographs is needed: true anteroposterior, West-Point axillary, and Stryker notch views. Each component of this "instability" series can provide information to guide management. A true anteroposterior view of the shoulder is obtained by having the patient stand at a 30-degree oblique angle to the X-ray beam so that the glenohumeral joint is well visualized and joint-space narrowing can be determined. The West-Point axillary view identifies any bony avulsion of the capsule from the anterior glenoid rim. The Stryker notch view is of assistance in defining the presence and size of a Hill-Sachs lesion.

Glenoid version is not a contributing factor to instability. Studies that hypothesized a correlation of glenoid version to instability are now thought to have been flawed by inconsistencies in the reference axes selected for determining the glenoid tilt. Evaluation by computed tomography has shown no difference in glenoid version between patients with recurrent anterior dislocations and a control population. Recently, the angle between the sclerotic margin of the glenoid and the posterior border of the acromion (as seen on a routine axillary view) has been suggested as a method by which glenoid version could be determined. With this technique, investigators found no differences when they compared a control group, a group with anterior instability, and a group with posterior instability.

Arthrography has been helpful in evaluating patients more than 40 years old who are more likely to have a rotator cuff tear with a dislocation. Computed tomographic arthrography can add significant information in confusing cases. Specifically, labral and capsular abnormalities can be identified with this technique. The role of magnetic resonance imaging in such cases has not yet been defined.

Anterior Instability

An important prospective study of 254 patients with five years of follow-up has better defined the risk factors for recurrent anterior dislocation in young adults. Patients 12 to 40 years old were randomly assigned to an immobilization group (three to four weeks in a sling and swathe) and an early motion group (sling used for comfort as needed.) Immobilization did not reduce the recurrence rate. Age at the time of initial dislocation was the most important factor with regard to prognosis. During the five-year follow-up, two or more recurrences occurred in 55% of patients 12 to 22 years old, in 37% of those 23 to 29 years old, and in 12% of those 30 to 40 years old. There was no difference in prognosis for athletes and nonathletes.

Outline 1. Classification of glenohumeral instability

Frequency
    Acute
    Recurrent
    Fixed
Cause
    Traumatic (single episode)
    Microtraumatic (repetitive use)
    Atraumatic
        Voluntary
        Involuntary
Direction
    Anterior
    Posterior
    Inferior
    Multidirectional
Degree
    Dislocation
    Subluxation

Approximately 20% of patients with two or more dislocations in the first two years had no further episodes during the following three years. Previous studies that found recurrence rates in young patients of 85% to 90% may have lacked the controls used in this study. Although longer follow-up may increase the recurrence rate, these statistics represent reasonable estimates of anticipated outcome after an initial anterior dislocation.

When surgical management is chosen, a number of procedures are generally successful in managing this condition. The goal is simple: to identify and correct the abnormality responsible for the symptoms without restricting motion. Extra-articular procedures can alter the joint's biomechanics, resulting in a restriction of motion and possible arthritis. A Magnuson-Stack procedure, for example, does not correct the abnormality found in a true Bankart lesion, and it may significantly limit external rotation. Procedures that use metallic implants about the shoulder are currently in disfavor because of the risks of loosening and articular damage.

In a retrospective review of the modified Bristow procedure in 207 patients, 62% responded to a questionnaire; of these, 34% had pain or discomfort in the shoulder. Postoperative instability was present in 9.7%. Only 16% of athletes whose dominant arm had been operated on returned to their preinjury level of throwing. Although neurologic compromise was not mentioned, the musculocutaneous nerve is at increased risk during the Bristow procedure. These factors should discourage the routine use of the modified Bristow procedure.

Arthroscopic management of anterior instability is in its infancy. Short-term follow-up data are available for two different methods. Using a staple in an arthroscopic capsulorrhaphy has the risks associated with metallic implants. Two centers using this technique had a 20% failure rate. A transglenoid absorbable suture technique avoids some complications related to metal staples, but this approach is technically demanding and may injure the infraspinatus branch of the suprascapular nerve.

The standard by which these newer surgical techniques must be judged is the Bankart repair, which has a success rate of approximately 95% without significant limitation of motion or subsequent arthritis.

Posterior Instability

Although posterior subluxation is now recognized more frequently, traumatic posterior dislocations continue to be uncommon. Perhaps 4% of shoulder dislocations are isolated posterior dislocations. This diagnosis is often missed by the physician who first sees the patient.

In a review of 41 locked posterior dislocations, the correct diagnosis was made between one and six weeks after injury in 13 cases, between six weeks and six months in 12 cases, and after six months in 16 cases. The mechanisms of injury included motor-vehicle accidents (16 cases), seizures (11 cases), electroshock treatments (eight cases), and alcohol-related injuries (six cases). The physical examination revealed an inability to rotate the arm externally. The average internal rotation deformity was 40 degrees (Fig. 1, left). Patients were frequently unable to supinate the forearm (Fig. 1, right). The axillary radiograph was diagnostic in all cases; in no case, however, was an axillary view taken initially. Further, anteroposterior radiographs were not diagnostic. (This again emphasizes the impor-

tance of the complete trauma series in the initial evaluation.) Various treatment techniques were used, depending on the duration of the dislocation, the size of the humeral head defect, the condition of the glenoid fossa, and the general health of the patient. Management of the dislocations included no treatment, closed reduction, transfer of the subscapularis tendon, transfer of the lesser tuberosity, hemiarthroplasty, and total arthroplasty. Suggested indications for arthroplasty were a humeral defect of more than 45% of the articular surface or a dislocation that had been present for an extended period. If there was destruction of the glenoid fossa, a total shoulder arthroplasty was used. It is recommended that the humeral component be placed in neutral version in these patients to decrease the tendency to posterior subluxation.

Recurrent Posterior Subluxation Because no reported series using a specific technique has shown a high success rate, surgeons tend to use an extensive course of rehabilitation in the management of recurrent posterior subluxation. Recent studies have shown that glenoid version apparently does not play a role in instability. Thus, the use of glenoid osteotomy in the surgical management of instability should be reconsidered. In a small group of eight patients treated by posterior capsulorrhaphy, infraspinatus advancement, and glenoid osteotomy, there were six good and two fair results. It is not clear if the osteotomy contributed significantly to the results. In light of reports of a 41% recurrence after glenoid osteotomy, this technique should be used only in secondary reconstruction techniques, at least for the present.

In cases that demonstrate an avulsion of the capsule-ligament complex posteriorly, a posterior Bankart type repair should be successful. A lax capsule can be managed by a capsular shift and infraspinatus reinforcement. Cases in which there is deficient tissue or bone may be best managed by the addition of a bone block (taken from the iliac crest or scapular spine) that is fashioned as an extension of the glenoid, increasing its depth.

The few studies dealing with this condition and the small numbers of patients in each study emphasize the lack of reliable guidelines in the management of posterior instability.

Multidirectional Instability

The term multidirectional instability implies a shoulder that has a component of symptomatic inferior instability in addition to anterior and/or posterior instability. Surgery in such cases has generally been less successful than surgery in unidirectional anterior instability, perhaps because of deficient capsular tissues, a mild connective tissue disorder resulting in increased laxity, or an unrecognized emotional disturbance manifested as voluntary instability.

Although many patients with multidirectional instability have evidence of generalized ligamentous laxity, most can recall a discrete episode that initiated the instability. The first step in the treatment of recurrent multidirectional instability is a rigorous physical therapy program to strengthen the internal and external rotators. This, in conjunction with educating patients about the condition, may eliminate symptoms. Only when a program such as this fails should surgery be considered.

Standard stabilization procedures have not been very successful. One investigator suggested a capsular shift pro-

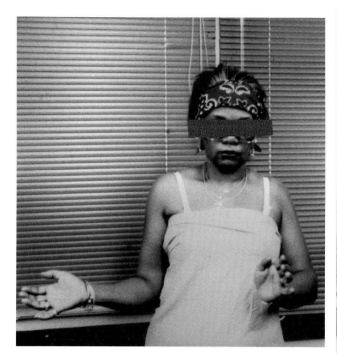 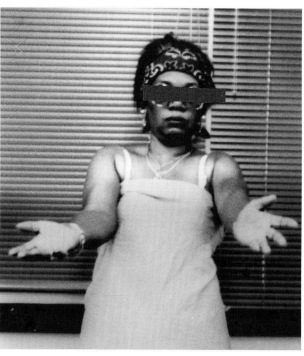

Figure 1

Fixed posterior dislocation that occurred during a seizure and was missed before referral. **Left**, Inability to rotate the arm externally. **Right**, Inability to supinate the arm.

cedure in which tension is introduced into the inferior and posterior portions of the capsule by advancing the anteroinferior capsule along its lateral attachment on the humerus. The anterosuperior capsule is then plicated over this tissue in an effort to reinforce and strengthen the repair. Another recent suggestion is performing a similar capsular plication on the medial side of the joint adjacent to the glenoid. This "T-plasty" technique has an important advantage in that it allows the surgeon to correct a Bankart lesion if one is present.

Rigid criteria regarding selection of patients for surgical management and the new technical modifications are expected to increase the percentage of satisfactory results in this difficult group of patients.

Acromioclavicular Joint

Acromioclavicular joint injuries have generally been divided into three grades. A grade I injury represents a true sprain of the acromioclavicular joint, with no observable instability clinically or radiographically. Grade II injuries show subluxation of the joint, implying disruption of the acromioclavicular ligaments with continuity of the coracoclavicular ligaments. Grade III injuries are dislocations of the joint with disruption of both the acromioclavicular and coracoclavicular ligament complexes.

This basic, understandable, and useful system is now being expanded to include uncommon injuries. Unfortunately, these more cumbersome classification schemes can be difficult to use. There are, however, certain acromioclavicular dislocations that involve a more extensive injury to the surrounding soft tissues and that require surgical intervention to allow reapproximation of the joint. The

expanded classification systems have tried to elaborate on these more extensive soft-tissue injuries. They are, therefore, useful in deciding whether or not surgery is indicated. Unless there is avulsion of the deltoid and/or the trapezius from the clavicle or muscle interposition prevents any reapproximation of the joint, the nonsurgical management of most acromioclavicular injuries continues to be recommended.

In an anatomic study of the acromioclavicular joint and its supporting ligaments, the coracoacromial ligament was found to have fibers confluent with the inferior capsule of the acromioclavicular joint. It was thought that these fibers may stabilize the acromioclavicular joint. The intra-articular fibrocartilaginous disk was a highly variable structure, with no disk found in 20% of specimens.

In a biomechanical study using biplane radiography and load-displacement testing before and after sequential sectioning of the ligaments, the acromioclavicular ligament was found to be the primary restraint to posterior displacement of the clavicle, contributing two thirds of the superior constraint at lower (physiologic) loads. The conoid portion of the coracoclavicular ligament provided the primary restraint to anterior and superior displacement of the clavicle at higher loads.

Of a group of 127 patients with grade III injuries reviewed after an average of ten years, 52 had undergone surgery (either a Bosworth screw or Steinmann pin fixation) and 75 were treated nonsurgically by various techniques. The radiographic appearance of those treated surgically or in a Kenny-Howard splint (11 patients) was better than that of those who were untreated (12 patients) or treated with a simple sling (43 patients). The clinical results, however, were equal. Patients who had undergone an attempted reduction and were then taped or placed in a cast had the worst results. Failures were evident within six months and were salvaged by distal clavicular resections with good results.

A prospective randomized study of 84 patients again showed no clinical difference between surgical and nonsurgical treatment of grade III acromioclavicular separations. The surgical technique involved an open reduction of the acromioclavicular joint, excision of the intra-articular disk, transfixation of the joint with two threaded pins, and a capsular and ligament repair (Phemister technique). Problems with the metallic fixation occurred in 16 of 39 cases. The rehabilitation period was shorter in the nonsurgical group. The authors of that study currently limit surgery to patients who do overhead work or who are thin and have very prominent clavicles.

Fractures

Proximal Humerus

An epidemiologic study showed statistical confirmation of long-standing beliefs about fractures of the proximal humerus: 77% occurred in women and the incidence increased exponentially in those more than 50 years old. The overall incidence in patients more than 50 years old was 3.7 per 1,000 per year. The fractures were generally minimally displaced and resulted from moderate trauma. These findings implicate osteoporosis as the significant cofactor. All patients sustaining this injury should be examined for osteoporosis and treated accordingly.

The Neer classification of fractures of the proximal humerus continues to be an appropriate basis for treatment. Generally, nondisplaced fractures (that is, less than 1 cm of displacement and less than 45 degrees of angulation) can be managed in a simple sling or sling and swathe until pain subsides and the humerus can be moved as a unit. Progressive therapy, initially passive and then active, is then instituted. As in all injuries about the shoulder, physiotherapy has a major role in the functional outcome. Aggressive therapy begun too early increases the risk of nonunion, and the neglected fracture is likely to end up with restricted motion because of adhesive capsulitis.

Two-Part Fractures Two-part neck fractures can usually be managed by closed reduction. If an appropriate reduction cannot be achieved, percutaneous or open reduction should be undertaken. Two-part fractures involving the tuberosities are associated with rotator cuff tears. If the tuberosity is significantly retracted, it should be reattached and the rotator cuff repaired.

Three-Part Fractures Perhaps because it is relatively uncommon, the three-part fracture is more frequently discussed. In general, the technique chosen depends on the quality of the bone, the demands of the patient, and the patient's ability to participate in a rehabilitation program. In a noncompliant or sedentary elderly patient with osteopenic bone, a closed reduction may be the treatment of choice. In more active, elderly patients with poor bone stock, the use of prosthetic replacements is increasing. This has the advantage that physiotherapy can be instituted rapidly. Care must be taken to restore appropriate soft-tissue tension and this may be better achieved with one of the newer modular designs. In younger, healthy, active individuals, open reduction and internal fixation should be

attempted. A technique recently popularized involves tension band wiring of the humeral head fragments to the shaft (Fig. 2). All 14 fractures treated by this technique united with a normal glenohumeral relationship. Osteonecrosis developed in two cases. Postoperative active motion was approximately 130 degrees of forward flexion, 80 degrees of abduction, 30 degrees of external rotation, and internal rotation to L-2. Physiotherapy was lengthy, and gains were seen as long as one year postoperatively.

Four-Part Fractures Four-part fractures are best managed by prosthetic replacement. Care must be taken to restore appropriate soft-tissue tensions in the rotator cuff and ensure that the tuberosities are attached to the prosthesis and the humeral shaft. In young, healthy patients, open reduction and internal fixation is occasionally attempted. If the fixation is tenuous, prosthetic replacement should be selected because immobilization will lead to limited motion.

Fracture-Dislocations In fracture-dislocations in which the humeral head fragment is below the coracoid (Fig. 3) and in severely displaced neck fractures, the neurovascular structures may be at risk. The sharp edges of the fracture can cause a thrombosis or lacerate the axillary artery. Care must be taken when extricating a humeral head fragment from a subcoracoid position because it may be tamponading a laceration. Preparations for improved exposure via release of the conjoined tendon or a coracoid osteotomy should be made before manipulating the humeral head fragment.

Humeral Shaft

Most humeral shaft fractures heal with nonsurgical management. Surgery increases the risk of nonunion, infection, and radial nerve palsy. However, closed reduction with intramedullary fixation or open reduction with compression plating can be used in a patient with multiple injuries or one with a "floating" elbow.

Adequate follow-up was available for 58 of 63 humeral diaphyseal fractures in patients with multiple trauma who were treated with intramedullary stabilization (Rush rods or Ender nails). A 94% union rate was achieved with immediate closed intramedullary fixation. Stabilization via antegrade insertion gave excellent results when the point of entry did not violate the rotator cuff. Impingement symptoms requiring device removal were common when the insertion portal was incorrect. Retrograde insertion through an epicondylar portal gave poor results and was not recommended. With the portal of entry proximal to the olecranon fossa, excellent results were achieved. Encroachment on the olecranon fossa must be avoided to prevent limitation of elbow extension. The authors still recommended nonsurgical management for isolated humeral shaft fractures.

Eighty-eight patients with humeral shaft fractures treated by Ender nails were prospectively studied. There was one nonunion in the 86 fractures available for follow-up. The average time to union was seven weeks. A distal entry portal proximal to the olecranon fossa was used in fractures of the proximal and middle thirds, and a proximal portal was used for fractures in the distal third. This wide distance between the portal and fracture decreases the risk of fracture propagation between these two points. Again, the au-

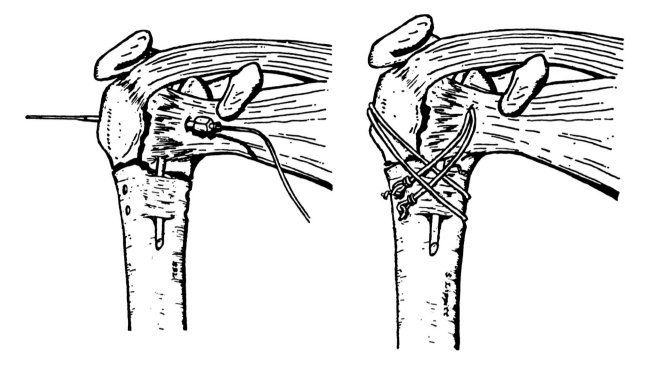

Figure 2

Tension-band wiring technique for three-part fractures of the proximal humerus. (Reproduced with permission from Hawkins RJ, Bell RH, Gurr K: The three-part fracture of the proximal part of the humerus: Operative treatment. *J Bone Joint Surg* 1986;68A:1410–1414.)

thors recommended this technique only for fractures that are recalcitrant to closed reduction and immobilization.

Although the rate of nonunion is generally thought to be higher in patients who have undergone surgery (as many as 13% in some series), an inappropriately applied hanging cast can also increase the risk of nonunion. In two series that included a total of 72 nonunions, the primary treatment had been a hanging cast in 42 cases, surgery in 13 cases, and various techniques in the remainder.

Of 39 humeral nonunions treated with electrical stimulation, only 17 (44%) healed. The protocol used constant direct-current with percutaneously inserted electrodes for 12 weeks and cast immobilization for a total of 24 weeks.

In another series, 24 of 26 nonunions (92%) healed when treated with bone grafts and rigid internal fixation. The average time to union was 5.6 months. These basic principles are recommended: resection of atrophic nonunions, drilling of sclerotic areas, apposition of bleeding diaphyseal surfaces, adequate autogenous cancellous iliac bone graft, compression across the nonunion, and rigid plate fixation with at least six points of cortical fixation above and below the nonunion.

Clavicle

A consecutive series of 150 fractures of the clavicle was evaluated to determine the mechanism of injury. Surprisingly, only 6% of the patients had fallen onto an outstretched hand. The remaining 94% sustained trauma to the shoulder (87% had fallen on the shoulder and 7% had sustained a direct blow). No evidence was found to support the theory that fractures at the proximal, middle, and distal thirds of the clavicle have different mechanisms of injury.

A prospective, randomized study was done to compare a simple sling to a figure-of-eight bandage in the treatment of midclavicular fractures. The study included 61 patients with an average age of 19 years. The functional and cosmetic results of the two groups were identical. There were no nonunions. Reduction of displaced fractures was not accomplished by either method of treatment. The authors noted that the simple sling may provide a more comfortable course of treatment and fewer skin problems.

Although nonunion of clavicular fractures is uncommon, three recent studies have been done. Clavicular nonunions may not require treatment because they are occasionally asymptomatic. Symptoms of the nonunions that required surgical management included limited shoulder motion, neurologic symptoms, thoracic outlet syndrome, and arterial ischemia. Various treatments, including external fixation, have been used successfully. However, rigid immobilization with a plate and supplemental iliac bone grafting seems the most efficacious (Fig. 4). Large clavicular defects have been managed successfully with a sculptured bicortical graft from the iliac crest.

Nerve Injuries

Suprascapular Nerve

One condition that is frequently overlooked as a cause of shoulder pain is suprascapular nerve entrapment. Patients complain of a deep, diffuse pain about the posterior and lateral aspects of the shoulder and radiating to the neck or down the arm. Chronic cases demonstrate atrophy and weakness of the supraspinatus and infraspinatus. Adduc-

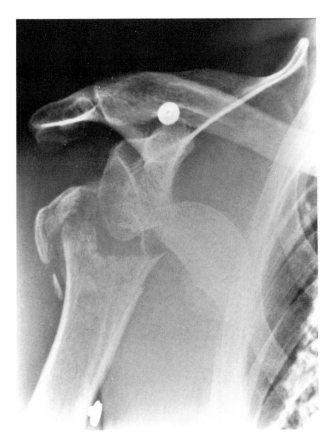

Figure 3

Fracture dislocation of the shoulder with humeral head fragment in a subcoracoid position. Extraction of the humeral head fragment resulted in an axillary artery laceration. The surgeon must be aware that the neurovascular structures are at risk in markedly displaced proximal humerus fractures and in fracture-dislocations.

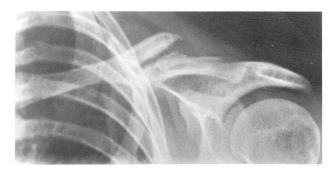

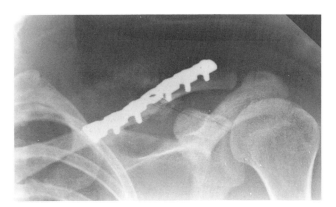

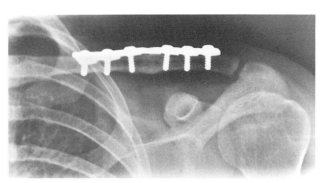

Figure 4

Middle-third clavicular nonunion that caused disabling symptoms. **Top**, Eighteen months after injury. **Center**, Postoperative film after open reduction. Internal fixation with a reconstruction plate and iliac crest bone graft. **Bottom**, Nine weeks postoperatively, the clavicle has healed. (Provided by Stephen M. Howell, MD.)

tion of the arm across the body may aggravate symptoms. Deep palpation over the suprascapular notch frequently causes severe pain. The diagnosis is confirmed by an electromyogram that shows increased latency. Anatomic variations of the suprascapular notch, the transverse scapular ligament, or postfracture changes may result in a predisposition to developing this syndrome.

Asymptomatic paralysis of the infraspinatus branch of the suprascapular nerve has been described in the dominant arm of 12 top-level volleyball players. None had a history of a specific injury or pain. All demonstrated atrophy of the infraspinatus and had weakness in external rotation by manual muscle testing and isokinetic evaluation. The authors theorized that the repetitive movements of the shoulder unique to the volleyball serve may be responsible for this condition. Because no player was aware of any impairment, no treatment was given.

Axillary Nerve

Anterior shoulder dislocations are known to put the axillary nerve at risk. The reported incidence of axillary nerve neuropraxia after dislocation ranges from 8% to 18%. If an axillary nerve injury occurs with a dislocation, recovery is generally complete. If a patient is unable to abduct the arm

after a dislocation and subsequent reduction, the treating physician may incorrectly assume the axillary nerve has been injured. In patients more than 40 years old, an inability to abduct the arm is more probably the result of a rotator cuff tear. An arthrogram and repair of the cuff tear, if present, is recommended.

Nerve injuries related to surgery do not have as favorable a prognosis as those associated with dislocations. Revision stabilization procedures are probably the most likely to put the axillary nerve in jeopardy, but injuries have been recently reported after capsular shifts and Putti-Platt procedures. An anatomic study has shown that articular branches to the inferomedial portion of the capsule can tether the nerve during translocation of the inferior capsule. If a postoperative deficit is noted, and the lesion does

Table 1. Distance between the entry point of the musculocutaneous nerve into the coracobrachialis and the inferior tip of the coracoid process

Distance (mm)	No. of Cadavers
0 to 15	0
16 to 20	1
21 to 25	2
26 to 30	1
31 to 35	7
36 to 40	9
41 to 45	8
46 to 50	12
51 to 55	9
56 to 60	4
61 to 65	4
66 to 70	2
71 to 75	1
76 to 80	0
81 to 85	0
86 to 90	1
Mean = 49	Total = 61

not rapidly, progressively, and completely recover, exploration should be undertaken. Suture material has been found encircling the axillary nerve on reexploration. Early nerve grafting has resulted in good return of muscle function but continued sensory loss.

Musculocutaneous Nerve

The musculocutaneous nerve is at increased risk during the Bristow procedure. Injuries have also been reported after a Putti-Platt procedure. An anatomic evaluation of 61 specimens identified the entry point of the musculocutaneous nerve as being as close as 20 mm from the coracoid process (Table 1 and Fig. 5). In three specimens, a proximal branch entered within 15 mm of the coracoid. Any manipulation of the coracoid-conjoined tendon complex can result in a nerve injury. Again, if a deficit is seen postoperatively and there is no evidence of rapid recovery, early exploration is in order.

Brachial Plexus

Injuries to the brachial plexus from malpositioning a patient during surgery are avoidable. Certain arm positions should be avoided because of undue stretch of the plexus: (1) extension of the arm and lateral flexion of the head; (2) allowing the arm to sag off the table in an abducted, externally rotated, and extended position; and (3) overdistraction of the glenohumeral joint.

Transient paresthesias occur in as many as 30% of patients after shoulder arthroscopy. A study of plexus strain during simulated arthroscopy found that increased forward flexion and adduction resulted in decreased strain. Extension and abduction increased strain. It has been suggested that this risk can be decreased by placing the patient in a sitting "beach-chair" position, without traction on the arm.

Controversies

Shoulder Arthroscopy

The role of the arthroscope in the diagnosis and treatment of shoulder disorders is a significant area of controversy. Some believe that shoulder arthroscopy may be used too

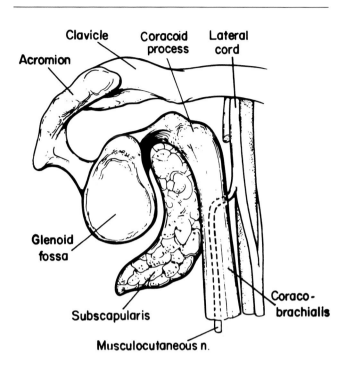

Figure 5

Anatomic drawing showing the entrance of the musculocutaneous nerve into the coracobrachialis. This nerve is at risk from retraction during open shoulder procedures and it may be tethered by transposition of the coracoid (Bristow procedure).

often, before its scientific benefits have been proven. Perhaps the fascination of this new technology will lead practitioners with inadequate training to perform both diagnostic and surgical arthroscopy despite the lack of long-term studies documenting any advantage of surgical arthroscopy over its open counterpart.

Surgical arthroscopy of the shoulder, however, does have a vast potential. In the next few years, diagnostic arthroscopy is expected to increase our understanding of the pathophysiology of shoulder instability, both acute and recurrent. Diagnostic arthroscopy will better identify the lesions involved in patients who have a combination of instability and impingement. This group of generally athletic individuals has been particularly difficult to manage. Only 15 of 35 athletes and four of 18 throwers were able to return to their preinjury status after an open anterior acromioplasty for impingement complaints. Low-grade instability from repetitive microtrauma may manifest itself as a cuff dysfunction, resulting in impingement. Diagnostic arthroscopies will define the abnormality better, thereby guiding treatment.

Surgical arthroscopy is a viable alternative in managing certain shoulder disorders, such as removal of intra-articular loose bodies, irrigation and debridement for septic arthritis, and obtaining a synovial biopsy specimen when rheumatoid arthritis or pigmented villonodular synovitis is suspected. Its use in recalcitrant subacromial impingement and acromioclavicular arthritis is being defined. Perhaps arthroscopy will eventually be used in the management of rotator cuff tears and recurrent shoulder instability. However, in light of a reported 21% redislocation rate after arthroscopic stabilization, we should hesitate before embracing these techniques prematurely.

Acromioclavicular Joint

The indications for surgical intervention in acromioclavicular joint disruptions remain controversial. More refined classification systems, which include significant soft-tissue injuries such as avulsion of the trapezius or the deltoid from the distal clavicle, can aid in clarifying this

particular controversy. Although not yet supported by scientific documentation, the trend in clinical practice is to operate on acromioclavicular disruptions that involve extensive soft-tissue avulsion. In grade III injuries, however, clinical studies have found that nonsurgical treatment is preferable. This controversy is unlikely to be resolved soon, because some of the pertinent data come from questionnaires or surveys from which no conclusions can be drawn.

Annotated Bibliography

Keywords

Acromioclavicular joint; Arthroscopy; Axillary nerve; Brachial plexus; Clavicle; Fracture; Glenohumeral instability; Humerus; Musculocutaneous nerve; Shoulder; Suprascapular nerve

General Considerations

Conn RA, Cofield RH, Byer DE, et al: Interscalene block anesthesia for shoulder surgery. *Clin Orthop* 1987; 216:94–98.
    A successful interscalene block was achieved in 82 of 100 patients undergoing shoulder surgery. Complications are uncommon but can be significant (seizure, respiratory depression). Interscalene block should be considered as anesthesia for shoulder surgery.

Glenohumeral Instability

Hawkins RJ, Neer CS II, Pianta RM, et al: Locked posterior dislocation of the shoulder. *J Bone Joint Surg* 1987;69A:9–18.
    Forty patients with 41 locked dislocations were reviewed. The initial physician missed the diagnosis in almost all cases. The axillary view, once obtained, was diagnostic in all cases. Various treatments were used, depending on the findings in each case.

Hernandez A, Drez D: Operative treatment of posterior shoulder dislocations by posterior glenoidplasty, capsulorrhaphy, and infraspinatus advancement. *Am J Sports Med* 1986;14:187–191.
    Eight patients with posterior instability were reviewed ten to 114 months after undergoing the above procedure. There were six good and two fair results. One patient had limited internal rotation and pain, and another had occasional instability symptoms and pain.

Hovelius L: Anterior dislocation of the shoulder in teenagers and young adults: Five-year prognosis. *J Bone Joint Surg* 1987;69A:393–399.
    Patients with 256 primary anterior dislocations were prospectively monitored for five years. Immobilization for three to four weeks did not alter the recurrence rate. Two or more recurrences occurred in 55% of patients 22 years old or younger.

Matthews LS, Vetter WL, Oweida SJ, et al: Arthroscopic staple capsulorrhaphy for recurrent anterior shoulder instability. *Arthroscopy* 1988;4:106–111.
    The first 25 consecutive patients undergoing this technique were monitored for an average of 36 months. Four patients

had postoperative instability requiring reoperation, and one additional patient had the staple removed. By Rowe's rating scale, 17 had good or excellent results.

Morgan CD, Bodenstab AB: Arthroscopic Bankart suture repair: Technique and early results. *Arthroscopy* 1987;3: 111–122.
    Twenty-five patients with recurrent traumatic anterior dislocations were treated arthroscopically with a transglenoid absorbable suture technique. At early follow-up (average, 17 months), no recurrences had yet occurred and all patients had lost their apprehension sign.

Mowery CA, Garfin SR, Booth RE, et al: Recurrent posterior dislocation of the shoulder: Treatment using a bone block. *J Bone Joint Surg* 1985;67A:777–781.
    Five patients with recurrent posterior dislocation were treated with an intracapsular bone block from the iliac crest. Four patients had excellent results and one had anterior instability postoperatively.

Randelli M, Gambrioli PL: Glenohumeral osteometry by computed tomography in normal and unstable shoulders. *Clin Orthop* 1986;208:151–156.
    Computed tomographic evaluations were performed on 50 normal subjects and 40 patients with recurrent anterior dislocation. There were no significant differences between the two groups in glenohumeral index, glenoid anteroposterior orientation, or humeral retrotorsion.

Torg JS, Balduini FC, Bonci C, et al: A modified Bristow-Helfet-May procedure for recurrent dislocation and subluxation of the shoulder: Report of two hundred and twelve cases. *J Bone Joint Surg* 1987;69A:904–913.
    Of 207 patients who had this procedure, 131 (63%) responded to a questionnaire. Thirty-four percent of these had pain or discomfort in the shoulder. Only 16% of athletes whose dominant arm had been operated on returned to their pre-injury level of throwing. Postoperative instability occurred in 20 shoulders.

Acromioclavicular Joint

Fukuda K, Craig EV, An KN, et al: Biomechanical study of the ligamentous system of the acromioclavicular joint. *J Bone Joint Surg* 1986;68A:434–440.
    Twelve cadaver shoulders underwent radiologic and load-displacement testing before and after sequential cuttings. Primary stabilizers varied with the amount of loading. With lower loads the acromioclavicular ligament provided the primary constraint

and at higher loads the conoid portion of the coracoclavicular ligament provided the primary constraint.

Larsen E, Bjerg-Nielsen A, Christensen P: Conservative or surgical treatment of acromioclavicular dislocation: A prospective, controlled, randomized study. *J Bone Joint Surg* 1986;68A:552–555.

Eighty-four patients with grade III injuries were randomly assigned to surgical or nonsurgical treatment and prospectively monitored for 13 months. Rehabilitation time was less in the nonsurgical group and there was no difference between the two groups in clinical results.

Skjeldal S, Lundblad R, Dullerud R: Coracoid process transfer for acromioclavicular dislocation. *Acta Orthop Scand* 1988;59:180–182.

Seventeen patients with grade III injuries were treated by transposition of the coracoid tip to the clavicle. After a mean follow-up of 7.5 years, only 12 patients had good function. The authors recommend against the use of this operation.

Taft TN, Wilson FC, Oglesby JW: Dislocation of the acromioclavicular joint: An end-result study. *J Bone Joint Surg* 1987;69A:1045–1051.

Of 127 patients with grade III injuries reviewed approximately ten years after treatment, 52 had undergone surgical and 75 nonsurgical treatment. The clinical results were equal. Poor results, which were evident by six months, were managed by distal clavicular resection.

Walsh WM, Peterson DA, Shelton G, et al: Shoulder strength following acromioclavicular injury. *Am J Sports Med* 1985;13:153–158.

Isokinetic evaluations were performed after recovery from acromioclavicular injuries. Grade III injuries treated nonsurgically had no strength deficits. Grade III injuries treated surgically had strength deficits in vertical abduction and grade II injuries had weakness in horizontal abduction.

Fractures

Proximal Humerus

Hawkins RJ, Bell RH, Gurr K: The three-part fracture of the proximal part of the humerus: Operative treatment. *J Bone Joint Surg* 1986;68A:1410–1414.

Fifteen patients who underwent surgical fixation of three-part fractures were reviewed. The only failure was one treated with a buttress plate. A tension band wiring technique gave good results. Two patients showed evidence of osteonecrosis.

Kristiansen B, Barfod G, Bredesen J, et al: Epidemiology of proximal humeral fractures. *Acta Orthop Scand* 1987; 58:75–77.

The fractures were more common in women (77%) and with increased age. In those more than 50 years old, the incidence was 3.7 per 1,000 per year. Osteoporosis was implicated as a major contributing factor.

Lim EV, Day LJ: Thrombosis of the axillary artery complicating proximal humeral fractures: A report of three cases. *J Bone Joint Surg* 1987;69A:778–780.

In three cases of displaced proximal humeral fractures, vascular surgery was required to manage an axillary artery thrombosis. Collateral circulation may result in a warm extremity. The authors recommend exploration of the artery immediately after fracture stabilization.

Humeral Shaft

Brumback RJ, Bosse MJ, Poka A, et al: Intramedullary stabilization of humeral shaft fractures in patients with multiple trauma. *J Bone Joint Surg* 1986;68A:960–970.

Sixty-three fractures in patients with multiple injuries were managed with Rush rods or Ender nails. Good results were achieved with antegrade insertion when the cuff was not violated and with retrograde insertion when the portal was proximal to the olecranon fossa. Epicondylar insertion and insertions through the cuff gave poor results.

Esterhai JL Jr, Brighton CT, Heppenstall RB, et al: Nonunion of the humerus: Clinical, roentenographic, scintigraphic, and response characteristics to treatment with constant direct current stimulation of osteogenesis. *Clin Orthop* 1986;211:228–234.

Of 39 humeral shaft nonunions treated with electrical stimulation, 17 healed. Electrical stimulation of humeral nonunions is not a panacea. Patient selection is critical.

Hall RJ Jr, Pankovich AM: Ender nailing of acute fractures of the humerus: A study of closed fixation by intramedullary nails without reaming. *J Bone Joint Surg* 1987;69A:558–567.

Eighty-five of 86 humeral shaft fractures healed with this technique at an average of 7.2 weeks. The technique is recommended in fractures not amenable to closed management.

Healy WL, White GM, Mick CA, et al: Nonunion of the humeral shaft. *Clin Orthop* 1987;219:206–213.

Twenty-four of 26 humeral shaft nonunions were managed successfully with resection of the nonunion, iliac crest bone grafting, and compression plating.

Clavicle

Andersen K, Jensen PO, Lauritzen J: Treatment of clavicular fractures: Figure-of-eight bandage versus a simple sling. *Acta Orthop Scand* 1987;58:71–74.

Sixty-one patients were randomly assigned to either a figure-of-eight bandage or a simple sling. Clinical and radiographic results were equal at three months.

Jupiter JB, Leffert RD: Non-union of the clavicle: Associated complications and surgical management. *J Bone Joint Surg* 1987;69A:753–760.

Of 19 patients who underwent bone grafting and plating, 17 achieved union. Four other patients were treated with partial or complete clavicular resection.

Stanley D, Trowbridge EA, Norris SH: The mechanism of clavicular fracture: A clinical and biomechanical analysis. *J Bone Joint Surg* 1988;70B:461–464.

Of 122 patients who were able to detail how they sustained their fracture, only 6% had fallen onto an outstretched hand. Ninety-four percent had direct trauma to the shoulder. A biomechanical model is presented that supports the clinical findings.

Nerve Injuries

Bach BR Jr, O'Brien SJ, Warren RF, et al: An unusual neurological complication of the Bristow procedure. *J Bone Joint Surg* 1988;70A:458–460.

After undergoing a Bristow procedure, a patient complained of pain and weakness in the ulnar distribution of the hand with abduction and external rotation. This was caused by traction on the lateral cord of the plexus because of a proximal insertion of the musculocutaneous nerve into the conjoined tendon. An anatomic study of the musculocutaneous nerve is presented.

Bryan WJ, Schauder K, Tullos HS: The axillary nerve and its relationship to common sports medicine shoulder procedures. *Am J Sports Med* 1986;14:113–116.

Cadaveric dissections demonstrated the precarious position of the axillary nerve in relation to the posterior arthroscopy portal, the anterior or posterior capsular shaft, and rotator cuff surgery.

Cooper DE, Jenkins RS, Bready L, et al: The prevention of injuries of the brachial plexus secondary to malposition of the patient during surgery. *Clin Orthop* 1988;228: 33–41.

A review of positions that should be avoided to decrease the risk of brachial plexus injuries.

Klein AH, France JC, Mutschler TA, et al: Measurement of brachial plexus strain in arthroscopy of the shoulder. *Arthroscopy* 1987;3:45–52.

Strain gauges were applied to different points along the brachial plexus of five cadavers. Traction was applied to the arm, simulating shoulder arthroscopy. Extension and abduction increased strain.

Richards RR, Hudson AR, Bertoia JT, et al: Injury to the brachial plexus during Putti-Platt and Bristow procedures: A report of eight cases. *Am J Sports Med* 1987;15: 374–380.

Eight cases of iatrogenic injury to the brachial plexus, primarily the musculocutaneous and axillary nerves, are presented. If an injury is noted postoperatively, and the lesion does not rapidly, progressively, and completely recover, the brachial plexus should be explored.

Skyhar MJ, Altchek DW, Warren RF, et al: Shoulder arthroscopy in the beach chair position. *Arthroscopy* 1988;4:238–242.

Shoulder arthroscopy in a sitting beach-chair position was carried out in 100 patients. No traction was required. There were no complications related to patient positioning.

26
Shoulder: Reconstruction

Basic research has improved our understanding of the glenohumeral articular surfaces, shoulder muscle function, the role of static restraints, and peripheral nerve anatomy. Glenohumeral arthroplasty has proven to be a reliable procedure for relieving pain and restoring function with a low complication rate. The indications for glenohumeral arthrodesis are less common. The use of flexible plates has improved fixation and the fusion rate. The refinement of new diagnostic techniques such as ultrasonography and magnetic resonance imaging has improved our ability to diagnose partial-thickness tears and the extent of full-thickness tears. Arthroscopic anterior acromioplasty has become an alternative to open acromioplasty for the treatment of impingement lesions.

Basic Science

Articular Surfaces

The articular surface area of the humeral head is three to four times that of the glenoid. Thus, the stability provided by the glenoid socket is minimal. Radiographs suggest that the glenoid surface tends to be significantly flatter than the surface of the humeral head. However, a recent quantitative study of glenohumeral joint surfaces using stereophotogrammetry found that both surfaces can be approximated by a sphere, and that the radius of the glenoid tends to be only slightly larger than that of the humeral head. The cartilage thickness is greater at the periphery of the glenoid, accounting for the discrepancy created by radiographs that outline only the subchondral bone.

A recent cadaver study found that the glenoid labrum roughly doubles the depth of the glenoid socket, but the biomechanical significance of this is as yet unclear. A previous study had found that complete excision of the glenoid labrum with the capsule left intact has no effect on glenohumeral stability. Additionally, several studies have noted that, with intact ligaments, the humeral head translates posteriorly in abduction and external rotation, the clinical position producing anterior instability. Therefore, the humeral head is not in contact with the anterior glenoid rim and labrum. Although many textbooks suggest that the labrum is a fibrocartilaginous structure analogous to the menisci of the knee, the labrum is mostly dense fibrous tissue and serves as the glenoid attachment of the glenohumeral capsule and ligaments. Usually there is only a small transition zone of fibrocartilage between the capsule and the glenoid cartilage (Fig. 1).

Studies at several centers have expanded our understanding of the subacromial articulation. Investigations have centered on the morphologic characteristics of the acromion, the histologic characteristics of the rotator cuff tendons, and pathologic changes associated with rotator cuff disease.

Static Restraints

The glenohumeral capsule contains thickenings that have been termed the superior, middle, and inferior glenohumeral ligaments. Varying positions of elevation and rotation tighten different regions of the capsule, implying a degree of functional specificity. Sequential cutting studies have established the inferior glenohumeral ligament as the prime static restraint against anterior instability. A recent histologic study suggested that the inferior glenohumeral ligament functions together with a thickening in the posterior axillary pouch to act as a "hammock" supporting the glenohumeral joint. The material properties and failure mechanisms of these tissues are largely unknown, and are the subject of current research.

The coracohumeral ligament has recently been studied by several groups. It connects the base of the coracoid with the rotator cuff tendon insertion at the rotator interval between the supraspinatus and the suscapularis. It may be shortened in pathologic conditions, limiting external rotation and elevation. It is important to release this structure adequately at the time of surgical reconstruction. A cadaver study noted that the coracohumeral ligament became taut with flexion, while the interior glenohumeral ligament became taut with abduction. Therefore, with both ligaments intact, the humerus is restricted to the scapular plane as it approaches full elevation. This explains in part the ligamentous origin of the zero position of Saha.

Muscles

The rotator cuff muscles guide and center the humeral head on the glenoid, and provide a dynamic fulcrum for the powerful deltoid muscle. Forces applied to the posterior cuff tendons have been shown to decrease strain in the inferior glenohumeral ligament when stressed in the anterior apprehension position. This suggests that strengthening of the infraspinatus and teres minor is indicated in the treatment of anterior instability. Stabilization of the humeral head is also provided by the tendon of the long head of the biceps. A recent cadaver study noted significant migration of the superior head on sectioning of this tendon. Also, another study of unrestricted arm motion showed increasing electromyographic activity of the anterior and middle deltoid with elevation, supporting its role as a prime mover. The activity of the suprapinatus was more constant, suggesting a stabilizing role. Another study, utilizing selective block of either the axillary or the suprascapular nerve, found that the deltoid and the supraspinatus contributed equally to producing torque for glenohumeral elevation. However, the infraspinatus was also paralyzed by the suprascapular block. If only the branch to the infraspinatus is blocked, there is a 25% reduction in torque. More significantly, external-rotation torque is reduced by 70%, confirming the prime role of the infraspinatus in external rotation.

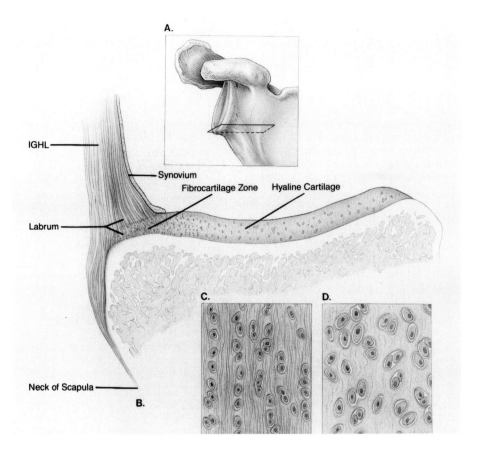

Figure 1

The glenoid labrum is a wedge-shaped fibrous structure that serves as the attachment site of the glenohumeral capsule and ligaments. Fibrocartilage is generally present only in a small transition zone, as shown in this diagram based on recent histologic studies.

An anatomic study noted that the superior subscapular nerve tends to innervate the upper and middle portions of the subscapularis, while both the axillary and inferior subscapular nerves innervate the lower portion. This research suggests that transferring the upper 70% of the subscapularis for massive cuff tears preserves innervation of both segments.

Investigators recently reported separate blood supply and innervation to the clavicular and sternal heads of the pectoralis major. They concluded that the clavicular head can be employed as an active muscle transfer for massive cuff tears. This work also supports the isolated transfer of the sternal head for subscapularis deficiency at revision surgery. The sternal head has the advantage of a better vector for head depression.

Nerves

Musculocutaneous nerve injury has been reported after anterior approaches for shoulder replacement and other procedures. A recent study found that the frequently cited range of 5 to 8 cm below the coracoid for the level of penetration of the nerve into the coracoid muscles cannot be relied on as a "safe zone," because 29% of the nerves enter proximal to 5 cm below the coracoid, and motor twigs to the coracobrachialis may enter even higher. Another investigator has examined in a systematic way the distor-

tions in musculocutaneous nerve position produced by coracoid transfer. These must be kept in mind should revision be necessary.

The suprascapular nerve is at risk in arthroscopic procedures that involve transglenoid pin placement, as well as in attempts at rotator cuff mobilization beyond the glenoid rim. A recent series of 89 cadaver dissections found that the nerve was closest to the posterior rim of the glenoid at the level of the scapular spine, with an average of 1.8 cm between the nerve and the glenoid rim.

Arthroplasty

Indications and Evaluation

Total shoulder replacement has become established in the treatment of glenohumeral arthritis. Initially, constrained replacements were thought to be necessary to substitute for a deficient rotator cuff. However, they have been associated with a high incidence of mechanical failure, and do not reliably reproduce cuff function. Additionally, the majority of shoulders for which a replacement is indicated have intact or repairable rotator cuffs. Therefore, constrained replacements are rarely indicated and unconstrained replacements are preferred.

Infection or loss of both rotator cuff and deltoid function

is a contraindication to unconstrained replacements. In the evaluation of an arthritic glenohumeral joint it is essential to have a complete shoulder series, including anteroposterior views in the plane of the scapula in internal rotation, neutral, and external rotation, a supraspinatus outlet view, and an axillary view. The anteroposterior rotational views outline humeral head incongruities and inferior osteophytes. The axillary view is crucial to evaluating the glenoid for loss of joint space and erosion of the bone stock. In osteoarthritis, it is important to identify posterior glenoid wear, and in rheumatoid arthritis central erosion or subsidence to the base of the coracoid must be recognized. If routine radiographs are not adequate, computed tomography or magnetic resonance imaging may be helpful in evaluating the glenoid. The acromioclavicular joint must always be evaluated clinically and radiographically for tenderness and excrescences. A peristently painful acromioclavicular joint with unrecognized damage will compromise the result of a total shoulder replacement.

Technique

Several technical and design modifications of unconstrained replacements have occurred. Clinically, a small percentage of plastic glenoid components have shown wear, deformation, or stem breakage. Therefore, metal backing has been added. Biomechanical testing has shown that loosening and fracture of the plastic glenoid component can occur under excessive loads (Fig. 2), and that metal backing improves fixation strength. Finite-element analyses have suggested that metal backing may slightly improve stress transfer to cortical bone. Cement is still required, although some centers are clinically testing a cementless glenoid component. Long-term results are not available. Several centers have introduced modular humeral head components to allow a greater choice of head sizes and facilitate revision surgery if needed. However, the results and potential benefits of this modification remain unclear. A press-fit uncemented humeral component should be attempted if there is good bone stock, especially if the patient is young. The incidence of humeral component subsidence or loosening is extremely low. Cement is indicated when there is deficient or poor-quality humeral bone.

A long deltopectoral approach with preservation of the deltoid origin is recommended. In osteoarthritis, an internal-rotation contracture may be present, requiring lengthening of the subscapularis tendon to allow adequate external rotation.

Glenoid bone loss may be significant, especially in patients whose arthritis is secondary to instability repairs or old dislocations, or whose component requires revision. Mild glenoid wear can be corrected by a combination of lowering the prominent side, accepting a small shift in glenoid component version, and adjusting humeral component version as needed. More severe defects may require custom implants or bone grafts. A recent series of 20 large, internally fixed glenoid bone grafts reported this to be a worthwhile procedure for supporting a glenoid implant.

Properly supervised rehabilitation is essential for a successful result, and must be adapted to the status of the soft tissues at surgery and the stability of the implant. Passive motion is started early, usually within 48 hours. If the deltoid and rotator cuff are intact, as in osteoarthritis, active use may begin when pain and spasm have subsided,

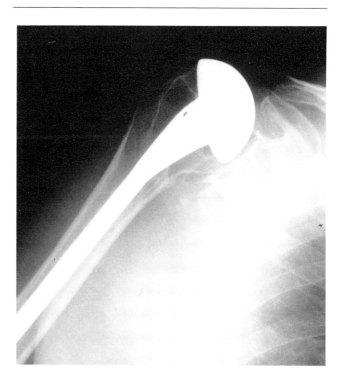

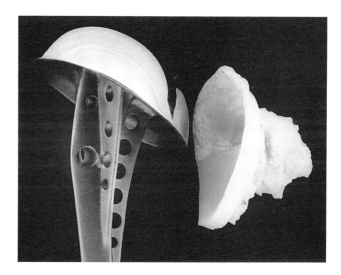

Figure 2

This patient had a Neer I humeral component used with a Neer II glenoid. **Top,** There was superior migration of the humeral component and the inferior edge of the humeral component had eroded the superior aspect of the glenoid component. **Bottom,** Glenoid component recovered at revision shows marked erosion and wear.

generally within two weeks. If a cuff or tuberosity repair was performed, active use is delayed until healing can be expected, generally six to eight weeks.

Results

Several series are now available that evaluate unconstrained total shoulder replacement, and the overall results have been encouraging. As would be expected, resurfacing

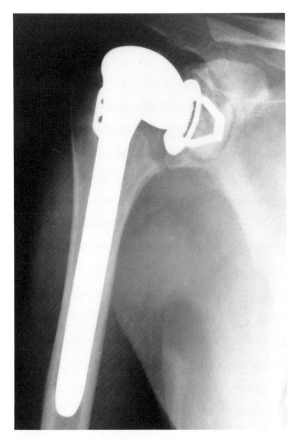

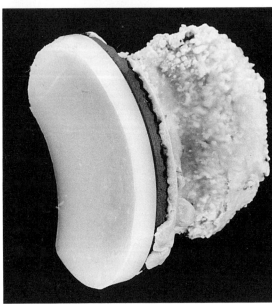

Figure 3

Symptomatic glenoid loosening. **Top,** There is a complete, progressive glenoid lucent line. **Bottom,** The glenoid component was grossly loose at revision and easily removed.

of deformed and incongruous glenohumeral articular surface has been associated with consistently good relief of pain. Good or excellent results with respect to pain relief have ranged from 80% to 96% in recent series. However,

range of motion and function have been variable and dependent on diagnosis. The best functional results are associated with osteoarthritis because the rotator cuff is usually intact and of good quality. In cases resulting from old trauma or failed surgery, there may be extensive soft-tissue scarring and tuberosity retraction that compromises reconstruction, leading to stiffness and weakness.

Rheumatoid disease is associated with rotator cuff deficiency, but this may not always be severe. In three recent series that included 116 rheumatoid shoulders undergoing total shoulder replacement, 28 had normal cuffs, 76 had cuff attenuation or small tears, and only 12 had major tendon defects. Therefore, in most cases the cuff is normal or repairable. In severe rheumatoid cases with large rotator cuff tears as well as extensive glenoid bone loss, a hemiarthroplasty may be a better alternative than total joint replacement. Several investigators have reported satisfactory pain relief with this approach. Ipsilateral shoulder and elbow arthroplasties may be required in patients with rheumatoid arthritis. The more painful joint should be done first. A recent series of rheumatoid patients undergoing replacement of the ipsilateral shoulder and elbow reported good results in reference to pain and function.

The longevity and durability of total shoulder replacements are as good as or better than those of other joint replacements. Five recent series of total shoulder replacements totaling 329 arthroplasties with an average follow-up of 46 months had a revision rate of only 8.2% for all causes. One additional series with long-term follow-up included 615 total shoulder replacements and reported a 3.6% revision rate. More than one half the patients in this series were under 60 years of age.

Radiolucent lines around the glenoid component are common. However, there has not been a direct correlation of radiolucent lines to clinical loosening. A radiographic follow-up study of 69 total shoulder replacements found that 48 patients had lucent lines present before hospital discharge. However, only six of these progressed, and none were symptomatic after an average follow-up of five years. A recent series of 71 total shoulder replacements followed up for five to 11 years noted a complete lucent line of 1.5 mm or more around one third of glenoids, yet only three revisions were necessary for glenoid loosening. Another series reviewing 140 total shoulder replacements in rheumatoid patients reported that 82% had glenoid radiolucent lines, yet only 1% were definitely loose and 8% were thought to be probably loose. No glenoid revisions were performed in this series. The overall glenoid loosening rate in five recent series was 4.3% (Fig. 3).

An association between rotator cuff deficiency and glenoid loosening was recently reported; this was thought to be the result of a "rocking-horse" effect on the glenoid component produced by the upwardly unstable humeral component. If the cuff cannot be adequately repaired at the time of total shoulder replacement, consideration should given to not using a glenoid component (Fig. 4).

Clinically significant heterotopic bone after total shoulder replacement for glenohumeral arthritis has been uncommon in most reports. However, a series from Denmark had some ectopic ossification in 45% of cases. In 10% of the cases the ossifications roentgenographically bridged the glenohumeral and/or the glenoacromial space and were associated with limited range of motion.

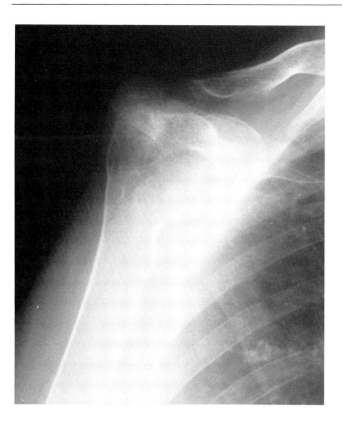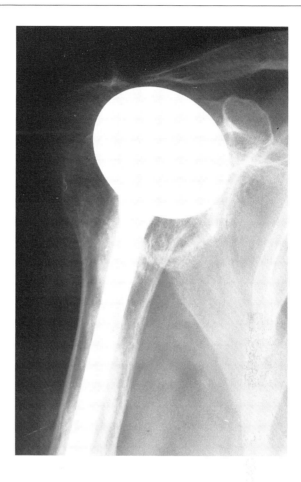

Figure 4

This patient had advanced rheumatoid disease. **Left,** Extensive glenoid bone loss and a massive tear of the rotator cuff. **Right,** The shoulder was reconstructed with a large humeral head replacement without a glenoid. The patient had excellent pain relief and good use below the horizontal.

Rotator Cuff Disease

Etiology

Subacromial impingement lesions and rotator cuff tears continue to be common causes of shoulder pain and disability. Through the years several causes have been proposed for these lesions. Any pathologic process that decreases the space between the rather rigid coracoacromial arch and the greater tuberosity results in impingement of the rotator cuff and bursa. The subacromial space is normally between 1 and 1.5 cm in width. A recent radiographic study reported abnormal superior humeral head migration in patients with impingement before complete tendon tearing. It was thought that this upward displacement perhaps resulted from intrinsic rotator cuff dysfunction, and that this may have initiated the impingement. This cuff weakness may account for the clinical success of treating impingement with a rehabilitation program emphasizing strengthening of the rotator cuff muscles. Another investigator has stressed the role of intrinsic tension overload in the supraspinatus tendon and noted pathologic findings of angiofibroblastic hyperplasia in rotator cuff tears.

Most impingement lesions are secondary to abnormalities in the coracoacromial arch. A recent study of 140 cadaveric shoulders classified the acromion's morphologic characteristics into three types: flat, curved, and hooked (Fig. 5). Only 39% of the shoulders had hooked acromions but these had 70% of the full-thickness cuff tears, whereas the 17% of shoulders with flat acromions had just 3% of the cuff tears. Several clinical series of rotator cuff repairs have reported spurs and irregularities of the anterior acromion with sclerosis and excrescences of the greater tuberosity, as well as adjacent flattening and wear of the long head of the biceps tendon.

Whether impingement is the initiating cause or merely a continuing factor in cuff degeneration has been the subject of controversy. Some have thought that the frequent location of partial tears on the articular side is inconsistent with impingement; however, a tendon compressed and sheared between two bones (acromion and humerus) may fail on either side or in midsubstance. One histologic study of 200 cadaveric shoulders found attritional changes in the anterior acromion in all shoulders with complete cuff tears as well as in those with bursal-side partial tears, but not in shoulders with articular-side partial tears. The authors concluded that impingement was not the initiating factor in these tears. However, several reports have noted good results from treating partial-thickness tears with acromioplasty alone. If impingement were purely secondary to superior humeral migration caused by cuff "dysfunction,"

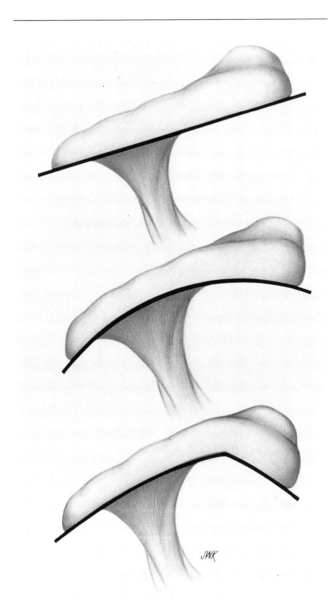

Figure 5

Three acromial types: type I (at top) is flat, type II (at middle) is curved, and type III (at bottom) is hooked.

surgical alteration of the acromion's morphologic characteristics would not be expected to have a beneficial effect.

Recently, it was observed at several centers that there may be an association between glenohumeral instability and subacromial impingement, especially in young, athletic patients. These patients are usually involved in overhead sports, and subtle changes in glenohumeral stability can alter the excursion of the greater tuberosity under the rigid coracoacromial arch. Treatment must be directed at the instability, as acromioplasty has a high failure rate in this group. Diagnosis in these patients can be extremely difficult because of the lack of objective radiographic findings. The impingement injection test, the relocation test (removing the pain from an anterior apprehension maneuver by applying posterior pressure to the humeral head), examination with the patient under anesthesia, and arthroscopy (comparing capsular and labral abnormalities

with subacromial abnormalities) may all be useful. If a diagnosis of primary impingement resistant to conservative treatment is established in a young patient, acromioplasty can be effective. A recent series of 26 patients less than 40 years old (average age, 32 years) undergoing acromioplasty had 81% good or excellent results. It should be emphasized that anterior acromioplasty is an uncommon procedure in patients under 40 years of age.

Trauma can be responsible for a full-thickness rotator cuff tear, especially if there is an anterior dislocation in an older patient. However, many patients found to have a cuff tear after trauma often have had shoulder pain before the injury, signifying preexisting rotator cuff abnormality.

Imaging

Routine radiographs of patients with impingement syndrome may be normal, but in chronic cases may show cysts, sclerosis, or irregularity at the greater tuberosity, and spurs and sclerosis of the anterior acromion. Furthermore, in one recent study, radiographs of patients with small complete tears of the rotator cuff were often normal.

Large or massive rotator cuff tears may demonstrate a decreased acromiohumeral interval. The sensitivity of this finding is increased by stress views, in which active deltoid contraction causes superior humeral migration. This would normally be prevented by the head-depressing function of an intact cuff. One study evaluated a maneuver in which the patient holds the arm at 30 degrees of abduction while holding a 2-kg weight. This stressed view revealed a diminished acromiohumeral distance in 74% of patients with arthrographically proven rotator cuff tears, although conventional radiographs were abnormal in only 47%. Similar findings were reported in another study in which superior humeral migration was elicited by having the patient "push up" out of a chair.

The supraspinatus outlet view is helpful for evaluating the acromion's morphologic characteristics. Spurs and abnormal sloping of the acromion are better visualized. This view is a lateral one in the scapular plane (tangential "Y" view) with the beam directed caudad approximately 5 to 10 degrees. Preoperative and postoperative acromial characteristics can be compared (Fig. 6). A prospective study of arthroscopic acromioplasty in 24 patients found that better results were associated with adequate bone removal documented with this view. Significantly, all excellent results occurred in patients with flat acromions postoperatively.

The axillary view allows identification of persistent unfused anterior acromial epiphysis. A recent review of 26 such cases stressed the value of the axillary view. A computed tomographic scan can be helpful in some cases.

Single- and double-contrast arthrography continues to be a highly accurate test for the diagnosis of full-thickness tears of the rotator cuff. It is less useful in the diagnosis of partial tears. Some articular-side partial tears may be demonstrated, but intrasubstance and bursal tears are not. Subacromial bursography has been advocated for the diagnosis of bursal-side partial tears, but is difficult to interpret.

Several recent series have reported encouraging results with ultrasonography in the diagnosis of rotator cuff tears. Advantages include comfort, the opportunity to compare both shoulders, economy, and the ability to image abnormal anatomy dynamically. Additionally, various parts of the tendon can be examined to delineate the extent of ten-

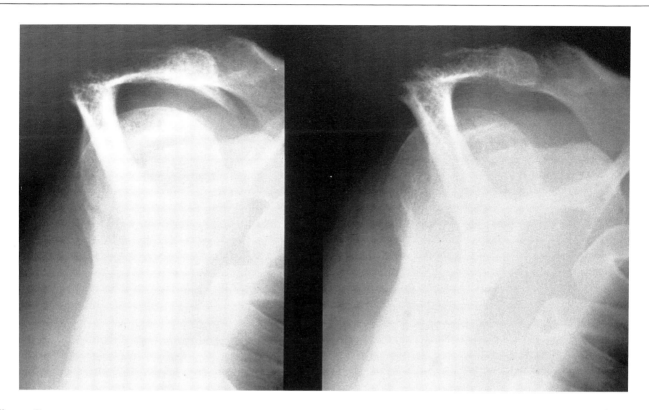

Figure 6

The preoperative supraspinatus outlet view (**left**) demonstrated a large anterior acromial spur extending into the coracoacromial ligament in this patient with a partial-thickness rotator cuff tear. The spur was removed arthroscopically, as confirmed by a postoperative view (**right**). (Reproduced with permission from Bigliani LU, Flatow EL: History, physical examination, and diagnostic modalities, in McGinty J, Caspari R, Jackson D, et al (eds): *Operative Arthroscopy.* New York, Raven Press, in press.)

don tearing. Accuracy has been improved with more modern equipment and the addition of dynamic scanning. Recent data have suggested that the use of focally increased echogenicity as a criterion for partial-thickness tears was associated with a high rate of false-positive findings. Ultrasonography has been reliable in detecting full-thickness tears in most reports, but less valuable in detecting defects of less than 1 cm and partial-thickness tears. Although ultrasonography is more difficult to interpret in the postoperative shoulder, one study reported a high degree of accuracy in assessing the integrity of the rotator cuff in a series of patients with recurrent symptoms after acromioplasty with or without cuff repair. Operator dependence has been noted as a drawback to this diagnostic modality.

Magnetic resonance imaging is also proving to be useful in the diagnosis of rotator cuff disease (Fig. 7). However, it is currently expensive, time-consuming, and difficult for claustrophobic patients. There appears to be less operator dependence than in ultrasound. It produces precise, readily understandable images of the bones and soft tissue. The coracoacromial arch can be visualized in different planes, allowing improved correlation with conventional radiographs. Partial-and full-thickness tears can be differentiated and the extent of tears can be visualized. Initial studies reported a high sensitivity, but also a tendency to confuse partial-thickness tears with lesser degrees of tendon damage. Clinical experience and newer equipment appears to be improving the specificity of this test.

Arthroscopy continues to be useful for direct visualization of both bursal- and joint-side partial-thickness cuff tears.

Acromioplasty

The majority of subacromial impingement lesions can be successfully treated conservatively; if they become chronic, however, open or arthroscopic (closed) acromioplasty may be necessary. Resection of the coracoacromial ligament alone has not been shown to be effective. The rationale of acromioplasty is to enlarge the space for the rotator cuff tendon. Investigators used a microcapillary infusion technique to measure pressure in the subacromial bursa with active elevation. Pressure at rest averaged 8 mm Hg and rose to 39 mm Hg with arm elevation. A cadaver study using a balloon catheter noted a similar increase in subacromial pressure with arm elevation. This was significantly reduced after anterior acromioplasty.

Since its introduction in 1972, open anterior acromioplasty for impingement with an intact rotator cuff has been consistently associated with good results. Three recent series totaling 173 patients reported excellent results in 144. Adequate bone removal from the entire undersurface of the anterior acromion is essential for success. Also, several studies have implicated the acromioclavicular joint as a source of impingement and pain. The indication for complete acromioclavicular resection is preoperative tenderness. If the acromioclavicular joint is not tender but there

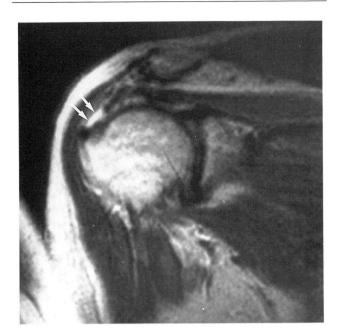

Figure 7

This T$_2$-weighted image shows a bright area (arrows) at the supraspinatus insertion that is caused by fluid, suggesting a rotator cuff tear. This was confirmed at surgery. (Reproduced with permission from Bigliani LU, Flatow EL: History, physical examination, and diagnostic modalities, in McGinty J, Caspari R, Jackson D, et al (eds): *Operative Arthroscopy*. New York, Raven Press, in press.)

are prominent inferior osteophytes, a partial resection of the undersurface of the distal clavicle is preferred.

Arthroscopic (closed) acromioplasty is a new procedure first described in 1984 with the same indications as the open procedure. It minimizes deltoid injury and expedites rehabilitation. As in open acromioplasty, adequate bone removal is important for success. A recent quantitative cadaver study of bone removal failed to note any significant difference in adequacy between anterior acromioplasty done in an open fashion vs arthroscopically. A two- to five-year follow-up series of arthroscopic acromioplasties included 65 patients without full-thickness cuff tears. Fifty-nine patients achieved satisfactory results. Several other series with shorter follow-up have also reported satisfactory results, but have emphasized that it is a demanding technique. Two separate reports of arthrosopic acromioplasty, each with a minimum two-year follow-up, together contained 37 patients with full-thickness rotator cuff tears. Eighteen had unsatisfactory results and both reports concluded that open repair was preferable for most of these cases.

Rotator Cuff Repair

The majority of partial-thickness tears do not require repair. If there is significant thinning, the involved segment can be resected and the edges repaired. Most investigators favor surgical repair of full-thickness rotator cuff tears. The goals of repair are to provide dynamic stability, to restore the strength of external rotation, to improve head depression (reestablishing the force couple with the deltoid), and to seal the synovial cavity for articular nutrition. Pain re-

lief, provided by anterior acromioplasty, may improve function, but cuff repair is thought to be important for restoring strength and functional activity.

Small and medium-sized tears can be repaired by tendon-to-tendon and tendon-to-bone techniques. Nonabsorbable sutures are biomechanically superior to staples. Further, staples can lead to impingement or migration into the glenohumeral joint (Fig. 8). Large and massive tears are more difficult to repair because of retraction and scarring. Often the tear is chronic, and the quality of the tissue is poor. The best results have been reported with mobilization and transposition of existing cuff tissue. This may include release of the coracohumeral ligament and rotator interval, capsular release at the glenoid margin, biceps incorporation, and, if needed, transfer of the upper portion of the subscapularis. Mobilization of retracted tendons is important for reestablishing a functional muscle-tendon unit for adequate range of motion.

The results of muscle transfers, fascial grafts, and synthetic implants have not been encouraging. However, one report noted good early results after latissimus dorsi transfer in a small group of patients. Another investigator has advocated subacromial decompression and cuff debridement for patients with irreparable, massive tears. Early results have been encouraging, but cuff repair is still recommended whenever possible. A report of a similar procedure noted only 40% good results with very large tears, and progressive glenohumeral arthritis and superior subluxation with follow-up of more than ten years.

A well-supervised postoperative rehabilitation program is important. Passive exercises should be started early, generally within 48 hours. Active exercises are delayed for at least six weeks, and resistance is slowly increased.

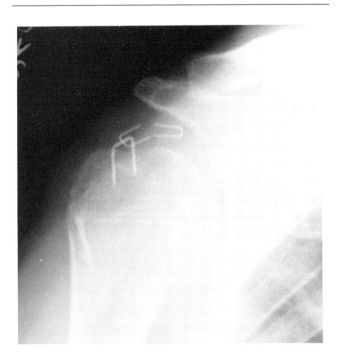

Figure 8

This patient had undergone rotator cuff repair in which staple fixation failed. Several of the staples had migrated into the glenohumeral joint.

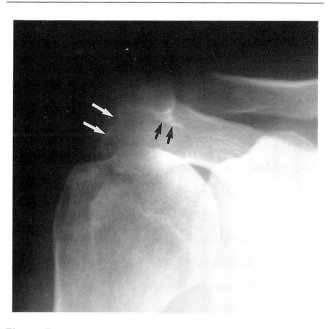

Figure 9

This patient had continuing pain after previous lateral acromionectomy and rotator cuff repair. Despite resection of the lateral acromion (curved arrows), there was a persistent anterior acromial spur (arrows). After revision with anterior acromioplasty, the patient experienced dramatic pain relief.

The results of acromioplasty and tendon repair in several large series with follow-up extending to 14 years and averaging between three and six years have been satisfactory in 84% to 91%. These results did not deteriorate with time. Pain relief was more predictable than improved function in massive tears, and compliance with rehabilitation was essential.

Revision Surgery

Several factors have been identified with failure of impingement and rotator cuff surgery. A review of 51 patients with continuing pain and disability after acromioplasty noted persistent impingement (Fig. 9), missed diagnoses (especially acromioclavicular pain and cervical spondylosis), and worker's compensation status as the most common factors associated with the failure of initial surgery.

Reoperation after failed rotator cuff repair is technically more demanding and has less predictable results than initial repair. Rerepair should be considered for pain relief rather than for functional improvement. Better results have been reported in patients with an intact deltoid origin and good-quality cuff tissue. Previous lateral or total acromionectomy, deltoid retraction (Fig. 10), and soft, friable residual cuff tissue make reconstruction more difficult. Procedures that deform the acromion or deltoid origin should be avoided.

Attempts to restore deltoid function after it has been lost have been frustrating. Of ten patients in whom the latissimus dorsi was rotated on its pedicle to replace a paralyzed anterior deltoid, only six could elevate their arms above 90 degrees.

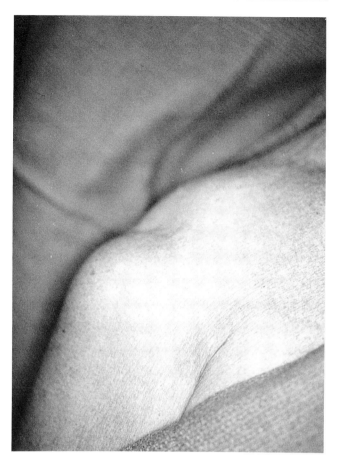

Figure 10

This patient had undergone rotator cuff surgery with a scarred, detached deltoid origin. In this setting, revision is rarely able to restore active elevation. (Illustration provided by Stephen J. McIllveen, MD).

Miscellaneous Considerations

Arthrodesis

Shoulder fusion is an infrequently performed procedure in the arthroplasty era. Recent studies have emphasized that loss of glenohumeral rotation produces greater functional deficits than had been appreciated previously. Additionally, pain relief is unreliable, and pseudarthrosis is not uncommon. In a series of 17 shoulder arthrodeses, nine had moderate to severe pain after an average follow-up of four years. Severe functional deficits were common, even with the recommended fusion position (25 to 40 degrees of abduction, 20 to 30 degrees of flexion, and 25 to 30 degrees of internal rotation). One report found the results of hemiarthroplasty to be superior to those of arthrodesis in patients with rheumatoid arthritis.

Currently, the indications for shoulder fusion are painful glenohumeral joint incongruity in the presence of infection, and unreconstructable loss of both rotator cuff and deltoid function. Modern internal fixation may reduce the incidence of pseudarthrosis. In a recent series of 11 arthrodeses, solid fusion was reported in all after use of a carefully contoured pelvic-reconstruction plate. Spica cast immobilization was used postoperatively for six weeks.

Acromioclavicular Joint

Acromioclavicular arthritis can cause pain directly or contribute to impingement symptoms if the undersurface of a hypertrophied joint diminishes the space under the coracoacromial arch. Acromioclavicular degeneration is common in older patients in whom there is an overlap between cervical spine disease and rotator cuff abnormality. Diagnostic selective local anesthetic injection is of great value, particularly because radiographs may underrepresent acromioclavicular disease. A recent study compared radiographs with pathologic findings in 108 cadaveric acromioclavicular joints. Early osteoarthritic changes were frequently missed by radiographs. Clinically, the ability of an acromioclavicular lidocaine injection to eliminate shoulder pain aids diagnosis, helps to predict the possible value of surgical resection of the distal clavicle, and may be of therapeutic value if a steroid preparation is added. Multiple steroid injections should be avoided.

The role of a painful acromioclavicular joint in rheumatoid arthritis has received increased attention. Acromioclavicular pain and tenderness were present in one third of a series of rheumatoid patients with painful shoulders. Another study of rheumatoid patients used selective lidocaine injections of the acromioclavicular joint, subacromial space, and glenohumeral joint to differentiate the sources of painful symptoms. It was suggested that isolated acromioclavicular resection may be indicated in patients in whom the acromioclavicular joint is the most painful area. However, in most instances, this is a procedure secondary to glenohumeral replacement.

When nonsurgical management has failed, resection of the distal clavicle has been associated with good results. This procedure can be performed arthroscopically, either through a bursal approach or through a superior portal. Adequate bone removal is possible and allows proper contouring of the distal clavicle (Fig. 11).

Biceps Tendon

Tenderness over the tendon of the long head of the biceps brachii in its groove accompanies many conditions that inflame the shoulder because an extension of the glenohumeral synovial lining surrounds the tendon in the bicipital groove for varying distances. Additionally, in the superior part of the groove the tendon is in the impingement area and may be involved in the impingement syndrome.

Most investigators now believe that most cases of biceps tendinitis are secondary to other shoulder abnormalities. Therefore, isolated tenodesis in the groove has limited value. A recent study of 54 tenodeses of the biceps for chronic tendinitis noted early good results, but the results deteriorated with time; only 50% had satisfactory results after an average of seven years.

Another study reported 94% satisfactory results (average follow-up, 29 months) in 17 patients undergoing biceps tenodesis or transfer for primary biceps tendinitis. Careful patient selection by excluding other shoulder abnormalities contributed to the high rate of success. It was emphasized that primary bicipital tendinitis is uncommon, and that biceps tendinitis was secondary to other disorders in 95% of the cases.

If the biceps tendon is found to be flattened and inflamed by impingement at the time of rotator cuff repair, it should be left intact and decompressd by anterior acromioplasty.

If it is torn or displaced from its groove, then tenodesis as part of the overall procedure is recommended.

Calcific Tendinitis   Most patients with calcific tendinitis respond to nonsurgical management, which includes needling and steroid injections. Open excision has been associated with postoperative stiffness. Encouraging results were reported after arthroscopic calcium removal in 16 patients, but the follow-up was short. Localization of the calcium arthroscopically is aided by needles and humeral rotation but can be difficult.

Suprascapular Nerve Entrapment

Suprascapular nerve entrapment is an uncommon cause of weakened external rotation. The more common causes include rotator cuff tears, cervical radiculopathy, stroke, and brachial plexus injuries. Entrapment of the nerve in the suprascapular notch is difficult to diagnose. Pain and tenderness over the notch and atrophy and weakness of the supraspinatus and infraspinatus are characteristic. Temporary relief with local injection may aid evaluation. Confirmation of the diagnosis by electromyography is essential.

Surgical release may relieve symptoms. A recent study reported satisfactory results after division of the transverse scapular ligament in seven of nine patients. Two patients had compromised results because of coexisting cervical and mechanical shoulder disorders, emphasizing the need for careful evaluation of all sources of pain.

Anesthesia

Interscalene brachial and cervical plexus block has been successfully used for both arthroscopy and major open reconstruction. A recent study reported the use of an interscalene catheter for continuous brachial plexus block as needed. General anesthesia offers a greater degree of muscle relaxation for examination under anesthesia.

Frozen Shoulder

Frozen shoulder is a symptom that can be caused by many conditions and results in painful restriction of shoulder motion. The term adhesive capsulitis has been applied to a syndrome of pain and stiffness associated with capsular contracture, especially in the axillary recess. A series of clinical, arthrographic, histologic, and arthroscopic investigations has suggested that this is a primary inflammatory condition involving the capsule and synovium. Whether primary or secondary, there is a large group of patients with painful restricted shoulder motion for whom no other diagnosis can be established, and whose symptoms resolve as motion is restored.

The patients are frequently women between the ages of 40 and 60 years. An increased incidence has been reported in diabetes mellitus, thyroid disease, and Parkinson's disease. One study in diabetics noted that shoulder symptoms were associated with insulin treatment, diabetes lasting more than ten years, and retinopathy.

The majority of cases resolve with a properly supervised rehabilitation program. Gentle stretching exercises performed at least three times daily are essential. Excessive force should not be used and will only discourage the patient. Refractory cases may improve after manipulation under anesthesia. A prolonged regional block and arthro-

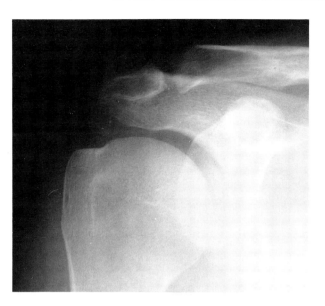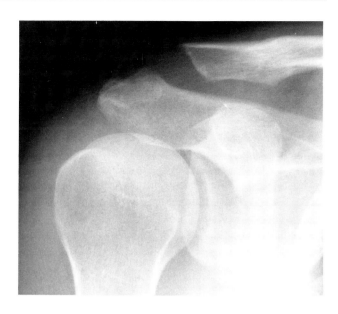

Figure 11

Left, This patient had osteolysis of the distal clavicle refractory to nonsurgical treatment. **Right**, The patient underwent arthroscopic resection of the distal clavicle via a superior portal. Precise contouring is possible, and there is minimal swelling since the subacromial bursa is not violated.

scopic debridement may also be useful in the treatment of this problem. Open release is rarely indicated, and is associated with a high degree of residual stiffness. It may be indicated when there is severe osteopenia on radiographs, a history of dislocation, or failure of simple manipulation. Hydraulic distension of the glenohumeral joint has been reported to be efficacious in reducing pain and improving motion. Local anesthesia is used and postdistension physiotherapy may be, in effect, manipulation under local anesthesia. Studies have suggested that distension itself often ruptures the subcoracoid recess and other areas, rather than the critical axillary fold.

Controversies

Open vs Arthroscopic (Closed) Acromioplasty

Since it was first described in 1972, open anterior acromioplasty has been a reliable procedure for the treatment of subacromial impingement lesions, with a high percentage of success. Recently, arthroscopic (closed) acromioplasty has been introduced as an alternative. The advantages of this approach include avoiding an incision, minimizing deltoid injury, facilitating rehabilitation, shortening postoperative recovery, and performance as an outpatient procedure. Adequate bone removal can be achieved, but it is difficult and depends on adequate hemostasis.

Early results were satisfactory, but not as good as those with open acromioplasty. A few series have reported results approaching those of open acromioplasty. Results were good in patients with partial-thickness cuff tears, but unsatisfactory in patients with full-thickness tears. Complications included inadequate or inappropriate bone removal, excessive bleeding, acromial fracture, and

instrument breakage. In some patients the postoperative recovery was as long as that after an open procedure.

Arthroscopic acromioplasty is a reasonable technique for decompression of partial-thickness tears, and results improve with experience. Open acromioplasty is a proven procedure that should not be abandoned, and is preferred in patients with full-thickness rotator cuff tears.

Glenoid Replacement in the Patient With Rotator Cuff Deficiency

Glenoid component loosening has been associated with superior migration of the humeral head secondary to a deficient rotator cuff. Massive cuff defects are most common in patients with severe rheumatoid arthritis and cuff-tear arthropathy. If sufficient cuff is not available for adequate head coverage and stabilization, a hemiarthroplasty may be a reasonable alternative. Hemiarthroplasty has produced satisfactory pain relief in arthritic patients. Pain relief in itself may produce a limited improvement in function. Avoiding the use of a glenoid component may facilitate cuff repair because lateral displacement of the humerus is less. The primary indication for surgery in these patients is pain relief; functional considerations are secondary.

Rotator Cuff Repair vs Debridement

Rotator cuff debridement has been described as an alternative to cuff repair in a group of patients with massive, scarred, retracted cuff tears. The early results in a small group of patients were encouraging. A similar study reported less satisfactory results with long-term follow-up, including progressive glenohumeral arthritis and superior head subluxation. The rationale for this procedure is that cuff debridement and decompression remove impingement and relieve pain. Functional improvement is secondary to pain relief. The majority of rotator cuff tears can and should be repaired. Mobilization and transposition of existing cuff tissue have been associated with satisfactory results in massive rotator cuff tears.

Annotated Bibliography

Keywords

Acromioclavicular joint; Acromioplasty; Arthrodesis; Arthroplasty; Arthroscopy; Biceps tendon; Calcific tendinitis; Coracohumeral ligament; Frozen shoulder; Glenoid; Humeral head; Nerve injury; Rotator cuff; Suprascapular nerve

Basic Science

Flatow EL, Bigliani LU, April EW: An anatomic study of the musculocutaneous nerve and its relationship to the coracoid process. *Clin Orthop* 1989;244:166–171.

Ninety-three shoulders were dissected. The frequently cited range of 5 to 8 cm below the coracoid for the level of penetration cannot be relied on to describe a safe zone, as 29% of the nerves entered the coracobrachialis proximal to 5 cm below the coracoid. Small nerve twigs to the coracobrachialis entered proximal to the main nerve trunk, tethering the nerve at an additional level.

Gagey O, Bonfait H, Gillot C, et al: Anatomic basis of ligamentous control of elevation of the shoulder (reference position of the shoulder joint). *Surg Radiol Anat* 1987;9:19–26.

A cadaver study investigated the ligamentous restraints on shoulder motion. The coracohumeral ligament and the inferior glenohumeral ligament combined to restrict the humerus to the scapular plane as it approached full elevation.

Howell SM, Imobersteg AM, Seger DH, et al: Clarification of the role of the supraspinatus muscle in shoulder function. *J Bone Joint Surg* 1986;68A:398–404.

Selective suprascapular and axillary nerves blocks were performed in volunteers, and abduction torque was measured with an isokinetic dynamometer. The supraspinatus and deltoid were found to be equally responsible for abduction power at all degrees of abduction.

Kumar VP, Satku K, Balasubramaniam P: The role of the long head of biceps brachii in the stabilization of the head of the humerus. *Clin Orthop* 1989;244:172–175.

In a cadaver study, there was a significant decrease in the acromiohumeral interval on tensing the short head of the biceps, but not on tensing either the long head or both heads of the biceps brachii. Severing the tendon of the long head while both the heads were tensed caused a significant upward migration of the head of the humerus.

Soslowsky LJ, Ateshian G A, Bigliani LU, et al: Sphericity of glenohumeral joint articulating surfaces. *Trans Orthop Res Soc* 1989;14:288.

Analytic stereophotogrammetry and computer graphics were used to determine precisely the surface geometry of cadaveric glenohumeral joints. Normal shoulder articular surfaces can be approximated by a sphere with standard deviations less than 1% of the radius.

Arthroplasty

Barrett WP, Franklin JL, Jackins SE, et al: Total shoulder arthroplasty. *J Bone Joint Surg* 1987;69A:865–872.

Fifty total shoulder replacements in 44 patients were followed up for an average of 3.5 years (range, 2.0 to 7.5 years). Eighty-eight percent had no significant pain at follow-up. The revision rate was 8%. Four patients had loosening of the glenoid component.

Barrett WP, Thornhill TS, Thomas WH, et al: Nonconstrained total shoulder arthroplasty in patients with polyarticular rheumatoid arthritis. *J Arthrop* 1989;4:91–96.

Ninety-three percent of 114 patients with polyarticular rheumatoid arthritis who underwent 140 total shoulder arthroplasties had excellent pain relief. Improvement in function was compromised in advanced disease. Early shoulder replacement to preserve bone stock and rotator cuff tissue is recommended.

Franklin JL, Barrett WP, Jackins SE, et al: Glenoid loosening in total shoulder arthroplasty: Association with rotator cuff deficiency. *J Arthrop* 1988;3:9-46.

Seven cases of total shoulder arthroplasty with deficient rotator cuffs exhibited major glenoid radiolucent lines or actual translation of the glenoid component. The amount of superior migration of the humeral component was closely correlated with the degree of glenoid loosening, and was observed to cause superior tipping of the glenoid component—a "rocking-horse" glenoid.

Fukuda K, Chen CM, Cofield RH, et al: Biomechanical analysis of stability and fixation strength of total shoulder prostheses. *Orthopedics* 1988;11:141–149.

Various total shoulder replacement designs were tested for joint subluxation resistance and glenoid component fixation strength. Joint subluxation resistance increased with axial compressive force applied, and with the amount of curvature of the glenoid articulating surface. Most glenoid components had sufficient fixation strength against normal shoulder joint forces. Loosening and fracture of the plastic glenoid component occurred under high load.

Neer CS II, Morrison DS: Glenoid bone-grafting in total shoulder arthroplasty. *J Bone Joint Surg* 1988;70A:1154–1162.

Nineteen shoulders given a large, internally fixed bone graft for glenoid deficiency were followed up for two years or more (average, 4.4 years). The clinical results were judged to be excellent in 16 and satisfactory in one. None of the glenoid components clinically loosened or migrated, and no patient has needed further surgical treatment.

Orr TE, Carter DR, Schurman DJ: Stress analyses of glenoid component designs. *Clin Orthop* 1988;232:217–224.

Finite-element analyses were performed to determine the stress fields in the natural glenoid and to calculate the change in bone stresses after implantation of glenoid components of various designs. Metal-backing of the glenoid component may produce a slight improvement in stress transfer to cortical bone. Superior restraints on the component, intended to prevent subluxation, increase stresses and may cause earlier loosening than encountered with unconstrained components.

Rotator Cuff Disease

Etiology

Bigliani LU, Morrison DS, April EW: The morphology of the acromion and its relationship to rotator cuff tears. *Orthop Trans* 1986;10:228.

Three types of morphologic characteristics were identified in 140 cadaveric shoulders: type I, flat; type II, curved; and type III, hooked. Only 39% of shoulders had a type III acromion, but these had 70% of the rotator cuff tears.

Ozaki J, Fujimoto S, Nakagawa Y, et al: Tears of the rotator cuff of the shoulder associated with pathological changes in the acromion: A study in cadavera. *J Bone Joint Surg* 1988;70A:1224–1230.

A study of 300 cadaveric shoulders noted pathologic changes on the undersurface of the anterior acromion in all complete tears but not in all partial tears. The uniform finding of attritional changes once a full tear is present suggests that impingement is at least a continuing factor in cuff degeneration, and supports routine acromioplasty at the time of tendon repair.

Imaging

Cotty P, Proust F, Bertrand P, et al: Rotator cuff tear: Roentgen diagnosis. *J Radiol* 1988;69:633–638.

The radiographs of 105 patients undergoing arthrography were reviewed. The presence of radiographic findings was correlated with rotator cuff tears. "Leclerq's maneuver," abducting the arm while holding a weight, elicited a diminished acromio-humeral distance on radiographs in shoulders with a cuff tear with greater sensitivity than did nonstressed views.

Crass JR, Craig EV, Feinberg SB: Sonography of the postoperative rotator cuff. *AJR* 1986;146:561–564.

The finding of a gap or defect in the tendon is the only accurate sign of recurrent cuff tear. Postoperative changes distort the sonographic pattern.

Mack LA, Gannon MK, Kilcoyne RF, et al: Sonographic evaluation of the rotator cuff: Accuracy in patients without prior surgery. *Clin Orthop* 1988;234:21–27.

In 139 consecutive shoulders for which ultrasonographic and surgical findings were correlated, the overall accuracy of ultrasonography was 95%.

Seeger LL, Gold RH, Bassett LW, et al: Shoulder impingement syndrome; MR findings in 53 shoulders. *AJR* 1988;150:343–347.

Magnetic resonance imaging depicted the pathologic changes in impingement. T_2-weighted images allowed differentiation of tendinitis from small tears. Subacromial arch abnormalities were well visualized.

Acromioplasty

Bigliani LU, D'Alessandro DF, Duralde XA, et al: Anterior acromioplasty for subacromial impingement in patients younger than 40 years of age. *Clin Orthop* 1989; 246:111–116.

Only 11 patients had partial-thickness cuff tears and one had a full-thickness tear, in contrast to the patient population over 40 years of age in whom a longer duration of impingement was associated with a higher rate of complete tears. After an average follow-up of 33 months, 81% had good or excellent results.

Chard MD, Sattelle LM, Hazleman BL: The long-term outcome of rotator cuff tendinitis: A review study. *Br J Rheumatol* 1988;27:385–389.

Of 137 patients treated nonsurgically, only 40% had no pain or persistently active tendinitis at follow-up. Rotator cuff tendinitis was found not to be a self-limited condition.

Ellman H: Arthroscopic subacromial decompression: Analysis of one- to three-year results. *Arthroscopy* 1987; 3:173–181.

This study reviewed the one- to three-year results of 50 arthroscopic subacromial decompressions. Eighty-eight percent had good or excellent results. Eight of ten patients with full-thickness tears had good results; excellent results were not obtained in this group.

Gartsman GM, Blair ME Jr, Noble PC, et al: Arthroscopic subacromial decompression: An anatomical study. *Am J Sports Med* 1988;16:48–50.

A cadaver study compared arthroscopic acromioplasty with the open procedure. Critical measurement of bone removal failed to demonstrate any significant differences between the two groups.

Hawkins RJ, Brock RM, Abrams JS, et al: Acromioplasty for impingement with an intact rotator cuff. *J Bone Joint Surg* 1988;70B:795–797.

A total of 108 patients with intact rotator cuffs underwent acromioplasty for chronic impingement syndrome. After an average follow-up of five years, 87% had satisfactory results. Results were less successful in women, in patients with preoperative shoulder stiffness, in worker's compensation cases, and when trauma was involved.

Rotator Cuff Repair

Ellman H, Hanker G, B ayer M: Repair of the rotator cuff: End-result study of factors influencing reconstruction. *J Bone Joint Surg* 1986;68A:1136–1144.

The long-term follow-up of 50 rotator cuff repairs revealed satisfactory results in 84%. Tear size and reconstructive difficulty correlated with length of preoperative pain symptoms. Significant preoperative weakness was associated with poorer results.

Hawkins RJ, Misamore GW, Hobeika PE: Surgery for full-thickness rotator-cuff tears. *J Bone Joint Surg* 1985; 67A:1349–1355.

One hundred patients were evaluated after rotator cuff repair. Significant reduction in pain was achieved in all patients and function was improved in most.

Neer CS II, Flatow EL, Lech O: Tears of the rotator cuff: Long-term results of anterior acromioplasty and repair. *Orthop Trans* 1988;12:673–674.

Of 233 cuff repairs followed up for one to 13 years (average, 4.6 years), 91% had good or excellent results that did not deteriorate with time. Unsatisfactory results were associated with long-standing, massive tears and lack of compliance with rehabilitation.

Neviaser RJ, Neviaser TJ, Neviaser JS: Concurrent rupture of the rotator cuff anterior dislocation of the shoulder in the older patient. *J Bone Joint Surg* 1988;70A: 1308–1311.

Thirty-one patients who were unable to abduct the involved arm after reduction of a primary anterior dislocation of the glenohumeral joint were found to have a ruptured rotator cuff. All of the patients were more than 35 years old. The incidence of injury to the axillary nerve was 7.8%.

Revision Surgery

Hawkins RJ, Chris T, Bokor D, et al: Failed anterior acromioplasty: A review of 51 cases. *Clin Orthop* 1989; 243:106–111.

Thirty-four patients had residual impingement and 23 patients had other diagnoses contributing to failure. Worker's compensation cases had poorer results.

Miscellaneous Considerations

Arthrodesis

Hawkins RJ, Neer CS II: A functional analysis of shoulder fusions. *Clin Orthop* 1987;223:65–76.

No patient could work overhead or with the arms abducted as required for activities such as hammering, house painting, or climbing a ladder. Fifty-three percent had moderate to severe pain. The position of rotation was crucial: 25 to 30 degrees of internal rotation.

Jonsson E, Brattstrom M, Lidgren L: Evaluation of the rheumatoid shoulder function after hemiarthroplasty and arthrodesis. *Scand J Rheumatol* 1988;17:17–26.

Five shoulder arthroplasties were compared with five arthrodeses. All had satisfactory pain relief. Functional results were superior in the arthroplasty group.

Richards RR, Sherman RM, Hudson AR, et al: Shoulder arthrodesis using a pelvic-reconstruction plate: A report of eleven cases. *J Bone Joint Surg* 1988;70A:416–421.

All 11 cases fused without bone graft. Careful plate contouring was important. A spica cast was used for six weeks postoperatively. Plate removal was not required in any case.

Acromioclavicular Joint

Petersson CJ: The acromioclavicular joint in rheumatoid arthritis. *Clin Orthop* 1987;223:86–93.

The acromioclavicular joint was clinically and roentgenographically examined in 49 rheumatic patients with painful shoulders. Roentgenographically, acromioclavicular changes were encountered in 85% of the shoulders, but the joint was tender and painful in only one third. Resection of the distal clavicle gave predictable pain relief.

Stenlund B, Marions O, Engstrom KF, et al: Correlation of macroscopic osteoarthrotic changes and radiographic findings in the acromioclavicular joint. *Acta Radiol* 1988;29:571–576.

In 108 cadaveric acromioclavicular joints examined pathologically and radiographically, only moderate to severe arthrosis was detected on the radiographs. Tomography did not improve the sensitivity.

Biceps

Becker DA, Cofield RH: Tenodesis of the long head of the biceps brachii for chronic bicipital tendinitis: Long-term results. *J Bone Joint Surg* 1989;71A:376–381.

Fifty-four shoulders were followed up for an average of 13 years after tenodesis of the tendon of the long head of the biceps brachii for chronic tendinitis. Early good results deteriorated with follow-up; a satisfactory result was achieved in only one half the patients. Biceps tenodesis is not recommended as an isolated procedure.

Suprascapular Nerve Entrapment

Post M, Mayer J: Suprascapular nerve entrapment: Diagnosis and treatment. *Clin Orthop* 1987;223:126–136.

Ten cases of suprascapular nerve entrapment were identified in 2,520 patients with painful shoulder symptoms. Response to decompression was gratifying. Electromyography is important for diagnosis.

Anesthesia

Conn RA, Cofield RH, Byer DE, et al: Interscalene block anesthesia for shoulder surgery. *Clin Orthop* 1987; 216:94–98.

Interscalene brachial and cervical plexus block was successful in 82 of 100 patients undergoing major shoulder surgery. The block lasted an average of eight hours. Complications were infrequent and included seizure, respiratory depression, and loss of consciousness.

Frozen Shoulder

Fareed DO, Gallivan WR: Office management of frozen shoulder syndrome: Treatment with hydraulic distension under local anesthesia. *Clin Orthop* 1989;242:177–183.

Twenty patients with frozen shoulder were treated with hydraulic distension. Pain and stiffness were reliably relieved within four weeks of distension. There were no complications.

Hill JJ Jr, Bogumill H: Manipulation in the treatment of frozen shoulder. *Orthopedics* 1988;11:1255–1260.

Of 118 frozen shoulders, 17 did not respond to nonsurgical treatment, and underwent manipulation with the patient under anesthesia. Seventy-five percent had no pain and full motion at follow-up, and the rest were only mildly impaired.

27

Elbow and Forearm: Trauma

The elbow and forearm are frequent causes of traumatic disability to the upper extremity. Complicated injuries to the elbow joint frequently result in loss of elbow motion or painful arthritis that reduces the functional strength and positioning of the upper extremity. Forearm fractures when not properly treated lead to loss of forearm rotation and associated nerve and vessel injuries that can have a serious detrimental effect on the hand. There is continuing controversy about how aggressively surgeons should treat intra-articular fractures of the elbow, radial head fractures, and open fractures of the forearm.

Anatomy and Biomechanics

Basic research studies continue to provide important information regarding normal elbow and forearm anatomy and mechanics. Functional evaluations demonstrate that 30 to 130 degrees of flexion-extension of the elbow is needed for daily activities and 50 degrees of pronation and supination is required for most activities (normal elbow flexion-extension, 0 to 150 degrees; normal pronation, 80 degrees; normal supination, 85 degrees).

The anatomy of the elbow, which functions as a classical hinge or pin-type joint, has been clarified by recent studies of the collateral ligaments (Figs. 1 and 2), the joint surface contact area, and contribution of the proximal olecranon to elbow stability. The medial collateral ligament is the prime stabilizer of the elbow (Fig. 2). It consists of anterior and posterior wings that stabilize the elbow to valgus stresses. The humeral origin is posterior to the center of rotation, creating a cam effect and resulting in increased ligament tension with elbow flexion.

The anterior portion of the ligament appears to be more important than the posterior portion. The lateral collateral ligament is the main stabilizer to varus stress (Fig. 1). The proper collateral ligament extends from the base of the lateral epicondyle and inserts through the annular ligament around the radial head onto the proximal ulna. The annular ligament is believed to tighten from pull of the supinator muscle during forearm supination. An accessory "lateral ulnohumeral ligament" forms the inferior border of the collateral ligament with an origin from the inferior lateral epicondyle and an insertion onto the crista supinatoris. Recent studies suggest that this ligament plays an important role in lateral stability, especially after radial head excision. Laxity or insufficiency of the lateral ulnohumeral ligament can be demonstrated by a positive "lateral pivot-shift" of the proximal ulna on the humerus.

The articular anatomy is an important contributor to elbow stability. The elbow is one of the most congruous joints in the body. The semicylindrical trochlea and olecranon are firmly seated together under compressive loads from contraction of the biceps and brachialis muscles and

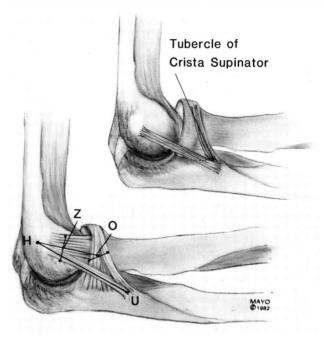

Figure 1

Lateral collateral ligament complex. The radial collateral ligament is line H to O. O is the midportion of the annular ligament. H-U is the lateral ulnar collateral ligament. Fibers from the lateral ulnar collateral ligament and annular ligament insert on the ulna at the crest of the supinator. (Reproduced with permission from Morrey BF, An KN: Functional anatomy of the ligaments of the elbow. *Clin Orthop* 1985; 201:84–90.)

provide important anteroposterior stability, especially during lifting. Recent studies of force transmission across the elbow have shown that the force across the radial head is greatest in the first 0 to 30 degrees of flexion and decreases with further flexion. Force across the radiocapitellar joint is greater during forearm pronation (30% to 40% of the total) than during forearm supination (15% to 20%). During valgus stress, the radial head carries 30% of the initial load and the medial collateral ligament and anterior capsule share the remaining stress equally. In flexion, however, the medial collateral ligament carries more than 60% of valgus force and the radiocapitellar contact becomes less important. With varus stress (in extension), the anterior capsule carries 30%, the joint surface 50%, and the radial collateral ligament 15% of the applied load. In flexion, the joint surface supports 75% of the load and the radial collateral ligament only 10%.

When excision is considered after radial head fractures or when stability is being tested after elbow dislocations, it is important to keep in mind the importance of both ligamentous and bone supports for elbow stability. Injury

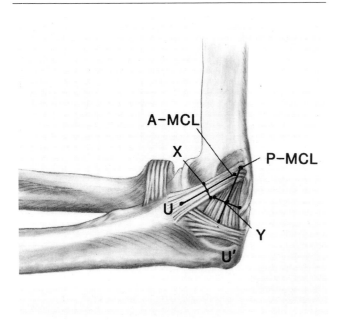

Figure 2

Medial collateral ligament complex. Anterior portion, A-MCL; anterior width, line X; posterior portion, P-MCL; posterior width, line Y; accessory portion, U-U'. (Reproduced with permission from Morrey BF, An KN: Functional anatomy of the ligaments of the elbow. *Clin Orthop* 1985;201:84–90.)

to the elbow with the forearm in pronation increases radial head-capitellar contact forces and explains the mechanism of radial head fractures and dislocations. With the elbow in extension, the force across the proximal radius is greatest with valgus stress. With the elbow in flexion, the force across the ulnohumeral joint is greatest with varus stress. These factors help to explain the probable mechanism of elbow joint fractures in flexion and elbow dislocation in extension.

Elbow Dislocations

Elbow dislocations result from a fall with the elbow extended, the arm abducted, and the forearm in supination. Less commonly, elbow dislocation results from a direct blow. Biomechanical studies indicate that it is difficult to dislocate a flexed elbow. Ligament load studies explain why posterior or posterolateral dislocations are the most common. These injuries produce extensive soft-tissue injury, including soft-tissue avulsion of collateral ligaments. Both nerve and vessel damage can result from the initial injury or when these structures are trapped within the elbow joint. Loss of elbow extension, which is the result of damage to the anterior capsule and brachialis muscles, is a common sequela of this injury.

Closed reduction of elbow dislocations with an early return to protected motion is the recommended treatment. Reduction should be performed only after radiographs are obtained to rule out associated fractures and interposition of the medial epicondyle within the joint. Longitudinal traction with gradual flexion and downward pressure on the forearm reduces posterior or posterolateral dislocations. To prevent further damage to the anterior capsule and brachialis muscles, hyperextension should be avoided.

A full range of motion should be confirmed after the reduction, mediolateral stability tested, and radiographs reviewed to rule out any mechanical block. Although some recent European studies suggest that an open reduction with primary ligament repair should be considered for elbow dislocations, Swedish investigators demonstrated that closed reduction produced superior results. Recurrent dislocations were not present in either group of patients and both groups lost an average of 15 to 20 degrees of extension. The patients with open reductions, however, lost more elbow flexion. Simple elbow dislocations, therefore, should be treated by simple techniques—closed reduction and an early stable range of motion.

Fracture-Dislocations Fracture-dislocations of the elbow are the exception to treatment by closed reduction. In most cases these require surgical treatment. A fracture of the medial epicondyle, in particular, is a warning sign that bone or soft tissue may be trapped within the elbow joint. After fracture-dislocation of the elbow, any evidence of median nerve deficit associated with limited passive elbow motion should alert the surgeon to the possibility of nerve entrapment. Delayed union and lack of anatomic reduction of the medial epicondyle are associated with nerve entrapment. If nerve entrapment in the elbow is suspected but the diagnosis remains in question, early surgical exploration is indicated to settle the issue.

Fractures of the Elbow

Radial Head Fractures

Radial head fractures are common in adults. They can occur alone or in association with elbow dislocations. Radial head and neck fractures are associated with nerve injuries, tearing of the interosseous membrane, and injuries to the distal radioulnar joint. There is disagreement regarding the treatment of radial head fractures.

The radial head is entirely intra-articular and makes contact with both the capitellum and the proximal ulna. The radial head supports as much as 40% of the joint's contact force. Mason's classification of radial head fractures provides treatment guidelines (Table 1). Mason type I fractures with less than 25% of the radial head involved should be treated conservatively, that is, by nonsurgical methods including early range of motion with splint support. Mason type II fractures can be treated by conservative methods (protection and early motion), open reduction and internal fixation, or excision of the radial head. Results of treatment are about the same for each of these methods. If conservative methods fail, moreover, the results of late excision of the radial head are just as good as those for early excision

Table 1. Mason classification of radial head fractures*

Fracture	Description
Type I	Undisplaced
Type II	Marginal, with displacement (including angulation, impaction, and depression)
Type III	Comminuted, involving the entire radial head
Type IV	Associated with dislocation of the elbow

*Data taken from DeLee JC, Green DP, Wilkins KE: Fractures and dislocations of the elbow, in Rockwood CA Jr, Green DP (eds): *Fractures in Adults*, ed 2. Philadelphia, JB Lippincott, 1984, vol 1, pp 559–652.

(until recently the preferred method of treatment). Late excision should be delayed for at least three weeks after the injury to avoid complications related to myositis ossificans. Conservative treatment initially does not affect the end results.

Open treatment of Mason type II fractures is recommended when at least one half of the radial head remains to provide stable fixation. Kirschner wires or small Herbert screws provide adequate internal fixation, although both must be buried beneath the articular cartilage to avoid soft-tissue impingement (Figs. 3 and 4).

For Mason type III injuries, excision of the radial head is recommended. The level of excision should be just distal to the annular ligament. Dangers include division of the posterior interosseous nerve and injury to the ulnohumeral ligament. A direct lateral approach is preferred to an anconeous approach to spare the lateral ulnohumeral ligament, and the radial head should be excised with the forearm in pronation so that the supinator muscle is not stretched.

For Mason type IV injuries (posterior dislocation with radial head fracture), the radial head should be excised (if comminuted) or retained (if internal fixation is possible) (Fig. 5). If the radial head is resected, some investigators believe that prosthetic replacement is indicated. Despite these recommendations, long-term studies of complicated fracture-dislocations of the elbow and Essex-Lopresti lesions demonstrated poor function associated with Silastic radial head replacement. In one series of patients monitored for an average of 3.4 years after silicone radial head replacement, the results were unsuccessful in 56% and there were degenerative changes in the elbow and prosthesis fractures.

The question of elbow function after radial head excision has been studied, and it is clear that this is a relatively safe procedure. Follow-up studies done eight to 46 years after radial head excision demonstrated that the patients had few complaints and only occasional mild pain. Range of motion was nearly normal. The distal radioulnar joint was rarely symptomatic and proximal migration averaged only 2 mm.

Late excision of the radial head for Mason type II and type III injuries produced good to excellent results in 80% of cases. Because the results of late excision are favorable, preservation of the radial head has been recommended for all Mason types I and II fractures and for most Mason types III and IV fractures whenever feasible.

Olecranon Fractures

Fractures of the olecranon can have little influence on normal elbow function or can contribute to late instability and arthritis. Most olecranon fractures are caused by a direct blow to the elbow. A few result from a fall onto the outstretched hand that produces incomplete elbow dislocation or an avulsion fracture from sudden contraction of the triceps.

The diagnosis of olecranon fracture is based on the inability to extend the elbow and radiologic evidence of a fracture with or without displacement. True lateral and oblique radiographs are recommended. The classification of olecranon fractures has been updated to distinguish the different levels of intra-articular involvement and degrees of fracture displacement. The olecranon process (distal

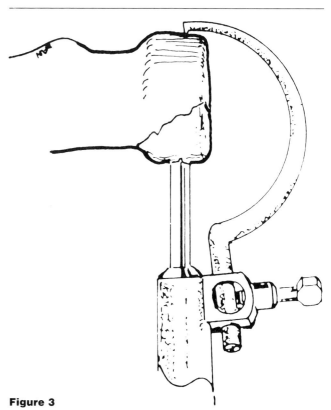

Figure 3

Technique of Huene alignment guide placement for Herbert screw fixation of marginal radial head fractures.

and proximal thirds) has been studied, and its mechanical importance emphasized.

For treatment of displaced olecranon fractures, it appears that the best results occur with a combination of intramedullary screws combined with a figure-of-eight wire. The final results were mixed when an intramedullary screw or Rush rod alone was used. Some authors favored a tension-band wire (AO technique), whereas others found that the tension-band wire alone produced unacceptable results. Skin problems and displacement of the wire through osteoporotic bone were complications. If tension-band wires are selected for olecranon fractures, a 20-gauge wire in a figure-of-eight configuration plus two longitudinal K-wires is recommended. Open reduction with neutralization plate and screw fixation has strong advocates and can be used in most displaced fractures with good results. Regardless of the fixation technique, fractures with more than 60% articular surface involvement or a residual displacement of more than 2 mm had poor results.

In elderly patients with excessive comminution, excision of as much as 50% of the olecranon, along with repair of the triceps aponeurosis, has been recommended. Elbow motion is frequently not limited but ulnohumeral joint resistance to anteroposterior displacement may be compromised (at least according to recent biomechanical studies); therefore, caution must be used when deciding on the extent of olecranon excision. Patient selection is important.

Supracondylar and Intra-articular Fractures

Fractures of the distal humerus can be supracondylar, transcondylar, or intercondylar (T-shaped or Y-shaped) in-

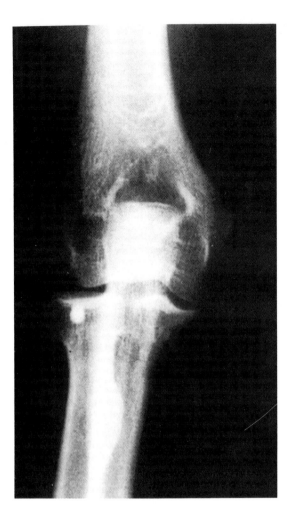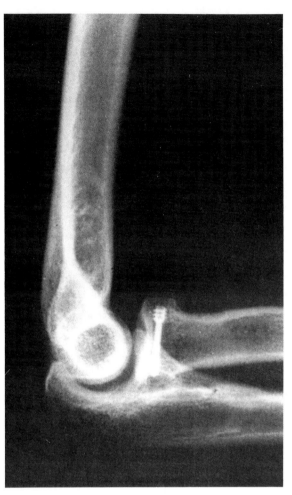

Figure 4

Postoperative results of Herbert screw fixation of radial head fracture (marginal fracture, mild displacement). (Reproduced with permission from McArthur RA: Herbert screw fixation of fractures of the head of the radius. *Clin Orthop* 1987;224:79–87.)

juries. Isolated articular surface fractures of the medial or lateral condyle are less common.

Supracondylar Fractures Supracondylar fractures are usually extension injuries in which the distal component is pulled proximally and posteriorly by the pull of the triceps muscle. Flexion injuries are less common and usually result from a direct blow to the back of the elbow. A supracondylar fracture can be clinically distinguished from elbow dislocation by palpation of the medial and lateral epicondyle and the olecranon process, which maintain their normal triangular relationship in supracondylar fractures.

Treatment of supracondylar fractures requires a careful reduction by traction with the forearm in extension. The patient should be given general anesthesia. Once full length is obtained, gradual flexion helps lock the fragments in place. Flexion, which should not be excessive, is limited by palpation of the radial pulse. With medial displacement, pronation is recommended to tighten the lateral periosteal attachments; with lateral displacement, supination is rec-ommended to tighten the medial periosteum. When it is difficult to maintain the reduction, percutaneous pins or open reduction and a lateral compression plate should be used.

Intra-articular Fractures Intra-articular fractures of the elbow have been divided into types I to IV depending on the degree of displacement, rotation, and comminution. Type I, undisplaced fracture, can be treated conservatively with a cast or splint. Types II and III fractures, which are classified by displacement alone or with rotation, require open reduction and internal fixation. The surgical procedure consists of initial reduction of the intra-articular fractures, followed by stabilization of the distal humerus to the proximal humeral shaft (Fig. 6). Type IV fractures, fractures with comminution, are difficult treatment problems. Both closed and open treatment programs have been advocated. A comparative study of 42 patients, however, demonstrated improved results with open treatment; 22 of the 29 fractures treated with open reduction and internal fixation had good to excellent results (76%) whereas only

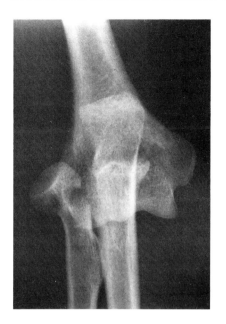
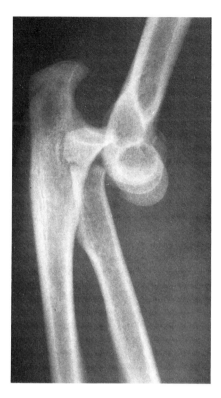
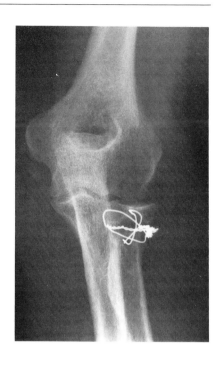

Figure 5

Fracture dislocation of the elbow-radial neck fracture. **Left,** Anteroposterior view. Angulated radial neck fracture with posterior lateral elbow dislocation. **Center,** Lateral view. Unreduced posterior lateral elbow dislocation. **Right,** Tension-band wire (90-90 double loop) fixation of radial neck fracture with reduction of elbow dislocation.

one of 13 fractures given closed treatment in traction had satisfactory results (8%). Rigid internal fixation and bone grafting is used to maintain the anatomic reduction of the distal humerus. Most surgeons prefer a posterior approach that reflects the triceps medially (Bryan approach) or a transolecranon osteotomy. Both approaches provide excellent exposure of the distal humerus. Olecranon osteotomy reportedly has a higher complication rate (nonunion). Early joint motion is advised.

Fractures of the Radius and Ulna

In the adult, fractures of the radius and ulna should be treated by open reduction and internal fixation. The only exceptions are isolated fractures of the shaft of the ulna that are undisplaced or minimally displaced. The surgical approach to the radius depends on the location of the fracture. A fracture of the proximal radius can be exposed through either the posterior midforearm (Thompson approach) or by medial dissection between the flexor carpi ulnaris and the extensor carpi ulnaris (Boyd approach). A fracture of the midshaft or distal radius is best exposed through an anterolateral (Henry) approach centered over the flexor carpi radialis with plate fixation on the anterior surface. The ulna is exposed medially, and the compression plate should be placed on the dorsal surface of the ulna.

In Galeazzi fractures or Monteggia fractures, open reduction and internal fixation of both the fracture and the joint dislocation should be considered. If joint instability is still present after plate fixation, closed reduction and K-wire fixation or open ligament repair of the distal and proximal radioulnar joint should be performed.

Forearm fractures require anatomic alignment to maximize the postoperative results. Fracture union and restoration of full forearm rotation are the treatment goals. Angulation of as much as 20 degrees can be accepted, but rotational malalignment is not acceptable. Internal fixation plates should have screws across a minimum of six cortices. Intramedullary rods are less satisfactory than internal fixation plates for forearm fractures. An exception is the unusual circumstance of a pathologic fracture of the radius or ulna.

The role of internal fixation of open wounds remains a controversial subject. In general, internal fixation hardware is not recommended for open wounds. In forearm fractures, however, where the tolerance for error in forearm alignment is small, plate fixation for Gustilo type I wounds (clean wound, open less than 1 cm) or type II wounds (clean wound, open more than 1 cm but with little soft-tissue damage) is acceptable provided that the wound edges are not closed primarily. For type III wounds (dirty wound with neurovascular and extensive soft-tissue injury) most surgeons favor external fracture fixation. One study suggested that immediate plate fixation, leaving the wound open for delayed closure, can be considered for type III wounds that can be debrided clean and in which wound cultures grow less than 10^3 colonies. In a series of 57 fractures given open plate treatment, however, there were six

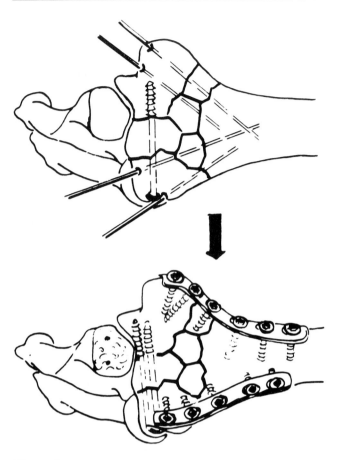

Figure 6

Techniques to achieve stable internal fixation of intercondylar fracture of the humerus. Internal fixation of articular components by Kirschner wires and interfragmentary screws followed by plate fixation of articular construct to the medial and lateral columns of the distal humerus. (Reproduced with permission from Jupiter JB, Neff U, Holzach P, et al: Intercondylar fractures of the humerus. *J Bone Joint Surg* 1985;67A:226–239.)

nonunions and two infections in the 11 type III wounds (Fig. 7).

Pediatric Fractures and Dislocations

Elbow Dislocations

Elbow dislocations in children most commonly occur in a posterior or posterolateral direction. Medial and lateral collateral ligament injuries are less frequent in children; as a result, many elbow dislocations involve an avulsion fracture of the medial epicondyle. Because ossification of the medial epicondyle can be delayed until the age of 5 or 6 years, elbow dislocations must be carefully assessed to ensure that there are no associated injuries and that the joint is congruent after reduction.

Elbow dislocations in children can be confused with physeal injuries that involve the distal humerus. Recent studies using single- or double-contrast arthrography of the elbow demonstrated that these techniques can be helpful in distinguishing physeal injuries from elbow dislocations, particularly before ossification of the growth centers of the elbow. Clinical examination can also provide information

because the triangular relationship of the two epicondyles and the olecranon process is distorted in elbow dislocations and the medial and lateral epiphysis do not remain aligned with the olecranon in physeal fractures.

Once elbow dislocation has been diagnosed, reduction is done with the patient under general anesthesia. Longitudinal traction with the elbow in extension unlocks the distal and proximal components and the reduction can be achieved with flexion. A smooth range of motion with a stable and congruent joint is confirmed by postoperative radiographs taken to evaluate the joint alignment and exclude associated fractures. Immobilization for three weeks in a long arm cast is recommended; this is followed by active assisted range-of-motion exercises. Vigorous physical therapy is not needed to restore normal elbow motion in a child.

If a congruent elbow reduction is not achieved, the interposition of soft tissue or bone must be suspected. Several cases of overlooked median nerve incarceration have been reported. The usual radiographic appearance of bone interposition, in fact, may not be present in children in whom ossification of the medial epicondyle has not occurred. Therefore, joint alignment and the ulnohumeral articular space, in particular, must be reviewed for possible soft-tissue or bone entrapment. The absence of mediolateral stability of the elbow is a clue that the medial epicondyle may be avulsed as a consequence of the dislocation.

Supracondylar Fractures

Displaced supracondylar fractures in children present some of the most difficult evaluation and treatment decisions. Obtaining an anatomic reduction and preventing late deformity are important considerations. Previous studies have demonstrated the need for an algorithm or programmed approach to treatment based on the presence of normal circulation to the distal extremity, intact neurologic status, and maintaining the supracondylar fracture reduction by closed reduction vs percutaneous or open treatment techniques. In general, closed reduction is sufficient for nearly all supracondylar fractures. The reduction, however, must be performed in a safe, efficient manner. Options include manual reduction with an assistant providing countertraction; straight lateral or Dunlop traction (skin traction); or skeletal traction through the olecranon.

Extension supracondylar fractures result from a fall onto the outstretched hand. Neurovascular entrapment is not uncommon as a consequence of the injury or as a result of the reduction. For this reason, lateral traction is preferred to other forms of fracture reduction. With manual reduction using countertraction, the goal is to restore length first and then to flex the elbow gradually while maintaining proximal countertraction. Medial or lateral displacement is corrected after the posterior position of the distal segment is realigned with the humeral shaft. For very unstable fractures that cannot be maintained except by full elbow flexion, the traction is best maintained with the elbow in extension and the forearm in pronation. Gradual flexion, while traction is maintained, is begun once the fracture appears more stable. If there is initial medial displacement, the forearm should be immobilized in pronation to tighten the medial hinge. If the initial displacement is lateral, supination of the forearm is recommended. Radiographic correlation is essential in two planes (anter-

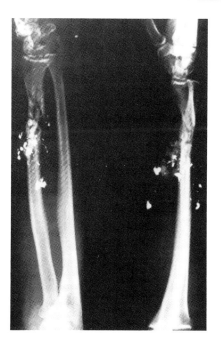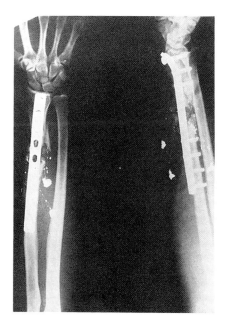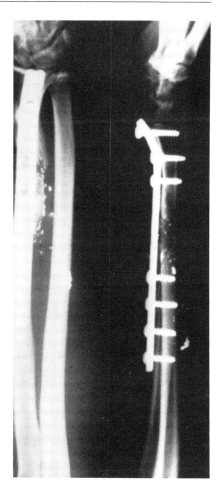

Figure 7

Immediate plate fixation of open fracture of the radius. Delayed wound closure. **Left**, Initial radiographs demonstrating a grade IIIB gunshot wound of the forearm. **Center**, Postoperative radiographs. **Right**, Nonunion of the radius with loss of initial bone graft. Delayed autogenous cancellous bone grafting of open fractures of Gustilo wound type III is recommended to augment fracture healing. (Reproduced with permission from Moed BR, Kellam JF, Foster RJ, et al: Immediate internal fixation of open fractures of the diaphysis of the forearm. *J Bone Joint Surg* 1986; 68A:1008–1017.)

oposterior and lateral), and any malalignment must be corrected. Rotational malposition, in particular, does not improve with time and will result in secondary varus or valgus deformity.

Cubitus varus is the most common complication of supracondylar fractures in children. For this reason, lateral traction is recommended for severely displaced or delayed treatment cases. Lateral traction (and not overhead traction with the elbow in flexion) allows careful radiographic assessment because the carrying angle is visible throughout the treatment period. For more resistant cases, pin fixation of the supracondylar fracture should be considered.

Closed reduction and percutaneous pinning of supracondylar fractures of the humerus in children was first reported in 1948. In the 1970s several articles were written concerning these cases. In the 1980s this has become a popular method of treatment.

The procedure consists of closed reduction with the patient under anesthesia. Two K-wires are inserted, usually either two parallel wires beginning at the lateral epicondyle and extending proximally and medially, or two crossed wires, one from the lateral epicondyle extending proxi-

mally and one from the medial epicondyle extending proximally and laterally. General anesthesia and sterile surgical techniques are usually employed. The procedure is best accomplished with the help of image intensification, and it must be remembered that percutaneous pinning is not a method of reduction but solely a method of maintaining reduction. Thus, if satisfactory reduction is not obtained, percutaneous pinning should not be performed. In this instance, traction or other reduction is more appropriate. The procedure is much easier to perform if it is done shortly after the fracture, before swelling has developed. Swelling obscures bony landmarks and greatly increases the likelihood of improper pin placement. It is not an easy technique to learn or to teach. The ability to conceptualize three-dimensional relationships is beneficial.

The primary indication for the procedure is an unstable supracondylar fracture that can be reduced but in which the reduction cannot be maintained. Reduction and percutaneous pinning enhance stability and make postoperative management easier and safer. This technique is also indicated when reduction can be obtained but maintained only with the arm in marked flexion, which in turn occludes vascularity of the forearm and hand. In this instance, the fracture can be percutaneously pinned and the elbow extended to a safe zone to allow reestablishment of arterial flow and venous return. It is useful in cases with concomitant fractures of the ipsilateral forearm because it stabilizes the elbow. Another advantage of the stabilization is that it allows flexion and extension of the elbow so that the carrying angle can be evaluated at the time of reduction. A splint or cast can be safely applied with the elbow in 90 degrees of flexion, and hospitalization time is significantly reduced in comparison with closed reduction and observation, traction, and open reduction.

Two types of postoperative management can be used. If the pins are well seated and have no drainage about them, the cast can be removed at three weeks and motion begun, with the pins left in place for another three weeks. The other method is to remove the pins at three weeks and apply a second cast for another two to three weeks.

The disadvantages of the procedure include the need for excellent radiographic control during the pinning, which may be prolonged, and pin problems including migration of pins, pin-tract infections, and nerve impingement. A pin placed from the medial side entering the medial epicondyle must be far enough anterior to avoid the ulnar nerve. Another disadvantage is that it is easier to pin the distal fragment erroneously in complete extension rather than with its normal 35 to 45 degrees of forward angulation. When the fracture heals in this position, elbow flexion is incomplete. This is usually temporary, and elbow extension gradually returns with remodeling.

Undisplaced fractures or fractures with mild extension malalignment can usually be safely treated by elbow flexion and immobilization in a splint or cast. Displaced fractures can often be reduced and held by closed methods, particularly if they can be treated soon after the fracture, before the appearance of swelling. Displaced fractures that can be reduced but not held and those that can be reduced and held only in marked flexion are best treated by closed reduction and percutaneous pinning. The technique of open reduction and internal fixation is best used when the fracture cannot be reduced, when there is neurovascular compromise uncorrected by the reduction, and in open fracture.

Radial Head Fractures

Fractures through the articular surface of the proximal radius are rare. Fractures of the proximal radius in children involving the neck of the radius or the proximal radial physis, that is, separation through the physis, are common. The average age of the patient at the time of injury is 10 to 11 years. Of the physeal separations, the majority are Salter-Harris type II. Displacement of the radius can be mild to severe. The mechanism is a fall onto the outstretched hand that transmits the force through the radial shaft, driving the proximal radius against the capitellum. Lateral displacement is usual. Posterior displacement also occurs and is believed to be secondary to posterior elbow dislocation in which there is spontaneous reduction of the elbow at the expense of separation of the radial head beneath the capitellum. A forceful elbow reduction has been implicated in these types of radial head separations.

Treatment of fractures of the proximal radius is determined by the extent of the initial angulation. Most fractures of the proximal radius or physeal separations can be

treated by closed reduction and cast or splint immobilization. When angulation is greater than 15 degrees, closed reduction is necessary. Displacement of more than 45 degrees or the inability to reduce the angulation to less than 15 degrees in a closed fashion requires open reduction. Poor results are associated with angulation of 30 degrees or more.

To hold displaced fractures or separations of the radial head, crossed K-wires are recommended. Recent reports have noted problems when the pins cross the humerus into the radial head, and obliquely directed K-wires into the proximal radius only are now preferred.

Internal fixation of the proximal radius has not been associated with significant complications. Deformity of the radial head, capsulitis, and periarticular ossification are potential sequelae leading to poor results. Surgical intervention has not been shown, however, to increase the potential for these complications and may, in fact, help to minimize them by avoiding repeated closed reductions. Premature physeal closure is also a potential risk. This can be avoided by gentle fracture or physeal reduction.

Fractures of the Lateral Condyle and Epicondyle

Fractures of the lateral condyle and epicondyle are fairly common fractures about the elbow in children. A fracture of the lateral condyle usually constitutes a Salter-Harris type IV injury and is a potentially serious intra-articular fracture. The fracture line begins within the distal humerus, splitting obliquely from lateral to medial and entering the elbow joint between the trochlea and the capitellum. Displacement results from the initial injury and can be difficult to reduce because of the continued pull of the wrist extensor tendons originating from the epicondyle. Rotation of as much as 90 degrees can occur.

For undisplaced fractures, immobilization in a long arm cast (elbow in flexion, wrist in extension, and forearm in supination) is recommended. Radiographs are needed after ten to 14 days to ensure that late displacement of initially undisplaced fractures has not occurred.

Displaced fractures of the lateral condyle require open reduction and internal fixation. Through a lateral extended Kocher approach to the elbow, the fracture fragment is derotated and internally fixed with K-wires. Intraoperative concerns include incomplete reduction of the articular joint surface and premature physeal closure or arrest. A technique of atraumatic reduction and limited internal fixation with smooth K-wires apparently limits these potentially serious complications.

Fractures of the Medial Condyle and Epicondyle

Medial Condyle Fractures of the medial condyle are uncommon (less than 1.5% of elbow injuries in children). They result from a fall on the flexed elbow that can cause the edge of the semilunar notch of the olecranon to split the trochlea. Avulsion fractures are even less common and usually involve the medial epicondyle (physeal separation). Because the trochlea's ossification center is delayed until after the age of 9 years, fractures of the medial condyle can be difficult to diagnose. Careful clinical examination and radiographs of the opposite elbow provide the most assistance in arriving at the correct diagnosis.

Kilfoyle's classification divides condylar fractures into three types: type I is undisplaced with the fracture line extending from the medial metaphysis to the medial condylar physis; type II is displaced with the fracture line extending from the medial metaphysis through the medial physis; and type III is displaced with rotation and displacement producing elbow instability. Treatment is nonsurgical for type I (undisplaced), consisting of four weeks in a cast. Treatment for type II (displaced) and type III (displaced and rotated) is surgical, with open reduction and K-wire fixation plus cast immobilization for four weeks. (A Campbell posteromedial approach is preferred.)

The results in a small series of fractures were excellent for types I and II. Type III fractures were associated with decreased range of motion and growth disturbance. Fracture nonunion and osteonecrosis have not been reported.

Medial Epicondyle Fractures of the medial epicondyle are either isolated injuries or are associated with dislocations of the elbow. The medial collateral ligament originates from the interior surface of the medial epicondyle, lateral to the attachment of the epiphysis. In elbow dislocations, the medial epicondyle and median nerve can be incarcerated within the elbow joint.

When a fracture of the medial epicondyle is suspected from clinical examination, careful review of the radiographs is necessary to determine whether displacement of the epicondyle has occurred and, if so, the extent of displacement. Before the ossification of the medial epicondyle occurs (usually at 5 years of age), comparison views of the opposite elbow are helpful in assessing the alignment of the elbow and ensuring that entrapment within the elbow joint has not occurred. When there is a question regarding displacement, arthrography of the elbow joint is useful.

Treatment of injuries to the medial epicondyle is conservative unless the displacement is greater than 5 mm, the medial joint line is unstable, or the epicondyle itself becomes intra-articular. For undisplaced or minimally displaced fractures, conservative treatment in a long arm cast is sufficient and fibrous union is usually asymptomatic. For displaced fractures of the epicondyle, open reduction and K-wire fixation to the opposite cortex is necessary. This is followed by cast immobilization (elbow in flexion and forearm in pronation). Good function and normal range of motion can be expected.

Forearm Fractures

Most forearm fractures in children are managed by closed reduction and cast immobilization. The main complications resulting from forearm fracture are related to rotational malalignment and crossunion. Treatment is designed to maintain forearm length and restore full forearm rotation. When these prerequisites are not met, the results are unsatisfactory. In children less than 12 years old, no more than 15 degrees of angular deformity and no more than 5 degrees of rotation are acceptable if loss of forearm rotation is to be prevented. From the age of 12 years to maturity, angular deformity and rotational deformity are not acceptable. When either of these factors cannot be corrected, open reduction and internal fixation should be done.

With respect to overall forearm length, there is controversy about whether bayonet apposition is acceptable or whether end-to-end bone contact is essential. In young children (less than 10 years old), side-to-side apposition is acceptable because of future longitudinal growth. In older children, the ability to correct for malalignment and shortening is not available and anatomic reduction is strongly encouraged.

Crossunion of the forearm is a second major complication associated with both-bone forearm fractures. It is more frequent when the fractures occur at the same level. The risk is increased by excessive surgical trauma to the soft tissues between the radius and ulna. Separate surgical approaches are, therefore, recommended when internal fixation with plates is chosen. The loss of forearm rotation that follows crossunion is not easily treated despite interpositional use of fat, fascia, and silicone spacers. Using an atraumatic technique and avoiding multiple attempts at closed reduction helps to prevent crossunion. Fortunately, crossunion is uncommon in children and the results after treatment are better than in adults.

A satisfactory outcome is a forearm with less than 20 degrees of rotational loss, a normal clinical appearance, and freedom from pain. In one review, results were satisfactory in 85% of patients more than 12 years old who were treated with open reduction and plate fixation and those less than 12 years old who were treated with closed reduction and cast or percutaneous pins. Problems included unacceptable shortening, abnormal bowing, and malrotation. Younger patients had a higher percentage of satisfactory results than older children when a less-than-anatomic reduction was obtained, whereas the older children had unsatisfactory results when more than 20 degrees of angulation was accepted, rotational alignment was not perfect, or when there was a proximal shaft fracture that responded less to remodeling.

Malunion of forearm fractures can be corrected by open osteotomy or by a semiopen technique. When the patient is 5 to 12 years old, drill osteoclasis is recommended. In this procedure, percutaneous drilling through a 5-mm incision of the malunion site is performed with a 3.2-mm drill bit. Closed manipulation of the fracture to improve the reduction can be done with the periosteal hinge remaining intact. Rotational and angulation corrections can be made. For children older than 12 years, in whom the potential for remodeling is less, open reduction and internal fixation after the corrective osteotomy is preferred so that the alignment is anatomic, forearm bowing is corrected, and the interosseous membrane is preserved.

In children, ipsilateral forearm fractures and either elbow injuries or humeral fractures are an indication for open reduction and internal fixation. Management of the proximal injury can be improved when the forearm fracture is stable.

Associated Problems

Soft-Tissue Coverage

When significant trauma to the elbow and forearm causes injury to bone and soft tissue, soft-tissue coverage can be difficult. In the last several years, a number of new cutaneous and myocutaneous flaps have been used to provide soft-tissue coverage. Pedicle flaps that can be transferred include the latissimus dorsi as a muscle flap alone or in combination with skin as a myocutaneous flap; the brachioradialis as a muscle rotation flap; and, from the lateral chest wall, the external oblique fasciocutaneous pedicle flap. For smaller defects, fasciocutaneous forearm flaps (the

Chinese radial forearm flap or ulnar forearm flap) can be rotated on the radial or ulnar arteries. Free tissue transfer can be performed if the local tissues are damaged. Successful transfers to the elbow and forearm include cutaneous groin flaps, the scapular flap, and the lateral arm flap. Free muscle flaps include the rectus abdominis, gracilis, latissimus dorsi, tensor fascia femoris, and serratus anterior muscles based on the principal arteriovenous pedicles.

In severe fractures around the elbow or forearm, external fixation of the fractures combined with free tissue transfers or pedicle flap transfers can make a difference in limb salvage. In addition, when there has been a complete amputation of the extremity, free tissue transfer (including tissue from the amputated part) can be used to maintain limb length and, in some cases, to convert a potential above-elbow amputation into a below-elbow amputation, thus preserving the elbow joint, which greatly enhances function and the ability to wear a below-elbow prosthesis.

Nerve Injury

Injury to the peripheral nerves in association with elbow and forearm trauma usually involves the median or ulnar nerves. Recently, the anterior interosseous nerve has been implicated in both closed reduction and open reduction of forearm fractures. Repeated attempts at closed reduction of proximal forearm fractures and elbow fracture-dislocations can increase neurologic damage and should be avoided if there is evidence of neurologic damage. With open reduction of fractures, the deep nerves (anterior and posterior interosseous) that are closely related anatomically to the area of fracture can be damaged by bone-holding forceps. Identification and protection of these structures before applying plates or bone clamps is advised.

Radiologic Imaging

Advances in radiologic imaging have improved the identification of specific kinds of elbow and forearm trauma. Computed tomographic scans comparing both extremities provide the optimum method of assessing malrotation of the radius or ulna. It is also extremely helpful in assessing associated proximal and distal radioulnar joint subluxation or dislocations (for example, Galeazzi and Monteggia fractures or Essex-Lopresti fracture-dislocations of the forearm).

For elbow dislocations and fracture-dislocations, the radial head-capitellum view is accurate in demonstrating a displaced radial head, capitellum, and coronoid fractures and displaying the articular surface of the distal humerus. This view is now preferred over the external oblique view. The anteroposterior, lateral, medial oblique, and radial head-capitellum views are now recommended as part of the elbow trauma series.

For dislocations or physeal fractures about the elbow in a young child with incomplete ossification centers, arthrography of the elbow (single- or double-contrast) can provide information about the injured tissues. Arthrography is recommended, along with comparative radiographs of the opposite elbow, for fractures of the lateral condyle, supracondylar fractures, Salter-Harris type II and type III intra-articular fractures, physeal separations, and elbow dislocations. Clear visualization of the cartilaginous portions of the elbow joint permits the specific injury to the elbow to be identified.

Controversies

Elbow Dislocations

Dislocation of the elbow involves a significant injury to the collateral ligaments and may include fractures of the medial epicondyle, radial head, or coronoid process. Soft-tissue interposition and entrapment of the medial epicondyle have been reported. As a result of these fractures, there has been a controversy regarding recommendations to treat elbow dislocations by open reduction and repair of the collateral ligament injuries in contrast to closed reduction and splinting. The treatment plan of open reduction and ligament repair comes primarily from European countries. The emphasis on anatomic repair of the ligament injuries and attention to any associated fractures has been a natural extension of the concept of open repair of knee and ankle ligament injuries. Precise repair of the torn or avulsed collateral ligament, when performed early, should provide the proper tension and alignment of the ligaments and prevent late instability.

In North America and Great Britain, a more conservative approach to elbow dislocations has been recommended and followed. Closed reduction and early motion appears to avoid the problems of elbow flexion contractures and heterotopic bone formation and late elbow instability is uncommon. A report in which 34 elbow dislocations treated in a closed fashion were compared with 28 dislocations treated in an open fashion should end whatever controversy remains with respect to open treatment of elbow dislocations. Simply stated, the results were identical with the exception that open reduction was associated with more complications and a relative loss of elbow flexion. The results failed to support any contention that open reduction of elbow dislocation should be performed except in the case of intra-articular entrapment of bone or soft-tissue structures.

Radial Head Fractures

A second controversial subject is treatment of radial head fractures. There are differences of opinion regarding open vs closed reduction, excision vs retention of the radial head, early vs late resection (if radial removal is chosen), and Silastic prosthetic replacement vs no replacement. Choosing the optimum treatment plan requires consideration of the different types of radial head fractures and the long-term results of a number of different treatment plans.

Mason type I fractures (undisplaced or involving less than 25% of the radial head) are fairly straightforward with conservative (nonsurgical) treatment leading to an almost full range of motion without pain. Mason type II fractures (marginal fractures with displacement of the radial head and including angulation, impaction, and depression) can be treated by open reduction and internal fixation if the fragments are large (noncomminuted) or by excision of the radial head (either early or late) without affecting the prognosis. For example, if open reduction is chosen but at surgery internal fixation is not possible, then excision of the radial head should be chosen. If the radial head is comminuted and closed treatment is chosen, results of late excision of the radial head are equal to those of early excision and it is only necessary to avoid excision between three days and three weeks.

For many Mason type II fractures, nonsurgical treatment is now preferred initially to avoid lateral elbow instability and problems of proximal migration of the radius and because late excision has been successful. Symptoms at the distal radioulnar joint or interosseous membrane can also affect the decision-making process. It is probably better to make these decisions later when the degree of adjacent joint injuries may be less difficult to access. However, there is a definite opinion that early evaluation and repair of injured structures at both the proximal and distal radioulnar joints is the procedure of choice.

Silastic prosthetic replacement of the radial head remains controversial. Indications have included radial head fractures with elbow dislocations, Monteggia fracture-dislocations, and Essex-Lopresti lesions (tearing of the interosseous membrane and ligaments of the distal radioulnar joint with radial head fracture). The question remains whether a silicone prosthesis (or any radial head prosthesis for that matter) can provide the stability needed to resist the forces transmitted across the forearm to the elbow. For Mason types III and IV fractures, a prosthetic replacement may be needed, but to date no effective device is available. The current recommendation is to use a silicone prosthesis, but very selectively. Further studies on the problems of silicone synovitis may in fact show this recommendation to be incorrect and silicone prostheses of many types may become obsolete.

Olecranon Fractures

The controversy regarding olecranon fractures is the debate on the best method of internal fixation. The best results are obtained by open reduction and internal fixation with an intramedullary screw or rod, alone or in combination with a figure-of-eight wire. For significant intra-articular involvement, open reduction and plate fixation has been suggested as the best method of maintaining a congruent joint surface. Finally, there is a good study demonstrating that the tension-band wire technique can be very effective in preventing fracture displacement and that it may be preferred in comminuted fractures. Other than skin and subcutaneous irritation caused by the tension-band wires, there is actually little strong evidence to recommend one technique over the others because the reports did not compare different techniques. The surgeon must, therefore, examine the olecranon fracture pattern, consider the treatment alternatives, and then select the method that fits the fracture and that will work the best in each individual case.

Excision of the olecranon remains the final alternative in comminuted fractures. Clinical studies have demonstrated that this method can be effective, although recent biomechanical studies demonstrated a loss of anteroposterior elbow stability. It appears safe to say that olecranon excision limited to the proximal 30% to 40% in elderly patients is acceptable but in the younger, more active patients, olecranon excision should be avoided unless some loss of mechanical stability and probable weakness of elbow extension strength can be accepted.

Annotated Bibliography

Keywords

Elbow; Forearm; Fracture; Fracture-dislocation; Olecranon; Radius; Ulna

Anatomy and Biomechanics

Morrey BF, An KN: Functional anatomy of the ligaments of the elbow. *Clin Orthop* 1985;201:84–90.
The important elements of medial and lateral collateral ligaments are reviewed with respect to elbow stability. The lateral ulnohumeral ligament, a previously unrecognized structure, is described as essential for lateral stability.

Stormont TJ, An KN, Morrey BF, et al: Elbow joint contact study: Comparison of techniques. *J Biomech* 1985;18:329–336.
The contact area of the trochlea and olecranon fossa of the proximal ulna were studied with pressure-sensitive film and silicone casting. The load distribution occurs among the four facets of the proximal ulna. Radiocapitellar contact occurred only after valgus stress.

Elbow Dislocations

Boe S, Holst-Nielsen F: Intra-articular entrapment of the

median nerve after dislocation of the elbow. *J Hand Surg* 1987;12B:356–358.
A case report of a man who had closed reduction of an elbow dislocation entrapping the median nerve without a fracture of the medial epicondyle. The authors postulate that the nerve passed behind the humeral epicondyle after the medial capsule and the flexor pronator origin were stripped.

Josefsson PO, Gentz CF, Johnell O, et al: Surgical versus nonsurgical treatment of ligamentous injuries following dislocations of the elbow joint. *Clin Orthop* 1987;214:165–169.
Surgical repair of the collateral ligaments and nonsurgical closed reduction had equal long-term results. Loss of flexion-extension was greater in the repair group. The findings fail to support any superiority of ligament repair over conservative treatment.

Mehlhoff TL, Noble PC, Bennett JB, et al: Simple dislocation of the elbow in the adult: Results after closed treatment. *J Bone Joint Surg* 1988;70A:244–249.
A long-term review of 52 elbow dislocations demonstrated residual symptoms in 60%, with flexion contracture in 15%, residual pain in 45%, and pain on valgus stress in 35%. The authors stress that early active motion was the most important factor in complete rehabilitation.

Fractures of the Elbow

Radial Head Fractures

Broberg MA, Morrey BF: Results of delayed excision of the radial head after fracture. *J Bone Joint Surg* 1986; 68A:669–674.

Late excision of the radial head (four weeks to 20 years) produced satisfactory results with improved motion and complete pain relief. The authors concluded that unless the arm is symptomatic, surgeons should reconsider the need for early radial head excision of Mason type I and type II fractures.

Carn RM, Medige J, Curtain D, et al: Silicone rubber replacement of the severely fractured radial head. *Clin Orthop* 1986;209:259–269.

Silicone replacement of the radial head was associated with complications that included degenerative arthritis of the elbow in 56% of cases followed up for a minimum of 3.4 years. There is doubt about whether a silicone prosthesis can adequately transfer the dynamic forearm forces across the elbow.

Coleman DA, Blair WF, Shurr D: Resection of the radial head for fracture of the radial head: Long-term follow-up of seventeen cases. *J Bone Joint Surg* 1987; 69A:385–392.

Seventeen patients with closed radial head fractures were reviewed eight to 46 years after resection of the radial head. Few patients complained of pain. Ulnar variance had changed, however, to a positive variance, averaging 2 mm (range, 0 to 8 mm) in 15 patients.

Goldberg I, Peylan J, Yosipovitch Z: Late results of excision of the radial head for an isolated closed fracture. *J Bone Joint Surg* 1986;68A:675–679.

A retrospective review of Mason types II and III closed radial head fractures demonstrated satisfactory results in 86% after late excision. With such good results with late (delayed) excision, the authors now recommend nonsurgical early treatment.

McArthur RA: Herbert screw fixation of fracture of the head of the radius. *Clin Orthop* 1987;224:79–87.

Herbert screw fixation of displaced fractures of the radial head was effective in maintaining fracture reduction without impeding elbow or forearm motion.

Schwartz N: Dislocation of fragments and indications for operative therapy in segmental radial head fractures. *Handchir Mikrochir Plast Chir* 1986;18:319–322.

The authors found that 70% of fresh isolated radial head fractures did well with conservative treatment and that another 20% had only minimal dysfunction. Ten percent had poor results. The authors concluded that nonsurgical treatment was justified and that surgery offered no specific advantage.

Olecranon Fractures

An KN, Morrey BF, Chao EY: The effect of partial removal of proximal ulna on elbow constraint. *Clin Orthop* 1986;209:270–279.

In a biomechanical study, ulnohumeral joint resistance decreased with increasingly larger olecranon excisions. The authors showed that excision of the proximal half of the olecranon affects elbow stability, contradicting reports that as much as 80% of the olecranon can be excised without complication.

Fyfe IS, Mossad MM, Holdsworth BJ: Methods of fixation of olecranon fractures: An experimental mechanical study. *J Bone Joint Surg* 1985;67B:367–372.

For earlier mobilization of the injured elbow, better internal fixation was tested with five different methods. Tension-band wire fixation with a double knot was strongest and was pre-ferred for oblique fractures whereas a five-hole plate was best for comminuted fractures.

Murphy DF, Greene WB, Dameron TB Jr: Displaced olecranon fractures in adults: Clinical evaluation. *Clin Orthop* 1987;224:215–223.

Intramedullary screw plus wire combinations were superior to tension-band wires in the treatment of displaced olecranon fractures. Symptomatic wire prominence complicated AO tension-band wiring. Intra-articular displacement of 2 mm or more should not be accepted.

Wolfgang G, Burke F, Bush D, et al: Surgical treatment of displaced olecranon fractures by tension-band wiring technique. *Clin Orthop* 1987;224:192–204.

Excellent results were reported in 78% of patients with displaced olecranon fractures using AO tension-band wire. The authors noted that excision of as much as 50% of the olecranon was effective in comminuted fractures.

Supracondylar and Intra-articular Fractures

Dushuttle RP, Coyle MP, Zawadsky JP, et al: Fractures of the capitellum. *J Trauma* 1985;25:317–321.

Fractures of the capitellum were reviewed in 17 patients and the final results showed little difference in range of motion with various modes of management. For a single large fragment, a trial of closed reduction followed by open reduction is recommended. Comminuted fractures of the capitellum should be excised.

Henly MB, Bone LB, Parker B: Operative management of intra-articular fractures of the distal humerus. *J Orthop Trauma* 1987;1:24–35.

Surgical stabilization of intracondylar fractures of the distal humerus gave good or excellent results in 23 of 25 patients. Anatomic reduction was consistently achieved but complications were noted with the transolecranon approach (27%).

Jupiter JB, Neff U, Holzach P, et al: Intercondylar fractures of the humerus: An operative approach. *J Bone Joint Surg* 1985;67A:226–239.

Controversy regarding the best approach for intracondylar fractures is addressed in this review of 34 patients. The AO classification (types C1, C2, and C3) and open reduction with careful surgical technique gave good or excellent results in 27 cases.

Richards RR, Khoury GW, Burke FD, et al: Internal fixation of capitellar fractures using Herbert screws: A report of four cases. *Can J Surg* 1987;30:188–191.

Four patients with displaced fractures of the capitellum were treated with open reduction and internal fixation with Herbert screws. This allowed rigid fixation and early joint motion. The Herbert screw can compress the fracture site, and its head is buried beneath the articular surface so that removal can be avoided.

Zagorski JB, Jennings JJ, Burkhalter WE, et al: Comminuted intra-articular fractures of the distal humeral condyles: Surgical vs nonsurgical treatment. *Clin Orthop* 1986;202:197–204.

Forty-two patients with comminuted intra-articular fractures of the distal humerus were studied. Only 8% of those treated nonsurgically had satisfactory results. Anatomic restoration by open reduction and internal fixation is recommended through a posterior "U" incision with extra-articular transolecranon osteotomy.

Fractures of the Radius and Ulna

DeLuca PA, Lindsey RW, Ruwe PA: Refracture of bones of the forearm after the removal of compression plates. *J Bone Joint Surg* 1988;70A:1372–1376.

Sixty-two plates were removed in 37 patients. Seven forearm bones had refractured. Contributing factors were major trauma producing the injury, radiolucency at the fracture site, and fractures of both the radius and ulna.

Lange RH, Foster RJ: Skeletal management of humeral shaft fractures associated with forearm fractures. *Clin Orthop* 1985;195:173–177.

In a series of nine ipsilateral fractures of the humerus and forearm, results improved after open reduction and rigid internal fixation. Aggressive management of both fractures is recommended in the patient with multiple injuries.

Moed BR, Kellam JF, Foster RJ, et al: Immediate internal fixation of open fractures of the diaphysis of the forearm. *J Bone Joint Surg* 1986;68A:1008–1016.

Open reduction and internal fixation is advocated for types I and II and selected type III open forearm fractures. The results were good to excellent in 85%. Deep infections occurred in two cases (4%) and nonunion in seven cases (14%).

Vince KG, Miller JE: Cross-union complicating fracture of the forearm: Part I. Adults. *J Bone Joint Surg* 1987; 69A:640–653.

Twenty-eight cases of crossunion and complication of forearm fractures were separated into proximal third, middle third, and distal third. Excision was successful in 12 of 17 patients. Fractures at the same level had an increased risk of crossunion; crossunion is less common in children.

Pediatric Fractures and Dislocations

Elbow Dislocations

Floyd WE III, Gebhardt MC, Emans JB: Intra-articular entrapment of the median nerve after elbow dislocation in children. *J Hand Surg* 1987;12A:704–707.

Two cases of median nerve entrapment occurred after closed elbow dislocations. Early surgical exploration is recommended when a median nerve deficit is present after closed reduction, especially in fractures of the medial epicondyle.

Fowles JV, Kassab MT, Douik M: Untreated posterior dislocation of the elbow in children. *J Bone Joint Surg* 1984;66A:921–926.

Open reduction was successful in 14 of 15 patients treated three weeks to four years after elbow dislocation. A posterior approach to remove fibrous tissue, release contracture, and reduce the elbow is recommended.

Supracondylar Fractures

Gerardi JA, Houkom JA, Mack GR: Treatment of displaced supracondylar fractures of the humerus in children by closed reduction and percutaneous pinning. *Orthop Rev* 1989;18:1089–1095.

This was a retrospective study of 25 displaced supracondylar fractures treated by closed reduction and percutaneous pin fixation with average follow-up 16 months. Excellent and good results were obtained in all except one, and no complications were reported.

Ippolito E, Caterini R, Scola E: Supracondylar fractures of the humerus in children: Analysis at maturity of fifty-three patients treated conservatively. *J Bone Joint Surg* 1986;68A:333–344.

Long-term follow-up of 53 patients from an initial pool of 131 fractures demonstrated significant varus or valgus deformity in only seven patients treated with overhead skeletal traction, followed by shoulder spica cast at one week. Complications were not observed.

Nacht JL, Kassab MT, Chung SMK: Supracondylar frac-

tures of the humerus in children treated by closed reduction and percutaneous pinning. *Clin Orthop* 1983;177: 203–209.

This was a retrospective review of five patients with displaced supracondylar fractures with an average follow-up of 38 months. Excellent results were obtained in 19. Three patients had mild cubitus varus and three had loss of flexion. There were no neurologic or vascular complications.

Pirone AM, Graham HK, Krajbich JI: Management of displaced extension-type supracondylar fractures of the humerus in children. *J Bone Joint Surg* 1988;70A:641–650.

In the treatment of displaced supracondylar fractures, the best results were achieved by percutaneous K-wire fixation, skeletal fixation, or open reduction with internal fixation. Closed reduction and cast had the lowest percentage of excellent results and had a higher percentage of early and late complications.

Radial Head Fractures

Fowles JV, Kassab MT: Observations concerning radial neck fractures in children. *J Pediatr Orthop* 1986;6:51–57.

A review of 23 fractures of the radial neck demonstrated that angulation of more than 60 degrees was best treated by open reduction and internal fixation with transarticular K-wires. Fractures of the wires occurred in three cases and oblique wire fixation is now recommended.

Roberts JA: Angulation of the radius in children's fractures. *J Bone Joint Surg* 1986;68B:751–754.

Fractures of the proximal radius demonstrated that little radial deviation deformity is acceptable and that rotational deformities remodel little if at all. If adequate fracture reduction cannot be obtained or maintained, closed percutaneous pin fixation or open reduction and K-wire fixation should be performed.

Steinberg EL, Golomb D, Salama R, et al: Radial head and neck fractures in children. *J Pediatr Orthop* 1988;8:35–40.

In a review of 42 consecutive fractures of the radial head and neck, analysis of initial and final results demonstrated that when the angulation exceeds 30 degrees open reduction should be performed and internal fixation with K-wires is recommended.

Walsh HP, McLaren CA, Owen R: Galeazzi fractures in children. *J Bone Joint Surg* 1987;69B:730–733.

Although uncommon, Galeazzi fractures in children require careful evaluation for instability of the distal radioulnar joint. In this series, only seven of 17 cases had good results when joint injury was not recognized.

Fractures of the Lateral Condyle and Epicondyle

Herring JA, Fitch RD: Lateral condylar fracture of the elbow. *J Pediatr Orthop* 1986;6:724–727.

Open reduction through a lateral approach is described with K-wire internal fixation for fractures of the lateral condyle of the humerus. Growth disturbance and cubitus valgus deformity were minimized by accurate fracture reduction and precise articular surface alignment.

Josefsson PO, Danielsson LG: Epicondylar elbow fracture in children: 35-year follow-up of 56 unreduced cases. *Acta Orthop Scand* 1986;57:313–315.

Displaced medial epicondyle fractures are best treated by open reduction and internal fixation whereas minimally displaced fractures (<5 mm) respond to conservative (nonsurgical) treatment. Pseudarthrosis in minimally displaced fractures did not influence functional results.

Fractures of the Medial Condyle and Epicondyle

Fowles JV, Kassab MT, Moula T: Untreated intra-articular entrapment of the medial humeral epicondyle. *J Bone Joint Surg* 1984;66B:562–565.

The authors report six cases of entrapment of the medial epicondyle after elbow dislocation treated by closed reduction and casting. Good results were obtained by excising the fragment or by reattachment to the medial condyle.

Papavasiliou V, Nenopoulos S, Venturis T: Fractures of the medial condyle of the humerus in childhood. *J Pediatr Orthop* 1987;7:421–423.

The authors classified medial condyle fractures into three types (Kilfoyle), and recommended cast immobilization for type I and open reduction and fixation with K-wires for types II and III. Supracondylar closing wedge osteotomy was satisfactory for correction of cubitus varus.

Forearm Fractures

Creasman C, Zaleske DJ, Ehrlich MG: Analyzing forearm fractures in children: The more subtle signs of impending problems. *Clin Orthop* 1984;188:40–53.

Results were unsatisfactory in 15% of 56 patients treated by closed reduction and casting. Abnormal bowing and angulation, shortening, and malrotation—especially in proximal forearm fractures—had a higher incidence of poor results.

Kalamchi A: Monteggia fracture-dislocation in children: Late treatment in two cases. *J Bone Joint Surg* 1986;68A:615–619.

Successful open reduction of the proximal ulna and corrective osteotomy and open reduction of the radial head are described in two patients. Both patients had a greenstick fracture of the proximal ulna and the radial head distribution was initially unrecognized.

Vince KG, Miller JE: Cross-union complicating fracture of the forearm: Part II. Children. *J Bone Joint Surg* 1987;69A:654–661.

Ten crossunions of the forearm were collected from seven hospitals, indicating the relatively rare occurrence of this problem. Resection of crossunion in children had better results than in adults.

Wiley JJ, Galey JP: Monteggia injuries in children. *J Bone Joint Surg* 1985;67B:728–731.

Conservative treatment of Monteggia fractures in children produces satisfactory results. The authors propose a simple classification that includes all variants.

Associated Problems

Soft-Tissue Coverage

Dell PC, Sheppard JE: Vascularized bone grafts in the treatment of infected forearm nonunions. *J Hand Surg* 1984;9A:653–658.

Wide local excision, control of sepsis, and external fixation are combined with a vascular fibular reconstruction to treat osteomyelitis and restore length and stability to the forearm.

Foucher G, van Genechten F, Merle N, et al: A compound radial artery forearm flap in hand surgery: An original modification of the Chinese forearm flap. *Br J Plast Surg* 1984;37:139–148.

The Chinese radial forearm flap is a versatile, robust skin flap that can include skin, bone, tendon, and nerves. The flap can be rotated proximally or distally to achieve soft-tissue coverage.

Jones NF, Hardesty RA, Goldstein SA, et al: Upper limb salvage using a free radial forearm flap. *Plast Reconstr Surg* 1987;79:468–471.

A radial forearm flap from a nonreimplantable upper limb provided soft-tissue coverage of the amputation stump and salvaged the elbow joint.

Lovie MJ, Duncan GM, Glasson DW: The ulnar artery forearm free flap. *Br J Plast Surg* 1984;37:486–492.

A forearm flap based on the ulnar artery can include the flexor carpi ulnaris muscle for added bulk. The authors describe 20 surgical and cadaveric dissections.

Sbitany U, Wray RC Jr: Use of the rectus abdominis muscle flap to reconstruct an elbow defect. *Plast Reconstr Surg* 1986;77:988–989.

A superiorly based rectus abdominis flap was successfully transferred to reconstruct an infected elbow with exposed bone and metal screws.

Nerve Injury

Hope PG: Anterior interosseous nerve palsy following internal fixation of the proximal radius. *J Bone Joint Surg* 1988;70B:280–282.

Three cases of anterior interosseous nerve palsy were recognized after internal fixation of the proximal radius. A bone-holding forceps should be used with caution in these injuries.

Mirovsky Y, Hendel D, Halperin N: Anterior interosseous nerve palsy following closed fracture of the proximal ulna: A case report and review of the literature. *Arch Orthop Trauma Surg* 1988;107:61–64.

Closed reduction of a fracture of the proximal ulna that required repetitive reduction attempts was complicated by anterior interosseous nerve palsy.

Radiologic Imaging

Akbarnia BA, Silberstein MJ, Rende RJ, et al: Arthrography in the diagnosis of fractures of the distal end of the humerus in infants. *J Bone Joint Surg* 1986;68A:599–602.

Arthrography can be helpful in differentiating traumatic dislocation in the elbow from displaced physeal fractures of the distal humerus. In children less than 10 years old, arthrography of the elbow is recommended in addition to plain radiographs.

Greenspan A, Norman A: Radial head-capitellum view: An expanded imaging approach to elbow injury. *Radiology* 1987;164:272–274.

An improved technique of evaluating traumatic conditions of the elbow, particularly radial head-capitellum and coronoid process fractures. It is very effective in displaying the extent of fracture displacement.

28

Elbow and Forearm: Reconstruction

This chapter reviews recent information regarding the basic science of elbow and forearm function as well as various pathologic conditions and their treatment. Controversies surrounding these issues are particularly common with regard to the elbow because it poses such difficult clinical problems and because the outcome of treatment is so unpredictable. There is, however, a difference between truly controversial areas and those in which uncertainty exists simply because the available information is inadequate.

Diagnostic and Anatomic Studies

The fat-pad sign is generally accepted by clinicians as demonstrating the presence of a fracture or a significant intra-articular abnormality. This accepted dictum was recently challenged in a study specifically addressing the accuracy and significance of the fat-pad sign. After 820 radiographs were reviewed and 244 known fractures were excluded, anterior fat-pad signs were found in 56 patients. Posterior fat-pad signs were also present in 34 of the 56, despite the absence of an identifiable fracture. Intra-articular abnormality was defined as the cause of hemarthrosis in five of the 56 patients. A fracture was later found in only six of the remaining 51 patients. Four of the six fractures were undisplaced radial head fractures. Hence, the clinician should recognize that the fat-pad sign, particularly posteriorly, may represent significant intra-articular injury but that it represents an otherwise unrecognized fracture only about 10% of the time. Radial head fracture is most common. Hence, unless there are clinical findings of significant intra-articular abnormality, the elbow should not be overtreated by prolonged immobilization.

Other diagnostic studies have assessed the role of contrast-enhanced computed tomography on the assumption that elbow abnormalities are difficult to image by routine tomography. There is no proof of this hypothesis, and many clinicians would disagree with it. Sophisticated imaging techniques have a relatively limited role in elbow studies. Routine plain films and tomograms are sufficient in more than 90% of cases.

The absence of olecranon bursitis in young patients has now been explained. Dissection of 63 randomly selected cadavers and the use of the methylene blue injection technique demonstrated that the bursa does not exist in children less than 7 years of age. The size of the bursa increases as a function of age, and all individuals more than 10 years old do have some form of olecranon bursa. The bursa was found to be greater in volume on the right side than on the left, suggesting that dominance and, therefore, activity are important in the development of the bursa or at least of its characteristics.

Radial Head Function and Abnormalities

Basic Science Studies

A better understanding of the force-transmission characteristics and stabilizing role of the radial head has been achieved during the last three years. This has provided an improved rationale for the management of radial head fractures and the design of joint replacements.

Investigators employed a static model that provided a discrete 20-N load while testing the stabilizing role of the radial head in resisting valgus stress. They demonstrated a 24% to 32% increase in valgus laxity between 0 and 90 degrees of elbow flexion when the radial head was removed (Fig. 1). Interestingly, a Silastic implant did not alter the valgus instability pattern. The anterior bundle of the medial collateral ligament was found to be the most important stabilizer of valgus stress. The elbow was too unstable to test when this structure was sectioned. Another experiment using a similar model also demonstrated that the radial head contributes about 28% of valgus stability. These investigators, however, demonstrated that a Silastic implant restored stability to about 78% of normal.

The actual amount of force transmitted by the radial head under normal loads has also been investigated. In a simulated active-motion model, a force transducer placed

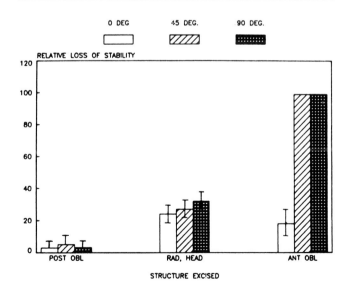

Figure 1

The posterior oblique and anterior oblique portions of the medial collateral ligament and radial head as valgus stabilizers of the elbow. Note that the radial head contributes 25% to 35% of the valgus stability, depending upon the position of the elbow. (Reproduced with permission from Hotchkiss RN, Weiland AJ: Valgus stability of the elbow. *J Orthop Res* 1987;5:372–377.)

between the radial tuberosity and the radial head showed that the greatest force transmission occurs in the first 30 degrees of elbow flexion. These investigators also demonstrated that radiohumeral force transmission is greater when the forearm is in pronation than when it is in supination (Fig. 2). Additionally, muscle activity generates a force of less than one body weight across the radiohumeral joint. This calculation is markedly less than that suggested previously.

Elbow Synovectomy

Synovectomy of the rheumatoid elbow continues to be an accepted treatment, particularly in the early refractory stages of disease. Concern about loss of motion after elbow synovectomy prompted a technique modification that includes a release of the common flexor and extensor tendons from the medial and lateral epicondyles in association with radical synovectomy in patients with rheumatoid arthritis. In a study of 23 synovectomies, ten elbows had mild (stage I) osseous involvement, 12 had moderate (stage II) involvement, and one had extensive (stage IV) involvement. After one to eight years of follow-up, 21 patients reported improved range of motion and only two showed deterioration. The average postoperative arc of motion was 102 degrees. All patients functioned better in the activities of daily living. Three patients were reported to have slight instability and one developed an ulnar nerve paresthesia postoperatively. Results were considered to be satisfactory in all cases despite the diverse spectrum of preoperative involvement.

The generally accepted role of synovectomy in the hemophilic patient was recently restated to include recurrent hemorrhages not responding to medical management. After a follow-up ranging from 18 to 70 months, nine of 23 patients had increased pronation and supination and 14 had improved flexion-extension. Importantly, only four patients experienced recurrent bleeding after synovectomy. These findings support the accepted position that synovectomy is a valuable adjunct in the control of recurrent hemarthrosis when nonsurgical management fails in hemophilic patients with involvement of the elbow. These results also indicate that the radial head should be excised

in adults if it has undergone secondary degenerative changes.

Traumatic Conditions of the Elbow

Although elbow dislocations are seldom ignored or overlooked, such cases occasionally occur. A surgical procedure designed to reduce the chronically dislocated elbow and provide stability for the reduced position uses the medial collateral ligament and an intra-articular component somewhat analogous to an anterior cruciate ligament (Fig. 3). In 11 cases the average postoperative arc of motion was 38 to 105 degrees, but the average varus-valgus instability was 13 degrees. In many instances, the chronically dislocated elbow may function as well as one that has been reconstructed and, thus, late reconstructive procedures may not benefit the patient.

Ligamentous repair for acute elbow dislocation was prospectively studied in 30 cases. The medial collateral ligament was disrupted in all 30 elbows and 16 had lateral instability as well. At follow-up, repair of the ligament demonstrated no advantage over nonsurgical treatment. Thus, acute repair of ruptured collateral ligaments is not indicated for elbow dislocation.

An uncommon but difficult problem with respect to distal humeral nonunion is limitation of motion or gross instability. Even a flail elbow does not always produce pain. In a group of 20 patients ranging in age from 68 to 84 years, there were 13 extra-articular and seven intra-articular fractures. The time from fracture to nonunion averaged 20 months (range, three to 120 months). Nineteen patients had pain with instability and 15 had a decreased range of motion after additional surgery. Union was achieved in 19 patients (94%) with the AO technique (Fig. 4), but, importantly, function was rated excellent in only one case and good in only six, yielding a satisfaction rate of only 35%. Seven results were fair and six were poor. Extra-articular fractures did best because of the greater amount of bone stock with which to provide rigid stability and early motion. Obtaining a successful union is not, therefore, necessarily synonymous with achieving a satisfactory functional result in a patient with distal humeral nonunion.

The most common residual effect of elbow trauma is

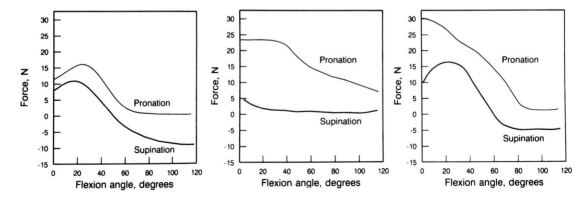

Figure 2

Force transmission across the radial head is consistently greater when the forearm is in pronation than in supination. (Reproduced with permission from Morrey BF, An K-N, Stormont TJ: Force transmission through the radial head. *J Bone Joint Surg* 1988;70A:250–256.)

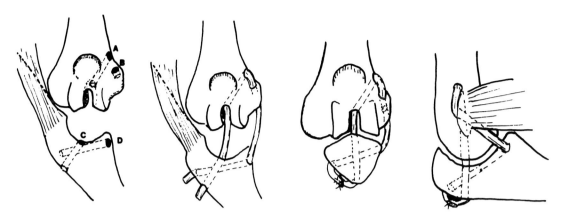

Figure 3
Reconstructive procedure for the chronically dislocated elbow consists of reconstructing the medial collateral ligament and producing an intra-articular checkrein effect with the graft. (Reproduced with permission from Arafiles RP: Neglected posterior dislocation of the elbow: A reconstruction operation. *J Bone Joint Surg* 1987;69B:199–202.)

stiffness with or without pain. There is almost no new information concerning this issue. One report discussed 58 cases of stiff elbow in which a modified Köcher approach was used for lysing anterior and posterior adhesions. The specific modification, which has significant value, consisted of releasing the triceps in continuity from the tip of the olecranon, thus leaving the extensor mechanism as a continuous sheet of muscle and retinacular tissue (Fig. 5). Although the surgical procedure is primarily a soft-tissue release, a fascial interposition arthroplasty was also performed in approximately 20% of these cases. The results were satisfactory (defined as more than 70 degrees of flexion-extension) in 51 cases. This degree of improvement may seem modest, but even modest improvement in an ankylosed elbow can be quite significant functionally.

The use of distraction arthroplasty as an adjunct to an ankylosis release in 20 of 26 patients has recently been reported (Fig. 6). The results were gratifying as the range of flexion-extension motion improved from a mean of 32 degrees (range, 60 to 92 degrees) preoperatively to a mean of 95 degrees (range, 30 to 125 degrees) after surgery. The complication rate was 30%. The complications included infection (4%), ulnar nerve irritation (8%), and triceps rupture (4%). The procedure is technically difficult and the goals and risks involved must be carefully assessed.

The difficult issue of postoperative management of the stiff elbow by continuous passive motion has been considered. In three patients with simple extension loss who were treated with anterior capsulectomy, the contracture decreased from more than 40 degrees preoperatively to only 5 degrees postoperatively. These cases do not prove the value of continuous passive motion, but do suggest that it is a helpful adjunct. For flexion contractures to resolve to such an extent, the elbow joint must be essentially normal. If intrinsic (intra-articular) abnormalities are present, flexion contracture rarely improves beyond 20 degrees of extension.

Management of massive bone loss remains a difficult clinical problem. No new data have appeared in the last three years. Although allografts have been used to replace entire joints and parts of joints, experience is limited. The technique is demanding and the complication rate is high.

This subject was discussed in *Orthopaedic Knowledge Update 2.*

The role of elbow arthrodesis continues to be discussed but no new data have been reported. It is indicated only for refractory infections. For patients with massive bone loss, solid fusion is difficult to achieve and functional loss is always significant.

Semi-anatomic implants have worked exceptionally well in older patients undergoing revision procedures.

Total Elbow Arthroplasty

A number of recent reports dealing with elbow joint replacement have demonstrated the value of this procedure for patients with significant bone loss and as a revision procedure.

Basic Science Studies

An anatomic study replicated the contour of the distal humerus and correlated it with the axis of elbow rotation, providing a more scientific basis for designing elbow resurfacing replacements. In addition to the design, the study also provided information for improving surgical techniques. Biomechanical data, design characteristics, and surgical technique are vital factors in decreasing or eliminating instability problems in the resurfacing devices.

Resurfacing Devices

Resurfacing replacement remains popular in the United Kingdom and the United States (Fig. 7). After three to nine years of follow-up on at least two resurfacing design modifications, the failure rate was high. In 60 procedures, 42 of which were done for rheumatoid arthritis, 15 devices required revision, six because of deep infection and nine because of loosening. Interestingly, seven of the nine that loosened involved the ulnar component. The high infection rate has been noted previously, but loosening of resurfacing devices is not often reported. Twenty-two of the 60 devices demonstrated some lateral instability and five demonstrated posterior instability. In three cases the instability was severe enough to require revision surgery. In

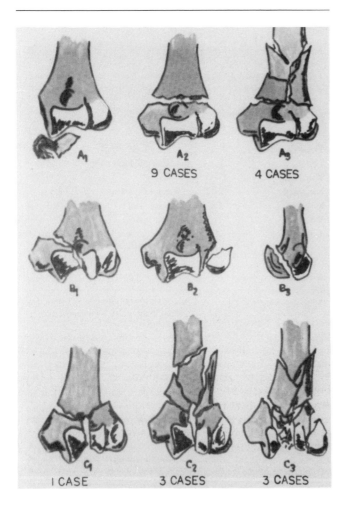

Figure 4

AO principles of rigid fixation are sought in treating the distal humeral nonunion. Osteoporosis of the distal fragment can make rigid fixation particularly difficult. (Reproduced with permission from Ackerman G, Jupiter JB: Non-union of fractures of the distal end of the humerus. *J Bone Joint Surg* 1988;70A:75–83.)

sharp contrast to most previous reports, these investigators observed that patients with degenerative disease did better than those with rheumatoid arthritis. Overall, 27% of the procedures were classified as major failures and complications developed in an additional 10%.

Another review of 16 resurfacing procedures for rheumatoid arthritis had a limited follow-up of only 26 months. Two prostheses had already loosened and required additional surgery, three had become infected, and three had ulnar nerve complications. These data underscore the difficulty of the surgical technique and of determining the optimum design for this difficult joint.

A study of capitellocondylar procedures in patients with rheumatoid arthritis also found a high complication rate. After two to eight years of follow-up, 20 of 35 cases (57%) had complications. Nine had transient ulnar nerve palsy, three developed infection, and three were unstable. Significantly, 12% of the humeral components and 34% of the ulnar components demonstrated some interface lucency on radiographic study. Overall, the functional result and patient satisfaction were acceptable. Nonetheless, the devel-

opment of radiolucent lines is potentially worrisome, particularly in light of continued problems with instability.

Semiconstrained Devices

Experience with more constrained devices, on the other hand, continues to be somewhat favorable (Fig. 8). After 30 months of follow-up in 45 patients, a third modification of the Mark III GSB prosthesis produced 87% good results, 7% fair results, and 4% poor results. Importantly, there was no loosening and only a 2% incidence of lucent lines. The improvement in surgical technique was demonstrated by a 3% infection rate and a 3% incidence of ulnar neuropathy. Most of the complications were related to the design (four of the 45 prostheses became uncoupled). Because 15% of these cases were posttraumatic, it is possible that joint replacement may be a viable treatment option in selected patients with arthritis after trauma. One recent report was devoted to replacement of marked bone loss. Of 16 such patients, ten had posttraumatic problems and six had flail elbows. The average follow-up was four years (range, two to 9.6 years). After replacement, 14 of the 16 elbows were rated as excellent or good but three underwent reoperation, one because of infection, one because of articular problems, and one because of a protruding humeral stem and nerve palsy. In this very difficult group of patients, a semiconstrained device is considered to be a viable salvage option preferable to indefinite bracing or other less attractive possibilities.

Both of these studies involved devices with some play or looseness of the articular mechanism. In contrast, one device used in the United Kingdom for marked bone loss employs a more constrained coupling mechanism. This experience was less gratifying. Although a functional arc of motion was obtained in most, deep infection occurred in three of 26 cases and there were 36 complications. This underscores the value of appropriate prosthetic design and the need for meticulous surgical technique in this difficult population.

In a study of reimplantation for revision of failed elbow arthroplasty, 33 procedures followed up for at least three years (average, six years), had 55% satisfactory results with the first procedure and 75% satisfactory results after some additional revision. Three of the 33 became infected. In addition, six of the initial 33 revisions became loose and required additional reimplantation. The modified semiconstrained Coonrad device holds significant promise in total elbow arthroplasty and in the reconstruction of distal humeral and proximal ulnar bone loss (Fig. 8).

Other Issues

Additional issues with regard to joint replacement includes the timing of procedures in the patient with concurrent shoulder and elbow involvement. After a review of 35 cases (minimum follow-up, two years), using the criterion of a longer interval between procedures when the elbow was done first, it was concluded that treating the elbow restored more function than treating the shoulder and thus the elbow should be replaced first. These investigators pointed out, however, that the more symptomatic joint should be replaced initially. Only in instances in which the shoulder and elbow are equally involved and both provide functional impediments did they recommend that the elbow replacement be performed first.

The anticipated change in strength after elbow replace-

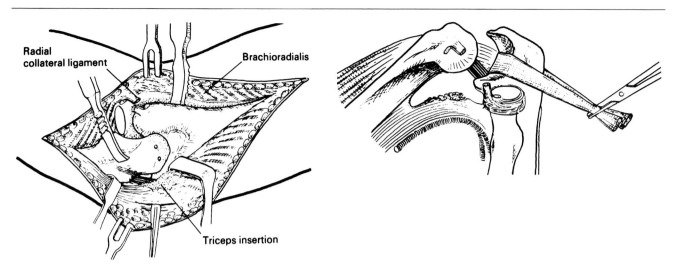

Figure 5

Exposure of the posterolateral aspect of the elbow. **Left,** The triceps is reflected from the olecranon in continuity. **Right,** The entire soft-tissue envelope (anterior, posterior, and lateral) is released. The medial collateral ligament is retained if at all possible. The joint is then resurfaced or otherwise fashioned depending on the abnormality.

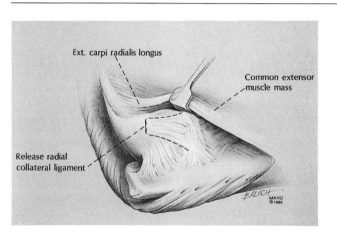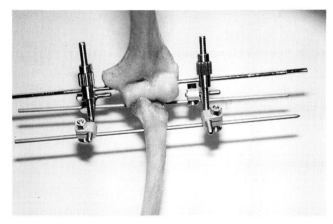

Figure 6

Modified Kocher exposure allows (1) triceps reflection, (2) olecranon removal, (3) posterior capsule release, and (4) anterior capsule release (**left**). The distraction device allows motion about the axis of rotation while the ulna is separated from the humerus (**right**).

ment surgery has also been studied recently. In general, strength improves approximately 70% in patients with rheumatoid arthritis. A more modest 25% improvement occurs in posttraumatic patients. On the basis of limited data, this improvement appears to be independent of the design of the prosthesis. Importantly, extension strength is not improved after surgery and, in some instances, increased weakness in extension has been observed after elbow replacement because of violation of the triceps during the surgical approach.

Sports-Related Injuries

The number of studies of elbow function has increased, but most relate to muscle and exercise physiology. One recent investigation of note, however, attempted to explain the common phenomenon of muscle stiffness and pain after exercise. By correlating electromyographic tracings with

symptoms of muscular pain during elbow flexion, these investigators demonstrated no electromyographic evidence of abnormal muscular activity. This led them to conclude that muscle pain after exercise is a response to damage to the connective tissue. This damage increases the mechanical sensitivity of muscle receptors, which in turn gives rise to the pain.

Tennis elbow continues to be the subject of both clinical and basic investigation because this is probably the most common elbow complaint. In a careful study of anatomic dissections, the variation of the common extensor muscle tendon origin was defined. It was shown that the extensor carpi radialis brevis muscle consists of a keel-shaped tendon with attachments to both the extensor carpi radialis longus and extensor digitorum communis as well as to the supinator muscle. In addition, attachments to the radial collateral ligament, to the anular ligament, and to the capsule itself were observed. In approximately 22% of the specimens, a prolongation of the extensor carpi radialis brevis

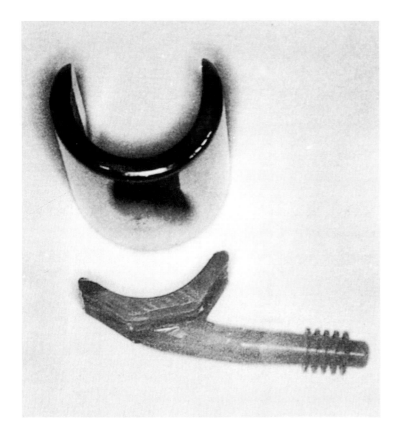
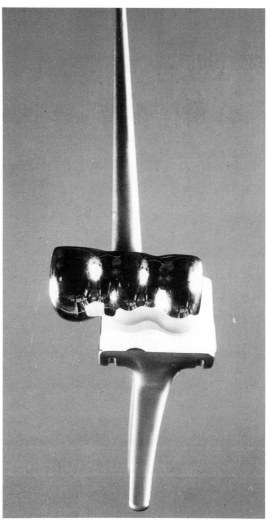

Figure 7

Various resurfacing designs include the Liverpool from the United Kingdom (**left**) and the capitellocondylar most commonly used in the United States (**right**).

muscle was attached to the lateral epicondyle. In about 8%, a bursa was present between a capsule at the head of the radius and the overlying soft tissue; this was the so-called radiohumeral bursa. Importantly, the neurovascular anatomy showed little variation. This study supported the emerging hypothesis that tennis elbow is primarily a mechanically induced condition and that this condition is primarily related to the extensor carpi radialis brevis.

The surprising possibility of lateral elbow pain caused by a compartment syndrome of the anconeus muscle has been documented. A clinical case report revealed pressures of as much as 130 mm Hg after exercise in this muscle. After fasciotomy, the pressure decreased to 30 mm Hg. In addition, this patient had complete cessation of pain six months after fasciotomy of the anconeous muscle. The possibility of an anconeus compartment syndrome should, therefore, be kept in mind when dealing with unusual presentations of lateral elbow pain after exercise.

Disruption of the distal biceps tendon has been reported by several investigators. However, a partial rupture of the distal biceps tendon, which occurred after an acute injury, has now been shown to consist of elongation of both the laceratus fibrosus and the biceps tendon with decreased flexion and supination strength. A Z-shortening of both structures returned strength to normal. Histologic studies demonstrated a scar but no degenerative tissue.

The Forearm

Basic Science Studies

There have been only a few investigations of the function of the interosseous membrane or the mechanical interrelationship of the distal radioulnar and the proximal radioulnar joints. The issue of forces transmitted across the radial head after alterations at the distal radioulnar joint was addressed in an experimental study. In intact specimens, approximately 17% of the normal axial load was transmitted by the ulna when the forearm was in neutral

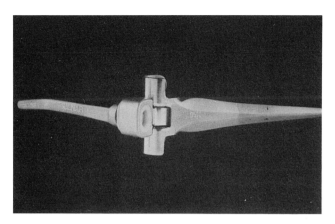

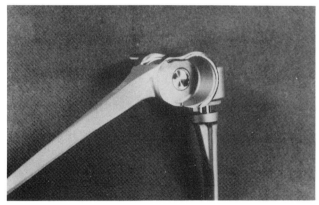

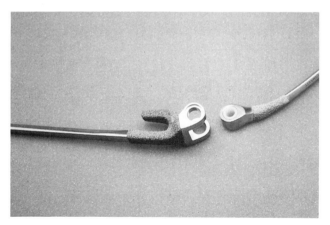

Figure 8

Semiconstrained devices allow some play at the articulation. **Top**, The modified GSB device. **Center**, The triaxial device. **Bottom**, The Mayo modified Coonrad device.

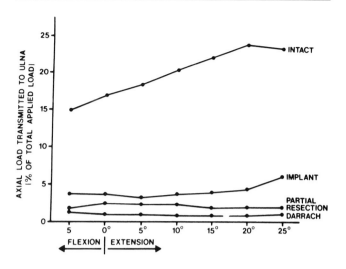

Figure 9

Dramatic decrease of axial load after resection of the distal ulna. This is not appreciably changed by the introduction of the Silastic implant. (Reproduced with permission from Trumble T, Glisson RR, Seaber AV, et al: Forearm force transmission after surgical treatment of distal radioulnar joint disorders. *J Hand Surg* 1987;12A:196–202.)

The axis of forearm rotation lies in the center of the radial head proximally and the ulnar head distally. Further, in the distal fourth of the forearm, the axis of rotation coincides with the attachment of the interosseous membrane to the ulna. This is also the strongest attachment of the interosseous membrane. The obvious implication is that angular deformities in this region may have less of an effect because they are close to the axis of rotation. Deformities in the proximal three fourths of the forearm have a greater impact on the effective length of the fibers available to rotate, possibly causing more limitation of forearm rotation.

Further study of the anatomy and mechanics of the fibers of the interosseous membrane of the forearm revealed that a dense central band of type II collagen tissue, approximately twice the thickness of the rest of the interosseous membrane, is present in almost all anatomic specimens. It was further shown that this central band constituted approximately 71% of the longitudinal stiffness of the interosseous membrane after the radial head was excised. Further, the contribution of the triangular fibrocartilage to the longitudinal stiffness of the complex was only 8%, less than that previously reported (Fig. 10). These investigators also demonstrated that when the forearm is in supination, the interosseous membrane assumes a configuration that exhibits greater stiffness and thus may possibly accommodate the increased loads placed in an axial direction. This observation is consistent with other force transmission data for the radial head. Finally, it was shown that displacement of as much as 1 cm is required for the stiffness of the system to be comparable to that of the intact interosseous membrane.

Clinical Studies

One of the most vexing questions facing the practicing orthopaedic surgeon is the advisability of removing plates after fixation of a forearm fracture. One study revealed an inordinately high incidence of refracture (seven of 23 cases)

rotation. When the distal ulna was resected, force transmission proximally decreased to an almost imperceptible 1% to 2%. Adding a distal ulnar Silastic implant did not change the mechanics; the mean proximal ulnar force transmission was only 4% after the implant was inserted. However, when the implant lengthened the ulna by 4 mm, the proximal ulnar load increased to approximately 75% of the initial normal force. The findings of this study thus tended to agree with the data that failed to demonstrate the biomechanical suitability of Silastic implants in accommodating the functional loads of the normal radial head (Fig. 9).

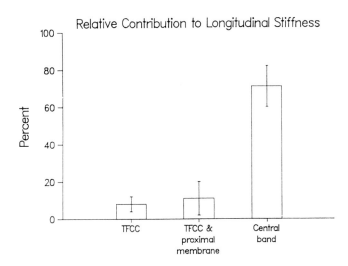

Figure 10

The relative contribution of the central band to longitudinal stiffness of the forearm. The proximal membrane refers to the portion proximal to the central band and to the triangular fibrocartilage (TFC). (Reproduced with permission from Hotchkiss RN, An K-N, Sowa DT, et al: An anatomic and mechanical study of the interosseous membrane of the forearm: The pathomechanics of proximal migration of the radius. *J Hand Surg* 1989;14A:256–261.)

after removal of the hardware. A repetition of this study in 37 patients found that seven (19%) sustained refractures of the bone through a screw hole. The time from plate removal to refracture ranged from 42 to 121 days. The clinical implications of these findings are identical to those previously reported, that is, the removal of plates from the forearm must be done with great caution and the patient must be clearly informed of the risk of this complication. Protective splints may be beneficial. The risk does seem to lessen with time, but some risk still exists as late as two years after plate removal.

Neurologic Dysfunction and Entrapment Syndrome

A host of articles have appeared on specific causes of various entrapment phenomena about the elbow. More generally, however, a prospective study of 6,500 patients attempted to identify the cause of postoperative ulnar nerve palsy. The 17 patients who developed this complication (0.26%) were examined an average of 3.5 years after the surgery. The electromyographic studies showed slowing of the conduction time in the normal extremity, suggesting the important clinical possibility of a predisposition to the condition. These investigators concluded that many patients may have a subclinical ulnar neuropathy that becomes symptomatic as a result of surgical maneuvers and tourniquet application. Similarly, a review of compression neuropathies in the anterior forearm emphasized that bilateral nerve entrapment should prompt the physician to consider a systemic process such as diabetes or cervical arthritis rather than a local origin. Importantly, it should also be noted that the bilateral entrapment syndromes respond less predictably to surgical decompression.

A most interesting study of the blood supply to the ulnar nerve demonstrated that dissection of the ulnar nerve and

anterior translocation do not disrupt the intraneural vascular pattern. Intraneural neurolysis does, however, disrupt the circulation of the nerve, and the intraneural vessel plexus is destroyed after interfascicular neurolysis. Ulnar nerve translocation was assessed clinically in a long-term study in which the nerve was translocated anteriorly into the muscular groove. Of 27 procedures followed up for an average of nine years in which motor deficit was the primary finding, 21 (78%) were considered satisfactory on the basis of electromyographic evaluation. These investigators further demonstrated that results were less gratifying if symptoms had been present for longer than one year.

Among the many reported causes of posterior interosseous nerve compression at the elbow are synovial chondromatosis and bicipital bursa. The radial sensory nerve may be compressed by a ganglion cyst arising from the elbow joint. A case of median nerve compression causing the so-called pronator syndrome was reportedly the result of a persistent median artery in the region of the elbow joint.

Soft-Tissue Coverage

Significant attention has been given to soft-tissue coverage about the forearm and elbow in the nonorthopaedic literature. A free radial forearm flap has become a popular method of treating some soft-tissue defects in the proximal forearm and elbow. However, providing asymptomatic secondary coverage of the donor site has proven to be a problem. Covering the donor site with a split-thickness skin graft and then immobilizing the forearm and wrist for ten days effectively decreased this secondary effect in 14 of 16 patients.

In another study of the radial forearm flap in 15 patients at two centers, complications include delayed healing, prolonged swelling, persistent pain and stiffness in the hand, and measurably reduced hand and wrist strength. Nonetheless, a free radial forearm flap can be a valuable adjunct in a variety of soft-tissue problems and can help salvage a short, below-elbow amputation.

Controversies

Diagnostic and Anatomic Studies

As new imaging technologies are developed, their usefulness and application to various anatomic parts and pathologic conditions must be investigated. Computed tomography and magnetic resonance imaging are rarely indicated for elbow conditions because almost all elbow abnormalities can be diagnosed by means of a careful examination and routine tomography or radiography. The relative ease with which elbow conditions can be diagnosed is one of the reasons that elbow arthroscopy has a definite although limited place in the diagnostic armamentarium. Nonetheless, investigators should continue to explore the applications of the newer imaging techniques. These techniques should not be overused or employed as an alternative to a careful and thoughtful routine examination.

Elbow Synovectomy

Synovectomy of the elbow prompts as many controversies, or at least questions, as any reconstructive procedure about the elbow. Differences in opinion exist with regard to whether the single lateral incision is adequate or whether a supplemental medial incision is needed to allow more complete synovial removal. To date, the lateral incision appears to be completely sufficient.

The question of whether or not a synovectomy can be redone should the first procedure fail has been addressed only occasionally. This does not seem to be a relevant issue if the initial procedure is done in the more advanced stages. If the synovectomy is performed in the earlier course of the disease, a second synovectomy may be appropriate if the patient has symptoms that would justify an initial procedure.

Another issue is whether synovectomy should be chemically induced with agents such as yttrium or osmic acid or should continue to be surgically performed either by an open procedure or arthroscopically. There are no data on the merits or disadvantages of arthroscopic synovectomy and the data on nonsurgical chemical synovectomy are incomplete. As those who are knowledgeable about elbow abnormalities and arthroscopic techniques perform and report the results of arthroscopic synovectomies, this particular issue may be resolved.

Another relevant question is how severe joint involvement must be before synovectomy (with or without radial head excision) ceases to be beneficial. In Europe the procedure is being done for more advanced stages of the disease, perhaps because of poor results obtained with the alternative procedure, joint replacement. Because elbow joint replacement is becoming a reliable operation in the United States, most surgeons in this country reserve synovectomy with radial head excision for less severe disease. Since a more severely damaged joint is even more unstable after synovectomy and radial head excision, joint replacement is usually done in such cases.

There is some controversy as to whether or not a radial head implant should be used after synovectomy with radial head excision. If the synovectomy is performed in the earlier stages of the disease, the radial head is sometimes relatively uninvolved. However, if the radial head is removed in early-stage disease, the medial collateral ligament tends to be adequate and the implant is not needed. Because synovectomy should not be performed in the later stages of the disease when the medial collateral ligament is deficient, the need for an implant is again questionable. Although there are anecdotal reports with regard to the value of radial head implant with this procedure, to date the data do not support its routine use.

Total Elbow Replacement

Probably no greater controversy exists with regard to the elbow than joint replacement arthroplasty. Clinicians' opinions vary greatly with respect to the optimum design for elbow joint replacement. The disappointing early results with constrained joint replacements have prompted some to recommend the use of resurfacing designs or synovectomy for severely involved joints. Others, however, have taken a more moderate approach, believing that there is a spectrum of abnormality that may be best addressed by a spectrum of options. Unfortunately, because most surgeons are familiar with only a single design or only one

is available to them, a need for a single optimum design seems to be emerging. Clearly, there is a trade-off between elbow instability and implant loosening with any resurfacing design. The recent data continue to demonstrate that resurfacing implants have an instability rate of about 10%. Conversely, data appearing (to date) only in unrefereed journals suggest that semiconstrained devices have significantly decreased the incidence of loosening, shown no instability, and may be successful in joints with more damage, including those undergoing difficult revision procedures.

Surface coatings for biologic fixation are being used on several available implants but their value has not yet been demonstrated. Although uncemented devices are not generally suitable for patients with rheumatoid arthritis, this is the most common condition meriting elbow replacement. Hence, this technology may have limited application for the elbow. Currently, the experienced surgeon has several options that can be offered with confidence in cases of rheumatoid arthritis and with optimism in posttraumatic and difficult salvage cases. It is obvious, however, that elbow joint replacement should be performed only by experienced surgeons who have determined that no other options are suitable for the patient with severe elbow dysfunction.

The Forearm

The optimum management of distal radioulnar problems remains one of the more difficult issues. The effect of distal ulnar resection on the mechanics of the elbow has not been completely studied but what is known does help to explain the complications associated with a so-called Essex-Lopresti injury. Because distal radioulnar dissociation or disruption virtually eliminates the ability of the proximal ulna to transmit forces, radial head resection is followed by proximal radial migration. The stiffness characteristics of the interosseous membrane and its load-absorbing quality provide some explanation of the biomechanical unsuitability of the Silastic implant. Nonetheless, studies have demonstrated the importance of the radiohumeral joint and of preserving the radial head whenever possible. Thus, emphasis should probably be placed on open reduction and internal fixation for radial head fractures whenever possible. Present data seem to suggest that a radial head implant of a material other than Silastic may be beneficial. Nonetheless, because of the relative infrequency of concurrent injuries of the wrist and elbow, which result in such difficult management problems, a new-generation radial head implant fabricated from a more suitable material is not likely in the near future.

The issue of whether or not to remove plates from the forearm remains controversial. The recent data clearly support leaving the plates in place unless there is some compelling reason for their removal. It should be noted that fractures proximal to the plate, one of the stated reasons for removal, are very uncommon. If the implant must be removed, the patient must be warned and, ideally, the forearm protected with a splint (although in fact the protective value of forearm splints has not been clearly demonstrated). A splint may at least remind the patient to limit the amount of lifting forces applied to the extremity.

Annotated Bibliography

Keywords

Arthroplasty; Elbow; Entrapment syndrome; Forearm; Grafting; Prostheses; Radial head; Rheumatoid arthritis; Sports medicine; Synovectomy

Diagnostic and Anatomic Studies

Chen J, Alk D, Eventov I, et al: Development of the olecranon bursa: An anatomic cadaver study. *Acta Orthop Scand* 1987;58:408–409.

No olecranon bursa was found in individuals less than 10 years old.

Quinton DN, Finlay D, Butterworth R: The elbow fat pad sign: Brief report. *J Bone Joint Surg* 1987;69B:844–845.

Without clinical evidence suggesting fracture, a positive fat-pad sign represents significant intra-articular abnormality in only about 10% of patients. This usually involves a missed radial head fracture.

Singson RD, Feldman F, Rosenberg ZS: Elbow joint: Assessment with double-contrast CT arthrography. *Radiology* 1986;160:167–173.

Little evidence is presented to justify the use of double-contrast computed tomography in the routine assessment of the elbow.

Elbow Synovectomy

Le Balc'h T, Ebelin M, Laurian Y, et al: Synovectomy of the elbow in young hemophiliac patients. *J Bone Joint Surg* 1987;69A:264–269.

Confirms the role of synovectomy in decreasing the number of recurrent hemorrhagic episodes in the elbow, as was done previously with regard to the knee.

Saito T, Koshino T, Okamoto R, et al: Radical synovectomy with muscle release for the rheumatoid elbow. *Acta Orthop Scand* 1986;57:71–73.

This previously unreported release of the common flexor and extensor tendons appears to improve the arc of motion after radical synovectomy for rheumatoid arthritis of the elbow.

Traumatic Conditions of the Elbow

Ackerman G, Jupiter JB: Non-union of fractures of the distal end of the humerus. *J Bone Joint Surg* 1988;70A:75–83.

This excellent study demonstrated that surgery led to modest (35%) objective satisfaction despite a very successful rate of union.

Arafiles RP: Neglected posterior dislocation of the elbow: A reconstruction operation. *J Bone Joint Surg* 1987;69B:199–202.

A surgical approach for reconstructing the medial collateral ligament supplemented with an intra-articular "anterior cruciate" type of reconstruction for the ignored or missed chronic posterior dislocated elbow.

Breen TF, Gelberman RH, Ackerman GN: Elbow flexion contractures: Treatment by anterior release and continuous passive motion. *J Hand Surg* 1988;13B:286–287.

Case reports emphasizing, without actually proving, the value of continuous passive motion after anterior capsule release for posttraumatic elbow flexion contracture.

Josefsson P, Gentz C, Johnell O, et al: Surgical versus nonsurgical treatment of ligamentous injuries following dislocation of the elbow. *J Bone Joint Surg* 1987;69A:605.

This careful prospective study demonstrated the clinically accepted impression that surgical reconstruction of the collateral ligaments is of no clinical value in acute elbow dislocation.

Morrey BF: Treatment of the posttraumatic stiff elbow: Distraction arthroplasty. *J Bone Joint Surg*, in press.

This technique, which is described in detail, improved motion from a preoperative range of 60 to 90 degrees to 30 to 125 degrees in 26 patients.

Tsuge K, Murakami T, Yasunaga Y, et al: Arthroplasty of the elbow: Twenty years' experience with a new operation. *J Bone Joint Surg* 1987;69B:116–120.

This work is of significant merit as regards the description of the surgical technique. This is an important contribution to a better understanding of the surgical technique of restoring motion to the posttraumatic stiff elbow.

Total Elbow Arthroplasty

Bell S, Gschwend N, Steiger U: Arthroplasty of the elbow: Experience with the Mark III GSB prosthesis. *Aust NZ J Surg* 1986;56:823–827.

Supports the emerging data suggesting that semiconstrained devices are performing much more satisfactorily than the more constrained designs. This report of 45 patients demonstrated 87% satisfactory results after an average follow-up of 2.5 years. The complication rates are decreasing and there was no instability.

Figgie HE III, Inglis AE, Ranawat CS, et al: Results of total elbow arthroplasty as a salvage procedure for failed elbow reconstructive operations. *Clin Orthop* 1987;219:185–193.

The authors demonstrated that a semiconstrained implant can be an effective salvage procedure for failed total joint or other elbow reconstructive procedures. The results were encouraging.

Friedman RJ, Ewald FC: Arthroplasty of the ipsilateral shoulder and elbow in patients who have rheumatoid arthritis. *J Bone Joint Surg* 1987;69A:661–666.

A retrospective review led the authors to conclude that elbow joint replacement somehow protects the extremity from requiring a shoulder replacement in a more advantageous fashion than if the shoulder procedure is done first. Emphasis is placed on the fact that the most symptomatic joint should be done first.

Morrey BF, Askew LJ, An K-N: Strength function after elbow arthroplasty. *Clin Orthop* 1988;234:43–50.

Strength improves an average of 70% after joint replacement in patients with rheumatoid arthritis and 25% in those with nonrheumatoid diseases. Extensor strength may be improved in the patients with rheumatoid arthritis but is often weak in the posttraumatic patient.

Morrey BF, Bryan RS: Revision total elbow arthroplasty. *J Bone Joint Surg* 1987;69A:523–532.

Of 33 reimplant revision procedures, 55% were satisfactory after the first procedure and 75% were considered satisfactory after an additional revision operation. The complication rate was high but acceptable for this type of difficult case. The semiconstrained modified Coonrad implant appears to be a promising salvage procedure.

Roper BA, Tuke M, O'Riordan SM, et al: A new unconstrained elbow: A prospective review of 60 replacements. *J Bone Joint Surg* 1986;68B:566–569.

Several resurfacing designs were used over a nine-year period. The complication failure rate was similar to those in early reports on other designs. The study emphasizes the inherent complication rate and technical difficulty of doing elbow joint replacement.

Ross AC, Sneath RS, Scales JT: Endoprosthetic replacement of the humerus and elbow joint. *J Bone Joint Surg* 1987;69B:652–655.

The major value is the historical description of a constrained implant for difficult distal humeral problems. The complication rate of 150% serves to indicate the difficulty of such cases.

Sourmelis SG, Burke FD, Varian JP: A review of total elbow arthroplasty and an early assessment of the Liverpool elbow prosthesis. *J Hand Surg* 1986;11B:407–413.

The study provides little additional information regarding the early experience with resurfacing implants but again emphasizes the high complication rate (10% with loosening, 14% with infection, and 20% with ulnar nerve complications).

Trancik T, Wilde AH, Borden LS: Capitellocondylar total elbow athroplasty: Two- to eight-year experience. *Clin Orthop* 1987;223:175–180.

A report of 35 capitellocondylar resurfacing protheses used in patients with rheumatoid arthritis demonstrated a complication rate of more than 50% but many did not compromise the final result, which was satisfactory in approximately 90%. A radiolucent line around the ulnar component was noted in as many as 30% of the patients.

Wevers HW, Siu DW, Broekhoven LH, et al: Resurfacing elbow prosthesis: Shape and sizing of the humeral component. *J Biomed Eng* 1985;7:241–246.

The major value of this work is the care with which these investigators defined the humeral contour and axis of rotation. This will permit accurate replication with resurfacing designs and has implications for surgical technique and soft-tissue balance.

Sports-Related Injuries

Abrahamsson S-O, Sollerman C, Söderberg T, et al: Lateral elbow pain caused by anconeus compartment syndrome: A case report. *Acta Orthop Scand* 1987;58:589–591.

The authors documented increased compartment pressure in the anconeus that is relieved by fasciotomy. This provides an additional explanation for lateral elbow pain that is not caused by epicondylitis.

Briggs CA, Elliott BG: Lateral epicondylitis: A review of structures associated with tennis elbow. *Anat Clin* 1985;7:149–153.

A worthwhile review of possible anatomic causes of "lateral epicondylitis." This study supports the hypothesis that tennis elbow is primarily a mechanically induced condition and describes the varied anatomic distribution of the extensor carpi radialis brevis origin. It helps explain why it tends to be the primary site of involvement.

Jobe FW, Stark H, Lombardo SJ: Reconstruction of the ulnar collateral ligament in athletes. *J Bone Joint Surg* 1986;68A:1158–1163.

Demonstration of a reconstructive procedure for medial collateral ligament deficiency of the elbow in the athlete. The results (approximately 60% satisfactory) in the 16 patients treated were impressive because this population consists of high-performance throwers.

Jones DA, Newham DJ, Clarkson PM: Skeletal muscle stiffness and pain following eccentric exercise of the elbow flexors. *Pain* 1987;30:233–242.

On the basis of electromyographic data, the authors concluded that pain after exercise is a response to damaged connective tissue rather than an inherent abnormality of the muscle itself.

Nielsen K: Partial rupture of the distal biceps brachii tendon: A case report. *Acta Orthop Scand* 1987;58:287–288.

This case report of a stretched distal biceps tendon rupture is the first of its kind. It was treated effectively by Z-shortening of the biceps tendon and laceratus fibrosus.

Sisto DJ, Jobe FW, Moynes DR, et al: An electromyographic analysis of the elbow in pitching. *Am J Sports Med* 1987;15:260–263.

Simultaneous electromyography of the forearm musculature failed to demonstrate differences of activity for curve and fast balls. Hence, muscle activity is not related to the known chronic medial elbow problems associated with throwing a breaking ball.

The Forearm

DeLuca PA, Lindsey RW, Ruwe PA: Refracture of bones in the forearm after removal of compression plates. *J Bone Joint Surg* 1988;70A:1372–1376.

The high incidence of refracture through holes in bone after plate removal (19%) confirmed previous findings.

Hidaka S, Gustilo RB: Refracture of bones of the forearm after plate removal. *J Bone Joint Surg* 1984;66A:1241–1243.

Refracture in seven of 23 patients after plate removal prompts reconsideration of the value of removing the metallic implants in a routine manner in such patients.

Hotchkiss RN, An K-N, Sowa DT, et al: An anatomic and mechanical study of the interosseous membrane of the forearm: The pathomechanics of proximal migration of the radius. *J Hand Surg* 1989;14A:256–261.

A thickening in the middle third of the interosseous membrane was identified. The Silastic radial head implant was unable to compensate for the lost stiffness on axial load.

Mori K: Experimental study on rotation of the forearm: Functional anatomy of the interosseous membrane. *Nippon Seikeigeka Gakkai Zasshi* 1985;59:611–622.

Forearm rotation axis goes through the radial head and the center of the distal ulna. This axis coincides with the ulnar attachment of the interosseous membrane in the distal quarter of the forearm. This has implications for forearm angular deformity.

Trumble T, Glisson RR, Seaber AV, et al: Forearm force transmission after surgical treatment of distal radioulnar joint disorders. *J Hand Surg* 1987;12A:196–202.

Resection of the distal ulna results in virtual loss of proximal ulnohumeral force transmission with axial load. A distal ulnar Silastic implant does not restore this lost force-transmission capacity.

Neurologic Dysfunction and Entrapment Syndrome

Altissimi M, Pecorelli F, Pimpinelli G: Ulnar nerve compression at the elbow. *Ital J Orthop Traumatol* 1986;12:395–399.

This was a long-term study of the results of anterior translocation of the ulnar nerve into the muscular groove. Results were considered satisfactory in 78% on the basis of motor evaluation at follow-up. The results were less gratifying when the symptoms had been present for longer than one year.

Alvine FG, Schurrer ME: Postoperative ulnar-nerve palsy: Are there predisposing factors? *J Bone Joint Surg* 1987;69A:255–259.
Interesting study of more than 6,500 patients demonstrated ulnar nerve palsy after upper-extremity tourniquet procedures in only 0.26%. A long-term electromyographic evaluation of the group with palsy demonstrated that possible familial abnormalities predispose to this complication.

ei-Hadidi S, Burke FD: Posterior interosseous nerve syndrome caused by a bursa in the vicinity of the elbow. *J Hand Surg* 1987;12B:23–24.
A patient with posterior interosseous nerve syndrome had difficulty extending the metacarpophalangeal joint of the fifth finger. A bicipital bursa was identified and recovery followed decompression of the bursa.

Gainor BJ, Jeffries JT: Pronator syndrome associated with a persistent median artery: A case report. *J Bone Joint Surg* 1987;69A:303–304.
A case report of this condition.

Graf P, Hawe W, Biemer E: Gefassversorgund des N. ulnaris nach Neurolyse im Ellenbogenbereich. [A vascular study of ulnar nerve following neurolysis in the area of the elbow.] *Handchir Mikrochir Plast Chir* 1986;18:204–206.
This interesting study demonstrated that the blood supply to the nerve was not disturbed after decompression or after dissection of the nerve. After infrafascicular neurolysis, the intraneural vessel plexus was destroyed.

Hermansdorfer JD, Greider JL, Dell PC: A case report of a compressive neuropathy of the radial sensory nerve caused by a ganglion cyst at the elbow. *Orthopedics* 1986;9:1005–1006.
A case of a ganglion cyst from the elbow joint causing compression of the radial sensory nerve.

Howard FM: Compression neuropathies in the anterior forearm. *Hand Clin* 1986;2:737–745.
The author emphasizes that bilateral nerve entrapment is most commonly caused by diabetes mellitus or cervical arthritis. Such bilateral entrapment responds less predictably to surgical decompression.

Jones JR, Evans DM, Kaushik A: Synovial chondromatosis presenting with peripheral nerve compression: A report of two cases. *J Hand Surg* 1987;12B:25–27.
Synovial chondromatosis caused median nerve compression at the wrist and posterior interosseous nerve compression at the elbow. As in previously reported cases, recovery follows decompression.

Soft-Tissue Coverage

Jones NF, Hardesty RA, Goldstein SA, et al: Upper limb salvage using a free radial forearm flap. *Plast Reconstr Surg* 1987;79:468–471.
A case report in which the free radial forearm flap was used to salvage a very short below-elbow amputation.

McGregor AD: The free radial forearm flap: The management of the secondary defect. *Br J Plast Surg* 1987;40:83–85.
A split-thickness skin graft is used to cover the donor site of the free radial forearm flap. This technique decreases the morbidity of this procedure.

Timmons MJ, Missotten FE, Poole MD, et al: Complications of radial forearm flap donor sites. *Br J Plast Surg* 1986;39:176–178.
Documents the various complications in 15 patients from two centers who were treated with the free radial forearm flap. Despite the complication rate, this is considered to be a valuable reconstructive procedure for soft-tissue defects about the elbow.

29

Wrist and Hand: Trauma

Cumulative trauma and occupationally induced overuse syndromes are receiving intense study from hand surgeons, industry, and compensation carriers. It is now generally recognized that surgical treatment, although often effective in the short run, is not itself curative for this type of injury. Modification of the work environment is often required.

Carpal instability is a major focus of basic and clinical investigation. Early diagnosis and anatomic repair are crucial for consistent long-term results.

Fractures of the distal radius continue to attract attention. Anatomic restoration of the articular surface, by open reduction if necessary, is needed for a lasting satisfactory functional result.

The technical evolution of small plates, screws, and external fixators, coupled with careful surgical technique and early motion, now allow good results in a higher percentage of unstable and complex finger fractures.

The technical application of microsurgical repair to the hand and wrist continues to expand. Although the cost-effectiveness and patient acceptance of single-digit reconstruction continue to arouse controversy, emergency free flap coverage of severe open injuries is gaining acceptance.

In acute flexor tendon repairs, the "finishing" stitch has assumed more importance and improved techniques of early controlled mobilization are now also advocated for some extensor injuries as well.

Occupational Disorders

De Quervain's tenosynovitis is often part of a complex of work-related syndromes. In one recent series, 27 women with de Quervain's tenosynovitis had 31 associated diagnoses; in the 19 surgically treated patients, there were 14 complications.

Epidemiologic studies have shown a strong correlation beween high-frequency (more than 2 cycles per minute) and high-force (more than 6 kg) work exposure with a variety of conditions, including de Quervain's tenosynovitis, trigger finger, and other forms of tenosynovitis. The combination of high repetition and high force increased the likelihood of developing these symptoms 29-fold. Job modifications and improved work-station design have the potential to reduce job-related overuse syndromes. In one study, adding a five-minute exercise break every 90 minutes significantly improved hand blood flow in assembly workers. Ergonomic studies have shown that tool handles should be roughly 6 cm in diameter and extend completely across the palm. In general, tools should weigh no more than 1.5 kg and the center of mass should be in the grip area. Work space should be tailored to the worker's height; shoulder flexion or abduction beyond 60 degrees should be avoided and in general the elbow should be comfortably flexed, the forearm in midpronation, and the wrist in neu-

tral or slight extension. Jobs that deviate from these specifications have been shown to have an increased risk for cumulative trauma disorders.

Wrist Injuries

Fractures of the Distal Radius

Some studies have suggested that postural instability may predispose to the falls that are associated with Colles' fractures in the elderly. Thus, a combination of postural instability and osteoporosis may be responsible for the high incidence of Colles' fractures in elderly women. Treatment of both problems may be necessary to reduce the risk of this injury. Follow-up studies of Colles' fracture continue to belie the dictum that "perfect freedom" of motion and function result when malunion is accepted. Patients whose fractures healed with 5 mm or more of shortening had, on average, only 75% of the grip strength present in patients whose fractures healed with 1 mm or less of shortening. Experimental work with pressure-sensitive film has shown that small angular changes in the carpal face of the radius produce significant changes in the location of load-bearing areas. Dorsal angulation of 30 degrees increased the load on the ulna from 21% of the total radioulnar load to 50%. This abnormal loading may predispose to the ulnocarpal impingement syndrome, a triad of pain, triangular fibrocartilage tear, and lunotriquetral instability. In addition, proximal carpal row motion is reduced by the radial malalignment and cannot respond to load from the capitate-metacarpal unit. Midcarpal motion may become erratic, painful, and unstable.

In young adults particularly, accurate reduction of the articular surface appears critical to achievement of a good result after Colles' fracture. In one study of 24 young adult patients whose intra-articular Colles' fractures healed with more than 1 mm of articular incongruity, 91% had post-traumatic arthritis and 57% had unsatisfactory clinical function after a minimum follow-up of two years. External fixation alone is often not sufficient to achieve or maintain reduction of severely comminuted intra-articular fractures; in another series of 76 such patients, complications occurred in more than 50% and malunion in 15%. One classification of intra-articular fractures emphasized the lunate impaction "die-punch" fracture of the distal radius. These fractures are the result of violent forces and separate the medial half of the radius into dorsal and volar fragments. Often in such fractures articular congruity cannot be achieved or maintained by closed reduction. For such fractures, open reduction is advised. Depending on comminution, fixation may be best achieved with plates and screws, Kirschner wires, external fixation, or some combination of these. Bone grafting is often necessary as well.

Scaphoid Fractures

In scaphoid fractures with displaced or angulated proximal fragments that do not respond to the usual reduction maneuver, associated scapholunate ligament disruption should be suspected. If proper alignment of the scaphoid is maintained but the remainder of the proximal row is not correctly aligned, then scapholunate ligament disruption is again likely. In one study of 20 patients with scaphoid nonunions, 13 had a scapholunate ligament rupture confirmed at surgery. Carpal malalignment after scaphoid fracture, whether from nonunion, malunion, or untreated intercarpal ligament injury, has a clear and prejudicial effect on functional outcome. Because of the importance of scaphoid alignment to the result, a more accurate way to view the scaphoid than routine radiography is needed. Computed tomography in the plane of the scaphoid long axis can be helpful.

The long-term sequelae of scaphoid nonunion were outlined in *Orthopaedic Knowledge Update 2*. Recent work has shown that malunion is similarly detrimental. In experimental osteotomies, scaphoid angulation of 15 degrees or more significantly impaired wrist motion; healed fractures with dorsal carpal instability showed 47% poor functional results in one series. If symptomatic malunion wih dorsal carpal instability is treated by open reduction, including osteotomy of the malunited scaphoid, improved motion and strength can result.

Carpal Instability

The diagnosis and appropriate treatment of carpal instability remain problematic. Two reports on the long-term follow-up of lunate and perilunate dislocations indicate that poor outcome depended more on the presence of a scapholunate gap at the end of treatment than it did on delay in treatment. Experimental studies have shown that the resulting malalignment dramatically alters wrist joint loading. Patients with scapholunate dissociation may be more likely to have negative ulnar variance than normal subjects. This may further increase the loading of the distal radius. The causative significance of the association of scapholunate dissociation and negative ulnar variance is unclear. Scapholunate dissociation is also suspected of playing a role in scaphoid nonunion, as an injury at both ends of an intra-articular segment would probably result not only in altered vascularity but also in altered control of the proximal scaphoid segment by wrist positioning.

The injury producing a newly described instability pattern—posttraumatic ulnar translation—is thought to occur in a pronated forearm with the wrist hyperextended and ulnarly deviated (Fig. 1). This stretches the radial volar carpal ligaments. Ligament failure results in a slowly developing ulnar translation of the entire carpus. This is actually a type of radiocarpal dislocation and can be accompanied by other ligament ruptures such as scapholunate ligament rupture. The diagnosis of ulnar translation instability is often delayed, repair is difficult, and the results of treatment have so far been disappointing. Early arthroscopy may help make the diagnosis at a time when treatment might be more effective.

Treatment of complex carpal instabilities remains difficult. The optimum treatment would allow accurate early diagnosis with secure fixation in as normal a position as possible. Early diagnostic maneuvers now include arthroscopy to assist in visualization. For complex fracture-dis-locations, external fixation can be a useful adjunct to reduction, as well as to supplement internal fixation postoperatively. In one recent series, seven of ten patients had good results after open reduction and combined internal and external fixation.

Fractures and Dislocations in the Hand

Metacarpal and Phalangeal Fractures

The emphasis on managing unstable fractures continues to be on early, accurate, stable reduction. In general, for hand fractures the simplest form of fixation consistent with satisfactory reduction and early mobilization is preferred. For most fractures, simple cast or splint protection suffices; for many others, percutaneous or open fixation with K-wires provides the requisite stability. In selected cases, more rigid internal fixation may be indicated. In one report, miniature plates and screws were used to treat 52 fractures that were irreducible or for which acceptable reduction could not be maintained while still permitting mobilization of adjacent joints. Final total active motion in this selected group of patients was more than 90% of normal, and there was only one major complication. The technique of open reduction and internal fixation is critical to the end result when this method of treatment is chosen, however; in another report, five of 17 metacarpal fractures and three of six phalangeal fractures treated by open reduction and plate fixation were complicated by stiffness, malunion, or nonunion.

For severely comminuted or contaminated fractures, miniature external fixators (Fig. 2) can maintain length and alignment while permitting wound access for debridement or bone grafting. Joint stiffness can be a problem, however, particularly at the level of the proximal interphalangeal joint.

Nonunions of metacarpals and phalanges, although rare, do occur; a recent review of 25 nonunions showed unstable internal fixation with K-wires to be a factor in most cases. Rigid internal fixation with plates and screws and supplemental bone grafts provided the best results, with both sound union and greatly improved motion.

Ligament Injuries

A new classification of injury to the ulnar collateral ligament of the thumb has been proposed and correlated with a treatment program. The diagnosis and treatment scheme are based on a stress test of the metacarpophalangeal joint in full flexion and standard radiographs (Table 1). Seventy percent of the patients with type IV injuries had a displaced collateral ligament (Stener lesion). Early identification of surgical candidates seems worthwhile in these injuries; in one report patients whose surgery was delayed three weeks or more did worse than those with more immediate repairs.

The failure mechanism of the lateral ligaments of the proximal interphalangeal joint appears to begin with a separation from the proximal phalanx, with the tear proceeding distally along the interface between the proper and accessory collateral ligaments. It then progresses by the "critical corner" of the base of the middle phalanx to the distal volar plate (Fig. 3). Angulation of more than 20 degrees on stress testing indicates complete ligament rupture. Infolding of the ligament is rare; usually the ligament returns to its normal anatomic position. On the basis of this

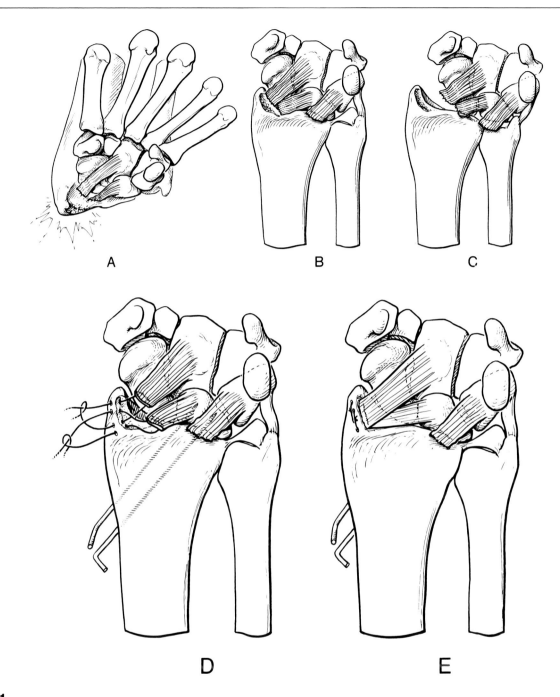

Figure 1
Posttraumatic ulnar translation. **A**, The injury force. **B**, Failure of early ligament healing. **C**, Translation to ulnar side. **D** and **E**, Repair and pin fixation. (Reproduced with permission of the Mayo Foundation from Rayhack JM, Linscheid RL, Dobyns JH, et al: Posttraumatic ulnar translation of the carpus. *J Hand Surg* 1987;12A:180–189.)

evidence, nonsurgical treatment seems appropriate for ligament injuries that do not show angulation of more than 20 degrees on stress, and possibly also for complete tears without deformity suggesting ligament infolding.

Microsurgery

Microsurgical applications in the hand continue to expand. An emergency free flap is one that is applied within the first few days after a severe injury. Basic principles of wound management must be strictly followed. Severely contaminated wounds require several debridements before the surgeon can be sure that all contaminated tissue has been removed. A wide excision of damaged and contaminated tissue, along oncologic principles, is the goal. If, after debridement, local cover is not possible, an emergency free flap can be considered. Such tissue can be a source not only of skin and soft-tissue cover, but also, depending on the source, vascularized bone, nerve, and tendon segments

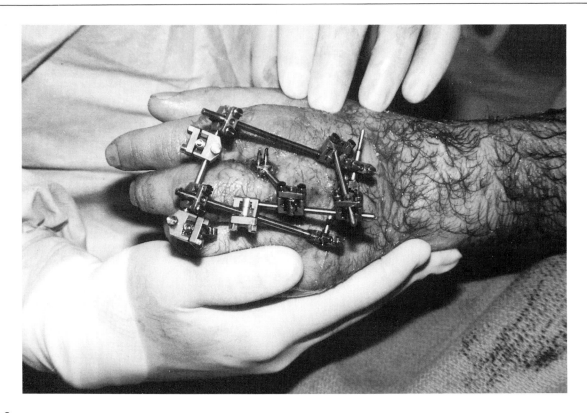

Figure 2
A miniature external fixator can be useful in maintaining the length of severely comminuted bony segments while permitting mobilization of adjacent uninjured joints.

as well. Early free flap coverage can reduce the infection rate, hospital stay, and the need for further surgery. Also, in one study the success rate of emergency free flaps was actually greater than that of delayed free flap coverage of similar wounds.

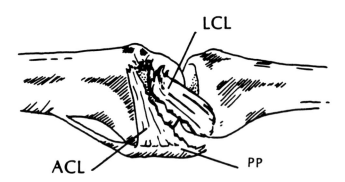

Figure 3
The sequence of proper collateral ligament rupture. The lateral collateral ligament (LCL) remains attached to the middle phalanx while the accessory collateral ligament (ACL) and palmar plate (PP) remain attached to the proximal phalanx. The palmar plate may be avulsed with a fragment of bone from the palmar aspect of the middle phalanx as well. (Reproduced with permission from Kiefhaber TR, Stern PJ, Grood ES: Lateral stability of the proximal interphalangeal joint. *J Hand Surg* 1986;11A:661–669.)

Table 1. Classification of injuries to the ulnar collateral ligament of the metacarpophalangeal joint of the thumb

Injury	Fracture	Examination	Treatment
Type I	Undisplaced	No stress	Cast
Type II	Displaced	Not needed	ORIF
Type III	None	Stable	Cast
Type IV	None	Unstable	Repair
Type V	Volar plate	Stable	Cast

Tendon Injuries

Flexor Tendon

The techniques of flexor tendon repair and rehabilitation continue to be refined. Primary repair calls for a core-grasping suture, generally followed by a circumferential finishing suture to finish or "tidy" the repair. A recent laboratory investigation suggested that the finishing suture may have more than a cosmetic importance. The holding power of a running Lembert "tidying" stitch alone exceeds 1 kg. The force needed to produce a gap at a repair fixed with a standard core-grasping suture increased from 1 kg to 3 kg when a running Lembert tidying suture was added.

Rehabilitation after repair continues to emphasize early controlled mobilization. When closely supervised, passive motion and rubber-band flexion-active extension exercises are combined with a splint having a palmar pulley to increase the joint flexion possible from the rubber band. Total active motion in excess of 180 degrees can be obtained in as many as 95% of patients. Strength may be more difficult to restore; after repair the mean grip of the injured hand may be only 75% of that of the uninjured side.

With any method of tendon rehabilitation, tendon rupture may complicate the recovery. Early recognition and rerepair using the same technique as the primary repair can salvage a good or excellent result in approximately 60% of patients.

Flexor tendon advancement as a technique of flexor restoration may have some advantage over end-to-end repair if employed within strict limits. Because of the combined muscle belly for the four flexor digitorum profundus tendons, however, advancement of one tendon affects the other three. This is known as the "quadriga effect." Cadaver studies suggest that advancement results in loss of less than 20 degrees of extension in the injured digit and less than 1 cm of flexion lag in adjacent digits if the advancement is no more than 1.5 cm in the index finger or 1.0 cm in the other fingers.

Extensor Tendon

Controlled mobilization has become the standard rehabilitation method for flexor injuries in the hand. This method is now gaining favor for extensor injuries as well. Two recent series showed good results with this technique for extensor injuries between the midproximal phalanx and the wrist; central slip injuries fared less well. It appears that 5 mm of repair-site excursion is sufficient to reduce adhesions clinically. This can be obtained with 30 to 40 degrees of metacarpophalangeal joint motion in a dynamic extension splint (Fig. 4).

Nerve Injuries

Recent cadaver studies have confirmed the anatomic basis of grouped fascicular repair for the median and ulnar nerves at the wrist. The internal topography of these nerves is consistent between individuals and for lengths of 10 cm or more along the course of the nerve. As an adjunct to topographic nerve maps, biochemical identification of motor and sensory axoplasm may soon be possible within the time constraints of a surgical procedure to aid fascicular matching. Choline acetylase is present in motor axoplasm at eight times its concentration in sensory axoplasm. It can be assayed in 70 to 80 minutes and remains increased for as long as five months after injury. Convincing clinical evidence of improved results for nerve repair using improved fascicle-matching techniques, however, has yet to be produced.

Infections

Human bites, infections secondary to intravenous drug abuse, septic flexor tenosynovitis, and other serious hand infections are often polymicrobial and susceptible to complications. One recent comparative study showed improved results for such infections when they were treated by a protocol including hospitalization, drainage in the operating room, intravenous antibiotics, open wound management, and early mobilization. Readmissions dropped from 10% to 1%, reoperations from 34% to 1%, and chronic arthritis from 10% to 3%, compared with the nonstandardized treatments used before institution of the protocol.

Infection with *Mycobacterium marinum* is uncommon, and may be confused with nonseptic tenosynovitis. The most common history for this infection is a puncture wound from contact with a fish or crustacean. Delay in diagnosis is common, and local steroid injections may exacerbate the symptoms. Diagnosis depends upon culture of fluid or tissue in specific media at 31 C. Treatment with oral rifampin and ethambutol is often successful; recalcitrant cases usually respond to surgical debridement.

Burns

Hydrofluoric acid is used widely in industry in the manufacture of fluorocarbons, aluminum, and semiconductors, and in oil refining. Hydrofluoric acid burns differ from other chemical burns in that the fluoride ion easily penetrates the skin, and can cause deep tissue damage that can continue for days. Treatment requires the neutralization and precipitation of the absorbed fluoride ion. In the past, iced benzalkonium chloride solutions were recommended as treatment, but a risk of cold injury exists and the treatment is often painful. More recently, calcium gluconate has gained favor in the treatment of hydrofluoric acid burns. After copious irrigation of the burned area, a 2.5% calcium gluconate gel is massaged into the affected area. A glove may be used to hold the gel in place on the hand. For fingertip burns, nail removal can aid penetration of the gel into the nail-bed. If calcium gluconate treatment is begun within a few hours after the onset of the burn, pain is often dramatically relieved, and no further treatment is usually necessary. Persistent symptoms can be treated by local injection of 10% calcium gluconate solution into the burned area, and debridement or fasciotomy as necessary.

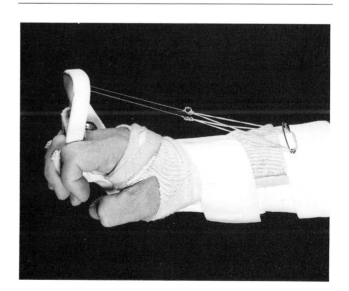

Figure 4

A dynamic metacarpophalangeal extension splint with metacarpophalangeal flexion block at 40 degrees can provide controlled mobilization for extensor tendon injuries.

Controversies

Mallet Fracture

Most mallet fractures are small and minimally displaced; these can be successfully treated nonsurgically by splinting for six to eight weeks in extension. Controversy exists over treatment of fractures that are displaced, make up more than one third of the articular surface, and do not reduce when the joint is splinted in extension, especially when there is associated volar subluxation of the distal phalanx. Although closed treatment of such fractures often results in posttraumatic arthritis, flexion averaged 65 degrees and extension deficit 5 degrees in one long-term study, with minimal symptoms in patients treated without surgery. This series and other series found high complication rates for open reduction and internal fixation of mallet fractures, explaining the poor functional results. To balance the picture, a recent report described a specific technique of open reduction and internal fixation in which one collateral ligament was divided to aid exposure. A K-wire was used to reduce the joint and the fracture fragment was fixed with an additional 0.028-inch K-wire. The digit was then splinted for four weeks with the proximal interphalangeal joint in 30 degrees of flexion. The pins were then removed and the joint resplinted for another four weeks. With this technique, after an average follow-up of 46 months, 32 of 33 patients had satisfactory results with an average of 70 degrees of distal interphalangeal joint motion and 1 to 2 degrees of extension deficit. Posttraumatic arthritis developed in only 30%.

Although this most recent report introduced some controversy into the treatment of mallet fractures, it is possible that the controversy can be resolved. For most fractures and most patients, closed treatment provides the simplest and most reliable approach. Patients should be cautioned that a dorsal bump from the malunited fracture is common and that radiographs are likely to show posttraumatic arthritis, but that function is likely to be satisfactory. Patients who have fracture-subluxations that cannot be reduced by closed means and are perhaps younger, with occupations that require normal or near-normal distal interphalangeal joint motion, particularly in extension, may be considered candidates for open reduction and internal fixation, provided also that the surgeon is experienced in the fixation of small intra-articular fractures.

Sheath Closure After Zone 2 Flexor Tendon Repair

Nearly all hand surgeons agree that the annular pulley portions of the flexor tendon sheath should be preserved at the time of flexor tendon repair. There is less agreement on the management of the membranous portions of the sheath. In the past, sheath resection was advised to reduce the risk of adhesions between tendon and sheath. More recently, sheath preservation and closure has been recommended, with several theoretical justifications. Synovial nutrition is known to be important in both human and animal experimental models of tendon healing. Sheath closure may also have a mechanical benefit in that the tendon repair may be able to glide more easily beneath a repaired sheath, and less likely to catch on the free edge of a pulley. Some have even recommended reconstruction of the sheath by grafting to ensure a closed sheath after the repair.

Several recent studies have raised questions regarding the necessity of sheath closure after flexor tendon repair in the finger. Recent experimental studies have shown no difference in tendon nutrient uptake in closed-sheath and open-sheath groups. Several recent clinical studies also failed to demonstrate a benefit from sheath closure, although one did show improved results when vincular blood supply was not damaged. All these studies agreed that there was no detriment to ultimate finger motion from sheath closure.

Thus, it appears that sheath closure can be left to the surgeon's preference. Elaborate efforts to obtain sheath closure by sheath grafts are probably not necessary.

Microsurgical Reconstruction of Severe Single-Digit Injury

As microsurgical techniques improve, smaller and smaller amputated parts can be salvaged. Several recent reports discuss successful reimplantation of free flap coverage of fingertip and distal finger amputations. The question arises as to whether this represents an advantage over stump closure by nonmicrosurgical means. In one recent report, 11 of 17 fingertips were successfully reimplanted, but five required distal interphalangeal joint arthrodesis and only one regained measurable two-point discrimination. The average hospital stay was 13 days and surgical time ranged from six to 20 hours. In another report, 51 of 59 reimplanted single digits survived. Total active interphalangeal joint motion averaged 82 degrees in amputations distal to the proximal interphalangeal joint but only 35 degrees in amputations proximal to that level. Surgical time averaged six hours and the average patient returned to work after 2.3 months. In a third report, free toe pulp transfer was used to reconstruct fingertip amputations in nine patients with good cosmetic results. On the other side of the ledger, in one recent report 20 patients had devascularizing injury to the index finger. Ten fingers were amputated and only one patient was functionally dissatisfied, because of cold sensitivity. Ten digits were revascularized. Of the revascularized digits, eight had cold sensitivity, five were painful, and four patients specifically regretted not having the finger amputated initially. No study has yet demonstrated a functional advantage to fingertip or single-digit reimplantation over wound closure. A cosmetic benefit is usually obvious, but there is a cost in terms of the intensity of medical service required. Satisfactory finger motion is preserved in distal reimplantations, but this is largely the result of the function of the amputation stump and not of the reimplanted part. There is no easy answer to this controversy, but it is clearly important to discuss these issues with patients before reimplantation or revascularization of single digits or fingertips, so as to best determine the specific needs of and most appropriate treatment for each patient.

Annotated Bibliography

Keywords

Burns; Carpal instability; Extensor tendon; Flexor tendon; Fracture; Infection; Ligament; Mallet fracture; Metacarpal fracture; Nerve injury: Phalangeal fracture; Radius; Scaphoid; Tendon; Tenosynovitis

Occupational Disorders

Arons MS: De Quervain's release in working women: A report of failures, complications, and associated diagnoses. *J Hand Surg* 1987;12A:540–544.
Twenty-seven patients with de Quervain's tenosynovitis also had a total of 31 additional diagnoses. Fourteen of 19 who underwent surgery had complications.

Blair SJ, Armstrong TJ, Louis DS, et al (eds): Occupational disorders of the upper extremity. *J Hand Surg* 1987;12A:821–970.
This special issue highlights the medical, social, and, to some extent, political issues surrounding a group of disorders that have been variously called "overuse syndromes," cumulative trauma syndromes, and repetitive motion disease and discusses the many factors to be considered in their prevention and treatment.

Hansford T, Blood H, Kent B, et al: Blood flow changes at the wrist in manual workers after preventive interventions. *J Hand Surg* 1986;11A:503–508.
After 90 minutes of manual labor, hand blood flow was significantly reduced from initial values in 16 factory workers. A five-minute exercise program produced greater increases in flow than a five-minute rest period, but both were effective in restoring flow to normal levels.

Wrist Injuries

Burgess RC: The effect of a simulated scaphoid malunion on wrist motion. *J Hand Surg* 1987;12A:774–776.
In a cadaver study, loss of radiocarpal extension occurred at 15 degrees of scaphoid flexion angulation. Loss of midcarpal extension occurred at 30 degrees of angulation.

Condamine JL, Le Bourg M, Raimbeau G: Nonunion of the carpal navicular (scaphoid) and the Matti Russe procedure. *Ann Orthop Ouest* 1986;18:23–31.
In this review of 106 fractures, persistent radiolunate angles of more than 20 degrees had a 50% nonunion rate; 60% of malunions also had radiolunate angles of more than 20 degrees. Functional results were very good in only 23% of patients with malunion compared with 56% in patients with anatomic union.

Crilly RG, Delaquerrière Richardson L, Roth JH, et al: Postural stability and Colles' fracture. *Age Ageing* 1987; 16:133–138.
Both anteroposterior and lateral postural sway were significantly greater in 19 postmenopausal women with Colles' fractures than in 24 postmenopausal women without Colles' fractures.

Czitrom AA, Dobyns JH, Linscheid RL: Ulnar variance in carpal instability. *J Hand Surg* 1987;12A:205–208.
The presence of negative variance was significantly increased in patients with scapholunate dissociation. There was no association of negative variance with lunotriquetral instability or the scapholunate advanced collapse wrist.

Fernandez DL, Ghillani R: External fixation of complex carpal dislocations: A preliminary report. *J Hand Surg* 1987;12A:335–347.
The authors used this technique in ten cases and found it helpful in surgical reduction and fixation maneuvers and excellent for postoperative cast-free immobilization.

Knirk JL, Jupiter JB: Intra-articular fractures of the distal end of the radius in young adults. *J Bone Joint Surg* 1986;68A:647–659.
Analysis of 43 fractures showed that an accurate articular reduction with ulnar styloid union was the factor most productive of a good result. The restoration of articular tilt and radial length were usually not critical to a good outcome after 6.7 years of follow-up.

Melone CP Jr: Open treatment for displaced articular fractures of the distal radius. *Clin Orthop* 1986;202:103–111.
The classification emphasizes that the two medial fragments most associated with poor results are not usual in Colles' or Smith fractures but are associated with violent-force injuries.

Minami A, Ogino T, Ohshio I, et al: Correlation between clinical results and carpal instabilities in patients after reduction of lunate and perilunar dislocations. *J Hand Surg* 1986;11B:213–220.
Ten patients, average age 27 years, were followed up for 26 months. Poor results were correlated with the presence of a scapholunate gap but not with delay in treatment.

Monsivais JJ, Nitz PA, Scully TJ: The role of carpal instability in scaphoid nonunion: Casual or causal? *J Hand Surg* 1986;11B:201–206.
Of 20 patients with nonunion of the scaphoid, 13 had scapholunate dissociation confirmed by surgical exploration. The surgical repair of nonunion should include assessment of scapholunate dissociation and a plan for its repair.

Nakamura R, Hori M, Horii E, et al: Reduction of the scaphoid fracture with DISI alignment. *J Hand Surg* 1987;12A:1000–1005.
Eight cases of malunion or nonunion achieved excellent results with the anterior wedge graft used to correct the humpback deformity associated with DISI alignment. Fixation employed the Herbert screw in all cases.

Rayhack JM, Linscheid RL, Dobyns JH, et al: Posttraumatic ulnar translation of the carpus. *J Hand Surg* 1987; 12A:180–189.
Seven men and one woman were treated after an average delay of 7.3 months. The injury was associated with other ligament disruptions. Delayed repairs were difficult and the results of repair disappointing. The authors present a technique of early repair along with a plea for early diagnosis.

Short WH, Palmer AK, Werner FW, et al: A biomechanical study of distal radial fractures. *J Hand Surg* 1987;12A:529–534.
As dorsal angulation of the articular face of the distal radius increased, the load shifted significantly from radial to ulnar and volar to dorsal. The load also shifted significantly to the distal radioulnar joint as the dorsal tilt increased.

Villar RN, Marsh D, Rushton N, et al: Three years after Colles' fracture: A prospective review. *J Bone Joint Surg* 1987;69B:635–638.
Intra-articular fractures and residual shortening were directly related to weakness and loss of motion. Angular deformities

directly correlated with motion loss. Fractures with the least anatomic deformity of union had the best functional results.

Weber SC, Szabo RM: Severely comminuted distal radial fracture as an unsolved problem: Complications associated with external fixation and pins and plaster techniques. *J Hand Surg* 1986;11A:157–165.

Complications occurred in 52% of cases in which pins and plaster were used and in 62% in which external fixation was used. Ipsilateral carpal or forearm fractures increased the risk of complications.

Fractures and Dislocations in the Hand

Dabezies EJ, Schutte JP: Fixation of metacarpal and phalangeal fractures with miniature plates and screws. *J Hand Surg* 1986;11A:283–288.

Fifty-two unstable fractures in 48 patients were treated with excellent results. Careful technique made early motion possible.

Helm RH: Hand function after injuries to the collateral ligaments of the metacarpophalangeal joint of the thumb. *J Hand Surg* 1987;12B:252–255.

Twenty-two patients underwent immediate repair; at follow-up, strength was normal and pain minimal. Eight patients with delayed repair (three weeks or more) had an average pinch strength only 60% of normal and pain.

Kiefhaber TR, Stern PJ, Grood ES: Lateral stability of the proximal interphalangeal joint. *J Hand Surg* 1986; 11A:661–669.

This excellent experimental study of the lateral stability of the proximal interphalangeal joint offers new information about the sequence of rupture of the collateral ligament when it is stressed in the position of extension. Joint opening of more than 20 degrees on stress was considered to represent a complete rupture.

Louis DS, Huebner JJ Jr, Hankin FM: Rupture and displacement of the ulnar collateral ligament of the metacarpophalangeal joint of the thumb: Preoperative diagnosis. *J Bone Joint Surg* 1986;68A:1320–1326.

A classification relating to unstressed radiographic findings and the clinical stress test of the metacarpophalangeal joint of the thumb is presented. This classification improved the likelihood of finding a Stener lesion at surgery by more accurately eliminating as surgical candidates patients with partial ligament injuries.

Meals RA (ed): Problem fractures of the hand and wrist. *Clin Orthop* 1987;214:2–152.

An excellent review of the current state of osteosynthesis, external fixation, and nonsurgical treatment of hand fractures.

Seitz WH Jr, Gomez W, Putnam MD, et al: Management of severe hand trauma with a mini external fixateur. *Orthopedics* 1987;10:601–610.

The Hoffman external mini-fixator was successfully used in 25 open comminuted fractures, achieving the goals of good early wound care and fracture stability.

Stark HH, Gainor BJ, Ashworth CR, et al: Operative treatment of intra-articular fractures of the dorsal aspect of the distal phalanx of digits. *J Bone Joint Surg* 1987; 69A:892–896.

Of 36 fractures, 35 had congruent reductions with minimal arthritic change after an average of 46 months of follow-up. Mean extension lag was 2 degrees; flexion was 71 degrees.

Microsurgery

Lister G, Scheker L: Emergency free flaps to the upper extremity. *J Hand Surg* 1988;13A:22–28.

At one major hand center, 31 emergency free flaps were used over a four-year period. Only two flaps failed.

Tendon Injuries

Allen BN, Frykman GK, Unsell RS, et al: Ruptured flexor tendon tenorrhaphies in zone II: Repair and rehabilitation. *J Hand Surg* 1987;12A:18–21.

Eight of 61 primary repairs ruptured an average of five weeks after surgery. The rerepair gave 60% excellent or good results. This complication may possibly be avoided by a longer restriction on full active flexion against resistance.

Amadio PC, Hunter JM, Jaeger SH, et al: The effect of vincular injury on the results of flexor tendon surgery in zone 2. *J Hand Surg* 1985;10A:626–632.

In a study of 82 fingers, mean total active motion was 221 degrees when vincula were intact, and 176 degrees when they were not. The difference was statistically significant (P < .01). Total active motion with sheath closure was 204 degrees; with the sheath unrepaired, it was 187 degrees. This difference was not significant.

Chow JA, Thomes LJ, Dovelle S, et al: A combined regimen of controlled motion following flexor tendon repair in "no man's land." *Plast Reconstr Surg* 1987;79:447–455.

Forty-three of 44 fingers had excellent or good motion results with a treatment program of controlled active and passive motion in a "palmar pulley" splint.

Evans RB, Burkhalter WE: A study of the dynamic anatomy of extensor tendons and implications for treatment. *J Hand Surg* 1986;11A:774–779.

Motion of 5 mm at the extensor repair site may successfully avoid tenodesis. This can be achieved by allowing 30 to 40 degrees of motion at the metacarpophalangeal joints, which may obviate joint stiffness as well.

Gault DT: Reduction of grip strength, finger flexion pressure, finger pinch pressure and key pinch following flexor tendon repair. *J Hand Surg* 1987;12B:182–184.

In 67 patients followed up for an average of two years, pinch and grip in the injured hand averaged 75% of that in the uninjured hand.

Malerich MM, Baird RA, McMaster W, et al: Permissible limits of flexor digitorum profundus tendon advancement: An anatomic study. *J Hand Surg* 1987;12A:30–33.

If 1 cm of advancement is exceeded in the long, ring, and little digits, there is a predictable loss of extension in the digit. The "quadriga effect" may reduce flexion power in the adjacent digits as well. The index profundus may be safely advanced as much as 1.5 cm because of its limited communication with other flexors.

Saldana MJ, Ho PK, Lichtman DM, et al: Flexor tendon repair and rehabilitation in zone II open sheath technique versus closed sheath technique. *J Hand Surg* 1987;12A:1110–1114.

This well-controlled, prospective study seems to provide evidence that sheath repair is not a factor in zone 2 injuries when careful postoperative mobilization is employed. In 48 fingers, open sheath repair gave 96% good or excellent results, compared with 88% in 42 with closed sheath repair. The difference was not statistically significant.

Wade PJF, Muir IFK, Hutcheon LL: Primary flexor tendon repair: The mechanical limitations of the modified Kessler technique. *J Hand Surg* 1986;11B:71–76.

This study provides good data suggesting that the "finishing" stitch is important in preventing gap formation at the repair site when the repair is stressed. This stitch probably has holding power and may add integrity to the repair.

Nerve Injuries

Chow JA, Van Beek AL, Bilos ZJ, et al: Anatomical basis for repair of ulnar and median nerves in the distal part of the forearm by group fascicular suture and nerve-grafting. *J Bone Joint Surg* 1986;68A:273–280.

Internal topography of distal forearm nerves appears to be consistent with regard to fascicular group arrangement. On the basis of this anatomic study, it should be possible with the operating microscope to readily identify, match, and align separate fascicular groups for repair or grafting.

Ganel A, Engel J, Rimon S: Intra-operative identification of peripheral nerve fascicles: Use of new rapid biomechanical assay technique. *Orthop Rev* 1986;15:85–88.

Choline acetylase can be assayed in 70 to 80 minutes by biochemical methods. In normal peripheral nerve, this enzyme is eight times more prevalent in motor axoplasm than in sensory axoplasm. It rapidly increases in the proximal stump and decreases in the distal stump after surgery. Precise identification of motor versus sensory fascicles can be obtained as long as five months after injury.

Infections

Chow SP, Ip FK, Lau JHK, et al: *Mycobacterium marinum* infection of the hand and wrist: Results of conservative treatment in twenty-four cases. *J Bone Joint Surg* 1987;69A:1161–1168.

In 24 patients, diagnosis was delayed an average of 3.5 months. Eleven healed with antitubercular therapy. Three given steroid injections had delayed healing of biopsy sites. Ten patients, eight of whom had had steroid injections, required surgical debridement.

Spiegel JD, Szabo RM: A protocol for the treatment of severe infections of the hand. *J Hand Surg* 1988;13A: 254–259.

Sixty-nine consecutive patients were treated with a protocol of incision and drainage in the operating room, broad-spectrum intravenous antibiotics, and open wound management wih early motion. Compared with 107 consecutive patients treated before the protocol was begun, the readmission rate dropped from 10% to 1%, the reoperation rate from 34% to 1%, and healing time from 34 to 22 days. Thirty-six percent of the infections were mixed aerobic and anaerobic.

Burns

Anderson WJ, Anderson JR: Hydrofluoric acid burns of the hand: Mechanism of injury and treatment. *J Hand Surg* 1988;13A:52–57.

Prompt treatment with 2.5% calcium gluconate gel resulted in pain relief and satisfactory function in 12 cases. Two patients with delayed treatment had permanent impairments.

Controversies

Lescalie F, Fouque PA, Saint-Cast Y, et al: Les réimplantations distales des extrémités [Distal reimplantations of extremities]. *J Chir* 1987;124:236–240.

Logan A, Elliot D, Foucher G: Free toe pulp transfer to restore traumatic digital pulp loss. *Br J Plast Surg* 1985; 38:497–500.

Urbaniak JR, Roth JH, Nunley JA, et al: The results of replantation after amputation of a single finger. *J Bone Joint Surg* 1985;67A:611–619.

30

Wrist and Hand: Reconstruction

Reconstruction of the hand and wrist has been improved by increasing knowledge of biomechanics and the recognition of different instability patterns secondary to ligamentous injury in the wrist. New diagnostic techniques, various arthroplasties and arthrodeses of the wrist, and tendon reconstruction are now being used. Other developments have occurred in the areas of osteonecrosis of the scaphoid and lunate, arthritis, Dupuytren's contracture, and carpal tunnel syndrome.

Biomechanics of the Wrist

Wrist motion, as determined by a triaxial electrogoniometer, is 50 degrees of flexion, 30 degrees of extension, 10 degrees of radial deviation, and 15 degrees of ulnar deviation. Electromyographic studies of wrist motion have demonstrated a large burst of activity about 40 ms before the onset of movement in the agonist and a large burst of activity by the antagonist at the onset or just after onset of movement.

Recent studies have shown that the scaphoid contact area is 1.47 times that of the lunate, and that each area of contact between the scaphoid and the lunate and the distal radius and triangular fibrocartilage complex was separate and distinct. In these studies, the contact areas were localized, accounting for approximately 20% of the available joint surface, and shifted from a palmar location to a more dorsal location as the wrist moved from flexion to extension (Fig. 1). The contact area was greatest with the scaphoid more horizontally oriented in ulnar deviation, and the contact area of the scaphoid and lunate with the distal radius and triangular fibrocartilage complex increased as the wrist moved from radial to ulnar deviation and/or from flexion to extension. Under functionally applied loads in the range of 103 N, the average contact pressures were fairly low, ranging from 2 to 5.6 MPa (Fig. 2). Studies of load changes in cadaveric extremities with perilunate instabilities demonstrated that the scaphoid contact area decreased as the amount of perilunate instability increased. In all stages of perilunate instability, the contact areas remained a relatively small part of the overall joint surface. Pressures were significantly increased in wrists with stage III instability (section of the palmar and dorsal scapholunate interosseous ligaments, radiocapitate ligament, and radioscapholunate ligament) compared with normal wrists. With increasing instability, the contact area of the lunate shifted palmar and ulnar. The distance between the scaphoid and lunate contact areas changed little except when the wrist was placed in 20 degrees of extension, neutral radioulnar deviation, and 90 degrees of supination.

Physiology of the Tendons of the Hand

Recent studies on the intrinsic healing of flexor tendons have shown that not only do the fibroblasts in the central

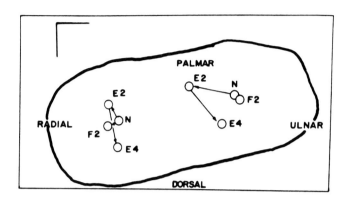

Figure 1

Scaphoid and lunate, pressure centroids of the wrists (normalized to be plotted as right wrists) show typical pattern of centroid shift moving from 20 degrees of flexion (F2), to neutral (N), to 20 degrees of extension (E2), to 40 degrees of extension (E4). Pronation-supination and radioulnar deviation postures remain constant. An averaged coordinate joint outline is used for orientation. (Reproduced with permission from Viegas SF, Tencer AF, Cantrell J, et al: Load transfer characteristics of the wrist: Part I. The normal joint. *J Hand Surg* 1987;12A:971–978.)

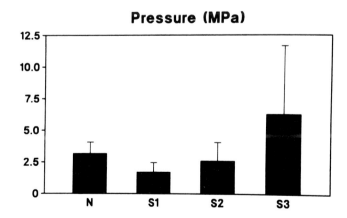

Figure 2

Average high-pressure zone pressure for normal and destabilized wrists. N, normal; S1, stage I; S2, stage II; S3, stage III. (Reproduced with permission from Viegas SF, Tencer A, Cantrell J, et al: Load transfer characteristics of the wrist: Part II. Perilunate instability. *J Hand Surg* 1987;12A:978–985.)

endotenon core of the tendon produce collagen at the cut end of the tendon but also that the outer layer of the epitenon cells appear to produce more collagen during tendon repair. It has also been suggested that the rate of healing may differ in different tendons.

Since the publication of *Orthopaedic Knowledge Update 2*, there has been an increased interest in the integrity of the flexor tendon sheath and its effect on nutrition and adhesion formation. The flexor tendon sheath consists of both a visceral synovial layer and a parietal synovium that are in continuity with the annular and cruciate pulleys (Fig. 3). Both components of the sheath are continuous at the tendon insertions, at the vincula, and at the proximal tendon sheath cul-de-sac (Fig. 4). Synovial cells constitute each portion of the sheath.

A study of 61 fresh human cadaveric fingers supported a significant addition to the pulley system (Fig. 5). This is the palmar aponeurosis pulley, which has an average width of 9 mm and is located 1 to 3 mm distal to the cul-de-sac of the synovial sheath in the palm. It is anchored by vertical septi and appears to be important in preventing loss of flexion of the digit.

The common clinical practice for fixing tendons is to pass them through tunnels in the metaphyseal bone. Two recent studies demonstrated that firm fixation does not occur. Osseous integration of the tendon did not occur, and an area of sclerotic bone surrounded the tendon. Ultimate fixation appears to be limited to the tendon healing to itself and to the scarring between the tendon and periosteum.

Diagnostic Evaluation

Radionuclide Imaging

The etiology of wrist pain can be elusive. In one study evaluating the use of tomography, wrist arthrography, computed tomography, magnetic resonance imaging, and bone scintigraphy, it was found that bone scans were abnormal in 95% of cases involving fractures and intrinsic ligament ruptures and normal in 96% of patients with no definable injury. Bone scan findings correlated poorly with partial intrinsic ligament injury and synovitis. Development of a wrist pain algorithm was recommended. Because abnormal bone scans are generally nonspecific, positive findings necessitate further clinical and diagnostic evaluation (Algorithm 1).

Arthrography

Of 100 patients who underwent wrist arthrography, 77 had abnormal arthrograms. In 29 instances, abnormalities were demonstrated by injection either into the distal radioulnar joint or the midcarpal joint but not by radiocarpal joint injection. In 38 instances, abnormalities were identified by radiocarpal joint injection but not by either distal radioulnar joint injection or midcarpal joint injection. Some cases of triangular fibrocartilage complex detachments were demonstrated by distal radioulnar joint injections and not

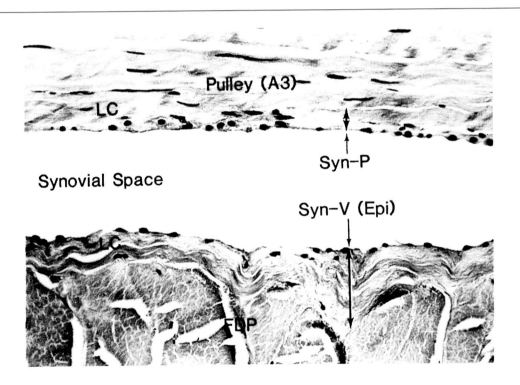

Figure 3

The surfaces of the A3 pulley and the flexor digitorum profundus are lined respectively by parietal synovium (Syn-P) and visceral synovium (Syn-V). The latter constitutes the epitenon (Epi) of the flexor tendons. Each synovial surface is supported by laminated collagen (LC). They are morphologically identical to each other and to the surfaces of the palmar plates that line the fibro-osseous tunnel. (Reproduced with permission from Cohen MJ, Kaplan L: Histology and ultrastructure of the human flexor tendon sheath. *J Hand Surg* 1987;12A:25–29.)

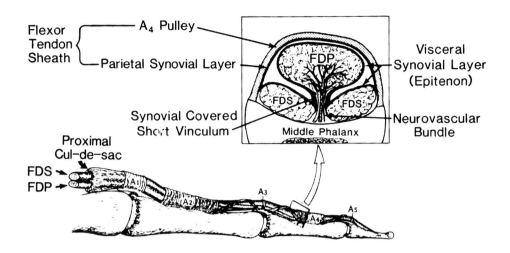

Figure 4

The parietal synovial sheath of the digital flexor tendon typically extends from the level of the metacarpal heads to the insertion of the flexor digitorum profundus. The annular pulleys (A1 to A5) are closely applied over this layer, as are the variable cruciform fibers shown but not labeled. Between the annular pulleys this layer is termed the membranous portion of the sheath. The flexor digitorum profundus (FDP), the flexor digitorum superficialis (FDS), and their vincula are separately covered by a layer of visceral synovium that is continuous with the parietal layer at the proximal cul-de-sac, the vincula origins, and the tendon insertions. (Reproduced with permission from Cohen MJ, Kaplan L: Histology and ultrastructure of the human flexor tendon sheath. *J Hand Surg* 1987;12A:25–29.)

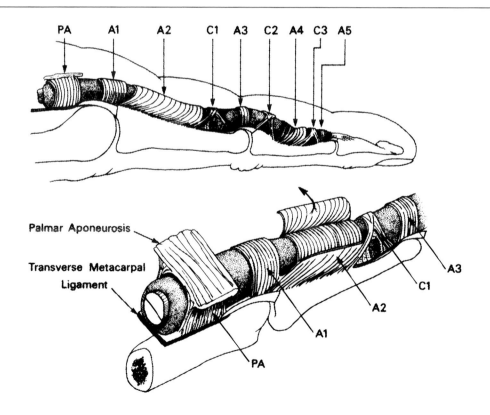

Figure 5

Composite of the flexor tendon synovial sheath and pulleys, including the palmar aponeurosis pulley, five annular pulleys, and three cruciform pulleys. (Reproduced with permission from Doyle JR: Anatomy of the finger flexor tendon sheath and pulley system. *J Hand Surg* 1988;13A:473–484.)

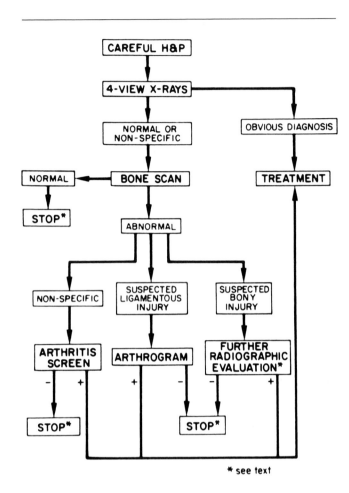

Algorithm 1

Strategy for evaluating unexplained wrist pain. "Further radiographic evaluation" consists of one or more of the following: instability series, spot films, magnified views, fluoroscopy, computed tomography, or magnetic resonance imaging. (Reproduced with permission from Pin PG, Semenkovich JW, Young VL, et al: Role of radionuclide imaging in the evaluation of wrist pain. *J Hand Surg* 1988;13A:810–814.)

by midcarpal or radiocarpal joint injections. Thus, all three injections are necessary for a complete diagnostic evaluation of the wrist.

An analysis of the prevalence of complex perforations in the triangular fibrocartilage showed them to be present in 39 of 162 patients (24%). The tear was most common at the radial aspect of the triangular fibrocartilage complex; small defects also appeared in either the proximal or distal surface of the triangular fibrocartilage complex. These perforations did not correlate with pain, carpal instability, ulnar variance, or other diagnostic findings.

Magnetic Resonance Imaging

Magnetic resonance imaging is superior to standard radiography and computed tomography for evaluating the wrist. Early studies supported its use in diagnosing ganglia, rheumatoid arthritis, arteriovenous malformations, carpal fractures, and carpal tunnel syndrome and in evaluating the zone of soft-tissue injury related to fractures and, importantly, osteonecrosis. In 13 patients thought to have osteonecrosis of either the proximal fracture fragment of the scaphoid or the lunate in Kienböck's disease, the mag-

netic resonance imaging findings correlated with the histologic findings. Magnetic resonance imaging may detect osteonecrosis before the onset of carpal collapse.

In addition, magnetic resonance imaging appears to be a highly accurate method of diagnosing traumatic disruptions of the triangular fibrocartilage complex. Some investigators have reported a consistent correlation between the location and the extent of the triangular fibrocartilage complex injury and the magnetic resonance imaging findings.

Computed Tomography

In most clinical situations, coronal computed tomographic images are superior to transaxial images because of their increased detail and ease of interpretation. For specific problems, such as radioulnar subluxation and fractures of the hook of the hamate, transaxial images were superior.

Posttraumatic Problems of the Wrist

Kienböck's Disease

Little new information has been reported on Kienböck's disease since the publication of *Orthopaedic Knowledge Update 2*, which stated that resection with tendon or silicone replacement could be used for patients with stage III disease. However, in patients with advanced collapse (stage III and stage IV), progression of collapse of the carpus, progression of osteoarthritis, and subluxation of the prosthesis were common.

Recent clinical and biomechanical studies support the use of radial shortening in stage II and stage III disease in the presence of ulnar minus variance. In ulnar neutral variance, a medial closing or lateral opening radial wedge osteotomy is recommended. Each of these three procedures unloads the lunate fossa and redistributes the load to the scaphoid fossa and the ulnar column. Scaphotrapeziotrapezoid fusion and scaphocapitate fusion unload the lunate fossa and transfer all the load to the scaphoid fossa. Capitohamate fusion does not unload the lunate fossa.

Scaphoid Nonunion and Osteonecrosis

Untreated or persistent nonunion results in a high incidence of periscaphoid arthritis, especially in the radioscaphoid joint. Degenerative changes in the radioscaphoid joint were reported in 75% of patients in whom scaphoid nonunion persisted for four years. Sixty percent also had midcarpal changes nine years after initial fracture with persistant nonunion. Trispiral tomography is a useful technique for visualizing subtle fractures, comminution, angulation, cysts, sclerosis, and erosions involving the scaphoid or other carpal bones. Russe bone grafting leads to a high rate of union (92%). Other methods include the use of percutaneous pinning and the use of the Herbert screw. With percutaneous pinning, the complications are low and the reported union rate is 77%. Recent reports indicate a union rate of 84% with the Herbert screw. Advantages of the Herbert screw include decreased immobilization time and improved wrist motion, improvement in any associated collapse deformity, and early return to function. However, there is a learning curve and a higher complication rate with initial use of the device. Other disadvantages are the technical demands of insertion and possible damage to articular cartilage in the scaphotrapezial joint.

Factors associated with nonunion include carpal instability, displacement, volar angulation, osteonecrosis, and fractures of the proximal third. Patients in whom bone grafting has failed and who have early posttraumatic arthritic changes often remain symptomatic after additional procedures to achieve union. Salvage procedures may be reasonable alternatives to continued attempts at bone grafting in such cases.

Arthritis of the Wrist

Total Joint Replacement

More than 90% of patients who receive silicone rubber wrist replacements obtain significant relief of pain. An average of 24 degrees of wrist flexion and 21 degrees of wrist extension is possible with these implants. In one series, however, the implant subsided in all cases and fractured in 65%. In another series of 53 Swanson silicone implants followed up for more than 30 months, the breakage rate was 9.4%. Progressive radiographic deterioration occurred in 70% and 25% required reoperation. Only 61% had good or excellent results. In a third series of 71 silicone wrist replacements, 20% of the implants fractured; an additional 5% required revision for pain and/or deformity. Prosthetic fracture often leads to increasing pain, stability of deformity, and diminished function. Excessive wrist motion, overuse, and inadequate surgical technique appear to contribute to this high rate of failure. For severely deformed or unstable wrists, fusion is the procedure of choice. In patients with severe bilateral involvement, arthrodesis on one side and a silicone implant on the opposite side may be required. Because of the high fracture rate of these implants, they are recommended only for patients with rheumatoid arthritis and are not recommended for those with posttraumatic arthritis.

Two reviews of the Volz total wrist replacement demonstrated significant relief of pain and patient satisfaction in a high percentage of cases. The new single-pronged metacarpal component gave good or excellent results in 77% of one series. Despite resorption of bone underneath the collar of the radial component in 79% and metacarpal component loosening in 24%, these patients had little or no discomfort. Complications occurred in 12 cases. In another series, however, the overall complication rate was 44%; the complications included loosening of the components, muscle imbalance, and dislocation. Loosening of the components was more common in patients with osteoarthritis. In cases in which extensor tendons are inadequate or there are severe deformities of the fingers, other types of arthroplasty or arthrodesis should be used. Preliminary results of trispherical total wrist arthroplasty in patients with advanced rheumatoid arthritis showed improvement in all patients (23 excellent, ten good, three fair, and two poor outcomes). The average arc of motion was 38 degrees. In three cases the metacarpal stem migrated and in nine cases lucency developed about the stems. There were no implant failures. This total wrist arthroplasty is recommended for class III and class IV rheumatoid disease.

Limited Arthrodesis

Limited arthrodesis has become increasingly popular, and many varieties have been reported. In one laboratory study of the amount of motion lost with limited wrist arthrodesis, fusions that crossed the radiocarpal joint lost 55% of the arc of flexion and extension, fusions that crossed the intercarpal joint lost approximately 27% of the arc, and fusions within a single carpal row that did not cross either joint lost approximately 12% of the arc.

In 17 patients who had limited wrist fusions for diseases other than rheumatoid arthritis, the overall results were excellent in five wrists, good in seven, fair in two, and poor in three. Patients who had midcarpal joint fusion did better than those who had radiocarpal joint fusion. Thirteen of the 17 wrists had a postoperative range of motion 30% or more than that of the opposite wrist. Interestingly, postoperative arthritic changes developed around the arthrodesis in three wrists. Scaphocapitate arthrodesis has been used to treat rotatory instability of the scaphoid and persistent scaphoid nonunion and to prevent carpal collapse with osteonecrosis of the lunate. In 16 patients who underwent scaphocapitate arthrodesis, the scaphocapitate fusion reduced radial deviation by an average of 10 degrees and ulnar deviation by an average of 4 degrees. Dorsiflexion was reduced by an average of 18 degrees and palmar flexion by an average of 5 degrees. Lunate excision in addition to scaphocapitate fusion diminished the functional end result. Nonunions required reoperation in two cases. Seven patients noted mild discomfort with heavy use.

One group evaluated four different types of intercarpal limited arthrodesis for volar intercalary segment instability. These included capitate-lunate-triquetrum-hamate fusion, lunate-triquetrum fusion, lunate-triquetrum-hamate fusion, and triquetrum-hamate fusion. The one patient with a lunate-triquetrum fusion had a poor result. Wrist pain was relieved in five of six patients in whom the arthrodesis crossed the midcarpal joint. Postoperatively, the active flexion and extension arc was 63% of that of the opposite wrist, the radioulnar deviation arc of motion was 57% of that of the opposite wrist, and grip strength was 74% of that of the opposite wrist. Only stabilizing the proximal to the distal row prevented the "clunking" phenomenon. These investigators recommended capitate-lunate-triquetrum-hamate arthrodesis for volar intercalary segment instability.

Scaphotrapeziotrapezoid (triscaphoid) arthrodesis has been used in the management of rotatory instability of the scaphoid and to prevent carpal collapse in advanced osteonecrosis of the lunate. One group reported five nonunions in 19 wrists and another reported 18 nonunions in 77 wrists. Postoperative reflex sympathetic dystrophy developed in 11 of the 77, and there was one radial nerve neuroma. Almost one third of the patients underwent additional surgery, and ten ultimately required wrist arthrodesis. Four patients required carpometacarpal joint arthroplasty on the thumb. One study of results after triscaphoid fusion showed only one nonunion in 20 cases but 75% of the patients had pain at the extremes of motion. Because radial styloid impingement resulting in pain and limited motion occurred in 33 of 99 cases of triscaphoid arthrodesis, one group now recommends that radial styloidectomy be a routine component of the triscaphoid arthrodesis procedure. A kinematic study of triscaphoid and scaphocapitate fusions found a decrease in wrist motion and a significant change in normal intracarpal kinematics with each type of fusion.

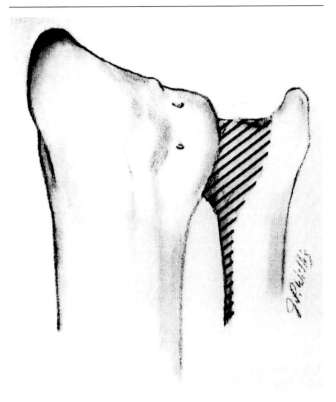

Figure 6

The ulna is resected in a convex curve, matching the concave radial metaphysis but retaining the full ulnar length and ulnar styloid process. (Reproduced with permission from Watson HK, Ryu JY, Burgess RC: Matched distal ulnar resection. *J Hand Surg* 1986;11A: 812–817.)

Proximal Row Carpectomy

Proximal row carpectomy is indicated in late scapholunate dissociation, dorsiflexion instability with secondary arthritis, carpal instability secondary to nonunion of the scaphoid, failed silicone lunate implant arthroplasty, and old unreduced transscaphoid perilunate dislocations. In one study, the outcome was successful in 13 of 15 cases, with an average range of motion of 39 degrees of dorsiflexion and 43 degrees of volar flexion. Grip strength of the dominant hand averaged 83% of that of the opposite side and grip strength of the nondominant hand averaged 41% of that of the opposite side. Strength increased steadily for as long as one year postoperatively.

Proximal row carpectomy has also been used in patients with arthrogryposis multiplex congenita, but the results are sometimes unpredictable. In 27 patients with an average follow-up of four years, motion remained stable or improved over preoperative measurements. Pain was relieved in 26 of the 27 patients, and 24 patients returned to their previous activity status. Grip strength improved to an average of 80% of that of the opposite side. Biomechanical analyses of the capitate radius articulation after proximal row carpectomy have shown a decrease in the radius curvature of the lunate fossa, suggesting wear deformation and predicting that clinical results may deteriorate with time. It has been suggested that proximal carpectomy is contraindicated if there is evidence of arthritic change in the lunate fossa and/or distal involvement of the head of the capitate.

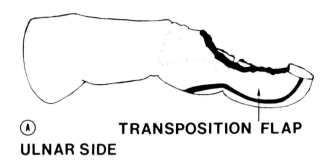

TRANSPOSITION FLAP
ULNAR SIDE

Figure 7

Distal digital transposition flap. (Reproduced with permission from Fleegler EJ, Weinzweig N: The versatile axial pattern digital transposition flap. *J Hand Surg* 1988;13A:494–500.)

Many procedures are being performed for distal radioulnar joint dysfunction. Radiographs of 20 patients with limited function and pain after Darrach resection arthroplasty could not be distinguished from those of an equal number of patients whose procedures were successful. Most of those in whom the procedure failed underwent two or more additional operations without success. Thus, reoperation after a failed Darrach procedure is probably not indicated. The procedure may not be suitable for younger patients and patients with lax ligaments.

Because of problems with the Darrach procedure, some use a "matched" resection arthroplasty of the distal ulna that leaves the styloid, the triangular fibrocartilage complex, and the distal ulnar ligaments intact distally and the ulnar shaft intact proximally (Fig. 6). The radial portion of the ulna is removed to match the opposite surface of the radial metaphysis so that the distance between the radius and the ulna remains stable from full pronation to full supination. Painless motion was achieved in all 44 patients, with pronation averaging 80 degrees and supination 88 degrees six years postoperatively.

Posttraumatic Problems of the Hand

Soft-Tissue Defects

An axial-pattern digital transposition flap can be used to reconstruct complex tissue loss involving the distal finger, especially the dorsum, with exposure of the distal joint (Fig. 7). The longitudinal axis of the flap is designed to include the digital artery. Both the digital artery and the nerve are identified distally. The nerve is left in its position, and the artery is dissected with the flap after it is ligated distally. After the flap has been transposed to cover the dorsal defect, a skin graft is used to resurface the donor site. This flap has been described as predictable, versatile, and valuable in salvaging severe injuries involving the distal portion of the finger. A radial artery fasciocutaneous flap is useful in crushing injuries of the hand in which there is exposed bone, tendon, or nerves that require subcutaneous resurfacing as well as skin.

An alternative to the radial artery fasciocutaneous flap is the vascularized temporoparietal fascial flap. This flap permits large defects in the hand to be resurfaced in a one-stage procedure.

Tendon Transfers

Transfer of the flexor carpi ulnaris to the extensor carpi radialis longus and/or brevis in patients with cerebral palsy benefits those who can actively extend their fingers to neutral with the wrist extended or flexed. Patients unable to extend the fingers to neutral, regardless of wrist position, do not benefit from this transfer. Function does not improve in patients unable to extend the fingers without flexing the wrist. Extension posture with contraction of the wrist developed in this group of patients. Tendon transfers also fail to improve function in patients with underlying problems of proprioceptive sensibility and cognition. Transfer of the flexor carpi ulnaris to the wrist extensors is indicated only in patients whose sole problem is weak grasp. In such patients, there may be impairment of the ability to release.

Improvement in extension of the fingers and opening of the hand without loss of grasp strength can be obtained by transferring the flexor carpi ulnaris into the extensor digitorum communis. In one study, functional levels were improved in spastic patients with volitional control of the wrist and finger flexors by means of brachioradialis muscle transfer to the extensor digitorum communis.

A long-term follow-up of the Moberg key grip procedure (release of the A1 pulley, tenodesis of the flexor pollicis longus tendon to the radius, and percutaneous pin fixation of the interphalangeal joint of the thumb) noted bowstringing of the flexor pollicis longus. This necessitated extending the wrist further to pinch small objects and, therefore, the A1 pulley probably should not be released. When a simultaneous tenodesis of the extensor tendons to the thumb was done, there was progressive flexion of the metacarpophalangeal joint and stretching of the extensor tenodesis. If a brachioradialis muscle transfer is done to improve extension, this procedure should be performed first and the key grip procedure performed later and only if the wrist's extension strength is at least 3+.

Tendon Injuries

Primary repair of flexor tendon injuries in zone 1 produces excellent results in children. A review of isolated flexor digitorum profundus and combined flexor digitorum profundus and flexor digitorum superficialis repairs in zone 2 in children less than 15 years old showed that an early passive range-of-motion program and a four-week immobilization program led to similar results. Total active range of motion averaged approximately 70% to 75% and there was little difference between age groups.

Late repair of flexor tendon injuries within zone 2 also presents a problem. In one series in which the average interval between the laceration and repair of the flexor tendon was six weeks, a total active-motion program produced excellent results in 21 cases, good results in seven cases, fair results in four cases, and poor results in ten cases (67% satisfactory results). The poor results were in patients less than 16 years old. Thus, delayed repair is a good alternative to tendon grafts in selected patients.

Two-stage flexor tendon reconstruction is still necessary in selected cases. In two large series in which most patients had Boyes grade 5 or grade 6 injuries, approximately 54% of the results were good to excellent. At final follow-up one group had a mean active range of motion of 176 degrees and a mean grip strength that was 79% of normal; the second group had a final active range of motion of more than 180 degrees. Rupture occurred in 4% in one series and in 14% in the other. Obviously, two-stage flexor tendon reconstruction is a salvage procedure. Postoperative therapy is important. Better results were reported in zone 4 and zone 5 injuries and poorer results in patients who were less than 10 years of age. In one series the severity of the final flexion contracture was related to the severity of the preoperative flexion contracture. Additional procedures were required in 15% of the fingers; these included production of a "superficialis finger" (elimination of active flexion at the distal interphalangeal joint by reinserting the distal end of the tendon graft into the middle phalanx) in 7%, amputation of the proximal interphalangeal joint in 3%, and other combinations of tenodesis and arthrodesis. There was no correlation between the number of intact or reconstructed pulleys and the amount of bowstringing postoperatively. Bowstringing was associated with flexion deformities. An evaluation of "belt loop" technique of pulley reconstruction in cadaveric fingers showed that range of motion was excellent when bowstringing was absent but that there was a 40% loss of power in the fingers.

An early controlled-motion rehabilitation program has been recommended for extensor tendon injuries. To achieve 5 mm of passive tendon glide, the metacarpophalangeal joint must have 28 to 40 degrees of flexion.

Extensor tendon ruptures are common in rheumatoid arthritis. Sixty patients with single or double tendon rupture were successfully treated with a variety of tendon transfers. Early treatment of distal radioulnar joint derangements is recommended in these cases. Rupture of three or more extensor tendons is often associated with impairment of overall function and extensor lag. Because flexion is not a problem and extensor lag is common in such cases, it is better to err on the side of increased tension when completing the tendon transfer.

Arthritis of the Hand

Joint Replacement

A 44-month follow-up study of silicone rubber implants in the metacarpophalangeal joints of patients with rheumatoid arthritis showed significant relief of pain in 27 of 32 patients. Twenty-eight patients were happy with the cosmetic improvement, and 27 believed that hand function had improved. The implant fractured in one case, ulnar deviation of more than 10 degrees recurred in ten cases, and active motion of the metacarpophalangeal joint averaged 34 degrees. Bone resorption and migration of the implant occurred in eight cases.

A five-year follow-up study of 133 digits with silicone implants at the metacarpophalangeal joint showed bone remodeling, with a cortical bony shell about the implant stems and thickening of the cortical bone at the metacarpal and phalangeal metaphyses. The proximal phalanx did not shorten and the average shortening of the metacarpal was 9%.

A study of 210 silicone rubber metacarpophalangeal joint implants in 55 hands showed an initial improvement in ulnar drift from 25 degrees to 5 degrees. This gradually worsened to 12 degrees during the follow-up period (from two to eight years). The average extension deficit decreased from 56 degrees preoperatively to 10 degrees postoperatively, but increased to 22 degrees at long-term follow-up.

Average range of motion initially improved from 17 to 51 degrees but gradually decreased to 39 degrees at long-term follow-up. Tension and grip strength did not improve. The procedure remains useful in treating painful arthritis and/or deformity of the metacarpophalangeal joints but initial improvement is followed by gradual deterioration.

Twenty-three patients underwent silicone interpositional arthroplasty at the distal interphalangeal joint. Pain was relieved in all cases and range of motion averaged 33 degrees. Extension lag was common, averaging 12 degrees. One prosthesis fractured, and only one joint had lateral instability. The procedure retains motion while preserving stability in painful degenerative joint disease.

Arthrodesis

Union occurred in 170 of 171 arthrodeses of the small joints in the hand (Fig. 8). The joint surfaces were resected back to medullary bone, tightly coapted, and fixed with Kirschner wires. Bone grafting was used when necessary. Proximal interphalangeal joint arthrodesis using the Herbert screw for compression was successful in 50 of 51 joints (Fig. 9). The joints fused within six weeks and required only minimal external protection.

For arthrodesis of the digital joints in children without interference with growth, the articular cartilage is removed down to the ossific nucleus (Fig. 10). Subchondral bone is carefully removed to expose cancellous bone on each side of the joint. The surface is coapted and held with crossed K-wires. This technique produced no detectable growth disturbance after an average follow-up of three years.

Trapeziometacarpal Joint

Because silicone synovitis is becoming increasingly common, alternatives to the use of silicone as a replacement for the trapezium have been sought. *Orthopaedic Knowledge Update 2* noted that comparative studies were lacking. Since then, however, long-term results comparing tendon interposition arthroplasty and silicone implant arthroplasty for trapeziometacarpal arthritis have been reported. After an average follow-up of four years with silicone replacement, there was a 25% failure rate with subluxation, loss of implant height (nearly 50%) resulting in shortening of the thumb, and silicone synovitis (Fig. 11).

Tendon interposition arthroplasty has become accepted for surgical management of severe osteoarthritis of the trapeziometacarpal joint. Several techniques have been described but only one report included a comparison with silicone implant arthroplasty. In this series of 25 cases followed up for an average of two years, the initial arthroplasty space collapsed in only three cases, subluxation averaged 7% of the width of the metacarpal (compared with 35% with the silicone implant), and excellent results were obtained in 23 cases. No revisions were necessary. The technique is similar to that in which the distally based radial half of the flexor carpi radialis is used to reconstruct the ligamentous support for the metacarpal (Fig. 12). Two additional steps are performed: (1) A supporting ligamentous sling is made by passing the tendon through the center of the base of the metacarpal and its ulnar cortex. This maintains length and prevents radial subluxation. (2) The remaining tendon is folded and placed into the area of the absent trapezium as a spacer. In one series of 89 cases, 65 patients were satisfied after resection arthroplasty and use

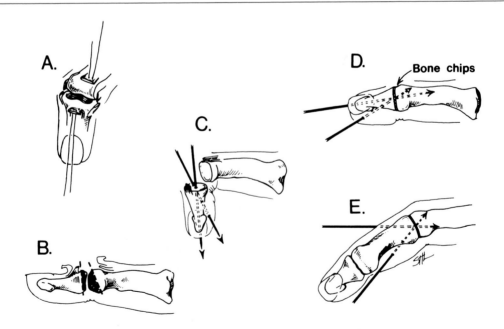

Figure 8

The basic technique for small-joint fusion in the hand is simple, with similar principles for the distal interphalangeal, proximal interphalangeal, and metacarpophalangeal joints. **A**, Exposure. **B**, Resection of proximal and distal joint surfaces back to medullary bone, creating two flush medullary surfaces that, when accurately and tightly coapted along cortical margins, result in the desired alignment for the planned fusion. **C**, Insertion of crossed Kirschner pins through the distal surface. **D** and **E**, Total contact; accurately aligned apposition of two flush surfaces with nonparallel Kirschner pins driven into proximal bone. (Reproduced with permission from Burton RI, Margles SW, Lunseth PA: Small-joint arthrodesis in the hand. *J Hand Surg* 1986;11A:678–682.)

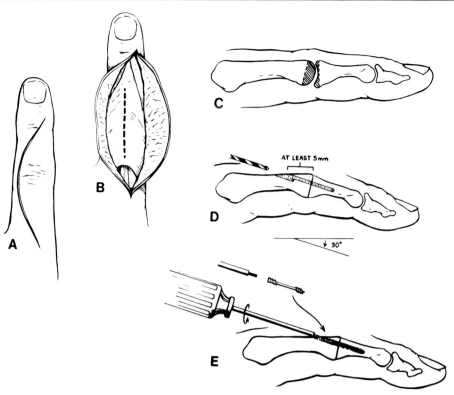

Figure 9

Proximal interphalangeal joint arthrodesis. **A**, A 5-cm dorsal curvilinear incision is centered over the joint. **B**, The dorsal apparatus is longitudinally split in a midline incision reflecting the apparatus radially and ulnarly. **C**, The shaded portions reflect the proposed osteotomies. **D**, The dorsal proximal phalangeal cortex and middle phalangeal medullary canal are sequentially drilled and tapped. **E**, The Herbert screw is inserted carefully to ensure that the proximal threads are completely sealed. (Reproduced with permission from Ayres JR, Goldstrohm GL, Miller GJ, et al: Proximal interphalangeal joint arthrodesis with the Herbert screw. *J Hand Surg* 1988;13A:600–603.)

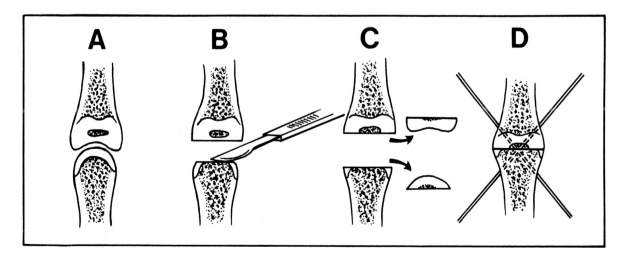

Figure 10

The surgical procedure at a digital joint. **A**, The articular surface after incision of the joint capsule and release of collateral ligaments. **B**, Sequential removal of articular cartilage. **C**, Exposure of the ossification center and removal of subchondral bony surfaces. **D**, Coaptation of subchondral surfaces and internal fixation with Kirschner wires. (Reproduced with permission from Kowalski MF, Manske PR: Arthrodesis of digital joints in children. *J Hand Surg* 1988;13A:874–879.)

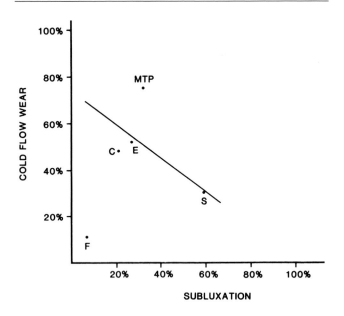

Figure 11

The inverse relationship between silicone wear and implant subluxation. C, condylar implant; E, Eaton cannulated trapezium implant; F, fascial arthroplasty of the LRTI type; MTP, metatarsophalangeal implant; S, Swanson trapezium implant. (Reproduced with permission from Pellegrini VD JR, Burton RI: Surgical management of basal joint arthritis of the thumb: Part I. Long-term results of silicone implant arthroplasty. *J Hand Surg* 1986; 11A:309–324.)

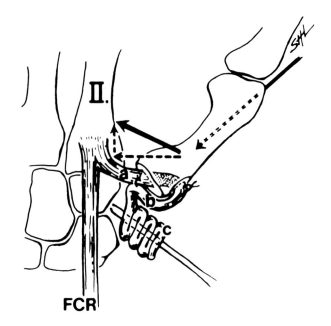

Figure 12

Schema of ligament reconstruction with tendon interposition arthroplasty. The forces producing proximal migration and radial subluxation of the metacarpal are neutralized. Schema shows ligament reconstruction (a), metacarpal resurfacing (b), and tendon arthroplasty spacer (c). (Reproduced with permission from Burton RI, Pellegrini VD Jr: Surgical management of basal joint arthritis of the thumb: Part II. Ligament reconstruction with tendon interposition arthroplasty. *J Hand Surg* 1986;11A:324–332.)

of the flexor carpi radialis tendon. A strip of tendon was wrapped around the main portion of the flexor carpi radialis and the abductor pollicis longus. Adduction contracture was relieved in only one half of the cases.

Reports of silicone or reactive synovitis to particulate debris from worn or fractured silicone implants have been increasing. This process has been seen with silicone finger joints and trapezial, scaphoid, lunate, ulnar head, and wrist implants.

Radiographic changes occur in as many as 75% of the scaphoid implants and 55% of the lunate implants. They are not common in the finger-joint implants. Patients with radiographic changes frequently have pain (56% of cases). The process appears to worsen with time and can be prevented by removing the implant, synovectomy, curettage of the lytic lesions, and bone grafting the defects if they are large enough. Because of this condition, patients with silicone implants should be monitored regularly.

Carpal Tunnel Syndrome

Intracarpal canal pressure is increased in patients with carpal tunnel syndrome compared with normal control patients. These pressures increased even further with exercise and remained increased for a longer period than did those of the control patients. Carpal tunnel syndrome can be an occupational disease, but it cannot be determined whether or not an individual case of carpal tunnel syndrome is occupationally related. Occupations that offer the greatest risk are those that require repetitive motions, especially those requiring flexion and ulnar deviation of the wrist while the hand is used.

Carpal tunnel release produces an average widening of the transverse arch of 2.7 mm. There is a direct relationship between widening of the canal and decreased grip strength but no relationship among range of motion, residual pain, or forearm circumference. There are five indications for carpal ligament release: symptoms lasting longer than ten months, age over 50 years, a positive Phelan test within 30 seconds, constant paresthesias, and the presence of flexor tenosynovitis. The indication for surgery was persistence of these factors despite trials of nonsurgical treatment such as splinting, nonsteroidal anti-inflammatory medication, and steroid injections.

Dupuytren's Contracture

A recently reported statistical relationship between cigarette smoking and Dupuytren's disease suggests that cigarette smoking may produce microvascular occlusion and subsequent fibrosis and contracture.

Other studies of the long-term results of palmar fasciotomy suggest that the deformity tends to recur. A review of 83 cases of Dupuytren's disease in women recommended only a limited fasciectomy, that is, removal of the diseased fascia. Women are more than twice as likely as men to have a flare reaction after surgery. The investigators noted that finger flexion was diminished in 76% of patients who had a flare reaction and 35% of those without a flare reaction. Thus, women tend to have a worse result than men. Women are more likely to have a flare reaction if they undergo a carpal tunnel release when the palmar fascia is excised. Therefore, these procedures should not be done simultaneously. If the symptoms persist, carpal tunnel release should be carried out later.

Controversies

Wrist Arthroplasty vs Arthrodesis

Arthrodesis of the wrist is currently used in posttraumatic conditions, destruction of the wrist after infection, paralytic conditions, spastic cerebral palsy, certain tumors, degenerative arthritis, failed arthroplasty, and rheumatoid arthritis. Most wrist arthrodeses are performed in patients with rheumatoid arthritis. In these patients, freedom from pain, ability to function, and stability of the wrist are important. Initial enthusiasm for silicone implant arthroplasty of the wrist has waned because of an increased fracture rate, bone resorption with sinking of the prosthesis, and recurrent deformity. However, there are also disadvantages with arthrodesis. Many activities of daily living require some wrist motion, and patients with arthrodeses who have rheumatoid involvement in other upper-extremity joints often find it difficult to write, dress, eat, and perform other activities around the house. Therefore, in cases of multiple joint involvement, preservation of some wrist motion can be a major benefit to the patient. In 20 consecutive patients who were treated with wrist arthrodesis (Fig. 13), average time to fusion was 11 weeks. The patients with solid fusion obtained relief of pain and had satisfactory functional results. In a later functional assessment in patients with bilateral wrist arthrodeses, the Jebsen-Taylor function test gave normal results 38% of the time and abnormal results 62% of the time. Of nine patients, two thought function remained unchanged and seven thought function had improved. Rayan and associates concluded that grip strength improved even in patients with rheumatoid arthritis and that bilateral wrist arthrodeses did not adversely affect upper extremity function.

Some authors favor arthroplasty. Other surgeons have been unable to duplicate the results obtained by Volz. His prosthesis is currently undergoing design changes, and future trials will be necessary to evaluate its success. A suggested combination of fusion and a condylar silicone implant to replace the capitate allows motion at the midcarpal level. The pain was relieved in a small series of cases, and average postoperative range of motion was 42 degrees of extension and 23 degrees of flexion. These early results are encouraging but, because rheumatoid arthritis involves all the joints of the carpus, progression of the disease process is possible in these cases.

In a comparison of 33 patients with rheumatoid arthritis who underwent wrist fusion with 37 who underwent silicone wrist implant arthroplasty, results were good or excellent in 97% of the arthrodesis cases and 78% of the arthroplasty cases. Postoperative flexion averaged 32 degrees and extension averaged 29 degrees; most patients reported that dexterity and strength were adequate. Arthroplasties on dominant hands gave better results than those on the nondominant side. There were no pseudarthroses in their group, and the complication rate in the fusion group was 18%. In the arthroplasty group, 25% required revisions. Interestingly, bone resorption was noted about the implants in 14%, and subsidence was noted in

11%. Swanson predicted that the use of titanium grommets would lead to minimal resorption and settling. The grommets also theoretically protect the surface of the implant from debriding by bone that could result in the development of silicone synovitis. Arthroplasty results were not predictable in patients with class IV rheumatoid arthritis who had anterior wrist dislocations, in patients receiving long-term steroids, and in patients using ambulatory aids. Wrist fusion is recommended for patients with marked osseous destruction and in patients whose wrist extensor tendons are absent. Previous infection that has resolved is also an indication for fusion rather than arthroplasty.

In patients with rheumatoid arthritis who have severe bilateral wrist involvement, the preferred treatment is arthrodesis in a neutral position on the nondominant side for functions that require more strength and arthroplasty on the dominant side so that the patient has some wrist motion for performing the activities of daily living. Arthroplasties may be inappropriate for young patients because of the progressive nature of the disease and the obvious possibility that they may require ambulatory aids as they get older.

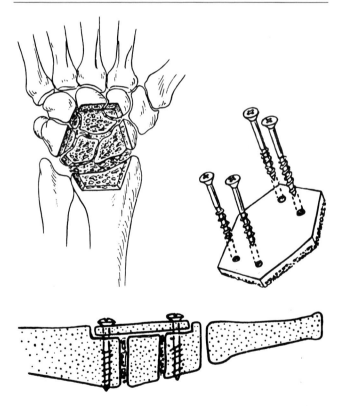

Figure 13

Wrist arthrodesis. **Top left**, The articular cartilage of the radiocarpal and intercarpal joints is removed. A cancellous bed is made by removing the dorsal cortex of the radius and carpal bones. **Top right**, An inner table iliac corticocancellous bone graft is shaped like the decorticated bed, drilled, and tapped for interfragmentary screw fixation. **Bottom**, The corticocancellous bone graft is fixed in its bed with four 4-mm cancellous screws and the spaces are filled with cancellous bone graft material. (Reproduced with permission from Rayan GM: Wrist arthrodesis. *J Hand Surg* 1986;11A:356–364.)

Distal Radioulnar Joint

The Darrach procedure remains the classic treatment for distal radioulnar joint derangement. Careful minimal bone resection and soft-tissue reconstruction are essential for good results. In a study of 20 patients with limited function and pain after the Darrach procedure, the authors were unable to identify any radiographic differences between these patients and patients who had successful Darrach resections. They concluded that the Darrach procedure can lead to serious disability in young patients and in patients with lax ligaments.

Others have supported this concept by stating that the triangular fibrocartilage complex is functionally disabled by the Darrach procedure. Obviously, excessive bone resection with the Darrach procedure leads to distal instability of the ulna with pain, prominence of the distal ulna, and mechanical impingement against the radius with rotation. A previously described technique called "hemiresection-interposition arthroplasty" produced stable, painless motion in 85% of patients with rheumatoid arthritis and in 100% of those with degenerative or posttraumatic arthritis.

Another type of arthroplasty preserves ulnar length, the styloid process, and the triangular fibrocartilage complex. In this "match distal ulnar resection," the radial side of the distal ulna is resected to match the opposing surface of the radius throughout the arch of forearm rotation. After an average follow-up of six years, each of the 44 wrists had a stable distal ulna and painless rotation averaging 80 degrees of pronation and 88 degrees of supination. No patient required additional surgery.

Hagert reported success with a corrective osteotomy and reconstruction of the radioulnar ligament in a malunited distal radius in cases of derangement of the distal radioulnar joint. His results were excellent in 17 cases, good in 19, fair in two, and poor in one. He noted a good correlation between the radiographic results and the functional results.

Another procedure that maintains the function of the triangular fibrocartilage complex while restoring forearm rotation is the Lauenstein procedure. Although the clinical results are limited, it has the advantage of preserving the triangular fibrocartilage complex as well as maintaining the normal anatomic configuration of the wrist. However, if excessive bone is resected, a distal portion of the proximal ulna may be unstable. If inadequate bone is resected, reactive bone may form at the osteotomy site, limiting motion. Each of these procedures has its advocates, and the results vary in different clinical series. In elderly patients, a carefully performed Darrach procedure is recommended. In younger patients with distal radioulnar joint dysfunction, the treatment of choice appears to be resection arthroplasty of the distal radioulnar joint with preservation of ulnar length, the ulnar styloid, and the triangular fibrocartilage complex and, possibly, interposition of tissue between the distal radius and the ulnar. In cases of malunion of the distal radius with involvement of the ulnar joint, the recommended treatment is corrective osteotomy and soft-tissue reconstruction of the ligamentous support of the distal radioulnar joint.

Annotated Bibliography

Keywords

Arthritis, Arthrodesis; Carpal tunnel; Dupuytren's contracture; Hand reconstruction; Osteonecrosis; Proximal row carpectomy; Tendon transfer; Wrist reconstruction.

Biomechanics of the Wrist

Burgess RC: The effect of a simulated scaphoid malunion on wrist motion. *J Hand Surg* 1987;12A:774–776.
   Wrist extension is diminished in malunion of the scaphoid.

Short WH, Palmer AK, Werner FW, et al: A biomechanical study of distal radial fractures. *J Hand Surg* 1987;12A:529–534.
   Load distribution is concentrated in the radial and articular surfaces and increasing angular deformities of the distal radius increases load transmission through the ulna.

Viegas SF, Tencer AF, Cantrell J, et al: Load transfer characteristics of the wrist: Part I. The normal joint. *J Hand Surg* 1987;12A:971–978.
   The contact areas of the scaphoid and lunate against the distal radius and triangular fibrocartilage complex are located on the palmar aspect. When the wrist is in extension, the contact areas are on the dorsal surface.

Viegas SF, Tencer AF, Cantrell J, et al: Load transfer characteristics of the wrist: Part II. Perilunate instability. *J Hand Surg* 1987;12A:978–985.
   Perilunate instability decreases the contact area with the scaphoid. Pressures increased with stage III instability.

Physiology of the Tendons of the Hand

Cohen MJ, Kaplan L: Histology and ultrastructure of the human flexor tendon sheath. *J Hand Surg* 1987;12A: 25–29.
   The flexor tendon sheath consists of a parietal component and a visceral component. These are qualitatively similar and form a synovium-lined space.

Doyle JR: Anatomy of the finger flexor tendon sheath and pulley system. *J Hand Surg* 1988;13A:473–484.
   The author continues to use his original descriptive terminology for the pulley system with the addition of the palmar aponeurosis pulley.

Hausman M, Rubin C, Littler JW, et al: Morphologic and radiographic analysis of transferred tendon-bone junctions. *Proc Am Soc Surg Hand* 1988;43:3-5.
   Tendon does not heal directly to bone when passed through a metaphyseal tunnel. A sclerotic wall surrounds the tendon. Healing occurs at the periosteum.

Manske PR: Flexor tendon healing. *J Hand Surg* 1988; 13B:237–245.

Excellent review article on the current state of knowledge on the healing of flexor tendons.

Russell JE, Manske PR: Collagen synthesis during tendon repair: Epitenon impact. *Trans Orthop Res Soc* 1989;14:274.

Epitenon cells produce more collagen during flexor tendon repair in the macaque monkey than does the central endotenon core of fibroblasts. Both are apparently important in matrix synthesis during flexor tendon healing.

Diagnostic Evaluation

Radionuclide Imaging

Pin PG, Semenkovich JW, Young VL, et al: Role of radionuclide imaging in the evaluation of wrist pain. *J Hand Surg* 1988;13A:810–814.

Bone scans were used successfully in patients with wrist pain. When the bone scans are positive, additional clinical and diagnostic studies may be necessary to establish the diagnosis.

Arthrography

Zinberg EM, Palmer AK, Coren AB, et al: The triple-injection wrist arthrogram. *J Hand Surg* 1988;13A:803–809.

Only injection of all three joints (radiocarpal, midcarpal, and radioulnar) permitted accurate diagnosis of lesions in each of these three joints.

Magnetic Resonance Imaging

Trumble TE, Desser TS, McCarthy S, et al: Magnetic imaging in the diagnosis of avascular necrosis with clinical and histologic correlation. *Trans Orthop Res Soc* 1989;14:447.

Thirteen cases of osteonecrosis of the lunate or proximal scaphoid were diagnosed by magnetic resonance imaging. In each case, the diagnosis was substantiated by biopsy.

Computed Tomography

Biondetti PR, Vannier MW, Gilula LA, et al: Wrist: Coronal and transaxial CT scanning. *Radiology* 1987; 163:149–151.

Coronal images are superior to transaxial images except in fractures of the hook of the hamate and distal radioulnar subluxation.

Posttraumatic Problems of the Wrist

Kienböck's Disease

Imbriglia JE, Goldstein S, Brourman S, et al: Radial shortening for Kienböck's disease. *Proc Am Soc Surg Hand* 1988;43:5–9.

Radial shortening averaging 3 mm significantly relieved pain, allowed patients to return to work, and promoted revascularization (shown by radiographic evidence) in 21 patients with Kienböck's disease.

Kato H, Usui M, Minami A: Long-term results of Kienböck's disease treated by excisional arthroplasty with a silicone implant or coiled palmaris longus tendon. *J Hand Surg* 1986;11A:645–653.

Both the silicone implant and the palmaris longus tendon arthroplasty were unsuccessful in treating Kienböck's disease when advanced collapse was present.

Palmer AK, Werner FW: A biomechanical evaluation of operative procedures performed for the treatment of Kienböck's disease. *Proc Am Soc Surg Hand* 1988;43: 3–7.

In cadaveric wrists, the lunate fossa was unloaded by a change in ulnar variance of 2 mm or a change of 5 degrees of radial inclination. Capitohamate fusion was not recommended.

Scaphoid Nonunion and Osteonecrosis

Adams BD, Blair WF, Reagan DS, et al: Technical factors related to Herbert screw fixation. *J Hand Surg* 1988;13A:893–899.

Nonunion was present in 78% of cases secondary to technical factors such as poor scaphoid reduction, inaccurate jig placement, or improper screw length.

Cosio MQ, Camp RA: Percutaneous pinning of symptomatic scaphoid nonunions. *J Hand Surg* 1986;11A:350–355.

Thirteen patients with symptomatic nonunion of the scaphoid were treated by percutaneous pinning. Union occurred in ten patients.

Cooney WP, Linscheid RL, Dobyns JH, et al: Scaphoid nonunion: Role of anterior interpositional bone grafts. *J Hand Surg* 1988;13A:635–650.

An anterior wedge graft combined with a Herbert screw was used to treat angulated nonunions of the scaphoid. After correction of the deformity and union, both the scapholunate and the capitolunate angles improved.

Osterman AL, Bora FW, Maiting E: Herbert screw fixation for scaphoid nonunion. *Proc Am Soc Surg Hand* 1988;43:4.

In a large series of patients with scaphoid nonunion, a union rate of 84% was achieved with the Herbert screw without supplemental bone graft.

Vender MI, Watson HK, Wiener BD, et al: Degenerative change in symptomatic scaphoid nonunion. *J Hand Surg* 1987;12A:514–519.

In 64 patients, persistent nonunion led to a significant number of wrists with radioscaphoid degenerative changes but sparing of the radiolunate joint.

Arthritis of the Wrist

Total Joint Replacement

Brase DW, Millender LH: Failure of silicone rubber wrist arthroplasty in rheumatoid arthritis. *J Hand Surg* 1986;11A:175–183.

Twenty percent of the implants fractured with 12 of 14 requiring revision. Two of the revised implants also fractured.

Dennis DA, Ferlic DC, Clayton ML: Volz total wrist arthroplasty in rheumatoid arthritis: A long-term review. *J Hand Surg* 1986;11A:483–490.

Complications occurred in 12 of 23 patients but 86% reported pain relief and satisfaction with the outcome.

Fatti JF, Palmer AK, Mosher JF: The long-term results of Swanson silicone rubber interpositional wrist arthroplasty. *J Hand Surg* 1986;11A:166–175.

Results were satisfactory in only 35 of 53 cases after an average follow-up of 3.4 years. Radiographic deterioration was progressive in 75%.

Figgie HE III, Ranawat CS, Inglis AE, et al: Preliminary results of total wrist arthroplasty in rheumatoid arthritis using the trispherical total wrist arthroplasty. *J Arthrop* 1988;3:9–15.

Thirty-four of 38 patients were significantly improved beyond the level of an arthrodesis. Total wrist arthroplasty is recommended in patients with stage III and stage IV rheumatoid arthritis.

Menon J: Total wrist replacement using the modified Volz prosthesis. *J Bone Joint Surg* 1987;69A:998–1006.

In each series there was significant relief of pain but a high complication rate. The prosthesis is recommended for use in the low-demand patient with rheumatoid arthritis and not in those with osteoarthritis.

Limited Arthrodesis

Bax JC, Sproul JT, Klug MS, et al: Triskaphe arthrodesis: Solution or problem? *Proc Am Soc Surg Hand* 1988;43:3–3.

Nonunion occurred in 23% and reflex sympathetic dystrophy in 14% of 77 cases.

Frykman EB, Ekenstam FA, Wadin K: Triscaphoid arthrodesis and its complications. *J Hand Surg* 1988;13A: 844–848.

There were five nonunions in 19 patients.

Garcia-Elias M, Cooney WP, Linscheid RL, et al: STT vs. SC limited intercarpal fusions: A kinematic study. *Proc Am Soc Surg Hand* 1988;43:4–9.

Neither type of limited fusion is superior to the other. Both substantially change intracarpal kinematics.

Kraemer BA, Young VL, Weeks PM: Functional results after scaphoid-trapezium-trapezoid fusion. *Proc Am Soc Surg Hand* 1988;43:2–3.

Pain persisted postoperatively at the extremes of motion in 15 of 20 patients.

Meyerdierks EM, Mosher JF, Werner FW: Limited wrist arthrodesis: A laboratory study. *J Hand Surg* 1987;12A: 526–529.

The authors measured the passive arc of motion in cadaver wrists after three types of limited arthrodesis.

Minami A, Ogino T, Minami M: Limited wrist fusions. *J Hand Surg* 1988;13A:660–667.

The authors describe their results with radiocarpal and midcarpal joint fusions.

Pisano S, Peimer CA: Scaphocapitate intercarpal arthrodesis. *Proc Am Soc Surg Hand* 1988;43:3–1.

Scaphocapitate fusion is useful as a salvage procedure for advanced stages of Kienböck's disease, instability of the scaphoid, or persistent scaphoid nonunion.

Trumble T, Bour CJ, Smith RJ, et al: Intercarpal arthrodesis for static and dynamic volar intercalated segment instability. *J Hand Surg* 1988;13A:384–390.

Lunate-triquetrum-hamate-capitate fusion is recommended for a symptomatic volar intercalary segment instability deformity.

Proximal Row Carpectomy

Bieber EJ, Linscheid RL, Dobyns JH, et al: Failed distal ulna resections. *J Hand Surg* 1988;13A:193–200.

There were 20 cases of persistent pain and limited function after Darrach resection. No identifiable abnormalities were found.

Broudy AS, Imbriglia JE, Hagberg WC, et al: Proximal row carpectomy: A clinical evaluation. *Proc Am Soc Surg Hand* 1988;43:3–12.

Pain was relieved in 26 of 27 patients followed up for an average of four years. Motion and grip strength improved, with final results achieved at four to five months postoperatively.

Green DP: Proximal row carpectomy. *Hand Clin* 1987;3: 163–168.

Pain was relieved in 13 of 15 patients. Motion and grip strength improved with time (three to six months).

Watson HK, Ryu JY, Burgess RC: Matched distal ulnar resection. *J Hand Surg* 1986;11A:812–817.

A new technique for partial resection of the distal ulna gives predictable results in derangement of the distal radioulnar joint.

Posttraumatic Problems of the Hand

Soft-Tissue Defects

Fleegler EJ, Weinzweig N: The versatile axial pattern digital transposition flap. *J Hand Surg* 1988;13A:494–500.

This is a useful flap based on a digital artery for salvage of severe composite tissue loss of the distal finger.

Kleinman WB, O'Connell SJ: The versatility and effectiveness of the radial artery fasciocutaneous forearm flap in upper extremity soft tissue coverage. *Proc Am Soc Surg Hand* 1988;43:4–6.

The authors used this flap in 22 cases.

Upton J, Rogers C, Durham-Smith G, et al: Clinical applications of free temporoparietal flaps in hand reconstruction. *J Hand Surg* 1986;11A:475–483.

Vascularized temporoparietal fascia may be used as an alternative in soft-tissue coverage of large defects in the hand.

Tendon Transfers

Hoffer MM, Lehman M, Mitani M: Long-term follow-up on tendon transfers to the extensors of the wrist and fingers in patients with cerebral palsy. *J Hand Surg* 1986;11A:836–840.

Finger extension and release improved after transfer of the flexor carpi ulnaris to the extensor digitorum communis.

Rieser TV, Waters RL: Long-term follow-up of the Moberg key grip procedure. *J Hand Surg* 1986;11A:724–728.

The authors recommend transfer of the brachioradialis for wrist extension before procedures on the thumb. If 3+ wrist extension is achieved, they then carry out the Moberg procedure but do not suggest release of the A1 pulley in order to avoid bowstringing of the flexor pollicis longus tendon.

Wenner SM, Johnson KA: Transfer of the flexor carpi ulnaris to the radial wrist extensors in cerebral palsy. *J Hand Surg* 1988;13A:231–233.

Patients benefited from this transfer who were able to extend the fingers actively to neutral with the wrist in flexion or extension. Patients who could not actively extend the fingers to neutral did not benefit from this transfer.

Tendon Injuries

Amadio PC, Wood MB, Cooney WP III, et al: Staged flexor tendon reconstruction in the fingers and hand. *J Hand Surg* 1988;13A:559–562.

A two-stage reconstruction gave acceptable results in severely damaged fingers. Complication rates were high, flexion contractures common, and postoperative rehabilitation critical to the final result.

Green SM, Posner MA: Secondary flexor tendon repair. *Proc Am Soc Surg Hand* 1988;43:343.

Results were satisfactory in 67% of patients undergoing delayed or secondary flexor tendon repair in zone 2. Children had poorer results.

Moore JR, Weiland AJ, Valdata L: Tendon ruptures in

the rheumatoid hand: Analysis of treatment and functional results in 60 patients. *J Hand Surg* 1987;12A:9–14.

Treatment of single or double tendon ruptures with tendon transfers was highly successful. Extensor lag was common after reconstruction for three or more tendon ruptures.

O'Connell SJ, Moore MM, Dell PC, et al: Primary repair of zone I and II flexor tendon injuries in children. *Proc Am Soc Surg Hand* 1988;43:2–1.

A large three-center review study demonstrated excellent results with primary repair of zone I injuries in children under the age of 15 years. Digital motion was approximately the same after immobilization and passive motion treatment.

Wehbé MA, Mawr B, Hunter JM, et al: Two-stage flexor-tendon reconstruction: Ten-year experience. *J Bone Joint Surg* 1986;68A:752–763.

Mean active motion in 136 patients was 176 degrees. Complications included flexion contracture in 41%, tendon rupture in 14%, and infection in 4%.

Arthritis of the Hand

Joint Replacement

Bieber EJ, Weiland AJ, Volenec-Dowling S: Silicone-rubber implant arthroplasty of the metacarpophalangeal joints for rheumatoid arthritis. *J Bone Joint Surg* 1986;68A:206–209.

Silicone arthroplasty led to relief of pain and a high degree of patient satisfaction. However, active range of motion decreased and recurrent ulnar drift increased with time.

Swanson AB, Poitevin LA, de Groot Swanson G, et al: Bone remodeling phenomena in flexible implant arthroplasty in the metacarpophalangeal joints: Long-term study. *Clin Orthop* 1986;205:254–267.

A cortical shell formed about the stems of the implant and the metaphyses of the metacarpal and proximal phalanx thickened.

Vahvanen V, Viljakka T: Silicone rubber implant arthroplasty of the metacarpophalangeal joint in rheumatoid arthritis: A follow-up study of 32 patients. *J Hand Surg* 1986;11A:333–339.

Patient satisfaction was high with this operation. Bone resorption about the stem and migration of the implant were found in 24% of the fingers.

Zimmerman NB, Suhey P, Clark GL, et al: Silicone interpositional arthroplasty of the distal interphalangeal joint. *Proc Am Soc Surg Hand* 1988;43:3-7.

In selected cases this procedure offers pain relief with stability and improved motion.

Arthrodesis

Ayres JR, Goldstrohm GL, Miller GJ, et al: Proximal interphalangeal joint arthrodesis with the Herbert screw. *J Hand Surg* 1988;13A:600–603.

Compression arthrodesis by means of the Herbert screw resulted in a 98% union rate.

Burton RI, Margles SW, Lunseth PA: Small-joint arthrodesis in the hand. *J Hand Surg* 1986;11A:678–682.

Union was achieved in 99% of cases by means of tight coaptation of metaphyseal bone and fixation with crossed Kirschner wires.

Kowalski MF, Manske PR: Arthrodesis of digital joints in children. *J Hand Surg* 1988;13A:874–879.

Successful arthrodesis can be achieved in children without interference with growth of the digits.

Trapeziometacarpal Joint

Burton RI, Pellegrini VD Jr: Surgical management of basal joint arthritis of the thumb: Part II. Ligament reconstruction with tendon interposition arthroplasty. *J Hand Surg* 1986;11A:324–332.

This technique, which uses tendon graft as a spacer with ligament reconstruction, is a successful alternative to silicone implant arthroplasty.

Hay EL, Bomberg BC, Burke C, et al: Long-term results of silicone trapezial implant arthroplasty. *J Arthrop* 1988;3:215–223.

Overall results were good after an average four-year follow-up although degenerative changes involving the implant increased with time.

Nishijima N, Ueba Y, Yamamuro T: Growth of autografted tendons: An experimental study in vivo. *J Hand Surg* 1988;13A:234–237.

The initial growth in length of transplanted flexor digitorum profundus tendons in young chickens was similar to that of control tendons. At 15 weeks experimental growth was less than control growth but by 20 weeks there was no statistical difference.

Nylén S, Juhlin LJ, Lugnegard H: Weilby tendon interposition arthroplasty for osteoarthritis of the trapezial joints. *J Hand Surg* 1987;12B:68–72.

Another type of resection arthroplasty that avoids the risks of implant dislocation and silicone synovitis.

Peimer CA: Long-term complications of trapeziometacarpal silicone arthroplasty. *Clin Orthop* 1987;220:86–98.

Wear particles of silicone less than 15 µ in size cause destructive synovitis.

Peimer CA, Medige J, Eckert BS, et al: Reactive synovitis after silicone arthroplasty. *J Hand Surg* 1986;11A:624–638.

Silicone synovitis secondary to particulate debris of the implants can occur. The process can be stopped by removal of the implant, synovectomy, and curettage of any lytic lesions.

Pellegrini VD Jr, Burton RI: Surgical management of basal joint arthritis of the thumb: Part I. Long-term results of silicone implant arthroplasty. *J Hand Surg* 1986;11A:309–324.

An excellent review demonstrating significant silicone implant wear with ligamentous reconstruction. Reactive synovitis and bone resorption increased with time.

Carpal Tunnel Syndrome

Gartsman GM, Kovach JC, Crouch CC, et al: Carpal arch alteration after carpal tunnel release. *J Hand Surg* 1986;11A:372–374.

There is a direct relationship between widening of the transverse carpal arch and decreased grip strength after carpal tunnel release.

Kaplan SJ, Glickel SZ, Eaton RG: Prognostic factors in carpal tunnel syndrome. *Proc Am Soc Surg Hand* 1988; 43:2–3.

The presence of stenosing flexor tenosynovitis was a strong indication for surgical release. Nonsurgical management often failed.

Szabo RM, Chidgey LK: Stress carpal tunnel pressures

in carpal tunnel patients and normal patients. *Proc Am Soc Surg Hand* 1988;43:4–1.

Patients with carpal tunnel syndrome had higher intracarpal pressures than normal patients. Their pressures also increased more and remained increased longer than those of the control subjects.

Dupuytren's Contracture

Zemel NP, Balcomb TV, Stark HH, et al: Dupuytren's disease in women: Evaluation of long-term results after operation. *J Hand Surg* 1987;12A:1012–1016.

Palmar fasciectomy produced poorer results in women than in men. Only the contracted fascia should be removed and prophylactic carpal tunnel release, which was associated with a postoperative flare reaction, should not be done.

Controversies

Wrist Arthroplasty vs Arthrodesis

Rayan GM: Wrist arthrodesis. *J Hand Surg* 1986;11A: 356–364.

Rayan GM, Brentlinger A, Purnell D, et al: Functional assessment of bilateral wrist arthrodeses. *J Hand Surg* 1987;12A:1020–1024.

Taleisnik J: Combined radiocarpal arthrodesis and midcarpal (lunocapitate) arthroplasty for treatment of rheumatoid arthritis of the wrist. *J Hand Surg* 1987;12A:1–8.

Vicar AJ, Burton RI: Surgical management of the rheumatoid wrist: Fusion or arthroplasty. *J Hand Surg* 1986; 11A:790–797.

Distal Radioulnar Joint

Bieber EJ, Linscheid RL, Dobyns JH, et al: Failed distal ulna resections. *J Hand Surg* 1988;13A:193–200.

Hagert CG: The distal radioulnar joint. *Hand Clin* 1987; 3:41–50.

Watson HK, Ryu JY, Burgess RC: Matched distal ulnar resection. *J Hand Surg* 1986;11A:812–817.

III
Spine

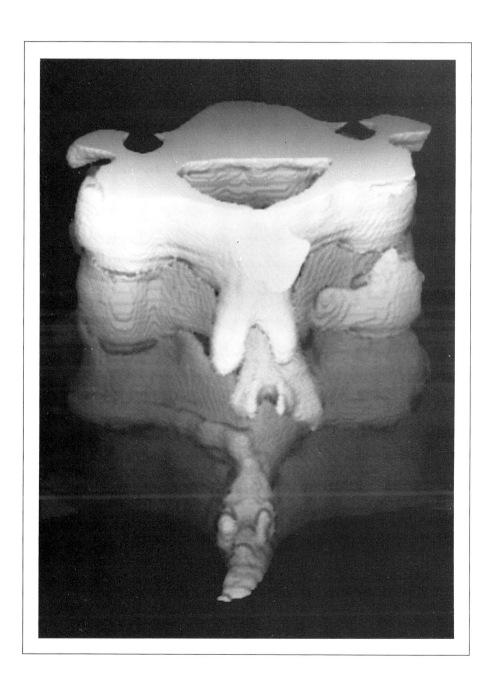

31

The Cervical Spine: Pediatric and Reconstructive Aspects

The surgical management of the cervical spine in the patient with rheumatoid arthritis is often controversial. Surgical intervention in patients with severe rheumatoid arthritis may be associated with a significant rate of morbidity and mortality. The surgical approach in a patient with cervical spondylotic myelopathy is frequently debated. Similarly, the use of methylmethacrylate to stabilize the cervical spine can be questioned.

Congenital Anomalies

Tethering of the cord can result from disparity between the longitudinal growth of the cord and the bony canal. However, differential growth does not explain why symptoms typically occur long after longitudinal growth has ceased. Tethering is often associated with a fibrous, cartilaginous, or osseous cleft that results in a longitudinal split in the spinal cord known as diastematomyelia. This dysraphic condition may originate from a persistent neurenteric canal originally formed during the embryonic development of the notochord. Most of the lesions occur in the lumbar spine and less than 5% occur in the cervical spine. Cervical spine radiographs in such cases may show a widened interpedicular distance in the lower (C-5 to C-7) cervical spine. Gradual impairment of bowel and bladder control can occur. Tethering of the cord should be considered when there is neurologic deficit along with midline cutaneous abnormalities and underlying spina bifida occulta. It is important to recognize this condition to avoid progressive neurologic deficit. Computed tomography with intrathecal contrast is an effective method of diagnosis.

Congenital anomalies of the cervical spine are relatively uncommon and neurologic compromise secondary to them is even less common. Typically, such anomalies are incidental findings; however, when they are associated with neurologic deficit, they may be the source of neural compromise. Patients with congenital anomalies who show evidence of root and/or cord compromise may require further neurodiagnostic studies to delineate the source of the neural compression and provide the basis for treatment.

Pediatric Conditions Involving the Cervical Spine

Abnormalities of the Atlantoaxial Articulation

The atlantoaxial articulation is a unique structure both anatomically and functionally. Approximately one half of all cervical spine rotation occurs at this level. Because of this, many of the deformities are rotatory in nature. Traumatic atlantoaxial rotatory subluxation or dislocation is perhaps the most common problem involving this segment. However, other conditions that can cause rotatory instability include inflammatory diseases such as rheu-

matoid arthritis or ankylosing spondylitis, congenital disorders such as Down's syndrome, pyogenic infection (particularly in the pharyngeal region), and tumors. Patients typically have torticollis. All these conditions must be considered in the differential diagnosis. Atlantoaxial rotatory subluxation may become fixed and pose a long-term management problem. Prompt recognition of acute subluxation or dislocation may avoid a later fixed deformity or potential instability. Patients can be treated with a short period of traction to achieve reduction; after an appropriate period of immobilization, they can return to function.

In addition to rotatory abnormalities of the atlantoaxial articulation, anteroposterior displacement can result from congenital, traumatic, infectious, or inflammatory factors. As in cases of atlantoaxial rotatory dislocation, pharyngitis of viral, bacterial, or granulomatous origin can lead to laxity of the supporting ligaments, producing atlantoaxial displacement in the anteroposterior plane. When significant instability is present, stabilization, typically a posterior fusion of C-1 and C-2, may be needed. The sagittal diameter of the cervical canal is a good predictor of the risk of neurologic damage. As the predens interval increases, the space available for the cord is compromised. When this interval is greater than 7 to 9 mm, the cord may be at risk.

Atlantoaxial instability is common in patients with Down's syndrome (trisomy 21) (Figs. 1 and 2). Significant instability with the spinal cord at risk may require stabilization. In many late cases, complete reduction is not possible and decompression along with stabilization may be necessary, particularly if signs of myelopathy are present. Combined rotatory and anteroposterior subluxation of the atlantoaxial complex can also occur. In addition, instability of the occipitocervical junction is possible and this level should also be evaluated. Attention has been focused on cervical instability since the advent of screening for patients who participate in the Special Olympics. Children should be screened with dynamic lateral flexion-extension radiographs. Mild to moderate instability (a predens interval of less than 7 to 9 mm) is often managed by observation, a cervical orthosis, and avoidance of contact sports, tumbling, or other activities likely to load the neck. In patients with significant instability and/or neurologic signs or symptoms, surgical stabilization should be considered.

Other Conditions

Hemophilia Although patients with hemophilia may have cervical spine involvement, instability is less common than it is in the peripheral joints. A recent report showed no correlation between the severity of peripheral joint involvement and the cervical spine radiographic changes. Compared with the peripheral joints, the cervical articulations have a smaller ratio of synovium to joint surface area and are less susceptible to direct trauma. In addition,

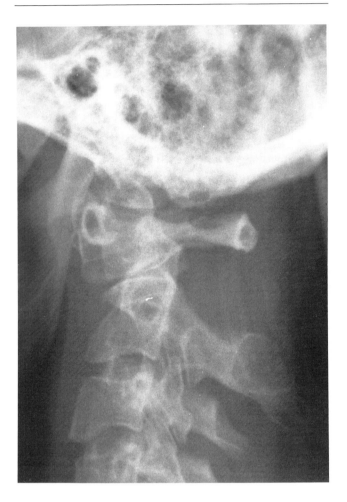

Figure 1

Lateral radiograph demonstrates significant atlantoaxial instability in a patient with Down's syndrome.

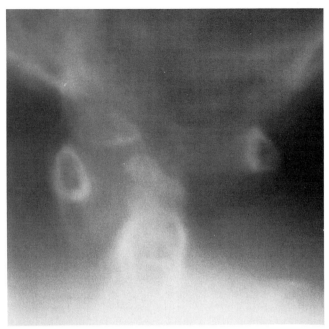

Figure 2

Lateral tomogram of the patient shown in Figure 1 demonstrates an ossiculum terminale in addition to the instability. Tomography is useful in quantitating the degree of subluxation.

stresses on the weightbearing joints may be much greater than those in the neck.

Juvenile Rheumatoid Arthritis Juvenile rheumatoid arthritis can involve the cervical spine. Patients with polyarticular involvement (more than four joints) or systemic onset frequently complain of stiffness, and radiographic changes in the cervical spine are common (Fig. 3). Even in the presence of extensive radiographic involvement, neck pain is not common. The presence of severe neck pain and/or torticollis, therefore, warrants investigation for other causes such as fracture or infection.

Cervical Kyphosis Cervical kyphosis tends to be problematic in children. One common cause of this condition is extensive laminectomy for a tumor. In patients who undergo additional radiation therapy, a rapidly progressive kyphosis leading to neurologic involvement may develop. Kyphosis can also occur in patients with intact posterior elements as a result of congenital, traumatic, metabolic, or neoplastic processes. The more horizontal orientation of the facets in young children compared with that in adults may partially explain the greater propensity for kyphotic instability in this age group. Early recognition and treat-

ment are the keys to arresting the progression and improving the neurologic signs and symptoms.

Disk Calcification Calcification of the cervical intervertebral disk is a self-limited disorder in children. The calcification typically occurs in the anulus fibrosus. The patient typically experiences the spontaneous onset of neck pain and stiffness. This is often misdiagnosed as a fracture. Treatment usually includes rest and cervical immobilization.

Child Abuse Unfortunately, child abuse is a common clinical entity. One problem is the "shaken baby syndrome." A recent report stated that a history of actual shaking is often lacking and the diagnosis is usually based on a constellation of clinical and radiographic findings. Clinical findings include either retinal hemorrhages with subdural or subarachnoid hemorrhage. A computed tomographic scan often confirms these findings. In fatal cases, there may be signs of blunt impact to the head, frequently first noted at the time of autopsy. A study using models of 1-month-old infants found that blunt force, as well as shaking, is needed to cause serious injury. Shaking alone in an otherwise normal baby is unlikely to cause the shaken baby syndrome.

Tumors and Metabolic Conditions

Primary neoplasms of the spine can cause neck or back pain and, although relatively rare, must be considered in the differential diagnosis. Benign lesions include osteochondromas, hemangiomas, and osteoblastomas. Primary osseous lesions should be carefully defined by means of arteriography, tomography, bone scans, computed tomography with or without myelography, magnetic resonance imaging, or some combination of these.

The goals of treatment include definitive diagnosis, surgery appropriate for the tumor type, and maintenance or restoration of neural function and spinal stability (Algorithm 1).

Younger patients tend to have benign tumors and to survive without symptoms after treatment, whereas older patients are more likely to have malignant neoplasms that result in death. Surgery, nonetheless, can provide years of painless and productive function.

Primary malignant lesions include chordomas and solitary plasmacytomas. An interlesional—rather than total—excision of suspected malignant lesions can be used to decompress the neural and/or vascular structures; this is followed by an arthrodesis for stability. Anterior resection is indicated for tumors involving the anterior column; a posterior approach is used for tumors involving primarily the posterior elements. Both anterior and posterior excisions should be combined with arthrodesis. Patients with two-column involvement are typically treated by staged anterior and posterior resection and arthrodesis.

Most malignant lesions involving the adult cervical spine are metastatic rather than primary. Common sources of metastatic lesions are the breast, prostate, renal cell, and lung. Many of these lesions can be treated with radiation and/or chemotherapy and an orthosis. Pain not relieved by such measures and progressive instability and/or progressive neurologic involvement are indications for surgical intervention. Pathologic fractures of the cervical spine are a difficult management problem because of instability and the potential for neural compromise. Quality of life issues are an important additional consideration for patients with limited life expectancies. Surgical intervention may allow them to be managed outside the hospital with less supportive care. An overriding concern in management is the overall general medical status of the patient, including the expected length of survival.

Renal Osteodystrophy

Renal osteodystrophy can involve the cervical spine. Dialysis and renal transplantation has resulted in longer survival of patients with uremia and renal failure. The classic findings of renal osteodystrophy of the spine include the "rugger-jersey" spine, but osteopenia without accompanying sclerosis of the end plate may be seen. Such osteopenia is thought to result from a complex combination of abnormalities including hyperparathyroidism, osteomalacia, osteoporosis, and direct complications of dialysis such as aluminum toxicity. Ligament rupture has been reported in these patients; this phenomenon is probably related to metabolic acidosis, which eventually results in an abnormal ratio of elastin to collagen.

Adult Conditions of the Cervical Spine

Rheumatoid Arthritis

Rheumatoid arthritis often involves the cervical spine. The incidence of cervical involvement in patients with polyarticular rheumatoid arthritis has been reported to be higher than 80%. Fortunately, most patients with rheumatoid arthritis with cervical involvement do not have significant instability. The patient with more severe cer-

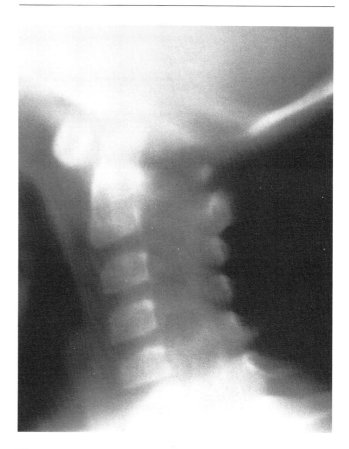

Figure 3

Lateral radiograph of a 6-year-old child with juvenile rheumatoid arthritis. The child has mild atlantoaxial subluxation.

vical involvement often has multiple joint involvement with significant destruction of the joints and resultant deformity. In addition, such patients typically are weakened by chronic disease and may also have peripheral neuropathies, making the diagnosis of cervical involvement difficult. Cervical spine involvement typically includes one or more of the following patterns: atlantoaxial subluxation, cranial settling, or occipitoatlantoaxial impaction and subaxial subluxation.

Progressive destruction of the ligaments, cartilage, and bone in the cervical spine may produce significant instability and, ultimately, neural compression. Early signs and symptoms include pain and neck stiffness. The severity of the neurologic involvement does not necessarily correspond with the degree of subluxation. Such cases can usually be managed with a cervical orthosis and intermittent follow-up examinations that include lateral flexion-extension radiographs of the cervical spine. Dynamic radiographs are also recommended to rule out undetected instability in patients who are to be given a general anesthetic. Progressive neurologic impairment and/or progressive instability are indications for surgical intervention. Intractable pain may be a further indication in rare cases. The goals of surgery are to stabilize the spine, relieve neurologic compression, and relieve pain.

Surgical management typically consists of stabilization procedures alone (Fig. 4). When significant neural compromise is unrelieved by skeletal traction, a decompressive

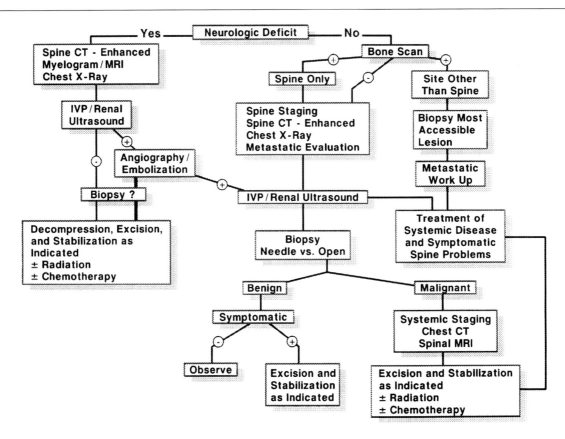

Algorithm 1

The approach to spine tumors. (Adapted with permission from Weinstein JN, McLain RF: Primary tumors of the spine. *Spine* 1987;12:843–851.)

procedure may also be indicated (Figs. 5 and 6). Atlantoaxial subluxation is typically managed with a posterior fusion of C-1 and C-2. Occipitocervical fusion may be considered when the posterior arch of C-1 is deficient because of erosion by rheumatoid pannus or congenital factors. Cranial settling is managed by a posterior occipitocervical fusion, but when cord compromise is significant, a transoral resection of the odontoid may be necessary. For patients with subaxial subluxation that is progressing or causing neurologic compromise, a posterior cervical arthrodesis is the most common procedure. Anterior fusion techniques may increase instability and are rarely warranted as isolated procedures.

A recent preliminary report detailed the use of somatosensory evoked potentials in the evaluation of the unstable rheumatoid spine. They may prove to be useful in monitoring the clinical status of patients with rheumatoid arthritis and may provide further insight regarding the indications for surgical intervention.

Ankylosing Spondylitis

Complications of ankylosing spondylitis include fracture and the chin-on-chest deformity. A cervical fracture is often associated with severe neurologic complications (Fig. 7). Fractures typically involve the lower cervical spine, which is often obscured by overlapping shadows on a lateral radiograph. A history of even minor trauma and neck pain should lead the physician to suspect an undetected fracture. Cervical radiographs should be obtained; tomography and/or computed tomography may be necessary to

establish the diagnosis. These fractures often result in a large epidural hematoma, causing neurologic deficits. They are also extremely unstable. Prompt rigid immobilization with a halo applied to maintain alignment of the preexisting kyphosis is important in preventing neurologic complications. In carefully selected cases, the fracture may provide a serendipitous opportunity to correct the flexion deformity, but the risk of epidural bleeding must be considered.

Neuromyopathic Conditions

Neuromyopathic conditions can also cause severe flexion deformities of the cervical spine similar to those seen in ankylosing spondylitis. Treatment involves an anterior surgical release of the contracted sternocleidomastoid muscles, halo dependent traction, posterior bony element resection, and spinal fusion supplemented with internal fixation. When extensive correction involves wide vertebral-body separation anteriorly, the addition of an anterior keystone strut graft may be necessary.

Infection

Differentiating between aseptic and bacterial meningitis after spinal surgery can be difficult. Traditionally the diagnosis is based on clinical findings and cerebrospinal fluid analysis. According to a recent report, standard cerebrospinal fluid testing may not be reliable in all cases. High fever, new neurologic deficits, active cerebrospinal fluid leak, and elevated leukocyte counts in the cerebrospinal

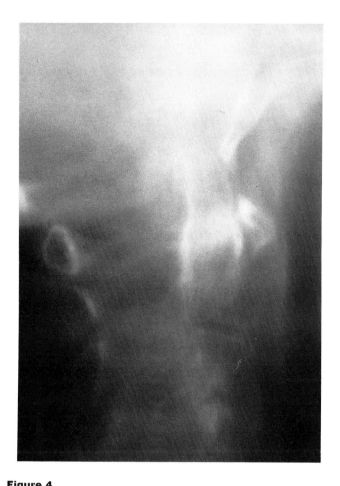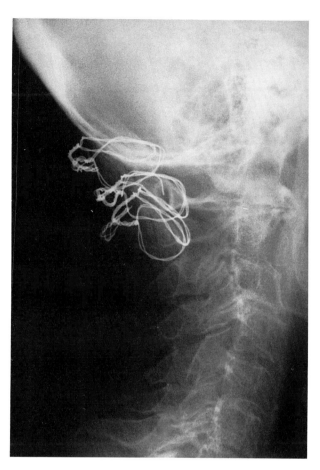

Figure 4

A patient with rheumatoid arthritis. **Left,** Lateral tomogram shows moderate cranial settling. **Right,** Postoperative lateral radiograph demonstrates occipitocervical arthrodesis.

fluid and peripheral blood tended to predict a bacterial cause. The cerebrospinal fluid glucose level and differential leukocyte count were less helpful criteria. No criterion or combination of criteria was sensitive and specific enough to reliably differentiate aseptic from bacterial meningitis in all patients. Further accuracy may be obtained by newer evolving tests such as cerebrospinal fluid levels of lactate, ferritin, total amino acids, and C-reactive protein.

Rabbit models have been useful in studying the pathogenesis and treatment of various spinal infections. A recent study evaluated antibiotic penetration in the nucleus pulposus. In adult humans, the intervertebral disk space is avascular and antibiotics must penetrate through a process of diffusion. The rabbit intervertebral disk is a reasonable model because of its anatomic and biochemical similarities to the human intervertebral disk. Clindamycin and tobramycin achieved therapeutic levels in the nucleus pulposus and both were present at levels above 50% of the serum concentrations. Cephalothin was not detected in the nucleus pulposus. The condition may be different in younger children because the intervertebral disk is somewhat vascular and antibiotic penetration is less of a problem. In adults with established infection, neovascularization in the involved tissue may provide a route for antibiotic penetration.

Cervical Spondylosis

Pain In a recent long-term follow-up, patients with neck pain who had suspected soft-tissue injuries and initially severe pain were the most likely to have an unsatisfactory outcome. No other clinical features were of value in predicting the final result in this series. There was no relation to degenerative changes, the sagittal diameter of the spinal canal, or the degree of cervical lordosis. Thus, caution is necessary when predicting outcome on the basis of the initial signs and symptoms (other than pain) and radiographs alone.

Cervical manipulation has been used to treat various neck pain syndromes. Such manipulations have been reported to cause serious neurologic injury. Vertebral artery damage has also been reported after cervical manipulation. The vertebral arteries are susceptible to trauma within the neck. Thus, a change in neurologic function after manipulation requires accurate diagnosis and prompt treatment.

Radiculopathy An anatomic study in cadavers demonstrated the intradural connections between adjacent cervical spinal roots. Intradural intersegmental connections between sensory nerve roots occur frequently in the cervical region and have been shown to have clinical and surgical significance. Posterior rootlet connections are the

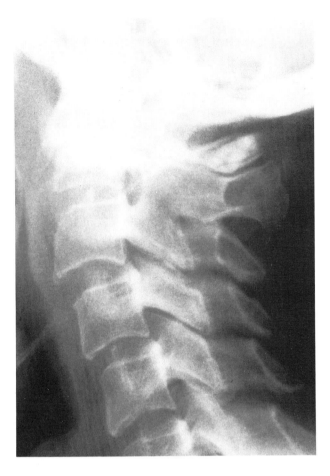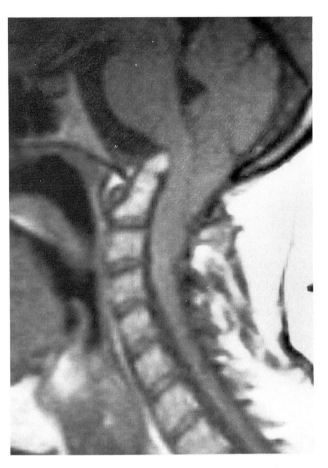

Figure 5
A patient with rheumatoid arthritis. **Left,** Lateral radiograph suggests severe cranial settling. Note that the anterior arch of the atlas is adjacent to the body of the axis. **Right,** Sagittal-plane magnetic resonance imaging confirms severe cranial settling with neural compression.

most common. These anatomic interconnections may explain the sensory or motor overlap observed in neurologic examinations. These anatomic differences may explain in part why clinical findings may appear to arise from an adjacent rather than the actual level.

Cervical disk herniation typically occurs at the posterolateral corner of the disk space between the posterior edge of the uncinate process and the lateral edge of the posterior longitudinal ligament. Herniations can also occur posteriorly (central herniation) or anteriorly. Anterior cervical disk herniation may manifest symptoms entirely different from those of radiculopathies caused by classic posterolateral herniation. An anterior herniation can cause esophageal impingement with resultant dysphagia. Herniated disk material can also become sequestered within the spinal canal and migrate around the surface of the cord, resulting in myelopathy. Sequestered fragments can be multiple. Treatment is based on accurate localization of the herniated material by imaging studies that dictate the appropriate surgical approach.

Internal disk derangement has been reported to be a source of unrelenting neck pain, but this diagnosis is controversial. Symptomatic levels are determined by the reproduction of the patient's symptoms at the time of injection. The cervical diskogram should be the last diagnosis technique—following myelography, computed tomography, and/or magnetic resonance imaging. This technique should only be considered when symptoms have been present for longer than a year. Positive surgical results have been reported in approximately two thirds of patients when the pain pattern is reproduced and specific guidelines followed.

Cervical Spondylotic Myelopathy

Anatomy and Pathophysiology The blood supply of the spinal cord consists of three major longitudinal arteries. A large anterior spinal artery and two dorsal lateral arteries supply the cord. These vessels are regionally fed by medullary vessels of segmental origin. The location of the anterior spinal artery makes it vulnerable to direct compression by osteophytes and degenerative disk material. In addition, the medullary feeder vessel may be compressed as it traverses the foraminal opening to the midventral surface of the cord.

Spinal canal size is a second anatomic factor in the development of cervical spondylotic myelopathy. The spinal canal may be small because of congenital and/or developmental factors. Further compromise can result from protrusion of disk material, buckling of the ligamentum fla-

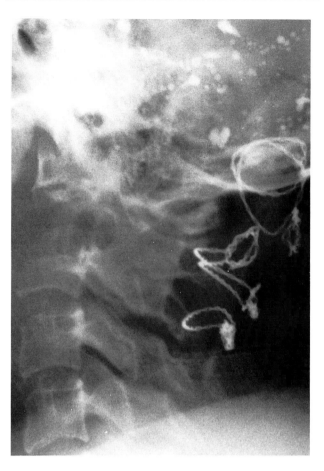

Figure 6

Lateral radiograph of the patient shown in Figure 5 after transoral resection of the dens and posterior occipitocervical arthrodesis.

vum, and the development of osteophytes. Reports on the biomechanics of cervical spondylotic myelopathy indicate that abnormal stresses and strains on the spinal cord are caused by dynamic factors in addition to static factors. These factors include normal and abnormal motion, normal and abnormal loads applied, and the mechanical properties of the spinal cord and the spinal column.

Lateral radiographs are typically used to estimate canal size. Radiographs must be obtained with the X-ray source at the standard distance from the patient and the film so that direct measurements can be made. When the spondylotic anteroposterior diameter of the canal is less than 11 or 12 mm, significant compression is likely to be present. Canal and cord size can be measured most accurately with a contrast-enhanced computed tomographic scan.

Myelopathy is multifactorial in origin. Patients typically have a variation of the anterior cord syndrome (preservation of posterior-column position and vibration), implying that the early major pathologic changes are anterior cord compression and ischemia in conjunction with a narrow canal. Electrophysiologic changes occur and the evoked potentials alter as the disease progresses. Intrinsic changes within the spinal cord include blockage of axoplasmic flow, distortion of cord tissue, and stretching of intrinsic transverse terminations of the anterior spinal artery. Tissue destruction with demyelination of white mat-

ter occurs in severe cases. The pathologic findings appear to correlate with clinical severity.

Diagnosis The primary diagnosis of cervical spondylotic myelopathy is made clinically. Patients may have involvement of the upper and lower extremities as well as gait and bladder disturbances. The neurologic pattern tends to be consistent with a lower motor neuron lesion at the level of the spondylotic compression and upper motor neuron findings below that level. Therefore, the upper-extremity findings include weakness and decreased reflexes at the level of the lesion and hyperreflexia below that level. There may be an abnormal Hoffmann's reflex. The lower extremities tend to be weak with hyperreflexia and Babinski reflexes may be late. The gait is classically broad-based.

Neuroradiographic investigation typically includes plain films to determine sagittal diameters and the presence of osteophytes and computed tomographic scanning and myelography to determine the presence and location of sites of compression. In addition, magnetic resonance imaging may provide information regarding myelopathic changes within the spinal cord itself. Magnetic resonance imaging and delayed computed tomography and myelography are complementary diagnostic studies that can assist in determining the extent of abnormal spinal cord alterations as well as suggesting the prognosis.

Spinal cord monitoring can be useful in monitoring the clinical course of patients with spondylotic myelopathy. Serial radiologic surveys, combined wih electromyography and spinal cord monitoring, offer a way to measure the risk of progressive neurologic abnormalities developing in an individual patient. Somatosensory evoked potentials and motor evoked potentials evaluate white-matter function within the cord (medial posterior columns and posterolateral segment of lateral columns). The development of an H-reflex on electromyographic studies provides evidence of spinal cord compromise.

Treatment There are two major surgical approaches to the management of patients with cervical spondylotic myelopathy: anterior and posterior. The anterior procedures, which are the most frequently used, include the Smith-Robinson procedure (excision of the intervertebral disk with or without removal of osteophytes and a horseshoe-shaped graft) and the Cloward procedure (removal of a dowel of bone at the level of the interspace and bone grafting). Proponents of the Cloward procedure believe that there is better visualization for decompression but others believe that the integrity of subchondral bone is interrupted and that there is a greater potential for late collapse. A third anterior approach is multilevel subtotal vertebrectomy with preservation of the lateral walls of the vertebrae followed by application of a longitudinal strut graft.

There are two basic types of posterior procedures: laminectomy and laminoplasty. The indication for surgery is progressive impairment of function without sustained remission. The best results are obtained in patients who have had symptoms for less than six months. Laminectomy is often performed in patients with involvement of more than two levels and narrow spinal canals. Laminoplasty, which was originally developed for the treatment of ossification of the posterior longitudinal ligament, has the potential to provide a wider spinal canal while, at least in theory, preserving the stability of the vertebral column.

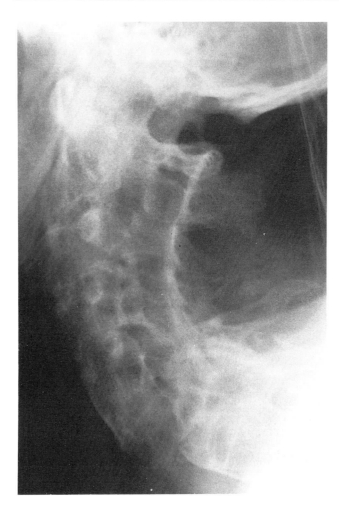
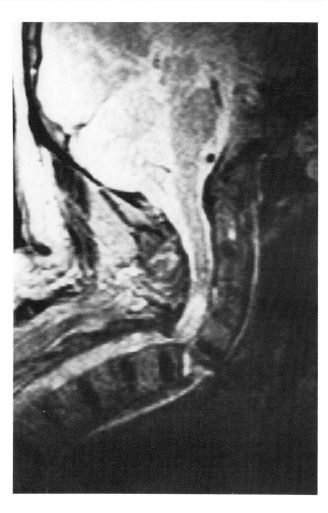

Figure 7

A 58-year-old quadriplegic patient with ankylosing spondylitis. **Left**, Lateral radiograph shows a fracture-dislocation of C-6 and C-7. **Right**, Sagittal-plane magnetic resonance imaging shows high-grade compression at the level of the fracture-dislocation.

Diagnostic Techniques

Evaluation of problems involving the occipitoatlantoaxial complex is often difficult because of the complexity of the anatomy and overlapping radiographic shadows. One measure of potential problems in this region is the predens angle. This is the angle between the posterior aspect of the arch of C-1 and the anterior surface of the dens (Fig. 8). A V-shaped predens interval is not an indication of injury to the transverse ligament and a tilted dens does not necessarily indicate trauma.

During the past decade "dynamic" imaging became popular. Certainly flexion-extension radiographs have been used for some time, but dynamic computed tomographic and magnetic resonance imaging scans are now being done. The functional diagnosis of rotatory instability of the atlantoaxial complex can be made by measuring the range of motion on computed tomographic images after maximum rotation to both sides.

"Dynamic" magnetic resonance imaging of the cervical spine has been particularly useful in the diagnosis of cord compression in patients with cervical spondylotic myelopathy and in rheumatoid arthritis (Fig. 9). Measuring the transverse area of the spinal cord or dural sac is useful in patients with cervical spondylotic myelopathy. The obliquity of computed tomographic scan cuts affects anatomic measurements of the spinal canal. An angulation of the scan cut enlarges the area but this enlargement does not exceed 4% if the angulation of the cut is less than 15 degrees.

Intraoperative detection of the adequacy of a surgical decompression is often difficult. One report described a technique of instilling water-soluble contrast medium intraoperatively to evaluate the extent of anterior cervical diskectomy. This technique may indicate the adequacy of the margin of dissection and prevent a poor outcome resulting from inadequate decompression.

Surgical Techniques

Extensive exposure of the anterior aspects of the occipitoatlantoaxial complex can be extremely difficult. A retropharyngeal approach to the upper part of the cervical spine provides anterior access to the neural elements from the clivus to the body of C-3 without the need for dissection

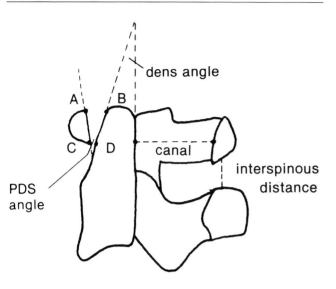

Figure 8

The predens angle (PDA) is formed by lines AC and BD.
(Reproduced with permission from Bohrer SP, Klein A, Martin W III: "V" shaped predens space. *Skeletal Radiol* 1985;14:111–116.)

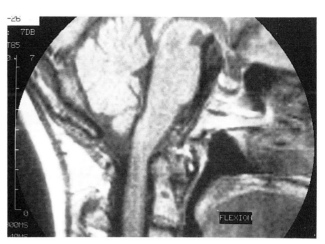

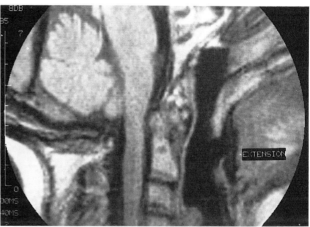

Figure 9

A patient with rheumatoid arthritis and atlantoaxial subluxation. **Top,** Flexion sagittal-plane magnetic resonance imaging. Note the "tenting" of the spinal cord around the dens. **Bottom,** Extension sagittal-plane magnetic resonance imaging.

of the carotid sheath or entrance into the oral cavity. Other surgical options in this region of the spine include dislocation of the temporomandibular joints, osteotomy of the mandible with splitting of the tongue, the transoral approach, and the anterolateral approach. The transoral approach to the upper cervical spine is indicated in problems involving the anterior elements of the upper cervical spine as well as in cases of compression of the medulla and spinal cord at the craniovertebral junction. Stabilization of the craniovertebral junction is most commonly performed posteriorly, using an autogenous bone graft between the occiput and upper cervical spine. In selected cases with significant instability, internal fixation devices and supplemental methylmethacrylate have been used. Internal fixation may be more advantageous than bone grafting alone because it provides rigid stabilization that allows early mobilization. This may contribute to eventual bony union. Such devices are currently being investigated.

Spinal Cord Monitoring

The status and integrity of the spinal cord during surgery is an important concern. The wake-up test, which was primarily developed in conjunction with scoliosis surgery, has been a popular technique but its false-positive and false-negative results have created problems. Somatosensory evoked potentials and motor evoked potentials, recorded either in the spine or the cerebral cortex, have become a popular technique for monitoring the integrity of the spinal cord. For cervical spine surgery, both tibial nerve and median nerve somatosensory evoked potentials have been used. Typical stimulus rates have been in the range of 5.1 to 6.1 Hz. In severe incomplete spinal cord injury, the higher rates of stimulus preservation commonly used may result in failure to obtain waveforms adequate for spinal evoked potentials. Unconventionally low stimulus rates (4.1 Hz or less) may greatly facilitate monitoring in such situations (Fig. 10).

Experimental data and clinical experience (primarily in scoliosis surgery) suggest that the motor action potentials and spinal evoked potentials reflect two independent functions of the spinal cord. The motor action potential measures the function of the lateral part of the cord and the spinal evoked potential reflects the function of the posterior columns. The ability to monitor both sensory and motor pathways during surgical procedures on the spine or spinal cord may allow better detection of spinal cord injury at the time when it may still be reversible.

The surgeon should be aware that both false-positive and false-negative evoked potentials occur. False-negative findings are less common, but they may have more severe consequences. Factors reported to alter potentials include the depth of anesthesia, the metabolic status of the patient, and defective equipment.

Spinal evoked potentials have also been used to evaluate cord function in patients with cervical spondylotic myelopathy. This technique may be useful in evaluating the function of the cervical cord, diagnosing the level and severity of cord lesions, and monitoring progression in myelopathy. In addition, evoked potentials may have a role in

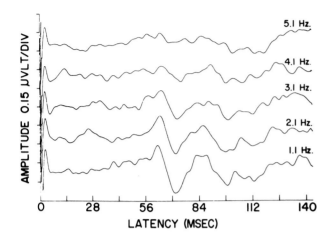

Figure 10

Deterioration of evoked potential waveform with increasing stimulus frequency. The waveform recorded at 5.1 Hz has deteriorated sufficiently to preclude adequate intraoperative monitoring. (Reproduced with permission from Schubert A, Drummond JC, Garfin SR: The influence of stimulus presentation rate on the cortical amplitude and latency of intraoperative somatosensory-evoked potential recordings in patients with varying degrees of spinal cord injury. *Spine* 1987;12:969–973.)

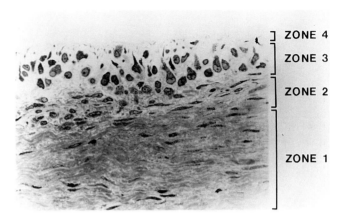

Figure 11

Photomicrograph of tissue at the bone-cement interface, divided into zones. In zone 1, the cells are fusiform and immersed in a coarse matrix. In zone 2, the cells are plumper and the matrix is finer. In zone 3, the cells are teardrop-shaped. Zone 4, which was directly apposed to the cement in vivo, is acellular and amorphous (toluidine blue, × 500). (Reproduced with permission from Whitehill R, Drucker S, McCoig JA, et al: Induction and characterization of an interface tissue by implantation of methylmethacrylate cement into the posterior part of the cervical spine of the dog. *J Bone Joint Surg* 1988;70A:51–59.)

monitoring patients at risk for the development of epidural compression secondary to neoplasm.

Halo Device

The halo device has been the most widely used orthosis for the stabilization of the cervical spine made unstable by trauma, surgery, inflammatory disease, congenital abnormalities, or other causes. Despite widespread use of many years, there have been continued problems related to the device. The common recommendation for the torque used to tighten the halo pins was 0.68 N·m. A recent study suggested that a higher torque, 0.90 N·m, may be more effective. Despite the recommendation that the torque screwdriver be used only once, a recent study found that the accuracy and dependability of the torque screwdriver was maintained after repeated use.

The biomechanics of halo fixation has also been evaluated, including the effect of halo vest length on stability in the cervical spine. Shorter vests may one day play a role in upper cervical lesions. The advantages of such a vest include improved comfort, ease of nursing care, and the ability to provide cardiopulmonary resuscitation without removing the vest. The halo device effectively controls rotation of the cervical spine regardless of the length of the vest.

The halo device may fail to immobilize the cervical spine and the treating physician must be aware of this possibility. Frequent monitoring should be done with serial radiographs. The mere application of the halo device does not always guarantee cervical immobilization.

Motion within the spine in patients wearing halo vests is also a clinical concern. Investigators have found that flexion-extension motion occurs in each cervical motion segment. They compared the motion patterns to a "curling

snake." The motion was greatest in the upper cervical spine and decreased further down.

A biomechanical analysis of the halo device in children raised concerns regarding the thinness of the skull in children less than 6 years of age. Computed tomographic scanning of the skull is recommended before elective application in young children to ascertain the safest location for pin placement.

Controversies

Methylmethacrylate Stabilization

Although methylmethacrylate can be a useful adjunct in the treatment of malignant disease, it is controversial. There are extensive basic science and clinical reports on the use of methylmethacrylate for stabilization of the spine. Methylmethacrylate predictably fails with time because of fatigue fracture and, therefore, long-term stability must be provided by bony arthrodesis. Animal studies of various types of constructs, including bone fusion alone, methylmethacrylate fusion alone, and various combinations of methylmethacrylate, wire, and bone, revealed that fusions remained inferior in mechanical strength when the acrylic was used alone. In patients with metastatic disease (other than those with extremely short life expectancies), combination constructs should be considered. Despite their greater mechanical strength, these combination constructs should be protected with an orthosis in the early postoperative period.

Methylmethacrylate should only be considered as an adjunct to stabilization in patients with tumors and severe instability secondary to rheumatoid arthritis. Traumatic and degenerative conditions are usually best managed with conventional techniques using bone graft. Errors with the use of methylmethacrylate include inappropriate indications and improper application. A common error is to apply too much cement; this has been reported to cause major problems with wound closure and to result in wound infection. In addition, the "bonding" of the cement to adjacent bone is poor.

The interface tissue surrounding methylmethacrylate implanted in the posterior part of the cervical spine in dogs has been recently characterized (Fig. 11). The tissue formed at the bone-cement interface is morphologically similar to that associated with the bone-cement interface in loose aseptic total hip replacements. This raises concern regarding potential flaws. Thus, methylmethacrylate must be viewed solely as a temporary splint that may adversely affect bone graft maturation and survival.

Surgical Management of the Rheumatoid Cervical Spine

Definitive long-term studies of the natural history of cervical spine involvement are not available, and thus the indications for surgical management of this condition remain controversial.

Zoma and associates described a series of 32 patients who underwent 40 operations. The overall success rate was 57%. Thirty-five percent were considered failures and there was an 8% mortality rate. Their indications for surgery were progressive neurologic impairment, progressive instability, and, occasionally, intractable pain. The authors found that the most important factor determining outcome was the severity of neural involvement. When there was a severe neurologic deficit, 87% of the operations resulted in either failure or death. When there was minimal or no neural involvement, 80% achieved good clinical results. These findings led the authors to question the wisdom of operating on such patients. They thought that early recognition and treatment of potentially serious instability was the most important factor in preventing poor results.

Santavirta and associates, Heywood and associates, and Clark and associates all described rheumatoid patients managed surgically with more positive outcomes. Santavirta and associates concluded that fusion of an unstable rheumatoid cervical spine relieves pain and prevents progression of existing neurologic lesions without undue risk for the patient. They acknowledged, however, that the indications for surgical intervention are not yet clear.

A similar positive experience with cervical arthrodeses in patients with rheumatoid arthritis was recently described by Heywood and associates. They found that most of their cases could be managed by stabilization alone and recommended early intervention when there was significant instability.

Indications for surgery in the series reported by Clark and associates included progressive instability with neurologic deficits or severe pain. In addition, the authors thought that "impending" neural deficit was a valid indication for surgery. "Impending" deficit was defined as severe instability combined with cord or thecal sac compression on neuroradiographic studies. Instability at additional levels may occur after an arthrodesis, and patients should be monitored by periodic dynamic radiographs.

A comparison of these series shows that Zoma and associates had more patients with serious neurologic deficit at the time of surgical intervention, and thus a higher percentage of adverse results. The patients described by San-

tavirta and associates and Clark and associates appeared to have less neurologic involvement and therefore a more favorable prognosis. Indeed, Zoma and associates had a high percentage of good results (80%) in patients with lesser neurologic involvement. Therefore, it appears that in patients with significant instability from rheumatoid involvement of the cervical spine and early progressing neurologic deficit and/or severe pain, surgery is best performed before the neurologic deficit becomes severe and possibly irreversible.

Surgical Management of Cervical Spondylotic Myelopathy

The way to treat a patient with cervical spondylotic myelopathy is frequently debated. There are advocates of anterior and posterior surgical approaches to this condition. The posterior procedures include laminectomy and laminoplasty, and there is a debate among the advocates of each. The anterior approach has the advantage of decompressing the spinal cord and nerve roots at the usual site of compression. Anterior procedures, however, are limited by the amount of decompression that is technically feasible laterally (that is, decompression of neuroforamina), as well as the number of levels. Most authors prefer an anterior approach when two interspaces (three vertebral levels) or less are involved.

Advocates of the posterior approach point to the relative ease of the surgical exposure and the ability to decompress the neuroforamina adequately as well as achieving decompression at multiple levels. A concern regarding potential postoperative instability in a patient with multilevel laminectomy was partially responsible for the development of the laminoplasty procedure, of which there are many variations. Advocates cite the following advantages: it is technically easy to perform, it provides stability, it is safer than midline laminectomies because the dissection is done laterally, and the limited postoperative range of motion may prevent recurrence.

Hirabayashi and Satomi reported a significant rate of instability in a series of patients who underwent laminectomy compared with patients treated by laminoplasty. Nakano and associates, however, found no significant difference between laminectomy and laminoplasty from the standpoint of symptomatic improvement or the development of postoperative instability in patients with cervical spondylotic myelopathy or ossification of the posterior longitudinal ligament, although patients were mobilized faster and recovered more quickly after laminoplasty.

Herkowitz compared anterior cervical fusion, cervical laminectomy, and cervical laminoplasty in the treatment of multilevel spondylotic radiculopathy. He concluded that an anterior cervical fusion provided the best results and that laminoplasty was an effective alternative to the anterior procedure. He further concluded that laminectomy was the least useful option in multilevel disease, and that laminoplasty restricted cervical motion the most.

Thus, when the cervical spondylotic condition is limited to two interspaces (three vertebral bodies) or less, the anterior approach provides the most effective decompression. When there is significant stenosis and/or three or more interspaces (four vertebral body levels), the posterior approach may be most advantageous. Although a laminoplasty may avoid the potential problem of postoperative instability, laminectomy nevertheless continues to have a definite role in the primary management of multilevel cervical spondylotic myelopathy.

Annotated Bibliography

Keywords

Ankylosing spondylitis; Arthritis; Atlantoaxial articulation; Cervical spine; Child abuse; Congenital anomalies; Halo traction; Hemophilia; Infection; Intervertebral disk; Juvenile rheumatoid arthritis; Kidney; Kyphosis; Methylmethacrylate; Neoplasm; Radiculopathy; Renal osteodystrophy; Spinal cord; Spondylosis

General Considerations

The Cervical Spine Research Society: *The Cervical Spine*, ed 2. Philadelphia, JB Lippincott, 1989.
An excellent review of all aspects of the cervical spine.

Congenital Anomalies

Eller TW, Bernstein LP, Rosenberg RS, et al: Tethered cervical spinal cord: Case report. *J Neurosurg* 1987;67: 600–602.
Computed tomography with metrizamide intrathecal contrast is the most useful method of diagnosis. Interoperative somatosensory evoked potentials correlate well with clinical improvement after surgery.

Okada K, Fuji T, Yonenobu K, et al: Cervical diastematomyelia with a stable neurological deficit: Report of a case. *J Bone Joint Surg* 1986;68A:934–937.
Cervical diastematomyelia is associated with abnormalities of the laminae in 85% of patients. Signs and symptoms are present in more than 50% of patients and are often related to problems with the lower extremity, gait, and posture.

Pediatric Conditions Involving the Cervical Spine

Duhaime AC, Gennarelli TA, Thibault LE, et al: The shaken baby syndrome: A clinical, pathological and biomechanical study. *J Neurosurg* 1987;66:409–415.
This is a review of 48 cases. A history of shaking was often lacking. Thirteen children who died all had signs of blunt impact to the head.

Francis WF, Noble DP: Treatment of cervical kyphosis in children. *Spine* 1988;13:883–887.
A single-stage anterior release and strut graft fusion may be necessary when the posterior elements are absent. Patients with intact posterior elements often require preoperative traction and initial posterior osteotomies with interoperative traction followed by an anterior release and strut grafting.

Hensinger RN, DeVito PD, Ragsdale CG: Changes in the cervical spine in juvenile rheumatoid arthritis. *J Bone Joint Surg* 1986;68A:189–198.
A review of 121 patients with juvenile rheumatoid arthritis. Patients with pauciarticular disease rarely have cervical symptoms or radiographic changes. Clinical stiffness and radiographic changes are more common in patients with polyarticular or systemic onset.

Kerns S, Pope TL Jr, de Lange EE, et al: Annulus fibrosus calcification in the cervical spine: Radiologic-pathologic correlation. *Skeletal Radiol* 1986;15:605–609.
Interarticular disk calcification can be secondary to a variety of a pathologic processes. The differential diagnosis includes various metabolic disorders such as hyperparathyroidism, ochronosis, gout, and pseudogout as well as ankylosing spondylitis, tumor, and trauma.

Kobori M, Takahashi H, Mikawa Y: Atlanto-axial dislocation in Down's syndrome: Report of two cases requiring surgical correction. *Spine* 1986;11:195–200.
Patients may have associated ossiculum terminale in addition to the dislocation. The combination of ligamentous laxity and anomaly of the dens places the patient at higher risk for spinal cord compression.

Romeyn RL, Herkowitz HN: The cervical spine in hemophilia. *Clin Orthop* 1986;210:113–119.
Although mild instability of C-1 and C-2 was noted in a few patients, soft-tissue thickening and fibrosis may protect the atlantoaxial complex from progressive laxity. Long-term follow-up is necessary to determine the patterns of degenerative change and instability in patients with hemophilia.

Tumors and Metabolic Conditions

Bohlman HH, Sachs BL, Carter JR, et al: Primary neoplasms of the cervical spine: Diagnosis and treatment of twenty-three patients. *J Bone Joint Surg* 1986;68A:483–494.
A review of 23 primary benign or malignant osseous neoplasms of the cervical spine. The approach to a primary neoplasm is presented, including diagnostic and surgical management.

Goldman AB, Abrahams TG: Multiple findings of renal osteodystrophy reflected in the vertebral bodies and apophyseal joints of the cervical spine. *Skeletal Radiol* 1986;15:308–312.
The authors describe the clinical findings in a patient with renal osteodystrophy. Since the advent of renal dialysis and transplantation, survival has been improved and this clinical problem is more frequently recognized.

Kostuik JP, Errico TH, Gleason TF, et al: Spinal stabilization of vertebral column tumors. *Spine* 1988;13:250–256.
A report of 100 consecutive cases of vertebral tumors that were surgically stabilized. The authors recommend specific treatment of neurologic deficits based on (1) tumor type and sensitivity to treatment, (2) rapidity of onset, (3) relative stability of the vertebral column, and (4) location of dural compression.

Weinstein JN, McLain RF: Primary tumors of the spine. *Spine* 1987;12:843–851.
A review of 82 primary neoplasms of the spine, including six benign cervical lesions. Many of the benign lesions were aggressive and had an overall five-year survival of 86%. The authors present an excellent algorithm describing the approach to such patients.

Adult Conditions of the Cervical Spine

Rheumatoid Arthritis

Clark CR, Goetz DD, Menezes AH: Arthrodesis of the cervical spine in rheumatoid arthritis. *J Bone Joint Surg* 1989;71A:381–392.
The authors describe a consecutive series of 41 patients with rheumatoid arthritis who were treated surgically. Overall the authors reported an 88% rate of bony arthrodesis, a 5% rate of fibrous union, and a 7% rate of nonunion. All problems with union occurred in patients who underwent isolated atlantoaxial arthrodesis. Preoperative neurologic status was unchanged or improved in all patients. There were no deaths in the immediate postoperative period. Four patients died later but all deaths were unrelated to cervical involvement.

Heywood AWB, Learmonth ID, Thomas M: Cervical spine instability in rheumatoid arthritis. *J Bone Joint Surg* 1988;70B:702–707.

The authors reported their findings in 26 patients who underwent 30 procedures. There were two deaths in the immediate postoperative period in patients who underwent anterior cervical fusions for subaxial subluxation. The authors consequently advise against this procedure in such patients.

Lachiewicz PF, Schoenfeldt R, Inglis A: Somatosensory-evoked potentials in the evaluation of the unstable rheumatoid cervical spine: A preliminary report. *Spine* 1986;11:813–817.

The presence or absence of evoked potentials and their latencies are the major features used in clinical interpretation. Short-latency somatosensory evoked potentials are recorded after electrical stimulation of peripheral sensory nerves. Fifty-eight percent of those with irreducible atlantoaxial subluxation and/or cranial settling demonstrated cervical cord conduction latencies.

Santavirta S, Slatis P, Kankaanpaa U, et al: Treatment of the cervical spine in rheumatoid arthritis. *J Bone Joint Surg* 1988;70A:658–667.

This series included 18 patients who were treated surgically and 14 treated nonsurgically. Procedures included 13 atlantoaxial fusions and five occipitocervical fusions. Pain was relieved in 12 of 15 patients treated surgically compared with only one in eight treated nonsurgically. Neurologic status was either unchanged or improved in the surgical group but slightly worse in the nonsurgical group.

Zoma A, Sturrock RD, Fisher WD, et al: Surgical stabilisation of the rheumatoid cervical spine: A review of indications and results. *J Bone Joint Surg* 1987;69B:8–12.

The goals were to stabilize the spine, relieve cord compression and associated neurologic impairment, and relieve pain. The authors found that the results for pain relief were superior to those for neurologic improvement. Their series of patients included 16 posterior fusions and 13 occipitocervical fusions. The complications included four wound infections and nine graft fractures and/or reabsorptions.

Ankylosing Spondylitis

Broom MJ, Raycroft JF: Complication of fractures of the cervical spine and ankylosing spondylitis. *Spine* 1988;13:763–766.

Five patients who suffered severe neurologic compromise after fractures of the cervical spine developed delayed neurologic complications (two to 35 days after injury). Diagnosis was delayed in four cases and three of these delays resulted in significant morbidity.

Simmons EH, Bradley DD: Neuro-myopathic flexion deformities of the cervical spine. *Spine* 1988;13:756–762.

This report details the surgical management of six patients with severe chin-on-chest deformity secondary to neuropathic or myopathic disease.

Infection

Eismont FJ, Wiesel SW, Brighton CT, et al: Antibiotic penetration into rabbit nucleus pulposus. *Spine* 1987;12:254–256.

The authors used a rabbit model to evaluate antibiotic penetration. Four antibiotics were evaluated. Clindamycin and tobramycin achieved therapeutic levels. Cephalothin was not detected in the nucleus pulposus and the data on oxycillin were inconclusive.

Ross D, Rosegay H, Pons V: Differentiation of aseptic and bacterial meningitis in postoperative neurosurgery patients. *J Neurosurg* 1988;69:669–674.

This study evaluated various criteria for differentiating bacterial aseptic meningitis in a postoperative group of patients. The type of surgery, the presence of foreign bodies, the use of steroids, the day on which postoperative symptoms developed, a change in mental status, neck stiffness, and nausea were not helpful in differentiating between the two. No criterion was sensitive and specific enough to differentiate reliably between the two in all patients.

Cervical Spondylosis

Fast A, Zinicola DF, Marin EL: Vertebral artery damage complicating cervical manipulation. *Spine* 1987;12:840–842.

This report describes a patient who underwent cervical manipulation and had resultant damage to the vertebral artery and temporary brain-stem signs and symptoms. The vertebral arteries are susceptible to trauma at three locations: the transverse foramen, the atlantoaxial joint, and the occipitoatlantal joint.

Gore DR, Sepic SB, Gardner GM, et al: Neck pain: A long-term follow-up of 205 patients. *Spine* 1987;12:1-5.

A long-term follow-up of 205 patients with neck pain (minimum follow-up, ten years) revealed that 79% had decreased pain and 43% were pain-free. However, 32% had moderate or severe residual pain.

Marzo JM, Simmons EH, Kallen F: Intradural connections between adjacent cervical spinal roots. *Spine* 1987;12:964–968.

The authors performed a series of anatomic dissections and found 54 intraneural connections. The typical pattern is a peripheral dorsal or ventral rootlet joining the central portion of the next rostral or caudal root and passing together through the foramen into the spinal cord.

Whitecloud TS III, Seago RA: Cervical discogenic syndrome: Results of operative intervention in patients with positive discography. *Spine* 1987;12:313–316.

This is a review of 34 patients who underwent cervical arthrodesis because of a positive diskogram. Symptomatic levels were selected by reproduction of the patients' symptoms at the time of injection. The authors reported 70% good or excellent results provided that appropriate guidelines were followed.

Cervical Spondylotic Myelopathy

Cervical Spine Research Society: Cervical spondylotic myelopathy. *Spine* 1988;13:828–880.

A series of articles by several authors provides an excellent review of this condition describing the anatomy, pathophysiology, biomechanics, clinical findings, and treatment.

Herkowitz HN: A comparison of anterior cervical fusion, cervical laminectomy and cervical laminoplasty for the surgical management of multiple level spondylotic radiculopathy. *Spine* 1988;13:774–780.

The author reviewed a series of 45 patients who underwent one of these three procedures for the treatment of cervical spondylotic radiculopathy. Eighteen patients underwent anterior fusion, 12 underwent laminectomy, and 15 patients were treated with laminoplasty. The overall success rates for the various procedures were 92% for anterior fusion, 66% for laminectomy, and 86% for laminoplasty.

Hirabayashi K, Satomi K: Operative procedure and results of expansive open-door laminoplasty. *Spine* 1988;13:870–876.

Of a series of 90 patients who underwent extensive open-door laminoplasty for the treatment of cervical spondylotic myelopathy, 75% had excellent results and 25% were without change. There was no postoperative malalignment such as swan-neck deformity.

Mefty O, Harkey LH, Middleton TH, et al: Myelopathic cervical spondylotic lesions demonstrated by magnetic resonance imaging. *J Neurosurg* 1988;68:217–222.

This report of myelopathic changes demonstrated by magnetic resonance imaging found two types of lesions: (1) localized spinal cord changes at the level of compression consistent with myelomalacia, which are best revealed on the T_2-weighted image as a high-intensity signal; and (2) lesions consistent with either cystic degeneration or secondary syrinx, which were noted locally and/or extending longitudinally inside the cord. These were best seen on T_1-weighted images and as signal voids on T_2-weighted images.

Nakano N, Nakano T, Nakano K: Comparison of the results of laminectomy and open-door laminoplasty for cervical spondylotic myeloradiculopathy and ossification of the posterior longitudinal ligament. *Spine* 1988;13: 792–794.

Of 89 patients, 14 underwent laminectomy and 75 open-door laminoplasty. There were no significant differences in the results of these two procedures.

Diagnostic Techniques

Dvorak J, Hayek J, Zehnder R: CT-functional diagnostics of the rotatory instability of the cervical spine: An experimental study on cadavers. *Spine* 1988;13:197–205.

The authors evaluated 12 specimens. When an alar ligament was missing, there was an increase of 10.8 degrees in rotation to the opposite side.

Monu J, Bohrer SP, Howard G: Some upper cervical spine norms. *Spine* 1987;12:515–519.

An investigation of the predens angle in 175 normal individuals found that 98% of the patients had angles of more than 6 degrees. The overall range for the group was 0 to 13 degrees.

Schonstrom N: The significance of oblique cuts on CT scans of the spinal canal in terms of anatomic measurements. *Spine* 1988;13:435–436.

This study revealed that the magnitude of enlargement from oblique cuts of computed tomographic scans can be determined by a simple mathematical equation (x = y/cos a).

Walker J, Gillespie, Davis J, et al: Water-soluble contrast medium for intra-operative evaluation of anterior cervical discectomy. *J Neurosurg* 1988;68:491–492.

The authors describe their technique of instilling nonionic contrast medium into the disk space before obtaining anteroposterior and lateral radiographs after simple diskectomy using the Cloward technique to evaluate the adequacy of decompression.

Surgical Techniques

Bonney G, Williams JP: Trans-oral approach to the upper cervical spine: A report of 16 cases. *J Bone Joint Surg* 1985;67B:691–698.

A review of 16 patients who underwent decompression and stabilization through a transoral approach that included tracheostomy and splitting of the soft palate. Infection was a problem in cases in which the posterior pharyngeal wound broke down. There were three cases of delayed healing and one death in the immediate postoperative period.

McAfee PC, Bohlman HH, Riley LH Jr, et al: The anterior retropharyngeal approach to the upper part of the cervical spine. *J Bone Joint Surg* 1987;69A:1371–1383.

Results of 12 patients followed up for two years or longer revealed solid anterior fusion in all cases without subsequent loss of stability and with relief of neck pain. Complications included injuries to the hypoglossal nerve and 12th nerve neuropraxia.

Spinal Cord Monitoring

Kotani H, Saiki K, Yamasaki H, et al: Evaluation of cervical cord function in cervical spondylotic myelopathy and/or radiculopathy using both segmental conductive spinal-evoked potentials (SEP). *Spine* 1986;11:185–190.

This review of 73 patients found that somatosensory evoked potentials were useful in determining the type of myelopathy present: central cord; central cord with posterior lateral column involvement; or central cord, posterior column, and anterior lateral column involvement.

Schubert A, Drummond JC, Garfin SR: The influence of stimulus presentation rate on the cortical amplitude and latency of intraoperative somatosensory-evoked potential recordings in patients with varying degrees of spinal cord injury. *Spine* 1987;12:969–973.

The authors found a marked detrimental influence at the higher stimulus rates (6.1 and 5.1 Hz) commonly used. These findings were most pronounced in patients with antecedent spinal cord injury.

Siegal T, Siegal TZ, Sandbank U, et al: Experimental neoplastic spinal cord compression: Evoked potentials, edema, prostaglandins and light and electron microscopy. *Spine* 1987;12:440–448.

The authors used an experimental model of cord compression in Fischer rats and reported a progressive increase in latency of cervical responses that preceded the onset of clinical signs. Such monitoring may have a clinical role in identifying patients at risk for cord compression.

Halo Device

Botte MJ, Byrne TP, Garfin SR: Application of the halo device for immobilization of the cervical spine utilizing an increased torque pressure. *J Bone Joint Surg* 1987; 69A:750–752.

The authors evaluated the effect of torque loosening and infection in 42 patients. Compared with the control of 0.68 N·m, the loosening was decreased from 36% to 7% and the infection rate was decreased from 20% to 2% in the group of patients with the higher torque of 0.90 N·m.

Garfin SR, Botte MJ, Woo SL, et al: Reliability after repeated use of a torque screwdriver employed for halo pin fixation. *J Orthop Res* 1985;3:121–123.

The authors evaluated the reliability after repeated use of a torque screwdriver. They found that after cycling for 1,600 times, the accuracy was maintained within 7% to 9%.

Letts M, Kaylor D, Gouw G: A biomechanical analysis of halo-fixation in children. *J Bone Joint Surg* 1988;70B: 277–279.

The use of prolonged halo stabilization in a child is increasingly indicated because of trauma and congenital instability of the cervical spine. However, complications of pin fixation in this age group are frequent.

Lind B, Sihlbom H, Nordwall A: Forces and motions across the neck in patients treated with halo-vest. *Spine* 1988;13:162–167.

The authors evaluated 31 consecutive patients treated with a halo device and noted a variation in force depending on the position of the body as well as the type of exercise being performed.

Wang GJ, Moskal JT, Albert T, et al: The effect of halo-vest length on stability of the cervical spine: A study in normal subjects. *J Bone Joint Surg* 1988;70A:357–360.

This study involved 20 normal individuals who were studied with a halo device connected via an experimental headband. The authors concluded that lesions in the upper cervical spine could be effectively treated with a shorter vest. The lesions below C-4 required a vest extending caudal to the level of the 12th rib.

Controversies

Methylmethacrylate Stabilization

Whitehill R, Cicoria AD, Hooper WE, et al: Posterior cervical reconstruction with methylmethacrylate cement and wire: A clinical review. *J Neurosurg* 1988;68:576–584.

Whitehill R, Drucker S, McCoig JA, et al: Induction and characterization of an interface tissue by implantation of methylmethacrylate cement into the posterior part of the cervical spine of the dog. *J Bone Joint Surg* 1988;70A:51–59.

Surgical Management of the Rheumatoid Cervical Spine

Clark CR, Goetz DD, Menezes AH: Arthrodesis of the cervical spine in rheumatoid arthritis. *J Bone Joint Surg* 1989;71A:381–392.

Heywood AWB, Learmonth ID, Thomas M: Cervical spine instability in rheumatoid arthritis. *J Bone Joint Surg* 1988;70B:702–707.

Santavirta S, Slatis P, Kankaanpaa U, et al: Treatment of the cervical spine in rheumatoid arthritis. *J Bone Joint Surg* 1988;70A:658–667.

Zoma A, Sturrock RD, Fisher WD, et al: Surgical stabilisation of the rheumatoid cervical spine: A review of indications and results. *J Bone Joint Surg* 1987;69B:8–12.

Surgical Management of Cervical Spondylotic Myelopathy

Herkowitz HN: A comparison of anterior cervical fusion, cervical laminectomy and cervical laminoplasty for the surgical management of multiple level spondylotic radiculopathy. *Spine* 1988;13:774–780.

Hirabayashi K, Satomi K: Operative procedure and results of expansive open-door laminoplasty. *Spine* 1988;13:870–876.

Nakano N, Nakano T, Nakano K: Comparison of the results of laminectomy and open-door laminoplasty for cervical spondylotic myeloradiculopathy and ossification of the posterior longitudinal ligament. *Spine* 1988;13:792–794.

32
Cervical Spine and Cord: Trauma

The advent of trauma centers and spinal cord injury referral centers has had a dramatic impact on the care of patients with cervical spine injuries. Even so, injuries to the cervical spine and cord are a major source of a long-term disability. Despite major advances in treatment, at this point physicians have only a limited effect on the neurologic outcome and recovery of patients with spinal cord injuries. It is, therefore, extremely important to identify these patients early, and to control the incidence of neurologic deterioration once they have been admitted to the treatment center. The incidence of neurologic deterioration in spinal cord injuries has been estimated at 2% to 10% in various series. In addition, aggressive care of these patients not only prevents neurologic deterioration but also minimizes the almost inevitable multiple complications of spinal injury (deep venous thrombosis, urinary tract infections, decubitus ulcers, and the like). New types of imaging, such as computed tomographic scanning and magnetic resonance imaging, have recently made the evaluation of bone, ligamentous, and cord injuries more precise. The effective use of these techniques can aid in the recognition of injuries and, thus, the prevention of complications.

During the last ten years, spinal surgery has been marked by a rapid proliferation of various types of instrumentation. First used in the thoracic and lumbar spine, instrumentation for both the anterior and the posterior cervical spine is now available. It is important to develop a rational approach to using a variety of techniques for evaluating and treating cervical spine injury. The use of decompression as well as nonsurgical and surgical stabilization (with wires, bone-plate, screw, or screw-plate fixation and fusion) are part of the armamentarium of the surgeon treating cervical injuries. It must be remembered that initial enthusiasm for a technique is eventually tempered by respect for its complications and a realistic assessment of its effectiveness in particular injuries.

Patient Evaluation

The clinical evaluation of cervical spine trauma requires a meticulous and organized approach if pertinent findings are not to be missed. The initial assessment should concentrate on the evaluation of the spinal injury and an evaluation of the patient's general condition. The initial priority must be stabilization of the hemodynamically unstable patient. Therefore, in patients with multiple injuries, there must be simultaneous treatment of shock and cardiac or thoracic injuries, stabilization of massive pelvic injuries, and assessment of intra-abdominal injuries. Current data indicate that 20% of patients with cervical cord trauma are hypotensive when they reach the trauma center (systemic blood pressure, <100 mm Hg). Of these, approximately

30% have intraperitoneal or severe pelvic or extremity injuries that account for the shock. However, 70% have only neurogenic shock.

Precautions for stabilization of the cervical spine begin at the accident site. Patients with any history of trauma to the head and neck or conscious patients who report any neurologic symptoms, such as momentary loss of feeling or motor power, are immobilized in a collar and on a spine board until appropriate evaluation at the treating institution can be initiated. This immobilization should not be discontinued until the cervical spine has been assessed and found to be uninjured.

Assessment of the cervical injury should begin with an accurate and precise history of the mechanism of injury and, in the conscious patient, a complete history of motor and sensory changes at the scene of the accident. Cervical spine injuries occasionally result from direct blows to the neck but are more frequently the result of trauma to the head (that is, falling objects, diving into a pool, falls, or motor-vehicle accidents). A history of a particular portion of the head being struck, with resultant bruises, quickly delineates a possible mechanism of injury. Delineation of the mechanism of injury helps to direct subsequent clinical and radiographic examinations of the spine.

Physical Examination

The physical examination of the patient consists initially of observation of bruises and abrasions about the head and neck and determination of areas of tenderness. The neurologic examination delineates neurologic impairment and helps to focus the radiographic investigation. The neurologic examination should be extremely precise, beginning with cranial nerves, because fractures involving the occipital condyles can involve cranial nerve injuries, and fractures of the C-1 arch often result in greater occipital nerve dysesthesias. If gross motor paralysis is evident, it is critical to check the perianal region carefully for any sacral sparing, as may be the case in incomplete spinal cord injury. Findings from a rectal examination and a bladder sensation to the balloon of a Foley catheter may be the only clues that indicate an incomplete spinal cord injury. The period of spinal shock may last for a few hours, but usually resolves within 48 hours. The return of the bulbocavernosus reflex is generally accepted as the sign that the patient is out of spinal shock. If there is no function below the level of injury at that time, little recovery of useful motor function can generally be expected. However, root function may recover one or two levels below the level of injury, or the patient may retain root function after an injury. This does not change the ultimate prognosis for distal cord recovery.

Classification of Spinal Injury

Incomplete spinal cord injuries are often subdivided into a number of groups. These include (1) isolated nerve root

395

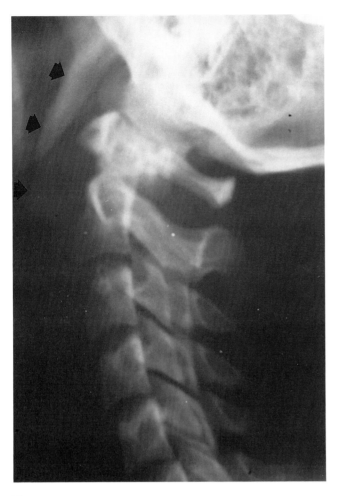

Figure 1

This lateral roentgenogram demonstrates a significant soft-tissue shadow, resulting from fracture of the anterior portion of the ring of C-1. Although there is little evidence of the lateral roentgenogram of fractures, the presence of this soft-tissue shadow (arrows) suggests that a fracture of the anterior portion of the upper cervical spine is present.

injuries, (2) anterior cord syndrome, (3) central cord syndrome, and (4) the Brown-Séquard syndrome. In addition, spinal cord injury can be classified by functional and quantitative criteria.

The Frankel classification is often quoted as a means of evaluating functional recovery from spinal injury. It is commonly used to compare functional recovery among therapeutic methods. The levels of injury are defined as Frankel A, which is complete paralysis, Frankel B, which is sensory preservation below the level of injury but no voluntary motor function, Frankel C, which is incomplete but useless motor function (trace), Frankel D, which is incomplete but useful voluntary motor function below the level of injury and generally fair to good motor strength, and Frankel E, which is normal function.

Currently, a more quantitative evaluation of motor and sensory function has been proposed to measure function more objectively for evaluation of different therapeutic methods. It is based on standardized muscle-testing techniques, with points allowed for both motor and sensory preservation. This allows more precise evaluation of func-

tion and recovery, but is more time-consuming because it evaluates individual muscle groups and assigns individual scores.

Radiographic Evaluation

The accurate assessment of skeletal as well as soft-tissue injuries involving the cervical spine is critically important. Generally, any patient who is admitted to a trauma center with a history of major skeletal trauma, a fall, head or facial injury, neurologic symptoms, or loss of consciousness should undergo a lateral screening roentgenogram of the cervical spine. This can provide a great deal of information about the bony architecture and integrity of the cervical spine. However, a "negative" lateral cervical spine roentgenogram should not preclude further testing in patients in whom cervical spine injury is strongly suspected (those with neck pain or paresthesia or momentary paralysis at the accident scene). In addition, the lateral screening roentgenogram should be carefully evaluated for an increased retropharyngeal soft-tissue shadow (Fig. 1). This may be the only evidence of an anterior upper cervical spine injury.

In addition, the overall alignment of the cervical radiograph should be evaluated so that any patient with kyphosis or rotational malalignment, even without evidence of a fracture, should undergo further evaluation. In patients with neurologic injury, the radiographic evaluation should be directed at the specific level of injury. This is critically important for patients with injuries at the cervical-thoracic junction (C7-T1) where roentgenograms showing the upper portion of C-7 may appear normal, but the injury is hidden by the shoulders. In any patient in whom the entire cervical spine to the C7-T1 interspace cannot be seen, another technique such as swimmer's view radiograph, tomogram, computed tomographic scan, or magnetic resonance imaging may be necessary.

Several techniques are available for more intensive investigation of both spinal column and spinal cord injuries after the initial localization of the lesion. These include conventional tomography, myelography, and/or computed tomography and magnetic resonance imaging. Before additional studies are undertaken, the goal of the study must be clarified to assess which study will give the most information. Although the role of conventional tomography has diminished significantly since the advent of computed tomography, there are still specialized situations in which conventional tomography gives valuable information (in fractures in which the plane of the fracture is parallel to the conventional axial cuts of a computed tomography). Conventional tomography, in most instances, gives more reproducible images than midsagittal or oblique-sagittal computed tomographic reconstructions. Specifically, in fractures of the dens, anteroposterior and lateral tomographs generally give more satisfactory information than the sagittal and frontal reconstructions of the computed tomographic scan (Fig. 2). Adequate images can be obtained if the patient's head can be kept absolutely motionless, and 1.5-mm slices can be obtained. In a patient with acute trauma, this is sometimes difficult to achieve.

Another instance in which tomography is valuable is the delineation of facet fractures and dislocations in the cervical spine. Again, the plane of the fracture is parallel to the axial cuts of the computed tomographic scan, thus requiring oblique-sagittal reconstructions to define facet in-

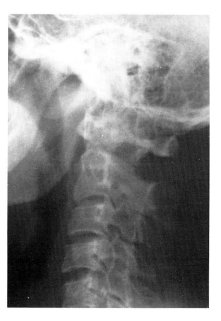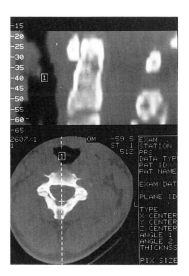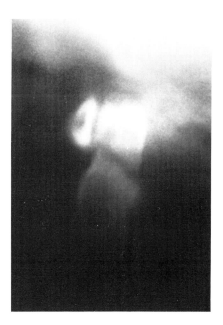

Figure 2

This patient sustained a fracture of the dens that was not clearly visible on a lateral roentgenogram (**left**). Because the fracture was parallel to the plane of the axial cuts, it was not visualized on that portion of the computed tomographic scan (3-mm cuts), and required lateral reconstruction. The lateral reconstruction (**center**) showed the fracture line but much less clearly than the lateral tomogram (**right**).

juries fully. Lateral tomography alone can help to elucidate the type of the facet injury (inferior or superior facet fracture, involvement of the pedicle dislocation). Newer computed tomographic technology such as three-dimensional reconstructions may eventually surpass linear tomography (Fig. 3).

Associated laminar fractures are not as well defined with conventional computed tomography. Care must be taken to ensure that the axial cuts are angled absolutely parallel to the arch of C-1 (Fig. 4). In cases in which this is difficult to achieve, or in which there is an associated dens fracture, lateral tomography to visualize the posterior arch fractures and anteroposterior tomography to visualize the anterior portion of the ring of C-1 provides satisfactory delineation. For most bone injuries in the cervical spine, however, conventional computed tomography achieves excellent delineation. It allows precise visualization of the posterior wall of the vertebral body and accurate assessment of canal size and impingement by bone fragments.

Thus, in patients in whom the primary consideration is to assess bone integrity, the position of bony fragments, and spinal column abnormalities, computed tomography provides a more accurate assessment than magnetic resonance imaging. When the goal of the radiologic study is assessment of cord abnormalities, magnetic resonance imaging is more effective than computed tomography (Fig. 5). This is especially helpful in the acute phase when there is a neurologic deficit that cannot be explained by the evident bony abnormality, or when the level of the spinal cord lesion differs from that of the obvious bone lesion. The "minimyelogram" or "cervical myelograph" has been combined with computed tomography in many patients who had incomplete neurologic deficits. The combination was used to define the degree of initial compression and verify the effectiveness of indirect decompression. The second technique that can be used for this is magnetic resonance imaging, which demonstrates soft-tissue encroachment (such as a disk herniation or hematoma) with great reproducibility. Magnetic resonance imaging does not detect a hematoma in the first six hours after surgical injury and is not completely diagnostic during the first 24 hours. Magnetic resonance imaging and computed tomography are not competing technologies, but complementary imaging techniques. Currently, magnetic resonance imaging does not define bony abnormalities as accurately as computed tomography and both may be necessary for elucidating cord and structural damage. Patients with cervical spondylosis, in whom a central cord syndrome develops after trauma, may have the injury documented by magnetic resonance imaging. In addition, on the T_2-weighted image, a low-intensity signal within the cord usually represents hematoma. The age of the injury can be determined by the presence of high-intensity signal around it in the acute phase.

Similarly, for patients with cervical facet fractures and dislocations, in whom the integrity of the intervening disk is suspect, the use of magnetic resonance imaging to evaluate the involved disk can be quite effective. Magnetic resonance imaging of acute spinal cord trauma also shows a number of different anatomic patterns of cord injury. The recognition of various patterns of cord injury on magnetic resonance imaging may permit the degree of eventual spinal cord recovery to be estimated. Finally, magnetic resonance imaging in the late phases of spinal cord injury is helpful in delineating posttraumatic syringomyelia.

Treatment of Cervical Spine Injuries

The four major treatments for spinal injury are (1) external immobilization in an orthosis, (2) prolonged traction, with

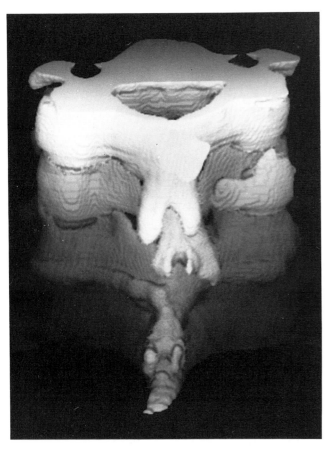

Figure 3
Although plain tomography remains the optimal method of visualizing fractures that require reconstruction in the cervical spine, three-dimensional reconstructions, as in this unilateral facet fracture, will probably supercede the use of plain tomography.

the use of orthosis, (3) surgical decompression of the spinal cord or roots, and (4) surgical spinal realignment and stabilization. Whether treatment should be surgical or nonsurgical depends on defining the goals of the treatment and identifying the methods most likely to achieve those goals.

Injury to the spinal cord and roots may be a result of a variety of different pathologic conditions caused by the traumatic event. There may be reversible soft-tissue lesions that compress the cord or roots. Disk herniation occurs in a significant number of patients. Epidural hemorrhage occurs in some patients, especially those with ankylosing spondylitis and cervical spine injuries. The more common irreversible or partially reversible spine injuries are probably related to cord contusion by bone or disk, as well as distortion of the cord by kyphosis of the surrounding spine. These result in contusion of the central cord, with ischemia, edema, and central necrosis.

Because these changes are not reversible, some investigators strongly believe that no surgical treatment can effect recovery in any way and therefore nonsurgical treatment should prevail. Others suggest that decompressive laminectomy may "decompress the cord" and perhaps augment recovery. Posterior compression may be caused by epidural hemorrhage (especially in patients with ankylosing spondylitis), or by a depressed laminar fracture. In this limited

number of cases, posterior laminectomy may be considered. However, with the possible exception of patients with severe spondylitis over multiple levels and central cord syndromes, patients with spinal injury usually have cord compression as a result of anterior abnormalities. In most patients in whom there is documented compression from the anterior disk or bone fragments, decompressive procedures should be done from an anterior approach. In patients with incomplete spinal lesions and in those with complete lesions without root function at or below the level of the injury, an anterior decompressive procedure can be considered. Even late anterior decompressive surgery has achieved recovery of root function in approximately 50% of patients. This may be critically important to function in the quadriplegic patient. The goals of those procedures, however, should be clearly defined.

A completely different set of surgical and nonsurgical interventions can be directed at injuries to the spinal column. In patients with severe malalignment of the spine secondary to injury, reduction of the malalignment is the primary goal. In other patients who have instability in any plane (rotatory, flexion-extension), the correction of the instability may be the specific goal. In patients with severe ligamentous disruption, restoration of stability can be achieved only by stabilization and fusion of that particular level. Significant ligamentous healing does not occur predictably, although spontaneous fusion at the level of injury can occur. However, in selected patients with bone disruption resulting in instability, nonsurgical treatment may produce results similar to those of surgery. The relative risks and benefits of the types of treatment must be individualized for the particular patient. Therefore, if the goals of treatment are clearly defined for each injury, and divided into goals related to the spinal cord vs those related to the spinal column, an appropriate treatment plan can be worked out for each patient.

Injuries to the Upper Cervical Spine

There are seven major types of injury to the upper cervical spine. Most are not associated with spinal cord injury and can be treated adequately by nonsurgical external immobilization. However, there are a number of exceptions.

Atlanto-occipital Dislocations

Atlanto-occipital dislocations are relatively rare. Most patients die immediately as a result of the complete respiratory arrest, with brain-stem involvement. These injuries result in total disruption of all ligamentous structures between the occiput and C-1, and may involve fractures of the posterior aspects of the atlanto-occipital joint (Fig. 6). Cervical traction is contraindicated in these patients, as it may stretch the brain stem. Immediate application of a halo vest to maintain stability of the spine without traction and attention to the patient's respiratory and neurologic status are critical. Although surgical stabilization has not been universally advocated, it is clearly the most predictable method of treatment of these injuries. The region from the occiput to C-1 or C-2 must be stabilized in these purely ligamentous injuries. This treatment should be undertaken regardless of the patient's neurologic status.

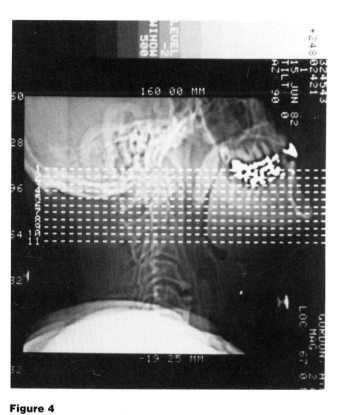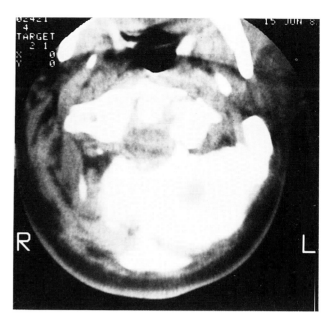

Figure 4

Visualization of the ring of C-1 requires angling the gantry so that it is parallel to the ring. Unfortunately, in the trauma patient, the gantry is frequently at an angle with the ring of C-1 and, therefore, the fractures within the ring cannot be visualized clearly **(right)**.

Fractures of the Lateral Mass and Occipital Condyle

Fractures of the occipital condyles, as well as the lateral masses of C-2, generally occur in combined axial loading and lateral bending injuries. Most fractures of the occipital condyle are relatively stable, but they can be associated with severe head trauma or with cranial nerve palsies. These are generally of two types—avulsion fractures or severely comminuted compression fractures. Similarly, the lateral masses of C-2 can be injured by bilateral bending forces and stellate comminution. These are generally stable injuries initially, and can be treated with orthotic immobilization, although a small percentage require late arthrodesis because of persistent symptomatic degeneration.

Atlas Fractures

Atlas fractures constitute about 25% of all injuries within the C1–2 complex and 10% of all cervical spine injuries. These injuries result from impaction of the skull on the arch of C-1. This commonly causes the arch to fail at the groove for the vertebral arteries, with either symmetric or asymmetric comminution of the anterior portion of the ring. With the exception of patients with severe intracranial damage, patients with C-1 ring fractures rarely have a neurologic deficit.

There are four major types of atlas fracture. The first is the posterior arch fracture, which is the result of hyperextension. Notably, 50% of patients with this injury have another cervical spine injury, either within the C1–2 complex or elsewhere. The most common associated injuries are traumatic spondylolisthesis of the axis and posteriorly

displaced dens fractures. Posterior arch fractures are stable injuries and can be treated by a cervical orthosis. They heal reliably.

The second type of fracture is a lateral-mass fracture (Fig. 7). This fracture occurs on one side of the neural arch with fracture lines generally passing anterior and posterior to the articular surfaces of the C-1 lateral mass. There may or may not be a second fracture on the opposite side of the posterior arch. Occasionally, these fractures pass directly through the articular surface of the lateral mass. On an open-mouth view, there is markedly asymmetric displacement of the lateral masses. The treatment is similar to that for Jefferson fractures.

The third type of fracture is the bursting or Jefferson fracture (Fig. 8). This results from pure axial load, with the force causing lateral bursting of the ring. Neurologic injury is exceedingly rare, as the available space for the spinal cord is generally opened by the lateral displacement of the lateral masses. There are two common misconceptions associated with Jefferson fractures:

(1) It has been demonstrated that a total lateral displacement of more than 6.9 mm produces rupture of the transverse ligament. However, this has not been shown to cause flexion-extension instability between C-1 and C-2 of more than 5 mm. Although some have suggested that arthrodesis is necessary to prevent the occurrence of late instability in significantly displaced Jefferson fractures, this has not been demonstrated. The rupture of the transverse ligament associated with Jefferson fractures differs from a rupture caused by flexion force, which is a pure soft-tissue injury and in which there is an associated disruption of the alar

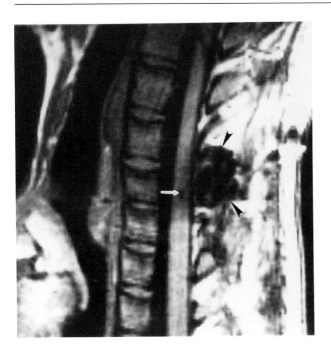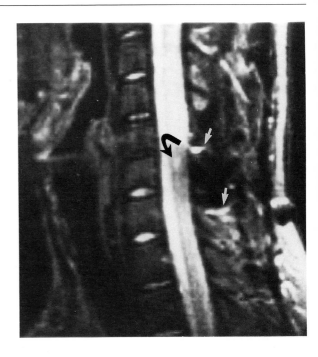

Figure 5

Magnetic resonance imaging after posterior cervical fixation with titanium wire. **Left,** T_1-weighted image (500/17) obtained in the midsagittal plane in an 18-year-old with mild central cord syndrome after a C5-6 bilateral face dislocation. Focal central area of decreased signal at the upper border of C-6 (arrow) was believed to represent an area of myelomalacia or a small cyst. A region of decreased signal surrounds the titanium wires placed posteriorly at C5-6 (arrowheads). This produced a slight uniform decrease in signal in the posterior cervical canal. **Right,** T_2-weighted image (2500/90) reveals focal increased signal intensity in same region (curved arrow) with only minimal interference (straight arrows) from adjacent titanium fixation wire. (Reproduced with permission from Mirvis SE, Geisler F, Joslyn JN, et al: Use of titanium wire in cervical spine fixation as a means to reduce MR artifacts. *AJNR* 1988;9:1229–1231.)

ligaments and C-1 and C-2 facet capsules. In Jefferson fractures, the alar ligaments, as well as a portion of the C-2 capsules, remain intact; once the ring fracture has healed, gross instability (more than 5 mm) does not generally occur. Surgical stabilization of these fractures is rarely indicated.

(2) The second misconception concerns the role of the halo vest in the reduction of these fractures. Long-term follow-up studies have shown that nonunions of Jefferson fractures are uncommon. The application of a halo vest does not aid in the reduction of these fractures because the halo vest cannot apply axial distraction to the cervical spine and, in certain instances, can result in axial compression of the cervical spine. To reduce Jefferson fractures (or lateral mass fractures), which are axial compressive injuries, prolonged distraction must be applied. This can be achieved only with prolonged halo traction (Fig. 9). Although the displacement is reduced initially by traction, once a halo vest is applied the reduction is generally lost, unless traction is applied for longer than six weeks (when preliminary healing of the fragments can occur). Therefore, in minimally displaced Jefferson fractures, consideration should be given to prolonged axial traction (six weeks or longer) to maintain reduction of the fracture and allow preliminary healing before the application of a halo vest. This may eliminate nonunions. At the conclusion of treatment, lateral flexion-extension roentgenograms should be obtained to ensure that significant atlantoaxial subluxation is not present. If a patient has more than 5 mm of atlan-

toaxial subluxation, a late stabilization of C-1 and C-2 should be undertaken.

The fourth type of fracture is an avulsion from the anterior portion of the ring (Fig. 10).

Rupture of the Transverse Ligament (Atlantoaxial Subluxation)

These pure ligamentous injuries result from a severe flexion injury. The injury involves rupture of the transverse ligament, rupture of the alar ligaments, and disruption of the facet capsules of C-1 and C-2. There is a marked increase in the atlantodens interval (Fig. 11) that may be difficult to diagnose. These patients often have severe spasms of the neck muscles that reduce the atlantodens interval. As a result of the spasms they cannot flex to demonstrate the increase in the atlantodens interval. However, they may also have a significant increase in the retropharyngeal soft-tissue shadow, and this may be helpful in delineating the injury. These are pure ligamentous injuries and, therefore, there is agreement that surgical stabilization is necessary. This is achieved by a fusion of C-1 and C-2, often with a wire passed around the arch of C-1 and the spinous process of C-2. This narrows the atlantodens interval. A bone graft permits fusion and restores stability.

Atlantoaxial Rotatory Fixation

This injury in adults is most often related to vehicular accidents. Neurologic injury is rare, and should be differentiated from atlantoaxial subluxations, which are self-lim-

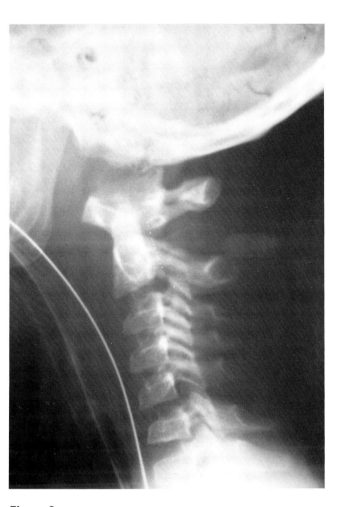

Figure 6
This patient sustained a complete occiput C-1 dislocation as a result of a motor-vehicle accident, with paralysis of all respiratory function and immediate death.

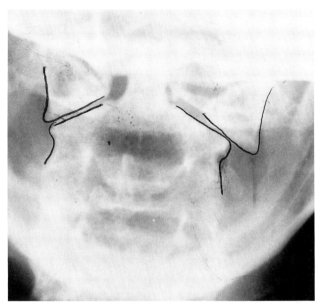

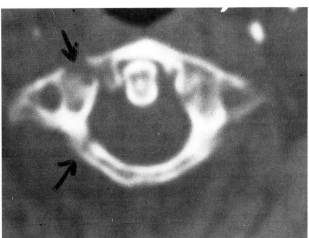

Figure 7
Lateral mass fracture of the atlas. **Top,** The open-mouth view shows no displacement of one lateral mass and marked displacement of the opposite side. **Bottom,** The computed tomographic scan through the ring of the atlas shows the fractures (arrow) anterior and posterior to the lateral mass on one side with no fractures in the posterior arch on the second side. (Reproduced with permission from Levine AM, Edwards CC: Traumatic lesions of the occipito-atlantoaxial complex. *Clin Orthop* 1989;239:53–68.)

ited and occur predominantly in children. There are four types of atlantoaxial rotatory fixation. The classification is based on the degree and direction of displacement and the presence or absence of increase in the atlantodens interval. The critical problem in these patients is early recognition of the injury. The injury is often not recognized initially, since it is difficult to get roentgenograms parallel to the plane of both C-1 and C-2 because of torticollis. Open-mouth roentgenograms help diagnose the injury by demonstrating a "wink sign." The computed tomographic scan is most helpful in delineating the direction and the rotation of C-1 and C-2 (Fig. 12).

Because delayed diagnosis and treatment is common, there has been controversy over the appropriate type of treatment. Most investigators believe that cervical traction with the use of a halo is indicated to reduce the deformity. However, in older fixed deformities there may be little or no reduction of the malrotation. In patients with acute injuries, skeletal traction may begin at relatively low weights, but progress to as much as 14 to 16 kg in a controlled fashion. It is possible to palpate the anterior ring of C-1 and the rotatory dislocation in the posterior oro-

pharynx. This is helpful in achieving a reduction. With gentle traction on the head, direct pressure can be applied to the anteriorly displaced C-1 arch, and reduction occurs with a "pop." Direct palpation is also helpful in determining the relative stability of the joint at the conclusion of manipulation. These are saddle-type joints, and rely to some extent on ligamentous restraint for stability. Therefore, although a reduction can be achieved, it may not be stable. Atlantoaxial arthrodesis is the treatment of choice for patients who have sustained neurologic deficit with the injury or in cases in which there is transverse ligament rupture associated with an increase in the atlantodens in-

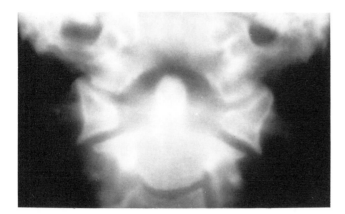

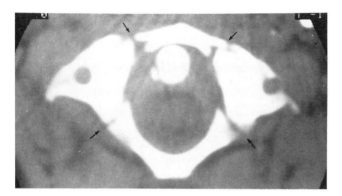

Figure 8

Roentgenograms of a patient who sustained a Jefferson fracture while diving into a pool. **Top,** Anteroposterior tomogram demonstrates splaying of the lateral masses of C-1. **Bottom,** Computed tomographic scan in the plane of C-1 demonstrates all four fractures of the ring, two in the anterior arch and two in the posterior arch (arrows). (Reproduced with permission from Levine AM, Edwards CC: Treatment of injuries in the C1-C2 complex. *Orthop Clin North Am* 1986;17:31–44.)

terval of more than 5 mm. In addition, fractures that have been reduced and maintained in a halo vest and in which there is either pain or instability after three months of immobilization should undergo fusion of C-1 and C-2. The passage of the sublaminar wires at C-1 may help achieve a reduction of C-1 on C-2 at the time of surgery. After reduction, a standard atlantoaxial arthrodesis can be done.

Dens Fractures

Treatment for type II fractures of the dens has remained an area of relative controversy. The type II injury, which occurs at the junction of the dens and the body of the axis, has several variations, which have become more important with the closer scrutiny of treatment results. Specifically, there have been reports of a number of cases of "high type II" dens fracture (Fig. 13). The limited reported experience to date has shown a slightly worse prognostic result for spontaneous union. Also, there are anteriorly and posteriorly displaced type II dens fractures. These are important for two reasons. Patients with posteriorly displaced dens fractures have a higher incidence of associated fractures of the ring of C-1. Failure to recognize this fracture may complicate treatment. In addition, posteriorly displaced type

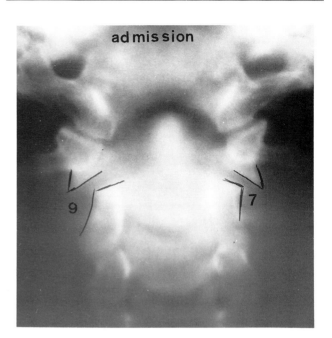

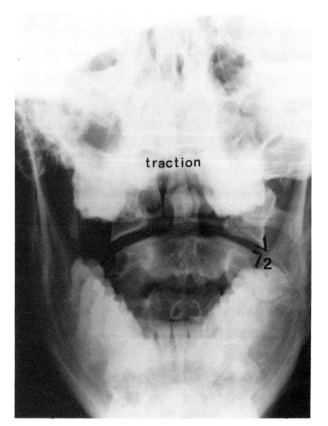

Figure 9

Jefferson fracture of the ring of C-1 demonstrating on the initial tomogram that the patient has 9 mm of displacement on one side and 7 mm of displacement on the opposite side, for a total of 16 mm of displacement. **Top,** Because there was disruption of the transverse ligament and wide splaying of the lateral masses, the patient was placed in 25 lb of traction and the splaying and apposition of the bony fragments was significantly decreased, with a total residual displacement of 2 mm on each side. This was maintained in longitudinal traction. The patient was kept in traction for six weeks and then mobilized in a halo vest to maintain the reduction.

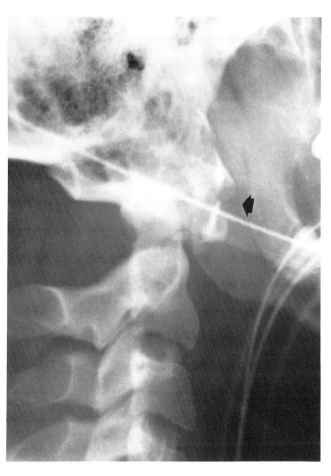

Figure 10

A lateral roentgenogram shows a horizontal fracture of the anterior arch of C-1 (arrow), most probably an avulsion fracture of the anteroinferior portion of the arch of C-1. (Reproduced with permission from Levine AM, Edwards CC: Traumatic lesions of the occipito-atlantoaxial complex. *Clin Orthop* 1989;239:53–68.)

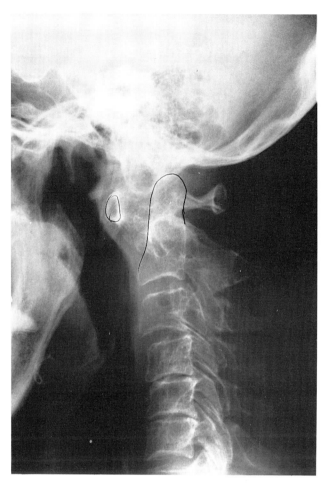

Figure 11

A lateral flexion roentgenogram demonstrates an atlantodens interval of 12 mm, diagnostic of complete rupture of the transverse ligament, the alar and apical ligaments, and a disruption of some fibers of the C1-2 joint capsule. (Reproduced with permission from Levine AM, Edwards CC: Traumatic lesions of the occipito-atlantoaxial complex. *Clin Orthop* 1989;239:53–68.)

II dens fractures have been noted to be more unstable when treated with "Gallie-type" wiring (a construct with a sublaminar wire beneath the ring of C-1 and a spinous process wire around C-2). This tends to displace these fractures posteriorly.

Reported rates for nonsurgical unions have ranged from 20% to 80%. Part of the problem has been the lack of uniformity among the nonsurgical treatments. A recent combined study demonstrated that type II fractures had a 68% union rate when treated with a halo vest. However, there was a 96% healing rate with posterior cervical fusion. The prerequisite for nonsurgical treatment should be halo vest treatment for three months (not a cervical collar). A number of studies have suggested that 5 mm of initial anterior or posterior displacement is associated with a lower healing rate. In addition, in displaced type II dens fractures in which anatomic reduction cannot be achieved and/or maintained, the nonunion rate is higher. There are some data suggesting that older patients also have a lower rate of union, although this may be related in part to reluctance to use halo vests as primary immobilization for elderly patients.

Type III dens fractures can either be impacted or dis-

placed. The displacement in most cases is anterior with an oblique fracture line. Most fractures unite when treated in an external orthosis, although the nonunion rate has been said to be as high as 11%.

In view of the incidence of nonunion, a reasonable treatment approach for type II dens fractures with more than 5 mm of initial displacement or in which an anatomic reduction cannot be achieved and maintained with a halo vest is primary surgical stabilization with an atlantoaxial arthrodesis. In less displaced fractures or in those in which a stable anatomic reduction can be achieved with a halo vest, external immobilization in a halo vest for three months achieves a reasonable degree of union. Current data suggest that an increase in the application of torque from 0.68 to 0.9 N·m decreases the loosening rate of pins from approximately 36% to 7%. A halo vest requires attention to detail and proper pin maintenance to minimize the complications of pin-site infection, skin problems beneath the vest, and disfiguring scars.

In patients who require surgical stabilization, anteriorly displaced dens fracture must be differentiated from pos-

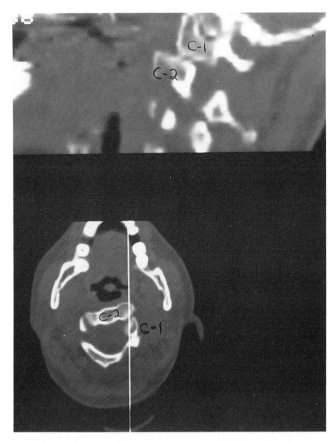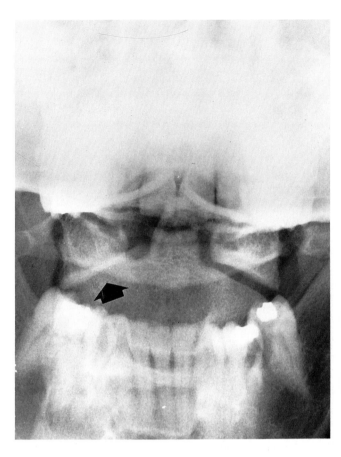

Figure 12

Left, The computed tomographic scan shows a traumatic, posteriorly displaced rotatory fixation after an automobile accident. The right lateral mass of C-1 is posteriorly displaced in reference to the right lateral mass of C-2, causing neurologic deficit. This is well demonstrated on the sagittal reconstruction of that side. The opposite side is nondisplaced. **Right,** This open-mouth roentgenogram shows a wink sign, in which the lateral mass of C-1 overlaps the lateral mass of C-2 on the affected side. (Reproduced with permission from Levine AM, Edwards CC: Traumatic lesions of the occipito-atlantoaxial complex. *Clin Orthop* 1989;239:53–68.)

teriorly displaced dens fracture. In posteriorly displaced dens fractures, a "Gallie-type" wiring construct tends to displace the fracture further (Fig. 14). Using a bone block and double sublaminar wires to maintain the distance between the posterior arches of C-1 and C-2 achieves a stable configuration more effectively.

In addition, care should be taken to exclude a posterior arch fracture in association with the posteriorly displaced type II dens fracture. In an unstable, severely displaced dens fracture with an associated posterior arch fracture and multiple injuries, some early data suggest that an anterior dens screw may be effective. Concern about complications and the accuracy of screw placement are paramount. A second technique is posterior arthrodesis with bilateral posterior screw fixation of C-1 and C-2. At this point, there are only limited indications for the use of a dens screw. If this is not done, the patient should be immobilized in a halo vest to allow healing of the ring of C-1 and a delayed fusion of C-1 and C-2 undertaken.

For displaced type III dens fractures, stabilization in a halo vest can limit the degree of malunion. However, these are generally oblique fractures and are likely to translate minimally; because of the cancellous surfaces, however, they unite with great frequency. Only patients with non-

displaced, impacted type III injuries should be treated in a cervical orthosis.

Traumatic Spondylolisthesis of the Axis (Hangman's Fractures)

Bipedicular fractures of the axis can be subdivided into types, which is helpful in selecting treatment alternatives. Although many different classifications have been proposed, there are four basic types and treatment is related to the fracture pattern. Only type III fractures are frequently associated with neurologic deficit and require any surgical intervention. Type I fractures are minimally displaced and generally result from hypertension and axial load, with failure of the neural arch in tension. Most of these fractures heal satisfactorily with simple orthotic immobilization.

Type II fractures have both significant angulation and translation. These generally result from hyperextension and axial load, causing the neural arch to fail with a predominantly vertical fracture line, followed by severe flexion, resulting in stretching of the posterior anulus of the disk and anterior translation and angulation. The majority of these fractures heal adequately with orthotic immobi-

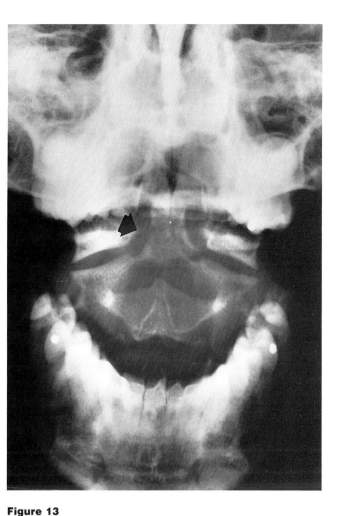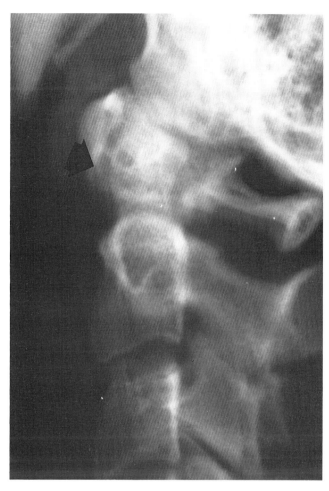

Figure 13

This 18-year-old woman sustained a high type II fracture, as seen on the anteroposterior (**left**) and lateral (**right**) roentgenograms. The fracture line starts well above the base of the dens and is through the midportion. Since the surface area of contact is small, anatomic reduction is critical to healing.

lization. However, in fractures with significant displacement (more than 5 mm) delayed union or nonunion may occur. Because immobilization in a halo vest does not achieve or maintain reduction, halo traction and slight extension for three to six weeks may be necessary to maintain an anatomic reduction (Fig. 15). The patient can then be mobilized in a halo vest for the remainder of the three-month period.

Type IIA fractures are a flexion-distraction variant of type II fractures, which can be recognized by two different criteria: (1) They demonstrate severe angulation between C-2 and C-3 with minimal angulation. (2) They generally have a more horizontal than vertical fracture line through the C-2 arch. Recognition of these injuries is important, in that application of traction can cause marked widening of the C2–3 disk space and increase displacement. Treatment is a halo vest with slight compression applied under image intensification to achieve an anatomic reduction.

Type III injuries combine facet injuries with a bipedicular injury. In these cases, the facet dislocations are irreducible, because the unilateral or bilateral facet dislocation is associated with a bilateral transpedicular fracture sep-

arated from the vertebral body (Fig. 16). These are also more frequently associated with neurologic deficit. Recognition of this injury is critical because these fractures require open reduction of the facet component of the injury to achieve stability, followed by halo immobilization for the bipedicular fracture. These are relatively rare, and constitute only 10% of all hangman's fractures.

Injuries to the Lower Cervical Spine

Injuries to the lower cervical spine differ from those involving the upper cervical spine. With the decreasing ratio of canal area to cervical cord, there are proportionally more patients sustaining injuries to the lower cervical spine who have some degree of neural compression. In those patients with lower cervical spine injuries (both fractures and dislocations) who have no neurologic deficit, the primary concern is the presence or absence of instability (flexion-extension or rotatory instability). Flexion-extension instability is primarily a result of disruption of the interspinous ligament, the ligamentum flavum, the facet cap-

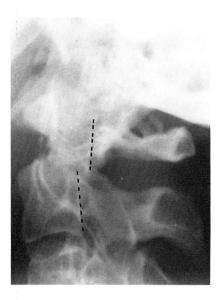
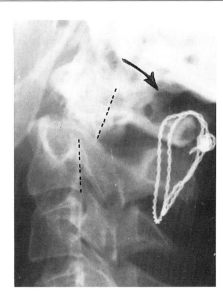
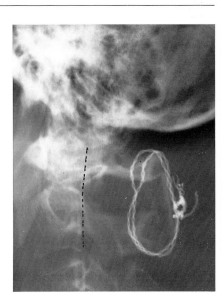

Figure 14

This 36-year-old man sustained a posteriorly displaced type II dens fracture (**left**). As a result of the instability of the fracture and the inability to obtain and maintain a reduction, surgical stabilization was selected. Initially, Gallie wiring was done, which further displaced the fracture posteriorly as well as angulating it posteriorly (**center**). This was later revised to a bone-block fusion with sublaminar wires around C-1 and C-2, increasing stability and orienting the ring of C-1 parallel to the ring of C-2, thus aiding in maintaining the reduction and resisting posterior angulation and displacement (**right**).

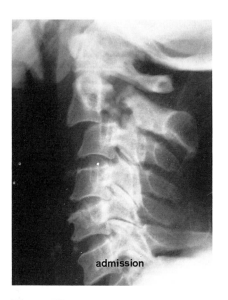
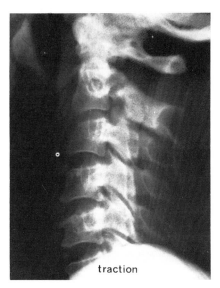
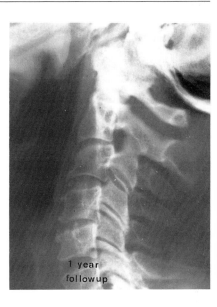

Figure 15

Left, Type II traumatic spondylolisthesis of the axis. **Center,** The initial displacement was 12 mm. The patient was placed in halo traction (20 lb) with slight extension of the neck over a roll to achieve anatomic reduction. (Reproduced with permission from Levine AM, Edwards CC: Treatment of injuries in the C1-C2 complex. *Orthop Clin North Am* 1986;17:31–44.) **Right,** Follow-up roentgenograms at one year demonstrate maintenance of reduction and healing of the traumatic spondylolisthesis in an anatomic position.

sules (fracture of the facet joints), the disk, or the anterior longitudinal ligament. Rotatory instability in the lower cervical spine results primarily from cervical facet injuries.

A second group of patients consists of those with injuries between C-3 and C-7 who have a neurologic deficit on the initial physical examination. These patients require immediate skeletal traction to realign the spine, stabilize the instability, and restore the dimensions of the canal for de-

compression of the damaged cord. Skeletal traction allows adequate realignment in many cases.

The application of cervical traction should be done in a sequential, standardized fashion. Weight should be added in defined increments and roentgenograms taken at appropriate intervals to ascertain that a particular segment is not overdistracted. Although the use of steroids to "decrease cord swelling" has had some advocates, there are

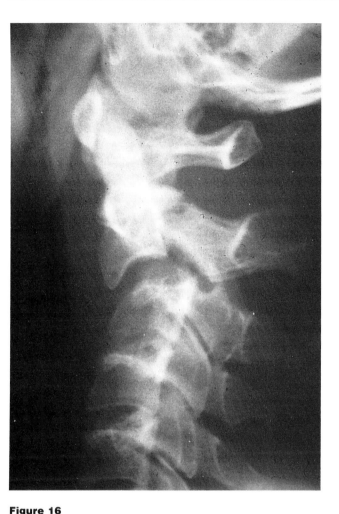 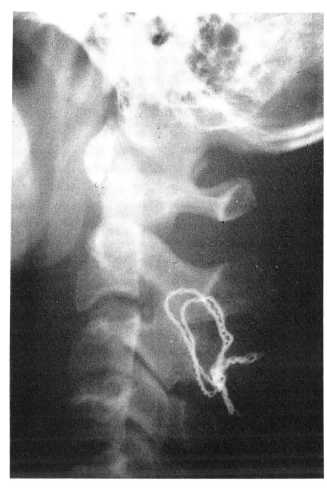

Figure 16

Left, This patient sustained a type III traumatic spondylolisthesis of the axis with a dislocation of the C2–3 facet joints, as well as a fracture of the pedicle of C-2. This could not be reduced in traction, because the facet could not be relocated. **Right,** The patient was, therefore, treated by open reduction and internal fixation of the bilateral facet dislocation, followed by external immobilization for healing of the traumatic spondylolisthesis in an anatomic position.

no data proving their effectiveness. When neurologic deficit is present, there are two major considerations: (1) the definition of cord compression and the strategy for decompression and (2) the determination of the presence or absence of instability and requirements for stabilization.

The timing of surgical procedures for lower cervical spine trauma varies. The decision is based on two major considerations. If the patient has cord compression that can be relieved by reduction of a dislocation or some other maneuver in cervical traction, then the decision regarding surgical intervention can be delayed until the patient's condition has stabilized. Conversely, should a patient with an incomplete deficit have severe compression that cannot be relieved by realignment or traction, then direct decompression should be attempted as soon as the patient's general condition permits the surgery. Similarly, dislocations of the cervical spine can usually be reduced in traction. If there is cord compression that cannot be reduced nonsurgically, then urgent reduction of the deformity is necessary to effect a relative decompression of the canal. The "minimyelogram" or "cervical myelography" with computed tomography was used to define the degree of initial compression and verify

the effectiveness of indirect decompression in many patients with incomplete neurologic deficits. Today, metrizamide myelography can be replaced by magnetic resonance imaging in the evaluation of compression of the dural sac and the effectiveness of indirect decompression. In the absence of gross instability, a more conservative program without immediate surgical intervention can be instituted. As in the upper cervical spine, there are a number of discrete injury types. The major types are minor compressions and avulsions, facet fractures and dislocations, burst fractures, and teardrop injuries.

Minor Compressions and Avulsions

Many isolated fractures of the cervical spine that include compression fractures can be treated with an external cervical orthosis. Fractures with less than 25% compression and an intact posterior wall can be treated nonsurgically with an orthosis. Compression of more than 50% without compression of the posterior wall of the vertebral body may indicate undetected posterior ligamentous instability. In the absence of neurologic deficit, flexion-extension roentgenograms can help to delineate this condition. Interspinous wiring and fusion restore the stability of the disrupted posterior ligamentous complex. Similarly, minor avulsion fractures associated with whiplash injuries of the anterior portion of the vertebral body heal, although disruption of the disk or scarring within the paravertebral musculature may have long-term sequelae.

Facet Injuries (Fractures and Dislocations)

The two major types of injury to the facets produce significantly different instabilities. Both fractures and dislocations can be associated with neurologic deficit in the cervical spine. These can be divided into unilateral facet fractures, unilateral facet dislocations, bilateral facet fractures, bilateral facet dislocations, and combined injury of one fracture and one dislocation. Because facet fractures result in fracture of the bony buttress, even with reduction in traction there is residual rotatory instability. Unilateral facet fractures may be accompanied by single-root deficits, the Brown-Séquard syndrome, or mixed neurologic patterns. Application of traction generally reduces the deformity immediately (Fig. 17). Although a number of investigators have suggested that facet fractures could be controlled in a halo vest, this has not been substantiated in recent studies. In the absence of neurologic deficit, some have argued that the injury will heal in an unreduced position, and that reduction is not needed. The residual rotatory instability of a facet fracture, however, is not well controlled with a halo vest, and thus nonsurgical treatment always results in malrotation, although union may occur. A root deficit, in particular, makes a stable reduction of the rotatory component mandatory. This can be achieved by oblique wiring from the inferior facet of the upper level to the spinous process of the lower level (Fig. 18). Several posterior plating techniques (hook-plate) have also shown effectiveness in the control of these rotatory instabilities, although the role of posterior cervical plating and its attendant risks are still undefined.

The unilateral facet dislocation, conversely, represents a purely ligamentous injury. These are often difficult to reduce and pure longitudinal skeletal traction is not sufficient. Since the buttress of the facet is intact, a reduction maneuver must be undertaken to unlock the dislocated facet and reduce it back to normal position. This reduction is successful in slightly less than 50% of patients. A recent study compared 20 patients with facet dislocations; ten dislocations were allowed to heal in the displaced position and ten underwent open reduction and one-level posterior interspinous fusion. Of the ten left in the displaced position, seven produced residual pain and five of the seven underwent secondary posterior fusion. Of the ten that underwent single-level posterior fusion, none were painful at follow-up. Therefore, reduction and single-level fusion give a better long-term clinical result. Therefore, if reduction can be achieved by manipulation and traction, and there is no neurologic deficit, the patient can be given the alternative of three months of halo immobilization and the possibility of spontaneous fusion. If the dislocation cannot be reduced in this manner, open reduction and single-level posterior interspinous wiring can be done. If a neurologic deficit is present, posterior interspinous wiring must be done even if reduction can be achieved by manipulation and traction.

The facet injury that most often produces neurologic deficit is bilateral facet dislocation. These are also pure ligamentous injuries, with disruption of the posterior lig-

amentous complex, including the interspinous ligament, ligamentum flavum, and both facet capsules. In addition, in severe cases there is disruption of the disk; this can be accompanied by severe translation and spinal cord injury. The overall alignment of the spine can usually be reduced rapidly by segmental increase in tong traction (Fig. 19). If there is significant disruption of the entire ligamentous complex, distraction and extension allows reduction of the injury in a closed fashion in an awake but sedated patient. This must be undertaken with caution. Six of 68 patients with unilateral and bilateral facet injuries demonstrated disk herniation. Disk herniation is often associated with bilateral facet dislocations and may be exacerbated by the reduction maneuver, leading to neurologic deficit. The disk herniation can be identified by either myelography or magnetic resonance imaging, and requires an anterior diskectomy to evacuate the disk material before single-level interspinous wiring and fusion. Failure to recognize this can result in catastrophic neurologic deficit.

The incidence of bilateral facet fractures, or fracture combined with dislocation, is extremely small. The resultant instability is either bidirectional rotational instability (in the bilateral facet fractures) or a combination instability (in the combination injury). Posterior wiring techniques can be used to counteract the instabilities. Aside from the evacuation of disk material from a soft disk herniation, anterior surgery plays little part in facet injuries of the cervical spine. Overall, the increasing evidence of unfavorable results with prolonged halo immobilization suggests that single-level posterior stabilization and fusion is a better choice for facet injuries of the cervical spine.

Vertebral Body Burst Fractures

Axial loading and flexion injuries of the cervical spine can produce severe comminution of the vertebral body with or without posterior-element involvement and with significant kyphosis. These usually result in spinal cord damage, with complete neurologic deficit. The posterior portion of the vertebral body is retropulsed into the spinal canal, impacting on the cord and causing severe disruption. Initial treatment of these injuries is longitudinal traction, which can pull these fragments back into more acceptable alignment and decrease the compression on the cord and roots by ligament axis and stretching of the anterior and posterior longitudinal ligament. The effectiveness of the decompression can be checked with myelography or magnetic resonance imaging while the patient is in traction. If the radiologic studies demonstrate continued compression, anterior surgical decompression may be indicated. This is especially true in the early management of incomplete paraplegia and in the late management of failure of root function to return at the level of the injury or, occasionally, at the level below.

In patients without residual compression, a halo vest may allow secondary collapse and residual compression. These patients may well be candidates for anterior corpectomy and stabilization even in the absence of severe compression. Before anterior surgery is done, the integrity of the posterior ligamentous complex should be assessed. In severe laminar fractures or ligamentous instability, an anterior strut graft alone may not be adequate. If the posterior ligamentous complex is intact, an anterior corpectomy of the affected body can be done. Either corticocancellous iliac crest graft or a fibular strut can be used to bridge the defect. The iliac crest graft is incorporated more

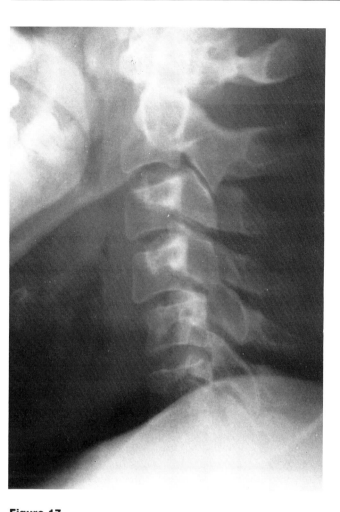 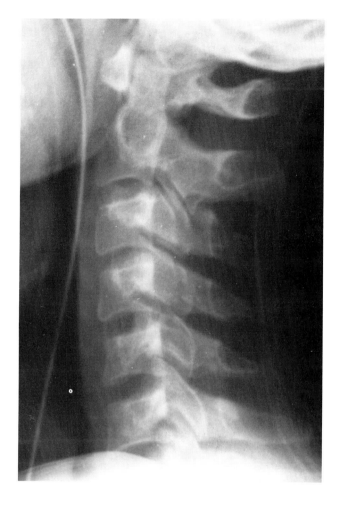

Figure 17

This 49-year-old man had acute neck pain and radicular symptoms after an automobile accident. A lateral roentgenogram (**left**) demonstrated a translational deformity between C-4 and C-5. Application of 20 lb of skeletal traction using Gardiner-Wells tongs achieved an immediate anatomic reduction (**right**), demonstrating that this was a unilateral facet fracture, which is easily reduced in longitudinal traction; however, the reduction is lost immediately on releasing the traction. This is in contradistinction to unilateral facet dislocations, which require a manual reduction maneuver to unlock the locked facet.

rapidly than the fibular strut. Currently, there is preliminary evidence, especially from Europe, that anterior-plate fixation may be of value. However, the extremely high risk of bicortical screw fixation, as well as the disastrous complications when anterior cervical hardware loosens, should temper enthusiasm for this hardware except in carefully selected situations. Biomechanical data have shown that anterior plates act like a tension band. With combined anterior and posterior disruption, anterior-plate fixation cannot resist flexion forces. Combined anterior and posterior procedures may be necessary. In patients with minimal displacement and relative stability, halo immobilization may produce a satisfactory long-term outcome. If the ligamentous complex is disrupted, halo vest immobilization or a secondary posterior construct can add to the relative stability.

Teardrop Fractures

Teardrop fractures of the cervical spine are a particular group with a complex instability pattern. The teardrop fracture should be differentiated from the anterior avulsion fracture. True teardrop injuries are flexion and rotation injuries in which the inferior tip of the upper body is driven down into the lower body by compression and flexion; a fracture line proceeds from superior to inferior, and exits through the disk space, totally disrupting the disk, as well as disrupting to varying degrees the facet capsules, ligamentum flavum, and interspinous ligament. This results in a grossly unstable injury in which the inferior portion of the superior body impinges on the canal and the dural sac (Fig. 20). It is frequently accompanied by partial or complete neurologic involvement.

These injuries have proven very difficult to stabilize because the posterior ligamentous complex is also disrupted to some degree. Although many investigators have used anterior corpectomies and fibular or iliac strut grafts, the posterior disruption has resulted in dislodgement of grafts, late kyphotic deformities, and unsatisfactory results. The injury can often be reduced satisfactorily in longitudinal halo traction, but the reduction cannot be maintained in a halo vest. Mobilization in a halo vest leads to kyphosis and recurrence of retrolisthesis of the vertebral body, caus-

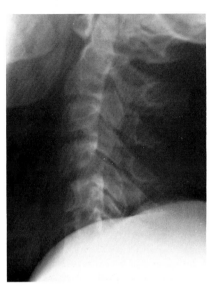
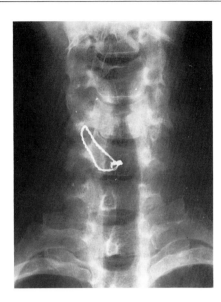
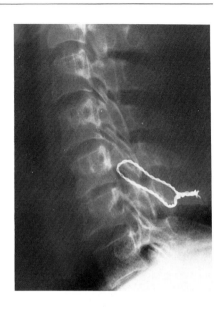

Figure 18

A lateral roentgenogram (**left**) demonstrates the unreduced facet fracture at C4–5 as seen in Figure 17. Because this is a rotational deformity, a rotational force is required to achieve reduction. The oblique wiring technique (**center**) reduces the rotatory component of the displacement, achieving anatomic alignment (**right**). Note, however, that the disk space has lost height at follow-up as a result of the significant disruption to the disk by this rotatory injury.

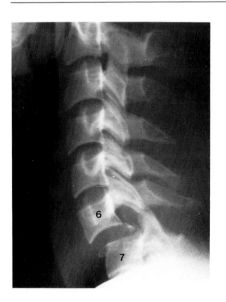
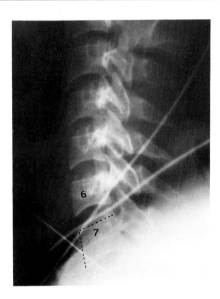
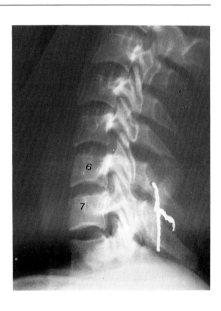

Figure 19

Left, A 19-year-old man sustained a bilateral facet dislocation at C6–7 without neurologic deficit. **Center,** Application of 40 lb of traction was necessary to disengage the facets; this was followed by slight extension of the neck, which achieved reduction, after which the traction was reduced to 15 lb. **Right,** Because all the posterior ligamentous structures were completely disrupted, single-level interspinous wiring and fusion was done to restore stability and allow mobilization of the patient.

ing secondary cord compression. A combination of anterior and posterior surgery may be effective in stabilizing the lesion. Most commonly, the canal can be fully decompressed by simple traction realignment of the spine. There are early reports of satisfactory stabilization in a small number of patients with this complex injury by anterior-plate fixation. These data are experimental, but suggest a possible future approach to this most unstable injury.

Gunshot Wounds

Gunshot wounds to the cervical spine are generally treated nonsurgically unless the wound transects the esophagus, thus contaminating the neck. Unless a bullet lies within the canal and compresses the dural sac in an incomplete injury, its presence causes little further harm. It has been suggested that a bullet left within the canal may increase the patient's lead level. However, most injuries can be

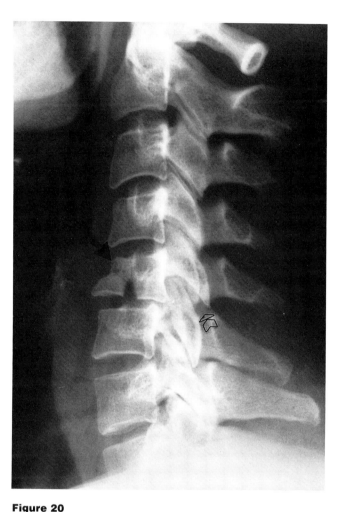

Figure 20

This 45-year-old woman sustained a flexion-rotation injury to C-5. This resulted in a teardrop fracture with disruption of the facet joint capsules (arrowhead), interspinous ligament, and disk. This allowed rotation of the posteroinferior portion of the body into the canal.

treated nonsurgically by skeletal traction and/or halo immobilization until the bone injuries heal.

Controversies

Methylmethacrylate Stabilization

Although there is a significant body of evidence demon-strating the usefulness of methylmethacrylate "stabilization" in traumatic injuries of the cervical spine, many disagree. In a recent report on the long-term use of posterior screws applied to the articular pillars, accompanied by methylmethacrylate columns over the heads of the screws, without a bone graft, the rationale was the decreased surgical time and "the immediate stability." The obvious disadvantage, however, is that the methylmethacrylate fatigues wih time. Biomechanical studies have shown that the interface between the methylmethacrylate and the bone is the point of potential failure. In addition, the methylmethacrylate occupies a large amount of space, and it may be difficult to reapproximate the soft tissue. Finally, the risk of catastrophic infection is particularly high. Another recent series demonstrated the catastrophic complications that can occur with methylmethacrylate fusions in the cervical spine. At this time, the use of methylmethacrylate in a posterior location for the "fusion" of cervical spine trauma is contraindicated. The technique uses the material in a biomechanically disadvantageous position (tension) and the multiple complications cannot be justified when standard wiring and bone graft fusion techniques have lower complication rates.

Cervical Spine Instrumentation

Although cervical spine instrumentation has been popular in Europe for a number of years, the proliferation of cervical spine instrumentation in the United States is relatively new. Anterior dens screw fixation is clearly experimental, but may serve a useful purpose in very difficult situations (severely unstable, posteriorly displaced dens fracture with fracture of the C-1 arch). Similarly, the use of anterior cervical plates should not be advocated at this time because of the necessity of bicortical screw fixation and precise application. In addition, loosening of the hardware can result in catastrophic neurologic complications. Even the investigational use of this hardware should be restricted to gross instability, which requires anterior corpectomy for direct decompression of anterior abnormalities. Reduction and stabilization of posterior abnormalities by means of anterior surgery with or without plates should be contraindicated. The recent use of bands and plates to replace wire constructs for posterior stabilization is also investigational. Early studies have not found that posterior plate fixation produces more stability than a wire construct. The appropriate use of wire constructs directed at counteracting instabilities produces a stable construct and maintains satisfactory reduction. Finally, the placement of screws from the posterior direction in the cervical spine has the disadvantages of insufficient holding power and possible root impingement.

Annotated Bibliography

Keywords

Atlantoaxial subluxation; Cervical spine; Facet joint; Fracture; Hangman's fracture; Methylmethacrylate; Spinal cord; Spinal instrumentation; Spondylolisthesis; Vertebra

Patient Evaluation

Cottler HB, Kulkarni MV, Bondurant FJ: Magnetic resonance imaging of acute spinal cord trauma: Preliminary report. *J Orthop Trauma* 1988;2:1–4.

Forty-three magnetic resonance imaging studies were done on 28 patients. Three patterns of magnetic resonance signals were seen in association with cord injuries, which may demonstrate potential for predicting neurologic recovery.

Harris JH Jr, Edeiken-Monroe B, Kopaniky DR: A practical classification of acute cervical spine injuries. *Orthop Clin North Am* 1986;17:15–30.

This article presents a practical classification of acute cervical spine injuries based on terminology with generally accepted and understood definitions, published results of experimentally produced acute injuries to the cervical spine, and the correlation of the radiographic and pathologic characteristics of the laboratory models with acute clinical injuries.

Lucas JT, Ducker DP: Motor classification of spinal cord injuries with mobility, morbidity and recovery indices. *Am Surg* 1979;45:151–158.

These authors demonstrate the use of a motor index for evaluation and classification of recovery of patients with spinal cord injuries. Although it is more complex than the Frankel classification, it gives a more precise evaluation of root recovery.

Marshall LF, Knowlton S, Garfin SR, et al: Deterioration following spinal cord injury. *J Neurosurg* 1987;66: 400–404.

This was a retrospective study of the course of 283 patients admitted to five trauma centers. Of the 283 patients, 14 deteriorated neurologically during the hospital stay. In 12 of the 14, the neurologic decline was associated with some specific management event; most involved cord injuries.

Soderstrom CA, McArdle DQ, Ducker TB, et al: The diagnosis of intra-abdominal injury in patients with cervical cord trauma. *J Trauma* 1983;23:1061–1065.

A review of 288 patients showed that 58 had shock (blood pressure, <100 mm Hg). Forty of the 58 patients (69%) had neurogenic shock and the remaining 18 had shock on the basis of intra-abdominal or other major injuries.

Templeton PA, Young JW, Mirvis SE, et al: The value of retropharyngeal soft tissue measurements in trauma of the adult cervical spine: Cervical spine soft tissue measurements. *Skeletal Radiol* 1987;16:98–104.

Widening of the retropharyngeal soft-tissue space has been interpreted as a sign of cervical spine trauma. The authors measured this space at the C2-C4 level on lateral cervical spine radiographs of 318 patients with histories of cervical trauma.

Injuries to the Upper Cervical Spine

Anderson LD, D'Alonzo RT: Fractures of the odontoid process of the axis. *J Bone Joint Surg* 1974;56A:1663–1674.

This is the original article classifying dens fractures into three major categories.

Böhler J: Anterior stabilization for acute fractures and non-unions of the dens. *J Bone Joint Surg* 1982;64A:18–27.

The initial concept of the anterior dens screw was devised simultaneously by Böhler and Aebi. This is the first reported series of the results of anterior dens screw fixation.

Botte MJ, Byrne TP, Garfin SR: Application of the halo device for immobilization of the cervical spine utilizing an increased torque pressure. *J Bone Joint Surg* 1987; 69A:750–752.

This study demonstrated the decreased loosening and infection rate with the increase in the amount of torque applied to halo pins from the previous standard of 6 in-lb (0.6 N/m) to 8 in-lb (0.9 N/m). The infection rate decreased from 20% to 2% and the loosening rate from 36% to 7%.

Clark CR, White AA III: Fractures of the dens: A multicenter study. *J Bone Joint Surg* 1985;67A:1340–1348.

The Cervical Spine Research Society conducted a multicenter survey of the treatment of dens fractures. Type II fractures went on to successful union in 68% of patients treated in a halo vest, and posterior cervical fusion was successful in 98% of patients with that injury. Treatment with orthoses was less successful. Significant displacement of more than 5 mm were evident in patients who went on to nonunion of a type II dens fracture. Type III dens fractures went on to successful union in 86% of patients, and it was recommended that halo vest immobilization be used in all patients with displaced type III fractures, because less effective immobilization led to higher rates of nonunion and malunion.

Garfin SR, Botte MJ, Waters RL, et al: Complications in the use of the halo fixation device. *J Bone Joint Surg* 1986;68A:320–325.

Pin loosening occurred in 36% of 179 patients and pin-site infection in 20%. Other complications also occurred. This suggested that it is safe to retighten loosened pins and to treat low-grade infections aggressively with systemic antibiotics and local wound care. Guidelines for the care of a halo orthodosis in adult patients can decrease complications.

Huelke DF, Nusholtz GS: Cervical spine biomechanics: A review of the literature. *J Orthop Res* 1986;4:232–245.

This article reviews the many clinical and laboratory investigative research reports on the frequency, causes, and biomechanics of human cervical spine impact injuries and tolerances.

Karlström G, Olerud S: Internal fixation of fractures and dislocations in the cervical spine. *Orthopedics* 1987;10: 1549–1558.

This article describes some of the new techniques and provides examples of, indications for, and methods of performing stable internal fixation.

Levine AM, Edwards CC: The management of traumatic spondylolisthesis of the axis. *J Bone Joint Surg* 1985; 67A:217–226.

Fifty-two cases of traumatic spondylolisthesis of the axis were evaluated and classified into four different types of fractures. Types I, II, and IIA were rarely associated with neurologic deficit, and could be treated nonsurgically. Type III fractures were more commonly associated with neurologic deficit and facet disruption, and required surgical stabilization.

Levine AM, Edwards CC: Traumatic lesions of the occipitoatlantoaxial complex. *Clin Orthop* 1989;239:53–68.

This article reviews less common injuries to the upper cervical spine, including fractures of the occipital condyle, occipitoatlantal dislocation, atlas fractures, rotatory dislocations, and lateral mass fractures of C-2.

Levine AM, Edwards CC: Treatment of injuries in the C1-C2 complex. *Orthop Clin North Am* 1986;17:31–44.

This article reviews current treatment modalities and classifications of the five most common upper cervical spine injuries. These are fractures of the atlas, ruptures of the transverse ligaments, rotatory dislocations, fractures of the dens, and traumatic spondylolisthesis of the axis.

Injuries to the Lower Cervical Spine

Benzel EC, Larson SJ: Functional recovery after decompressive spine operation for cervical spine fractures. *Neurosurgery* 1987;20:742–746.

Ninety-nine patients with C-4 to C-7 injuries were operated on, most through anterior decompression. No patient with a complete injury recovered but those with incomplete injuries showed some improvement. This study is, however, deceiving as there were no controls and spontaneous improvement cannot be differentiated from the results of surgery. This makes interpretation of the data in the article difficult.

Bohlman HH: Acute fractures and dislocations of the cervical spine: An analysis of three hundred hospitalized patients and review of the literature. *J Bone Joint Surg* 1979;61A:1119–1142.
This very large study of cervical spine injuries contributes several important points. Laminectomy was associated with multiple complications, and the use of steroids did not improve neurologic function.

Cabanela ME, Ebersold MJ: Anterior plate stabilization for bursting teardrop fractures of the cervical spine. *Spine* 1988;13:888–891.
This report deals with eight patients with bursting teardrop fractures who underwent anterior corpectomy and strut grafting with stabilization by means of a plate. Early results suggest a satisfactory outcome.

Copen DA, Nelson RW, Zigler JE, et al: Decompressive laminectomy in cervical spine trauma: A review of early and late complications. *Contemp Orthop* 1988;17:21–29.
The authors review the myriad of complications associated with cervical laminectomies. Laminectomy should be restricted to very selected circumstances.

Rorabeck CH, Rock MG, Hawkins RJ, et al: Unilateral facet dislocation of the cervical spine: An analysis of the results of treatment in 26 patients. *Spine* 1987;12:23–27.
Of 26 patients with unilateral facet injuries, 12 had isolated dislocations and 14 had fractures of the facets or bodies. Closed reduction was accomplished in only six patients. Of the other 20, ten fractures were left in the unreduced position and ten had open reduction. Those patients who underwent open reduction and fusion had better results than those whose fractures were left unreduced.

Controversies

Duff TA: Surgical stabilization of traumatic cervical spine dislocation using methyl methacrylate: Long-term results in 26 patients. *J Neurosurg* 1986;64:39–44.

McAfee PC, Bohlman HH, Ducker T, et al: Failure of stabilization of the spine with methylmethacrylate: A retrospective analysis of twenty-four cases. *J Bone Joint Surg* 1986;68A:1145–1157.

33

Thoracolumbar Spine: Pediatric Aspects

Trends and controversies initiated early in the 1980s have become more clearly focused since the publication of *Orthopaedic Knowledge Update 2*. The natural history of idiopathic scoliosis during growth has been documented further and indications for nonsurgical treatment refined. The usefulness of electrical stimulation for treating idiopathic scoliosis has been questioned on the basis of longer follow-up. Newer surgical techniques for idiopathic scoliosis have focused on restoring normal thoracic kyphosis and maintaining lumbar lordosis. Controversy continues as to the severity of idiopathic scoliosis needing fusion and how far fusion should extend into the lumbar spine. In congenital scoliosis, interest has been renewed in fusion of the convex half of the curve. In developmental spondylolisthesis, the availability of several reduction techniques has made reduction and instrumentation feasible, but the issue is still controversial.

Congenital Deformity of the Spine

Improved techniques may make abdominal ultrasound preferable to the intravenous pyelogram as a screening technique for the asymptomatic renal anomalies that accompany approximately 20% of congenital spine deformities. Magnetic resonance imaging has become increasingly useful as an imaging technique for the intraspinal anomalies often associated with congenital spine deformities.

Congenital Scoliosis

The diagnosis and follow-up of congenital spine deformities were covered in *Orthopaedic Knowledge Update 1* and *2*. Progression of congenital deformities often parallels growth rate, dictating periodic radiologic follow-up starting in infancy. Although brace treatment can, in rare cases, be used in unusually flexible curves, fusion is generally indicated for progressive curves.

The traditional treatment for progressive congenital scoliosis is early posterior in situ fusion. Recent studies have led to interest in a technique involving epiphysiodesis of the convex half of the curve.

Congenital Kyphosis

The observations regarding mandatory early fusion for congenital kyphosis noted in *Orthopaedic Knowledge Update 1* and *2* have been confirmed in the recent literature. If left surgically untreated, nearly all cases of congenital kyphosis progress with growth. Progression of kyphosis caused by failure of formation of the anterior elements is associated with paraplegia.

Idiopathic Scoliosis

Etiology and Natural History

Although genetic factors, growth, and possible aberrations in the central nervous system have been implicated, the precise cause of idiopathic scoliosis remains obscure. *Orthopaedic Knowledge Update 1* and *2* reviewed the natural history and prevalence of idiopathic scoliosis, as well as techniques for the screening, evaluation, and follow-up of mild curves. The growth potential remaining, curve severity, and, to a lesser extent, curve type help predict the likelihood that a given curve will increase and require treatment. Estimation of the likelihood of progression has been made easier by the development of a nomogram (Table 1 and Fig. 1).

Nonsurgical Treatment

Early detection and nonsurgical treatment of progressive curves during growth remains the goal of scoliosis surveillance. Whether such curves are best treated by electrical stimulation or bracing is currently controversial.

Surgical Treatment

The surgical treatment of adolescent idiopathic scoliosis was discussed in depth in *Orthopaedic Knowledge Update 2*. Since then, several issues have continued to provoke discussion. Debate continues as to how severe a curve must be to need fusion in an adolescent at or near the end of growth. Although most authorities agree on the need for fusion for idiopathic curves exceeding 50 to 55 degrees, curves between 40 and 50 degrees fall into a "gray zone" in which either observation or fusion may be appropriate. The decision to fuse is based on the prediction of future difficulties if the curve is left unfused. Such predictions depend heavily on published natural history studies of untreated scoliosis in the adult, which have been scarce, although several such studies have been published in the last few years. Ultimately, the decision to operate must be based on the predicted behavior of the untreated curve, weighed against the short- and long-term risks of surgery.

Several reports have called attention to the fate of the unfused portion of lumbar spine below instrumented scoliosis fusions. An inverse relationship between the number

Table 1. Likelihood of progression of two curves*

Data	Curve 1	Curve 2
Cobb angle (degrees)	20	20
Risser sign	3	0
Age (yrs)	14	10
Likelihood of progression (%)	10	80

*Likelihood estimated by the nonogram of Lonstein.

415

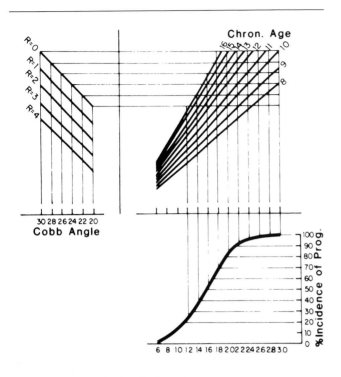

Nomogram devised using the formula:

$$progression\ factor = \frac{Cobb\ angle - 3 \times Risser\ sign}{chronological\ age}$$

Figure 1

Knowing the Cobb angle of the major curve, the Risser grade (0 to 5) of the iliac crest apophysis, and the patient's age permits the likelihood of progression to be estimated for curves between 20 and 29 degrees. To use the nomogram, start with the Cobb angle and follow the corresponding line vertically until the oblique line corresponding to the appropriate Risser value is encountered. Turn horizontally until the chronologic age line is met, then turn directly vertically downward until the curved line is encountered, then horizontally to the right to read the approximate percentage incidence of progression. (Reproduced with permission from Lonstein JE, Carlson JM: The prediction of curve progression in untreated idiopathic scoliosis during growth. *J Bone Joint Surg* 1984;66A:1061–1071.)

of remaining mobile segments and the incidence of low back pain after scoliosis fusion has been reported by some but not confirmed by others. Loss of lumbar lordosis, retrolisthesis below the fusion, and the postoperative "flat-back syndrome" have been blamed on the use of distraction instrumentation in the lumbar spine. Loss of lumbar lordosis has been reported even in cases in which the Harrington rod was contoured into lordosis. Although such reports emphasize the necessity of leaving the lumbar spine as mobile as possible, the standard criteria for selecting stable fusion levels when the curve involves the lumbar spine appear to remain valid. Different criteria for fusion levels may be necessary when Cotrel-Dubousset instrumentation is used.

Other studies of the three-dimensional nature of deformity in idiopathic curves have focused attention on the thoracic hypokyphosis (Fig. 2, *left*) and lumbar hypolordosis that typically accompany idiopathic curves in these locations. Newer segmental instrumentation techniques, such

as the Cotrel-Dubousset technique, have addressed these sagittal-plane deformities (Figs. 2, *right*, and 3). The Cotrel-Dubousset system, which allows multiple points of fixation and both compression and distraction on the same rod, is now becoming more popular for idiopathic scoliosis. The theoretical advantages of Cotrel-Dubousset instrumentation include improved correction of thoracic hypokyphosis and lumbar hypolordosis, preservation of lumbar lordosis when instrumentation extends into the lower lumbar spine, and cosmetic improvement in rib hump. Its potential disadvantages include its relatively high cost, that it is more technically demanding, and that it potentially is more invasive because of its multiple hook sites. Although recent short-term results are encouraging, longer series are needed to determine the optimal instrumentation for a given idiopathic curve. Conventional instrumentation for idiopathic scoliosis remains the Harrington rod or variations such as Wisconsin interspinous segmental fixation and Dwyer or Zielke anterior instrumentation for selected lumbar or thoracolumbar curves. Cotrel-Dubousset instrumentation, however, will probably supplant the Harrington rod for the treatment of flexible, moderate idiopathic thoracic and double curves in the near future.

Idiopathic Thoracic Hyperkyphosis (Scheuermann's Disease)

Idiopathic thoracic hyperkyphosis was discussed in *Orthopaedic Knowledge Update I* and *2*. Recent studies have better defined the range of deformity amenable to bracing, suggesting that kyphosis in excess of 75 degrees is less amenable to bracing. Natural history studies of untreated kyphosis are scarce, making the indications for prophylactic surgery on asymptomatic kyphoses controversial.

Spondylolysis and Spondylolisthesis

The diagnosis and management of spondylolysis and spondylolisthesis in children and adolescents were outlined in *Orthopaedic Knowledge Update I* and *2*. Several studies have cast light on the natural history of these disorders during growth. In one series, seven of 27 cases showed progression of slippage and in another series, only 5% showed more than 10 mm of further slippage with growth. Radiologic monitoring of spondylolysis and spondylolisthesis for potential progression is still indicated, particularly during periods of rapid growth.

Spondylolysis

Most spondylolysis is either asymptomatic or responds to conservative treatment. Recently attention has been called to the occurrence of symptomatic spondylolysis in gymnasts and other athletes. Although fusion remains the conventional treatment for the rare spondylolysis in need of surgery, interest in direct repair of the spondylolytic defect has been renewed. The technique of direct repair using cerclage wire or screws is potentially advantageous for midlumbar spondylolysis in which maximum preservation of mobility is desired, but simple fusion is still probably the conventional treatment.

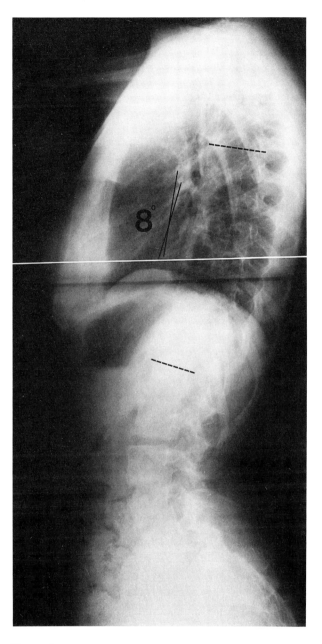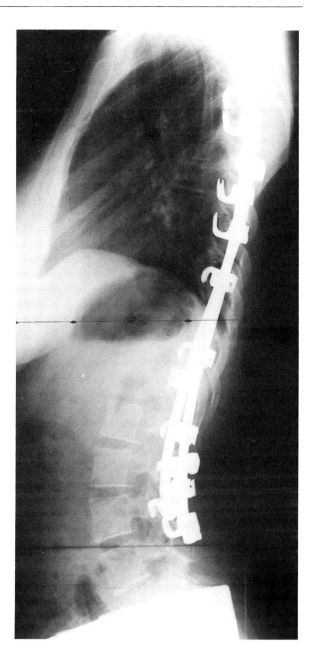

Figure 2

Thoracic idiopathic scoliosis. **Left**, Preoperative lateral radiograph of a typical 60-degree curve. Thoracic hyperkyphosis typically accompanies idiopathic thoracic curves. In this example, thoracic kyphosis is diminished to 8 degrees (normal, approximately 20 to 40 degrees). **Right**, Postoperative lateral radiograph. Cotrel-Dubousset instrumentation has helped restore more normal thoracic kyphosis.

Spondylolisthesis

The indications for surgical treatment of spondylolisthesis in children and adolescents have not changed in recent years. Renewed interest in reduction of severe spondylolisthesis has provoked discussion about the indications for reduction.

Low Back Pain

Orthopaedic Knowledge Update I and *2* outlined the clinical approach to low back pain in children and adolescents. Unlike back pain in adults, which is a common occurrence, back pain in adolescents and children suggests a significant spinal abnormality.

The recent availability of magnetic resonance imaging has led to the documentation of metabolic "degenerative" changes in the disks of children and adolescents with back pain. Although some changes seen on magnetic resonance imaging are clearly pathologic, no large studies of the incidence of changes detectable by magnetic resonance imaging in the asymptomatic adolescent population have been published. Until prevalence and follow-up studies are available, the prognosis and clinical significance of such changes noted on magnetic resonance imaging in adolescents must be speculative.

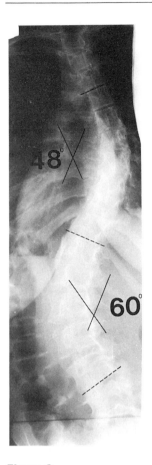
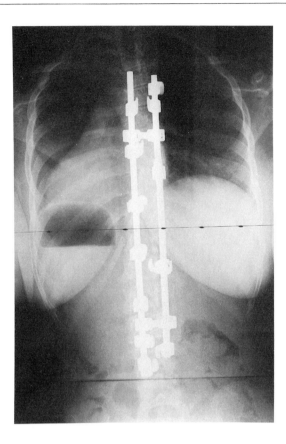
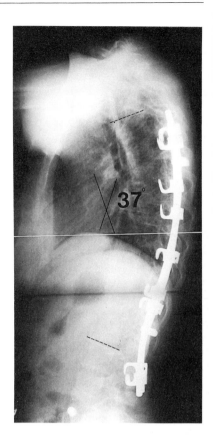

Figure 3

A 13-year-old child with adolescent idiopathic scoliosis. **Left**, Preoperative posteroanterior radiograph. **Center**, Postoperative posteroanterior radiograph. Cotrel-Dubousset instrumentation has provided a satisfactory correction of deformity in the coronal plane. Extension of the fusion to the lumbar spine was necessitated by the type and magnitude of curve. **Right**, Postoperative lateral radiograph. Cotrel-Dubousset instrumentation has successfully maintained normal lumbar lordosis.

Neuromuscular Deformities of the Spine

Little has changed in the treatment of spinal deformities caused by cerebral palsy, myelomeningocele, and other neuromuscular diseases. Segmental Luque sublaminar wire fixation continues to be the mainstay of surgical treatment for these conditions.

Controversies

Progressive Congenital Scoliosis: In Situ Fusion vs Anterior and Posterior Epiphysiodesis of the Convex Half of the Curve

In the younger child, isolated posterior fusion of a lordotic curve may act as a posterior tethering bar, producing more lordosis or even a rotatory lordosis-scoliosis as the unfused anterior vertebral bodies continue to grow. Most authorities, therefore, advise anterior as well as posterior fusion for progressive congenital scoliosis associated with lordosis. Stabilization of the progressive curve is generally achieved.

Recent published series have rekindled interest in fusion and epiphysiodesis of the convex half of progressive congenital curves in an attempt to gain correction of the curve with further growth. In this hemiepiphysiodesis technique, only the convex half of the posterior spine is fused; anteriorly, the convex half of the vertebral end plates and epiphyses are removed and fused. Some curve correction is achieved by a postoperative cast. Posterior fusion of the convexity alone has been associated with continued curve progression. However, two new reports of anterior and posterior fusion of the convex half of the curve and epiphysiodesis indicate that some curve correction as well as curve stabilization can be achieved. Only 50% of the patients achieved even a modest correction in the most optimistic report, but there were few failures of curve stabilization. There seems to be little additional risk in hemiepiphysiodesis, except the surgical risk of a thoracotomy and the theoretical disadvantage that a subsequent corrective osteotomy might be made more difficult by the presence of an anterior fusion mass.

Whether combined anterior and posterior fusion of the convex half of the curve should replace in situ posterior fusion (or in situ posterior and anterior fusion when the deformity includes lordosis) remains controversial and awaits larger series and further definition of which curves are likely to be corrected. Currently, the ideal candidate appears to be young, to have a short curve of less than 70 degrees, and to have no excessive kyphosis or lordosis.

Table 2. Guidelines for brace treatment of adolescent idiopathic scoliosis

Cobb Angle (degrees)	Nonsurgical Treatment
0 to 20	Observe for progression
21 to 25	Brace if substantial progression has been documented and much growth remains
26 to 30	Brace if progressive and growth remains
31 to 40	Brace if growth remains
41 to 45	If growth remains, consider bracing if all prognostic factors are favorable

Other progressive congenital curves are probably best treated by traditional techniques.

Progressive Adolescent Idiopathic Scoliosis: Electrical Stimulation vs Bracing

Natural history studies have led to recommendations that nonsurgical treatment be used for curves between 20 (or 25) and 30 degrees when significant progression has been demonstrated and substantial growth remains, and for those curves between 30 and 40 degrees if growth remains. Although some curves between 40 and 45 degrees can be treated successfully, most curves in excess of 45 degrees are not candidates for brace treatment (Table 2). Traditionally, treatment with a brace has continued until the end of skeletal growth, when the patient is slowly weaned from the brace. Although some patients achieve net correction, the average result of bracing is stabilization rather than significant correction of the curve. Curves with their apex in the midportion of the spine and those that show an initial reduction of 50% or more in the brace appear to do best. Lack of compliance with recommended brace wear continues to be a problem, and approximately 15% to 20% of curves increase despite bracing. Bracing during adolescence has been reported to have adverse psychological effects.

Enthusiasm for treatment of progressive curves by transcutaneous electrical stimulation was generated by preliminary successful reports and the desire to rid adolescents of the psychological and social burdens of brace wear. Transcutaneous electrical muscle stimulation systems using either laterally or paraspinally placed electrodes became popular. As more centers used electrical stimulation, negative findings began to be reported. Published series of electrical stimulation often included patients still in treatment or averaged results to include patients wih curves of less than 30 degrees at the inception of treatment, making it difficult to ascertain the effect of electrical stimulation on curves of more than 30 degrees, which are known to have a very high likelihood of progression. Reports comparing brace and electrical stimulation suggested similar results for mild curves treated by bracing and those treated by electrical stimulation, but indicated that bracing is probably more effective in controlling larger curves of more than 35 degrees. A recent study found no statistical difference in outcome between patients who had completed electrical stimulation treatment and patients who had no treatment at all.

A prospective comparison of no treatment, bracing, and electrical stimulation has been undertaken by the Scoliosis Research Society and may eventually give a definitive answer as to which, if any, is the most effective nonsurgical treatment. Until larger completed series of electrical stimulation patients are available, electrical stimulation must be viewed with caution. Traditional brace treatment is probably preferable for larger curves, and perhaps for all progressive curves.

Severe Spondylolisthesis: Indications for Reduction

Conventional surgical treatment for severe developmental L-5 spondylolisthesis consists of posterior fusion from L-4 to the sacrum with decompression and immobilization as needed. Relief of pain and prevention of further slippage can be expected if solid fusion is obtained, with several new large series continuing to document satisfactory results from in situ fusion and postoperative casting. Reduction to differing degrees of both the L-5 spondylolisthesis on the sacrum and the lumbosacral kyphosis that accompanies severe slips has been reported with increasing frequency and enthusiasm. Reduction has been accomplished by various means, including serial casting, traction, external fixators, and a variety of implanted posterior devices such as pedicle screws and rods. Advocates of reduction of severe slips cite documented instances of further progression of the severe slips after apparently solid fusion as one rationale for reduction and instrumentation. Reduction draws the transverse processes of L-4 and L-5 closer to the sacral ala, presumably making fusion more satisfactory and stability more likely. Another rationale cited for reduction is improvement in the cosmetic appearance of the trunk, but this is difficult to document objectively. In some series of in situ fusions, a common complaint was a residual distorted appearance of the trunk. However, many authors stress that most cosmetic disfigurement in severe spondylolisthesis is related to hamstring tightness and other muscle spasms that can be expected to improve greatly after fusion alone, without reduction.

Most series of reductions report new L-5 root deficits, some of which are permanent. One series reported three L-5 deficits in ten patients undergoing reduction of severe slips. New nerve root injury is rare when in situ fusion alone is undertaken, although others reported acute cauda equina syndrome after in situ fusion for severe dysplastic spondylolisthesis.

The indications for reduction of severe slips remain poorly defined, and await larger future series to define better the risks and potential gains involved. At the moment, for children and adolescents, in situ fusion and cast immobilization without instrumentation remain the customary treatment for severe slips.

Annotated Bibliography

Keywords

Congenital anomalies; Electrical stimulation; Epiphysiodesis; Kyphosis; Scheuermann's disease; Scoliosis; Spinal instrumentation; Spondylolisthesis; Spondylolysis; Thoracolumbar spine

Congenital Deformity of the Spine

Andrew T, Piggott H: Growth arrest for progressive scoliosis: Combined anterior and posterior fusion of the convexity. *J Bone Joint Surg* 1985;67B:193–197.
Thirteen cases of convex anterior and posterior fusion resulted in six apparent corrections and three failures.

McMaster MJ, David CV: Hemivertebra as a cause of scoliosis: A study of 104 patients. *J Bone Joint Surg* 1986;68B:588–595.
A longitudinal follow-up study of patients with hemivertebra alone indicated that incarcerated and semisegmented hemivertebrae usually do not require treatment. Fully segmented, nonincarcerated hemivertebrae may require treatment.

Winter R, Lonstein J, Denis F, et al: Convex growth arrest for progressive congenital scoliosis due to hemivertebrae. *J Pediatr Orthop* 1988;8:633.
A detailed description of the surgical technique is included in this article. Five patients showed correction as a result of the epiphysiodesis (average, 10 degrees) and only one curve progressed further. The absence of excessive kyphosis or lordosis, a short curve, and an age of less than 5 years were associated with postoperative correction.

Winter RB, Moe JH, Lonstein JE: The surgical treatment of congenital kyphosis: A review of 94 patients age 5 years or older, with 2 years or more follow-up in 77 patients. *Spine* 1985;10:224–231.
In this series of patients treated after the age of 5 years, the efficacy of early treatment is underlined. Traction is again noted to be dangerous in congenital kyphotic deformities.

Idiopathic Scoliosis

Etiology

Barack R, Wyatt M, Whitecloud T, et al: Vibratory hypersensitivity in idiopathic scoliosis. *J Pediatr Orthop* 1988;8:389.
Vibratory hypersensitivity was found to be significantly greater in children with scoliosis than in children without scoliosis. This strongly supports primary involvement of the central nervous system in the etiology of idiopathic scoliosis.

Deacon P, Archer IA, Dickson RA: The anatomy of spinal deformity: A biomechanical analysis. *Orthopedics* 1987;10:897–903.
The authors advance a biomechanical hypothesis for the progressive rotatory lordoscoliosis noted with idiopathic scoliosis.

Deacon P, Dickson RA: Vertebral shape in the median sagittal plane in idiopathic thoracic scoliosis: A study of true lateral radiographs in 150 patients. *Orthopedics* 1987;10:893–895.
The presence of true lordosis at the apex of all thoracic idiopathic scoliotic curves was noted in this analysis.

Lidstrom J, Friberg S, Lindstrom S, et al: Postural control in siblings to scoliosis patients and scoliosis patients. *Spine* 1988;13:1070.

This paper shows increased postural sway in both scoliosis patients and their siblings compared with controls, suggesting involvement of the central nervous system in the etiology of idiopathic scoliosis. The abnormality manifested in abnormal postural sway may be hereditary in origin.

Ohlen G, Aaro S, Bylund P: The sagittal configuration and mobility of the spine in idiopathic scoliosis. *Spine* 1988;13:413.
The authors call attention to the alteration in normal sagittal-plane configuration in patients with idiopathic scoliosis. Loss of the normal thoracic kyphosis and lumbar lordosis are clearly demonstrated in idiopathic scoliosis.

Pin LH, Mo LY, Lin L, et al: Early diagnosis of scoliosis based on school-screening. *J Bone Joint Surg* 1985;67A:1202–1205.
Examination of a group of 8,000 schoolchildren showed an incidence of scoliosis of 6.5% for 5 degrees and 2.4% for 10 degrees. This study confirmed the prevalence of mild scoliosis noted in other studies of childhood populations.

Sabato S, Rotman A, Robin GC, et al: Platelet aggregation abnormalities in idiopathic scoliosis. *J Pediatr Orthop* 1985;5:558–563.
The authors found statistically significant alterations in platelet aggregation in a group of scoliosis patients compared with controls. This observation has been both confirmed and denied in other studies. Its significance is unclear.

Natural History

Ascani E, Bartolozzi P, Logroscino CA, et al: Natural history of untreated idiopathic scoliosis after skeletal maturity. *Spine* 1986;11:784–789.
This series of patients included those with milder curves and showed that all curves progress after maturity is achieved. Thoracic curves were the most progressive, and double major curves the least progressive in this series. The incidence of back pain appeared to be similar to that in the general population. Pregnancy appeared to be associated with an increase in progression. Twenty percent of patients, particularly females with thoracic curves, had psychological disturbances. Overall disability, however, was minimal in this group of patients. Mortality was approximately double that in the general population.

Betz RR, Bunnell WP, Lambrecht-Mulier E, et al: Scoliosis and pregnancy. *J Bone Joint Surg* 1987;69A:90–96.
Although pregnancy has generally been considered to be associated with progression of adult scoliosis, this article argues that although progression may occur during pregnancy, it is not the result of pregnancy *per se*. No increase in back pain with pregnancy and no large difference in outcome of pregnancy were noted.

Bunnell WP: The natural history of idiopathic scoliosis before skeletal maturity. *Spine* 1986;11:773–776.
This is a carefully done review of 326 patients with untreated idiopathic scoliosis. Lack of correlation with family history, thoracic kyphosis and lordosis, and trunk imbalance with progression were noted. Curve severity and growth remaining correlated strongly with progression of the curve, as did, to a lesser extent, curve pattern.

Edgar MA: The natural history of unfused scoliosis. *Orthopedics* 1987;10:931–939.
In this series of 78 untreated patients with idiopathic scoliosis, the greatest progression after maturity occurred in tho-

racic curves and the least in double curves. Curves of more than 90 to 100 degrees tended to stabilize. Back pain appeared to be more common than in the general population.

Perdriolle R, Vidal J: Thoracic idiopathic scoliosis curve evaluation and prognosis. *Spine* 1985;10:785–791.

Although they included information on the progression of infantile and juvenile scoliosis, the authors contend that whether curves will progress in adolescence can be accurately predicted on the basis of the rotation and torsion of the individual vertebrae. It is their contention that the deformity was also present in childhood but to a lesser degree.

Weinstein SL: Idiopathic scoliosis: Natural history. *Spine* 1986;11:780–783.

A group of 54 patients with complete radiographs was selected from a previous series of adults with untreated scoliosis. In this series, lumbar and thoracolumbar curves in excess of 30 degrees showed the greatest progression during adulthood, whereas thoracic and double curves showed less progression.

Nonsurgical Treatment

Bassett GS, Bunnell WP, MacEwen GD: Treatment of idiopathic scoliosis with the Wilmington brace: Results in patients with a twenty to thirty-nine-degree curve. *J Bone Joint Surg* 1986;68A:602–605.

Of patients treated with a thoracolumbar spinal orthosis, only those patients with Risser grades 0 or 1 were selected for inclusion in this study. A 28% progression rate of 5 degrees or more despite bracing was noted. This higher-than-expected failure rate was probably attributable to the relative youth and high risk of the patients involved.

Bylund P, Aaro S, Gottfries B, et al: Is lateral electric surface stimulation an effective treatment for scoliosis? *J Pediatr Orthop* 1987;7:298–300.

In this small series, an extremely high failure rate was noted for large curves averaging 35 degrees. Electrical stimulation was considered a failure in this series of larger curves at high risk.

Carman D, Roach JW, Speck G, et al: Role of exercises in the Milwaukee brace treatment of scoliosis. *J Pediatr Orthop* 1985;5:65–68.

Twelve braced patients who did their prescribed exercises were compared with 12 who did not and the results were similar. This study has been used as an argument against the use of exercises in brace treatment of scoliosis. A larger prospective study is needed to address this question with statistical validity.

Clayson D, Luz-Alterman S, Cataletto MM, et al: Long-term psychological sequelae of surgically versus nonsurgically treated scoliosis. *Spine* 1987;12:983–986.

Similar psychological outcomes were noted in patients treated surgically compared with those treated nonsurgically.

Cochran T, Nachemson A: Long-term anatomic and functional changes in patients with adolescent idiopathic scoliosis treated with the Milwaukee brace. *Spine* 1985; 10:127–133.

The authors reviewed functional behavior in adults after Milwaukee brace treatment.

DiRaimondo CV, Green NE: Brace wear compliance in patients with adolescent idiopathic scoliosis. *J Pediatr Orthop* 1988;8:143.

Patients who had completed treatment were interviewed to determine their compliance with brace wear. Compliance was found to be about two thirds of that required and substantially less than had been reported to the physician.

Emans JB, Kaelin A, Bancel P, et al: The Boston bracing system for idiopathic scoliosis: Follow-up results in 295 patients. *Spine* 1986;11:792–801.

Bracing was approximately 85% successful, even for curves in excess of 30 degrees. Curves with apices in the midzone of the spine fared better than those at the cephalad or caudal ends. Part-time brace wear appeared to be as effective as full-time brace wear. Initial curve correction in the brace appeared to correlate best with final results.

Fisher DA, Rapp GF, Emkes M: Idiopathic scoliosis: Transcutaneous muscle stimulation versus the Milwaukee brace. *Spine* 1987;12:987–991.

Fifty patients treated with transcutaneous electrical stimulation were compared with controls treated with the Milwaukee brace. The mean pretreatment curve was less than 30 degrees. This study was flawed by the inclusion of many small curves and failure to report results for larger, high-risk curves separately.

Gardner A, Burwell R, Wozniak A, et al: Some beneficial effects of bracing and a search for prognostic indicators in idiopathic scoliosis. *Spine* 1986;11:779.

Although the supporting data are missing from this brief paper, a statistical comparison was made between braced and unbraced patients with similar curves. Correction while in the brace appeared to be a good indicator of final results.

Goldberg C, Cowling FE, Fogarty EE, et al: Electrospinal stimulation in children with adolescent and juvenile scoliosis. *Spine* 1987;12:482.

In this series of 41 patients, the failure rate was high, particularly in larger curves at high risk. The authors concluded that electrical stimulation cannot be recommended.

Hanks GA, Zimmer B, Nogy J: TLSO treatment of idiopathic scoliosis: An analysis of the Wilmington jacket. *Spine* 1988;13:626.

Successful bracing was achieved with a thoracolumbar spinal orthosis in 81% of patients. Part-time bracing appeared to be effective in this series.

McCollough NC III: Nonoperative treatment of idiopathic scoliosis using surface electrical stimulation. *Spine* 1986;11:802–804.

This study of a large series of patients with curves ranging from 20 to 40 degrees is still in progress. Although overall results are encouraging, many patients are still in treatment and many began with curves of less than 30 degrees.

Sullivan JA, Davidson R, Renshaw TS, et al: Further evaluation of the Scolitron treatment of idiopathic adolescent scoliosis. *Spine* 1986;11:903–906.

Combined early results from several centers documented an exceptionally high failure rate, particularly in curves of more than 30 degrees. Electrical stimulation is criticized in this article.

Winter RB, Lonstein JE, Drogt J, et al: The effectiveness of bracing in the nonoperative treatment of idiopathic scoliosis. *Spine* 1986;11:790–791.

This brief review attempts to dispel the notion that the outcome of brace treatment does not differ from that of untreated idiopathic scoliosis.

Surgical Treatment

Bergoyn M, Bollini G, Hornung H, et al: Is the Cotrel-Dubousset really universal in the surgical treatment of idiopathic scoliosis? *J Pediatr Orthop* 1988;8:45.

These authors reviewed their experience using several techniques. Cotrel-Dubousset instrumentation was thought to provide better correction in single thoracic and balanced double major curves. The Zielke VDS anterior procedure was still found to be preferable for lumbar and short thoracolumbar curves.

Casey MP, Asher MA, Jacobs RR, et al: The effect of Harrington rod contouring on lumbar lordosis. *Spine* 1987;12:750–753.

The use of Harrington distraction instrumentation in the lower lumbar spine was associated with loss of lumbar lordosis even when the rod was contoured into lordosis.

Denis F: Cotrel-Dubousset instrumentation in the treatment of idiopathic scoliosis. *Orthop Clin North Am* 1988;19:291–311.

This article provides an in-depth description of the application of Cotrel-Dubousset instrumentation to idiopathic scoliosis.

Dove J: Segmental wiring for spine deformity: A morbidity report. *Spine* 1989;14:229–231.

Substantially higher neurologic complication rates were associated with the use of segmental sublaminar wiring. Simple Harrington distraction instrumentation showed a 0.3% incidence of neurologic complications, and that for Harrington distraction with sublaminar wires was 4.6%.

Ecker ML, Betz RR, Trent PS, et al: Computer tomography evaluation of Cotrel-Dubousset instrumentation in idiopathic scoliosis. *Spine* 1988;13:1141–1144.

Computed tomography confirmed the widespread clinical impression that the rotational deformity of idiopathic scoliosis is corrected substantially wih Cotrel-Dubousset instrumentation. In addition, improvement of sagittal-plane deformities associated with idiopathic scoliosis (thoracic hypokyphosis) was documented. Lumbar lordosis was preserved with this technique.

Edgar MA, Mehta MH: Long-term follow-up of fused and unfused idiopathic scoliosis. *J Bone Joint Surg* 1988;70B:712–716.

Follow-up exceeded ten years in this group. Two thirds of unfused spines showed progression after maturity. Severe back pain was more common in unfused than in fused spines. There was a clear association between the distal extent of the fusion into the lumbar spine and the incidence of low back pain.

Fabry G, Van Meklebeek J, Bocky E: Back pain after Harrington instrumentation for idiopathic scoliosis. *Spine* 1989;14:620–624.

Four to 14 years after Harrington distraction instrumentation, 66% of patients had back pain but few had moderate or severe pain. In those with moderate to severe pain, there was a definite negative correlation between the number of free disks and the occurrence of pain. Whenever possible, the lower limit of fusion should end in the upper lumbar spine.

Hayes MA, Tomplins SF, Herndon WA, et al: Clinical and radiological evaluation of lumbosacral motion below fusion levels in idiopathic scoliosis. *Spine* 1988;13:1161–1167.

Increased translational motion and increased low back pain were noted in this series of 48 patients followed up for more than ten years. Both were increased when the more distal extent of the fusion mass was in the lumbar spine. A high incidence of retrolisthesis at the distal end of the fusion was also noted. However, there was no correlation between loss of lumbar lordosis and low back pain.

King HA, Moe JH, Bradford DS, et al: The selection of fusion levels in thoracic idiopathic scoliosis. *J Bone Joint Surg* 1983;65A:1302–1313.

This classic article provides guidelines for the selection of several types of idiopathic curves and provides the most commonly used classification system of idiopathic curves.

Lagrone MO, Bradford DS, Moe JH, et al: Treatment of symptomatic flatback after spinal fusion. *J Bone Joint Surg* 1988;70A:569–580.

Although this article concentrates on the reconstruction of symptomatic flatback after fusion, it also addresses its causes, noting a relationship with Harrington distraction instrumentation placed in the lower lumbar spine or sacrum. Avoidance of distraction instrumentation in the lower lumbar spine is advised.

Luk KD, Lee FB, Leong JC, et al: The effect on the lumbosacral spine of long spinal fusion for idiopathic scoliosis: A minimum 10-year follow-up. *Spine* 1987;12:996–1000.

A small series of patients followed up for more than ten years showed junctional kyphosis at the lower end of the distraction rod and fusion. Minimal low back pain was noted. The remaining unfused segments of the spine were hypermobile.

Luk KDK, Leong JCY, Reyes L, et al: The comparative results of treatment in idiopathic thoracolumbar scoliosis using Harrington, Dwyer and Zielke instrumentation. *Spine* 1989;14:275–280.

Anterior instrumentation, specifically Zielke instrumentation, appeared to produce results superior to those of instrumentation with a Harrington distraction rod alone.

Mason RJ, Betz RR, Orlowski JP, et al: The syndrome of inappropriate antidiuretic hormone secretion and its effect on blood indices following spinal fusion. *Spine* 1989;14:722–726.

The authors call attention to this syndrome that can follow extensive spine fusion. The diagnostic criteria and clinical features associated with this syndrome are reviewed.

Michel CR, Lalain JJ: Late results of Harrington's operation: Long-term evolution of the lumbar spine below the fused segments. *Spine* 1985;10:414–420.

In this very large series, followed up for more than ten years, patients who were treated with standard Harrington instrumentation had a low incidence of postoperative back pain. No correlation between the extent of the fusion into the lumbar spine and postoperative pain was noted.

Patel NJ, Patel BS, Paskin S, et al: Induced moderate hypotensive anesthesia for spinal fusion and Harrington-rod instrumentation. *J Bone Joint Surg* 1985;67A:1384–1387.

The use of moderate hypotensive anesthesia was associated with significantly less blood loss in this comparative series. No complications were attributable to the hypotensive anesthesia.

Richards BS, Birch JG, Herring JA, et al: Frontal plane and sagittal plane balance following Cotrel-Dubousset instrumentation for idiopathic scoliosis. *Spine* 1989;14:738–743.

This short-term review of postoperative results calls attention to postoperative trunk imbalance after Cotrel-Dubousset instrumentation and the occurrence of kyphosis at the junction between the instrumentation and unfused lumbar spine. Although the standard criteria for fusion levels were used, these rules may not be entirely applicable in type II curves when Cotrel-Dubousset instrumentation is used.

Shufflebarger HL, Clark CE: Cotrel-Dubousset instrumentation. *Orthopedics* 1988;11:1435–1440.

A review of the principles underlying Cotrel-Dubousset instrumentation is presented. Examples are given.

Thometz JG, Emans JB: A comparison of spinous process and sublaminar wiring combined with Harrington distraction instrumentation in the management of adolescent idiopathic scoliosis. *J Pediatr Orthop* 1988;8:129–132.

Harrington spinous process wiring (Wisconsin technique) and Harrington sublaminar wiring produced similar corrections in the coronal plane. For thoracic curvatures not requiring correction of thoracic lordosis, segmental spinous process wiring appeared to be a safe and effective alternative to sublaminar wiring.

Thompson GH, Wilber RG, Shaffer JW, et al: Segmental spinal instrumentation in idiopathic scoliosis: A preliminary report. *Spine* 1985;10:623–630.

An extremely high (22%) neurologic complication rate was noted in this series of patients with sublaminar wiring. Although the authors concluded that this incidence decreases with experience and the passage of time, the data can also be interpreted to suggest that sublaminar wiring should be avoided in idiopathic scoliosis.

Weatherley CR, Draycott V, O'Brien JF, et al: The rib deformity in adolescent idiopathic scoliosis: A prospective study to evaluate changes after Harrington distraction and posterior fusion. *J Bone Joint Surg* 1987;69B:179–181–182.

The rib hump associated with curves did not improve appreciably with Harrington distraction instrumentation and posterior fusion. A further increase in the magnitude of the rib hump was noted with the passage of time in most cases despite successful fusion.

Idiopathic Thoracic Hyperkyphosis (Scheuermann's Disease)

Gutkowski W, Renshaw T: Orthotic results in adolescent kyphosis. *Spine* 1988;13:485–489.

Results of orthotic treatment of moderate thoracic hyperkyphosis using a modified Milwaukee brace for the larger deformities were encouraging.

Sachs B, Bradford D, Winter R, et al: Scheuermann kyphosis: Follow-up of Milwaukee-brace treatment. *J Bone Joint Surg* 1987;69A:50–57.

Two thirds of patients treated with a modified Milwaukee brace showed substantial improvement over their original deformity. Control of curves of more than 75 degrees was less satisfactory.

Spondylolysis and Spondylolisthesis

Spondylolysis

Ogilvie JW, Sherman J: Spondylolysis in Scheuermann's disease. *Spine* 1987;12:251–253.

There was a high incidence of spondylolysis in patients with Scheuermann's thoracic hyperkyphosis, presumably secondary to the compensatory increased lumbar lordosis accompanying the thoracic hyperkyphosis.

Pedersen AK, Hagen R: Spondylolysis and spondylolisthesis: Treatment by internal fixation and bone-grafting of the defect. *J Bone Joint Surg* 1988;70A:15–24.

Direct repair of isthmic defects by internal fixation and grafting was generally successful when slippage was nonexistent or minimal. Highly specific indications are reviewed.

Spondylolisthesis

Freeman BL III, Donati NL: Spinal arthrodesis for severe spondylolisthesis in children and adolescents: A long-term follow-up study. *J Bone Joint Surg* 1989;71A:594–598.

A series of 14 patients confirmed the efficacy of in situ fusion for severe slips.

Harris IE, Weinstein SD: Long-term follow-up of patients with grade-III and IV spondylolisthesis: Treatment with and without posterior fusion. *J Bone Joint Surg* 1987;69A:960–969.

Patients with and without fusion were both remarkably symptom-free, although those with fusion showed some advantage. Both groups showed some further slippage.

Maurice HD, Moseley TR: Cauda equina lesions following fusion in situ and decompressive laminectomy for severe spondylolisthesis. *Spine* 1989;14:214.

This report chronicles the occurrence of perioperative cauda equina lesions in severe degrees of slippage. Caution in manipulation and decortication is urged, the presumed mechanism of nerve root injury being mechanical compression of roots during decortication.

Pizzutillo PD, Mirenda W, MacEwen GD: Posterolateral fusion for spondylolisthesis in adolescence. *J Pediatr Orthop* 1986;6:311–316.

Forty patients treated with posterolateral fusion and postoperative casting showed complete resolution of symptoms and neurologic defects. No pseudarthroses occurred. Two of 23 patients showed some further slippage before union occurred.

Saraste H: Long-term clinical and radiological follow-up of spondylolysis and spondylolisthesis. *J Pediatr Orthop* 1987;7:631–638.

In this large series, further slippage of more than 10 mm was noted in 11% of adolescents and 5% of adults. No factors were found to be predictive of further slippage.

Seitsalo S, Osterman K, Poussa M: Scoliosis associated with lumbar spondylolisthesis: A clinical survey of 190 young patients. *Spine* 1988;13:889–904.

The authors reviewed 92 patients with both significant, surgically treated spondylolisthesis and scoliosis. Lumbar curves tended to resolve whereas thoracic and thoracolumbar curves were not affected by spondylolisthesis fusion.

Seitsalo S, Osterman K, Poussa M, et al: Spondylolisthesis in children under 12 years of age: Long-term results in 56 patients treated conservatively or operatively. *J Pediatr Orthop* 1988;8:516–521.

Longitudinal follow-up of 32 preoperative and 24 nonsurgical cases showed a high incidence of further slippage with growth. Long-term results of in situ fusion for severe degrees of slip included five reoperations for nonunion and five persistent, asymptomatic nonunions. Nineteen percent showed further progression of slippage after surgery.

Stanton RP, Meehan P, Lovell WW: Surgical fusion in childhood spondylolisthesis. *J Pediatr Orthop* 1985;5:411–415.

Twenty cases of spondylolisthesis treated by posterolateral fusion and postoperative casting did well with resolution of symptoms, minimal further slip, and 10% pseudarthroses.

Low Back Pain

Blumenthal SL, Roach J, Herring JA: Lumbar Scheuermann's: A clinical series and classification. *Spine* 1987;12:929–932.

The diagnosis of "lumbar Scheuermann's" is reviewed and a classification proposed.

Gibson MJ, Szypryt EP, Buckley JH, et al: Magnetic resonance imaging of adolescent disc herniation. *J Bone Joint Surg* 1987;69B:699–703.

Magnetic resonance imaging abnormalities were seen in 20

adolescents with known disk herniation. Most showed abnormalities in more than one disk. Four of 20 asymptomatic adolescents also showed abnormalities. The significance of asymptomatic magnetic resonance imaging abnormalities is incompletely understood.

Greene TL, Hensinger RN, Hunter LY: Back pain and vertebral changes simulating Scheuermann's disease. *J Pediatr Orthop* 1985;5:1-7.

This series calls attention to the coexistence of Scheuermann-type radiographic changes (Schmorl's nodes, disk-space narrowing, vertebral wedging) in the thoracolumbar and lumbar spine associated with back pain. A relationship with trauma or excessive stress is postulated. Treatment by rest or bracing was successful.

van den Oever M, Merrick MV, Scott JH: Bone scintigraphy in symptomatic spondylolysis. *J Bone Joint Surg* 1987;69B:453-456.

In a series of patients with back pain and suspected spondylolysis, bone scintigraphy proved useful in detecting stress fractures and fresh spondylolysis and helped distinguish these from established spondylolysis.

Neuromuscular Deformities of the Spine

Boachie-Adjei O, Lonstein JE, Winter RB, et al: Management of neuromuscular spinal deformities with Luque segmental instrumentation. *J Bone Joint Surg* 1989;71A:548-562.

This is a comprehensive review of Luque segmental instrumentation used for cerebral palsy and other neuromuscular deformities. A detailed analysis of results showed the typical correction that can be expected with this technique.

Calvert PT, Edgar MA, Webb PJ: Scoliosis in neurofibromatosis: Natural history with and without operation. *J Bone Joint Surg* 1989;71B:2.

The natural history of the dystrophic form of scoliosis and kyphosis associated with neurofibromatosis is reviewed. The need for early surgical stabilization is stressed.

Cambridge W, Drennan JC: Scoliosis associated with Duchenne muscular dystrophy. *J Pediatr Orthop* 1987;7:436-440.

In a large number of patients with Duchenne's muscular dystrophy the progressive curve was related to an asymmetric contracture of the iliotibial band. The indications for fusion in Duchenne's muscular dystrophy are reviewed.

Kerat D, Bassett GS, Bunnell WP, et al: Scoliosis in Rett's syndrome. *J Pediatr Orthop* 1988;8:138-142.

Attention is called in this article to the progressive scoliosis that accompanies Rett's syndrome in most instances. A high percentage of cases progressed to requiring spine fusion.

McCarthy RE, Dunn H, McCullough FL: Luque fixation to the sacral ala using the Dunn-McCarthy method. *Spine* 1989;14:281.

An alternate to the Galveston technique of pelvic fixation is described. This technique appears to be particularly useful when soft bone or kyphosis is encountered.

McCarthy RE, Peek RD, Morrissy RT, et al: Allograft bone in spinal fusion for paralytic scoliosis. *J Bone Joint Surg* 1986;68A:370-375.

In this series, allograft bone provided fusion rates as good as those achieved with autogenous bone graft.

Miller F, Moseley CF, Koreska J, et al: Pulmonary function and scoliosis in Duchenne dystrophy. *J Pediatr Orthop* 1988;8:133-137.

The relationship between declining pulmonary function and advancing scoliosis is reviewed in this series. No difference in the rates of deterioration in fused and unfused spines was noted. The indications for fusion in Duchenne's muscular dystrophy are reviewed.

Sponseller PD, Whiffen JR, Drummond DS: Interspinous process segmental spinal instrumentation for scoliosis in cerebral palsy. *J Pediatr Orthop* 1986;6:559-563.

This article documents the successful use of spinous process segmental instrumentation rather than sublaminar wiring for moderate scoliosis associated with cerebral palsy. This appears to be an alternate technique for instrumentation of moderate curves.

Thometz JG, Simon SR: Progression of scoliosis after skeletal maturity in institutionalized adults who have cerebral palsy. *J Bone Joint Surg* 1988;70A:1290-1296.

Substantial progression of scoliosis associated with cerebral palsy was noted in this large group of patients.

Ward WT, Winder DR, Roach JW: Surgical correction of myelomeningocele scoliosis: A critical appraisal of various spinal instrumentation systems. *J Pediatr Orthop* 1989;9:262-268.

Combined anterior and posterior fusion provided a rate of fusion superior to that with single anterior and posterior fusion alone.

Winter RB, Pinto WC: Pelvic obliquity: Its causes and its treatment. *Spine* 1986;11:225-234.

This is an excellent review of the nomenclature and causative factors associated with pelvic obliquity.

34

Thoracolumbar Spine: Trauma

The primary goals in caring for patients who have sustained injuries to the thoracolumbar spine must include preserving life, protecting neurologic function, minimizing the risk of further spinal column or neurologic injury, and restoring and/or maintaining the stability and alignment of the spine.

Despite early and adequate decompression and the use of increasingly efficient internal immobilizing devices and fusions, neurologic recovery after traumatically induced incomplete spinal cord injury has not been consistent. The predominant major benefits of internal fixation of spinal fractures are decreased hospital stay, early rehabilitation,

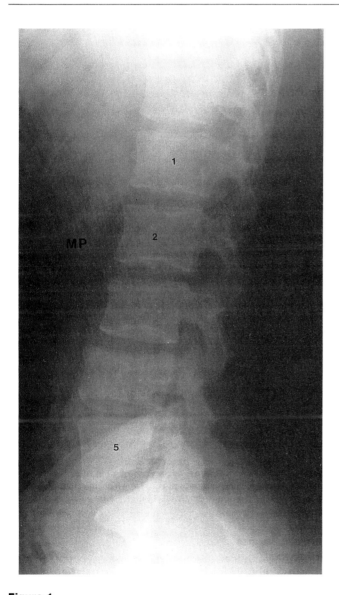
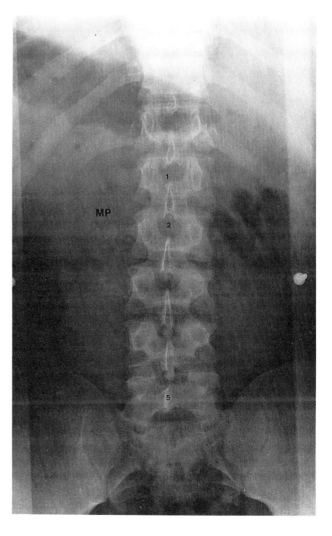

Figure 1

A 28-year-old man with compression fractures at L-3 and L-4. **Left**, Lateral radiograph of lumbosacral spine shows the fractures. L-4 is widened from anterior to posterior and narrowed from superior to inferior. A loss of lumbar lordosis is also apparent. **Right**, Anteroposterior radiograph of lumbosacral spine shows narrowing and lateral wedging of L-3 and L-4.

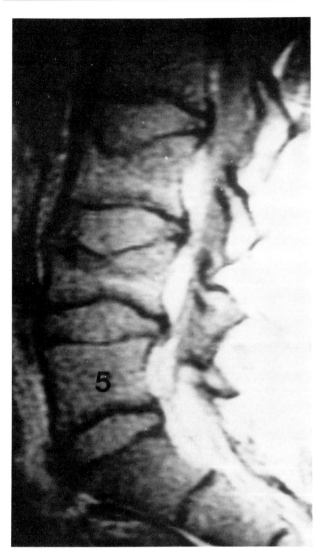

Figure 2
Magnetic resonance imaging of patient shown in Figure 1 reveals "classic" central and anterior compression of L-4.

and prevention of deformity. However, the statistics can be altered by an increasing awareness of (1) the timing of surgery related to the injury, (2) surgical approaches to maximize decompression and stabilization of the spine, (3) the instrumentation systems available and their mechanical constraints, and (4) the pathophysiology of spinal cord injury and its management.

Prehospital Care

Emergency personnel must maintain a high index of suspicion for spinal cord injury in victims of motor-vehicle crashes, falls, and recreational accidents that produce traumatic spine loading. Increased vigilance for spinal stabilization before evaluation for such injuries has in part contributed to a decline in complete spinal cord lesions from 50% to 39%.

Accident-scene investigation and injury-mechanism reconstruction can often aid in determining whether the victim is at risk for spinal column injury. For example, the lap seatbelt has been shown to produce a characteristic thoracolumbar flexion-distraction injury. Adding a shoulder harness helps decrease injuries to the thoracolumbar junction, but increases concern about cervical injuries. Without restraints, as in motorcycle accidents in which the victim is propelled over the handlebars and lands on the helmet or shoulder, thoracolumbar fracture-dislocation is frequent. Additionally, it is important to remember that a significant percentage of patients with spinal cord injury have concomitant head injuries. Until proven otherwise, all unconscious victims of falls or diving or motor-vehicle accidents should be treated as if they had spinal cord injuries.

Hospital Evaluation

The patient should be rigidly immobilized on a spine board or hard bed until spinal stability is definitively assessed. If instability is present, a kinetic rotating bed is useful to protect the spine and to decrease pulmonary and skin complications until surgical stabilization is done. Stryker frames are not as effective in immobilizing an injured spinal column.

History and Physical Examination

The history of the patient's injury and the neurologic and pain symptoms at the time of injury and at the time of hospital evaluation are critical.

In the physical examination, it is important that the back be inspected and palpated. Injuries to the skin over the back may dictate the time course of treatment.

The neurologic assessment should include deep tendon reflexes, tests for pathologic reflexes, and motor and sensory evaluation. The latter should be relatively root- and level-specific. Any sensory sparing is important to document, because this improves the prognosis of the patient. An absent bulbocavernosus reflex in the first 48 hours raises the possibility that the neurologic deficit is related to spinal cord contusion (frequently termed spinal shock) rather than to complete "functional" transection of the spinal cord. However, if the patient has complete paraplegia and the bulbocavernosus reflex is present, then spinal cord function is unlikely to improve.

Ten percent to 15% of patients sustaining spine fractures have associated major visceral disruption. Multiple-level spine injuries occur in 5% to 20% of all individuals with spine fractures. In patients with head and spinal cord injuries, the reported incidence of undetected fractures is 11% and the incidence of peripheral nerve injuries is 11%. Therefore, other injuries (extremity and truncal) must be excluded, particularly if the patient is insensate below a specific level and/or has a head injury, is noncompliant, or obtunded.

Radiographic Examination

Standard anteroposterior and lateral radiographs should be routinely obtained. At this time computed tomography is superior to other techniques in demonstrating bone impingement on the neural canal and for assessing stability.

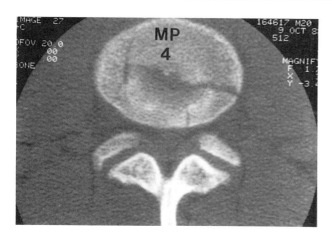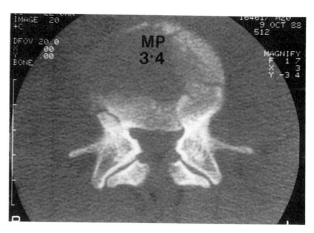

Figure 3

Computed tomography of patient shown in Figures 1 and 2. **Left**, Scan through inferior portion of L-4 shows "burst" nature of the fracture through the body. **Right**, Scan through the superior portion of L-4 shows fractures at the base of the pedicles and retropulsion of the L-4 body. Note that the facets are congruous.

A dural laceration can be anticipated (at surgery) if a patient with spinal cord injury has a burst fracture of the vertebral body combined with laminar fracture at the same level on the computed tomographic scan. Conventional polytomography should be reserved for evaluation of transverse-plane injuries, facet joints, and the like. However, with thin-slice, sagittal and/or coronal computed tomography reconstruction formats, tomograms may not be necessary. Computed tomography enhanced by intrathecal metrizamide is superior to myelography in localizing soft-tissue compromise of the spinal cord. Magnetic resonance imaging is probably the best way to evaluate soft tissues surrounding the spinal cord, the integrity of the disk at the level of injury (particularly as a possible cause of spinal cord injury), the extent of ligamentous disruption, and perhaps integrity of the facet joint capsule. At this point, it is complementary to computed tomographic scans.

Traumatic Injuries

Spinal Cord

Within seconds of injury to the spinal cord, deleterious metabolic and histologic changes occur. The spinal cord's microvasculature can be disrupted by mechanical deformation, edema, thrombosis, or vasoconstriction induced by local and circulating biochemical compounds. Maintenance of perfusion at the cellular level of the spinal cord, if possible, is important to protect remaining viable tissue and allow recovery. Many therapies have been tried to arrest or reverse ischemic insults. Despite encouraging experimental results, clinical efficacy has not been unequivocally demonstrated.

Steroids contribute to cellular membrane stabilization, reduce edema, and counteract sodium and potassium imbalance. Although impressive neurologic recovery has been shown in experimental models, clinical efficacy has not been adequately demonstrated. No change in neurologic status has been documented with steroids in complete lesions. Incomplete lesions, however, and particularly central cord syndromes, may benefit from their use. As a result, some recommend immediate steroid initiation as soon as spinal cord injury is detected. If a complete injury or any syndrome other than a central cord syndrome is apparent, medication should be discontinued. In general, however, routine use is not recommended, because the neurologic benefits are uncertain and the risks (gastrointestinal bleeding, osteonecrosis, and the like) are significant.

Endogenous opiates (endorphins) are released at the sites of spinal cord injury and may play a role in ischemia by decreasing spinal-cord blood flow. Naloxone, an opiate-receptor blocker, can reverse the circulatory effects of endorphins after spinal cord injury in some animal models. However, no statistically significant return of neurologic function has been observed in clinical studies. Thyrotropin-releasing hormone is an indirect opiate antagonist that improves cardiovascular function and spinal-cord blood flow. It does not reverse the analgesic effect of endorphins. Beneficial effects have been demonstrated in experimentally induced models of spinal cord injury. However, clinical efficacy has yet to be proven.

Other adjunctive investigational treatments that have not been substantiated clinically include hyperbaric oxygen, oxygenated fluorocarbons, and hypercarbia.

Central nervous system regeneration and recovery can occur in lower vertebrates, but has not been seen in birds, reptiles, or mammals. However, regeneration of axonal components has been demonstrated in mammals, principally by axonal sprouting from intact structures proximal to a lesion. Experimental manipulation of this process has been studied with electrical currents, endogenous compounds (including nerve growth factor), drugs, and hormones. Nerve grafting and transplantation have also been advocated as possible ways to restore function. These experimental techniques are not clinically useful at this time.

Thoracic Spine

The rib cage contributes to the biomechanics of the thoracic region. Coupled with the relatively sagittal orientation of the thoracic facets, the rib cage protects the thoracic spine against injury. Thus, significant force is required to fracture the thoracic spine, and rotational, ligamentous dis-

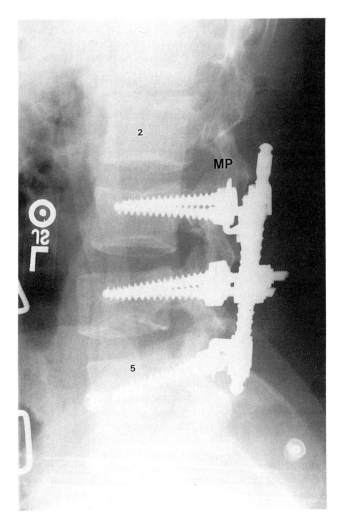
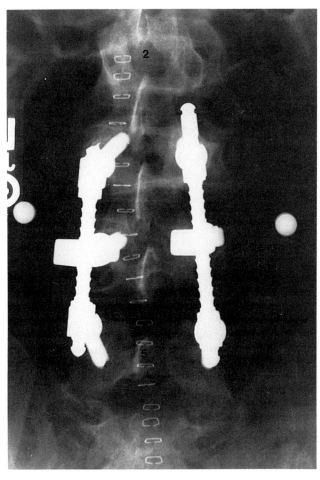

Figure 4

The patient shown in Figures 1 to 3 underwent surgical stabilization with the Edwards modular system. There are pedicle screws at L-2, L-3, and L-4. **Left**, Lateral radiograph. **Right**, Anteroposterior radiograph.

ruptions are rare. This is fortunate, because the canal in the thoracic region is relatively small in relation to the size of the spinal cord. However, ligament deformation within the elastic range may permit enough displacement to have a detrimental impact on the cord.

Anterior-wedge, lateral-wedge, and compression fractures of less than 30% are usually stable unless the posterior interspinous ligaments are torn. Compression fractures and fractures with wedging of more than 50% are often associated with posterior-element disruption and should be considered unstable. Dislocations and fracture-dislocations should also generally be considered unstable. Structural damage in the thoracic spine tends to be associated with neurologic deficits.

Lumbar Spine

The clinical instability of lumbar fractures presents unique problems to the physician. Only 3% of patients with lumbar spine fractures and/or fracture-dislocations have neurologic deficits. Neurologic injuries at this level tend to be less debilitating than those at higher levels, because roots are involved and not the spinal cord. The lumbar spine, however, must bear such high physiologic loads that subsequent pain and deformity are significant considerations in treating lumbar fractures.

Anterior-column stability in lumbar spine fractures depends largely on the well-developed anterior longitudinal ligament and anulus fibrosus. The posterior longitudinal ligament is less important in this region. The posterior column, particularly the facet joints, plays a critical role in maintaining stability. The interspinous ligaments are less important and are occasionally absent.

The association of a neurologic deficit with a lumbar fracture is a strong clinical indicator of instability. The presence of a neurologic injury within the relatively capacious and mobile lumbar spinal canal indicates that a large displacement must have occurred and significant bony or ligamentous damage taken place. Wedge fractures in the lumbar spine are common. As in other anatomic sites, compression of 40% or more usually implies instability. Furthermore, late complications of unstable lumbar compression fracture may include progressive deformity, pain, and perhaps neurologic compromise as a result of

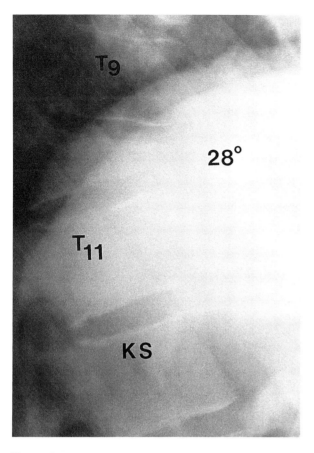
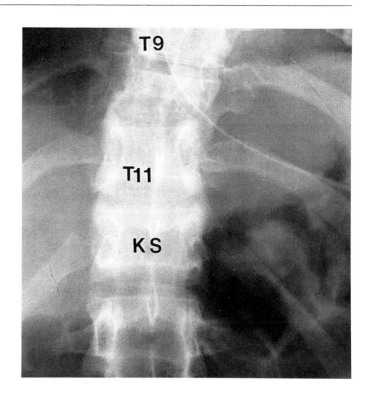

Figure 5

A 19-year-old man sustained a flexion injury to T-10 in a motor-vehicle accident. **Left**, Lateral radiograph shows marked anterior wedging and acute kyphosis at T-10. **Right**, Anteroposterior radiograph shows severe narrowing of T-10 and slight lateral subluxation of T-9 and T-10 on T-11.

the effects of gravity and weight on the spine above the kyphotic element. As the amount of compression increases, the bending moment at the body increases, and progressive deformity ensues as the tensile forces on the posterior interspinous ligaments exceed their capacities.

Mechanisms of Injury

Axial Compression Because of thoracic kyphosis, axial load in the thoracic spine generally results in an anterior flexion load to the vertebral body. Axial load in the more erect thoracolumbar region, however, results in more uniform compression to the vertebral body (Figs. 1 to 4). This may result in end-plate failure, followed by vertebral-body compression (wedge fracture). With additional force, a vertical fracture through the vertebral body occurs, producing a "burst" fracture. With even greater loading, there is centripetal displacement of bone and disk fragments. This results in the radiographic finding of interpedicular widening and a fracture of the lamina. The stability of these lesions is related to the amount of middle- and posterior-column disruption. Computed tomographic scans frequently demonstrate significant retropulsion of bone into the neural canal. This finding indicates instability in cases that might be considered to be stable on the basis of routine radiography.

Lateral Compression This loading produces injuries similar

to anterior-wedge compression injuries except that the deformities are asymmetric (Fig. 1, *right*). This pattern involves compression on one side and ligamentous tensile failure on the contralateral side. Lesions limited to bone are usually stable injuries. Combined (bone and ligament) lesions may be chronically unstable, leading to progressive pain and deformity.

Flexion These forces cause compression anteriorly at the vertebral bodies and disks, with tensile forces developed posteriorly (Figs. 5 and 6). The ligaments usually do not fail immediately (particularly with rapid loading rates), but posterior avulsion fractures can develop. As the bone fractures and more angulation develops, force is dissipated. With intact posterior ligaments (or an avulsion fracture), a stable fracture pattern most often results. However, facet capsule disruption may occur, leading to instability.

Flexion-Rotation These forces are similar to those in pure flexion, but the ligaments and facet capsules tend to fail as rotation increases, disrupting both anterior and posterior columns (shear injuries). These forces lead to fracture-dislocations (Figs. 7 to 9). Pure dislocations in the thoracic or lumbar spine are rare because of the size and orientation of the posterior facets, requiring a high degree of flexion for dislocations to occur. Thus, fracture-dislocations imply

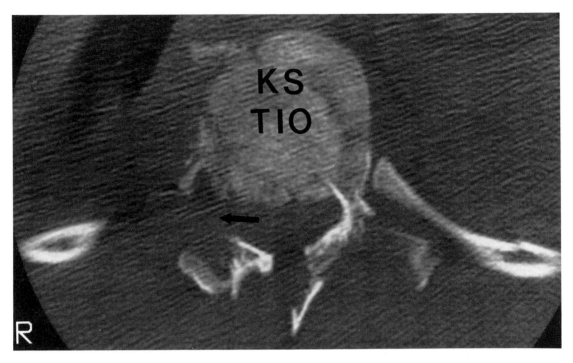

Figure 6

Computed tomographic scan of patient shown in Figure 5 demonstrates fracture of the body and posterior elements and slight canal impingement by retropulsed bone.

destruction of all three columns and a grossly unstable spine.

Distraction In this injury pattern, the fulcrum in flexion is moved anteriorly (usually to the abdominal wall), and the entire vertebral column is subjected to large tensile forces. The vertebrae and disks are torn or avulsed rather than crushed as occurs in most spinal fractures (Figs. 10 to 12). These are potentially very unstable injuries, especially if the anterior longitudinal ligament also fails. The radiographic appearance of this lesion was first described by Chance in 1948. These are often called "seatbelt" injuries, or Chance fractures if bone is involved. This injury can produce a pure osseous lesion, a mixed osteoligamentous lesion, or a pure ligamentous injury; typically all three columns are involved.

Extension When the head or upper trunk is thrust posteriorly, the forces developed are the reverse of those in pure flexion injuries. Tension is applied anteriorly to the strong anterior longitudinal ligaments and anterior portion of the anulus fibrosus and compression forces are transmitted to the posterior elements. This can result in laminar, spinous process, and perhaps pedicular fractures (Figs. 13 and 14). Avulsion fractures of the anterior portions of the vertebral bodies can occur. Normal lumbar lordosis can convert pure axial loads into an extension loading mechanism. This injury pattern, however, is uncommon, and is generally stable. When it is associated with posterior translation, however, the lesion can be presumed to be unstable.

These biomechanical mechanisms do not often occur as individual events in real life. Because forces are combined,

careful assessment is needed to determine which columns are involved, whether bone and/or ligaments have failed, and what remaining structures are intact and can be used in maintaining or obtaining a reduction. Only after making such an assessment can the physician intelligently plan surgical stabilization.

Treatment Methods

The treatment options for trauma to the spinal column are many and somewhat controversial. Initial experience with internal fixation (wiring of spinous processes, Meurig-William plates, and the like) proved less than ideal and led many physicians to advocate a nonsurgical approach. Today, however, improved surgical fixation systems and techniques, combined with increased knowledge of the biomechanics of injury and the need for better reduction of fractures, have made surgical intervention to stabilize, reduce, and fuse the traumatized spine widely accepted.

Postural reduction and recumbent treatment still has advocates and remains a treatment option. Good functional results do not necessarily depend on anatomic restoration. Although the incidences of neurologic recovery were similar in conservatively treated and surgically treated groups, the latter had significantly decreased residual spine pain and deformity, shortened hospitalization, and earlier rehabilitation.

During the mid-1970s a number of investigators reported excellent results for thoracolumbar fracture treatment with Harrington instrumentation. Anatomic reduction was obtained in 80% and patients could be mobilized

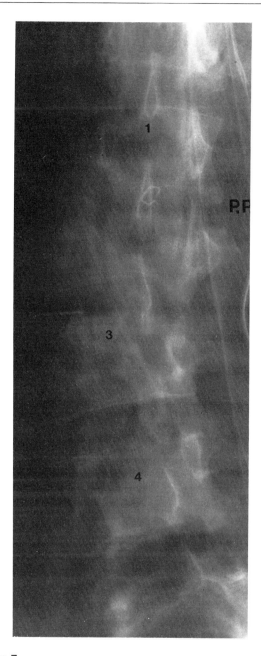

Figure 7
A 21-year-old patient sustained an L-2 on L-3 fracture-dislocation with incomplete spinal cord injury in a motor-vehicle accident. Anteroposterior radiograph shows the rotational component. This is apparent when one notes that L-1 is in a true anteroposition and L-3 is oblique. Also, note the lateral position of L-1 relative to L-3.

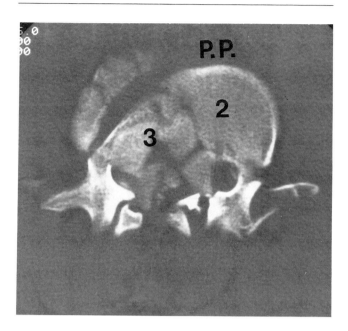

Figure 8
Computed tomographic scan of patient shown in Figure 7 displays L-2 and L-3 on the same cross-sectional cut. The severe disruption of the bone is apparent. The ligamentous disruption must be nearly complete for this degree of multiplane dislocation to occur (L-3 lies posterior and lateral to L-2).

Controversies

Spinal Stability

The overall concept of spinal stability after trauma is still evolving. Injury patterns and fracture types once seemed clear and easy to classify on the basis of radiographs. Later, a classification system based on a two-column construct—an anterior weightbearing column of vertebral bodies and a posterior column of neural arches resisting tension—was proposed. The prediction of late instability can be incorporated into this scheme with treatment directed towards prevention of predicted development of deformity, neurologic deficit, and/or pain.

More recently, computed tomography has led to the definition of a three-column system—with a middle osteoligamentous-neural element—consisting of the posterior longitudinal ligament, the posterior portion of the vertebral body, and the posterior anulus fibrosus, along with the spinal cord or cauda equina. Some believe that the integrity of the "middle" column is the key anatomic determinant of stability and should also be used to determine the surgical method used for fixation; however, this belief is not universally accepted.

Less rigid, nonmechanistic classifications of spinal instability are also useful. Neurologic deficits, as well as anticipated loading, must be individually assessed to determine spinal stability.

If significant deformity and/or significant translation or angulation is noted, and a neurologic deficit is or was present, early (acute) instability exists. In this case, the spine must be protected from further damage by some form of relatively rigid immobilization. If, however, the injury can be classified as "stable" and involves primarily bone with

with external support at two weeks (compared with 12 weeks with plating and 11 to 12 weeks with recumbency). The incidence of residual low back pain was low. Neurologic recovery, however, was not significantly different from that reported with recumbent treatment.

Posterior instrumentation remains the mainstay of treatment when instability is present. The burgeoning number of systems and innovative approaches, however, has led to some controversies.

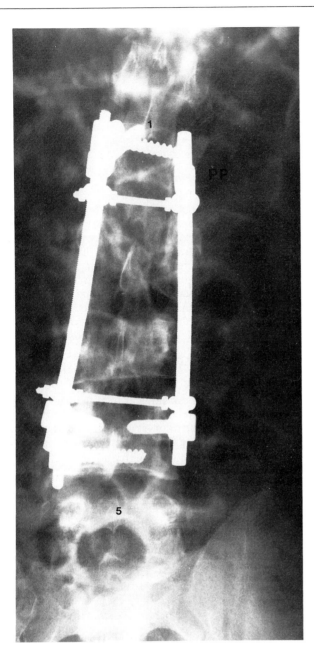
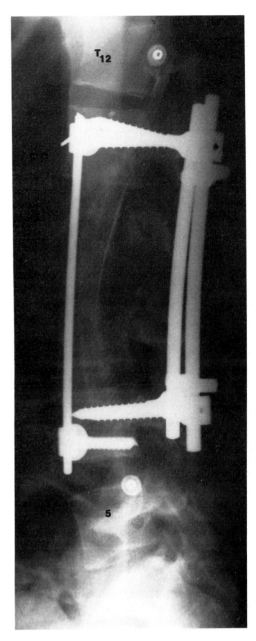

Figure 9

Postoperative radiographs of patient shown in Figures 7 and 8. The patient was treated "nonconventionally" in an attempt to correct and stabilize this severe injury. **Left,** Anteroposterior view shows a Kostuik-Harrington rod-screw anteriorly and Cotrel-Dubousset instrumentation with screws posteriorly. **Right,** Lateral view of single-rod Kostuik-Harrington device, allograft strut from L-1 to L-4, and Cotrel-Dubousset instrumentation posteriorly. The usual Kostuik-Harrington construct involves two sets of hook-screws and rods. Because of the severe rotational component, two screws in each body were not placed. Although claw hooks could have been used posteriorly with the Cotrel-Dubousset instrumentation, screws were used to avoid further injury to the cauda equina.

mild vertebral-body compression and isolated laminar or facet fractures, less rigid immobilization can be employed. Weightbearing, gravity, or other normal physiologic forces should not alter the configuration of these fractures.

The risk of chronic (late) instability should be considered in the evaluation of the acute injury. This includes "stable" compression fractures if compression is greater than 40% or if spinous process gaping or facet widening is noted.

If instability is present or the potential for late instability is significant, surgical stabilization and fusion are usually recommended. However, deformity does not always imply pain, and anatomic reduction does not always correlate with return of neurologic function. Opinions differ about the exact definition of stability (early or late) and the importance of stabilization and reduction with respect to eventual function.

Timing of Surgery

In the presence of a cauda equina syndrome or progressive neurologic deficit, emergency decompression is indicated.

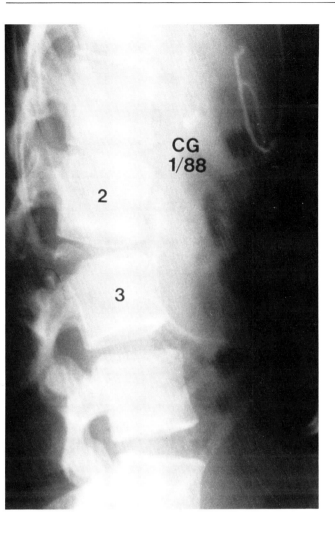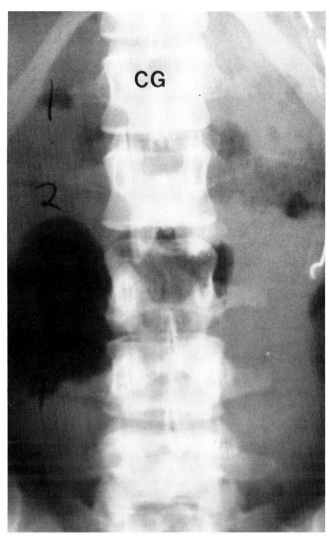

Figure 10

A 17-year-old girl sustained a flexion-distraction injury in a motor-vehicle accident. She was wearing a seatbelt but not a shoulder harness. **Left**, Lateral radiograph shows disruption through the L2-3 disk space, separation through the superior aspect of the L-3 body posteriorly and pedicles, and wide gaping between the posterior elements of L-2 and L-3. **Right**, Anteroposterior view shows marked widening between the laminae of L-2 and L-3.

In other patients with spinal cord injuries, the timing of surgery is controversial, with some recommending treatment as soon as the patient is stable and others advocating a delay of four or more days to allow posttraumatic swelling to resolve. There is no clear evidence that the results of decompression of neural structures are enhanced by early reduction, nor that they are significantly compromised by a one-week delay. In fact, significant functional recovery has been observed after anterior decompressions done more than one year after the spinal cord injury. A reasonable approach is to treat nonprogressive neurologic deficits on a semiemergency basis, with the patient taken to the operating room when medical and surgical conditions are optimal.

Decompression

There are three major ways to "decompress" the thoracic and lumbar spine. The indirect method is from the pos-

terior aspect, usually employing distraction instrumentation and three- or four-point fixation to realign the spine. These reductions usually are performed with hooks and contoured rods (Harrington, Cotrel-Dubousset) or hooks, rods, and sleeves (Edwards) to create distraction and provide an anterior vector force across the fracture. To reduce retropulsed bone from the canal requires a relatively intact posterior longitudinal ligament that will, when stretched, pull the bone out of the canal, anteriorly towards the body. The hook-rod or hook-rod-sleeve methods are familiar to most surgeons, and when properly used provide excellent anatomic realignment and are fairly effective in "decompressing" the spinal canal. These techniques are probably the methods of choice when there is a kyphotic deformity or posterior elements are disrupted, particularly if the posterior cortex of the body is intact. This technique is less reliable in reducing bone from the canal if there are several comminuted pieces of bone retropulsed against the cord

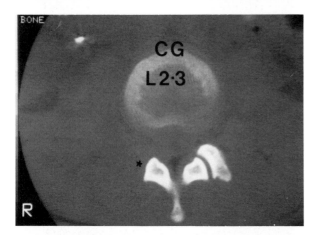

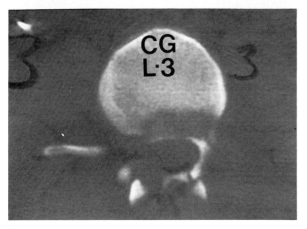

Figure 11

Computed tomographic scans of patient shown in Figure 10. **Top**, Sagittal reconstruction shows widening posteriorly. **Center**, Cut at L2-3 disk space. Asterisk, Place at which L-3 facet on right should articulate with L-2 facet (L-3 is distracted out of view). **Bottom**, Cut through L-3 shows disruption at base of pedicle and posterior cortex.

or cauda equina. However, with time there is remodeling; bone that is left within the canal resorbs, at least in part, if anatomic alignment is achieved. Although the immediate anatomic decompression may not be as good as the ultimate appearance after resorption, there is a dramatic improvement in neurologic function providing that at least two thirds to three quarters of the canal is free of bone.

A problem with posterior decompression, independent of the technique used, is the intraoperative assessment of the adequacy of decompression. A more generous laminectomy to enhance direct visualization may increase the instability, and intraoperative myelography lacks resolution. Intraoperative ultrasonography is one promising solution to this problem.

Three weeks or more after injury, spinal disruptions and deformities become difficult to reduce adequately by posterior instrumentation alone. To realign a burst fracture or compression injury that is more than three weeks old requires anterior decompression and fusion, supplemented by posterior instrumentation (usually compression rodding).

Other techniques for decompression involve more direct reduction of the bony fragments. A posterolateral decompression is performed through the same midline incision and is aided by initial reduction with hooks-rods or hooks-rods-sleeves. To accomplish the decompression, a laminectomy is performed and the pedicle slightly burred down. This allows a posterolateral evaluation of the retropulsed bone, anterior to the dural elements. With angled instruments, the bone can be tamped or curetted out of the canal back into the vertebral body. This procedure has been shown to be relatively safe and effective in the thoracolumbar junction and lumbar spine, but the risks increase in the thoracic spine, where there is less room available.

The other method of direct decompression is the anterior approach. This technique allows excellent decompression and strut fusion but has the most potential morbidity. If there is significant kyphotic deformity, the degree of correction of the alignment of the vertebral column may be less than with posterior techniques. After an anterior procedure, posterior compression instrumentation and fusion may be useful to increase the stability of the anterior graft, increase the probability of successful fusion, and help correct residual deformities. In most cases, anterior instrumentation is not used. Iliac crest or fibular grafts are locked into place by the compression forces supplied by the spine and supplemented by posterior instrumentation. Although anterior internal-fixation systems are available, their applications are limited. The Dwyer and Zielke instrumentation systems have been well studied, but were not designed to stabilize fractures. Although good for deformity surgery, rigid distraction for fracture treatment is not provided. Additionally, the screw-bone interface can be the site of weakening and loss of fixation, particularly in osteoporotic spines. The Kostuik-Harrington system allows significant corrections, provides more rigid internal fixation, and is useful in the treatment of acute injuries. However, experience with this device is limited to only a few centers.

The currently favored approach, therefore, is an anterior decompression and strut fusion (done as the first part of a two-stage procedure) with posterior compression rodding and fusion. If the spine surgeon is not familiar with the approach, including repair of vascular injuries, two or three surgical teams may be required, which can complicate scheduling and planning, particularly in an emergency situation. The decompression of the neurologic structures, however, is the most complete because the anterior approach is the most direct way to attack retropulsed bone against the spinal cord or cauda equina.

Laminectomy alone should not be used and is usually ineffective. Laminectomy does not relieve anterior compression, and frequently leads to increased late deformity, pain, and neurologic deficit.

Although anterior surgery is theoretically the optimum treatment, in most cases posterior instrumentation is adequate. If posterior instrumentation is combined with posterolateral decompression when more than 50% of the

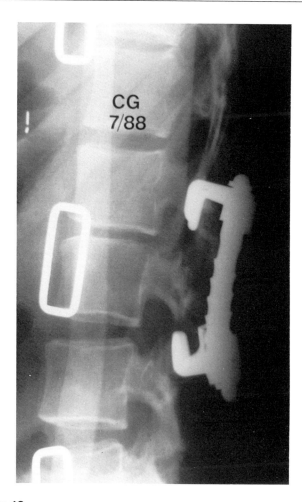 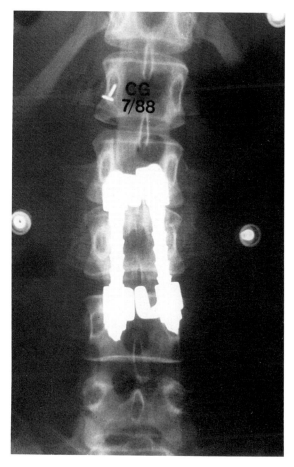

Figure 12

Postoperative radiographs of patient shown in Figures 10 and 11. **Left**, Lateral view shows Edwards compression instrumentation in place. Hooks are at L-2 and L-3 in a compression mode to reduce the posterior ligamentous injury. **Right**, Anteroposterior view. The L2-3 interlaminar space is reduced.

canal is compromised, anterior decompression is unlikely to be necessary. After posterior and/or posterolateral decompression, if a computed tomographic scan shows significant bone within the canal and the patient's neurologic symptoms warrant, an anterior decompression and fusion should be performed at a later date.

Posterior Instrumentation

Instrumentation Level There have been a great many recommendations concerning levels of instrumentation for Harrington rods and fusion. Decisions can be difficult because of the viscoelastic property of the spinal column and the rigidity of the rod, which create some problems in maintaining a reduction and may be related to the 10% incidence of hook "cut-out." Early recommendations were to instrument and fuse two levels above and two levels below the injury. Later, instrumentation for three levels above and three levels below the injury was recommended, along with a "short" fusion. The advantage of moving the upper hooks farther from the fracture is that the moment arm at the fracture site is increased and the reduction improved. This significantly reduces tilting of the upper ver-

tebra, and changes the mechanism of hook failure from slipout to one of complete laminar fracture. The biomechanical advantages of "rodding long and fusing short" are offset by accelerated degenerative changes occurring at the unfused but instrumented levels. Arthritic changes have been observed in the facet joints of instrumented but not fused levels in both canine models and in humans.

Harrington Instrumentation The Harrington rod was initially introduced for scoliosis. Application of the original straight rod to fractures was limited by poor lumbar reduction and rotational control. The square-ended rod-hook modification allows contouring as well as two-plane stability. Thus, distraction rodding using the three-point bending principle can be extended throughout the thoracolumbar spine. Distraction rods can be used successfully to stabilize and reduce flexion-rotation injuries, burst fractures, and compression fractures considered unstable because of posterior-column disruption. The rods require three- or four-point fixation to reduce the vertebral body anteriorly and to close the disruption posteriorly. Supplemental bone fusion, with either autograft or allograft material, is usually done.

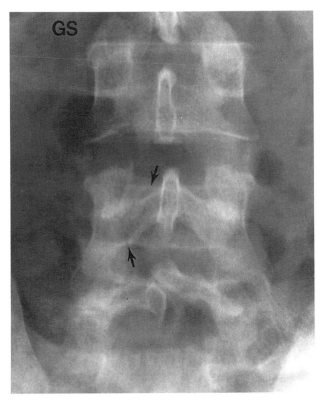

Figure 13

A 38-year-old man fell from a height, landing on his feet. Anteroposterior view. Arrows denote fractures through the lamina of L-4. Incidental spina bifida occulta can be seen at L-5.

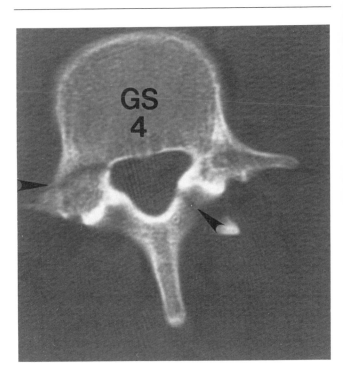

Figure 14

Computed tomographic scan of patient shown in Figure 13 reveals laminar and pedicular fractures at L-4 (arrowheads).

If healing does not occur, the internal-fixation device will eventually fail. If hook failure and dislodgement are to be avoided, external immobilization is essential. This can generally be provided by a rigid custom-molded thoraco-lumbar spinal orthosis or plaster body jacket. Harrington distraction systems tend to fail by dislodgement at the rod-hook site, hook-lamina separation, or fracture at the ratchet-smooth rod junction. Recommendations for preventing this include hook placement solidly under the lamina (both cortices), 2 cm of rod extension beyond the proximal hook, and minimizing the extent of the racheted rod between the hooks.

Compression rods, superior in resisting flexion and perhaps rotational forces, tend to fail by fracturing the laminae to which the hooks are attached. The site of bone-metal fixation is critical. Biomechanical studies have demonstrated that the lamina is stronger than the transverse processes and spinous processes. Additionally, the strength of the transverse process diminishes with progression toward its tip. Accurate hook-metal placement and choice of location are crucial factors in determining the success or failure of whatever system is employed.

The Harrington compression system (particularly the larger of the two compression rods) also plays a role in stabilizing flexion distraction injuries. Compression rods reduce the fracture and provide rigid stabilization while the fusion becomes solid. Compression rods fixed to hooks around the lamina provide more rigid stabilization and a stronger construct than the distraction system when tested against flexion loading.

Understanding the mechanism of injury and the nature of the particular instability makes possible the selection of the proper Harrington distraction or compression rod. Harrington instrumentation has proven to be successful over a number of years and has been the first choice of most surgeons. Reduction of anterior vertebral-body fractures depends not only on the distraction forces created by the device but on the three-point fixation obtained by contact with the rod and the lamina adjacent to the fractured and displaced vertebra.

Edwards Instrumentation This posterior instrumentation system modifies the three-point force system by using rod sleeves and a more "anatomic" hook design than the Harrington system (Figs. 15 to 17). The rod sleeves come in four sizes with increasing diameters for use in the high thoracic, low thoracic, thoracolumbar, and lumbar areas of the spine. The sleeves provide the central anterior bending force for sagittal-plane reduction. Improved sagittal-plane correction is provided by an inherent, elastic energy-storage capability that permits continuous correction during the period of stress relaxation. The sleeves, additionally, provide increased mediolateral stability because they are securely wedged between the central spinous process and the lateral facet joints. For fractures with intact posterior elements, the sleeve is placed at the superior face of the fractured vertebra. When the posterior elements are disrupted, a bridging technique can be used. The hooks are placed to obtain a mechanical advantage for the rod and sleeve and should be located 3 to 5 cm from the sleeve edges to provide the appropriate lever arm for corrective forces.

For most thoracic, thoracolumbar, and lumbar injuries,

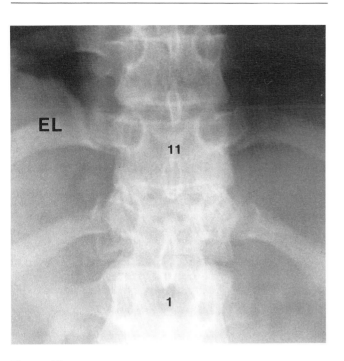

Figure 15
A 40-year-old woman sustained a T-12 burst fracture in a motor-vehicle accident. Anteroposterior radiograph shows narrowing of T-12. There is lateral comminution.

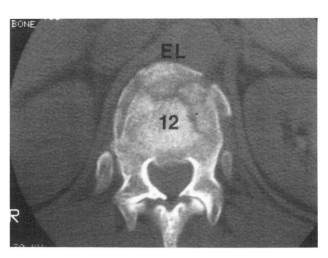

Figure 16
Computed tomographic scan of patient shown in Figure 15 reveals fracture of body and slight bone retropulsion. Note that facet at right is not congruous.

instrumentation techniques with hooks, rods, and sleeves to create three- or four-point fixation are the most commonly used, and are safe and effective. However, attention must be paid to obtaining alignment and attempting to decrease the number of motion segments to be instrumented and fused. With the Edwards system of anatomic hooks and polypropylene sleeves, the number of instrumented segments can be reduced to three or four, particularly in the lumbar spine. This system is relatively easy to use and effective.

Locking Hook System A locking hook system has recently been introduced. This system employs a 7-mm rod threaded at both ends to accommodate a modified Jacobs hook. These hooks allow exact rotational fixation, as well as a sliding cover that locks the upper lamina into the hook.

Segmental Instrumentation The use of segmental spinal instrumentation in the treatment of scoliosis was introduced in the 1970s. This system offers more rotational and translational control than Harrington rods. Segmental wiring provides a direct transverse force at each motion segment, thus decreasing dependency on the anterior longitudinal ligament for the maintenance of correction, as well as decreasing the viscoelasticity associated with hook cut-out by fixation at multiple levels. It does not, however, provide axial load-bearing or distractive forces. Subsequently, C-rods and rectangular rods were developed to resist these axial forces.

Because segmented wiring was successful in scoliosis, it was applied to the treatment of spinal trauma. In fractures, the standard 4.8-mm rods and 16-gauge wire are replaced with stiffer, 6.3-mm rods and 18-gauge wire. Because of

the higher potential for wire breakage, it is recommended that each level be doublewired.

The Luque system provides more rigid fixation than does Harrington instrumentation. Sublaminar wires are employed and fixed to a contoured Luque L-rod. A fusion is then performed posteriorly. Because the L-rod does not provide distraction, anatomic reduction of the fractured vertebral body and spinal column is less predictable. Although the fusion becomes solid posteriorly and the bone heals anteriorly, the deformity has not been corrected and the spinal canal remains compromised and narrowed.

This technique, however, may be the procedure of choice for thoracic or lumbar spinal fractures with complete neurologic injuries. Since no operation has been shown to reverse a complete neurologic deficit, rigid stabilization for rehabilitation becomes the most important objective. The Luque technique fulfills this objective and provides immediate stability. It does not require extensive external immobilization to maintain stability, and, therefore, rehabilitation can begin soon after surgery and medical stabilization, without external encumbrances.

To combine the advantages of the Harrington and Luque systems, a hybrid consisting of segmentally wired Harrington instrumentation was proposed. This technique offers the advantages of increased translational and rotational control, while maintaining an axial distractive force and reducing the problems of stress relaxation and hook cut-out. It increases the axial load-bearing capacity and resists flexion better than Harrington rods. The greatest improvement, however, is in rotational stability. Failure occurs at a site remote from the bone-metal interface. Sublaminar wiring to compression rods should be used cautiously, however, because the wiring may drive the sublaminar hook into the underlying spinal cord.

Biomechanical studies suggested initially that Luque instrumentation was indicated for translational injuries without comminution, fracture-dislocations, flexion-rotation injuries, and slice fractures. These biomechanical advantages, however, must be weighed against the higher morbidity associated with segmental instrumentation. This

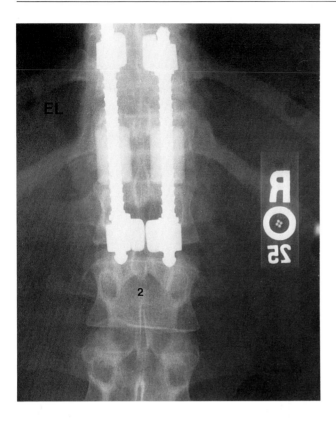

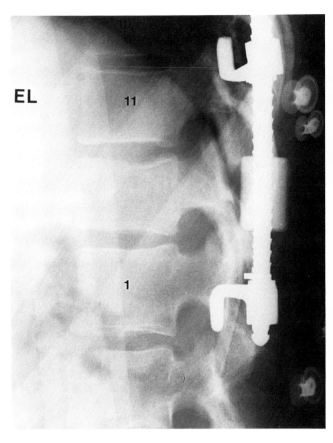

Figure 17

Postoperative radiographs of patient shown in Figures 15 and 16. **Left,** Anteroposterior view of reduction with Edwards distraction instrumentation. "Anatomic" hooks are under the laminae of T-10 and L-2. A polyethylene rod "sleeve" at the T11–12 junction provides anterior force for the reduction. **Right,** Lateral view.

technique requires more technical expertise, increases surgical time and blood loss, and significantly increases the risk of iatrogenic neurological sequela. Additionally, the passage of sublaminar wires is associated with an incidence of neurologic injury of as much as 25% (this includes subclinical changes on evoked potentials) and should be used cautiously in patients with spinal cord injuries. When evaluating the biomechanical benefits vs the neurologic risk of segmental instrumentation, the physician must also consider the patient's preference. Studies have shown that patients care most about the risk of nerve damage, followed by the risk of reoperation. The nature of aftercare (external immobilization) was the lowest priority.

Because of these risks, spinous process wiring has been used. The Wisconsin wiring technique offers the advantages of segmental fixation, without the risk of passing sublaminar wires. However, it is still difficult to maintain distraction and realign the height of a burst fracture.

Cotrel-Dubousset Instrumentation The Cotrel-Dubousset spinal instrumentation system is now being applied to trauma with increasing frequency. This system was developed for use in scoliosis and first applied clinically in 1981. The advantages of this system are that several hooks can be used in both distraction and compression modes, allowing correction of complex deformities while providing the stability of segmental instrumentation. The system is further enhanced by the use of a transverse traction device that converts the system to a fixed rectangular structure. Cotrel-Dubousset instrumentation, which uses the segmental concept with hooks, was thought to have an advantage over sublaminar wires in spinal trauma. It is technically difficult to use and maneuver in an unstable spine, and its indications for spinal trauma are still evolving. It does supply very rigid fixation; it can be used in distraction or compression, which should help realign the spine; and three-point fixation can be obtained by proper contouring of the rod. However, the manipulations necessary to secure multiple hooks to the rod and bend the rod, as well as inserting several sublaminar or pedicle hooks, appear to add a risk to the spinal cord that exceeds that of the more commonly used Harrington or Edwards hooks and rods. A 25% incidence of neurologic injury associated with this device has been reported.

Pedicle-Screw Instrumentation The application of multiple pedicle-screw fixation systems to thoracolumbar trauma is in its infancy. These systems improve sagittal-plane translational correction, as well as secure segmental bony fixation. Because of limitations imposed by pedicle diameter, these systems are best applied to lumbar fractures. Lumbar pedicles decrease in size proximally, and insertion into L-1 and L-2 may be difficult and lead to an increased risk of neurologic complications. The superiority of sacral screw fixation over hooks makes this the method of choice for treatment of low lumbar fractures. However, except for early mobilization, there is no proven advantage over extension casting and in situ fusion for L-4 and L-5 fractures compared with pedicle-screw instrumentation.

Many plate-screw, rod-screw, and internal-fixation systems are being evaluated, but have not yet been approved by the Food and Drug Administration for use in the spine. Pedicle screws can be connected to rods (Edwards, Long Beach), an internal fixator (AO, Vermont, Olerud), or to rigid plates (VSP, Luque, Louis, Roy-Camille). Pedicle-screw systems are particularly useful for fractures involving L-3, L-4, and L-5 in which conventional hooks and rods have a particularly high rate of failure inferiorly. However, the risks of pedicle-screw fixation include neurologic injury

and vascular injury from the screws. Additionally, if the system does not permit significant distraction and three-point contouring, then anatomic alignment may not be achieved and canal decompression may be less than ideal. The pedicle screw-plate systems and the internal fixator are extremely rigid devices; "windshielding" with loosening at the bone-screw interface has been noted, with a slight recurrence of deformity, while the fusion is being established. The major advantage of the internal fixator is that it limits disruption and fusion of the adjacent motion segment. A fundamental unresolved question is the appropriate rigidity for ideal fixation and which type of system supplies it. At this time, however, the indications for pedicle-screw fixation are just developing, except for lower lumbar fractures.

Annotated Bibliography

Keywords

Axial compression; Fracture; Lateral compression; Lumbar spine; Spinal cord; Thoracolumbar spine

Aebi M, Etter CHR, Kehl TH, et al: The internal skeletal fixation system. *Clin Orthop* 1988;227:30–43.
  Review of technique and indications for use of the AO internal fixator. The authors' surgical results are described.

Ashman RB, Birch JG, Bone LB, et al: Mechanical testing of spinal instrumentation. *Clin Orthop* 1988;227:113–125.
  Biomechanical testing of commonly used segmental instrumentation devices is described.

Benson DR: Unstable thoracolumbar fractures, with emphasis on the burst fracture. *Clin Orthop* 1988;280:14–29.
  A good review of the mechanistic approach to describing thoracolumbar fractures. This also describes the author's progression through various systems to arrive at his current treatment plan.

Berry JL, Moran JM, Berg WS, et al: A morphometric study of human lumbar and selected thoracic vertebrae. *Spine* 1987;12:362–367.
  A useful reference for determining the size and location of thoracic and lumbar pedicles in vertebral anatomy.

Bohlman HH: Treatment of fractures and dislocations of the thoracic and lumbar spine. *J Bone Joint Surg* 1985;67A:165–169.
  A review of the author's treatment for thoracic and lumbar spine injuries.

Bohlman HH, Freehafer A, Dejak J: The results of treatment of acute injuries of the upper thoracic spine with paralysis. *J Bone Joint Surg* 1985;67A:360–369.
  These authors have extensive experience with anterior decompression in incomplete injuries. The technique is useful and permits neurologic function to recover after incomplete injuries.

Bradford DS, McBride GG: Surgical management of

thoracolumbar spine fractures with incomplete neurologic deficits. *Clin Orthop* 1987;218:201–216.
  Significant experience with and current recommendations for the treatment of thoracolumbar spine fractures with spinal cord injury.

Cotrel Y, Dubousset J, Guillaumat M: New universal instrumentation in spinal surgery. *Clin Orthop* 1988;227:10–23.
  This article describes the Cotrel-Dubousset instrumentation and its many varied applications.

de la Torre JC: Spinal cord injury: Review of basic and applied research. *Spine* 1981;6:315–335.
  Excellent review article on the treatment of the neurologic component of spinal cord injury.

Eismont FJ, Green BA, Berkowitz BM, et al: The role of intraoperative ultrasonography in the treatment of thoracic and lumbar spine fractures. *Spine* 1984;9:782–787.
  The authors describe their extensive experience with intraoperative ultrasonography, the technique, and its utility.

Garfin SR, Katz MM, Marshall LF: Spinal cord, in Cales RH, Heelig RW Jr (eds): *Trauma Care Systems*. Rockville, Aspen Systems, 1986.
  A review article on the prehospital and hospital care of the patient with spinal cord injury, including an algorithm for treatment of a patient with thoracolumbar injury.

Guyer DW, Yuan HA, Werner FW, et al: Biomechanical comparison of seven internal fixation devices for the lumbosacral junction. *Spine* 1987;12:569–573.
  A biomechanical comparison of a number of internal fixation devices (anterior and posterior) for stabilization of the lumbosacral spine.

Hasday CA, Passoff TL, Perry J: Gait abnormalities arising from iatrogenic loss of lumbar lordosis secondary to Harrington instrumentation in lumbar fractures. *Spine* 1983;8:501–511.
  This article describes difficulties with gait encountered when a straight posterior instrumentation rod is used and lumbar lordosis is therefore lost.

Jacobs RR, Schlaepfer F, Mathys R Jr, et al: A locking

hook spinal rod system for stabilization of fracture-dislocations and correction of deformities of the dorso-lumbar spine: A biomechanic evaluation. *Clin Orthop* 1984;189:168–177.
This article describes the locking-hook posterior instrumentation system for thoracolumbar injuries.

Kahanovitz N, Arnoczky SP, Levine DB, et al: The effects of internal fixation on the articular cartilage of unfused canine facet joint cartilage. *Spine* 1984;9:268–272.
Degenerative changes at facet joints in instrumented but nonfused spinal segments are related to an animal model.

Kaneda K, Abumi K, Fujiya M: Burst fractures with neurologic deficits of the thoracolumbar-lumbar spine: Results of anterior decompression and stabilization with anterior instrumentation. *Spine* 1984;9:788–795.
An anterior-fixation device for stabilization and treatment of burst fractures is described. The device is not yet approved for use in the United States.

Karlstrom G, Olerud S, Sjostrom L: Transpedicular segmental fixation: Description of a new procedure. *Orthopedics* 1988;11:689–700.
This article describes a pedicular internal fixation system for thoracolumbar fractures.

Keene JS, Wackwitz DL, Drummond DS, et al: Compression-distraction instrumentation of unstable thoracolumbar fractures: Anatomic results obtained with each type of injury and method of instrumentation. *Spine* 1986;11:895–902.
This article provides an overview of different techniques for the treatment of thoracolumbar injuries. The Wisconsin technique for segmental fixation is described.

Kostuik JP: Anterior fixation for fractures of the thoracic and lumbar spine with or without neurologic involvement. *Clin Orthop* 1984;189:103–115.
The Kostuik-Harrington device for anterior fixation of fractures is described. This system is available, although experience outside of a single center is limited.

Krag MH, Weaver DL, Beynnon BD, et al: Morphometry of the thoracic and lumbar spine related to transpedicular screw placement for surgical spine fixation. *Spine* 1988;13:27–32.
A significant article in terms of pedicular-screw fixation strength and placement.

Levine A, Edwards CC: Lumbar spine trauma, in Camins M, O'Leary P (eds): *The Lumbar Spine*. New York, Raven Press, 1987, pp 183–212.
The Edwards system and techniques of application are described in this chapter. It also lists the authors' indications and timing for surgery.

Luque ER: Segmental spinal instrumentation of the lumbar spine. *Clin Orthop* 1986;203:126–134.
This article describes the author's extensive experience with segmental spinal instrumentation and the Luque technique of sublaminar wire fixation.

Luque ER: Interpeduncular segmental fixation. *Clin Orthop* 1986;203:54–57.
This article describes a new pedicle screw-plate system devised by the author.

McAfee PC: Biomechanical approach to instrumentation of thoracolumbar spine: A review article. *Adv Orthop Surg* 1985;313–327.
A useful review article for planning the surgical approach and type of instrumentation, based on biomechanical knowledge of the instrumentation system and the injury pattern.

McAfee PC, Bohlman HH: Complications following Harrington instrumentation for fractures of the thoracolumbar spine. *J Bone Joint Surg* 1985;67A:672–686.
This article details the authors' experience with referred cases in which Harrington instrumentation failed.

Rogers LF: The roentgenographic appearance of transverse or Chance fractures of the spine: The seat belt fracture. *Contemp Orthop* 1983;7:7.
A good review of the radiologic features of flexion-distraction injuries.

Rossier AB, Cochran TP: The treatment of spinal fractures with Harrington compression rods and segmental sublaminar wiring: A dangerous combination. *Spine* 1984;9:796–799.
This article lists a significant complication from combining sublaminar wires with Harrington compression rods. The proximal hook can be driven into the spinal cord, leading to a spinal cord injury. This technique is still useful in complete paraplegia in which the loss of one additional thoracic neurologic level might be balanced by the rigidity of the fixation.

Roy-Camille R, Saillant G, Mazel C: Plating of thoracic, thoracolumbar, and lumbar injuries with pedicle screw plates. *Orthop Clin North Am* 1986;17:147–159.
A new pedicle screw-plate fixation device is described. The authors' extensive experience is included. The authors have one of the longest and most complete follow-ups for any existing pedicle-screw system.

Stover SL: Spinal cord injury—Update. *J Am Parapl Soc* 1983;6:66–74.
A useful review regarding treatment of the neurologic components of spinal cord injury.

Wenger DR, Carollo JJ: The mechanics of thoracolumbar fractures stabilized by segmental fixation. *Clin Orthop* 1984;189:89–96.
A biomechanical analysis of sublaminar segmental wiring techniques for the treatment of thoracolumbar injuries.

Willen J, Lindahl S, Irstam L, et al: Unstable thoracolumbar fractures: A study by CT and conventional roentgenology of the reduction effect of Harrington instrumentation. *Spine* 1984;9:214–219.
This study showed a lack of complete reduction of retropulsed bone with posterior instrumentation. However, the clinical results did not necessarily correlate with the radiographic findings.

35

Thoracolumbar Spine: Reconstruction

Reconstructive surgery of the thoracolumbar spine has long been used for the management or prevention of deformity (postsurgical, posttraumatic, and developmental) as well as in the management of neoplasms, infections, and rheumatologic disorders. The standard method of reconstruction (in situ bone grafting and Harrington instrumentation) has proven successful in most circumstances but it does have some limitations. The Harrington system relies primarily on distraction with two points of fixation at either end of the rod to achieve correction of deformities in the frontal plane only. Frontal-plane correction is achieved at the expense of sagittal-plane contour, which is a particular problem in the lower lumbar spine because it produces loss of lordosis.

Major advances in reconstructive spinal surgery took place during the 1980s because the limitations of the older methods were recognized and new knowledge about the biomechanics of the thoracolumbar spine under normal and pathologic conditions was obtained. These efforts resulted in a technologic development of new instrumentation techniques that allow a greater emphasis on the three-dimensional correction of spinal deformities. However, as the ability to correct spinal deformity advances, it is important to remember that some deformities may still best be left alone. Spinal instrumentation and the indications for its use are still evolving, and many issues await clarification.

Diagnosis and Anatomy

Technologic advances in the imaging of the thoracolumbar spine have made possible a much more thorough understanding of the interrelationship of the spinal column and the neural axis and other adjacent soft-tissue structures. Steady improvement in the sensitivity and resolution of both computed tomography and magnetic resonance imaging has made contrast myelography unnecessary in many cases. Three-dimensional reconstruction programs for computed tomography have provided a sense of spatial orientation never before possible without direct dissection. Magnetic resonance imaging is a powerful tool for assessing the extent of vertebral tumor involvement and localizing infection.

These imaging advances have improved not only diagnostic capabilities but also preoperative planning. Undoubtedly, an inability to identify preexisting, adjacent abnormalities in bone or soft tissue contributed to some reconstructive failures in the past.

Deformity

Adult Scoliosis

As those who passed through adolescence before widespread educational and screening efforts and aggressive bracing management for scoliosis were common enter their fifth and sixth decades, symptomatic adult scoliosis has become increasingly common. In addition, it has been accepted that degenerative curves may form *de novo* in the adult; this is thought to be the result of disk degeneration and osteoporosis. In many respects, the surgical management and goals in adult scoliosis surgery differ greatly from those in adolescent scoliosis. In adolescent scoliosis the goal is partial correction of the deformity and prevention of further progression by the achievement of a solid fusion, whereas the goal in adult scoliosis surgery is primarily relief of pain through the achievement of a solid fusion. Correction of the deformity is a secondary issue and often is not even attempted.

Because the major problem in adult scoliosis is pain, the question in an individual case is to determine the exact origin of the pain. The presumption that pain is derived from degenerative facet joint disease is certainly plausible, but other conditions such as spinal stenosis, lumbar disk herniation, and lateral recess stenosis can also play major roles. Further investigation is warranted as part of preoperative planning. Because of the complex angles involved, computed tomographic scanning is not particularly informative unless particular attention is paid to gantry angle. Myelography probably remains the most sensitive diagnostic tool in the complex scoliosis curve and often localizes the source of the symptoms when other diagnostic studies cannot.

Diskography has also been advocated by some. If pain is provoked at a single level within the curve, a limited procedure with significantly less morbidity can be performed, that is, disk excision or single-level foraminotomy for nerve root decompression. More extensive decompression without fusion, particularly when facets are sacrificed, increases the risk of further deformity and should be addressed with a fusion procedure commensurate with the extent of surgical destabilization. Pedicular fixation systems are particularly well suited to this situation because they do not require intact posterior elements for rigid fixation and they spare motion segments above and below the decompression. The drawback to this use of pedicular fixation systems is the decreasing size of the pedicle and, therefore, the increasing risk of screw misplacement as one progresses cephalad through the thoracolumbar spine.

The development of Harrington instrumentation was a major advance in scoliosis surgery, improving fusion rates and significantly increasing the amount of correction. Although this system of instrumentation has been used in adults with scoliosis, the same predictably good results achieved in adolescents were never obtained. Adult scoliosis surgery was plagued by three persistent problems: instrumentation failure, pseudarthrosis, and, in the case of thoracolumbar curves, degenerative changes in the remaining mobile segments below the fusion. Attempts to prevent this last problem by fusion to the sacrum were accompanied by even higher rates of instrumentation failure and pseudarthrosis, in addition to significant flattening of the lumbar lordosis.

The introduction of the concept of segmental spinal instrumentation by Luque was the next major advance in scoliosis surgery and increased the predictability of fusion in adult scoliosis surgery to some extent but was not without occasional failure. The use of sublaminar wires has been associated with an increased incidence of neurologic complications but it certainly increases the mechanical strength of the fixation construct. Anterior fixation systems such as the Dwyer system made possible the correction of thoracolumbar curves with fusion of fewer segments, thus relieving much of the mechanical load on the lower lumbar spine and thereby avoiding the difficult problem of degenerative changes below the fusion. However, the Dwyer system tended to increase kyphosis and, thus, was not an ideal construct when extension into the mid and lower lumbar spine was necessary. The Zielke system, which uses a rigid rod rather than a flexible cable, overcame this problem to some extent. Once again, the increased incidence of pseudarthrosis with these systems remains a problem. The Kostuik modification of the Harrington distraction system for use in anterior thoracolumbar correction of deformity and fusion provides a stronger and more rigid construct and has further decreased the rate of instrumentation failure and pseudarthrosis, particularly in kyphotic deformities.

Combined anterior and posterior procedures further enhance results by decreasing the pseudarthrosis rate and improving correction, but the increased morbidity of two major surgical procedures must be kept in mind. Most recently, pedicular segmental fixation has allowed more rigid internal fixation with greater control over both sagittal and coronal deformities. These techniques are more technically demanding than their predecessors but appear to be very promising.

The Cotrel-Dubousset system offered a different approach to the surgical management of scoliosis by proposing that scoliosis deformities in children could be better corrected by derotation than by distraction alone. This system also uses segmental spinal instrumentation, thus providing a more rigid construct. The heart of this system is a solid rod with a knurled diamond point surface that allows placement of multiple hooks at any location along the rod in combinations of distraction and compression modes. In addition, application of pedicle-screw fixation is possible, adding to the versatility of the construct. Although derotation and correction of curvature may not be possible or even advisable in many adult scoliosis curves, a rigid, segmental fixation system theoretically offers advantages over previous systems (Figs. 1 and 2). Recent reviews of adolescent patients with scoliosis have suggested that this system may induce coronal decompensation, although this problem has not as yet been described in adults.

Postlaminectomy Deformity

Laminectomy has long been used to gain access to and expose the neural canal for a variety of reasons. This results from the relative ease of posterior spinal exposure compared with anterior exposure throughout the entire spine. However, the biomechanical consequences of laminectomy, particularly "wide" laminectomy including facet joint excision, often lead to progressive deformity. Most

often the primary deformity is kyphosis, but, in the severely degenerative adult spine, iatrogenic anterior or lateral horizontal displacement or progressive scoliosis can result from failure to protect the destabilized thoracolumbar spine from the biomechanical forces.

Prevention is the obvious key, and a realization of the biomechanical consequences of decompression and an adequate attempt at reconstruction at the time of laminectomy may save a great deal of effort in the future. Simple in situ posterolateral fusion suffices in many instances, particularly in the elderly patient with osteoporosis. Patients with advanced ankylosis may not require fusion at all. In younger patients, or when more extensive decompression involving facets and/or pedicles has been performed, internal fixation may be indicated. Before the onset of significant kyphosis, posterior instrumentation remains the procedure of choice but choice of instrumentation remains controversial. Although Harrington instrumentation has been the accepted method for reconstruction of the laminectomized thoracolumbar spine, many authorities now believe that distraction does not provide the ideal environment for fusion and may adversely alter the biomechanics of the spine. The Luque system requires an intact lamina for segmental fixation and, therefore, is not applicable after extensive laminectomy. Pedicle-screw systems are ideally suited to this use and probably offer the best solution to this problem (Figs. 3 to 5).

Once significant kyphotic deformity develops, posterior instrumentation may not be sufficient to correct and maintain reduction. Traditionally, anterior procedures have had a higher success rate for this particular problem. Kostuik-Harrington anterior fixation provides powerful mechanical corrective forces and has been successful in postlaminectomy kyphosis. This system uses cancellous screws with heads that accept standard Harrington distraction or compression rods. The screws are placed laterally through the vertebral body and distraction is used to correct the kyphosis. A second rod, usually a compression rod, is added to increase torsional stability. The increased morbidity and risk of anterior surgery must be balanced against the biomechanical advantages in each individual case.

Posttraumatic Kyphosis

The natural result of any destabilizing lesion of the thoracolumbar spine (whether caused by trauma, neoplasm, infection, or surgery) is the development of a kyphotic deformity because of the unbalanced biomechanical forces working on the spine. The anterior column of the spine is under compressive forces that cannot be resisted when the vertebral body and intervertebral disk are fractured or disrupted. The posterior column is under tension that cannot be resisted after ligament rupture or laminectomy. Late posttraumatic kyphosis often results in progressive neurologic dysfunction that requires decompression.

Anterior reduction of the kyphosis and stabilization gained increasing popularity but enthusiasm has been dampened somewhat by complications attributed to some of the devices. Although the concept of anterior stabilization is a sound one, further refinement of the implants is necessary to decrease complications and make the procedure more universally accepted.

Correction of chronic posttraumatic kyphosis presents a different set of problems. Goals must be clearly defined when surgical intervention is anticipated. In some patients,

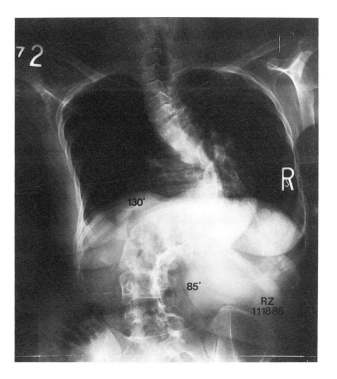

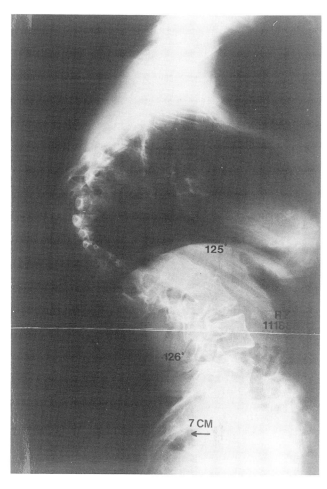

Figure 1

Preoperative radiographs demonstrate severe thoracolumbar kyphoscoliosis in a symptomatic adult patient.

correction of deformity to facilitate skin care or to improve sitting or standing posture is the sole goal. In other situations, neural decompression is also attempted in hopes of increasing neurologic recovery.

Kyphosis

Symptomatic kyphosis is relatively rare in adults. Severe Scheuermann's disease may evolve into a painful low back pain syndrome in the adult as a result of the increased biomechanical stress on the compensatory hyperlordotic lumbar spine. A similar condition can result from untreated congenital kyphosis. Surgical reconstruction of these conditions usually requires a two-stage procedure consisting of anterior release and bone grafting followed by posterior fixation and fusion.

Ankylosing spondylitis presents a special group of kyphotic deformities that require a different approach. Ankylosing spondylitis generally affects men in the second and third decades of life and may cause significant disability as a result of severe kyphosis, most commonly in the cervical and lumbar areas. Involvement of the hip and the resultant hip flexion contractures can contribute significantly to this overall problem. When this disease is fully expressed, patients are among the most functionally dis-

abled an orthopaedic surgeon is likely to encounter (Fig. 6). Because of the high neurologic risk of thoracic osteotomy, lumbar osteotomy, followed by cervical osteotomy, is often the surgical strategy. Most commonly, the osteotomy is carried out at L2-3, which avoids potential neurologic compromise of the cauda equina. This procedure has undergone very little modification since it was initially described in 1945. Essentially, the facet joints are resected at L2-3 in a diagonal fashion, at an angle of approximately 45 degrees to the longitudinal axis of the spine. The amount of bone resected is directly proportional to the amount of correction anticipated. Generally speaking, a correction of more than 45 to 50 degrees at any one level is probably unrealistic and increases the neurologic risks. Some physicians perform this surgery with the patient under local anesthesia to assure neurologic safety, but spinal cord monitoring and the "wake-up" test probably achieve the same goal. Harrington compression rodding was the procedure of choice in the past. Because of the nature of the disease, hook placement is usually accomplished by creating "slots" with a high-speed air drill in the approximate interspace two levels above and below the osteotomy. The advent of pedicle fixation, however, has added the advantage of segmental fixation with greater assurance of sagittal-plane stability and the possibility of increasing lumbar lordosis.

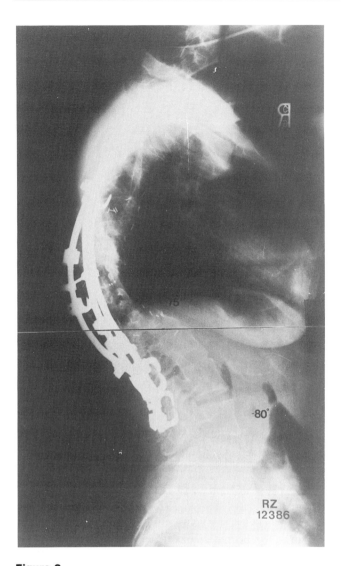

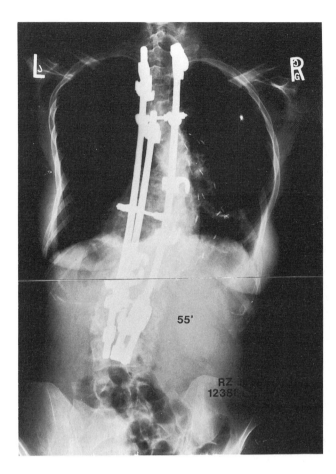

Figure 2

Postoperative radiographs of patient shown in Figure 1 demonstrate significant improvement of both frontal and sagittal plane deformities with the Cotrel-Dubousset system. The combined use of compression, distraction, and cross-linking not only allows greater mechanical advantages in the correction of deformity, but provides a much stronger construct.

Supplemental iliac crest bone grafting is used but fusion rarely fails in these patients. A hyperextension body cast or polypropylene jacket is usually worn to protect these patients because their relatively osteoporotic bone makes them susceptible to instrumentation failure. Dramatic improvement in functional status can be anticipated after a successful osteotomy.

Tumors

Tumors of the thoracolumbar spine present a great challenge. Although primary tumors of the spine are rare, advances in medical oncology have made metastatic tumors of the thoracolumbar spine an increasingly more common problem. Management of spinal tumors differs significantly from management of tumors of the appendicular skeleton. Radical excision in the sense applied to tumors of the long bones is impossible because of the spinal cord, nerve roots,

and, often, critical vascular structures that occupy the same anatomic "compartment." Nonetheless, the radical nature of the surgery can be among the orthopaedic surgeon's greatest technical challenges. First, a pathologic diagnosis must be made. If a known primary malignancy is present, the diagnosis can be accomplished inferentially. Biopsy may be necessary, however, if no primary lesion can be identified. Needle biopsy under computed tomographic control has been a major advance in this regard. It is important to realize, however, that the histologic characteristics of the tumor determine long-term survival and, therefore, to some extent the type of surgical construct required, but the anatomy or location of the lesion determines the surgical approach.

The second major principle in preoperative planning is the determination of the location and extent of the lesion. The bone scan and recently magnetic resonance imaging have been particularly helpful in this regard. Lesions that are radiosensitive should be irradiated and, with proper

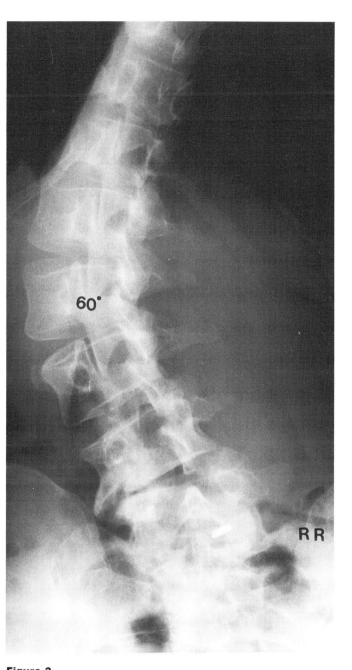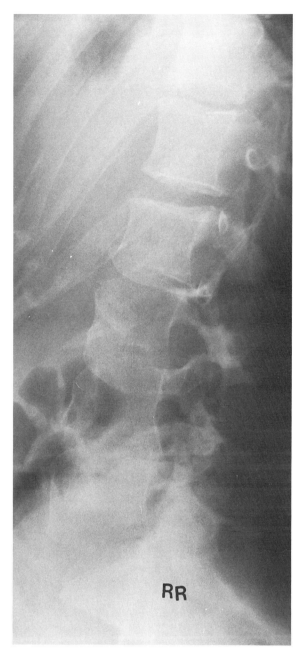

60°

R R

RR

Figure 3

A 40-year-old woman with a long history of moderate back pain demonstrated significant degenerative changes, particularly in the lower lumbar spine. Lateral views demonstrate relatively "flat" lumbar lordosis. The patient had a marked increase in pain, radiating into the left leg and accompanied by significant weakness of her left leg.

bracing, surgery can often be avoided entirely. However, lesions that are not radiosensitive or that are producing neurologic compromise are surgical candidates. It is convenient to group these patients into three categories in terms of preoperative planning.

The first group consists of those patients whose lesions occupy one specific anatomic location within the vertebra, that is, the body, the pedicle, or the lamina. These lesions should be approached on the basis of anatomic location; the stabilization accomplished depends on the degree of resection. The second category consists of patients in

whom the lesion involves both anterior and posterior elements of the same vertebra. These patients usually require both anterior resection and decompression and posterior stabilization with either Harrington or pedicle-screw fixation. Again, the choice of anterior construct is determined by the anticipated lifespan of the patient. The third category consists of patients with multiple-level anterior and posterior involvement (Fig. 7). Unless anterior decompression is indicated because of neurologic compromise, these patients are best treated with a "salvage" posterior fusion with internal fixation and generous margins above and be-

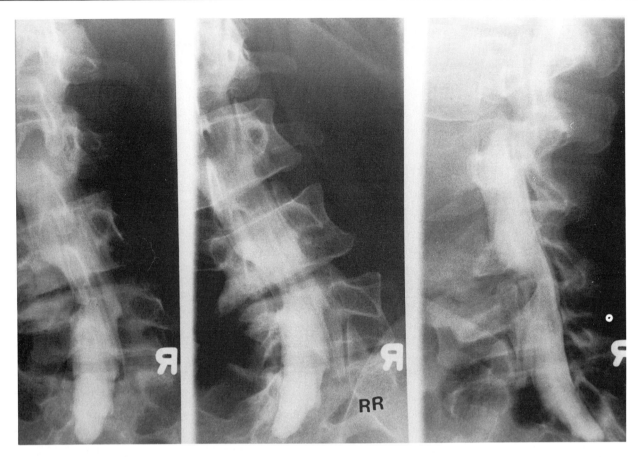

Figure 4

A total-spine myelogram (lumbar portion illustrated here) of the patient shown in Figure 3, in correlation with computed tomographic scanning, demonstrated a significant extradural defect at L4-5. This was thought to be a combination of a hypertrophic facet joint and an acute herniated disk at this level.

low the area of involvement (Figs. 7 and 8). Such a procedure usually results in dramatic relief of pain and usually circumvents kyphotic deformity and the resultant neurologic compromise.

Infection

Pyogenic infection of the thoracolumbar spine is relatively uncommon and is frequently misdiagnosed. Several series have documented delays in diagnosis of eight to 13 weeks and one series found that 25% of patients waited more than two years for a correct diagnosis. Many factors are responsible for this delay. Often patients with vertebral osteomyelitis have few systemic symptoms such as fever or sepsis and cannot localize pain accurately, and many have normal complete blood cell counts. In one series, three of seven patients with thoracic osteomyelitis underwent cholecystectomy for chronic pain before receiving a correct diagnosis. Additionally, symptoms may be attributed to concurrent infection or a disease process such as carcinoma.

The diagnosis can be made more expeditiously if a high index of clinical suspicion is maintained in patients with atypical or unexplained back pain, particularly when the pain is unrelenting and occurs at night. Plain roentgenography may not demonstrate early infection for several

weeks or longer, depending on the virulence of the infection. Technetium bone scans are said to have a sensitivity of more than 90% in patients whose symptoms have lasted more than two days. In an animal study, magnetic resonance imaging was found to be much more sensitive than bone scanning in the diagnosis of disk-space infection, making the diagnosis several days earlier. Gallium scanning is said to be significantly more sensitive than technetium scanning in the diagnosis of disk-space infection. The combination of gallium and technetium adds significantly to the ability to diagnose vertebral infections. Computed tomographic scanning may show destructive lesions of vertebral bodies much earlier than plain roentgenograms and are very accurate in demonstrating soft-tissue paravertebral diseases.

Initial treatment consists of definite identification of the bacterial organism through needle or open biopsy or inferential identification by means of positive blood, urine, or abscess culture. Appropriate intravenous antibiotics should be instituted along with spinal immobilization, including bed rest, bracing, or a combination of both. Clinical deterioration or the onset of neurologic compromise demands decompression and debridement. Because many patients in these circumstances are critically ill, the morbidity of any anticipated surgical procedure must be considered on an individual basis. Costotransversectomy is an ideal procedure in critically ill patients or in those in whom

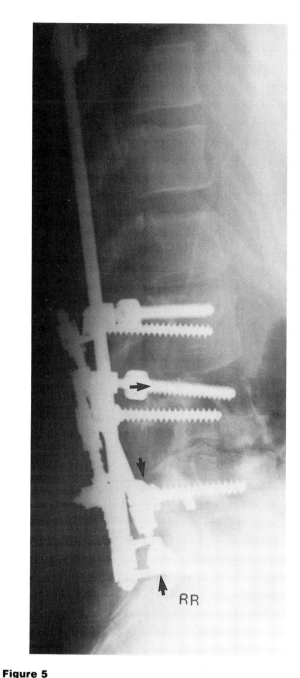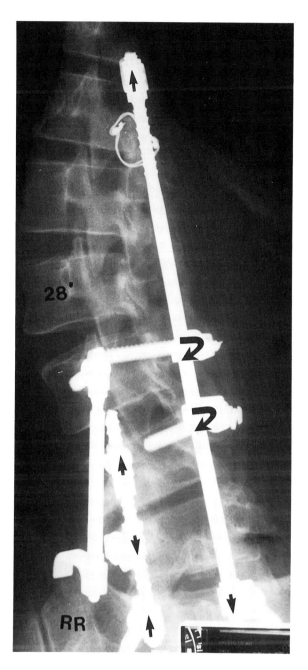

Figure 5

The surgical approach used in the patient shown in Figures 3 and 4 was directed at decompression of the L4-5 level with excision of the herniated disk and the hypertrophic facet joint as well as correction of the deformity. The latter was accomplished with the Edwards modular system. The use of rod connectors allowed sagittal and rotational control of the lower lumbar segments as well as compression between L-5 and the sacrum. A third rod was used to prevent decompensation. The force vectors applied to the deformity are indicated by arrows.

grossly purulent drainage is anticipated because it has the least morbidity while addressing the anterior anatomic site of the infectious process. Decompression and debridement through a transthoracic or retroperitoneal approach may offer wider exposure but this must be weighed against the increased morbidity of these procedures and the potential risk of bacterial contamination of these spaces. Autogenous bone grafting is generally appropriate as long as intravenous antibiotics are administered. Decompression via laminectomy has repeatedly been shown to be ineffective and

should be avoided except, possibly, in diffuse epidural empyema.

The development of neurologic complications in vertebral osteomyelitis is probably directly related to how soon treatment is initiated. The reported incidence varies from 3% to 40%. Several factors predisposing to neurologic compromise have been identified. These include increased age, more cephalad location of lesions, systemic disease (especially diabetes and chronic steroid therapy), and virulence of the organism, with *Staphylococcus aureus* being

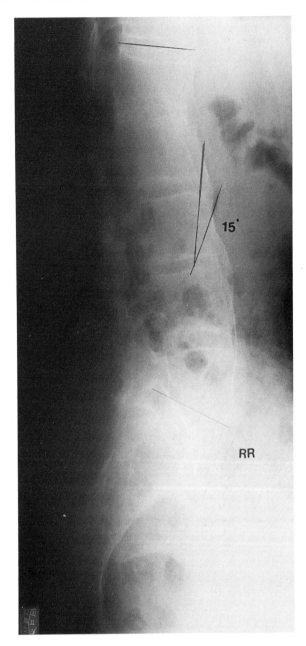
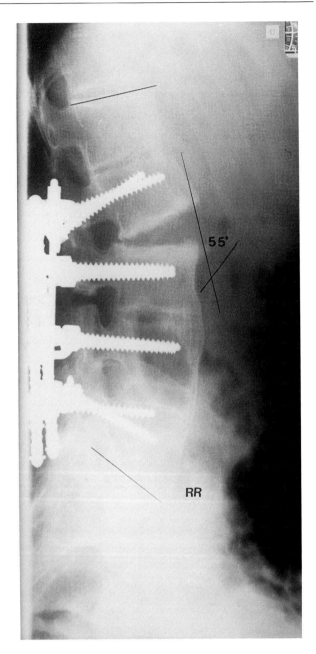

Figure 6

A 40-year-old man with ankylosing spondylitis. **Left**, He was becoming unable to work because of his progressive thoracic and lumbar kyphosis. **Right**, Osteotomies were performed at L2-3 and L3-4, but only completed at L2-3 because of the correction obtained. Pedicle-screw fixation was used over a wide margin because this was anticipated.

indicated most often. Treatment consists of decompression with appropriate intravenous antibiotic coverage, autogenous bone grafting, and appropriate spinal bracing. When neurologic deterioration occurs as a result of kyphotic deformity secondary to anterior infection, posterior fusion and Harrington rodding has proven to be safe and effective. Certainly, in the rare instance in which laminectomy has been performed for diffuse epidural empyema, reconstruction with internal fixation should be considered to avoid the late disastrous complications of postlaminectomy kyphosis.

Nonpyogenic vertebral osteomyelitis, principally tuberculosis, can be approached in a slightly different manner.

Early experiences in treating tuberculous osteomyelitis of the spine not only pioneered anterior spinal surgery of the thoracolumbar region but demonstrated that radical debridement, anterior strut graft fusions, and appropriate antituberculin drug therapy was extremely successful in the management of this difficult problem. The lower virulence of this organism, coupled with the usual multilevel presentation, makes direct anterior approach (transthoracic or retroperitoneal) the procedure of choice. The surgical management of tuberculosis of the spine has changed very little since then. Although tuberculosis of the spine is rare in residents of the United States, the disease remains endemic to Third World countries and the diagnosis must always

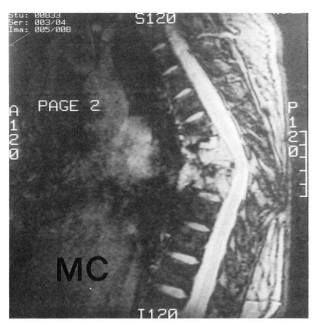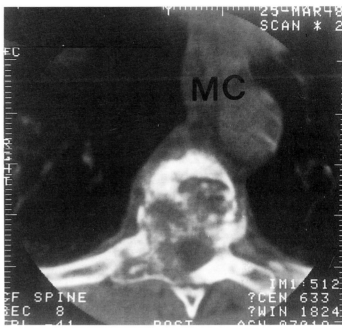

Figure 7

A 51-year-old woman had uncontrollable back pain and had a radical mastectomy ten years previously for breast carcinoma. **Left**, A magnetic resonance imaging scan demonstrated significant metastatic involvement of T-7 and T-8 with kyphotic deformity and early cord compression. Maximum radiation therapy had already been delivered. **Right,** A computed tomographic scan demonstrated tumor involvement of vertebral body, pedicle, and lamina at two levels.

be kept in mind. Similarly, the diagnosis of vertebral infection with *Brucella* and *Candida* organisms and coccidiomycosis should not be overlooked in individuals with a suggestive occupational history, impaired immunity, or exposure to an endemic area.

Spinal Cord Monitoring

Improved surgical techniques have facilitated the treatment of many thoracolumbar spinal problems. This increased capability, however, has also made it possible to correct the spine mechanically far beyond the physiologic limits of the spinal cord. It is, therefore, imperative to have a reliable and accurate means of monitoring spinal cord function during these lengthy and complex procedures. Limiting the risks of neurologic injury is of paramount concern. To be a clinically useful tool, spinal cord monitoring must fulfill certain criteria: (1) it must be accurate and sensitive; (2) it must be able to indicate a preinjury state or at least an injury to the cord that is reversible; and (3) it must not increase surgical time or risks.

The ideal form of spinal cord monitoring is not yet available. Several monitoring techniques, however, have been developed. These can be grouped into two major categories: (1) the wake-up test and (2) electrophysiologic monitoring. The wake-up test is effective and accurate. It does, however, have several major drawbacks: (1) only a limited number of muscles can be tested; (2) the technique tests motor function only; (3) results can be equivocal in certain cases; (4) it is not easily applied to patients with existing neurologic deficits; (5) it is not applicable to mentally retarded or very immature individuals because of their in-

appropriate or unreliable responses; and (6) it is indicative of an injury to the cord after the fact and, therefore, when it is not necessarily reversible.

These limitations have prompted the search for more sophisticated monitoring techniques. Electrophysiologic monitoring consisting of stimulation of neural tissue followed by the recording of evoked potentials has proved to be a useful tool. The use of somatosensory evoked potentials has had the widest application. This system is attractive because it can be performed repeatedly during the entire surgical procedure, it is applicable to patients with neurologic deficits, and, most importantly, it appears to be an indicator of impending spinal cord damage. Shortcomings do exist. This technique tests the dorsal columns of the cord (sensory paths). The status of the motor tracks is inferred. Evoked potential signals demonstrate considerable variation and can be affected by a number of variables in the operating room (for example, anesthetic agents, the depth of anesthesia, physiologic parameters, electrical interference, and technical errors). The mechanisms responsible for changes in evoked potentials have not been fully elucidated.

These shortcomings have prompted continued efforts to develop a more reliable, more sensitive, and more physiologically and anatomically accurate technique of spinal cord monitoring. Although not yet clinically available, motor evoked potential monitoring appears to be a promising alternative. This technique allows the stimulation of the motor cortex and the measurement of potentials from a distal site. These data more accurately depict the integrity of the motor tracks and, thus, are a more reliable measure of motor function.

Spinal cord monitoring is presently in an evolutionary

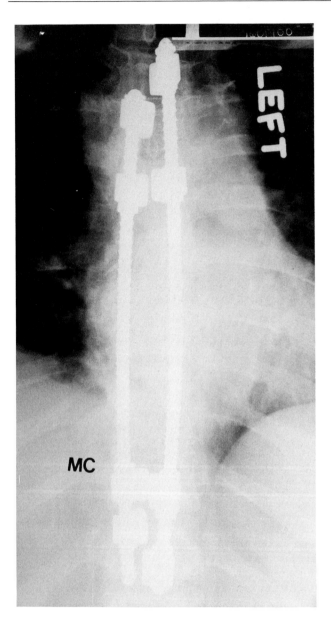
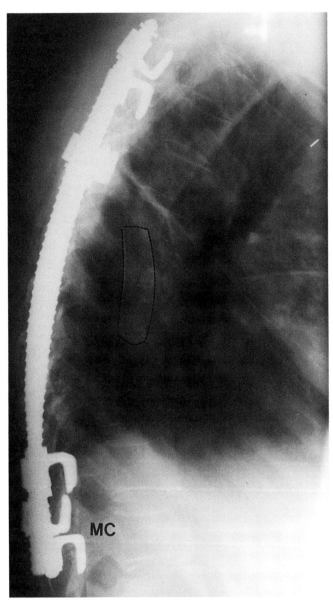

Figure 8

This patient underwent a combined anterior and posterior procedure. First, the posterior tumor involvement, including both pedicles, was resected, and correction of the kyphos deformity was achieved with the posterior Edwards modular system. The use of combined distraction and compression nodes on each rod results in a "claw" effect that significantly increases the mechanical strength of the construct. Next, transthoracic vertebrectomy resulting in total vertebrectomy at two levels was performed. Anterior reconstruction was achieved with a large iliac crest graft (dotted lines).

state. Both false-positive and false-negative evoked potentials have been reported. Although it is clear that no ideal method of spinal cord monitoring exists at present, some method should be used when intraoperative manipulation is employed in the management of spinal deformity.

Controversies

Adult Scoliosis

One of the major controversies in adult scoliosis is whether or not the results justify surgical reconstruction. All series concede a higher complication rate compared with adolescents, but there is a great deal of variability concerning reported relief of pain, functional capability, and self-image. Certainly these outcomes are not easily measured, depend on a large number of factors (many beyond the surgeon's control), and involve a large psychosocial component. Patient selection, therefore, assumes a much larger role in the surgical management of this problem, and may be the single most important determinant of successful outcome.

The second major controversy in the management of adult scoliosis is whether or not fusion of a lumbar curve should be extended to the sacrum. It is an accepted principle in adolescent scoliosis surgery to avoid fusing the sacrum if at all possible. This is based primarily on experience with the Harrington system, in which loss of lumbar lordosis or the "flatback" syndrome may occur. A high rate of pseudarthrosis or instrumentation failure also accompanies fusion to the sacrum. However, adolescent scoliosis and adult scoliosis are two distinct entities in terms of surgical management. Invariably, symptomatic lumbar curves in adults are the result of degenerative changes and these changes often involve the lumbosacral junction. In addition, it is often difficult to avoid decompensating a lumbar curve without fusion to the sacrum. Undoubtedly, ending a thoracolumbar fusion above a degenerative lumbosacral junction has contributed to poor pain relief in the past. With the advent of newer systems and techniques of lumbosacral fixation designed to eliminate the problem of loss of lordosis and decrease the rate of pseudarthrosis and instrumentation failure, this particular group of adult patients with scoliosis should achieve much better pain relief. The bias against fusion to the sacrum will no longer be automatically transferred from adolescent scoliosis to adult scoliosis.

Postlaminectomy Deformity

Controversy has arisen as to whether posterior fixation is as safe and efficacious as anterior techniques. In situ posterior fusion has a low probability of success because the fusion is under tension. Harrington compression instrumentation has been used in the treatment of postlaminectomy kyphosis in the past, but has the distinct disadvantage of increasing the number of motion segments that must be included in the surgical construct. In addition, once significant kyphosis has developed, distraction is counterproductive and the rod is really used as a long lever arm, which then places excessive loads on the points of hook fixation, leading to their failure. Although increasing familiarity with the mechanical corrective properties of pedicle-screw fixation has led some to conclude that successful results can be obtained with a posterior system with less risk and morbidity, more clinical experience is needed to determine whether this trend will prevail.

Posttraumatic Kyphosis

Controversies in the area of the surgical management of posttraumatic kyphosis center primarily on whether the anterior or the posterior approach is more appropriate. Before planning surgery, it is, therefore, essential to establish whether decompression is indicated and the degree of flexibility of the deformity. Situations requiring neural decompression are probably best treated anteriorly. Fixed kyphotic deformities require anterior release and fusion at the least and may require posterior fixation and fusion in addition. Flexible deformities not requiring decompression can best be accomplished with posterior fixation alone. Harrington compression instrumentation is sometimes adequate to achieve reduction but many of the newer devices offer more powerful and secure correction and fixation.

Tumors

One of the major controversies in spinal tumor surgery is whether or not such extensive surgery is warranted when it is only palliative and life expectancy is limited. Quality of life is the major issue, and reports indicate that significant relief of pain and neurologic recovery can be anticipated in properly planned surgical decompression and fusion.

The second controversial area in spinal tumor surgery is the choice of construct. The construct used should be determined by the projected life expectancy of the patient. For instance, for a lesion in the body of a vertebra, a vertebrectomy is performed and an iliac or rib strut graft is used if the patient's life expectancy is assumed to be longer than six months. Under the same circumstances, if the life expectancy is likely to be less than six months, a construct incorporating Steinmann pins placed into the intact vertebral bodies above and below the resection in retrograde fashion with methylmethacrylate is commonly used. However, the use of methylmethacrylate posteriorly predisposes to wound breakdown and infection and should be avoided if possible.

The choice of posterior fixation remains controversial as the newer fixation devices gain wider acceptance. Harrington compression rodding or Luque rodding remain the standards, but the increased biomechanical advantage of segmental pedicle fixation used in the Edwards modular system and the Cotrel-Dubousset system are becoming increasingly more accepted.

Infection

The major controversy in the treatment of spinal infection is whether or not to combine debridement with primary bone grafting and/or internal fixation with instrumentation. The success of primary bone grafting in nonvirulent infections such as tuberculosis and mycotic infections is well established. Recent reports have suggested similar results in more virulent infections. Primary placement of bone graft or instrumentation in the presence of gross infection and pus remains highly controversial and must be determined on a case-by-case basis.

Annotated Bibliography

Keywords

Infection; Kyphosis; Laminectomy; Neoplasms; Scoliosis; Spinal cord; Spinal instrumentation; Thoracolumbar spine

Diagnosis and Anatomy

Forristall RM, Marsh HO, Pay NT: Magnetic resonance imaging and contrast CT of the lumbar spine: Comparison of diagnostic methods and correlation with surgical findings. *Spine* 1988;13:1049–1054.

Thirty-two patients with suspected lumbar disk herniation underwent magnetic resonance imaging and computed tomographic evaluation of 100 disk levels and the results were compared with the surgical findings. Surgical findings supported the magnetic resonance imaging diagnosis in 90.3% of cases and the computed tomographic diagnosis in 77.4% of cases. The authors conclude that surface coil magnetic resonance imaging is superior to contrast-enhanced computed tomography in the diagnosis of disk herniation.

Zindrick MR, Wiltse LL, Doornik A, et al: Analysis of the mophometric characteristics of the thoracic and lumbar pedicles. *Spine* 1987;12:160–166.

This is the best available study on the morphometry of thoracolumbar pedicles from T-1 to L-5. Comparison of computed tomographic and roentgenographic measurements showed no significant difference. Pedicles were widest at L-5 and narrowest at T-5 in the transverse plane. In the sagittal plane, the widest pedicles were at T-11 and the narrowest at T-1. This is essential reading for those attempting pedicle-screw fixation.

Deformity

Adult Scoliosis

Betz RR, Bunnell WP, Lambrecht-Mulier E, et al: Scoliosis and pregnancy. *J Bone Joint Surg* 1987;69A:90–96.

The authors reviewed 335 skeletally mature women with scoliosis. One half of this group had been pregnant at least once and these women were compared with a similar group who had never been pregnant. The authors concluded that pregnancy does not increase the risk of progression of a mild to moderate curve. There was no significant adverse effect on a previously fused spine as a result of pregnancy. Mild to moderate scoliosis did not have a deleterious affect on pregnancy or delivery.

Grubb SA, Lipscomb HJ, Coonrad RW: Degenerative adult onset scoliosis. *Spine* 1988;13:241–245.

This study presents a series of adult patients with no history of scoliosis who developed deformity as a result of disk degeneration. In addition, they demonstrated progressive loss of lumbar lordosis. For the most part, the patients had symptoms consistent with spinal stenosis.

Gurr KR, McAfee PC: Cotrel-Dubousset instrumentation in adults: A preliminary report. *Spine* 1988;13:510–520.

This paper reviews 50 adult patients with scoliosis and other spinal disorders treated with Cotrel-Dubousset instrumentation. Curve correction was comparable to that with Harrington instrumentation. All cases progressed to a solid arthrodesis. Fewer motion segments were fused in tumor, trauma, and spondylolisthesis than with the Harrington or Luque systems.

Jackson RP, Simmons EH, Stripinis D: Incidence and severity of back pain in adult idiopathic scoliosis. *Spine* 1983;8:749–756.

This study compared a series of 197 adults with idiopathic scoliosis with 180 patients without known spinal deformity. The incidence of pain was the same, but the severity of pain was significantly greater in the scoliosis patients. Fifty-one percent of adult scoliosis patients had significant pain and 83% reported persistent and progressive pain, whereas 64% of the control group reported improvement in pain over time.

Sponseller PD, Cohen MS, Nachemson AL, et al: Results of surgical treatment of adults with idiopathic scoliosis. *J Bone Joint Surg* 1987;69A:667–675.

Forty-five patients with adult scoliosis were interviewed at least three years after surgery to determine the long-term results. There was a reduction in peak and constant pain, but no change in the frequency of peak pain. Similarly, functional im-

pairment caused by scoliosis was lessened and the ability to perform common activities of daily living was improved, but no important changes in occupation or recreational activity were recorded. A high complication rate and limited gains suggested that patient information and selection are important factors to be considered.

van Dam BE, Bradford DS, Lonstein JE, et al: Adult idiopathic scoliosis treated by posterior spinal fusion and Harrington instrumentation. *Spine* 1987;12:32–36.

Ninety-one adult patients with idiopathic scoliosis underwent posterior spinal fusion and Harrington rod instrumentation. Indications for surgery included pain, progressive deformity, and pulmonary symptoms. The average correction was 38% at the time of surgery and 32% at the time of follow-up (average, 3.5 years). Seventy-nine percent of the patients reported complete relief of the symptoms for which they underwent surgery. The complication rate was 33%, including a 15% pseudarthrosis rate and a 5% instrumentation failure rate.

Postlaminectomy Deformity

Johnsson KE, Willner S, Johnsson K: Postoperative instability after decompression for lumbar spinal stenosis. *Spine* 1986;11:107–110.

In this study of 45 patients with a mean age of 64 years and documented spinal stenosis, a higher incidence of postoperative slippage occurred in patients with degenerative spondylolisthesis (65%). A lower, but still significant, number of patients (20%) with acquired spinal stenosis demonstrated slippage. No attempt at fusion was made in this group.

Posttraumatic Kyphosis

Aebi M, Etter C, Kehl T, et al: Stabilization of the lower thoracic and lumbar spine with the internal spinal skeletal fixation system: Indications, techniques, and first results of treatment. *Spine* 1987;12:544–551.

This series of 30 patients with burst fractures was treated with the AO "internal fixator." The authors report anatomic reduction, early mobilization in a light orthosis, and two cases of instrumentation failure.

Bradford DS, McBride GG: Surgical management of thoracolumbar spine fractures with incomplete neurologic deficits. *Clin Orthop* 1987;218:201–216.

The results of surgical decompression in 59 patients with neurologic deficit secondary to thoracic or lumbar fractures were evaluated at a mean of 3.7 years after injury. More neurologic recovery occurred in patients who underwent anterior decompression (88%) than in those who underwent posterolateral or posterior decompression (64%).

Eismont FJ, Green BA, Berkowitz BM, et al: The role of intraoperative ultrasonography in the treatment of thoracic and lumbar spine fractures. *Spine* 1984;9:782–787.

This is a good description of the technique and interpretation of intraoperative ultrasonography in the assessment of the adequacy of decompression of the ventral neural canal after reduction.

Roberson JR, Whitesides TE Jr: Surgical reconstruction of late post-traumatic thoracolumbar kyphosis. *Spine* 1985;10:307–312.

Thirty-four patients underwent surgery for late posttraumatic kyphosis. This study emphasized biomechanical principles. Anterior fusion only, posterior fusion only, and combined procedures were performed according to these principles and solid fusion was achieved in all but one patient.

Kyphosis

Bradford DS, Ganjavian S, Antonious D, et al: Anterior strut-grafting for the treatment of kyphosis: Review of experience with forty-eight patients. *J Bone Joint Surg* 1982;64A:680–690.

This is a thorough description of surgical management of thoracic kyphosis. The series included 48 curves corrected from an average of 93 degrees to an average of 59 degrees postoperatively. Forty patients had combined anterior strut graft and posterior Harrington rodding.

Bradford DS, Schumacher WL, Lonstein JE, et al: Ankylosing spondylitis: Experience in surgical management of 21 patients. *Spine* 1987;12:238–243.

This was a relatively large series of patients with kyphotic spines managed by spinal osteotomy. The techniques of lumbar and thoracic osteotomy are described.

Cotler HB, Cotler JM, Stoloff A, et al: The use of autografts for vertebral body replacement of the thoracic and lumbar spine. *Spine* 1985;10:748–756.

A thorough presentation of techniques and their applications to a variety of kyphotic problems.

Tumors

DeWald RL, Bridwell KH, Prodromas C, et al: Reconstructive spinal surgery as palliation for metastatic malignancies of the spine. *Spine* 1985;10:21–26.

The authors present an aggressive approach to spine metastatic lesions using the analogy of prophylactic treatment of femoral lesions. They describe 17 patients and a classification for treatment purposes regardless of tissue type.

Kostuik JP, Errico TJ, Gleason TF, et al: Spinal stabilization of vertebral column tumors. *Spine* 1988;13:250–256.

The authors analyze the indications, techniques, and results of stabilization and reconstruction in 100 consecutive patients with spine tumors. A major indication for surgery was pain relief and 81% of the patients achieved this. Rigid stabilization was primarily responsible for pain relief. The complication rate was 4% and the average survival was 11.3 months.

Lee CK, Rosa R, Fernand R: Surgical treatment of tumors of the spine. *Spine* 1986;11:201–208.

The authors describe a series of 20 patients and propose several principles of management, including (1) an anterior approach for anterior lesions and a posterior approach for posterior lesions, (2) a one-stage anterior and posterior approach for extensive lesions, and (3) adequate fixation with the use of various internal fixation devices, bone graft, or cement. All their patients had satisfactory results.

Onimus M, Schraub S, Bertin D, et al: Surgical treatment of vertebral metastasis. *Spine* 1986;11:883–891.

The authors describe their series of 57 patients with metastatic disease who underwent 60 surgical procedures. They concluded that surgery is beneficial and should be preferred if direct cord compression or potential instability of the spine is noted preoperatively.

Infection

Abramovitz JN, Batson RA, Yablon JS: Vertebral osteomyelitis: The surgical management of neurologic complications. *Spine* 1986;11:418–420.

The authors describe 12 patients with neurologic complications of vertebral osteomyelitis. Adequate decompression with attention to stability was thought to be the key to success. Laminectomy alone produced delayed neurologic deterioration.

Eismont FJ, Bohlman HH, Soni PL, et al: Pyogenic and fungal vertebral osteomyelitis with paralysis. *J Bone Joint Surg* 1983;65A:19–29.

The authors present a retrospective review of 61 patients with vertebral osteomyelitis. Concurrent diabetes mellitus and rheumatoid arthritis, increased age, and more cephalad level of infection predisposed to paralysis. For patients with paralysis, the prognosis of isolated nerve root recovery is good with or without surgery. For patients with spinal cord compression, results are generally better with anterior decompression than with laminectomy.

Emery SE, Chan DPK, Woodward HR: Treatment of hematogenous pyogenic vertebral osteomyelitis with anterior debridement and primary bone grafting. *Spine* 1989;14:284–291.

The authors describe a series of 19 patients with pyogenic vertebral osteomyelitis who were treated with anterior debridement, primary bone grafting, and antibiotic coverage. After an average follow-up of four years, 18 were judged to have good results with no evidence of osteomyelitis or pseudarthrosis. One patient demonstrated pseudarthrosis.

Shitut RV, Goodpasture HC, Marsh HO: Diagnosing hematogenous vertebral pyogenic osteomyelitis. *Comp Orthop*, March-April 1987.

The clinical presentation and management of 21 patients with vertebral osteomyelitis were reviewed. The most common reasons for delay in diagnosis were nonspecific presentation, premature closure of diagnostic alternatives, and failure to consider hematogenous vertebral osteomyelitis as a complication of a previously recognized episode of infection at another site.

Szypryt EP, Hardy JG, Hinton CE, et al: A comparison between magnetic resonance imaging and scintigraphic bone imaging in the diagnosis of disc space infection in an animal model. *Spine* 1988;13:1042–1048.

A series of 33 rabbits was used to compare the efficacy of magnetic resonance imaging with that of scintigraphy in the diagnosis of pyogenic infection of the intervertebral disk. Magnetic resonance imaging was found to be more sensitive, particularly in the early stages of the disease. The overall results showed that magnetic resonance imaging had a sensitivity of 93%, a specificity of 97%, and an accuracy of 95%.

Spinal Cord Monitoring

Lieponis JV, Jacobs K, Bunch WH, et al: The effect of spinal cord blood flow on evoked potentials, in Ducker TB, Brown RH (eds): *Neurophysiology and Standards of Spinal Cord Monitoring*. New York, Springer-Verlag, 1988.

An overview of intraoperative spinal cord monitoring is presented. Altered primate spinal-cord blood-flow states demonstrated significant changes in evoked potentials. Study conditions mimicked actual operating room settings.

36
Lumbar Spine

Low back pain is the most costly musculoskeletal ailment. The exact cost is difficult to calculate, but estimates range from $16 billion to $50 billion for actual medical payments and lost productivity. Fifty percent of patients with back pain recover by two weeks and 90% have no pain by three months. Persistent symptoms are present in 7% at six months; by one year only 2% still have pain. The 7% of patients with pain after six months account for more than 85% to 90% of all the money spent on the treatment of and compensation for low back pain. In 1986 more than 11 million patients had low back impairments and 5.6 million patients were disabled by low back pain in the United States.

Epidemiology

Fifty percent to 80% of the population will experience one episode of low back pain during adult life that temporarily interferes with the ability to perform normal activities. Low back pain lasting at least two weeks has a cumulative lifetime prevalence in the United States of 13.8%. The typical age at onset is in the third decade of life; low back pain reaches its peak in individuals 55 to 64 years old and then decreases precipitously in those older than 65 years. Of all patients with low back pain, only 10% to 12% have concomitant sciatica. The peak age for the onset of sciatic pain is somewhat later (40 to 55 years). Only 1% to 2% of patients with sciatica secondary to a disk herniation require surgery. The peak age for surgical intervention is the early 40s.

Although the exact cause of 80% to 90% of all back pain is unknown, a variety of risk factors such as smoking, lower educational level, tension and anxiety, and cardiovascular symptoms are associated with a higher incidence of low back pain. Job-related risk factors include repetitive heavy lifting, particularly when a twisting posture is required, vibration, and consistently long periods of driving.

Diagnosis

Although the precise cause of pain is unknown in most cases, a complete medical history and physical examination are essential.

Medical History

The initial history is particularly important because it permits timely decision-making that prevents inappropriate or delayed treatment. Initial questioning should focus on the onset of pain and its initial location, that is, back, leg, or both, and whether the pain was acute or insidious in onset. Associated trauma, litigation, or worker's compensation claims are important components of the history because of their adverse effect on recovery.

Particular attention should be paid to the pattern of the pain. The effect of activity (walking, sitting, standing, lying) on the pain is helpful in differentiating between various spinal disorders (particularly spinal stenosis and disk herniation). The involvement of other joints and the general health of the patient may aid in the diagnosis of a variety of possible metabolic or rheumatologic disorders involving the spine. The history of medication use and effectiveness may also be helpful in evaluating potential therapeutic alternatives. Particular attention should be paid to the short- or long-term use of narcotic or addictive medication.

Probably the most important aspect of the history is differentiating the 90% of patients with low back pain alone from those with sciatic pain. True sciatic pain radiates below the knee into the respective anatomic branches of the sciatic nerve. It results from neurologic compression or irritation of one or more neural components of the sciatic nerve. Sciatic pain must be differentiated from the much more common referred pain patterns often seen in patients with low back pain without any neurologic involvement. Referred pain may radiate into the buttocks, hips, groin, and as far as the distal thigh; it is sometimes labeled sclerotomal pain. Few data are available on the causes and physiology of referred low back pain. This type of pain can be produced by injecting hypertonic saline into the interspinous ligaments and facet joints.

Patients should be questioned specifically about the distribution of the pain in the lower extremities as well as any concomitant weakness or numbness. L-4 nerve root compression typically results in pain radiating to the medial knee and the anterior thigh. Compression of the L-5 nerve root elicits pain and numbness over the lateral calf and the dorsum of the medial aspect of the foot, most notably in the first dorsal web space. Involvement of the S-1 nerve root results in pain and numbness radiating down the posterior calf to the lateral aspects of the foot and sole.

Patients complaining of nonanatomic ("stocking" or "glove") sensory loss or nonspecific motor loss through the entire lower limb or episodes of falling should be evaluated for other neurologic or psychosomatic conditions. It is highly unusual for solitary or even multiple lumbar root compression to result in episodic falling or "giving way," although "drop episodes" can occur in severe spinal stenosis.

Patients with neurologic compression in the lumbar spine occasionally have low back pain and sciatica with bowel or bladder dysfunction such as urinary retention or overflow incontinence. A history of incontinence, retention of urine, or frequent, small-volume urination is important because the cauda equina syndrome is one of the few surgical emergencies in patients with low back pain. It occurs in 1% to 2% of patients with lumbar disk herniations. These symptoms can also be produced by intradural and extradural tumors, infections, and epidural hemorrhage.

A complete medical history should elicit metabolic or systemic diseases, such as cancer, that may have a direct effect on the patient's spinal symptoms. A history of psychiatric illness, illicit or prescription drug abuse, or any recent change in the patient's psychosocial state (divorce, loss of job, and the like) can yield important information.

Physical Examination

The physical examination should begin with inspection of the entire spine. The presence of the normal cervical lordosis, thoracic kyphosis, and lumbar lordosis should be noted. Palpation and percussion of the spinal midline should be done to elicit any pain or malalignment. The paraspinal musculature and the sacroiliac region should be palpated to elicit any painful areas.

Forward flexion, extension, and right and left lateral bending should be performed so that lumbar motion as well as the type of pain provoked by motion (low back, referred, or sciatic pain) can be evaluated. Range of motion of the hips should also be measured to elicit any referred pain that might be misdiagnosed as spinal in origin. Restricted range of spinal motion, restricted hip motion, and restricted chest expansion are common in the spondyloarthropathies.

A neurologic examination should be performed. Abnormal gait patterns and the ability to heel-and-toe walk should be tested. Heel-walking principally measures L-4 and L-5 motor strength, while toe-walking is a gross measure of S-1 nerve root function. Plantar flexion and anteversion of the foot measure S-1 nerve root function. Ankle dorsiflexion strength is a measure of L-4 nerve root motor function; an extensor hallucis longus weakness is associated with abnormal L-5 nerve root function. Quadriceps strength may be decreased if the L-3 or L-4 nerve root is involved. Hip flexion strength is examined to demonstrate an alteration in L-1 or L-2 nerve root function. A rectal examination should be performed to assess sphincter strength.

Sensory examination will delineate loss of sensation in the anatomic dermatomal distribution of each specific nerve root. Both light-touch and pinprick responses should be tested. The lumbar nerve roots are distributed as follows: the S-1 nerve root, the lateral foot and sole; the L-5 root, the lateral calf and first dorsal web space; and the L-4 root, the medial knee region. Perineal and vaginal or scrotal sensation should be tested for S-2, S-3, and S-4 root function; sensation may be lost in the cauda equina syndrome. Proprioception of the lower extremity should be tested; proprioception is often lost in diabetic neuropathy.

Reflexes should be tested for evidence of asymmetry. Hyperreflexia, clonus, and Babinski reflexes are important signs of upper motor neuron involvement. An abnormal anal wink reflex is indicative of sacral root involvement. The knee jerk and ankle jerk represent L-4 and S-1 nerve root function, respectively. The posterior tibial reflex, innervated by L-5, is more difficult to elicit and is bilaterally absent in more than 50% of patients.

The most widely used test for neural irritability is the straight leg raising test. This can be done in the sitting or lying position. The knee is extended and the lower extremity flexed at the hip with the pelvis in a stable, fixed position. The straight leg raising test is positive only if sciatic pain radiating below the knee is reproduced. The test is not positive when only back pain or thigh pain is elicited.

The contralateral straight leg raising test is a much more specific measure of neural irritability. This test is performed by elevating the asymptomatic leg and eliciting sciatic pain radiating down the contralateral symptomatic leg. The bowstring test is performed in the same way as the straight leg raising test except that the knee is flexed until the sciatic pain is relieved. Manual compression of the neural elements in the popliteal fossa should normally cause minimal discomfort. However, if one of the component nerve roots is irritated, there will be proximal or distal radicular pain and/or paresthesias.

A reverse, prone straight leg raising test, or femoral stretch test, is done by extension of the straight leg at the hip. This specifically tests upper nerve root irritation (L-3, L-4).

Finally, it is important to examine the peripheral pulses and other physical signs of peripheral vascular disease. The symptoms of spinal stenosis and intermittent claudication caused by peripheral arterial disease are often indistinguishable. The presence of strong palpable pulses should preclude a diagnosis of vascular claudication.

Imaging Techniques

Radiography

Plain lumbosacral radiographs are the most commonly ordered diagnostic study for the patient with low back pain, but they rarely give pertinent diagnostic information. Most radiographic abnormalities correlate poorly with symptoms. The degenerative changes seen on these radiographs are more often those of the normal aging process of the lumbar spine.

The presence of disk-space narrowing and/or traction spurs at the L4–5 level has been associated with an increased incidence of lower-extremity symptoms (pain and neurologic loss) and low back pain in one study but not in others. The presence of transitional vertebrae, vacuum disk signs, disk-space narrowing at levels other than L4–5, claw spurs, and Schmorl's nodes has no documented correlation with an increased incidence or severity of back pain.

Although the diagnosis of spinal degeneration can be made on as many as 70% of radiographs, this should have little effect on management or treatment outcome. However, in one study, patients given the radiographic diagnosis of degenerative disease were treated with nonsteroidal or anti-inflammatory drugs three times more often than patients with normal radiographs regardless of the lack of clinical correlation. In addition, patients who were told the diagnosis was degenerative joint disease were far more satisfied with their treatment than those patients given a nonspecific diagnosis.

Thus, lumbosacral radiographs are not a necessary component of the initial examination. Indications for spinal radiographs are a clinical suspicion of neoplastic, infectious, metabolic, or traumatic disorder of the spine. Clinical judgment based on the history and physical examination should be used in these suspicious situations.

Myelography, Computed Tomography, and Magnetic Resonance Imaging

With the advent of water-soluble contrast myelography, contrast agents such as metrizamide now permit better visualization of the nerve roots, conus, and thoracic cord than did oil-based contrast. More recently, this technique has been superseded by computed tomographic scanning and magnetic resonance imaging in a majority of patients. There is continued controversy as to which is the best diagnostic technique. Several large studies have attempted to compare the sensitivity of myelography, computed tomographic scanning, and magnetic resonance imaging but the findings have been inconsistent.

In one study, the sensitivity of myelography was higher than that of the computed tomographic scan (82% vs 73%) in diagnosing a herniated lumbar disk. However, the specificity of myelography was lower (67% vs 77%). The positive predictive value of the two studies was essentially the same (93% vs 94%). In another study, the surgical findings agreed with myelographic findings in 94% of the cases and with computed tomographic findings in 92% of the cases.

In contrast, the surgical findings in patients with spinal stenosis and/or a herniated disk correlated better with the myelographic than the computed tomographic findings. Myelography was more accurate than computed tomographic scanning in the diagnosis of a herniated disk (83% vs 72%) and was also better in the diagnosis of spinal stenosis (93% vs 89%).

Another study comparing the surgical findings in patients undergoing decompression for spinal stenosis found the dimensions of the spinal canal measured on the computed tomographic scan to be accurate in only 20% of cases compared with 83% for myelographic measurements.

These studies demonstrate no clear-cut diagnostic superiority of one technique over the other. The invasive nature of myelography cannot be overlooked. Significantly more patients with no myelographic findings experience side effects than patients with myelographic abnormalities.

Another limitation of myelography is the presence of complete myelographic block when there is no visualization of the neural structures distal to the blockage. In one study, 59% of patients with a complete block were found to have intraspinal abnormalities caudally on computed tomographic scanning done after myelography. It is essential that patients with a complete myelographic block undergo computed tomographic scanning.

The major limitation of computed tomography without myelography is the inability to detect primary or secondary abnormalities beyond the vertebral levels scanned. The most frequently missed abnormalities are those of the conus and thoracic cord, which may often simulate lower lumbar lesions.

In the last several years, magnetic resonance imaging has improved tremendously, particularly because of the surface-coil innovations. Magnetic resonance imaging produces no toxic reactions, unlike myelography, and no radiation exposure, unlike both myelography and computed tomography. It has the capacity to identify intraspinal abnormalities proximal and distal to the primary lesion. The ability of magnetic resonance imaging to delineate early degenerative changes in the disk far exceeds the ability of either myelography or computed tomography. However, this sensitivity could lead to overdiagnosis and treatment, particularly of the degenerative changes that are part of normal aging. Forty percent of asymptomatic volunteers demonstrate abnormalities on magnetic resonance imaging.

The ability of magnetic resonance imaging to demonstrate specific types of disk herniations, particularly sequestered fragments, seems at least as good as or better than that of myelography or computed tomography (Fig. 1). In a study of patients undergoing surgery for lumbar disk herniations, magnetic resonance imaging had a sensitivity of 89%, a specificity of 82%, and an accuracy of 85% in distinguishing sequestered fragments from other forms of disk herniations. Its ability to diagnose central spinal stenosis appears to be equally promising. One drawback of magnetic resonance imaging is the difficulty of demonstrating lateral recess compression of nerve roots compared with the excellent visualization normally seen in the anteroposterior and oblique views of the metrizamide myelogram.

An important adjunct to the standard magnetic resonance imaging study is the use of intravenous paramagnetic contrast media such as gadolinium. This is particularly helpful in the patient in whom surgery has failed or who has recurrent symptoms and permits the differentiation of postoperative scarring from recurrent or retained disk herniations (Fig. 2). Preliminary reports suggest that this technique is superior to postoperative myelography and intravenous contrast-enhanced computed tomography.

Bone Scintigraphy

Bone scintigraphy is rarely necessary in the initial examination of patients with low back pain. It is most commonly used in the early detection of primary or metastatic disease involving the spine. Gallium and, more recently, indium scanning are more sensitive to infectious processes and should be used as adjuncts to standard bone scintig-

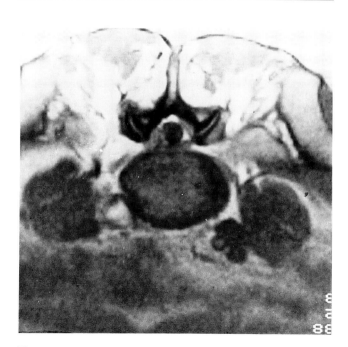

Figure 1

Magnetic resonance imaging demonstrates a large L4-5 disk herniation.

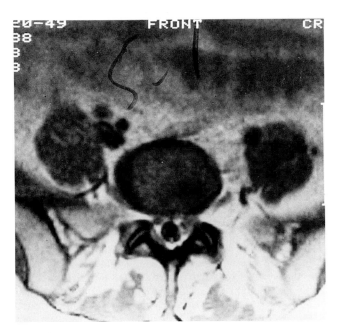

Figure 2
Magnetic resonance imaging enhanced with gadolinium demonstrates postoperative scarring but no recurrent disk herniation.

raphy. However, the indium scan's usefulness in the spine has not been confirmed.

Bone scintigraphy can also be helpful in evaluating the presence of pseudarthrosis, spondylolysis, and spondylolytic fractures.

Electrodiagnostic Studies

The role of electrodiagnostic testing in the diagnosis of low back pain and sciatica is not clearly established. There are conflicting reports on the reliability and diagnostic capability of these studies. Reports evaluating electromyography of the paravertebral muscles have shown that these studies have little value in clinical diagnosis, particularly after surgery in which denervation patterns are common.

Electromyography and spinal evoked potentials appear to be more helpful when used to measure neurologic abnormalities in the lower extremity. In difficult diagnostic situations, particularly in patients with chronic sciatica, these studies may be helpful. In a series of 100 patients with chronic low back pain and sciatica, the electrodiagnostic studies were found to be helpful in defining the radiculopathy in patients with otherwise equivocal clinical and computed tomographic findings. However, no single diagnostic factor, including electromyography, provided a conclusive diagnosis.

Spinal evoked potentials have been advocated as a diagnostic tool as well as a means of assessing adequate intraoperative decompression of the neural elements. Like electromyographic studies, the spinal evoked potentials appear to be helpful in arriving at a difficult diagnosis, but by themselves are not adequate for clinical decisions, particularly those involving surgical intervention. In general, electrodiagnostic studies are helpful in identifying patients with peripheral neuropathy from diabetes, demyelinating disorders, and a variety of metabolic diseases that include peripheral neurologic involvement. In most patients, a thorough physical examination may yield the same information as an expensive electrodiagnostic study.

Thermography

Thermography is an appealing diagnostic study because it is noninvasive, inexpensive, and relatively easy to interpret. The colorful images record changes in the skin temperature, theoretically "mapping" areas of "physiologic disturbance" and increased pain. Unfortunately, there are no studies that conclusively validate its use as a diagnostic tool in low back pain with or without sciatica. No clinical or treatment recommendation should be based on the results of thermography until further scientific studies are available. However, not all authorities agree, and some argue that this technique is important in objectifying the cause of low back pain.

Low Back Pain

The vast majority of patients with idiopathic low back pain have a self-limited course and improve spontaneously. Despite this overall excellent prognosis, a multitude of treatments have been used to influence the clinical course of idiopathic low back pain. Almost none of these have been scientifically validated.

In contrast to earlier recommendations, prolonged bed rest appears to be contraindicated in the patient with idiopathic low back pain. Two days appears to be as effective as a week of bed rest. Increased endurance and overall physical fitness have been documented as positively influencing the recurrence rate and natural history of idiopathic low back pain.

Activity level should be increased and exercises begun as quickly as possible. Proponents of both Williams flexion and McKensie extension exercise programs have maintained the superiority of their respective regimens. One study has shown that it does not matter which exercise regimen is used as long as the activity level is increased. Both groups of patients had significantly decreased pain, and neither group was statistically superior to the other.

The Back School approach, pioneered by the first Swedish Back School, appears to have a beneficial effect in decreasing the time away from work when used in an industrial setting. Away from the industrial setting, there appears to be good patient acceptance of the Back School approach, but its overall effect on the natural history of idiopathic low back pain, particularly chronic low back pain, is not clear.

Other treatments have met with less success. Although many are widely used and have been shown to provide short-term relief in varying degrees, most have not been shown in a scientific manner to be clinically effective in altering the long-term course of low back pain. These unproven modalities include traction, bracing, epidural steroids, facet joint injections, ultrasound, transcutaneous electrical nerve stimulation, massage, heat, and cold. Short-term manipulation does have some modest benefits but repetitive manipulation or its use in chronic low back pain is not valid. Until further studies prove their clinical usefulness, these techniques should not be used on a long-term basis because many are costly, time-consuming, and counterproductive.

The use of various medications has similarly shown no

significant benefit over aspirin or acetaminophen. Despite the popularity of the nonsteroidal anti-inflammatory drugs, none has been shown to be significantly better than aspirin or acetaminophen. Narcotic medications should be used with great caution because of their addictive and depressant side effects. Diazepam and similar medications have not been shown to affect the course of idiopathic low back pain, nor do they have a direct relaxing effect.

Chronic Low Back Pain

Patients with chronic, disabling low back pain have become a major socioeconomic factor in modern industrial society. Those few patients with persistent low back pain after six months account for a great percentage of the dollars spent on medical care and disability. Only recently has an organized, comprehensive approach been formulated to deal with this difficult problem.

These patients have been treated with a variety of therapeutic approaches. Pain clinics have used a variety of passive and invasive therapies, including manipulation, electrical stimulation, acupuncture, biofeedback, trigger-point injections, and epidural steroids. These measures have met with little success. Similar poor results have been found with repeated attempts at surgical intervention for the relief of chronic low back pain.

This complex psychosocial problem makes diagnosis and treatment extremely difficult. Recent studies have dealt with this dilemma with varying success. It is clear that patients receiving worker's compensation and those with ongoing litigation have a distinctly worse prognosis for recovery than other patients. One of the few variables that can reliably predict therapeutic success is the patient's age. Patients with chronic low back pain who are more than 50 years old are less likely to return to work than patients less that 50 years old.

The value of psychologic tests, and the Minnesota Multiphasic Personality Inventory, in particular, in predicting treatment outcome is now being questioned. However, there does seem to be some correlation of treatment success with the psychologist's and physician's impression of the patient at the initial interview.

With recent advances in ergonomic research, a great deal of information is now available pertaining to the trunk-strength and motion requirements of certain job-related tasks. Programs directed at restoring these normal trunk-strength parameters are the only therapies that have resulted in significant recovery in the chronically disabled. Prospective studies now available have documented the success of functional restoration programs in returning patients with chronic low back pain to a productive lifestyle. These programs appear to be the only type of comprehensive therapy with a significant degree of clinical success in improving the poor prognosis of patients with low back pain.

Herniated Lumbar Disk

Anular fractures or disruption of the normal concentric structure of the posterior anulus can result in protrusion of disk material that causes nerve root compression. The severity of this internal disruption determines the severity of the herniation. A partial tear or disruption of the outer anulus results in a bulging disk; complete disruption of the an-ulus and posterior ligament allows migration of the anular and nuclear material, resulting in a sequestered disk herniation.

It is important that a true disk herniation not be confused with a degenerative disk. Disk degeneration occurs normally as part of aging and is characterized by predictable biochemical, structural, and biomechanical alterations in the anulus and nucleus pulposus, resulting in disk-space narrowing and concentric disk bulging. This is distinctly different from a disk herniation with localized anular and nuclear abnormalities resulting in the herniation.

The disk herniation is clinically significant only if nerve root compression occurs. Back pain is often absent. Herniation of L3-4 causes impingement of the L-4 nerve root. Characteristic signs of an L3-4 herniation are quadriceps and anterior tibialis weakness, decreased knee jerk, sensory changes over the medial aspect of the knee, and a reverse straight leg raising test that is positive. Less than 10% of all lumbar disk herniations are at the L3-4 level.

Herniation of L4-5 compresses the L-5 nerve root. A very large or medial disk herniation can also result in compression of the S-1 nerve root. Compression of the L-5 nerve root produces decreased extensor hallucis longus strength and altered sensation over the lateral calf and first dorsal web space. Herniation of L5-S1 compresses the S-1 nerve root with decreased plantar flexion strength, sensation over the lateral foot, and a diminished ankle jerk. L4-5 and L5-S1 herniations together constitute more than 90% of all symptomatic lumbar disk herniations.

On rare occasions, extreme lateral or proximal disk herniations can compress the nerve root above the level of the herniation. A large disk herniation can compress the lower sacral roots, causing subsequent bladder or bowel dysfunction and resulting in cauda equina syndrome.

The most common misdiagnosis is mistaking referred low back pain for sciatica. It must be remembered that referred pain rarely radiates below the knee and has no associated objective neurologic findings. It is highly unusual for a lumbar disk herniation to cause bilateral sciatic pain. Patients with objective bilateral lower-extremity neurologic loss and sciatica should be examined thoroughly for the presence of an intraspinal lesion other than a disk herniation.

Initial treatment for most patients with sciatica should be conservative. Only cases involving bladder or bowel dysfunction (cauda equina syndrome) should be regarded as emergencies. These patients should undergo immediate magnetic resonance imaging or myelography to determine the cause of the neurologic dysfunction. Patients seen immediately after the onset of sciatic pain should have a brief period of bed rest. A return to restricted activities appears to be more beneficial than prolonged bed rest once the pain subsides.

Medication should be directed at pain relief without the depressant or addictive effects of narcotic medication. Nonsteroidal anti-inflammatory pain medication is preferable to narcotic medications, but may be no more helpful than aspirin or acetaminophen. Diazepam and similar central nervous system depressants have only a limited role in the treatment of the patient with low back pain or sciatica.

The use of epidural steroids to alleviate the sciatic pain caused by a herniated disk has been widely advocated. Prospective and retrospective studies have shown little long-term benefit of epidural steroid use in the patient with sciatic pain, but they may provide short-term relief in approximately 50% of patients. Further studies are needed before the use of epidural steroids in the treatment of sciatica from a herniated disk or spinal stenosis can be encouraged or condemned.

Manipulative therapy of various types has been advocated in the treatment of the herniated lumbar disk. These have included lumbar traction, autotraction, self-manipulation with various exercise regimens, immobilization, and manipulation. Although short-term success has been reported, none has been shown to have any long-term effect on symptoms. Prolonged hospitalization with bed rest and traction can no longer be recommended.

In the absence of significant, progressive neurologic loss, diagnostic testing can be delayed until four to six weeks after the onset of symptoms. Only 5% to 10% of patients with persistent sciatica will ultimately require surgical intervention. The ideal diagnostic procedure for evaluation of a suspected disk herniation is magnetic resonance imaging. Unlike myelography, it is noninvasive, requires no hospitalization, and is equally sensitive, specific, and accurate in delineating a lumbar disk herniation.

Myelography should be reserved for those few cases in which magnetic resonance imaging is equivocal and the objective clinical findings are strongly suggestive of nerve root compression. Computed tomography is also highly sensitive and specific and is a good alternative if magnetic resonance imaging is not available. Regardless of which test is used, it is of the utmost importance that the radiographic findings correlate with the patient's symptoms and findings. No invasive procedure should be recommended in the absence of this correlation. Inconsistencies between the clinical and radiographic findings warrant further diagnostic studies before definitive treatment is recommended.

Surgical Treatment of the Herniated Disk

A formal laminectomy seems unnecessary for the treatment of a simple herniated lumbar disk. Limited surgical disk excision is as effective and can be performed by removing only the ligamentum flavum on the affected side, accompanied by a minimal laminotomy and lateral recess decompression performed when necessary. The disk herniation should not be performed until adequate nerve root decompression is accomplished. Attempts to remove more disk material add little to the long-term results and increase the risk of vascular injury. Limited surgical disk excision in selected patients should result in a success rate of approximately 90%.

For many years spinal fusion was commonly performed along with the standard surgical disk excision. Recent studies have shown that at long-term follow-up patients undergoing disk excision and fusion do no better and perhaps less than patients undergoing only disk excision. Spinal fusion has only a limited role in lumbar disk excision.

Several factors can affect the success rate. Patients with motor weakness and severe sciatica appear to have diminished success if surgery is delayed longer than 12 weeks. Laborers and worker's compensation patients typically have lower success rates than other patients. Patients with exaggerated functional complaints and other measurable psychological disturbances do more poorly than well-adjusted patients. Despite the varied factors responsible for compromised surgical success, most postoperative failures are the result of inappropriate patient selection and a lack of correlative objective and abnormal radiographic findings.

Chemonucleolysis

Chemonucleolysis remains an alternative, albeit a controversial one, to surgical disk excision and has a success rate of approximately 75%. In a short-term retrospective study, the initial success rate was less than that expected with surgical disk excision, but follow-up at ten years revealed the results to be comparable.

Reports of neurologic complications after chymopapain injection have significantly reduced the routine use of chemonucleolysis. There appears to be both clinical and experimental evidence that the concomitant use of chymopapain and diskographic contrast agent inadvertently injected intrathecally may cause transverse myelitis and paralysis. Diskography must not be performed at the same time as the chemonucleolysis procedure.

The procedure should not be performed with the patient under general anesthesia. The use of local anesthesia is associated with a lower incidence of anaphylaxis.

Postoperative Rehabilitation

Postoperative rehabilitation appears to be important in the comprehensive care of the patient with a herniated lumbar disk. Recent studies have found significantly decreased postoperative isokinetic, isometric, and endurance strength. A combined flexion and extension program should be initiated three to six weeks after surgery to correct the strength loss.

Spinal Stenosis

The most common cause of spinal stenosis is degenerative changes in the lumbar disk and facet joint complex. It typically affects men and women over the age of 60 years and is more commonly found in the eighth decade of life. Spinal stenosis was thought to result primarily from bony impingement on the neural structures. However, with the advent of computed tomographic scanning, it became evident that the primary component of the stenosis was soft-tissue (ligamentum flavum, disk) compression of the dural sac. One study found the anteroposterior measurement of the bony canal to be far less accurate than the anteroposterior measurements of the dural sac on computed tomography or myelography. An anteroposterior diameter of 10 mm or a cross-sectional area of 100 mm^2 was the most accurate measure of lumbar spinal stenosis. Surgical decisions based on computed tomography alone are significantly less reliable than those using myelography as well. At this time, the diagnostic role of magnetic resonance imaging is increasing, but the procedure of choice is still the combination of myelography and contrast-enhanced computed tomography. With continued improvement in the diagnostic ability of magnetic resonance imaging, this is likely to change.

Although degenerative central spinal stenosis and/or lateral recess stenosis are the most common causes, other abnormalities can result in lumbar spinal stenosis. Congenital narrowing of the spine unassociated with achondroplasia or several of the other dwarfing syndromes has been shown to cause spinal stenosis. Spinal stenosis can be secondary to degenerative scoliosis and/or spondylolisthesis. Iatrogenic spinal stenosis can follow posterior lumbar spinal fusion, particularly at the level above the fusion. Other causes of spinal stenosis include primary and metastatic tumors and metabolic disorders, including Paget's disease and acromegaly.

The history and physical findings typical of spinal stenosis are distinctly different from and less consistent than those of a herniated lumbar disk. Patients with spinal stenosis frequently report claudication that is relieved by rest or bending forward. The symptoms can be re-created during the physical examination by extension of the lumbar spine and alleviated by forward flexion.

Symptoms do not always radiate into the usual dermatomal distribution, as would be expected in a disk herniation. The pain is often bilateral and may radiate into the buttocks, groin, thighs, or lower extremities. Paresthesias often accompany the pain and are relieved by changes in body posture. Although motor deficits are frequently absent, patients often complain of a feeling of heaviness in the lower extremities when walking. The positive neural tension signs are typically absent.

The most important element in the differential diagnosis is identifying the presence of peripheral vascular disease, which often resembles the symptoms of neural claudication.

Conservative treatment of spinal stenosis is relatively unsuccessful. Early symptoms can be treated with nonsteroidal anti-inflammatory medication. However, once claudication becomes pronounced, non-narcotic medication is rarely helpful. Narcotic medication must be used with great caution in elderly patients. Most elderly patients with spinal stenosis exhibit clinical signs of depression. Narcotic medication can exaggerate this depression.

There are no available data showing that any form of physical therapy, manipulation, or bracing has any significant prolonged effect on the symptoms of spinal stenosis. Epidural steroids can be helpful in the short-term relief of symptoms, but whether there is any significant long-term relief is controversial. Once the radiographic diagnosis has been established in a symptomatic patient, surgical decompression should be performed. Surgical decompression consists of alleviating all bony and soft-tissue compression present on the preoperative radiographs. Care should be taken to preserve the integrity of the facet joint complex when decompressing the lateral recess. Disk excision is not necessary and may add to postoperative morbidity in spinal stenosis unless there is actual herniation of the disk. Unnecessary excision of a degenerative disk is thought to predispose to further motion segment collapse and potential instability.

Overall, the results of spinal stenosis surgery are generally good. Reported good results range from 71% to 85%. The best results are in patients with lateral recess stenosis and/or central stenosis. Patients with other causes of spinal stenosis, particularly degenerative spondylolisthesis and/or scoliosis, do less well. According to one study, fewer than 10% of patients have increased symptoms postoperatively but approximately 5% will need additional surgery.

Postoperatively, patients should be encouraged to walk. This will improve lower-extremity strength and endurance as well as general cardiovascular conditioning, which is often compromised by the patient's prolonged preoperative immobility.

Spondylolisthesis

Degenerative spondylolisthesis, a focal type of spinal stenosis, results from degenerative changes involving the facet joints and intervertebral disk. These degenerative joint alterations produce abnormal segmental motion, resulting in spondylolisthesis, retrolisthesis, or lateral translational deformities. The resulting deformity may cause mechanical pain with or without sciatica or claudication.

Unfortunately, there are no definitive data correlating the radiographic presence of spondylolisthesis and clinical symptoms. Each case must be evaluated radiographically and clinically to ensure that the patient's symptoms correlate with the radiographic abnormalities. If it is determined radiographically and clinically that surgical intervention is indicated, preoperative planning is necessary. Adequate neurologic decompression is recommended when there is clinical and radiographic evidence of neural compression. Otherwise decompression is not necessary, and only a spinal fusion to stabilize the spondylolisthesis should be performed.

Regardless of the presence of neurologic involvement, a solid fusion must be obtained to prevent further mechanical symptoms and/or neurologic sequelae. During the last several years, the internal-fixation devices available for use in the lumbar spine have proliferated. They include Steffee plates, Luque and Edwards frames, Wiltse plates, and Cotrel-Dubousset instrumentation. The plate-fixation systems employ a rigid plate connected to the spine with pedicle-screw fixation. The Edwards and Cotrel-Dubousset instrumentation systems utilize a rod fixed to the spine with pedicular screws or more traditional spinal hooks. At this time, not all of these systems have been approved for general use in the lumbar spine by the Food and Drug Administration.

Several preliminary studies have reported encouraging results with supplemental internal fixation to stabilize and/or reduce degenerative spondylolisthesis. However, the risk of neurologic complications is significantly higher than with traditional bilateral lateral fusion, and some series report a higher infection rate. Before the new instrumentation is used, the advantages of reducing the spondylolisthesis must be weighed against the risk of the instrumentation. At this time, no long-term studies are available that prove that the results of fusion with internal fixation are superior to the results of bilateral lateral fusion with its lower risk of neurologic complications. Further studies are necessary to clarify this controversy, as well as to clarify which internal fixation systems are clinically superior.

Iatrogenic spondylolisthesis can also occur after laminectomy with bilateral facetectomy or pars interarticularis resection. If the pars interarticularis or facet joints are surgically excised, fusion of that level should be performed. Failure to recognize this potential cause of instability can result in a progressive spondylolisthesis not present preoperatively.

Regardless of the presence or absence of internal fixation, a meticulous bilateral lateral fusion should be performed to prevent pseudarthrosis. Midline posterior fusion should be avoided in the lumbar spine because of the increased risk of iatrogenic spinal stenosis. Clinical and experimental studies have shown that adjunctive electrical stimulation can decrease the risk of pseudarthrosis and enhance lumbar spinal fusion. However, this is not uniformly accepted and further prospective studies are needed before electrical stimulation can be recommended.

Lumbar Instability

No radiographic measurements or objective clinical signs are uniformly accepted as describing clinical or symptomatic lumbar instability. Investigators have used translations of 3 mm or more at L3–4 and L4–5 and 5 mm or more at L5-S1 or angulation of 10 degrees or more of a motion segment to document lumbar instability. However, a more recent report has shown that flexion-extension radiography was not useful in the diagnosis of lumbar instability. There was no statistical correlation between the abnormal flexion-extension motion noted on radiographs and the clinical symptoms. Unfortunately, studies such as this further confuse an area in which clear radiographic and clinical diagnostic criteria are needed but do not exist.

A new radiographic technique has recently been described to document clinically symptomatic lumbar instability. By using dynamic traction and compression radiography, clinically symptomatic instability was reportedly diagnosed more reliably than by conventional flexion-extension radiographs. As in previous studies, standard flexion-extension radiographs did not correlate with the degree of back pain experienced by these patients, but dynamic radiography did. Further studies and continued use of this diagnostic technique will determine its clinical practicality and effectiveness.

Although there are no accepted standards by which to measure lumbar instability, the suggestion of its presence either radiographically or clinically has been used to justify lumbar spinal fusion. Similarly, the presence of "internal disk derangement" on magnetic resonance imaging or computed tomographic diskography has been used as a criterion for recommending spinal fusion in patients with only low back pain. There are currently no prospective data documenting the clinical effectiveness of lumbar spinal fusion in patients with low back pain emanating from suspected lumbar instability or internal disk derangement. This lack of adequate scientific data should be considered before spinal fusion is recommended for a patient with chronic low back pain and radiographic "evidence" of lumbar instability. In a retrospective analysis, patients undergoing posterior fusion for a variety of diagnoses were found at follow-up to have more low back pain than the normal population, although most were not in severe pain. Despite this study's limitations, it did point out the need for clear, well-defined criteria for recommending spinal fusion for "instability" or internal disk derangement.

Pregnancy

During pregnancy, lumbar disk herniations are rare, but low back pain is relatively common. In one large study, 56% of pregnant women experienced low back pain during pregnancy. Most patients began to experience pain between the fifth and seventh months. The mother's weight gain, the baby's weight, or the number of previous pregnancies or children apparently did not have a significant effect on the incidence of low back pain. Although several theories have been proposed to explain the increased incidence of low back pain during pregnancy, including increased ligamentous laxity and change in spinal alignment, none have been conclusively proven to cause low back pain in pregnant women.

Coccygodynia

Treatment of coccygodynia is directed at relieving pain. Conservative measures, such as donut-shaped cushions, of-

fer temporary relief. There are no data to support the efficacy of local steroid injections.

Surgical excision of the coccyx for relief of pain is controversial. A large study of carefully selected patients with coccygodynia reported 88% good results in relieving preoperative symptoms. Despite these good results, coccygectomy is not widely accepted as the treatment of choice for persistent and painful coccygodynia, and there are data showing little benefit.

Lumbar Spine Osteolysis

Lumbar spine osteolysis has recently been described as a condition manifested by vertebral osteomyelitis and/or spinal stenosis. The cause is unclear. Lumbar spine osteolysis typically includes severe back pain and lower-extremity symptoms after radical decompressive procedures. Bone biopsy specimens are normal, as is the erythrocyte sedimentation rate. The radiographic appearance is one of progressive vertebral osteolysis in the presence of continued motion segment displacement (spinal instability). Appropriate treatment includes biopsy to exclude infection or tumor, followed by stabilization and fusion. Studies of its cause and natural history and the results of treatment are needed.

Controversies

Diskography

The popularity of diskography has waxed and waned over the last several decades. With the increased use of chemonucleolysis in the last decade, it has again been advocated as a diagnostic tool in patients with lumbar spine disease. Although diskography is an invasive procedure, the risk of infection is relatively low. Use of an 18-gauge needle without a stylet led to an infection rate of 2.7%. The incidence of diskitis can be reduced to 0.7% with the use of styletted needles and a two-needle technique at each level.

Diskography has a dual role as a diagnostic procedure. It has been used primarily to visualize the anatomic structure and integrity of the disk after the injection of a contrast agent. Originally this was done with anteroposterior and lateral plain radiographs, but more recently computed tomographic diskography has yielded superior imaging of the injected disk (Fig. 3). Classification systems have been devised in an attempt to correlate the symptoms, the anatomic severity of the degenerative disk disease, and the radiographic appearance of the diskogram.

Secondarily, the injected contrast agent has been used as a provocative test in an attempt to elicit or re-create the patient's pain and symptoms. A so-called positive provocation test is one in which the patient's back and/or radicular pain is re-created at the time of injection. It has also been postulated that a "normal" disk can accept less than 1 ml of fluid. There are no clinical data available to support this theory.

With the increased ability to recognize degenerative changes within the disk, the concept of "internal disk derangement" has evolved. It has been theorized that the internal disruption of the normal anatomic disk structure leads to pain and instability. Several studies have used abnormal computed tomographic diskography and provocation test data as criteria to recommend surgical diskectomy

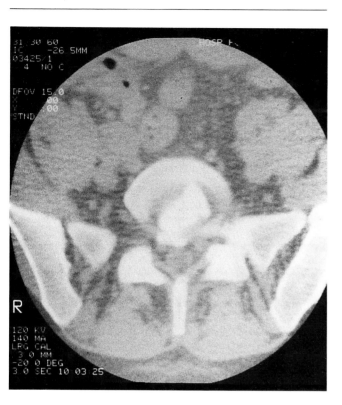

Figure 3

Computed tomographic diskography reveals anular disruption and accumulation of dye under the right nerve root.

debate about whether diskography is still needed at all. A study of magnetic resonance imaging and diskography in patients with low back pain was done to assess the relative accuracy of the two techniques in evaluating degenerative disk disease. Magnetic resonance imaging was 99% accurate in confirming abnormalities of the disk seen on computed tomographic diskography. Therefore, magnetic resonance imaging appears to be as effective as computed tomographic diskography but is less painful and invasive in evaluating early or long-standing degenerative disk disease. The remaining question is whether pain provocation yields enough clinical information to make diskography superior to magnetic resonance imaging.

Microdiskectomy

Proponents of microdiskectomy claim that the limited surgical exposure allows shorter hospitalization, less surgical trauma, and less postoperative scarring, thus resulting in improved success. Critics of microdiskectomy claim that the limited surgical approach increases the risk of missing sequestered disk fragments and decreases the ability to visualize and decompress a stenotic lateral recess. A recent comparative retrospective analysis of age-matched patients undergoing either limited surgical diskectomy or microdiskectomy found that neither procedure offered a clinical advantage over the other, except for decreased hospitalization in the microdiskectomy group. Microscopic magnification does not appear to have any clinical advantage over standard disk excision with respect to surgical success and resolution of preoperative symptoms.

Percutaneous Diskectomy

The latest in treatment alternatives to surgical diskectomy is percutaneous diskectomy. The first percutaneous diskectomy procedures were performed with modified pituitary rongeurs directed posterolaterally into the affected disk through a sheath or trochar. A portion of the disk was then removed manually with the rongeur. The latest innovation in this technique is the development of an automated suction device for removing a limited amount of disk material.

The procedure should be performed with the patient awake. Local anesthesia and sedation are used. The probe should be placed in the central portion of the disk under strict radiographic control to avoid improper placement of the device.

This procedure should only be performed in patients with a documented disk herniation and concomitant sciatic signs and symptoms who would otherwise be considered for surgical intervention. It should not be performed in patients with only back pain and mild disk bulging without sciatic symptoms. The presence of a sequestered fragment is a contraindication to this procedure, and magnetic resonance imaging should be performed to eliminate those patients.

Initial reports gave success rates of approximately 70% to 80%. A more recent study reported less favorable results, with only 55% of patients able to return to work after the procedure. Further studies are necessary to validate its use, long-term efficacy, complications, and precise indications.

and lumbar spinal fusion. Unfortunately, an almost equal number of studies have found diskography to be misleading because the significant number of false-positive and false-negative diskograms make appropriate recommendations difficult. In one prospective study of 137 patients in whom preoperative diskography showed abnormal images and a positive provocation test, 89% had significant postoperative relief of their symptoms. However, pain was relieved in only 52% of those with radiographic abnormalities but without a positive provocation test.

Other studies have shown no advantage of computed tomographic diskography over myelography and computed tomography. Comparisons of in vitro and in vivo diskography with histologic and surgical findings revealed an extremely high incidence of false-negative results. The diskograms were false-negative in 32% of patients with protruded disk herniations confirmed at surgery and 56% of patients with prolapsed disk herniations. Despite these confusing results, some authorities strongly advocate diskography as the diagnostic test of choice for low back pain that is chronic and disabling. Others argue that neither the test nor the syndrome is valid.

It is obvious from these conflicting studies that diskography cannot be relied on as the sole diagnostic test before disk excision or lumbar fusion. In fact, the improvement in the quality of magnetic resonance imaging has now led to

Annotated Bibliography

Keywords

Chemonucleolysis; Chronic pain syndrome; Coccygodynia; Computed tomography; Diskectomy; Intervertebral disk; Low back pain; Lumbar spine; Magnetic resonance imaging; Myelography; Percutaneous diskectomy; Pregnancy; Radiography; Scintigraphy; Spondylolisthesis; Stenosis; Thermography

Epidemiology

Deyo RA, Tsui-Wu YJ: Descriptive epidemiology of low-back pain and its related medical care in the United States. *Spine* 1987;12:264–268.

Epidemiologic data were derived from more than 10,000 responses to the National Health and Nutrition Examination Survey II. There were 1,763 positive respondents (only pain lasting two weeks was included as a positive response). The cumulative lifetime prevalence was 13.8%. This study also presents meaningful data relating to the age distribution and primary care of patients with low back pain.

Deyo RA, Tsui-Wu YJ: Functional disability due to back pain. *Arthritis Rheum* 1987;30:1247–1253.

A survey of 1,516 men and women attempted to correlate low back pain disability with socioeconomic factors. A variety of correlates emerged with various social and job-related factors affecting work performance and absenteeism. The most significant correlation (P <.001) was that more education correlated with fewer disability days.

Frymoyer JW, Cats-Baril W: Predictors of low back pain disability. *Clin Orthop* 1987;221:89–98.

This study presents a hypothetical model of a new method of predicting low back pain disability. The multiple variables affecting the chronicity of low back pain, including the physiologic, social, and psychological aspects of low back disability, are discussed.

Hadler NM: Regional musculoskeletal diseases of the low back: Cumulative trauma versus single incident. *Clin Orthop* 1987;221:33–41.

Review of the complex medical, social, vocational, and ergonomic aspects of low back pain.

Spitzer WO, et al: Scientific approach to the assessment and management of activity-related spinal disorders. *Spine* 1987;12:75.

This is a special supplement examining the current state of the epidemiology, diagnosis, and treatment of low back disorders containing an exhaustive bibliography (769 references).

Svenssonn HO, Andersson GB: Low back pain in 40- to 47-year-old men: Work history and work enviroment factors. *Spine* 1983;8:272–276.

A survey of 940 men 40 to 47 years old was done in an attempt to correlate work history and ergonomic factors with low back pain. Ten variables were found in a univariate analysis while three variables correlated with a covariance analysis. These were less overtime work, monotonous work, and a high degree of lifting.

Svensson HO, Vedin A, Wilhelmsson C, et al: Low-back pain in relation to other diseases and cardiovascular risk factors. *Spine* 1983;8:277–285.

The lifetime incidence of low back pain was found to be 61% with a prevalence of 31% in a random survey of 940 men aged 40 to 47 years. After analysis, four variables maintained a direct association with low back pain. They were calf pain on exertion, smoking, work involving high levels of physical activity, and frequent worry and tension. This study emphasizes the multisystem complexity of low back pain.

Imaging Techniques

Radiography

Frymoyer JW, Newberg A, Pope MH, et al: Spine radiographs in patients with low-back pain: An epidemiological study in men. *J Bone Joint Surg* 1984;66A:1048–1055.

A radiographic and clinical survey of 321 men attempted to identify any correlation between radiographic findings and symptoms. Only L4-5 disk-space narrowing and traction spurs correlated with low back pain and sciatica. No other radiographic abnormalities were found to have any correlation with symptoms.

Kaplan DM, Knapp M, Romm FJ, et al: Low back pain and x-ray films of the lumbar spine: A prospective study in primary care. *South Med J* 1986;79:811–814.

A prospective study of 96 men evaluated spinal radiographs and the incidence of pain and various treatment patterns. Seventy percent were found to have radiographic degenerative joint disease, but there was no correlation of radiographic abnormalities and symptoms. However, those diagnosed as having degenerative joint disease were more likely to be treated with anti-inflammatory medication and were more satisfied with their treatment.

Witt I, Vestergaard A, Rosenklint A: A comparative analysis of x-ray findings of the lumbar spine in patients with and without lumbar pain. *Spine* 1984;9:298–300.

There was no correlation of disk degeneration and spondylosis with symptoms in a series of 238 symptomatic patients and 66 patients with no low back pain.

Myelography, Computed Tomography, and Magnetic Resonance Imaging

Bell GR, Rothman RH, Booth RE, et al: A study of computer-assisted tomography: II. Comparison of metrizamide myelography and computed tomography in the diagnosis of herniated lumbar disc and spinal stenosis. *Spine* 1984;9:552–556.

This study of 122 patients undergoing surgery for spinal stenosis or a herniated disk compared myelography with computed tomographic scanning. Myelography proved superior in diagnosing both spinal stenosis and a herniated disk.

Bolender NF, Schönström NS, Spengler DM: Role of computed tomography and myelography in the diagnosis of central spinal stenosis. *J Bone Joint Surg* 1985;67A:240–246.

This analysis of 24 patients undergoing decompression for spinal stenosis compared preoperative myelography with computed tomographic scanning. The most reliable measurement was the dimensions of the dural sac on the lateral myelogram.

Bosacco SJ, Berman AT, Garbarino JL, et al: A comparison of CT scanning and myelography in the diagnosis of lumbar disc herniation. *Clin Orthop* 1984;190:124–128.

A group of 134 patients had computed tomographic scanning and myelography before surgery for lumbar disk herniations. No significant difference in diagnostic accuracy beteen the two techniques was found.

Herkowitz HN, Garfin SR, Bell GR, et al: The use of computerized tomography in evaluating non-visualized vertebral levels caudad to a complete block on a lumbar myelogram: A review of thirty-two cases. *J Bone Joint Surg* 1987;69A:218–224.

Of 32 patients with complete myelographic block, 59% had additional intraspinal abnormalities caudad to the block. These were visualized on postmyelogram computed tomography and confirmed at surgery.

Hueffle MG, Modic MT, Ross JS, et al: Lumbar spine: Postoperative MR imaging with GD-DTRA. *Radiology* 1988;167:817–824.

Thirty patients with recurrent disk herniations were evaluated with magnetic resonance imaging enhanced with gadolinium. Results were quite promising in differentiating postoperative scar and recurrent disk material.

Masaryk TJ, Ross JS, Modic MT, et al: High resolution of MR imaging of sequestered lumbar intervertebral disks. *AJR* 1988;150:1155–1162.

In this retrospective review of 20 patients with surgically documented sequestered disk her niations, magnetic resonance imaging had an 89% sensitivity, 82% specificity, and an 85% accuracy for diagnosing sequestered fragments.

Schipper J, Kardaun JW, Braakman R, et al: Lumbar disk herniation: Diagnosis with CT or myelography. *Radiology* 1987;165:227–231.

A series of 461 patients with disk herniations was evaluated with myelography and computed tomography. The authors concluded that computed tomography could have replaced myelography in as many as two thirds of the cases.

Bone Scintigraphy

van-den Oever M, Merrick MV, Scott JH: Bone scintigraphy in symptomatic spondylolysis. *J Bone Joint Surg* 1987;69B:453–456.

In a review of 66 patients with back pain and suspected spondylolysis, bone scintigraphy was shown to be useful in detecting active healing of the defect, established nonunion of the defect, and impending fractures of the defect.

Electrodiagnostic Studies

Ahern DK, Follick MJ, Council JR, et al: Reliability of lumbar paravertebral EMG assessment in chronic low back pain. *Arch Phys Med Rehabil* 1986;67:762–765.

Statistical analysis of electromyographic levels of the paravertebral levels in 40 postoperative patients and 30 nonsurgical patients showed no significant differences.

Haldeman S, Shouka M, Robboy S: Computed tomography, electromagnetic and clinical findings in chronic worker's compensation patients with back and leg pain. *Spine* 1988;13:345–350.

This was a comparative study of electromyographic, computed tomographic, and clinical findings in 100 patients with chronic sciatica and low back pain. Electromyographic findings were highly predictive of computed tomographic abnormalities but no diagnostic study was conclusive by itself.

Miller DJ: Comparison of electromyographic activity in the lumbar paraspinal muscles of subjects with and without chronic low back pain. *Phys Ther* 1985;65:1347–1354.

Paravertebral electromyography recordings done during normal activities in a group of asymptomatic subjects and a group of patients with chronic low back pain showed no differences between the groups.

Swash M, Snooks SJ: Slowed motor conduction in lumbosacral nerve roots in cauda equina lesions: A new diagnostic technique. *J Neurol Neurosurg Psychiatr* 1986; 49:808–816.

The authors reviewed the techniques and results of spinal stimulation and monitoring in 32 controls and ten symptomatic patients.

Thermography

Frymoyer JW, Haugh LD: Thermography: A call for scientific studies to establish its diagnostic efficacy. *Orthopedics* 1986;9:699–700.

A description of the methods of thermography and a call for scientific studies to validate its use.

Low Back Pain

Deyo RA, Diehl AK, Rosenthal M: How many days of bedrest for acute low back pain? *N Engl J Med* 1986; 315:1064–1070.

A randomized study of 203 patients with mechanical low back pain treated with either two or seven days of bed rest. Patients treated with two days of rest lost fewer days of work and had no difference in symptoms at follow-up.

Frymoyer JW: Back pain and sciatica. *N Engl J Med* 1988;318:291–300.

An excellent review of the treatment of nonsurgical and surgical low back disorders. An excellent bibliography covering all topics.

Hadler NM: Regional back pain. *N Engl J Med* 1986; 315:1090–1092.

Overview of the presentation, evaluation, and treatment of the patient with acute low back pain.

Jackson RP, Jacobs RR, Montesano PX: Facet joint injection in low-back pain. *Spine* 1988;13:966–971.

A prospective study of 454 patients with low back pain evaluated with facet joint injections. From the results of this study, it was not possible to identify clinical facet joint syndromes or predict patients responding well to the procedure.

Waddell G: 1987 Volvo award in clinical sciences: A new clinical model for the treatment of low-back pain. *Spine* 1987;12:632–644.

An extensive review of the conservative treatment of low back pain. Prolonged bed rest appears to be harmful and an early return to activity and exercises is strongly recommended to restore normal function.

Chronic Low Back Pain

Fredrickson BE, Trief PM, Van Bevern P, et al: Rehabilitation of the patient with chronic back pain. *Spine* 1988;13:351–353.

Prospective study of patients with chronic low back pain. A thorough analysis of risk factors and prognostic indicators to predict clinical success in patients undergoing rehabilitation for chronic back pain.

Mayer TG, Gatchel RJ, Kishino N, et al: Objective assessment of spine function following industrial injury: A prospective study with comparison group and one-year follow-up. *Spine* 1985;10:482–493.

Prospective study of 66 patients with chronic low back pain treated in a functional restoration program compared to 38 patients with chronic low back pain without similar treatment. Functional improvement was found in 80% of patients treated with twice as many treated patients able to return to work by one year.

Herniated Lumbar Disk

Cuckler JM, Bernini PA, Wiesel SW, et al: The use of epidural steroids in the treatment of lumbar radicular pain: A prospective, randomized, double-blind study. *J Bone Joint Surg* 1985;67A:63–66.

A prospective study of patients with sciatica secondary to a disk herniation or spinal stenosis. No significant difference in relief was found between the group treated with steroids and procaine and the group treated with procaine alone.

Fraser RD: Chymopapain for the treatment of the intervertebral disc herniation: The final report of a double-blind study. *Spine* 1984;9:815–818.

A prospective double-blind study of 60 patients undergoing either chymopapain or saline injections. Two years after injection, 77% of the chymopapain group were improved compared with 47% in the control group.

Haldeman S: Spinal manipulative therapy: A status report. *Clin Orthop* 1983;179:62–70.

A review of the various manipulative techniques and theories. Best results were obtained in patients with acute low back pain without sciatica. There does not appear to be any proven long-term benefit of manipulation.

Kahanovitz N, Viola K, McCulloch J: Limited surgical discectomy and microdiscectomy: A clinical comparison. *Spine*, in press.

A comparative analysis of matched groups of patients undergoing either limited surgical diskectomy or microdiskectomy for a herniated disk. There was no superiority of either technique in the relief of pain, symptoms, or return to work. Microdiskectomy patients were hospitalized fewer days than limited surgical diskectomy patients.

Kostuik JP, Harrington I, Alexander D, et al: Cauda equina syndrome and lumbar disc herniation. *J Bone Joint Surg* 1986;68A:386–391.

A retrospective review of 31 patients with cauda equina syndrome secondary to a herniated disk. Good results followed surgical decompression in 27 patients. Timing of surgery did not correlate with good results, although it was recommended that surgery be performed as quickly as possible after the onset of bladder symptoms.

McDermott DJ, Agre K, Brim M, et al: Chymodiactin in patients with herniated lumbar intervertebral disc(s): An open-label, multicenter study. *Spine* 1985;10:242–249.

A multicenter study of 1,498 patients with herniated disk treated wih chymodiactin. Success was attained in 79% to 88% of patients depending on the criteria. The incidence, etiology, and treatment of anaphylaxis and neurologic complications are discussed.

Onik G, Helms CA, Ginsburg L: Percutaneous lumbar discectomy using a new asperation probe. *Am J Radiol* 1985;144:1137–1140.

Descriptive review of the technique of and indications for percutaneous diskectomy.

Rosen C, Kahanovitz N, Viola K, et al: A retrospective analysis of the efficacy of epidural steroid injections. *Clin Orthop* 1988;228:270–272.

A retrospective analysis of 40 patients undergoing epidural steroid injections for the treatment of sciatica. Short-term relief was obtained but there did not appear to be any significant long-term benefit.

Spengler DM: Lumbar discectomy: Results with limited disc excision and selective foraminotomy. *Spine* 1982;7:604–607.

Description and results of limited surgical diskectomy in pa-tients with a unilateral disk herniation. Good results were found in 91% of patients.

Weber H: Lumbar disc herniation: A controlled, prospective study with ten years of observation. *Spine* 1983;8:131–140.

A prospective study of 280 patients with disk herniation. Surgically treated patients had significantly better results at one and four years, but the difference was no longer significant at ten years.

White AH, von Rogov P, Zucherman J, et al: Lumbar laminectomy for herniated disc: A prospective controlled comparison with internal fixation fusion. *Spine* 1987;12:305–307.

A prospective study of 69 patients treated by surgical diskectomy with and without fusion. Overall success was 87%, but results were better in patients without fusion. Fusion should not be done routinely in the patient with a disk herniation.

Yasuma T, Makino E, Saito S, et al: Histological development of intervertebral disc herniation. *J Bone Joint Surg* 1986;68A:1066–1072.

Histologic demonstration of the various physiologic and pathologic changes occurring in the herniated disk.

Spinal Stenosis

Hall S, Bartleson JD, Onofrio BM, et al: Lumbar spinal stenosis: Clinical features, diagnostic procedures and results of surgical treatment in 68 patients. *Ann Intern Med* 1985;103:271–275.

A review of 68 patients undergoing decompression for spinal stenosis. Eighty-four percent had good or excellent results.

Nasca RJ: Surgical management of lumbar spinal stenosis. *Spine* 1987;12:809–816.

A review of 80 patients treated surgically for spinal stenosis of various origins. Results were good in 71%, with the best results in those with central and/or lateral recess stenosis.

Spondylolisthesis

Hanley EN Jr: Decompression and distraction-derotation arthrodesis for degenerative spondylolisthesis. *Spine* 1986;11:269–276.

A review of 20 patients with symptomatic degenerative L4–5 spondylolisthesis. Satisfactory results were obtained in 85% of patients. No intraoperative complications were reported.

Johnson IP, Nasca RJ, Dunham WK: Surgical management of isthmic spondylolisthesis. *Spine* 1988;13:93–97.

Review of 44 patients undergoing fusion with and without decompression for spondylolisthesis. Results were good in 78%, fair in 18%, and poor in 4%. Only patients with documented nerve root compression should have a decompression with the fusion.

Kane WJ: Direct current electrical bone growth stimulation for spinal fusion. *Spine* 1988;13:363–365.

Two series of patients treated with adjunctive direct current electrical stimulation to enhance spinal fusion. The device appears to improve the fusion rate, particularly in difficult cases.

Sienkiewicz PJ, Flatley TJ: Postoperative spondylolisthesis. *Clin Orthop* 1987;221:172–180.

Iatrogenic spondylolisthesis was found in eight patients after inadvertent bilateral facetectomy or transection of the pars interarticularis. The L4–5 level appeared to be more susceptible to this postoperative complication. Fusion is recommended for all cases of suspected postoperative instability to prevent postoperative spondylolisthesis.

Steffee AD, Sitkowski DJ: Reduction and stabilization of grade IV spondylolisthesis. *Clin Orthop* 1988;227:82–89.
Descriptive review of the indications for and technique of internal fixation, reduction, and fusion of severe lumbar spondylolisthesis.

Lumbar Instability

Friberg O: Lumbar instability: A dynamic approach by traction-compression radiography. *Spine* 1987;12:119–129.
A description of a new dynamic radiographic study to demonstrate lumbar instability not apparent on routine flexion-extension radiographs.

Stokes IA, Frymoyer JW: Segmental motion and instability. *Spine* 1987;12:688–691.
A clinical and radiographic comparative analysis of 78 patients diagnosed as having degenerative instability of the lumbar spine. Despite previous reports, the flexion-extension radiographs in this study were not useful in the diagnosis of lumbar instability.

Pregnancy

Fast A, Shapiro D, Ducommun EJ, et al: Low-back pain in pregnancy. *Spine* 1987;12:368–371.
A review of 200 women shortly after childbirth found that 56% had back pain during pregnancy. Although 45% had sciatic pain, disk herniation requiring surgical diskectomy was rare.

Coccygodynia

Bayne O, Bateman JE, Cameron HU: The influence of etiology on the results of coccygectomy. *Clin Orthop* 1984;190:266–272.
The results of coccygectomy in 48 patients were analyzed with specific attempts to correlate surgical success with the etiologic cause of the coccygodynia.

Postacchini F, Massobrio M: Idiopathic coccygodynia: Analysis of fifty-one operative cases and a radiographic

study of the normal coccyx. *J Bone Joint Surg* 1983;65A:1116–1124.
A radiographic review of 120 asymptomatic subjects attempted to classify the anatomic configuration of the coccyx to correlate with treatment success. An additional review of patients with coccygodynia who underwent coccygectomy found an 88% success rate.

Lumbar Spine Osteolysis

Bradford DS, Gotfried Y: Lumbar spine osteolysis: An entity caused by spinal instability. *Spine* 1986;11:1013–1019.
Three cases of a new clinical entity are presented with diagnostic and treatment recommendations.

Controversies

Diskography

Abdelwahab IF, Gould ES: The role of discography after negative postmyelography CT scan: Retrospective review. *AJNR* 1988;9:187–190.

Colhoun E, McCall IW, Williams L, et al: Provocation discography as a guide to planning operations on the spine. *J Bone Joint Surg* 1988;70B:267–271.

Fraser RD, Osti OL, Vernon-Roberts B: Discitis after discography. *J Bone Joint Surg* 1987;69B:26–35.

Sachs BL, Vanharanta H, Spivey MA, et al: Dallas discogram description: A new classification of CT/discography in low-back disorders. *Spine* 1987;12:287–294.

Schneiderman G, Flannigan B, Kingston S, et al: Magnetic resonance imaging in the diagnosis of disc degeneration: Correlation with discography. *Spine* 1987;12:276–281.

Yasuma T, Ohno R, Yamauchi Y: False negative lumbar discograms: Correlation of discographic and histological findings in postmortem and surgical specimens. *J Bone Joint Surg* 1988;70A:1279–1290.

IV
Lower Extremity

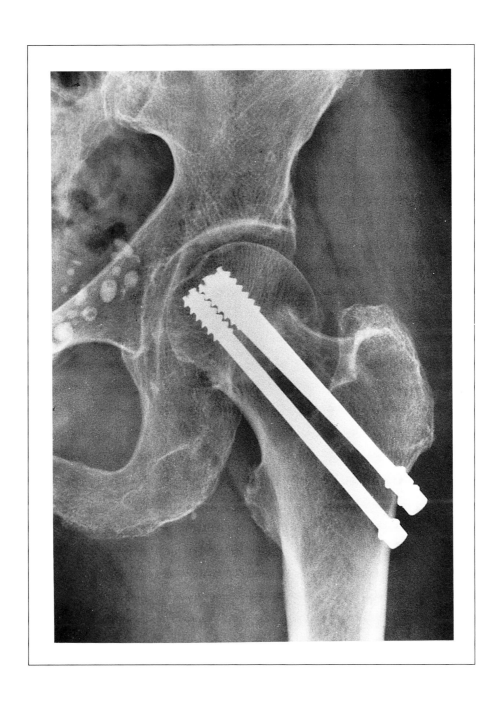

37

Hip and Femur: Pediatric Aspects

Pediatric concerns in regard to the hip and the femur include congenital conditions such as congenital dislocation of the hip and femoral anteversion, developmental disorders such as Legg-Calvé-Perthes disease, slipped capital femoral epiphysis, and transient hip synovitis, neuromuscular conditions such as cerebral palsy and spinal bifida, and neoplasms. Of particular interest is the recent suggestion that "missed" congenital hip dislocations are actually postnatal dislocations that are different from the neonatal variety.

Congenital Conditions

Congenital Dislocations of the Hip

Congenital dislocations of the hip can be broadly classed into either "typical" dislocations or teratologic dislocations. Although they are frequently similar in radiographic appearance, their treatment and prognosis are dramatically different.

Typical congenital dislocation of the hip constitutes a spectrum of deformity that includes complete dislocation (in which no cartilage contact exists between the femoral head and acetabulum), subluxation (in which there is cartilage-to-cartilage contact but a nonconcentric incongruous relationship), instability (either subluxation or dislocation), and dysplasia, which is generally thought to result from inadequate development of the acetabulum.

Causative factors include genetics (a multifactoral inheritance pattern), mechanical factors (prenatal and postnatal position), and hormones (maternal relaxins, for example, may affect the ligamentous support of the female infant's hip).

Identifiable risk factors in the infant include a positive family history (as much as a 36% risk if the infant's mother and a sibling have had congenital dislocation of the hip), breech position (a tenfold increase in risk), torticollis and plagiocephaly (approximately tenfold increase in risk), hyperextension and congenital dislocation of the knee (as much as a 50% incidence of congenital dislocation of the hip), and foot deformities.

Early diagnosis, that is, a positive Ortolani or Barlow sign, remains the cornerstone of diagnosis of an unstable hip in the first three months of life. Ultrasonography clearly has a role, but this technique is labor-intensive, and its ability to identify the unstable or stable but dysplastic hip depends on the expertise of the examiner. Radiographs are generally used only to confirm the position of a dislocated hip being treated, when a hip is suspect or has risk factors (in a child 3 months of age), or for follow-up of a treated dislocated or unstable hip. To date, no hip screening program has been 100% successful in eliminating late discoveries of dislocated hips. Whether these hips were "missed"

at birth or were normal at birth and later developed dislocations remains unresolved.

Early treatment of the dislocated or unstable hip is intended to maintain the hip in the concentrically reduced position. Although a number of abduction devices are available for this, the Pavlik harness is apparently the most versatile and the most popular. It must be emphasized that, regardless of the type of abduction device used, proof that the hip is being relocated is necessary. Similarly, extremes of position, especially abduction, should be avoided. The Pavlik harness fails to reduce the hip in as many as 8% of cases; osteonecrosis occurs in as many as 2.38%.

After the child is 6 months old, the harness is generally ineffective. At this point, closed reduction preceded by skin traction to lessen the likelihood of osteonecrosis is warranted. At what point this is no longer effective is open to question, but certainly there is evidence suggesting a high probability of success in children less than 3 years old.

Major indications for open reduction of the hip include failure to obtain a reduction and the need to place the hip in so extreme a position to maintain the reduction that there is risk of osteonecrosis. In children older than 3 years, it is generally accepted that primary open reduction with femoral shortening is the most prudent approach.

Once the femoral head is concentrically reduced, acetabular development continues until the age of 4 years and, to some extent, to the age of 8 years. Major causes of persisting acetabular dysplasia include failure to obtain a concentric reduction or early lateral migration of the femoral head after reduction. Osteonecrosis may also have an adverse affect.

The decision about reconstructive procedures after relocation of a congenitally dislocated hip must be based on either continuing subluxation or instability, or the failure of the acetabulum to develop adequately. If a varus rotation osteotomy is considered, it is best done before the child is 4 years of age because of the limited ability of the acetabulum to remodel after this age. After the age of 4 years, acetabular procedures are generally thought to be more effective than femoral procedures.

In late reconstruction of the congenitally dislocated hip it is advisable to attempt to maintain cartilage-to-cartilage contact rather than resort to salvage procedures such as Chiari or Colonna osteotomies. Although effective in improving hip function, they are clearly inferior to procedures in which the acetabulum itself is redirected.

Femoral Anteversion

Increased femoral anteversion is certainly the most common "hip problem" in most orthopaedists' offices.

Two recent studies have confirmed that femoral anteversion does not increase the risk of arthritis of the hip. Therefore, treatment to avoid future functional problems seems to be inappropriate.

Although femoral anteversion is a cosmetic problem, it can on occasion be a significant one. Bracing is ineffective. Spontaneous improvement in the anatomic problem can occur until the age of 8 years and spontaneous improvement in gait by "conscious override" can continue until adolescence. Therefore, surgery should be deferred.

Developmental Conditions

Legg-Calvé-Perthes Disease

Legg-Calvé-Perthes disease is osteonecrosis of the proximal femoral epiphysis caused by poorly understood nongenetic factors. It bears little, if any, relationship to transient synovitis of the hip. Unlike osteonecrosis in the adult, Perthes' disease almost always heals, but deformity of the femoral head is common.

The Catterall classification remains the most widely used classification system despite its significant limitations. Among these are the fact that the disease must reach the fragmentation and collapse stage before it can be classified and interobserver variability seriously limits its usefulness.

Plain radiographs remain the mainstay of classification. Bone scans and, more recently, magnetic resonance imaging appear to hold promise for the future in this regard.

The natural history of Perthes' disease is that as many as 50% of involved hips do well with no treatment. The vast majority of the other 50%, although having poor results by radiographic criteria (center edge angle, < 20 degrees; acetabular index, > 20 degrees; and Mose sphericity, > 2 mm out of round) do well functionally into the fifth decade.

Treatment The current goal of management is a spherical, well-covered femoral head; this is generally achieved by "containment." As yet, follow-up is insufficient to prove that the containment principle will have altered the natural history of the disease when the patient is 50 years old.

There are three types of Perthes' disease (Fig. 1):

(1) Round femoral heads contained in the acetabulum in the neutral position: These are generally in younger children with lesser degrees of involvement. Because they are already "contained," treatment should be aimed at restoring and maintaining motion with close follow-up throughout the healing process. It is generally thought that these hips have an excellent prognosis.

(2) Femoral heads that are nonspherical but can be "contained" by abduction with or without rotation: These are generally in older children and manifest higher percentages of femoral head involvement and clinical and radiographic "at risk" signs (prolonged stiffness, lateral subluxation, extensive metaphyseal change, lateral calcification, and Gage's sign). Arthrography may be useful in determining the sphericity of the cartilaginous femoral head as well as in assessing the degree of abduction and rotation necessary for complete containment.

Containment, after restoration of motion, has the most application in this group. Containment can be achieved by either abduction orthosis or surgery (pelvic or femoral). Both methods appear to have roughly comparable results in the short-term. Disturbingly, neither appears to benefit the older (more than 9 or 10 years old) child.

(3) The noncontainable hip: This is the hip with femoral head deformity severe enough that the femoral head on abduction impinges on the lateral acetabulum and hinge-abducts and subluxates. Treatment alternatives include Chiari osteotomy (to cover the extruded femoral head), cheilectomy (to remove the femoral head prominence that prevents containment), and valgus osteotomy (to bring more normal medial femoral head cartilage into weight-bearing position and to increase abduction). Short-term results suggest that last-mentioned procedure is the most useful for the symptomatic noncontainable hip.

Slipped Capital Femoral Epiphysis

Slipped capital femoral epiphysis appears to be the end result of physical and hormonal factors. Patients with slipped epiphyses as a group may manifest subtle endocrine changes but they do not have an endocrinopathy and preoperative endocrine testing is not generally recommended. Those slips resulting from endocrinopathy are generally recognizable because they appear in younger children and include characteristic features such as retarded bone age, short stature, and changes in the opposite epiphysis.

It has been shown that with removal of the perichondrial ring, the forces necessary to create a slipped epiphysis are approached by normal activities. More recently, it has been shown that the hips of patients with slips have a decreased neck-shaft angle and a relative retroversion that increases the shear across the proximal femoral epiphysis, suggesting that mechanical factors have an important role in slipped epiphysis.

Treatment of slipped epiphysis is designed to stabilize the epiphysis from further slipping and avoid complications (osteonecrosis and chondrolysis) at all costs. It is clear that in the absence of complications these hips do quite well; conversely, if either chondrolysis or osteonecrosis develops, early disabling arthritis is predictable.

Osteonecrosis results from manipulation of the epiphysis, open reduction of the epiphysis, and intracapsular osteotomies of the neck. In the acute or acute-on-chronic slip, reduction should be accomplished either by skeletal traction with internal rotation preoperatively or by a gentle manipulation at the time of surgery. Forceful manipulations must be avoided. In the chronic slip, no repositioning of the epiphysis should be attempted. When a slip is pinned, the pins should avoid the superolateral quadrant of the femoral head where the posterosuperior retinacular vessels enter. Chondrolysis results from pins penetrating the joint in more than 90% of cases.

Stabilization of the epiphysis can be accomplished by threaded pins, screws, or bone graft. Although bone-graft epiphysiodesis is a more extensive procedure, the published results make it a reasonable consideration in severe slips.

Because of the remodeling capability of the hip and the increased complication rate with osteotomies done acutely, osteotomies should be reserved for realignment of the hip after healing of the slipped epiphysis has taken place.

Transient Synovitis of the Hip

Transient synovitis of the hip is a benign, self-limited condition in children manifested by hip or knee pain, a limp, or limited motion of the hip, specifically a flexion contracture, limited abduction, or limited internal rotation.

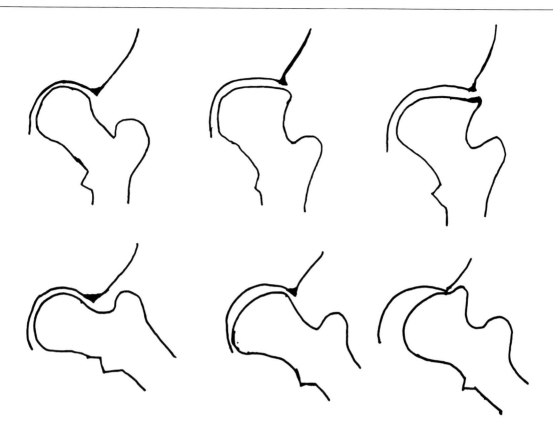

Figure 1

Three types of Perthes' disease. **Left,** Spherical femoral head contained equally well in neutral and abduction. **Center,** Flattened femoral head contained in abduction. The lateral portion "tucks into" the acetabular labrum. **Right,** Noncontainable femoral head. Abduction results in hinging and subluxation rather than containment.

Demographics and majority opinion favor a viral cause but this has not been proven.

The major concern is to differentiate this entity from septic arthritis of the hip and Perthes' disease. It can be distinguished from septic arthritis by the patient's temperature, leukocyte count, and erythrocyte sedimentation rate. If there is any question, aspiration arthrography of the hip should be performed. Perthes' disease may have a similar presentation. If there is a question on the initial radiographs, a bone scan or magnetic resonance imaging may be useful. The likelihood of this condition leading to Perthes' disease is small, no more than 3%. Routine follow-up radiographs are nevertheless recommended by many.

Treatment of transient synovitis should consist of traction and bedrest. Symptoms generally respond within a week. There is approximately a 5% recurrence rate with no change in the benign prognosis.

Cerebral Palsy

Children with cerebral palsy may have hip problems related to contractures, rotational malalignment, and subluxation or dislocation.

Contractures may limit functional ambulation. Adduction and flexion contractures are best treated by release. Care must be taken not to overlengthen the adductors because this makes ambulation more difficult.

Rotational deformities of the hip are common in the ambulatory patient with cerebral palsy. Although theoretically attractive, muscle transfers lack predictability. Definitive treatment is generally thought to be derotational osteotomy when the child is 8 to 10 years old. This can be done at either the intertrochanteric or the supracondylar level. If there is associated valgus or uncovering of the hip, the intertrochanteric level seems preferable.

Subluxation and dislocation of the hip are generally found in more severely affected patients. Pain is a major sequela in approximately 50%. Unilateral dislocations can result in pelvic obliquity and perhaps scoliosis, although the interrelationship of spine and hip is controversial.

The hip dislocation is caused by imbalance of the muscles, specifically the overpowering adductors and flexors. This produces coxa valga and anteversion, which in turn lead to acetabular dyplasia and ultimately hip instability and dislocation.

Early in this progression and in younger children with milder degrees of subluxation, muscle releases of the adductors and iliopsoas may be effective. Two cautions are in order. First, overzealous lengthening of the adductors, or release of the iliopsoas when the hamstrings or hip extensors are spastic may result in an extension-abduction contracture of the hip that is more debilitating and difficult to treat than the original problem. Additionally, one must be aware that in most of these children the neurologic involvement is relatively symmetric. Unilateral soft-tissue surgery has a definite untoward effect on the opposite hip in terms of progressive subluxation and contracture. Preoperative planning should address the issue of symmetry. Long-term bracing may improve the results of muscle releases.

In more severe deformity and older children, correction of the bony deformity—whether it is femoral or acetabular and femoral—should be considered. Before the corrective osteotomies are done, concentric reduction must be achieved.

Despite these surgical interventions, a significant number of patients with cerebral palsy in their adolescent and young adult years have hip pain sufficient to limit their function. Salvage alternatives include arthrodesis, total hip arthroplasty, and resection arthroplasty.

Published reports suggest that arthrodesis and total hip arthroplasty deserve consideration. The magnitude of these surgical procedures, the difficulties with postoperative immobilization, and the issues of ongoing spasticity and muscle imbalance, however, make these options less attractive.

The classic Girdlestone resection arthroplasty is ineffective in hip problems resulting from cerebral palsy. Proximal femoral resection (below the lesser trochanter) with interposition of the hip capsule, abductors, and proximal thigh musculature between the pelvis and distal fragment appears to be effective in alleviating pain and allowing pain-free sitting.

Neoplasms

Fibrous Dysplasia

Fibrous dysplasia is a benign condition that is perhaps better considered a congenital anomaly of bone-forming mesenchyme than an actual tumor. If untreated, fibrous dysplasia of the hip compromises the strength of the proximal femur and, because of repeated pathologic fractures, leads to a progressive varus or "shepherd's-crook deformity." Eradication of the fibrous dysplastic process is unlikely. A cancellous bone graft is quickly incorporated and becomes dysplastic. Treatment of the hip should furnish intrinsic structural support to prevent progressive deformity. This can be accomplished by large cortical bone grafts spanning the lesion or by means of metallic internal fixation.

Malignant Tumors

With improvements in preoperative assessment, intraoperative surgical techniques, and effective postoperative adjuvant therapies, tumors previously amenable only to hip disarticulation or hemipelvectomy can be removed safely and the distal limb spared. A prosthesis can replace the removed segment. Alternatively, rotationplasty—fusing the distal limb to the pelvis and using the ankle joint as a knee joint—and fitting the patient with a below-knee prosthesis can be considered instead of ablative surgery.

Controversies

Congenital Dislocation of the Hip

In the 1990s, the role of ultrasonography in the detection and evaluation of congenital dislocation of the hip will be better defined. The incidence of "developmental" late dislocation ("congenital" hip dislocation in children whose hips are known not to have been dislocated at birth) must be determined. Better terminology must be developed for idiopathic hip dislocation and subluxation. Discussion will continue about preoperative traction vs intraoperative femoral shortening in open reduction of congenital hip dislocation in older children.

Legg-Calvé-Perthes Disease

Although magnetic resonance imaging may improve the staging and evaluation of this condition, debate will continue about the relative efficacies of no treatment, bracing, and osteotomy. The results of a prospective controlled study comparing these modes of treatment will become available and are likely to generate considerable controversy.

Slipped Capital Femoral Epiphysis

The major debate in regard to this condition will continue to center around the desirability of cuneiform osteotomy of the femoral neck and open reduction for severe degrees of chronic slip. The recent renewal of interest in this topic should generate clinical series for discussion and indicate whether the rate of osteonecrosis after the procedure is low enough to justify it.

Spina Bifida

Dislocated hips in patients with spina bifida, unlike cerebral palsy, are rarely painful. It is clear that dislocated hips in patients unable to walk require no treatment. The issue in ambulatory patients is less clear. Studies can be quoted to support both treatment and nontreatment of the dislocated hip in such cases.

Annotated Bibliography

Keywords

Cerebral palsy; Congenital hip dislocation; Femoral anteversion; Fibrous dysplasia; Legg-Calvé-Perthes disease; Neoplasms; Osteonecrosis; Slipped capital femoral epiphysis; Spina bifida; Synovitis

Congenital Disorders

Congenital Dislocation of the Hip

Calvert PT, August AC, Albert JS, et al: The Chiari pelvic osteotomy: A review of the long-term results. *J Bone Joint Surg* 1987;69B:551–555.

Of 49 hips followed up for an average of 14 years after Chiari osteotomy, 75% had a positive Trendelenburg sign. Degenerative changes increased from 32% preoperatively to 85% at follow-up.

Castelein RM, Sauter AJM: Ultrasound screening for congenital dysplasia of the hip in newborns: Its value. *J Pediatr Orthop* 1988;8:666–670.
Eighty-two of 307 ultrasound examinations in newborns were abnormal; 79 of these became normal without treatment.

Grill F, Bensahel H, Canadell J, et al: The Pavlik harness in the treatment of congenital dislocating hip: Report on a multicenter study of the European Paediatric Orthopaedic Society. *J Pediatr Orthop* 1988;8:1–8.
A total of 3,611 children with dysplastic and dislocated hips were treated at an average age of 4.1 months. Higher grades of dislocation (Tonnis 3 and 4) had a failure rate of 14% or more and an osteonecrosis rate of 10% to 16%.

Høgh J, Macnicol MF: The Chiari pelvic osteotomy: A long-term review of clinical and radiographic results. *J Bone Joint Surg* 1987;69B:365–373.
A ten-year follow-up study of 94 Chiari osteotomies, 83 of which were done for pain, showed that function deteriorated slowly with time.

Ilfeld FW, Westin GW, Making M: Missed or developmental dislocation of the hip. *Clin Orthop* 1986;203:276–281.
The authors present 15 documented cases of subluxation or dislocation of the hip discovered after multiple previous examinations had given normal findings. The hypothesis is advanced that delayed subluxated or dislocated hips may constitute an entity not necessarily related to the neonatal condition.

Jensen BA, Reimann I, Fredensborg N: Collagen type III predominance in newborns with congenital dislocation of the hip. *Acta Orthop Scand* 1986;57:362–365.
Umbilical cord collagen was analyzed in newborns with congenital hip dislocation and controls. The findings suggest that alterations in collagen metabolism may explain joint hypermobility as a causative factor.

Powell EN, Gerratana FJ, Gage JR: Open reduction for congenital hip dislocation: The risk of avascular necrosis with three different approaches. *J Pediatr Orthop* 1986;6:127–132.
Comparison of hips treated with open reduction alone, open reduction and femoral osteotomy, and open reduction with innominate osteotomy suggest that the last-mentioned has the highest rate of complications.

Pozo JL, Cannon SR, Catterall A: The Colonna-Hey Groves arthroplasty in the late treatment of congenital dislocation of the hip: A long-term review. *J Bone Joint Surg* 1987;69B:220–228.
In 50 arthroplasties (mean follow-up, 20 years), symptomatic functional deterioration was noted.

Williamson DM, Benson MKD: Late femoral osteotomy in congenital dislocation of the hip. *J Bone Joint Surg* 1988;70B:614–618.
After the age of 5 years, femoral osteotomy alone was inadequate for true subluxation of the hip, unless there was already good acetabular development (acetabular angle, < 25 degrees).

Zionts LE, MacEwen GD: Treatment of congenital dislocation of the hip in children between the ages of one and three years. *J Bone Joint Surg* 1986;68A:829–846.
Of 51 congenitally dislocated hips, 75% were satisfactorily managed by traction, gentle closed reduction, and spica cast immobilization. Twenty-five percent required open reduction because of inability to obtain a stable closed reduction.

Femoral Anteversion

Hubbard DD, Staheli LT, Chew DE, et al: Medial femoral torsion and osteoarthritis. *J Pediatr Orthop* 1988;8:540–542.
Anteversion was measured by biplanar radiography in patients with idiopathic osteoarthritis and controls. No significant difference was found.

Developmental Conditions

Legg-Calvé-Perthes Disease

Christensen F, Søballe K, Ejsted R, et al: The Catterall classification of Perthes' disease: An assessment of reliability. *J Bone Joint Surg* 1986;68B:614–615.
Four experienced observers examining anteroposterior and lateral radiographs of 100 hips had an unacceptably low degree of interobserver agreement.

Evans IK, Deluca PA, Gage JR: A comparative study of ambulation-abduction bracing and varus derotation osteotomy in the treatment of severe Legg-Calvé-Perthes disease in children over 6 years of age. *J Pediatr Orthop* 1988;8:676–682.
In 36 patients, all more than 6.9 years old, bracing and femoral osteotomy gave similar results.

Hoikka V, Lindholm TS, Poussa M: Intertrochanteric varus osteotomy in Legg-Calvé-Perthes disease: A report of 112 hips. *J Pediatr Orthop* 1986;6:600–604.
Femoral osteotomy seldom helped in patients older than 9 years.

Quain S, Catterall A: Hinge abduction of the hip: Diagnosis and treatment. *J Bone Joint Surg* 1986;68B:61–64.
Twenty-seven hips with symptomatic hinge abduction were treated by valgus extension osteotomy. Short-term (average, three years) improvement in pain, deformity, and shortening was seen in 26.

Richards BS, Coleman SS: Subluxation of the femoral head in coxa plana. *J Bone Joint Surg* 1987;69A:1312–1318.
Closed reduction with muscle release and Petri casting was successful in obtaining reduction in 22 patients with lateral subluxation of the femoral head. Nevertheless, at follow-up 13 of the 22 hips showed nonspherical femoral heads.

Sponseller PD, Desai SS, Millis MB: Comparison of femoral and innominate osteotomies for the treatment of Legg-Calvé-Perthes disease. *J Bone Joint Surg* 1988;70A:1131–1139.
Objective ratings showed no difference between the two operations. Patients more than 10 years old had poor results with both procedures.

Slipped Capital Femoral Epiphysis

Gelberman RH, Cohen MS, Shaw BA, et al: The association of femoral retroversion with slipped capital femoral epiphysis. *J Bone Joint Surg* 1986;68A:1000–1007.
Analysis of 25 patients with slipped epiphyses showed diminished anteversion in comparison with controls. The authors hypothesized that this anatomic abnormality produces increased shear stresses across the growth plate, leading to slipping.

Lehman WB, Jofe M, Ehrlich MG: Chondrolysis following slipped capital femoral epiphysis. Presented at the meeting of Pediatric Orthopedic Society, Colorado Springs, Colorado, 1988.

A multicenter research study sponsored by the Pediatric Orthopedic Society of North America was undertaken to assess factors leading to chondrolysis. In 28 identified cases of chondrolysis, pins penetrating into the joint were implicated in 95%.

Mann DC, Weddington J, Richton S: Hormonal studies in patients with slipped capital femoral epiphysis without evidence of endocrinopathy. *J Pediatr Orthop* 1988; 8:543–545.

Twenty consecutive adolescent patients with slipped epiphyses were found to be endocrinologically normal. Routine endocrine evaluation would not seem indicated in these patients.

Pritchett JW, Perdue KD: Mechanical factors in slipped capital femoral epiphysis. *J Pediatr Orthop* 1988;8:385–388.

Three-dimensional force analysis of the hip in slipped epiphysis suggested that relative varus and retroversion leads to increased sagittal plane shear and results in growth plate failure.

Puri R, Smith CS, Malhotra D, et al: Slipped upper femoral epiphysis and primary juvenile hypothyroidism. *J Bone Joint Surg* 1985;67B:14–20.

In patients with slipped epiphysis, short stature, obesity, retarded bone age, or changes in the opposite epiphysis should alert the physician to the possibility of an endocrinopathy.

Stambough JL, Davidson RS, Ellis RD, et al: Slipped capital femoral epiphysis: An analysis of 80 patients as to pin placement and number. *J Pediatr Orthop* 1986;6: 265–273.

Best results were obtained with fewer than three pins, avoiding the superolateral epiphysis, and with the tips more than 2.5 mm away from the subchondral bone.

Szypryt EP, Clement DA, Colton CL: Open reduction or epiphysiodesis for slipped upper femoral epiphysis: A comparison of Dunn's operation and the Heyman-Herndon procedure. *J Bone Joint Surg* 1987;69B:737–742.

Although open reduction appeared to give a better result than epiphysiodesis in severe slips, it was associated with an 18% incidence of osteonecrosis.

Transient Synovitis of the Hip

Haueisen DC, Weiner DS, Weiner SD: The characterization of transient synovitis of the hip in children. *J Pediatr Orthop* 1986;6:11–17.

A review of 497 cases of transient synovitis of the hip found Legg-Calvé-Perthes disease in 2.5%. Recurrent synovitis occurred in 19 patients. The prognosis was benign. Follow-up radiographs after resolution of symptoms are recommended.

Kallio P, Ryöppy S, Kunnamo I: Transient synovitis and Perthes' disease: Is there an aetiological connection? *J Bone Joint Surg* 1986;68B:808–811.

Follow-up of 119 cases of transient synovitis found no cases of Perthes' disease.

Landin LA, Danielsson LG, Wattsgård C: Transient synovitis of the hip: Its incidence, epidemiology and relation to Perthes' disease. *J Bone Joint Surg* 1987;69B: 238–242.

A total of 294 cases of transient synovitis of the hip was diagnosed. The cumulative risk of suffering at least one episode was 3%. Perthes' disease was diagnosed in 3.4% of cases. Retrospectively, radiographic abnormalities were apparent in eight of ten in this group.

Cerebral Palsy

Baxter MP, D'Astous JL: Proximal femoral resection-interposition arthroplasty: Salvage hip surgery for the severely disabled child with cerebral palsy. *J Pediatr Orthop* 1986;6:681–685.

Comfortable sitting was achieved in five previously painful, spastic dislocated hips by this procedure.

Carr C, Gage JR: The fate of the nonoperated hip in cerebral palsy. *J Pediatr Orthop* 1987;7:262–267.

Unilateral soft-tissue procedures had a definite untoward effect on the contralateral hip, leading to progressive subluxation and pelvic deformity.

Cooperman DR, Bartucci E, Dietrick E, et al: Hip dislocation in spastic cerebral palsy: Long-term consequences. *J Pediatr Orthop* 1987;7:268–276.

Pelvic obliquity and scoliosis were present in 12 of 18 patients with unreduced unilateral hip dislocations, but in only two of seven with reduced, unilateral dislocations. One half of the dislocated hips were painful.

Lonstein JE, Beck K: Hip dislocation and subluxation in cerebral palsy. *J Pediatr Orthop* 1986;6:521–526.

In dependent sitters, the presence, absence, or magnitude of pelvic obliquity did not correlate with location, subluxation, or dislocation of the hip.

Houkom JA, Roach JW, Wenger DR, et al: Treatment of acquired hip subluxation in cerebral palsy. *J Pediatr Orthop* 1986;6:285–290.

Long-term postoperative abduction splinting improved the results of soft-tissue release in severely subluxated hips.

Matsuo T, Tada S, Hajime T: Insufficiency of the hip adductor after anterior obturator neurectomy in 42 children with cerebral palsy. *J Pediatr Orthop* 1986;6:686–692.

Hyperabduction of the hips in gait was noted after anterior branch obturator neurectomy, with functional deterioration in gait.

Root L, Goss JR, Mendes J: The treatment of the painful hip in cerebral palsy by total hip replacement or hip arthrodesis. *J Bone Joint Surg* 1986;68A:590–598.

Arthrodesis was successful in six of eight patients, and total hip replacement was successful in 13 of 15. One patient had deformation of the femoral component with trochanteric nonunion and pain, one had progressive femoral component loosening, and two had recurrent dislocations. Prolonged postoperative spica cast immobilization is necessary after both procedures.

Szalay EA, Roach JW, Houkom JA, et al: Extension-abduction contracture of the spastic hip. *J Pediatr Orthop* 1986;6:1–6.

Extension-abduction contractures of the hip can develop in severely involved patients either spontaneously or after adductor releases. When surgery is planned, assessment of all muscles about the hip is indicated.

Neoplasms

Enneking WF, Gearen PF: Fibrous dysplasia of the femoral neck: Treatment by cortical bone-grafting. *J Bone Joint Surg* 1986;68A:1415–1422.

Large cortical bone grafts, extending from normal bone proximal to normal bone distal to the fibrous dysplastic region successfully relieved pain, united the fracture, and prevented deformity.

Stephenson RB, London MD, Hankin FM, et al: Fibrous dysplasia: An analysis of options for treatment. *J Bone Joint Surg* 1987;69A:400–409.

In patients less than 18 years of age with symptomatic fibrous dysplastic lesions, internal fixation should be considered.

Winkelman WW: Hip rotationplasty for malignant tumors of the proximal part of the femur. *J Bone Joint Surg* 1986;68A:362–369.

As an alternative to ablative surgery for malignant disease, resection of the proximal femur (rotation of the distal segment and attachment to the pelvis so that the knee, which has been turned 180 degrees, serves as the hip joint and the ankle as the knee joint) allows the patient to be fitted with a below-knee prosthesis. Functional results suggest that this alternative deserves consideration.

Controversies

Spina Bifida

Weisl H, Fairclough JA, Jones DG: Stabilisation of the hip in myelomeningocele: Comparison of posterior iliopsoas transfer and varus-rotation osteotomy. *J Bone Joint Surg* 1988;70B:29–33.

Samuelsson L, Skoog M: Ambulation in patients with myelomeningocele: A multivariate statistical analysis. *J Pediatr Orthop* 1988;8:569–575.

38
Pelvis and Acetabulum: Trauma

The last decade has brought major advances in both the diagnostic assessment and the surgical stabilization of pelvic ring disruptions. New surgical approaches to the posterior pelvic ring have been developed to lessen the problems of nonunion, malunion, and leg-length discrepancy that so often accompany these major injuries.

Pelvic Fractures

Pelvic fractures typically occur in patients who have suffered high-energy trauma. The fracture is often associated with other injuries. Priorities in the initial management are similar to those for multiple trauma. Severe pelvic fractures can be associated with a high mortality rate from severe intrapelvic bleeding and also from the associated injuries. Severe bleeding results primarily from laceration of pelvic veins, although arterial bleeding also occurs. Injuries specifically associated with pelvic fractures include those of the neurologic, urologic, gynecologic, and gastrointestinal systems. Local injury to the skin and subcutaneous tissue is also common.

Control of Hemorrhage
Control of severe bleeding associated with a fracture is the primary initial concern. The severity of bleeding is highest in displaced and unstable disruptions of the posterior pelvic ring. Therapeutic measures for control of pelvic hemorrhage include: (1) intravenous crystalloid solution and whole blood; (2) external fixation of the pelvic ring; (3) internal fixation of the pelvic ring; (4) angiography, typically followed by transarterial embolization and possibly by repair of major blood vessels; and (5) use of military antishock trousers (MAST suit).

Crystalloid Solution and Whole Blood Resuscitation with crystalloid solution and whole blood is sufficient in most stable pelvic fractures. Stable pelvic fractures do not involve a significant disruption of the posterior pelvic ring. The initial displacement of the bone fragments is less. The addition of external fixation usually does little to control pelvic volume or enhance stability. Many unstable pelvic fractures can be managed by fluid resuscitation in the initial phase. The radiographic appearance alone, however, does not always indicate to the surgeon which patient can be managed with fluid resuscitation alone. One possible course is to monitor the patient, assessing the response to fluid resuscitation; if there is a problem with continued blood loss, other hemorrhage control measures can be undertaken.

External Fixation Unstable pelvic fractures are likely to require more than fluid resuscitation for hemorrhage control. External fixation has been shown to decrease initial blood loss in unstable pelvic ring fractures. Although simple fluid resuscitation may be successful even in unstable pelvic fractures, there is an argument for prophylactic external fixation very early in the treatment of these fractures. The initial control of pelvic volume and the addition of stability through an external fixator may prevent uncontrolled initial bleeding that might be difficult to control at a later time. The external fixation frame is typically applied to the anterior portion of both iliac crests. Many simple frame configurations provide adequate initial stability. With practice, the pins can be successfully placed through stab wounds along the iliac crest. External fixation is most effective in unstable fractures that increase the volume of the pelvic ring, such as injuries involving a wide separation of the symphysis pubis. External fixation does not control vertical translation of the pelvic ring nor does it truly immobilize the fracture site. External fixation can increase the risk of infection if later open reduction of the pelvis is contemplated. It can also provide an avenue for bacteria to invade subcutaneous hematomas that may be present after the injury. External fixation is not indicated for the initial management of patients with acetabular fractures.

Internal Fixation Internal fixation may be used in some cases during the acute phase. A good indication for anterior plate fixation is a dislocated symphysis pubis and either intra-abdominal or intrapelvic visceral trauma requiring surgical repair. Because internal fixation is much more effective in reducing and stabilizing the disrupted pelvic ring, it may ultimately have a role in the initial management of the patient with intrapelvic blood loss; however, at present this remains controversial and experimental.

Angiography If fluid resuscitation and external fixation fail, the surgeon should proceed to selective angiography. Although most bleeding is of venous origin, there are often small arterial bleeders that can be treated by angiographic embolization. The angiography should be localized as much as possible to the bleeding site to prevent aggravation of the circulatory injury. If angiography shows injury to major arteries of the pelvis, direct surgical repair is indicated. Angiographic embolization should not be performed unless there is good evidence that the patient's condition is unstable and a significant bleeding site has been identified. Adequate vascularization of muscle tissue with good collateral circulation is important if later surgical approaches to the pelvis or acetabulum for internal fixation are performed.

MAST Suit The MAST suit can be effective in controlling hemorrhage in unstable pelvic fractures. It can be applied by paramedical personnel and therefore serves as a resuscitative measure before the patient reaches the hospital. The MAST suit has some definite disadvantages, however, in that it prevents direct access to the patient for examination. It also prevents application of an external fixator. It may mask and complicate associated injuries to the lower extremities such as open fractures, vascular injury, or compartment syndrome.

Neurologic Injury

Neurologic injury is often associated with pelvic injury. It is more common in unstable fractures and typically results from a traction injury to the nerve roots and peripheral nerves as the pelvis undergoes severe displacement during the injury. The nerve fibers originating from L-5 to S-1 are most commonly involved, although nerve fibers anywhere from L-2 to S-4 can also be injured easily. The initial neurologic examination should include tests of sciatic, femoral, and obturator nerve function and a rectal assessment of the lower sacral nerve roots. Because of pain, it is usually not possible to test the superior and inferior gluteal nerves initially. The initial evaluation is particularly important because the neurologic picture can change during the course of treatment or as a complication of treatment.

Because the nerve injury results from traction to the peripheral nerves and nerve roots, surgical repair or attempts at decompression are rarely indicated. However, some sacral fractures unassociated with initial violent stretching of the nerve roots may result in neurologic deficits because of compromise of the spinal canal or neural foramina. These lesions may improve with neural decompression. In the case of displaced acetabular fractures, a displaced femoral head, posterior wall, or posterior column may occasionally compromise the sciatic nerve or the L-5 or S-1 nerve root. If the patient's neurologic condition worsens after the initial examination, emergency surgical reduction of the fracture is indicated.

In all cases the patient should be counseled as to the nature of the injury and the potential for recovery. If there is partial function of the injured nerve, improvement in function over a period of months can be expected. If there is a complete loss of function at the time of injury, return of some function is possible but normal function cannot be expected. Lower sacral nerve root injuries are associated with deficits in bowel, bladder, and sexual function. Bowel or bladder impairment is apparent very early. Impairment of sexual function must be evaluated during the first few months after the injury. Procedures such as tendon transfers for loss of the peroneal portion of the sciatic nerve should not be considered until three years have elapsed from the time of injury, after which neurologic function cannot be expected to return. Bowel, bladder, and sexual function sometimes returns slowly over a prolonged period.

Urologic Injury

Urologic injury in the form of injury to the bladder and urethra is common in pelvic fractures. The treatment of extraperitoneal bladder rupture is controversial among urologists; some advocate a primary repair of the bladder and others advocate treatment with a Foley catheter or suprapubic drainage. A patient with a pelvic fracture that requires internal fixation of the pelvic ring is best served by surgical repair of the bladder rupture. Urine from an unrepaired bladder contaminated by bacteria after a catheter is introduced freely communicates with a dislocated symphysis pubis or anterior pelvic ring or acetabular fracture sites.

Once a suprapubic catheter has been introduced, it becomes dangerous to approach an anterior pelvic ring fracture site for the purpose of internal fixation because of infection. In the case of a bladder rupture associated with a dislocation of the symphysis pubis, the best initial course is to repair the bladder surgically and to perform plate fixation of the symphysis pubis. A urologist may then proceed with postoperative Foley catheterization or suprapubic bladder drainage. In the case of a bladder rupture associated with an acetabular fracture, the bladder rupture should also be repaired initially. If the acetabular fracture is complex and requires a subsequent ilioinguinal approach, it is best to avoid drainage through a suprapubic catheter and to provide drainage through a Foley catheter. Although this increases the risk of urethral stricture, an infected hip joint after contamination of the ilioinguinal approach by a suprapubic catheter is a devastating and lifelong problem for the patient.

Disruption of the membranous urethra must always be managed by a suprapubic catheter. An urethral injury is best diagnosed by a dynamic retrograde urethrogram. This should be performed in patients with pelvic fracture before a urethral catheter is inserted because the catheter can aggravate a urethral tear. Any dislocation of the symphysis pubis should be plated initially, at the time of the suprapubic catheter insertion, because the catheter will be needed for several months and the opportunity for a definitive surgical reduction would otherwise be lost. The surgical approach to a fractured acetabulum may have to be modified accordingly. In any event, the orthopaedic surgeon should advise urologists about placement of suprapubic catheters or drains in the abdomen that might hinder the later internal fixation procedure.

Gynecologic Injury

Lacerations of the vagina often accompany symphysis pubis dislocation or fractures of the pubic rami. These injuries constitute open fractures of the pelvis. The pelvic fracture site is often palpable through the vaginal laceration. The diagnosis can easily be missed and too often blood in the vagina is attributed to menstruation. It is best to perform an irrigation and debridement of the fracture through a Pfannenstiel approach, using Hemovac drainage of the retropubic space and repair of vaginal lacerations more than 1 cm in length. The vagina is then irrigated twice daily at the patient's bedside with iodine solution. Large vaginal lacerations that involve the perineum and rectal area should be treated with a diverting colostomy. If the vaginal laceration is not extensive, it can probably be treated effectively after irrigation and debridement.

Gastrointestinal Injury

The most common gastrointestinal injuries involve lacerations of the rectum. Less often, there may be perforations of the large or small bowel. Again, these injuries constitute open fractures of the pelvis. Injuries to the large bowel and rectum are treated with diverting colostomy and irrigation and debridement of the fracture site. If the pelvic fracture is unstable, it should be stabilized with internal or external fixation. Initially, the surgeon can consider either an anterior external fixation frame or plating of a disrupted symphysis pubis. Because internal fixation is, in general, most effective in maintaining stability and reduction, this is usually preferred even in the presence of bacterial contamination. Some argue, however, that external fixation is indicated because it offers a lesser risk of infection.

Skin and Subcutaneous Injury

The violent force required to fracture the pelvic ring and acetabulum is transmitted through the surrounding skin and subcutaneous tissue. Lacerations of the skin can convert a closed fracture to an open one. More common is a closed degloving injury in which the fatty layer is avulsed from the underlying fascia. This is associated with necrosis of areas of the fatty tissue and a large cavity containing hematoma and liquified fat between the skin and subcutaneous tissue and the deep fascia. When these areas are large, they usually require surgical drainage and debridement. These large cavities can easily be infected with bacteria through the introduction of external fixator pins or trochanteric traction or distal femoral traction pins. They may also become infected spontaneously if not drained and debrided. Closed degloving injuries can compromise the surgeon's access for internal fixation and must always be considered in planning the incision. After drainage and debridement, a portion of the wound is left open for repeated packing of the subcutaneous cavity. It is safest not to attempt closure over drains but rather to allow closure through granulation and secondary wound healing. This occurs over a period of weeks and sometimes months after the injury. The resulting scar can be safely modified at a much later time with an elective surgical procedure if the patient desires.

Pelvic Ring Injuries

Classification

The most useful classification systems describe the anatomic site of injury and the stability of the pelvic ring.

Letournel's Classification This classification of pelvic ring injuries simply names the sites of injury anteriorly and posteriorly.

Anterior lesions can involve either a subluxation of the symphysis pubis or fractures of the pubic and ischial rami. Posterior lesions may involve transiliac fracture, dislocation of the sacroiliac joint, vertical fracture of the sacrum, or fracture-dislocation of the sacroiliac joint.

Anterior lesions are easily recognized but posterior lesions are sometimes difficult to detect. A transiliac fracture begins at the iliac crest and proceeds to the greater sciatic notch, avoiding the sacroiliac joint and acetabulum. A sacroiliac dislocation is a pure ligamentous injury that separates the attachments of the ilium to the sacrum. A vertical sacral fracture is usually minimally displaced and impacted, but can be widely displaced and possibly comminuted. Vertical sacral fractures can be lateral to the foramina, through the foramina, or medial to the foramina. A fourth pattern resembles an H, with a bilateral vertical component and a horizontal component crossing the sacral vertebral bodies and spinal canal. In the case of fracture-dislocation of the sacroiliac joint, the line of disruption proceeds partly through the bone of either the ilium or the sacrum and partly through the sacroiliac joint. The most

common form involves a fracture through the posterior iliac wing. This fracture line crosses the articular surface of the sacroiliac joint in an oblique pattern from proximal anterior to distal posterior. A posterior segment of the ilium remains stable in its attachment to the sacrum. The anterior segment of the ilium displaces, dislocating the anterior and inferior portions of the sacroiliac joint.

Bucholz Classification The classification of Bucholz divides pelvic ring injuries according to their stability (Fig. 1). Type I injuries have stable anterior and posterior pelvic ring lesions. A radiograph may show only fractures of the pubic rami anteriorly or may demonstrate an associated, non-displaced posterior fracture (most often of the sacrum). Type II injuries demonstrate anterior instability with partial posterior instability. These injuries usually result from an anteroposterior compression mechanism and typically have an "open-book" appearance. Type III injuries demonstrate both anterior and posterior pelvic ring instability. These injuries usually involve a proximal migration of the hemipelvis. If the symphysis pubis is dislocated, these injuries also demonstrate the open-book deformity. Although the instability is usually apparent from displacement on the plain films, at times it only becomes evident after examination of the computed tomographic scan. These injuries are common after a vertical shear mechanism.

Assessment of pelvic ring stability and proper classification of pelvic fracture must take into account the sites of bony injury visible on the radiographs and also the ligamentous injuries implied by the bony injuries and displacements. The soft-tissue injury to a large extent determines the stability of the pelvic ring after injury. Disruption of the sacrospinous and sacrotuberous ligaments of the pelvic floor or the strong posterior interosseous ligaments between the sacrum and ilium leads to instability. Bucholz type II injuries with diastasis of the symphysis pubis of 3 cm or more or type III injuries with more than 1 cm of proximal migration of the hemipelvis should be considered unstable.

A small category of injuries can be displaced but stable. Despite proximal displacement of 1 cm or even slightly more, some fractures of the sacrum are stable, in an impacted and displaced position. Another small category of injuries may appear minimally displaced but are unstable. Again, this is particularly true of sacral fractures, which may appear to be minimally displaced on the plain films although significant comminution or a gap at the fracture site may be evident on a computed tomographic scan.

Tile Classification This proposed new classification of pelvic ring disruptions is very useful in planning treatment. It consists of three major groups (Table 1). Type A, corresponding to Bucholz type I, is stable; type B, corresponding to Bucholz type II, is rotationally unstable but vertically stable; type C, corresponding to Bucholz type III, is rotationally and vertically unstable.

Radiology

Initial radiographic examination of a pelvic fracture includes anteroposterior, 40-degree caudad, and 40-degree cephalad projections. The anteroposterior view is indicated in all patients with significant trauma and provides the initial diagnosis of a pelvic fracture. The caudad projection inlet view shows the pelvis as a ring. It often best indicates

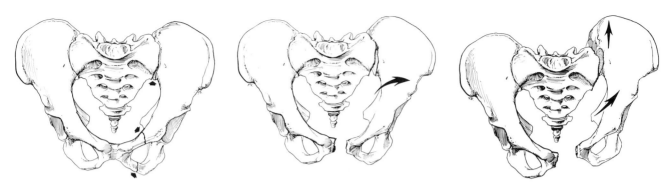

Figure 1

Bucholz classification of pelvic ring fractures. **Left**, Type I—stable anterior and posterior injuries. **Center**, Type II—anterior instability with partial posterior instability. **Right**, Type III—complete anterior and posterior instability.

Table 1. Tile classification of pelvic-ring disruptions

Classification	Description
Type A	Stable
A1	Fracture of the pelvis not involving the ring
A2	Stable, minimally displaced fracture of the ring
Type B	Rotationally unstable but vertically stable
B1	Open-book
B2	Lateral compression (ipsilateral)
B3	Lateral compression (contralateral)
Type C	Rotationally and vertically unstable
C1	Unilateral
C2	Bilateral
C3	Associated with an acetabular fracture

the true magnitude of displacement in cases of sacroiliac dislocation or sacral fracture. It also demonstrates the deformity of the pelvic inlet. With this projection, the X-ray beam roughly parallels the plane of the sacrum. The sacrum is seen on end with the sacral vertebral bodies anteriorly and the triangular formation of the sacral spinal canal posteriorly. The cephalad projection superimposes the anterior pelvic ring on the posterior pelvic ring. It is often the best indicator of a discrepancy in the position of the ischial tuberosities that could lead to later sitting problems for the patient. In this projection, the X-ray beam is directed roughly perpendicular to the plane of the sacrum and shows the sacrum in its longest dimension with the sacral foramina clearly visible (Fig. 2). The diagnostic radiographs can be supplemented with 45-degree oblique views of the pelvis. These views may disclose fractures of the acetabulum not seen on the other views as well as further defining lesions of the sacroiliac joint, iliac wing, and obturator foramen.

If the plain radiographs indicate that there is a possible displaced or unstable fracture of the posterior pelvic ring, a computed tomographic scan is indicated. The computed tomographic scan is particularly helpful in delineating sacral fractures and fracture-dislocations of the sacroiliac joint (Fig. 3). Three-dimensional reconstructions of computed tomographic scans are becoming more useful as the detail and quality of imaging improve. They are particularly useful in planning surgery for old malunions or nonunions of the pelvic ring (Fig. 4).

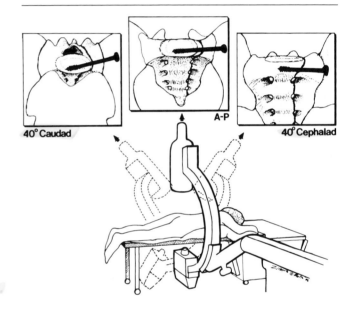

Figure 2

Positioning of the patient and use of the image intensifier for fracture fixation of the sacroiliac joint and sacrum. Anteroposterior, 40-degree caudad, and 40-degree cephalad views show proper positioning for a screw into the S-1 vertebral body.

Treatment Principles

The goals of orthopaedic management are to achieve bony union in a satisfactory position and to rehabilitate the patient as quickly as possible. A pelvic deformity can lead to leg-length inequality and sitting problems secondary to proximal displacement of one or both ischial tuberosities and possible dyspareunia or difficulties with parturition in women. Nonunion or late sacroiliac joint instability can cause pain and limit function. Most pelvic ring injuries are stable and can be treated by closed methods. This typically involves bedrest until the patient is comfortable and then allowing ambulation with external support and weightbearing as tolerated. Serial radiographs must be taken to ensure that an apparently stable lesion does not displace.

Fractures known to be unstable initially are best treated by open reduction and internal fixation. The strongest in-

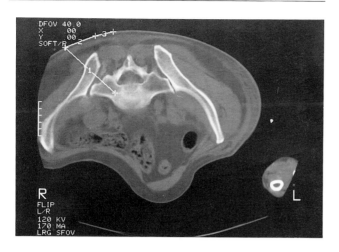

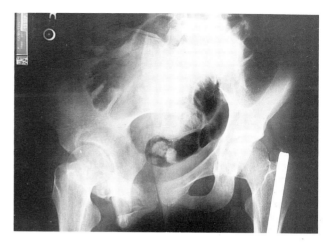

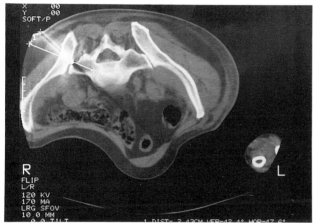

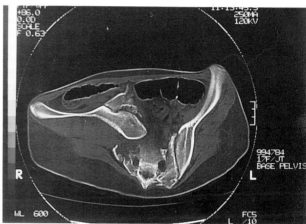

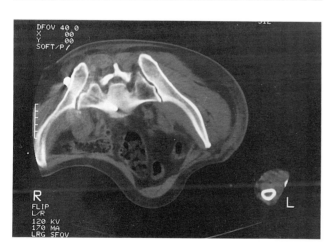

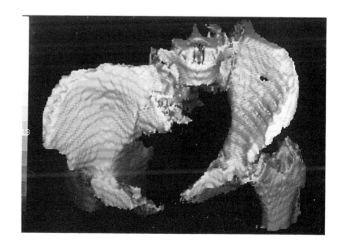

Figure 3

Computed tomography in fracture fixation of the sacroiliac joint and sacrum. **Top**, View through the sacral ala and S-1 vertebral body demonstrates sacroiliac joint widening without significant displacement. The technician draws a line on the screen to indicate a possible path for screw insertion. The patient is placed in the prone position under general or regional anesthesia in the computed tomographic suite. A laser beam directed at the patient indicates the entry point and direction for insertion to the surgeon. **Center**, A cannulated screw is partially inserted, but the placement is incorrect. A new line is drawn on the screen for another attempt. **Bottom**, Final correct placement of the cannulated screw is verified by the image.

Figure 4

Top, Anteroposterior radiograph of a 23-year-old woman three months after a motor-vehicle accident shows untreated fracture-dislocation of the sacroiliac joint and fractures of the pubic ramus. **Center**, Computed tomographic scan shows displacement of the ilium anterior to the sacrum. **Bottom**, Plastic model of the pelvis constructed from the computed tomographic data. Such models are often useful for old injuries requiring reconstruction.

dication for internal fixation is a displaced and unstable lesion of the posterior pelvic ring. Dislocations of the sacroiliac joint are pure ligamentous disruptions and cannot be expected to stabilize adequately after closed treatment. It is possible to treat some unstable sacral or iliac fractures or fracture-dislocations of the sacroiliac joint by closed reduction and maintenance of closed reduction through skeletal traction. The results, however, are less reliable and malunion and nonunion are common. This method also requires prolonged bedrest and immobilization of the patient, which can lead to debilitation and at least initial loss of motion in joints of the ipsilateral extremity. Skeletal traction should only be chosen if there is a bony injury anteriorly and posteriorly and a good reduction is apparent on the radiographs. Skeletal traction should be continued for eight to 12 weeks. At the completion of traction, it is best to document stability and union through stress radiographs and computed tomographic scans.

Bucholz type II injuries with a diastasis of the symphysis pubis of 3 cm or more are best treated by open reduction and plate fixation. It is difficult to justify pelvic sling treatment because of the ease and effectiveness of open treatment. Associated injuries increase the indications for internal fixation. This is particularly true if there are associated factures of the acetabulum or lower extremities.

Open Reduction and Internal Fixation

Displaced and unstable lesions of the posterior pelvic ring that are best treated by open reduction and internal fixation include fracture of the ilium, dislocation of the sacroiliac joint, fracture of the sacrum, and fracture-dislocation of the sacroiliac joint.

All posterior lesions except for the iliac wing fracture can be reached through a common posterior surgical incision. A vertical incision is made 2 cm lateral to the posterosuperior iliac spine. The incision starts proximal to the iliac crest and proceeds over the buttock distal to the greater sciatic notch. The gluteal muscles are reflected from their origins on the iliac wing laterally. The gluteus maximus is partially mobilized from its sacral origin. The erector spinae, as well as the multifidi, can be elevated from the sacrum in a medial direction if visualization of the sacral lamina is necessary. To assess reduction of sacral fractures or sacroiliac joint dislocations, the piriformis is mobilized at the greater sciatic notch so that a finger can be placed into the greater sciatic notch. It is best to palpate anteriorly along the sacrum and sacroiliac joint. Palpation through the greater sciatic notch also reveals the location of the sacral foramina and their accompanying sacral nerve roots. This posterior incision is normally performed with the patient in the prone position.

Fractures of the Iliac Wing

These fractures are usually approached through an incision paralleling the iliac crest. Exposure of the external or internal surface of the iliac wing can be accomplished as needed. An alternative approach to the sacroiliac joint is from the anterior. An incision is made along the iliac crest that continues slightly distal to the anterosuperior spine. The iliacus is mobilized from the internal iliac fossa and the anterior sacral iliac joint thereby exposed. An associated acetabular fracture or the positioning of the patient for surgery on other injuries may influence the choice of surgical approach. Local soft-tissue injuries such as contusions or abrasions or closed

degloving injury may also influence the choice of surgical approach.

Combined Injuries

Open reduction and internal fixation of the posterior pelvic ring displacement is done before other fixations in the pelvic ring. For example, a dislocation of the sacroiliac joint must be reduced and internally fixed before internal fixation of an acetabular fracture. This is true whether the acetabular fracture is ipsilateral or contralateral. If, however, a symphysis pubis dislocation is combined with an unstable posterior lesion and there are no fractures of the obturator foramen or either acetabulum, the symphysis pubis can be reduced and internally fixed first without hindering subsequent posterior internal fixation. Dislocation of the symphysis pubis combined with a sacral fracture or fracture-dislocation of the sacroiliac joint makes it necessary to operate on one lesion and then reposition the patient to operate on the other (Fig. 5). If the combined injury consists of a symphysis dislocation and a sacroiliac joint dislocation or fracture of the ilium, it is usually possible to use an anterior approach to both lesions, making repositioning unnecessary.

Fractures of the Ilium

After a fracture of the ilium is exposed, reduction is carried out with a two-screw technique by applying a reduction forceps to the heads of screws placed on each side of the fracture site or by applying a pointed reduction forceps either directly to the bone or with the points placed into drill holes in the bone. Fixation of an iliac wing fracture can be achieved with long screws placed between the two tables of the bone or with plates applied to the iliac crest or a flat surface of the bone. There should be at least two points of fixation, with fixation along the iliac crest as well as near the greater sciatic notch.

Fracture-Dislocations of the Sacroiliac Joint

These injuries should be approached via the normal posterior incision, perhaps one curving somewhat anteriorly at its proximal end. The patient is normally placed in a prone or lateral position on a radiolucent table. The reduction is carried out with the two-screw technique or with a pointed reduction forceps. Fixation is normally with long lag screws placed between the two tables of the ilium. Fixation can be obtained with a long lag screw 6.5 mm in diameter placed just above the superior border of the greater sciatic notch. In some cases, the ligamentous attachment of the posterior sacral fragment to the sacrum may be tenuous or this fragment may be comminuted. In either case, it is usually necessary to supplement the iliac fixation with fixation from the ilium into the sacrum.

Sacroiliac Joint Dislocations

These injuries are normally operated on with the patient in a prone position on a radiolucent table. The normal posterior vertical incision is made. Reduction is carried out with a pointed reduction forceps from the ilium to the sacrum. Screws are placed through the iliac wing and directed toward the S-1 sacral ala and S-1 vertebral body. During placement of the drill bit and screws, multiple oblique images of the sacrum are taken (anteroposterior 40-degree caudad and 40-degree cephalad views). An alternative method of reduction and fixation is from the anterior. For this the patient is positioned in a supine position on the radiolucent table. A pointed reduction forceps is used from the anterior portion of the sacral ala to the internal aspect of the ilium.

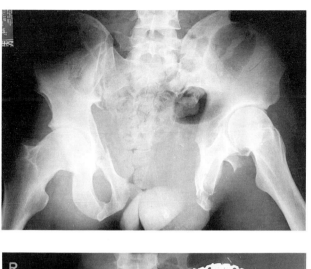
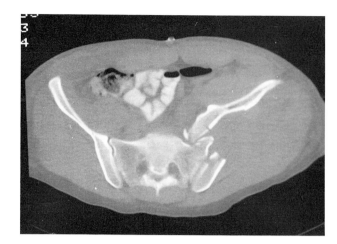
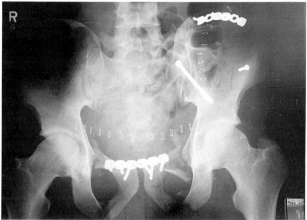
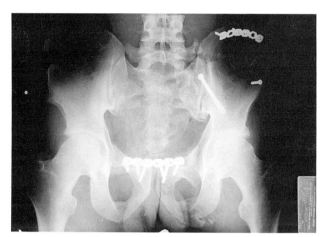

Figure 5

Top left, Anteroposterior radiograph of a 24-year-old man shows fracture-dislocation of the sacroiliac joint and dislocation of the symphysis pubis. The patient has an L-5 nerve root deficit. **Top right**, Computed tomographic scan demonstrates displacement of the ilium anterior to the sacrum. **Bottom left**, After open reduction and internal fixation of the fracture-dislocation of the sacroiliac joint by means of screws placed between the tables of the iliac wing and a plate, the patient was turned into the supine position and the symphysis pubis was plated. Note that the pubic ramus fractures were not plated despite moderate displacement. **Bottom right**, One year later, all fractures have healed. The patient has intermittent radiating pain in the L-5 nerve root distribution.

Fixation is normally by two three-hole plates from the anterior surface of the sacral ala to the internal iliac fossa. Care must be taken throughout the procedure to avoid a stretch injury to the L-5 nerve root as it traverses the anterior portion of the sacral ala. A variation of this procedure is to reduce the joint from anteriorly and then place a screw across the joint from the outer aspect of the iliac wing with a semiopen or percutaneous technique.

Fractures of the Sacrum Fractures of the sacrum are normally approached through a posterior vertical incision. If access is necessary for placement of fixation between the two iliac wings, an additional vertical incision can be made on the contralateral side. For this procedure the patient is positioned prone on the radiolucent table. Some authors have advocated a transverse incision that crosses both posterior iliac crests and the sacrum. The sacral fracture is initially distracted with a lamina spreader or distracting instrument placed between the two posterior iliac crests. This allows the sacral nerve roots to be inspected and the fracture site to be cleaned. The fracture is usually reduced

with a pointed reduction forceps from the spinous process of the sacrum to the iliac crest. As the reduction is performed, the sacral nerve root should be palpated through the greater sciatic notch to ensure that no injury occurs by bony compression.

The preferred method of fixation is a long lag screw 6.5 mm in diameter that traverses the iliac wing, the scroiliac joint, and the sacral ala and enters the S-1 vertebral body. The drill bit and screw must be carefully targeted with an image intensifier and anteroposterior caudad and cephalad projections (Fig. 6). The obvious danger in such internal fixation is direct trauma to the sacral nerve roots or cauda equina from a drill bit or screw. The safety of the procedure can be slightly enhanced by placement of a Kirschner wire before the drill bit is inserted or by using an oscillating drill. The primary guarantees of safety, however, are the surgeon's skill and knowledge of the three-dimensional relationships of the sacral anatomy.

Direct interfragmentary screw fixation provides the greatest fixation with the minimum of implant. However, because of technical difficulties and the potential for injury

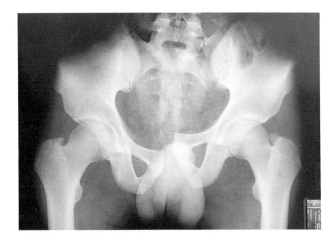

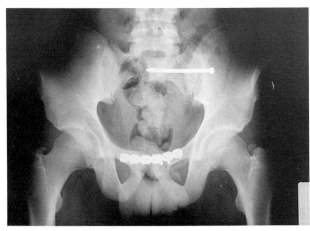

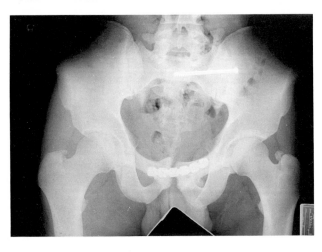

Figure 6

Top, Anteroposterior radiograph of a 17-year-old with a Bucholz type III pelvic injury. There is a fracture through the sacral ala that involves the L5-S1 facet joint. The symphysis pubis is dislocated. **Center,** After open reduction and internal fixation of the symphysis pubis, the sacrum is fixed with a screw inserted into S-1 under image intensifier control. **Bottom,** One year later, the fractures have healed and function is normal.

to the neurologic elements, some authorities have advocated fixation techniques that bridge the posterior iliac crests. One technique is to place large-diameter threaded Steinmann pins between the two posterior iliac crests with nuts applied to the Steinmann pins on the external aspect of the bone. Another technique is to use a transverse Double Cobra plate applied with multiple screws to both iliac wings. Fixation by one or two screws to the S-1 vertebral body can be supplemented by a long flexible plate applied transversely between the two iliac wings. To place this plate, the spinous process of the sacrum is osteotomized and the plate is slipped under the multifidi muscles on the posterior sacral lamina and the osteotomized spinous process. It is attached with cortical screws 3.5 mm in diameter to the two iliac crests.

Targeting of fixation screws for sacral fractures by computed tomographic scan has been described recently. The screws, however, must be placed in the computed tomography suite, which precludes open reduction of the fracture. This technique, therefore, must be reserved for cases with minimal displacement, an uncommon finding in the presence of true instability.

Dislocations of the Symphysis Pubis These injuries are approached through either a transverse or a vertical midline skin incision. The vertical incision can be extended proximally for treatment of intra-abdominal injury or bladder injury. The transverse incision is more cosmetic and is also satisfactory for bladder repair. Regardless of the direction of the skin incision, the deep dissection is the same, with a vertical splitting along the linea alba separating the two heads of the rectus abdominis. The rectus abdominis insertion may be avulsed from one side of the pubis. If it is firmly attached, it must be detached slightly from the undersurface of the attachment to facilitate exposure of the two sides of the pubis and superior pubic ramus. Reduction of a dislocated symphysis pubis is normally by a pointed reduction forceps applied to the outer aspect of the pubis. The two-screw technique can also be used for difficult cases.

The usual fixation is a six-hole or four-hole curved plate applied with screws 3.5 mm in diameter to the superior aspect of the pubis. The plate is placed posterior to the insertion of the rectus abdominis muscle. The screws are placed parallel to the long dimension of the bone. Use of a two-hole plate attached with 6.5-mm screws has been advocated and is adequate for a simple diastasis, although it is less effective than the four-hole or six-hole plate if there is a tendency toward vertical translation.

Fractures of the Pubic Ramus Fixation of a fracture of the superior pubic ramus is unusual and this procedure is limited to very widely displaced or gaping ramus fractures. Reduction and fixation is usually performed through the same incision used for the symphysis pubis, with the possible addition of partial or complete detachment of the rectus abdominis to facilitate more lateral exposure.

Postoperative Treatment Once stable internal fixation of the pelvic ring disruption has been achieved, it is beneficial to mobilize the patient as quickly as possible. Gait training is usually begun five to seven days after surgery. If the posterior injury is unilateral, partial weightbearing is allowed on the affected side. If the posterior injury is bilateral, the patient is usually permitted standing pivot transfers from bed to wheelchair and gait training is not started until six weeks postoperatively. Full weightbearing can usually be allowed six to eight weeks after surgical stabilization.

External Fixation

External fixation is useful to stabilize an acute displaced pelvic fracture to decrease the volume of the pelvis and help control blood loss (Fig. 7). The role of external fixation in definitive reduction and stabilization of unstable pelvic fractures is, however, limited. Closed reduction and fixation of a Bucholz type II injury with diastasis of the symphysis pubis and intact posterior sacroiliac ligaments is possible. Even with this injury, however, anterior plate fixation is more reliable and usually more acceptable to the patient than an external frame. When external fixation is chosen, it is usually applied with two 5-mm pins placed in each anterior iliac crest. The pins enter the bone just proximal to the anterosuperior spine and find good purchase in the thick anterior bone of the iliac wing. The pins should be directed in a posterior-distal and medial direction. The most common error in placement of external fixator pins is to orient them too vertically. This causes the tips of the pins to exit the external aspect of the ilium. The pins may then break free from the bone when they are used to manipulate the displaced pelvic fracture. The pins can usually be placed percutaneously with ease if the surgeon passes a spinal needle along the internal and external aspect of the ilium. This shows the direction for placement.

To control a simple anterior diastasis, any of a number of simple anterior frame configurations that apply an anterior tension band is sufficient. Some of the more rigid frame configurations provide some resistance to vertical translation, although this is usually insufficient to allow ambulation. External fixation is not indicated for vertically unstable disruptions of the posterior pelvic ring.

Complications of Pelvic Ring Disruption

Nonunion or malunion is not uncommon after a pelvic fracture that has a very unstable posterior ring disruption if primary internal fixation is not performed. The treatment of malunions and nonunions of the pelvic ring is much more difficult and dangerous to the patient than is the initial treatment of the injury. Surgical correction of nonunions and malunions must often be done in several stages. The risk of neurologic injury is high when proximal migration of the hemipelvis must be corrected or sacral nonunion sites containing nerve roots are immobilized. The bladder is easily injured when it is displaced into an old symphysis dislocation. The internal iliac vessels may lie in scar tissue very close to an old sacroiliac joint injury. The femoral artery or vein may be found in scar tissue adjacent to a nonunion of the pubic rami. Proper evaluation with three-dimensional computed tomographic scanning of the pelvis can be very helpful in these cases, as is construction of a plastic model of the deformed pelvis from the scan. Preoperative cystograms and arteriograms may assist in the assessment of the proximity of the bladder and vessels to nonunion sites. It is usual to use intraoperative cortical evoked potential monitoring to assist in preventing neurologic injury when old pelvic displacements are corrected.

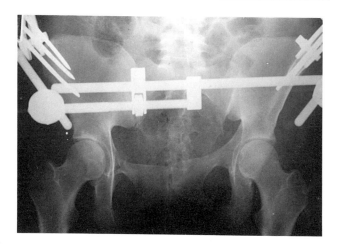

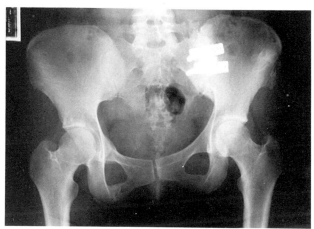

Figure 7

Top, Anteroposterior radiograph of the pelvis of a 23-year-old man after motor-vehicle trauma and external fixator placement. The patient has a Bucholz type III injury with a double vertical fracture of the right obturator foramen and dislocation of the left sacroiliac joint. The patient was hypotensive at admission and did not respond promptly to intravenous fluid and blood. Placement of the external fixator in the emergency room controlled the internal loss of blood. The sacroiliac joint was not reduced. The external fixator was removed after three days. After a one-week delay to permit the pin sites to heal, internal fixation was done. **Bottom**, One year after anterior fixation and fusion of the left sacroiliac joint, the clinical result is excellent and the patient has no pain.

Acetabular Fractures

Routine radiographic views for diagnosing acetabular fractures include anteroposterior views of the pelvis and hip and 45-degree oblique views of the pelvis. Understanding the normal radiographic landmarks of the acetabulum as well as the precise anatomy of the acetabular fracture is essential for proper decision-making and treatment. The plain radiographic views should be supplemented by computed tomographic evaluation.

The anteroposterior view of the acetabulum shows the iliopectineal line, which is a landmark of the anterior column, and the ilioischial line, which is the cortical margin of the quadrilateral surface and a landmark of the posterior column. The roof of the acetabulum is defined by its anterior and posterior rims, the iliac wing, the oburator foramen, and the roentgenographic "U" or teardrop. Careful examination of the anteroposterior views makes it possible to classify most acetabular fractures. The obturator oblique view rotates the uninjured side of the pelvis toward the X-ray beam and the obturator foramen appears large. The iliac wing appears on edge in its narrowest dimension. The pelvic brim, anterior column, and the posterior rim are profiled. The iliac oblique view shows the iliac wing in its largest dimension. The X-ray beam roughly parallels the plane of the obturator foramen. The greater and lesser sciatic notches, and thus the posterior column, and the anterior rim of the acetabulum are profiled.

The computed tomographic scan provides additional information and answers specific questions that the plain films cannot. The computed tomographic scan is useful for showing hidden fractures of the posterior pelvic ring such as minimally displaced sacral fractures. It may disclose minimally displaced fractures of the ilium as well as fractures of the quadrilateral surface. The rotational displacements of the anterior and posterior columns of the acetabulum are evident. Incarcerated fragments between the femoral head and the walls of the acetabulum and between the femoral head and the roof of the acetabulum are often best visualized on the plain films.

The classification advocated by Letournel is perhaps the most useful. Deciding which of the ten fracture types the injury can be classified as greatly assists in evaluating the indications for surgery and in selecting a surgical approach. This classification includes five simple fracture types—fractures of the posterior wall, the posterior column, the anterior wall, the anterior column, and transverse fractures.

Posterior-wall fractures involve the posterior articular surface, usually a portion of the retroacetabular surface, and sometimes the entire retroacetabular surface. The ilioischial line remains intact. Posterior-column fractures displace the posterior articular surface and also the ilioischial line. Anterior-wall fractures displace the central portion of the anterior column and the iliopectineal line. Anterior-column fractures involve a variable amount of the anterior column depending on whether the fracture is low or high. Again, the iliopectineal line is displaced. Transverse fractures cross the two columns of the acetabulum from anterior to posterior. They divide the innominate bone into two portions with a segment of roof attached to an intact ilium and a single ischiopubic fragment inferiorly.

Combined fracture types include associated posterior-wall and posterior-column fractures and associated posterior-wall and transverse fractures. A T-shaped fracture contains a transverse component and also a vertical component that separates the lower ischiopubic segment into anterior and posterior column segments. In associated anterior and posterior hemitransverse fractures, the anterior-column or anterior-wall pattern predominates in displacement and involvement of the roof. A low and usually minimally displaced posterior hemitransverse component is also present. Two-column fractures involve both columns of the acetabulum; however, unlike all other fracture types, all segments of the articular surface are detached from the intact portion of the ilium.

Treatment Principles

The goals of treatment are restoration of function and prevention of posttraumatic arthritis. Although articular car-

tilage can be damaged at the time of original injury or by unrecognized incarcerated osteochondral fragments, the most common cause of posttraumatic arthritis is residual joint incongruity from an imperfect reduction. With intra-articular displacement of more than 1 to 2 mm, especially in the weightbearing portion of the acetabulum, the articular cartilage cannot withstand the alteration in pressure distribution, and degenerative changes ensue.

Certain displaced intra-articular fractures can be treated successfully with skeletal traction. A two-column fracture without wide displacement and with apparent congruence on the three standard radiographic views can be treated in this manner. Similarly, a low transverse fracture not involving the weightbearing dome can usually be reduced with skeletal traction. Most displaced intra-articular fractures, however, require open reduction. The decision of whether or not to operate can usually be made on the basis of the initial plain radiographs and computed tomography. Of additional help is the use of a system to estimate the amount of acetabular dome that remains intact after the fracture. This system uses three measurements: the medial roof arc, the anterior roof arc, and the posterior roof arc.

These three measurements are made on the anteroposterior view, obturator oblique view, and iliac oblique view of the pelvis, respectively. The medial roof arc is measured by drawing a vertical line through the roof of the acetabulum to the geometric center of the femoral head. A second line is drawn from the fracture to the geometric center of the femoral head. The angle subtended by these lines is the medial roof arc. The anterior roof and posterior roof arcs are measured similarly. This method is most useful in posterior-column fractures, anterior-column fractures, transverse fractures, T-shaped fractures, and associated anterior-column and posterior hemitransverse fractures. Roof arc measurements have limited usefulness for evaluating two-column fractures and fractures of the posterior wall.

The following criteria should be met before nonsurgical treatment is selected: (1) the femoral head should remain congruent with the roof of the acetabulum when the patient is taken out of traction; (2) the anterior roof arc, medial roof arc, and posterior roof arc should all be greater than 45 degrees; and (3) the adequacy of the remaining acetabular rim in posterior-wall fractures should be assessed by plain radiographs and computed tomography because roof arc measurements are unreliable.

Neufeld-type roller traction is a useful form of nonsurgical treatment because it allows active lower-extremity exercises. Traction must be maintained for four to eight weeks to achieve bony union.

Surgical Treatment

Unless there is a coexisting anterior or posterior hip dislocation irreducible by closed means, open reduction and internal fixation of acetabular fractures is best undertaken no sooner than two to three days after injury. This allows the initial bleeding from the fracture site and pelvic vessels to subside. In the preoperative period, skeletal traction is usually provided through a distal femoral pin. This is particularly important in the case of a T-shaped or transverse fracture of the acetabular roof because the femoral head can be damaged by sharp fracture surfaces. To avoid difficulties in reduction, surgery should be performed within ten days of the injury. A bony callus is usually present by three weeks after the injury.

The most useful surgical approaches for open reduction and internal fixation of acetabular fractures are the Köcher-Langenbeck, the ilioinguinal, and the extended iliofemoral. A triradiate incision that can be extended to give an exposure similar to the extended iliofemoral approach has been advocated. No single surgical approach provides ideal exposure for all fracture types. Proper classification of the fracture configuration preoperatively is essential to selecting the best approach.

Köcher-Langenbeck Approach This is done with the patient in the prone position on a fracture table. Access is obtained to the retroacetabular surface as far distally as the ischial tuberosity. Only the most inferior portion of the iliac wing is accessible. Proximal access is limited by the superior gluteal vessels and nerve. The quadrilateral surface and pelvic rim are accessible by palpation through the greater sciatic notch. The greater and lesser sciatic notches are exposed by transecting the piriformis and obturator internus tendons in the trochanteric fossa. Exposure of the inferior aspect of the iliac wing is enhanced by osteotomy of the trochanter or transection of the gluteus medius tendon. Visualization of the interior of the joint can be obtained through a capsulotomy performed along the acetabular rim.

Ilioinguinal Approach This is done with the patient supine on a fracture table. This allows access to the internal aspect of the innominate bone and exposes the entire internal iliac fossa, anterior sacroiliac joint, pelvic brim, and quadrilateral surface. Limited access to the anterior portion of the external iliac wing is possible. The incision begins at a point two thirds of the way posterior along the iliac crest, proceeds forward to the anterosuperior iliac spine, and then moves transversely along the lower abdomen to a point 30 to 40 mm above the symphysis pubis. The abdominal wall muscles and the iliacus muscle are mobilized from the crest and internal iliac fossa. The inguinal canal is opened on both its roof and its floor to mobilize the abdominal muscles and transversalis fascia from the inguinal ligament. The structures passing across the inguinal ligament (including the spermatic cord, external iliac vessels, iliopsoas muscle, and the femoral nerve) are identified and retracted according to the segment of pelvis that is being reduced or internally fixed. This is primarily an approach to the anterior column; however, access to the posterior column can be gained by retracting the external iliac vessels medially and the iliopsoas and femoral nerve laterally. Open reduction and internal fixation is sometimes difficult through this exposure. Its advantages, however, include a cosmetically acceptable scar and lower incidences of surgical morbidity and postoperative heterotopic bone formation because of minimal muscle stripping from the innominate bone.

Extended Iliofemoral Approach This is done with the patient in the lateral position on the fracture table. This approach gives wide access to the entire external aspect of the iliac wing and the retroacetabular surface distal to the ischial tuberosity and limited access to the anterior column as far distally as the pectineal eminence. The incision begins at the posterosuperior iliac spine, proceeds anteriorly along the crest to the anterosuperior iliac spine, and then gently curves to follow the line of the anterolateral thigh distally almost to its midpoint. The incision follows a plane between nerves, reflecting the muscles innervated by the superior and inferior gluteal nerves posteriorly and the muscles innervated by the femoral nerve medially. The gluteal muscle and tensor fasciae latae are reflected from the external aspect of the iliac wing and their tendons are divided at their trochanteric insertions. The obturator internus and piriformis tendons are divided in the trochanteric fossa. Elevation of the iliacus from the internal iliac fossa and detachment of the rectus femoris origin from above the acetabulum and the anteroinferior iliac spine gives further access to the anterior column. Visualization of the internal aspect of the hip joint is possible by dividing the hip capsule next to the acetabular rim. This exposure provides the most commanding access to the innominate bone. The amount of dissection required, however, leads to a longer period of postoperative rehabilitation.

Triradiate Approach The triradiate approach offers an alternative way to expose the external aspect of the innominate bone. It gives almost the same exposure to the bone as the extended iliofemoral approach but the exposure to the posterior part of the ilium is not as good. The incision starts like that for the Köcher-Langenbeck approach, dissecting between the fibers of the gluteus maximus and splitting the fascia lata. The incision is then directed from the anterosuperior greater spine to the trochanter. The greater trochanter is osteotomized and the abductor insertion and the tensor fascia lata are retracted proximally. Further exposure to the iliac wing can be obtained by releasing fascia lata from the iliac crest, as in the extended iliofemoral approach. The incision can also be extended medially across the lower abdomen to obtain some exposure of the inner aspect of the bone.

Choosing the Approach The surgical approach is selected with the expectation that the entire operation can be performed through a single surgical incision. Intraoperative traction with a fracture table (preferably the Judet fracture table) stably positions the lower extremity and distracts the femoral head from its displaced position, allowing reduction of the acetabular fragments. The ASIF femoral distractor can be used as an alternative to the fracture table. When traction is used, it is important to flex the knee at least 60 degrees to relax the sciatic nerve.

An alternative advocated by other authorities is to place the patient in the lateral position on a standard table, permitting some mobility so that the patient can be rolled. This technique allows the option of simultaneous anterior and posterior approaches. Access to the bone is diminished and control of the fracture through the Köcher-Langenbeck and ilioinguinal approaches is less, however, with lateral positioning and no fracture table.

Reduction of Fragments Various reduction forceps are available for use in the reduction of fragments. A pointed reduction forceps can be applied directly to the bone. Other specialized reduction forceps are applied to the heads of screws temporarily placed on both sides of the fracture line. It is important to correct all components of the deformity, including diastasis, translational displacement, and rotational displacement. Rotation of the posterior column along its longitudinal axis is best controlled with a femoral head corkscrew-type extractor inserted into the ischial tuberosity. Rotation of a high anterior-column fracture can be controlled with a Farabeuf reduction forceps placed along the anteroinferior iliac spine. Fracture reduction usually cannot be achieved in a single step. It is often necessary to proceed by stepwise reduction of single fracture fragments to intact portions of the pelvis. In general, precise reduction of extra-articular fragments aids the final articular reduction. Incarcerated fragments and impacted articular surfaces must be recognized preoperatively to allow correction by manipulation.

Fixation Fracture fixation is achieved with a combination of interfragmentary screws and plates. Screw fixation alone is rarely satisfactory. Screws should be available in several diameters from 3.5 to 6.5 mm and in lengths up to 110 mm. Plates should be available in various lengths, and plate-bending devices are useful. Provisional fixation is with screws alone. Lag screws are preferred to provide interfragmentary compression, enhancing fracture stability. Fixation is completed with the application of plates, usually along the pelvic brim or paralleling the rim of the acetabulum. Although visualization of the reduction on the articular surface is desirable, it is not always possible.

The final articular reduction, therefore, is not always visualized and is often judged to be correct after precise reduction of the extra-articular cortex of the innominate bone.

Treatment of Specific Fractures

Posterior-Wall Fractures Fixation is performed through a Köcher-Langenbeck approach. The first steps are irrigation and debridement to ensure that there are no loose osteocartilaginous fragments in the hip joint. It is important to recognize any marginal impaction of the articular surface that can be corrected by elevation of the impacted segment. If significant impaction is present, additional bone grafting may be necessary. Free fragments consisting only of cartilage and cancellous bone should not be discarded unless they are very small. Fixation should use lag screws traversing the fragments and a curved posterior buttressing plate paralleling the posterior rim of the acetabulum.

Posterior-Column Fractures Isolated fractures of this type are exposed through a Köcher-Langenbeck approach with the patient in the prone position. Reduction is performed and visually assessed on the retroacetabular surface. Fixation is obtained by using a small reconstruction or dynamic compression plate applied from the ischial tuberosity to the lateral ilium along the retroacetabular surface.

Transverse Fracture Exposure is usually through the Köcher-Langenbeck approach with the patient prone. Reduction is carried out in a fashion similar to that for isolated posterior-column fractures, and fixation of the posterior column is carried out with a buttress plate. A long 6.5-mm cancellous screw is inserted across the anterior portion of the fracture into the superior pubic ramus. If the anterior component of the transverse fracture is situated high, exposure may be best obtained through the ilioinguinal approach.

Associated Transverse and Posterior-Wall Fractures Most of these can be exposed through the Köcher-Langenbeck approach with the patient prone on the fracture table. These fractures are often associated with posterior dislocation of the femoral head and incarceration of loose osteocartilaginous fragments. Distraction of the femoral head is necessary for thorough inspection of the interior of the joint and removal of these fragments. The transverse fracture is reduced and provisionally fixed, followed by reduction of the posterior-wall fracture and application of a buttress plate. The extended iliofemoral or triradiate approach may be necessary for particularly difficult or old associated transverse and posterior-wall fractures.

T-Shaped Fractures Most such fractures can be reduced and fixed through the Köcher-Langenbeck approach by reducing the posterior column in the usual manner and manipulating the anterior column either through the sciatic notch or from an intra-articular approach. If anterior-column reduction is not possible, a subsequent ilioinguinal approach is required. In many cases, initial use of the extended iliofemoral or triradiate approach may be preferred.

Anterior-Column and Anterior-Wall Fractures These are best exposed through the ilioinguinal approach, which provides access to the entire length of the anterior column. Fixation is accomplished with lag screws initially and completed by application of a plate along the pelvic brim.

Associated Anterior-Column and Posterior Hemitransverse Fractures The ilioinguinal approach with the patient supine on the fracture table is best. After anterior-column reduction and fixation, the posterior column is reduced by manipulation of the quadrilateral surface and fixed by passing long lag screws from the pelvic brim to the posterior column near the ischial spine.

Two-Column Fractures These are the most difficult acetabular fractures to reduce and fix satisfactorily. For the surgeon with significant experience, most of these fractures can be treated through the ilioinguinal approach. The anterior column is reduced and fixed to the ilium. The posterior column is then reduced; the reduction is judged by visualization of the quadrilateral surface. Fixation is performed with interfragmentary lag screws and supplementary reconstruction or buttress plate. The final articular reduction is not visualized but inferred by the reduction of the fracture lines on the inner aspect of the bone. The final reduction and implant position can be checked with the image intensifier. With the ilioinguinal approach, the incision is relatively cosmetic, the postoperative recovery rapid, and the incidence of significant ectopic bone formation negligible (Fig. 8). If a wound infection develops, it is typically intrapelvic and extra-articular.

The extended iliofemoral approach gives the most commanding access to the bone and should be used if a complex posterior-column fracture is present or if displaced fracture lines cross the sacroiliac joint.

Postoperative Management

Closed suction drainage is continued postoperatively for 48 hours. Antimicrobial agents are used for 48 to 72 hours after surgery. Passive motion of the hip is started on day 2 or day 3. Crutch walking, allowing up to 15 kg of weightbearing, is allowed on postoperative days 4 to 7, or when pain permits. Weightbearing is limited for the first eight weeks and then progressively increased.

Complications

The most common serious complications after surgical treatment of an acetabular fracture include surgical wound infection, iatrogenic nerve palsy, periarticular ectopic bone, and thromboembolic complications. Posttraumatic arthritis is the most common late complication.

Infection If the patient's general condition is good and no associated injuries are present, the risk of infection should not be higher than with other types of hip surgery. Unfortunately, however, most patients with fractures of the acetabulum have associated injuries that increase the risk of infection. These may include injuries to the abdominal or pelvic viscera or the extremities. A relatively common problem associated with acetabular fracture is local soft-tissue injury, including local wounds and abrasions or a closed degloving injury.

Closed degloving injuries must be drained and debrided either before or at the time of surgery to decrease the likelihood of infection. After drainage and debridement, it is almost always advisable to leave this area open either through the surgical incision or through a separate incision. Dressing changes and wound packing are necessary, sometimes for a prolonged period, until the wound closes secondarily. Primary excision of the necrotic fat and closure over drainage tubes has been unsuccessful.

Postoperative hematoma formation is likely in the large wounds necessary for acetabular surgery. Suction drains should be used liberally. The surgeon should always strive to preserve soft-tissue pedicles to all bone fragments to maintain the vascularity of the bone. If a fragment is devascularized, it usually vascularizes rapidly as long as no infection develops. However, in the presence of infection, bacteria rapidly colonize an avascular fragment and it usually requires debridement and excision. Some bloody drainage may come from the wound for the first one or two days after the operation, although this should subside quickly. A clear yellow serous fluid may drain from the wound for as long as ten days after surgery without infection being present. However, if the wound has not been draining for a number of days and then a bloody or cloudy yellowish discharge begins, the patient should be returned to the operating room immediately for irrigation and debridement of the wound.

If an infection is extra-articular, it can probably be controlled and function is not impaired. In the case of an intra-articular infection, however, the cartilage of the joint is invariably destroyed and hip function is significantly impaired.

Nerve Palsy Iatrogenic nerve palsy is caused almost exclusively by too vigorous or too prolonged retraction of the sciatic nerve. This occurs primarily with the Köcher-Langenbeck approach and involves primarily the peroneal branch of the sciatic nerve. There is a slight chance of a stretch injury to the sciatic nerve with the extended iliofemoral approach. There is also a slight possibility of stretch injury to the femoral nerve during the ilioinguinal approach. If a nerve palsy does develop, it is best treated with an ankle-foot orthosis. There is some chance that the sciatic nerve will recover during the first three years after the injury and tendon transfer procedures to correct a footdrop should not be performed during this period.

Ectopic Bone Formation Ectopic bone formation occurs al-

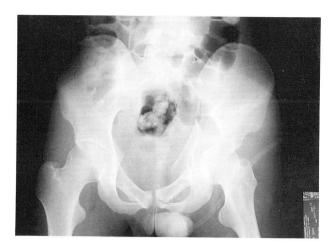
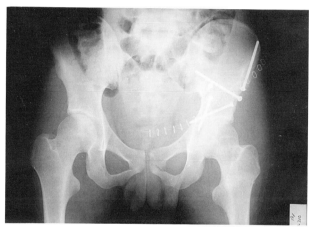
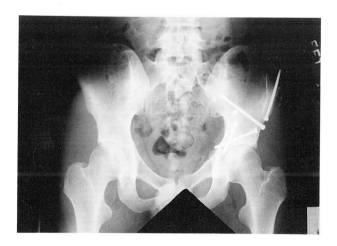

Figure 8

Top, Anteroposterior radiograph of the pelvis of a 19-year-old woman with a two-column acetabular fracture. **Center**, After open reduction and internal fixation through the ilioinguinal approach. **Bottom**, After two years, hip function is excellent.

most exclusively with lateral exposure of the innominate bone. The incidence of significant ectopic bone is highest with the extended iliofemoral approach, second highest with the Köcher-Langenbeck approach, and negligible with the ilioinguinal approach. Prevention of ectopic bone requires choosing the ilioinguinal approach whenever possible and attempting to limit muscle trauma during surgery by careful soft-tissue handling. Indomethacin, 25 mg three times a day, for several months after surgery may be helpful in decreasing the incidence and extent of ectopic bone. Postoperative radiation has been shown to be effective in decreasing the incidence of ectopic bone, but its long-term carcinogenic effects are unknown. Whenever possible, excision of ectopic bone should be delayed for 15 to 18 months after the injury. After this period, there is usually no problem with recurrence and motion can be expected to return to more than 80% of normal unless arthritis is present.

Thromboembolic Complications There is significant potential for deep venous thrombosis and pulmonary embolism with fractures of the acetabulum. Some authors recommend using pneumatic compression boots on both lower extremities from the time of admission until the patient is fully ambulatory. In older patients and patients considered to be at high risk, anticoagulation therapy is begun with heparin postoperatively. Home therapy with warfarin is continued for six to eight weeks. The prothrombin time is kept at about 150% of normal. Despite concern for possible thromboembolic complications, excessive anticoagulation must be avoided because a large wound hematoma can be devastating if a deep infection to the hip results.

Combined Acetabular and Pelvic Injuries

Occasionally, acetabular fractures are associated with significant injury to the posterior pelvic ring—that is, sacroiliac joint dislocation or sacral fracture. In these complex cases, reduction and stabilization of the posterior pelvic ring is required before reduction of the acetabular fracture. Precise reduction of a displaced acetabular fracture cannot be achieved when the pelvic ring is distorted. Fixation of the sacroiliac joint can often be done through a single surgical incision that also exposes the acetabulum. The sacroiliac joint can be exposed either by the Köcher-Lagenbeck approach with a cephalad extension or by an extended iliofemoral approach. The ilioinguinal approach can be used for access to both the anterior sacroiliac joint and the symphysis pubis.

Old Fractures

If surgery is delayed beyond three weeks after injury, an organized callus will be present about the fracture lines, impairing reduction. In younger patients with unacceptable displacement, especially those with simple fracture configurations, open reduction and internal fixation should be undertaken even if osteotomy of a partially or totally healed fracture is required. If the patient is older and has a complex fracture with minimal to moderate deformity, surgery can be deferred. Old posterior-column and posterior-wall fractures are operated on through the Köcher-Langenbeck approach. Old anterior-wall and anterior-column fractures are operated on through the ilioinguinal approach. All other old fractures are best operated on through the extended iliofemoral approach.

Controversies

External Fixation vs Arterial Embolization in the Management of Major Hemorrhage in Pelvic Ring Disruptions

There are no prospective studies that clearly show the superiority of either emergency application of external fixation or selective arterial embolization in the management of major hemorrhage after pelvic ring disruption. Although several retrospective studies demonstrated a clear decrease in hemorrhages after the application of an anterior fixator, the precise indications for its use remain unclear. Most traumatologists agree that patients with Tile type B1 and type C injuries and hemodynamic changes unresponsive to fluid resuscitation are good candidates for the emergency application of a fixator. Lateral compression injuries respond less well to this treatment. The role of selective embolization of bleeding vessels varies, depending on the availability of facilities and expertise at any given trauma center.

Indications for Open Reduction and Internal Fixation of Pelvic Ring Disruptions

The precise indications for open reduction and internal fixation of hemipelvic fractures and dislocations remain undefined. Most unstable pelvic ring disruptions, defined as those with more than 1 cm of shortening and gross mobility of the posterior elements of the pelvic ring, should be reduced and stabilized in young patients. The presence of pelvic ring instability is, however, often difficult to ascertain. Stress radiographs of the pelvis with and without longitudinal loads applied to the ipsilateral leg are useful in detecting hidden instability. Long-term follow-up studies are needed to determine whether the results of open reduction and internal fixation of unstable pelvic ring disruptions are superior to those of traditional nonsurgical methods.

Anterior vs Posterior Fixation of Sacroiliac Dislocations

Sacroiliac disruptions can be stabilized through either an anterior or a posterior approach to the joint. The posterior approach involves minimal dissection and has a low complication rate if there is no extensive soft-tissue contusion in the buttock area. Visualization of the joint is, however, limited and screw placement is often performed in a blind fashion. Fluoroscopic guidance of screw insertion has been advocated by several investigators. The anterior approach to the sacroiliac joint requires more dissection and moderate retraction on the L-5 nerve root. The joint, however, can be visualized easily and concomitant fusion can be performed without difficulty. The degree of rigidity of the fixation appears to be equivalent for the two approaches.

Most orthopaedic traumatologists currently prefer the anterior approach because of the ease of reduction and the potential for fusion at surgery. The direct placement of the plates and screws also minimizes the risk of inadvertent damage to the nerve roots during screw placement. Long-term follow-up studies are nonetheless needed to determine wheher this anterior approach yields better results than the more traditional posterior approach.

Indications for Open Reduction and Internal Fixation of Acetabular Fractures

Despite extensive work by many investigators, there is no consensus as to the exact indications for surgical repair of acetabular fractures. Gross hip instability, such as that following posterior fracture-dislocations, clearly warrants surgical repair. A minor degree of central subluxation, however, especially in elderly patients, is only a relative indication for surgery. The concept of roof arc measurements is a major advance in our assessment of the need for surgical repair. It is hoped that long-term follow-up studies substantiating the value of this measurement will be available soon.

Prevention of Heterotopic Ossification After Surgical Repair of Acetabular Fractures

Heterotopic ossification is one of the major complications of acetabular surgery involving dissection of the gluteal musculature. Brooker stage III and stage IV ossification can result in hip contracture and major functional disability. With present technology, it is impossible to determine in which patients this complication will develop.

Three approaches to this problem are currently available. Some surgeons recommend routine use of the ilioinguinal approach. The incidence of heterotopic ossification with this anterior approach to the pelvis is negligible. Adequate exposure of many acetabular fracture patterns, especially those involving the posterior wall and column, is impossible, however, and universal use of this single approach is not feasible. A second alternative is low-dose radiation immediately after surgery (approximately 10 to 20 Gy). Most acetabular fractures, however, occur in young patients and the long-term effects of this radiation, even with the use of selective portals and low dosage, is unknown. Most centers currently limit the use of radiation therapy to elderly patients with preexisting heterotopic ossification. A third approach is the use of indomethacin, 25 mg three times a day for four to six weeks after surgery. Retrospective data should soon be available to show that this is an effective treatment that avoids the risks associated with other forms of treatment. Prospective studies are, however, needed.

Annotated Bibliography

Keywords

Acetabular fracture; Dermatologic injury; Gastrointestinal injury; Gynecologic injury; Hemorrhage; Iliac wing fracture; Nerve injury; Pelvic fracture; Pelvic ring disruption; Sacral fracture; Sacroiliac joint; Shock; Urologic injury

Pelvic Fractures

Colapinto V: Trauma to the pelvis: Urethral injury. *Clin Orthop* 1980;151:46–55.
  Urethral injuries are reviewed and a classification outlined. Diagnostic techniques and therapeutic regimens are discussed.

Naam NH, Brown WM, Hurd R, et al: Major pelvic fractures. *Arch Surg* 1983;118:610–616.
  This review of pelvic fractures in 593 patients discusses factors influencing morbidity and mortality and outlines advanced treatment methods.

Perry JF Jr: Pelvic open fractures. *Clin Orthop* 1980;151: 41–45.
  In this series of 738 patients, there were 31 open fractures. These are reviewed in terms of complications, associated injuries, and mortality.

Saibil EA, Maggisano R, Witchell SS: Angiography in the diagnosis and treatment of trauma. *J Can Assoc Radiol* 1983;34:218–227.
  The role of angiography in the diagnosis of trauma is discussed. Transcatheter arterial embolization is described as possibly the definitive therapeutic procedure in pelvic bleeding.

Tile M: *Fractures of the Pelvis and Acetabulum.* Baltimore, Williams & Wilkins, 1984.
  This text details the radiologic study, classification, and surgical and nonsurgical treatments of fractures of the acetabulum and pelvis.

Pelvic Ring Injuries

Denis F, Davis S, Comfort T: Sacral fractures: An important problem. Retrospective analysis of 236 cases. *Clin Orthop* 1988;227:67–81.
  Sacral fractures, often undiagnosed and untreated, frequently result in neurologic symptoms and deficits in the lower extremities and urinary, rectal, and sexual dysfunction. This retrospective study included 236 patients with sacral fractures in a series of 776 patients with pelvic injuries. The sacral fractures were classified on the basis of their direction, location, and level. Injuries in zone I, the region of the ala, were occasionally associated with partial damage to the L-5 nerve root. Injuries in zone II, the region of the sacral foramina, were frequently associated with sciatica but rarely with bladder dysfunction. Injuries in zone III, the region of the central sacral canal, were frequently associated with saddle anesthesia and loss of sphincter function.

Lange RH, Hansen ST Jr: Pelvic ring disruptions with symphysis pubis diastasis: Indications, technique, and limitations of anterior internal fixation. *Clin Orthop* 1985;201:130–137.
  Twenty-four injuries associated with symphysis pubis diastasis were reviewed to compare two-hole and four-hole plate techniques for anterior internal fixation. The two-hole plate technique appears to be quite acceptable for maintaining reduction of the diastasis and, therefore, can be used to manage most anteroposterior compression injuries (those without complete posterior disruption). Vertical shear injuries, all of which are grossly unstable, can also be managed with anterior two-hole plates. However, this fixation method must be supplemented by some form of posterior stabilization to maintain pelvic ring reduction.

Matta JM, Saucedo T: Internal fixation of pelvic ring fractures. *Clin Orthop* 1989;242:83–97.

Fifty-four patients with unstable pelvic injuries were treated by one of three methods—skeletal traction, external fixation, or open reduction and internal fixation. A comparison of results demonstrated that internal fixation was superior for anatomic results, union rate, and functional results. Of 32 injuries treated by internal fixation, 22 were fixed initially and ten were fixed after failure of traction or external fixation. One deep wound infection was the only surgical complication. The authors describe current treatment protocols and fixation techniques.

Mears DC, Capito CP, Deleeuw H: Posterior pelvic disruptions managed by the use of the Double Cobra plate, in Bassett FH III (ed): American Academy of Orthopaedic Surgeons *Instructional Course Lectures, XXXVII.* Park Ridge, American Academy of Orthopaedic Surgeons, 1988, pp 143–150.

Five years of experience with 30 patients in whom the Double Cobra plate technique was employed for reconstruction of a variety of posterior pelvic injuries indicated that this method is apparently highly suitable for effective stabilization of both sacral fractures and bilateral sacroiliac dislocations. In late presentations and larger individuals, anterior reconstruction of the pelvic ring is strongly recommended.

Shaw JA, Mino DE, Werner FW, et al: Posterior stabilization of pelvic fractures by use of threaded compression rods: Case reports and mechanical testing. *Clin Orthop* 1985;192:240–254.

Threaded compression rods were placed between the posterosuperior spines as a means of posterior stabilization of pelvic fractures. Malgaigne fractures with sacroiliac disruptions were created in four cadaveric pelvises. Anterior frames alone provided little stabilization of the disrupted sacroiliac joints with either longitudinal or torsional loading. Markedly improved stabilization in both loading modes was achieved with posterior augmentation. Two typical cases are presented to demonstrate that posterior stabilization is as effective in clinical practice as in the biomechanics laboratory.

Simpson LA, Waddell JP, Peighton RK, et al: Anterior approach and stabilization of the disrupted sacroiliac joint. *J Trauma* 1987;27:1332–1339.

The authors describe their technique for and excellent results with anterior sacroiliac fixation.

Tile M: Pelvic ring fractures: Should they be fixed? *J Bone Joint Surg* 1988;70B:1–12.

Of 494 fractures treated over five years, only 19% needed stabilization (5% by internal means). External fixation should be used initially, followed by internal fixation posteriorly for unstable or unreduced fractures.

Acetabular Fractures

Aho AJ, Isberg UK, Katevuo VK: Acetabular posterior wall fracture: 38 cases followed for 5 years. *Acta Orthop Scand* 1986;57;101–105.

Thirty-eight patients with fractures of the posterior wall of the acetabulum were reviewed after an average of five years (range, two to 12 years). Results were good in 17 of 18 patients in whom manual reduction of a femoral head dislocation was successful, who had no sciatic nerve injury, and who did not undergo surgery. Of 20 patients who underwent surgery either because the fracture fragment was large or because of a persistent dislocation of the femoral head, six had poor results caused by femoral head necrosis. Skeletal traction seems unnecessary in the treatment of acetabular posterior-wall fractures.

Bosse MJ, Poka A, Reinert CM, et al: Heterotopic ossification as a complication of acetabular fracture: Prophylaxis with low-dose irradiation. *J Bone Joint Surg* 1988; 70A:1231–1237.

In a retrospective review of 37 patients who underwent surgery for 38 complex acetabular fractures, postoperative low-dose irradiation was administered to 17 patients (18 fractures) to suppress heterotopic ossification. All the operations were done through either an extended iliofemoral incision or a modified extended iliofemoral incision. Most received 10 Gy in 2-Gy increments, starting on the third postoperative day. The incidence of heterotopic ossification in the 18 irradiated limbs was much lower than that in the 20 patients in the control group (50% vs 90%). The difference in the incidence of severe (class III or class IV) heterotopic ossification between the two groups of patients was significant.

Bray TJ, Esser M, Fulkerson L: Osteotomy of the trochanter in open reduction and internal fixation of acetabular fractures. *J Bone Joint Surg* 1987;69A:711–717.

Osteotomy of the trochanter can enhance lateral and posterior exposures of the acetabulum and the retroacetabular space. During a two-year period, an osteotomy of the trochanter was done in ten patients in connection with open reduction and internal fixation of a displaced acetabular fracture. The trochanter was reattached with two 6.5-mm cancellous screws. All the osteotomies healed uneventfully.

Burk DL Jr, Mears DC, Kennedy WH, et al: Three-dimensional computed tomography of acetabular fractures. *Radiology* 1985;155:183–186.

Computer programs that produce three-dimensional surface reformations from sets of contiguous axial computed tomographic scans were used in evaluating various acetabular fractures in 20 patients. The three-dimensional images were easily correlated with plain radiographs, and new views were produced that provided a unique perspective not obtained by conventional radiography. The three-dimensional images were useful in complex displaced fractures. Plain radiographs and conventional computed tomography scans were more sensitive than the three-dimensional images in detecting undisplaced fractures.

Epstein HC: *Traumatic Dislocation of the Hip.* Baltimore, Williams & Wilkins, 1980.

Posterior dislocation of the hip combined with acetabular fracture leads to a high incidence of posttraumatic arthritis. The long-term results were best in those patients who underwent primary open reduction of the dislocation with removal of the intra-articular bone fragments and internal fixation of the fracture.

Hall BB, Klassen RA: Acetabular fractures in children: A long-term follow-up study. *Orthop Trans* 1982;6:355.

As in adults, posttraumatic arthritis is the most common problem after acetabular fracture in children. Two of 25 children had premature triradiate cartilage closure.

Harley JD, Mack LA, Winquist RA: CT of acetabular fractures: Comparison with conventional radiography. *Am J Radiol* 1982;138:413–417.

Computed tomography is recommended for routine evaluation of all acetabular fractures. Efficacy is greatest in demonstrating fractures of the roof, quadrilateral surface, and posterior wall and in diagnosing intra-articular free bony fragments.

Heeg M, Oostvogel HJ, Klasen HJ: Conservative treatment of acetabular fractures: The role of the weight-bearing dome and anatomic reduction in the ultimate results. *J Trauma* 1987;27:555–559.

A retrospective study of 57 conservatively treated acetabular fractures with an average follow-up of 7.9 years found that the overall functional results were satisfactory in 75%. The least satisfactory results were seen in fractures crossing the weightbearing dome of the acetabulum in which congruency could not be achieved. Fractures crossing the weightbearing dome that could be reduced by traction to less than 2 mm had good or excellent results in seven patients. The authors concluded that conservative treatment of acetabular fractures can be very successful, even in fractures crossing the weightbearing dome, provided that congruence is preserved during the period of traction.

Hesp W, Goris R: Conservative treatment of fractures of the acetabulum: Results after long-term follow-up. *Acta Chir Belg* 1988;88:27–32.

Of 79 patients with 81 fractures of the acetabulum, 83% had multiple injuries. The mean injury severity score was 34 (range, 9 to 75). Involvement of the dorsal column or roof of the acetabulum produced moderate or bad results in 79%. In such cases, surgical repositioning and fixation should be considered.

Johnson EE, Eckardt JJ, Letournel E: Extrinsic femoral artery occlusion following internal fixation of an acetabular fracture: A case report. *Clin Orthop* 1987;217:209–213.

Vascular injury is one of the drastic complications that can be caused by internal fixation of acetabular fractures. In one case, a large lag screw was malpositioned, so that it penetrated the superior pubic ramus at a point adjacent to the superficial femoral artery. Postoperative angiography revealed extrinsic compression of this vessel.

Judet R, Judet J, Letournel E: Fractures of the acetabulum: Classification and surgical approaches for open reduction. *J Bone Joint Surg* 1964;46A:1615–1646.

This classic article presents the initial findings in and techniques for open reduction and internal fixation of acetabular fractures. The anatomic classification provided continues to be the most useful acetabular fracture classification available.

Letournel E, Judet R: *Fractures of the Acetabulum*, Elson RA (trans-ed). New York, Springer-Verlag, 1981.

Thorough anatomic and radiographic descriptions of the ten major types of acetabular fractures are given. After analysis of an acetabular fracture and assignment of the classification, decision-making proceeds to selection of a surgical approach for open reduction and internal fixation. The long-term functional results are highly correlated with the accuracy of surgical reduction.

Matta JM, Anderson LM, Epstein HC, et al: Fractures of the acetabulum: A retrospective analysis. *Clin Orthop* 1986;205:230–240.

In this retrospective analysis of 64 major fractures of the acetabulum, a radiographic method of measuring the acetabular dome proved to have prognostic significance for those fractures that were treated nonsurgically or in which surgical reduction was inadequate. In fractures treated surgically, the accuracy of the reduction correlated significantly with the final clinical results.

Matta JM, Mehne DK, Roffi R: Fractures of the acetabulum: Early results of a prospective study. *Clin Orthop* 1986;205:241–250.

In a prospective series of major acetabular fractures, open re-duction and internal fixation was necessary in most. Accurate surgical reduction was possible in a large majority of the cases and the complication rate was acceptable. The early overall clinical results were satisfactory.

Matta J, Merritt P: Displaced acetabular fractures. *Clin Orthop* 1988;230:83–97.

The rate of satisfactory surgical reductions improved gradually over the first 50 operations in a prospective study of 121 displaced acetabular fractures. Overall, clinical results were satisfactory in 80% of this series. Complications included a 3% infection rate and 5% incidence of nerve palsy. Open reduction and internal fixation is indicated for most displaced fractures. However, closed treatment can produce satisfactory results in selected patients.

Mayo KA: Fractures of the acetabulum. *Orthop Clin North Am* 1987;18:43–57.

Open reduction and internal fixation is now the preferred treatment for most displaced fractures of the acetabulum. Long-term follow-up of a large number of cases operated on within the first three weeks of injury showed excellent clinical and radiographic results in about 74% of cases. The outcome after anatomic reduction is significantly better than in cases in which there is residual deformity. Reported complications included a 2% to 4% infection rate and nerve palsy in 3% to 6% of patients. Heterotopic bone formation occurred in almost one half of surgically treated cases, but required secondary resection in only 1% to 2%.

Mays J, Neufeld AJ: Skeletal traction methods. *Clin Orthop* 1974;102:144–141.

The technique of Neufeld roller traction is described. In this type of traction, the leg is suspended free while in traction and may be actively exercised in all directions while traction is maintained.

Miller ME, Allgower M, Schneider R, et al: *Manual of Internal Fixation*. Berlin, Springer-Verlag, 1979, pp 28–41.

The principle and technical application of the lag screw for internal fixation of fractures are described. With this technique a screw glides freely through the first bone fragment and is purchased only on the distal fragment.

Reinert CM, Bosse MJ, Poka A, et al: A modified extensile exposure for the treatment of complex or malunited acetabular fractures. *J Bone Joint Surg* 1988;70A:329–337.

A modification of the extended iliofemoral incision facilitates the surgical exposure of T-shaped, complex transverse, and two-column fractures and malunions. The modification includes the use of a T-shaped skin incision with large flaps and osteotomies of the iliac crest, greater trochanter, and antero-superior iliac spine.

Winquist RA: Open reduction and internal fixation of central acetabular fractures by anterior and posterior approaches. *Orthop Trans* 1982;6:93.

Simultaneous anterior and posterior approaches were used successfully to reduce and fix a series of centrally displaced fractures including transverse, T-shaped, and two-column fractures.

39
Hip: Trauma

Trauma to the hip, particularly hip fractures in the elderly, continues to be a major challenge to our healthcare system. Improved medical and surgical management of these patients has resulted in decreased mortality in the 1980s. Technical improvements in fracture fixation and prostheses have decreased the incidence of complications and improved functional outcomes. However, the increasing number of hip fractures that occur each year and the increasing age and frailty of the patients sustaining these fractures have made it difficult to keep pace with this growing healthcare problem.

Hip Dislocations

Hip dislocations are the result of high-energy trauma, usually from motor-vehicle accidents. They occur most often in young patients. Severe associated injuries occur in 35% to 95% of cases, and include craniofacial, chest, abdominal, and other musculoskeletal injuries. It is essential to obtain radiographs of the pelvis and the entire femur to identify the most commonly associated musculoskeletal injuries. These associated injuries occur in all types of hip dislocations.

Hip dislocations are divided into anterior and posterior types. Treatment principles include (1) careful evaluation of the patient for associated injuries, (2) immediate gentle, closed or, if necessary, open reduction with assessment of stability after reduction, (3) careful radiographic evaluation (including a computed tomographic scan), and (4) evaluation for congruency of reduction and any associated femoral head or acetabular fractures. In general, if a concentric, stable reduction is obtained, treatment should include a brief period of bedrest until symptoms subside; this is followed by protected weightbearing ambulation for four to six weeks, until soft-tissue healing occurs. The patient can then progress to full weightbearing. If the reduction is concentric but unstable and there are no associated fractures, traction should be maintained for four to six weeks until soft-tissue healing occurs. This is followed by progressive weightbearing ambulation. A nonconcentric reduction can result from intra-articular osteochondral fragments, interposed soft tissue, or malreduction of associated femoral head fractures. This is an indication for open reduction, joint exploration, and removal of osteochondral fragments. Treatment of associated femoral head or acetabular fractures depends on the location and size of the fragments and the stability of the reduction.

Complications of hip dislocation can be immediate or late. Femoral artery and femoral nerve injuries are rare and are associated with anterior dislocations. Sciatic nerve injuries are associated with approximately 10% of posterior dislocations. Acute neurovascular complications occur more often in elderly patients. Osteonecrosis can become evident as late as five years after injury. Delayed reduction increases the incidence of osteonecrosis. Posttraumatic degenerative arthritis after hip dislocation is more likely to occur when there are associated femoral head or acetabular fractures.

Anterior Dislocations

Anterior dislocations account for approximately 10% to 18% of all hip dislocations. They have been subdivided into superior (pubic) and inferior (obturator) types. Superior dislocations result from extension, abduction, and external-rotation forces. The femoral head is displaced anteriorly and may compress the femoral neurovascular bundle. Inferior dislocations, which are much more common, result from flexion, abduction, and external-rotation forces. Closed reduction can be accomplished by traction followed by extension and internal rotation. Femoral head fractures occur in 22% to 77% of cases and are either transchondral or indentation fractures. They may be difficult to identify without tomograms or computed tomographic scans. Transchondral fractures that result in nonconcentric reduction require open reduction and either excision or internal fixation of the fragment, depending on its size and location. Indentation fractures are more common, but no specific treatment is indicated. Osteonecrosis occurs in approximately 10% of cases and is associated with delayed reduction or repeated reduction attempts. Posttraumatic degenerative arthritis occurs in most cases and is associated with transchondral fractures, indentation fractures more than 4 mm in depth, and osteonecrosis.

Posterior Dislocations

Posterior dislocations account for as many as 90% of all hip dislocations. They have been classified by Epstein on the basis of associated femoral head and/or acetabular fractures (Table 1). In one series of patients with traumatic posterior dislocations, significantly decreased anteversion of the dislocated hips compared with controls was noted. Posterior dislocation occurs as a result of a force applied to the flexed knee along the axis of the femur. If the hip is in neutral or adduction, a simple dislocation occurs; if the hip is in abduction, an associated posterior acetabular

Table 1. Epstein's classification of posterior hip dislocations

Type	Description
I	No fracture or minor "chip" fracture
II	Large single fragment of posterior acetabular rim
III	Comminuted fracture of the posterior rim with or without major fragment
IV	Fracture of both acetabular rim and floor
V	Fracture of femoral head with or without other fracture

rim fracture occurs. Closed reduction can be performed by traction on the adducted and flexed hip.

If closed reduction with the patient under general anesthesia is unsuccessful, open reduction through a posterior approach is indicated. At that time, the joint should be explored to remove any osteochondral fragments. After reduction, radiographs should be evaluated carefully for concentricity of reduction. A computed tomographic scan should be performed in all cases to identify intra-articular fragments or associated fractures that may not have been evident on standard radiographs (Fig. 1). If the reduction is nonconcentric, open reduction with joint exploration, using a posterior approach, is indicated. Assessment of stability after reduction is essential. Associated acetabular fractures greatly increase the likelihood of instability. The risk of instability increases as the amount of posterior acetabular involvement increases. Unstable hips with large posterior acetabular fragments should undergo joint irrigation and debridement, followed by open reduction and internal fixation of the acetabular fragment to restore stability.

Osteonecrosis of the femoral head has been reported in 10% to more than 50% of posterior dislocations and fracture-dislocations. It usually occurs within two to three years of injury, but may develop as late as five years after the injury. The risk of osteonecrosis depends on the severity of the injury, delay in reduction, and repeated closed reduction attempts. The presence of a posterior acetabular fracture significantly increases the risk of osteonecrosis.

Delay of reduction for more than six to 12 hours after injury also increases the risk. Primary open reduction of all posterior dislocations and fracture-dislocations, along with internal fixation of acetabular fractures and removal of intra-articular fragments, has been reported in one large series to decrease the risk of osteonecrosis and posttraumatic degenerative arthritis, but this approach remains controversial. Posttraumatic degenerative arthritis occurs in most cases. Its occurrence depends on the severity of the initial injury, presence of a nonconcentric reduction, time between injury and reduction, the development of osteonecrosis, and the duration of follow-up. One series reported a 33% incidence of degenerative arthritis at ten years and a 75% incidence at 30 years.

Delayed diagnosis of posterior dislocations decreases the likelihood of a successful outcome. If the injury is three or more weeks old, closed reduction is usually not possible because fibrous tissue fills the acetabulum. Open reduction increases the risk of osteonecrosis in this situation, but is necessary. In young patients, open reduction and internal fixation of associated fractures is indicated. In elderly patients, primary replacement with a prosthesis is preferred.

Posterior Dislocations With Femoral Head Fractures Approximately 10% of posterior dislocations have associated fractures of the femoral head or heck. Epstein's type V injury was further categorized by Pipkin (Table 2 and Fig. 2). Femoral head fractures occur when a force is applied to the flexed knee with the hip adducted and flexed less than 50 degrees. The femoral head is driven into the posterosuperior portion of the acetabular rim, shearing off a fragment. Identification and sizing of the femoral head fragment may be difficult with standard radiographs. However, computed tomographic scanning usually provides this important information. Radiographs should be evaluated carefully before closed reduction is attempted so that a nondisplaced femoral neck fracture is not overlooked. A nondisplaced femoral neck fracture that becomes displaced as a result of attempted closed reduction significantly worsens the prognosis for this injury. Gentle, closed reduction should be attempted in Pipkin types I, II, and IV injuries; type III injuries require open reduction.

After reduction, radiographs, including computed tomographic scans, should be evaluated for concentricity and reduction of the femoral head fragment. If the reduction is concentric, skeletal traction should be used for six to eight weeks, followed by mobilization with protected weightbearing. If the reduction is not concentric, open reduction through a posterior approach is indicated.

Treatment depends on the type and the size of the fracture. Type I fractures, because of their caudad position, can generally be excised. Type II fractures involving less than one third of the articular surface should be excised. However, if more than one third of the articular surface is involved, open reduction and internal fixation is preferred. Type III fractures should be treated by primary

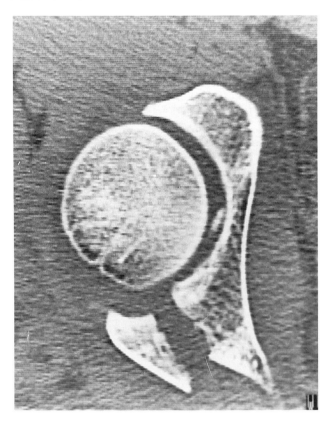

Figure 1
Computed tomographic scan after closed reduction of an Epstein type II posterior dislocation. A large displaced posterior acetabular fracture is evident, as is an intra-articular fragment.

Table 2. Pipkin's classification of femoral head fractures

Type	Description
I	Fracture of femoral head caudad to fovea
II	Fracture of the femoral head cephalad to fovea
III	Type I or type II plus femoral neck fracture
IV	Types I, II, or III plus fracture of acetabular rim

open reduction and internal fixation of the femoral neck fracture, followed by either excision or internal fixation of the femoral head fracture, depending on its size and location. When this injury occurs in elderly patients, primary replacement with a prosthesis is preferred. Treatment of type IV injuries depends on the stability and concentricity of the reduction. If the reduction is unstable or nonconcentric, open reduction, joint exploration, excision or fixation of the femoral head fracture, and internal fixation of the posterior acetabular fracture is indicated.

Posterior dislocations with femoral head fractures are at risk for osteonecrosis and posttraumatic degenerative arthritis. The incidence of osteonecrosis is decreased by prompt reduction (within six to 12 hours of injury). The prognosis for these injuries varies. Pipkin types I and II injuries are reported to have the same prognosis as simple dislocations. Pipkin type IV injuries have the same prognosis as posterior dislocations with acetabular fractures, but without femoral head fractures. Pipkin type III injuries have a poor prognosis.

Bilateral hip dislocations account for 1% to 2% of all hip dislocations. They result from high-energy trauma. Approximately 50% consist of bilateral posterior dislocations, 40% consist of anterior and posterior dislocations, and 10% consist of bilateral anterior dislocations.

Hip Fractures

Epidemiology

Hip fractures continue to be a major challenge to our healthcare system. More than 275,000 hip fractures occur annually in the United States at an estimated annual healthcare cost of over $3 billion. Of these fractures, 95% occur in patients more than 50 years of age. The number of hip fractures is increasing annually because of the increasing number of elderly in the population. Femoral neck fractures and intertrochanteric fractures occur with approximately equal frequency. The populations sustaining these two fractures have not shown any significant epidemiologic differences. By the year 2040, 22% of the population of the United States will be over 65 years of age, resulting in an estimated 500,000 hip fractures per year. However, on the basis of available data, controversy exists as to whether the incidence of hip fracture is increasing in the United States. Other countries (Sweden, Finland, Norway, England) have reported a definite increase in the incidence of hip fractures.

Healthcare Costs

Hip fractures represent a major component of healthcare costs in the United States. The annual cost of caring for these patients has been estimated to be as high as $7.3 billion. Hip fractures account for more than 30% of all patients hospitalized for the treatment of fractures and more than 50% of the hospital days for all patients with fractures. Recently, in an effort to control healthcare costs, a prospective payment system based on diagnosis-related groups has been instituted. Early reports have indicated a detrimental effect on elderly patients with hip fractures. One study showed that the hospital stay had decreased significantly. However, the percentage of patients discharged to a nursing home increased significantly (48% vs 21%), as did the number of patients residing in a nursing

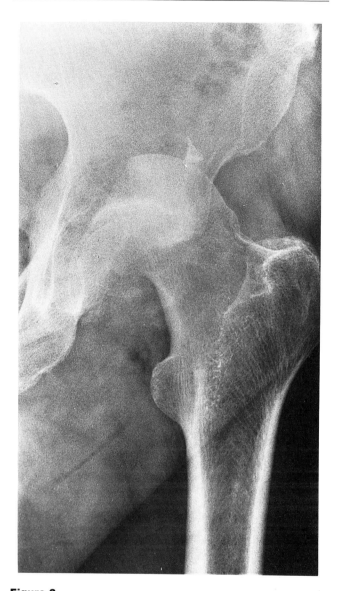

Figure 2

Posterior dislocation of the hip with associated displaced fracture of the femoral head (Epstein type V and Pipkin type I).

home six months after discharge (39% vs 13%). This has raised concerns about the current overall quality of patient care under this system. Another study showed that the current prospective payment system does not take into account the significant problems of comorbidities and postoperative complications frequently encountered in these patients. As the number of hip fractures continues to increase, it will become imperative to find effective ways of providing high-quality care while reducing healthcare costs.

Risk Factors

The incidence of hip fracture increases with increasing age. The incidence doubles for each decade beyond 50 years of age. Among patients 90 years and older, one third of women and one sixth of men have sustained a hip fracture. Females are affected more often, by a ratio of 2 or 3 to 1.

The incidence in white women is two to three times higher than those reported for black and Hispanic women. Urban populations have a higher incidence than rural populations; this may be related to the more sedentary urban lifestyle. The importance of a deterrent effect of physical activity on risk for hip fracture was further supported by one study showing that women who sustained hip fractures were significantly less physically active during their adult lives than women who had not sustained hip fractures. Excessive alcohol intake also increases the risk of hip fracture. Patients who have sustained a previous hip fracture are at an increased risk for a second hip fracture, which usually occurs on the contralateral side. Use of psychotropic medication (hypnotics or anxiolytics, tricyclic antidepressants, and antipsychotics) has been shown to increase the risk of hip fracture in patients 65 years or older. Patients with senile dementia, especially institutionalized patients, are at three times the risk for hip fractures compared with age- and sex-matched controls.

Approximately 90% of hip fractures occur as the result of a fall. The exceptions are hip fractures in young adults, which usually result from the high-energy trauma of motor-vehicle accidents. The frequency of falls increases markedly with age. Older women are much more likely to fall than older men. Medical conditions that predispose to falls include cardiac arrhythmias, seizures, and cerebrovascular insufficiency; disorders of vision, gait, and balance; and deficits of muscular strength and coordination. Environmental hazards (home safety) also cause falls. This may be particularly important, considering that approximately 75% of hip fractures occur as a result of a fall at home. A patient who sustains a hip fracture after an unexplained fall should be carefully evaluated for these predisposing conditions.

The contribution of osteoporosis and osteomalacia to the incidence of hip fractures has been studied extensively. Osteoporosis (decreased bone mass with normal bone mineralization) increases in frequency in women as they age. This frequency pattern is the same as that of hip fractures. Osteoporosis of the proximal femur results in decreased bone strength, which increases the likelihood of fracture from minor trauma. However, osteoporosis is not the cause of hip fractures in the elderly. Rather, it is a contributing factor that should be considered along with the other risk factors. Osteomalacia (decreased bone matrix mineralization with or without change in bone mass) was previously thought to predispose to hip fracture. However, recent studies have shown only a 2% incidence of osteomalacia in patients with femoral neck fractures.

Mortality

Different studies have reported a one-year mortality of as much as 50%. However, some of these studies reported the combined results of nonsurgical and surgical management, and others did not reflect a contemporary treatment approach. In a recent study reporting mortality for elderly patients who sustained hip fractures in the 1980s, the mortality was 20% for the first year after fracture and 13% for the second year after fracture. These findings agreed with previous reports that the impact of a hip fracture on mortality occurred primarily in the first year after injury. Longer follow-up studies have reported 50% overall mortality at three years, 60% at six years, and 77% after ten years.

Factors associated with increased mortality include advanced age, significant medical comorbidities, male sex, institutionalized living, and dementia. Disagreement exists as to whether fracture type, delay in surgical treatment, and type of surgical procedure are consistent risk factors for increased mortality.

Treatment Principles

It is generally accepted that surgical management, followed by early mobilization, is the treatment of choice for hip fractures in the elderly. Historically, nonsurgical management resulted in morbidity and mortality, as well as malunion and nonunion. However, nonsurgical management may be appropriate in selected elderly patients with dementia who were unable to walk before the fracture and who experience minimal discomfort from the injury. These patients should be mobilized as soon as possible to avoid the complications of prolonged recumbency. Nonsurgical management must be recommended judiciously in carefully selected patients.

Elderly patients with hip fractures should be stabilized medically before undergoing surgery. Most patients can undergo surgery within 24 hours of injury. Longer delays needed to stabilize medical problems have not been shown to increase morbidity or mortality. Rather, surgical treatment of medically unstable patients significantly increases the risk of mortality. Careful intraoperative cardiopulmonary monitoring has been shown to decrease hospital mortality. The choice of anesthesia (spinal vs general) has not been shown to have a significant effect on the incidence of postoperative confusion or mortality in elderly patients. The use of broad-spectrum antibiotics significantly decreases the incidence of postoperative infection. Currently, recommended regimens include the use of cephalosporins administered intravenously immediately before surgery and for 24 hours postoperatively. Prolonged use of prophylactic antibiotics has not been shown to be advantageous. Comparison of different cephalosporins has shown that cefazolin was more highly concentrated in the serum and in the surgical hematoma than cefamandole or cefoxitin after internal fixation of intertrochanteric fractures.

Postoperative management is directed at early mobilization to avoid the complications of recumbency. The ability to ambulate within two weeks of surgery has been shown to correlate with living at home one year after surgery. Prevention of pressure sores is extremely important. They have been reported to develop in approximately one third of patients with hip fracture, usually within the first week after admission. Patients who develop decubiti have a significantly longer hospital stay and higher mortality rate. Prevention of decubiti by meticulous nursing care remains the best teatment.

Functional Recovery

Successful treatment is often measured by those patients who are able to regain their prefracture level of function. Although this is the goal, it is quite difficult to achieve. Of patients who were functionally independent and living at home before the hip fracture, 15% to 40% require institutionalized care for more than a year after the fracture. Only 50% to 60% of patients regain their prefracture ambulatory status within a year. Approximately 50% to 83% of patients regain independent ambulation with assistive devices. Most patients require assistance in performing the activities of daily living. Of those who were independent before the fracture, only 20% to 35% regain the prefracture level of independence. Advances in fracture management have improved the outcomes for elderly patients with hip fractures, but improving the significant loss of prefracture ambulation, independence, and social function will require the development of innovative treatment approaches reflecting the combined efforts of orthopaedists, geriatricians, and physiatrists.

Pathologic Fractures

The proximal femur is a common site for metastatic lesions that result in pathologic fractures or impending fractures. The indications for stabilization of impending fractures include a painful lesion more than 2.5 cm in diameter or with destruction of 50% or more of the cortex of a long bone. Patients treated prophylactically for impending fractures have a lower surgical mortality, fewer complications, fewer stabilization failures, and more successful rehabilitation than those with pathologic fractures. In addition, stabilization of an impending fracture is easier and spares the patient the pain and disability associated with fracture. Life expectancy has been used as an indication for surgical treatment. Some have recommended that it be at least 90 days and others have suggested 30 days. Although there is no universal agreement, surgical treatment of impending and pathologic fractures is indicated in patients whose quality of life will be enhanced regardless of the anticipated life expectancy. Surgical management relieves pain and allows mobilization of the patient.

Preoperative evaluation and preparation of the patient must be meticulous because these patients are often quite debilitated. Particular attention should be given to serum calcium levels, since hypercalcemia is common. Metastatic lesions that are sensitive to radiation should undergo radiation therapy preoperatively or immediately after stabilization of the fracture. Radiation therapy has not been shown to decrease soft-tissue healing, but does interfere with incorporation of bone graft. Methylmethacrylate is an important adjunct in the stabilization of these fractures. It is used to fill defects that remain after tumor removal and for fixation of prostheses. Surgical management usually consists of internal fixation with adjunctive methylmethacrylate or replacement with a prosthesis. The choice depends on the location and size of the lesion and its sensitivity to radiation.

Femoral Neck Fractures

The Garden classification of femoral neck fractures (Table 3) is the one most commonly used. However, a recent study has shown the difficulty of differentiating the four types of fractures. Therefore, it may be more accurate to classify femoral neck fractures as nondisplaced (Garden types I and II) or displaced (Garden types III and IV).

The most significant complications of femoral neck fractures are nonunion and osteonecrosis. Increased intracapsular pressure resulting from a fracture hemarthrosis has been suggested as an important factor in the development of osteonecrosis. Different studies have reported increases in intracapsular pressure in both nondisplaced and displaced fractures. Positioning of the hip in internal rotation and extension consistently increased intracapsular pressure; external rotation and flexion consistently decreased

intracapsular pressure. Aspiration of the hemarthrosis has been reported to decrease pressure and improve blood flow in nondisplaced fractures of the femoral head. However, there are no reported studies of whether decompression of the hemarthrosis (by aspiration or capsulotomy) decreases the frequency of osteonecrosis.

The usefulness of radionuclide scanning performed immediately after fracture to predict the development of osteonecrosis remains controversial. Thus far, it has not been used to determine the choice of treatment (internal fixation vs prosthesis). However, sequential postoperative scanning has been used to predict the development of complications. In one study, scans performed within two weeks of fracture accurately predicted the development of healing problems in 91% of cases. Bone scanning has also been shown to be useful in identifying acute fractures in those elderly patients who have persistent hip pain after a fall but whose radiographs appear to be normal.

There is general agreement that treatment of nondisplaced femoral neck fractures (Garden types I and II) should consist of internal fixation with multiple pins or screws placed in parallel (Fig. 3). There is no consensus as to the optimal number of pins, although most authors report success with three or four pins or screws in both nondisplaced and displaced fractures. A laboratory study reported that there was no biomechanical justification for the use of more than three pins or screws, regardless of the implant chosen. Nonunion and osteonecrosis are uncommon after nondisplaced fractures. Most series report nonunion in less than 5% of cases and osteonecrosis in less than 8% of cases.

Treatment of displaced femoral neck fractures remains controversial. Most authors advocate closed reduction or open reduction and internal fixation in younger, active patients and primary replacement with a prosthesis in older, less active patients. Some authors have recommended primary total hip replacement. When internal fixation is used, there is general agreement that achieving an anatomic reduction is probably the most important factor in avoiding complications. An acceptable reduction may have as much as 15 degrees of valgus angulation and less than 10 degrees of anterior or posterior angulation. Prompt reduction of displaced fractures has been advocated, but has not consistently been shown to decrease the incidences of nonunion and osteonecrosis. After closed reduction, anteroposterior and lateral radiographs are necessary to determine the adequacy of the reduction. If a closed reduction is not acceptable, open reduction may be necessary. Internal fixation of displaced fractures most often uses multiple pins or screws placed in parallel. Sliding screw devices have been used but the results were found to be inferior. One prospective, randomized study reported a 64% union rate with a sliding screw-plate, compared with 84% for multiple screws. Excellent results have been reported with three 6.5-mm AO cancellous screws.

Nonunion and osteonecrosis continue to be problems.

Table 3. Garden's classification of femoral neck fractures

Type	Description
I	Incomplete fracture (impacted valgus fracture)
II	Complete fracture without displacement
III	Complete fracture with partial displacement
IV	Complete fracture with full displacement

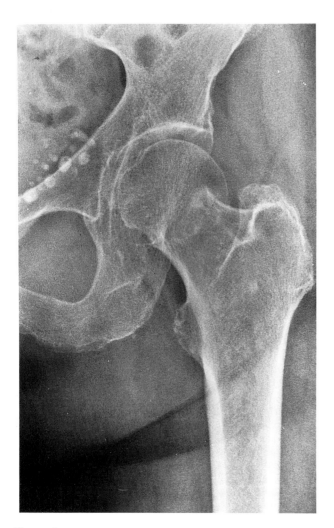 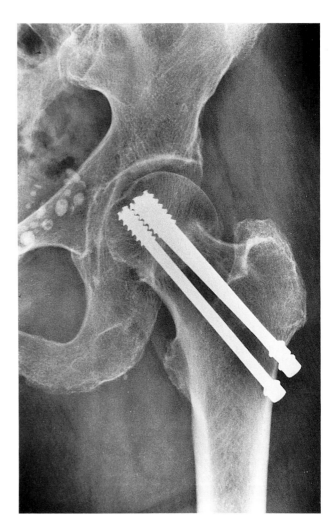

Figure 3
Left, An impacted valgus fracture of the femoral neck. **Right**, Treatment by multiple screw fixation.

The incidence of nonunion has ranged from 10% to 30% and that of osteonecrosis from 15% to 33%. Adequacy of reduction has consistently been reported as the most important factor affecting the development of these complications. Approximately one third of patients with osteonecrosis require additional surgery; approximately 75% of patients with nonunion or early fixation failure require early reoperation.

Weightbearing after internal fixation of femoral neck fractures remains controversial. Most series have used early mobilization of the patient with restricted weightbearing of the involved extremity until fracture healing was apparent. An earlier study did address this question and found that in adequately fixed fractures early weightbearing did not result in increased complications, morbidity, or fixation failure. However, subsequent studies have not addressed this issue and the question remains unanswered.

Primary replacement with a prosthesis has been advocated to avoid the problems of nonunion and osteonecrosis and to allow immediate weightbearing after surgery. In general, it has been advocated for older and less active patients, but whether the prosthesis should be of the fixed-

head type or a bipolar endoprosthesis has not been well defined. Most reports suppport the use of cement to secure the implant, no matter which type is selected. The incidence of acetabular migration is decreased with bipolar devices. The functional demands of this group of patients have led to the recommendation that a bipolar implant be used in more active patients. Patients whose ability to walk is limited do equally well with a cemented prosthesis with a fixed head. A recent study of 90 cemented bipolar endoprostheses for femoral neck fractures followed up for at least two years reported that 91% of patients were free of significant pain and 83% had returned to their preinjury level of function or required only a cane for ambulation. Acetabular erosion was minimal and none required revision to total hip replacement. Earlier bipolar designs produced technical complications related to disassembly of components. However, this has not been a problem with newer designs.

Earlier studies reported higher morbidity and mortality rates in patients undergoing primary total hip replacement than in patients undergoing internal fixation. Primary total hip replacement should be reserved for patients with femoral neck fractures with significant preexisting acetabular degeneration. Delayed total hip replacement for patients in whom complications develop after internal fixation or hemiarthroplasty can be expected to provide results comparable to those of elective primary total hip replacement.

Young Adults

In most cases, femoral neck fractures in young adults occur as a result of high-energy trauma (motor-vehicle accidents, falls from heights). However, in those that result from a simple fall, a predisposing factor is often present (alcoholism, medication use). When these fractures result from high-energy trauma, careful evaluation for other injuries should be performed. Specific consideration should be given to the possibility of ipsilateral femoral neck and shaft fractures.

Nondisplaced fractures should be treated by multiple pin or screw fixation. Nonunion and osteonecrosis are very uncommon after nondisplaced fractures, except in cases in which the diagnosis was delayed. Successful treatment of displaced fractures is related to achieving an anatomic reduction and stable internal fixation as soon as possible after the injury. A gentle, closed reduction should be attempted. If the reduction is unacceptable, an open reduction should be performed, followed by multiple pin or screw fixation. When the principles of prompt anatomic reduction and internal fixation are followed, the incidence of nonunion should be less than 10% and that of osteonecrosis 20% to 33%.

Treatment of acute displaced femoral neck fractures by means of muscle-pedicle graft, with or without bone graft, to decrease the incidence of nonunion and osteonecrosis remains controversial. Initial successful results have not been confirmed by later studies. A recent study reported that this procedure was useful in the treatment of ununited femoral neck fractures even when osteonecrosis was present.

Special Problems

Neurologic Impairment Neurologically impaired patients include those with Parkinson's disease, previous stroke, or severe dementia. For patients with Parkinson's disease who sustain femoral neck fractures, both internal fixation and primary replacement have been recommended. Earlier studies reported increased complications after primary replacement. However, this has not been supported by recent studies. The treatment chosen should be based on the patient's age, the fracture type, and severity of disease. All of these patients require meticulous medical and nursing care to avoid complications. If replacement is chosen, correction of a hip adduction contracture by tenotomy and an anterior surgical approach should be considered. Both measures may decrease the chance of dislocation.

Patients who have had strokes are at increased risk for hip fractures, primarily because of residual balance and gait problems and the osteoporotic changes in the paretic limb. The treatment approach depends on the fracture type and the patient's functional status. When the fracture occurs within one week of the stroke, poor functional recovery can be anticipated. If replacement is chosen, hip contractures may require tenotomy and an anterior approach may be preferred.

Institutionalized patients with severe dementia present a particular challenge. In-hospital mortality as high as 50% has been reported. Nondisplaced fractures should be treated by internal fixation. Displaced fractures requiring replacement should be performed through an anterior approach to decrease the risk of dislocation and infection from wound contamination. In nonambulatory patients with severe dementia who do not have significant discomfort from the injury, nonsurgical management with early bed-to-chair mobilization should be considered.

Rheumatoid Arthritis Femoral neck fractures in rheumatoid arthritis are associated with an increased incidence of complications. In general, nondisplaced fractures can be successfully treated by internal fixation. However, internal fixation of displaced fractures resulted in a 95% complication rate in one series. Therefore, for displaced fractures, arthroplasty is recomended. If significant acetabular degeneration is present, total hip arthroplasty is indicated. Femoral neck fractures are very uncommon in patients with underlying osteoarthritis of the hip. When they do occur, total hip arthroplasty is preferred.

Metabolic Disease Femoral neck fractures in patients with chronic renal disease or hyperparathyroidism are at increased risk for complications of internal fixation because of the associated metabolic bone disease. In these patients, cemented primary replacement is preferred.

Paget's Disease Femoral neck fractures in patients with Paget's disease should be evaluated carefully because of the likelihood of concomitant acetabular degeneration and deformity of the proximal femur. Nondisplaced fractures can be treated by internal fixation. For displaced fractures, primary replacement is preferred. If there was prefracture hip pain in the presence of acetabular degeneration, total hip arthroplasty is preferred; if acetabular degeneration is not present, a bipolar endoprosthesis may suffice. Deformity of the proximal femur and a tendency toward excessive bleeding are common.

Metastatic Disease Femoral neck fractures that occur as a result of metastatic disease require replacement. When the entire proximal femur is involved, a calcar or proximal femoral replacement may be necessary. For patients with acetabular involvement, a cemented acetabular component should be used. If acetabular involvement is extensive, portions of the ilium may have to be reconstructed with methylmethacrylate, wire mesh, and specialized acetabular components. It is important to identify any metastatic lesions in the femoral shaft before performing surgery. This decreases the risk of intraoperative fracture or shaft perforation.

Intertrochanteric Fractures

Intertrochanteric fractures occur with approximately the same frequency as femoral neck fractures in patients with similar demographic characteristics. The most important aspect of fracture classification is determination of stability. Stability is provided by an intact posteromedial cortical buttress of the distal fragment. Comminution of this area allows the fracture to collapse into varus. Unstable fracture patterns also include intertrochanteric fractures with subtrochanteric extension and reverse oblique fractures. Previously, most reports indicated that the majority of intertrochanteric fractures were stable. However, in recent series, unstable fractures accounted for 50% to 65% of all intertrochanteric fractures. The reasons for this changing pattern are uncertain.

Surgical treatment of intertrochanteric fractures has undergone an important evolution during the past 40 years. Surgical management using rigid nail-plate devices resulted in complications rates as high as 40% in unstable fractures. These devices did not allow impaction at the fracture site. Mechanical complications, including nail penetration, nail breakage, and superior "cut-out" resulted as unstable fractures impacted into more stable positions. In the 1960s, in an effort to overcome these mechanical problems, displacement osteotomies were developed to convert unstable fractures to more stable patterns. The Dimon and Hughston medial displacement osteotomy and the Sarmiento valgus osteotomy successfully decreased mechanical complications when rigid nail-plate devices were used. However, because additional impaction occurred after osteotomy and fixation, mechanical problems persisted when these devices were used.

In the 1970s, sliding nail and screw devices were developed. These devices provided secure fixation of the proximal (head and neck) fragment to the distal (shaft) fragment; more importantly, they allowed controlled impaction at the fracture site. Sliding screw devices were preferred over sliding nail devices because the screw provided better fixation in the proximal fragment. These sliding devices are "load-sharing" devices, unlike rigid nail-plates, which are "load-bearing" devices. They permitted early mobilization and weightbearing without the high risk of fixation failure associated with rigid nail-plate devices.

In the 1970s, intramedullary fixation of intertrochanteric fractures became popular. Condylocephalic nails were inserted in a retrograde manner, through an insertion point in the distal aspect of the femur. It was hoped that a less extensive surgical procedure that avoided exposure of the fracture site might decrease postoperative morbidity.

In the 1980s, calcar replacement endoprostheses have been used to treat selected, comminuted intertrochanteric fractures. At present, intertrochanteric fractures are most commonly treated by sliding hip screws, condylocephalic nails, or calcar replacement prostheses.

Sliding Hip Screws

These devices are commonly used for both stable and unstable intertrochanteric fractures (Fig. 4). They are avail-

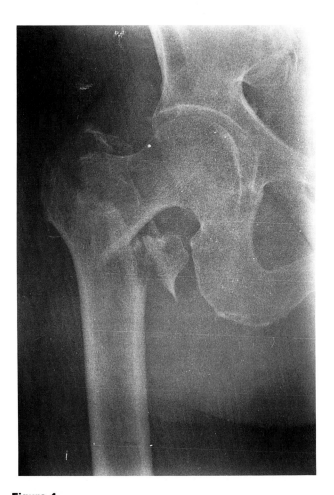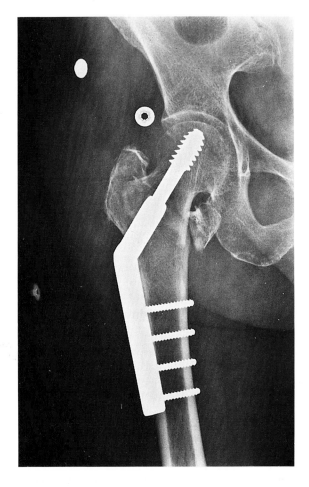

Figure 4
Left, Displaced intertrochanteric fracture, in varus, with posteromedial fragment. **Right**, Treatment consisted of anatomic reduction and fixation with an angled (135 degrees) sliding hip screw.

able in plate angles from 130 to 150 degrees in 5-degree increments. Plate angles of 135 and 150 degrees are usually used. There is no general agreement as to the optimal plate angle for these devices. Theoretically, a sliding device with the plate angle closest to the resultant force vector acting across the hip allows better sliding and impaction. The combined vector force across the hip acts at an angle of 159 degrees to the horizontal. Therefore, the larger the plate angle, the closer the angle is to the resultant force across the hip and the greater force that is available to aid impaction. Technically, a device with a plate angle of more than 150 degrees cannot be inserted properly.

The 150-degree plate angle has been shown to permit the best "sliding" in laboratory studies. However, it is difficult to insert a device with a 150-degree angle into the center of the femoral head and neck. Therefore, a valgus reduction has been recommended to avoid placement in the weakest superior portion of the head. The 150-degree device also has a smaller varus moment arm acting on the implant. This theoretically reduces the risk of implant failure. Despite these advantages, 135-degree devices are used more often. These devices are easier to insert in the desired central position of the femoral head and neck. In addition, the insertion point is in metaphyseal bone, while a diaphyseal insertion point is required for 150-degree devices. Clinical studies have not shown a significant difference in the amount of sliding and impaction for these two plate angles.

The most important aspect of insertion is secure placement of the screw within the proximal fragment. This requires insertion of the screw to within 1 cm of the subchondral bone. A central position within the femoral head and neck is most commonly recommended. If a central position is not possible, a posteroinferior position is preferred. Anterosuperior positions should be avoided because the bone is weakest in this area, increasing the likelihood of superior cut-out of the screw.

The necessity of medial displacement osteotomy with the sliding hip screw remains controversial. Because the sliding hip screw allows controlled collapse at the fracture site, anatomically reduced unstable fractures may impact spontaneously to a stable and often medially displaced position. This usually results in less shortening of the extremity than a formal medial displacement osteotomy. In a laboratory study of unstable intertrochanteric fractures treated with 135-degree sliding hip screws, anatomic reduction provided significantly higher compression across the calcar region and significantly lower tensile strain on the plate than medial displacement osteotomy. A recent clinical study comparing medial displacement and anatomic reduction for unstable fractures found that medial displacement had no advantage over anatomic reduction.

Sliding hip screw fixation for intertrochanteric fractures has resulted in a 4% to 12% incidence of loss of fixation. This usually occurs in unstable fractures. Most fixation failures can be attributed to technical problems of screw placement and fracture reduction. Although the sliding hip screw allows postoperative impaction at the fracture site, it is essential to obtain an impacted reduction at the time of surgery. This avoids excessive postoperative collapse that may exceed the sliding capacity of the device. If screw sliding brings the threads into contact with the plate barrel, additional impaction is not possible and the device be-

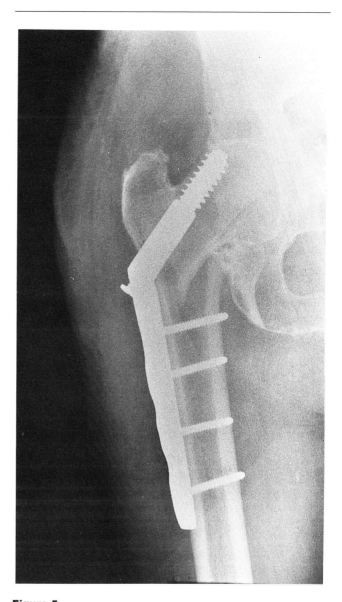

Figure 5

The sliding capacity of this sliding hip screw has been exceeded, resulting in superior "cut-out" with further impaction.

comes the biomechanical equivalent of a rigid nail-plate (Fig. 5).

Methylmethacrylate has been advocated as adjunctive fixation in extremely osteoporotic, unstable fractures treated by a sliding hip screw. One series reported fewer complications when adjunctive methylmethacrylate was used for fixation. However, currently, its routine use with sliding hip screw fixation for nonpathologic fractures is not recommended.

Intramedullary Devices

Intramedullary devices have been used extensively for intertrochanteric fractures (Fig. 6). The results have been variable and, in general, disappointing. The stated advantages of these devices were decreased surgical time and blood loss because of the remote insertion site and the ability to avoid exposing the fracture site. The procedure

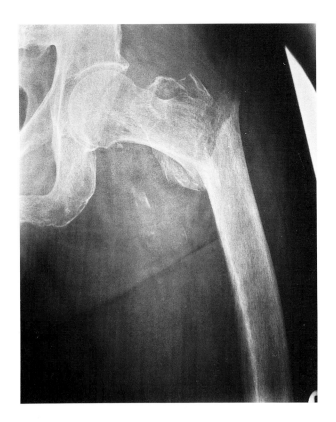
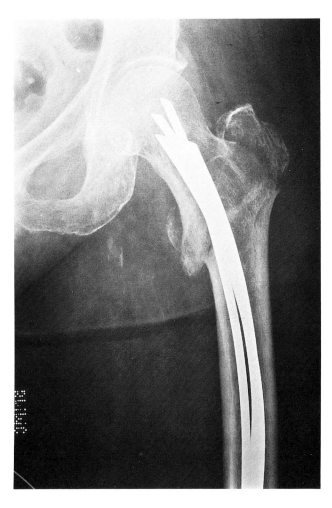

Figure 6
Left, Stable intertrochanteric fracture. **Right**, After treatment by closed reduction and retrograde Ender nailing.

is technically demanding and requires an image intensifier. In most series, the complication rates have ranged from 16% to 71%. The most common complications include varus deformity, knee pain caused by distal migration of the nails, and external-rotation deformity. Early reoperation has been necessary in as many as 19% of cases. The highest complication rates have been reported when these devices were used for unstable fractures. Although one large series using Ender nails had excellent results for both stable and unstable fractures, similar results have not been reported by other investigators.

A few clinical studies have directly compared Ender nails with sliding hip screws. In general, the complication rates for Ender nailing greatly exceeded those reported for sliding hip screws. At present, indications for Ender nailing of intertrochanteric fractures remain undefined. It is a technically demanding procedure that may be most useful in elderly, debilitated patients with stable fractures who can tolerate only minimal surgical intervention. An adequate number of nails must be used and they should be driven deeply into the femoral head with prebending into anteversion to prevent postoperative external-rotation deformity. They should not be used for unstable intertrochanteric fractures.

Replacement With Prostheses

Replacement has been used successfully to treat postoperative loss of fixation when repeat open reduction and internal fixation of intertrochanteric fractures is not possible or desirable. A calcar replacement hemiarthroplasty or bipolar endoprosthesis is necessary because of the level of the fracture. Primary replacement for comminuted, unstable fractures has also been successful in a limited number of patients. This procedure has the advantage of allowing early full weightbearing and rapid rehabilitation. The disadvantages include a more extensive surgical procedure and the potential for dislocation of the prosthesis. The indications for its use in the treatment of acute intertrochanteric fractures have not been defined. It does not appear to offer any advantages over a properly inserted sliding hip screw.

Special Situations

Trauma Intertrochanteric fractures in young patients generally result from high-energy trauma. Associated injuries are common, including ipsilateral femoral shaft fractures. These fractures should be treated by anatomic reduction

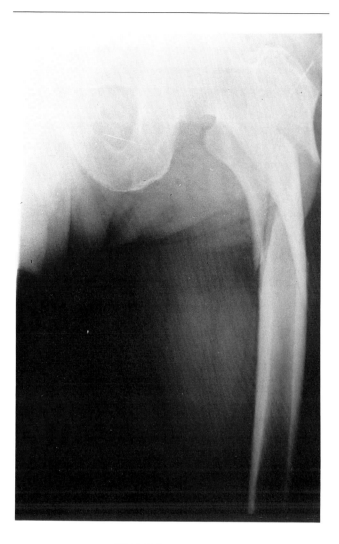

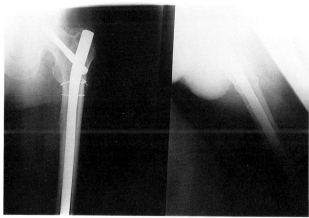

Figure 7

Top, Comminuted subtrochanteric fracture. **Bottom**, After treatment by open reduction, cerclage wiring, and insertion of a Zickel nail.

and internal fixation to avoid shortening of the extremity. Extension into the subtrochanteric area may require bone grafting.

Parkinson's Disease Patients with Parkinson's disease who sustain intertrochanteric fractures should be treated by sur-

gical stabilization of the fracture. These patients are, on the average, slightly younger than patients with Parkinson's disease who sustain femoral neck fractures. The incidence of complications and the mortality rate are higher than for patients without Parkinson's disease and rehabilitation is difficult and prolonged.

Paget's Disease Intertrochanteric fractures in patients with Paget's diease occur infrequently, but can pose special problems. Bone quality is variable, making internal fixation difficult. Intramedullary devices should be used cautiously because of the likelihood of canal compromise.

Metastatic Disease Pathologic fractures or impending pathologic fractures involving the intertrochanteric region should be treated by internal fixation, with adjunctive methylmethacrylate if necesary. Sliding hip screws and Ender nails have been used successfully in this often debilitated population. Because the incision site for Ender nailing is remote from the fracture, postoperative radiation therapy, if indicated, can be initiated immediately. Multiple rods are necessary to "stack" the canal. Avulsion fractures of the lesser trochanter in adults without a history of significant trauma should be regarded as indicative of metastatic disease. They are usually associated with an impending subtrochanteric pathologic fracture that should be treated by prophylactic internal fixation.

Subtrochanteric Fractures

Subtrochanteric fractures account for approximately 15% of all fractures of the proximal femur. These fractures start at or below the lesser trochanter and involve the proximal femoral shaft. They are generally seen in three groups of patients: (1) young patients with normal bones who experience high-energy trauma; (2) older patients with weakened bone whose fractures occur as a result of minor falls; and (3) older patients with pathologic or impending pathologic fractures from metastatic lssions. The subtrochanteric area experiences some of the highest biomechanical stresses in the body. The medial and posteromedial cortex is a site of high compressive forces, while the lateral cortex experiences high tensile stresses. This stress distribution has important implications for fracture fixation and healing.

Various classification systems have been proposed, but, as yet, none has been universally accepted. The determination of fracture stability is essential in planning treatment. In stable fractures, medial and posteromedial cortical support is intact or can be reestablished. In unstable fractures, comminution results in loss of continuity of the medial cortex. These fractures are at highest risk for complications and implant failure. Early use of fixed-angle nailplate devices for unstable fractures resulted in failure rates as high as 50%.

Surgical management of subtrochanteric fractures uses a variety of implants, including intramedullary devices, sliding hip screws, and plate-screw assemblies. Intramedullary devices were a significant improvement over previously used rigid nail-plates. Available devices include the Zickel nail, Ender nails, and interlocking rods. The Zickel nail has been used most extensively (Fig. 7). Insertion was initially described as an open procedure with exposure of the fracture site. For unstable fractures, supplemental fix-

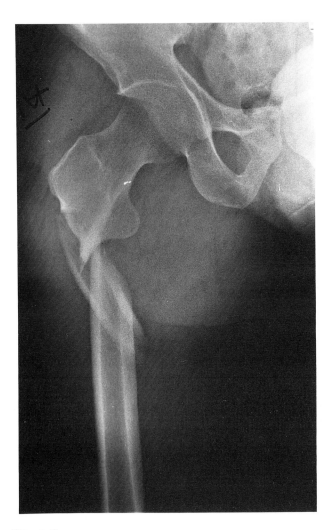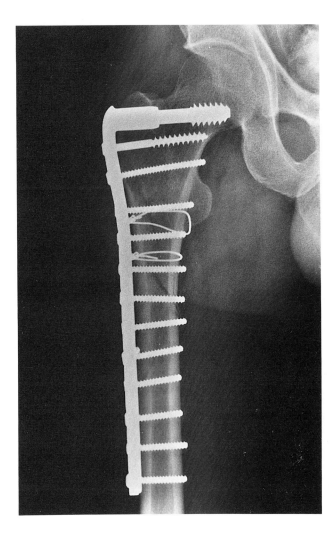

Figure 8
Left, Comminuted subtrochanteric fracture. **Right**, After treatment by open reduction and internal fixation using a dynamic compression screw.

ation (cerclage wires) is necessary to restore stability and prevent shortening. When significant medial comminution is present, bone grafting should be performed. One large series of subtrochanteric fractures treated by Zickel nailing reported satisfactory results in 90% of cases with only a 5% incidence of nonunion. This procedure can also be performed by a closed technique that avoids exposure of the fracture site. The closed technique requires a shorter operating time and decreases blood loss and postoperative morbidity.

Problems resulting from removal of the Zickel nail have been described. A small but significant number of patients have sustained a subtrochanteric fracture at the time of Zickel nail removal. The refracture is usually located approximately 4 cm distal to the lesser trochanter and in each case was different from the original fracture. These refractures occurred primarily in young patients undergoing nail removal because of local symptoms. In most cases, additional intramedullary fixation was necessary to treat the refracture. This complication may require reevaluation of the use of the Zickel nail in younger patients in whom eventual nail removal can be expected.

The results of Ender nailing of subtrochanteric fractures continue to be variable. A recent multicenter study reported that 10% of patients required reoperation within the first week for complications of fixation and 22% experienced significant knee pain. However, all fractures healed. Previous reports noted an early reoperation rate of as much as 32%. Interlocking nails have been used for subtrochanteric fractures when the lesser trochanter remained attached to the proximal fragment.

Sliding hip screws have also been used. One series reported a 95% rate of union. For this device to function optimally, the sliding component of the device must cross the fracture site. Therefore, only the most proximal subtrochanteric fractures and subtrochanteric-intertrochanteric fractures are suitable for this device. More distal fractures can be treated by use of a 95-degree blade plate or dynamic compression screw (Fig. 8). These devices provide improved fixation of the proximal fragment and act as a lateral tension band if the medial cortex is intact. If the medial cortex is comminuted, bone grafting should be performed.

Postoperative management depends on the fracture pattern and the method of fixation. For more proximal fractures treated with a sliding hip screw that allows impaction at the fracture site, early weightbearing can be permitted. Early weightbearing can also be allowed in stable fractures treated with intramedullary devices. Fractures with medial comminution or segmental comminution must be protected, regardless of the device used, for at least six to eight weeks until early healing is evident.

Pathologic fractures and impending pathologic fractures in the subtrochanteric region have been treated successfully with Zickel nailing, both with and without adjunctive methylmethacrylate. Insertion by a closed technique has been particularly beneficial in impending fractures. A recent series reported no fixation failures with this technique. The Zickel nail provides the benefits of proximal fixation with an intramedullary rod that can bridge more distal lesions.

Controversies

Femoral Neck Fractures: Osteonecrosis

The risk factors that may influence the development of osteonecrosis are the timing of the fixation, the effect of a manipulative reduction, and the influence of increased intracapsular pressure from hemiarthrosis. There are no recent reports clarifying the first two issues. In the last several years data have been presented to suggest that intracapsular pressure can be decreased by aspiration. However, there are no basic science studies demonstrating that this increased pressure can cause osteonecrosis and no clinical studies showing a decreased incidence of osteonecrosis after aspiration.

Femoral Neck Fractures: Internal Fixation vs Primary Replacement

The indications for internal fixation vs primary replacement with a prosthesis for displaced femoral neck fractures must be more clearly defined. This will require a more definitive identification of those patients at greatest risk for complications of internal fixation and the development of osteonecrosis. At present, the indications are somewhat vague, and often reflect the surgeon's preference. Resolving this issue would significantly decrease the need for reoperation after internal fixation procedures.

Femoral Neck Fractures: Early Weightbearing

The effect of early weightbearing after internal fixation of femoral neck fractures has not been satisfactorily established. Concern that early weightbearing might lead to fixation failure has led surgeons to restrict weightbearing. This can be exceedingly difficult for the elderly and a significant obstacle to their rehabilitation. One study has shown that fixation failure is not the result of early weightbearing in adequately stabilized fractures. However, as yet the orthopaedic community has not reached a consensus on this point.

Intertrochanteric Fractures: Reduction Techniques

The place of nonanatomic reduction techniques (medial displacement osteotomy, Sarmiento valgus osteotomy) in the treatment of unstable intertrochanteric fractures treated with the sliding hip screw remains to be established. The literature tends to support the use of anatomic reduction when the sliding hip screw is used, but formal medial displacement is thought by many to be necessary if a stable reduction is to be obtained. Proper insertion and use of the sliding hip screw may prove to be much more important than the specific reduction technique used.

Healthcare and Cost Containment

The problem of providing adequate healthcare for the increasing number of hip fractures that occur in the elderly each year may be one of the most significant challenges facing us today. Innovative treatment approaches directed at restoring these patients to their prefracture level of independence and function must be developed. Successful treatment of these patients will require the combined efforts of orthopaedists, geriatricians, and physiatrists. The problem appears to have been made worse by the advent of the prospective payment system and diagnosis-related groups. This effort to decrease healthcare costs may actually increase the cost of caring for these patients because of the increased need for nursing-home placement. Impact studies are needed to determine the effects of this system on the outcome of these patients. The results of these combined efforts must be directed at determining more effective treatment approaches that also facilitate control of rising healthcare costs.

Annotated Bibliography

Keywords

Femoral head fracture; Femoral shaft fracture; Healthcare costs; Hip dislocation; Hip fracture; Intertrochanteric fracture; Intramedullary fixation; Osteonecrosis; Paget's disease; Parkinson's disease; Pathologic fracture; Rheumatoid arthritis; Subtrochanteric fracture

Hip Dislocations

Calkins MS, Zych G, Latta L, et al: Computed tomography evaluation of stability in posterior fracture dislocation of the hip. *Clin Orthop* 1988;227:152–163.

This study found that joint stability depended on how much of the posterior acetabulum remained. Hips with less than 34% were unstable and those with more than 55% were stable. Seven of ten unstable hips had 0.5 mm or more of femoral head subluxation by computed tomography whereas none of the 21 stable hips had any demonstrable subluxation.

Epstein HC, Wiss DA, Cozen L: Posterior fracture dislocation of the hip with fractures of the femoral head. *Clin Orthop* 1985;201:9–17.

The authors report a series of 55 posterior hip dislocations with associated femoral head fractures after 55 years of follow-up. Specific treatment recommendations are discussed.

Hougaard K, Thomsen PB: Coxarthrosis following traumatic posterior dislocation of the hip. *J Bone Joint Surg* 1987;69A:679–683.

Ninety-eight patients with 100 hip dislocations were followed up for five to 26 years after injury. Long-term prognosis depended on the interval between injury and reduction.

Hougaard K, Thomsen PB: Traumatic posterior fracture-dislocation of the hip with fracture of the femoral head or neck, or both. *J Bone Joint Surg* 1988;70A:233–239.

Of 19 Epstein type V injuries, 13 were Pipkin types I or II fractures. The femoral head fracture did not affect the prognosis unless there was an associated femoral neck fracture.

Keith JE Jr, Brashear R Jr, Guilford WB: Stability of posterior fracture-dislocations of the hip: Quantitative assessment using computed tomography. *J Bone Joint Surg* 1988;70A:711–714.

The authors removed progressive increments of bone from the posterior part of the acetabular wall in 16 cadaveric hips. The hips were tested for stability and measured by computed tomography after each osteotomy. When less than 20% of the posterior part of the acetabular wall was removed, the hips remained stable. All hips became unstable after 40% of the wall was removed.

Suraci AJ: Distribution and severity of injuries associated with hip dislocations secondary to motor vehicle accidents. *J Trauma* 1986;26:458–460.

Thirty-eight patients had a 94.7% incidence of associated severe injuries that would have necessitated admission. Pelvic and extremity injuries occurred in 78.9% and 36.8% of patients, respectively.

Hip Fractures

Behr T, Dobozi WR, Badrinath K: The treatment of pathologic and impending pathologic fractures of the proximal femur in the elderly. *Clin Orthop* 1985;198:173–178.

Flexible intramedullary nails and other devices were used effectively for pathologic fractures of the proximal femur. Pain was relieved in 92% of patients; 84% became ambulatory; fracture union was obtained in 39% of patients surviving more than two months.

Davis FM, Woolner DF, Frampton C, et al: Prospective, multi-centre trial of mortality following general or spinal anaesthesia for hip fracture surgery in the elderly. *Br J Anaesth* 1987;59:1080–1088.

A prospective, randomized study of general vs spinal anesthesia for elderly patients with hip fracture showed no difference in 28-day postoperative mortality or one-year mortality. Other factors (age, postoperative arrhythmias, ischemic heart disease, congestive heart failure, increased anesthetic risk) were found to be more significant.

Elmerson S, Zetterberg C, Andersson G: Ten-year survival after fractures of the proximal end of the femur. *Gerontology* 1988;34:186–191.

In a series of 288 elderly patients who sustained hip fractures, mortality was 50% after three years, 60% after six years, and 77% after ten years. After ten years, only 1.4% of patients discharged to an institution were alive compared with 40% of the patients discharged to their homes. Age was the single most important factor determining long-term survival.

Falch JA, Ilebekk A, Slungaard U: Epidemiology of hip fractures in Norway. *Acta Orthop Scand* 1985;56:12–16.

The age- and sex-specific annual incidence of hip fractures in Oslo for 1978–1979 was the highest ever reported. The number of hip fractures in 1982 was five times greater than in 1950. This increase could not be explained only by the increasing number of elderly persons.

Finsen V, Benum P: Past fractures indicate increased risk of hip fracture. *Acta Orthop Scand* 1986;57:337–339.

Previous fractures (hip fractures or others) increased the probability of later hip fracture for women up to the age of 70 years and for men up to the age of 80 years.

Fitzgerald JF, Fagan LF, Tierney WM, et al: Changing patterns of hip fracture care before and after implementation of the prospective payment system. *JAMA* 1987;258:218–221.

Implementation of the prospective payment system resulted in a significantly decreased length of stay (10.3 vs 16.6 days). However, the number of discharges to nursing homes increased significantly (48% vs 21%), with most patients remaining in nursing homes six months after discharge (39% vs 13%).

Ions GK, Stevens J: Prediction of survival in patients with femoral neck fractures. *J Bone Joint Surg* 1987;69B:384–387.

In this series of 135 patients, the most important variable predicting survival was mental status. Other important variables were age and cerebrovascular disease.

Jensen TT, Juncker Y: Pressure sores common after hip operations. *Acta Orthop Scand* 1987;58:209–211.

In a comparison of patients undergoing hip surgery, 30% of patients with hip fracture developed pressure sores compared with 4% of patients undergoing selective total hip replacement. One half of the decubiti appeared within one week after surgery and occurred in patients more than 80 years of age.

Jette AM, Harris BA, Cleary PD, et al: Functional recovery after hip fracture. *Arch Phys Med Rehabil* 1987;68:735–740.

One year after hip fracture, only 33% of these elderly patients had regained prefracture function in the basic activities of daily living. An intensive rehabilitation program did not improve the results.

Jones S, DiPiro JT, Nix DE, et al: Cephalosporins for prophylaxis in operative repair of femoral fractures: Levels in serum, muscle, and hematoma. *J Bone Joint Surg* 1985;67A:921–924.

This prospective, controlled study compared antibiotic levels of cefazolin, cefamandole, and cefoxitin in serum, muscle, and postoperative hematomas. Cefazolin had significantly higher levels in serum and hematomas. The levels in muscle were similar for all three antibiotics.

Melton LJ III, O'Fallon WM, Riggs BL: Secular trends in the incidence of hip fractures. *Calcif Tissue Int* 1987;41:57–64.

The incidence of hip fractures in Rochester, Minnesota, was assessed for the years 1928 to 1982. Age-adjusted rates showed no overall increased incidence. However, increasing age-adjusted rates were noted for men. For women, the age-adjusted rates have remained fairly constant since the mid-1950s.

Menck H, Schulze S, Larsen E: Metastasis size in pathologic femoral fractures. *Acta Orthop Scand* 1988;59:151–154.

A series of pathologic fractures of the femur was evaluated to determine indications for prophylactic internal fixation. Prophylactic internal fixation was indicated if the ratio between width of metastasis and bone was 0.6 or more, if axial cortical destruction was 13 mm or more in the neck or was 30 mm or more in other parts of the femur, or if cortical destruction involved 50% or more of the circumference.

Ray WA, Griffin MR, Schaffner W, et al: Psychotropic drug use and the risk of hip fracture. *N Engl J Med* 1987;316:363–369.

The use of psychotropic drugs was found to increase the risk of falling and hip fractures in elderly persons. Use of hypnotics or anxiolytics having long half-lives, tricyclic antidepressants, and antipsychotics increased the risk of hip fracture; hypnotics and anxiolytics with short half-lives did not increase the risk of hip fracture.

Sexson S, Lehner J: Factors affecting hip fracture mortality. *J Orthop Trauma* 1988;1:298–305.

In a series of 283 patients, one-year mortality was 14.8%. Factors influencing mortality were age, number of preexisting medical conditions, postoperative level of ambulation, and delay of surgery for more than 24 hours in relatively healthy patients.

White BL, Fisher WD, Laurin CA: Rate of mortality for elderly patients after fracture of the hip in the 1980s. *J Bone Joint Surg* 1987;69A:1335–1340.

A series of 241 patients, average age 75.4 years, had a one-year mortality of 21.6%. In the second year after fracture, the mortality rate approached that of an age-matched population without fractures. Patients with significant medical problems (ASA III/IV) had a 49.4% one-year mortality compared with 8.0% for healthier patients.

Wilton TJ, Hosking DJ, Pawley E, et al: Osteomalacia and femoral neck fractures in the elderly patient. *J Bone Joint Surg* 1987;69B:388–390.

Iliac crest biopsies were performed in more than 1,000 elderly patients with femoral neck fractures. Osteomalacia was identified in only 2% of the specimens, indicating that osteomalacia is not a significant factor predisposing to femoral neck fractures.

Femoral Neck Fractures

Baksi DP: Internal fixation of ununited femoral neck fractures combined with muscle-pedicle bone grafting. *J Bone Joint Surg* 1986;68B:239–245.

Muscle-pedicle bone grafting and internal fixation were used to treat nonunions in patients with previously untreated femoral neck fractures. This procedure resulted in eventual union in 46 of 56 cases.

Bochner RM, Pellicci PM, Lyden JP: Bipolar hemiarthroplasty for fracture of the femoral neck. *J Bone Joint Surg* 1988;70A:1001–1010.

Of 90 patients followed up for at least two years after surgery, 91% were free of significant pain, 92% had satisfactory hip motion and muscle power, and 83% either returned to their preinjury level of function or used only a cane.

Bray TJ, Smith-Hoefer E, Hooper A, et al: The displaced femoral neck fracture: Internal fixation *versus* bipolar endoprosthesis. Results of a prospective randomized comparison. *Clin Orthop* 1988;230:127–140.

This prospective, randomized comparison found that bipolar endoprostheses resulted in less postoperative pain, greater mobility, fewer complications, and better functional results at two-year follow-up than internal fixation.

Crawfurd EJP, Emery RJH, Hansell DH, et al: Capsular distension and intracapsular pressure in subcapital fractures of the femur. *J Bone Joint Surg* 1988;70B:195–198.

Intracapsular pressure was increased in patients with nondisplaced and displaced femoral neck fractures; pressures were consistently higher in nondisplaced fractures. Capsular distension was confirmed by ultrasonography.

Delamarter R, Moreland JR: Treatment of acute femoral neck fractures with total hip arthroplasty. *Clin Orthop* 1987;218:68–74.

In this series of 27 patients with displaced femoral neck fractures and preexisting degenerative changes of the acetabulum, results after an average follow-up of 3.8 years were superior to those of hemiarthroplasty and comparable to those of elective total hip arthroplasty.

Fairclough J, Colhoun E, Johnston D, et al: Bone scanning for suspected hip fractures: A prospective study in elderly patients. *J Bone Joint Surg* 1987;69B:251–253.

Technetium scanning was a reliable method of identifying or excluding a femoral neck fracture in elderly patients with hip pain after a fall when standard radiographs were not helpful.

Frandsen PA, Andersen E, Madsen F, et al: Garden's classification of femoral neck fractures: An assessment of inter-observer variation. *J Bone Joint Surg* 1988;70B:588–590.

The authors describe the difficulty of delineating the various stages of Garden's classification. Forty-five percent of cases were classified as undisplaced (stages I and II) by some observers and displaced (stages III and IV) by other observers. Complete agreement on classification was present in only 22% of cases.

Greenough CG, Jones JR: Primary total hip replacement for displaced subcapital fracture of the femur. *J Bone Joint Surg* 1988;70B:639–643.

In this series of 37 elderly patients with displaced subcapital fractures without preexisting degenerative changes of the acetabulum, 19% required revision surgery after an average follow-up of 1.7 years and an additional 11% had radiographic signs of loosening.

Madsen F, Linde F, Andersen E, et al: Fixation of displaced femoral neck fractures: A comparison between sliding screw plate and four cancellous bone screws. *Acta Orthop Scand* 1987;58:212–216.

This was a prospective, randomized study of sliding hip and ASIF cancellous screws used for fixation of displaced femoral neck fractures. The two-year rate of union was 64% in the sliding hip screw group and 84% in the ASIF screw group.

Staeheli JW, Frassica FJ, Sim FH: Prosthetic replacement of the femoral head for fracture of the femoral neck in patients who have Parkinson disease. *J Bone Joint Surg* 1988;70A:565–568.

The authors report satisfactory results after prosthesis replacement for displaced femoral neck fractures in patients with Parkinson's disease of varying degrees of severity. Instability was not related to the surgical approach used. Adductor tenotomy may be helpful to enhance stability when contractures are present.

Strömqvist B, Hansson LI, Nilsson LT, et al: Prognostic precision in postoperative 99mmTc-MDP scintimetry after femoral neck fracture. *Acta Orthop Scand* 1987;58:494–498.

Technetium bone scanning performed within two weeks of femoral neck fracture predicted healing complications with a prognostic accuracy of 91%.

Strömqvist B, Kelly I, Lidgren L: Treatment of hip fractures in rheumatoid arthritis. *Clin Orthop* 1988;228:75–78.

Nineteen of 20 rheumatoid patients with displaced femoral neck fractures treated by internal fixation showed loss of reduction, nonunion, or superior segmental collapse compared with 50% of a matched nonrheumatoid group. Primary prosthesis replacement is recommended for rheumatoid patients with displaced femoral neck fractures.

Strömqvist B, Nilsson LT, Egund N, et al: Intracapsular pressures in undisplaced fractures of the femoral neck. *J Bone Joint Surg* 1988;70B:192–194.

Intracapsular pressure was more than 80 mm Hg in 16 of 50 patients with undisplaced femoral neck fractures. Extension and internal rotation consistently increased intracapsular pressure. Of 13 patients with decreased femoral head blood flow scintimetrically, nine showed significant increases in blood flow after aspiration of the hemarthrosis.

Swiontkowski MF, Harrington RM, Keller TS, et al: Torsion and bending analysis of internal fixation techniques for femoral neck fractures: The role of implant design and bone density. *J Orthop Res* 1987;5:433–444.

A biomechanical analysis evaluated fixation methods for femoral neck fractures. There was no benefit from the use of more than three pins or screws. Fracture stability was most closely correlated with bone density.

Tooke SM, Favero KJ: Femoral neck fractures in skeletally mature patients, fifty years old or less. *J Bone Joint Surg* 1985;67A:1255–1260.

Nonunion and osteonecrosis occurred in 5.5% and 33%, respectively, of displaced femoral neck fractures treated with a variety of internal fixation devices. The need for immediate and adequate reduction was stressed.

Yamagata M, Chao EY, Ilstrup DM, et al: Fixed-head and bipolar hip endoprostheses: A retrospective clinical and roentgenographic study. *J Arthrop* 1987;2:327–341.

A comparison of hemiarthroplasties and bipolar endoprostheses showed that acetabular erosion was more common after a hemiarthroplasty and loosening was more common after a bipolar endoprosthesis. Conversion to total hip replacement was performed more often after hemiarthroplasty (12.5% vs 7.2%).

Zetterberg C, Elmersson S, Andersson GB: Reoperations of hip fractures. *Acta Orthop Scand* 1985;56:8–11.

The incidence of reoperation after internal fixation of femoral neck and intertrochanteric hip fractures was analyzed for the years 1965 and 1981. The reoperation rate in 1981 was 29% for femoral neck fractures and 3.6% for intertrochanteric fractures. Compared with 1965, the incidence of reoperation decreased significantly only for intertrochanteric fractures.

Intertrochanteric Fractures

Bartucci EJ, Gonzalez MH, Cooperman DR, et al: The effect of adjunctive methylmethacrylate on failures of fixation and function in patients with intertrochanteric fractures and osteoporosis. *J Bone Joint Surg* 1985;67A:1094–1107.

Augmentation of fixation of intertrochanteric fractures with methylmethacrylate resulted in significantly fewer fixation failures than occurred in the uncemented group. However, hip function scores in the cemented group were significantly lower than those in the uncemented group.

Chang WS, Zuckerman JD, Kummer FJ, et al: Biomechanical evaluation of anatomic reduction versus medical displacement osteotomy in unstable intertrochanteric fractures. *Clin Orthop* 1987;225:141–146.

This laboratory study showed that anatomic reduction of unstable fractures resulted in significantly higher compression across the calcar region and significantly lower tensile strain on the plate than occurred with medial displacement osteotomy.

Cobelli NJ, Sadler AH: Ender rod versus compression screw fixation of hip fractures. *Clin Orthop* 1985;201:123–129.

In this study of 174 hip fractures, technical problems were encountered in 67% of those treated with Ender nails compared with 10% of those treated with compression screws. The technical complication rate was unacceptable for both stable and unstable fractures.

Mariani EM, Rand JA: Nonunion of intertrochanteric fractures of the femur following open reduction and internal fixation: Results of several attempts to gain union. *Clin Orthop* 1987;218:81–89.

Twenty patients with nonunions of intertrochanteric fractures underwent prosthesis replacement in nine cases and repeat open reduction and internal fixation in 11 cases, nine of which achieved union.

Phillips CD, Pope TL Jr, Jones JE, et al: Nontraumatic avulsion of the lesser trochanter: A pathognomonic sign of metastatic disease? *Skeletal Radiol* 1988;17:106–110.

Four adults with avulsion fractures of the lesser trochanter were found to have metastatic lesions in the intertrochanteric-subtrochanteric regions. This is a sign of metastatic disease and impending pathologic fracture.

Sernbo I, Johnell O, Gentz C-F, et al: Unstable intertrochanteric fractures of the hip: Treatment with Ender pins compared with a compression hip-screw. *J Bone Joint Surg* 1988;70A:1297–1303.

This was a prospective, randomized study with more than 100 patients in each treatment group. The Ender nail group had a significantly greater risk of reoperation, as well as frequent complications of external-rotation deformity, limb shortening, and knee pain.

Steinberg GG, Desai SS, Kornwitz NA, et al: The intertrochanteric hip fracture: A retrospective analysis. *Orthopedics* 1988;11:265–273.

The authors found that the preoperative character of an intertrochanteric fracture was an important determinant of postoperative stability in unstable fracture patterns. Medial displacement osteotomy had no advantage over anatomic reduction.

Stern MB, Angerman A: Comminuted intertrochanteric fractures treated with a Leinbach prosthesis. *Clin Orthop* 1987;218:75–80.

A calcar replacement hemiarthroplasty was used in 105 unstable intertrochanteric fractures. A total of 94% of the patients regained their prefracture ambulatory status. The length of hospital stay was also decreased.

Waddell JP, Czitrom A, Simmons EH: Ender nailing in fractures of the proximal femur. *J Trauma* 1987;27:911–916.

In this series of 723 intertrochanteric fractures, Ender nails were used successfully for both stable and unstable fractures. The complication rate decreased significantly as experience with the procedure increased.

Subtrochanteric Fractures

Bergman GD, Winquist RA, Mayo KA, et al: Subtrochanteric fracture of the femur: Fixation using the Zickel nail. *J Bone Joint Surg* 1987;69A:1032–1040.

A series of 131 patients with subtrochanteric fractures treated by Zickel nailing was divided into four groups: young patients after high-energy trauma, elderly patients after minor falls, patients with pathologic fractures, and those in whom previous treatment had failed. Results were satisfactory in 90% and nonunions occurred in 5%.

David AD, Meyer RD, Miller ME, et al: Closed Zickel nailing. *Clin Orthop* 1985;201:138–146.

A closed insertion technique was used successfully in this small group of patients. This resulted in significantly reduced operating time and blood loss. Fractures that do not require supplementary fixation can be treated with this technique.

Duobozi WR, Larson BJ, Zindrick M, et al: Flexible intramedullary nailing of subtrochanteric fractures of the femur: A multicenter analysis. *Clin Orthop* 1986;212:68–78.

Of 76 subtrochanteric fractures treated by flexible intramedullary (Ender) nailing, 10% required reoperation within one week. Knee discomfort developed in 22% of the cases. All fractures healed.

Ovadia DN, Chess JL: Intraoperative and postoperative subtrochanteric fracture of the femur associated with removal of the Zickel nail. *J Bone Joint Surg* 1988;70A:239–243.

Twelve subtrochanteric fractures occurred at the time of Zickel nail removal. These fractures differed from the original fracture and were located an average of 4.3 cm distal to the lesser trochanter. All fractures required reinsertion of internal fixation.

Ruff ME, Lubbers LM: Treatment of subtrochanteric fractures with a sliding screw-plate device. *J Trauma* 1986;26:75–80.

A sliding hip screw device was used to treat a variety of subtrochanteric fractures. Union was achieved in 95% of cases. Impaction of approximately 1 cm occurred in fractures with medial comminution.

Sangeorzan BJ, Ryan JR, Salciccioli GG: Prophylactic femoral stabilization with the Zickel nail by closed technique. *J Bone Joint Surg* 1986;68A:991–999.

Insertion of the Zickel nail with a closed technique was successful in this series of 43 impending pathologic fractures. No implant failures or infections reoccurred.

Yelton O, Low W: Iatrogenic subtrochanteric fractures: A complication of Zickel nails. *J Bone Joint Surg* 1986;68A:1237–1240.

The authors report four cases of subtrochanteric fracture occurring at the time of Zickel nail removal. The mechanism postulated is that the anterior and valgus angulation of the nail places excessive stress on the proximal femur during removal. All fractures required reinsertion of internal fixation.

40

Femur: Trauma

A fracture of the femoral shaft in an adult almost always requires surgical treatment and stabilization. Failure to perform this surgery promptly and accurately, allowing an early return to function, can lead to many complications.

Femoral Shaft Fractures

Patients With Multiple Injuries

Increasing evidence supports the proposition that early stabilization of femoral shaft fractures is a vital aspect of the management of patients with multiple injuries. The procedure significantly decreases the incidence of pulmonary complications (adult respiratory distress syndrome, fat emboli, pneumonia, and pulmonary failure) by allowing the patient to assume an upright position. Early fracture stabilization also decreases medical and orthopaedic complications in patients with both complete and incomplete spinal cord injuries. In addition to all the proven clinical benefits of early stabilization of femoral shaft fractures, the procedure significantly decreases healthcare costs for these patients.

Vascular Injury

Vascular injuries are relatively uncommon in association with femoral shaft fractures and occur at a rate of 2%. However, recent evidence suggests that the incidence of undetected injury to the femoral artery may be higher than previously thought. Arteriography is necessary when penetrating trauma of sufficient energy to cause a fracture occurs in proximity to the femoral artery. Blunt trauma causing a fracture of the distal fourth of the shaft of the femur can cause an arterial injury by tearing the femoral artery at the level of the adductor canal, where it is tethered. This injury may be an intimal tear and the patient may have normal distal pulses. Complete occlusion of the artery may occur later. Any question of an arterial injury with penetrating or blunt trauma should be resolved by arteriography. This may be delayed for as long as 24 hours if distal pulses are present.

Treatment of arterial injuries depends on the severity of vascular compromise and the amount of time that has elapsed since the injury. If distal pulses are present, indicating normal flow, femoral fractures can be stabilized initially and an arteriogram obtained after stabilization. If arterial compromise is severe, as in complete laceration, arterial flow must be reestablished within six hours. This can be done by temporarily shunting the artery, then stabilizing the femoral fracture by internal fixation, followed by arterial repair, all in a single procedure. When ischemia of the lower extremity lasts longer than several hours, four-compartment fasciotomy should always be performed. Arterial repair is usually accomplished by interposition of a vein graft or synthetic graft. Whenever femoral artery repair is performed, femoral vein repair must also be done. Sciatic nerve injuries in conjunction with arterial injury are generally caused by ischemia, contusion, or stretching and seldom require surgical repair.

Classification of Injuries

Fractures of the femoral shaft can be classified by their location, fracture pattern, degree of comminution, whether they are open or closed, and/or their causes. Fractures can occur in the subtrochanteric region, the shaft or diaphysis, or the distal third or supracondylar areas. Fractures in the proximal and distal thirds of the femur can heal with malrotation because of the transition in the area from diaphyseal to metaphyseal bone. Spiral and oblique fracture patterns, which are common in elderly patients, occur as a result of low-energy injuries in patients with large intramedullary canals and osteoporotic bone. Comminuted fractures have been classified by Winquist (Fig. 1) into types I through V. These result from high-energy absorption in young, healthy bone. They can heal with shortening and malrotation, as can spiral and short oblique fractures. The use of interlocking intramedullary nails has gained wide acceptance in this group of femoral fractures.

A type I comminuted femoral fracture consists of a small butterfly fracture that covers less than 25% of the width of the bone. A type II comminuted fracture is a larger butterfly fracture that covers 50% or less of the width of the bone. These fractures can be relatively stable in length and rotation if there is good contact between the major proximal and distal fragments and if the fracture occurs away from the distal or proximal metaphyseal flare. Type III comminuted fractures consist of a large segment (more than 50% of the width of the bone) with only a small spike of remaining proximal and distal fragments in contact. These fractures are always unstable in length and rotation. Type IV comminuted fractures consist of segmental comminution with no contact between the major proximal and distal fragments. These fractures are always unstable in length and rotation. The final fracture type (type V) consists of segmental bone loss and is always an unstable open fracture.

Femoral shaft fractures can also be classified into pathologic fractures and stress fractures. Pathologic fractures occur with minimal trauma and can often be diagnosed before the occurrence of a displaced fracture because of the pain caused by microscopic infraction. Pathologic fractures resulting from metastatic malignant tumors are common in the proximal femur (with breast carcinoma being most common). Fractures resulting from benign tumors occur as well, and are more commonly primary lesions (examples are solitary cyst, fibrous dysplasia, and enchondroma). Metabolic bone disease (Paget's disease, osteo-

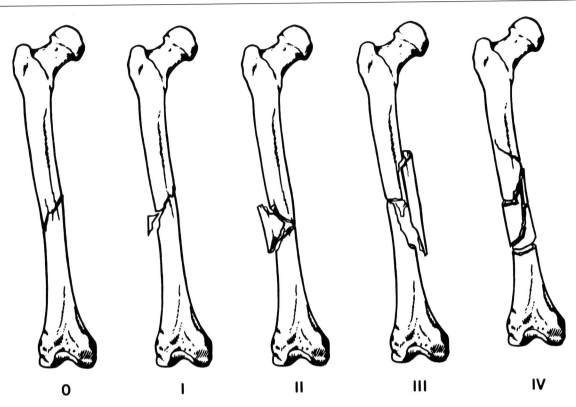

Figure 1
Winquist classification of comminuted femoral shaft fractures.

porosis, and osteomalacia) can also cause pathologic fracture. The femur is the bone most often fractured in patients with Paget's disease, and there may be a significant deformity that makes treatment difficult. Stress fractures caused by fatigue failure can be a significant problem in the femur. They may be asymptomatic in the femur until a displaced fracture occurs. Stress fractures of the femur may be more common than metatarsal stress fractures in military recruits. Exertional bone pain in a military recruit or long-distance runner should be treated with a high index of suspicion for stress fracture. Bone scans should be obtained and, if positive, the patient should be treated even if radiographs appear to be normal.

Open Fractures

Open femoral shaft fractures are less common than open tibial fractures because the size of the bone and soft-tissue mass surrounding the femur require more energy to fracture. All open fractures in the femur require irrigation and debridement. Surgical extensions of wounds for the purpose of irrigation and debridement can be closed but the compounded portion is left open.

Fracture management has long been a topic of controversy in these injuries. The traditional standard of care, consisting of initial debridement with delayed wound closure after five to seven days and surgical stabilization of the fracture after ten to 14 days, is quite acceptable in patients with isolated open femoral shaft fractures. Unfortunately, this protocol is unacceptable in the patient with multiple injuries, who requires immediate fracture stabilization. Recent studies have shown that immediate

intramedullary nailing can be safely accomplished by experienced surgeons in such cases with little or no difference in infection rates after thorough irrigation and debridement. This allows mobilization of the patient as well as easy access to the wound. External fixation in open femoral fractures should be reserved for large, severely contaminated wounds caused by close-range shotgun blasts or farm injuries and Gustilo grade IIIB injuries. Problems with external fixation include pin-tract infection, loss of joint motion, loss of fracture reduction, and poor access to the wound for wound management.

Ipsilateral Fractures

Hip and Shaft Ipsilateral hip fractures occur in as many as 5% of all femoral shaft fractures and this incidence may be increasing. This fracture is most commonly a femoral neck fracture, but can be an intertrochanteric fracture. These are always the result of high-energy trauma. Hip fractures are missed in 20% to 30% of cases. These fractures are usually overlooked because a radiograph was not obtained or because external rotation of the proximal femur masked the hip fracture. All patients with femoral shaft fractures, as well as all trauma patients, should have an anteroposterior radiograph of the pelvis done as part of the initial diagnostic evaluation. Possible femoral neck fracture must be excluded in all cases of femoral shaft fracture because of the severe complications that can occur with this injury.

Complications of femoral neck fractures include osteonecrosis of the femoral head (5% of cases) and nonunion of the femoral neck (5% of cases). This percentage is significantly less than the rate of osteonecrosis in isolated femoral neck fractures and may be the result of dissipation of energy through the shaft fracture. However, this reported rate may be falsely low because minimum follow-up is one year in most series. In young patients, there is no satisfactory treatment for osteonecrosis. Therefore, prompt diagnosis and proper initial treatment of this injury are important. The ideal treatment is early anatomic reduction and stable internal fixation. This requires surgery on an emergency basis and open reduction if anatomic reduction cannot be obtained in a closed fashion. The best stabilization for the femoral neck is multiple lag screws inserted parallel to allow interfragmentary compression.

In these fractures, management of one fracture significantly affects management of the other. In all reported series, surgical stabilization of both hip and shaft fractures has led to the best results. Management of the femoral shaft fracture should not compromise optimum management of the femoral neck fracture. Femoral shaft fractures have been managed successfully by compression plating and bone graft, by retrograde Küntscher nailing, and by interlocking nailing.

Preliminary stabilization of the femoral neck with pins or a screw, followed by nailing of the femoral shaft and then placement of parallel compression screws into the femoral neck, has been recommended. The use of one device to fix both fractures simultaneously, such as Ender nails or contralateral locked nails, has been tried but abandoned because of inadequate stabilization of the femoral neck.

Femoral Shaft and Tibial Shaft Ipsilateral fracture of the femoral shaft and tibia occurs in about 10% of all femoral fractures. The mortality is reported to be 5% to 15%, and "fat emboli syndrome" occurs in 9% to 13% of patients. One series of patients with multiple injuries noted that more than one half of the 132 patients had this combined injury. Therefore, resuscitation, diagnosis, and treatment of life-threatening injuries take precedence. This combined injury is a limb-threatening one and should be addressed next. Femoral fractures should be stabilized by internal fixation in the first 24 hours. Most major complications (fat emboli, pulmonary emboli, and death) occur when stabilization is delayed.

The best outcome of this injury has been reported with early stabilization of the femur and tibia and early restoration of the range of motion of the knee.

Good to excellent results have been reported in 85% of cases in which this approach was used. Open fractures are common in this injury (20% femur, 50% tibia). Therefore, internal fixation of the tibia alone carries a high risk. Ideally, the femur is stabilized with closed locked intramedullary nailing whenever possible; however, the treatment of the tibia must be individualized. Immobilization of the knee for no more than six weeks can give a good result. Closed tibial fractures that are undisplaced can be treated in a closed fashion with a patellar tendon cast that allows early knee motion. Low-grade open or displaced closed tibial fractures are best treated by intramedullary nailing with reamed or unreamed nails. Unreamed, locked tibial nails can be used in more comminuted open fractures without contamination or vascular injury. High-grade open or severely contaminated fractures of the tibia should be treated by external fixation. A recent report of five patients treated with external fixation of both the femur and tibia

has demonstrated that this method can be successful in open or contaminated fractures of both the femur and tibia. Intra-articular fractures (distal femur, proximal or distal tibia) should be managed by primary anatomic reduction and stable internal fixation that allows active range of motion as soon as possible.

Femoral Shaft and Knee Ligaments Ipsilateral knee ligament injury should be suspected in all patients with femoral shaft fractures. The actual occurrence rate is 5% and the injury is often undiagnosed throughout the course of treatment. After femoral fracture stabilization, the knee should be thoroughly reexamined to assess ligamentous stability. If indicated, arthroscopy can be performed at the same time as femoral fracture stabilization.

Methods of Treatment

The ideal treatment for femoral shaft fractures allows early mobilization of the patient and early range of knee motion to prevent joint stiffness. The treatment should allow anatomic restoration of length and alignment (angulation and rotation) with a high rate of union and low rate of complications (<1%).

Traction and Cast Brace Traction and some form of cast or brace have traditionally been the standard treatment for fractures of the femur. This is no longer the case. Although this method has a high rate of union with a low risk of infection, the results are too often unacceptable because of excessive knee stiffness and malalignment. Newer traction methods, such as roller traction and the use of cast bracing, have improved results by allowing earlier mobilization and knee motion. However, the time spent in traction in the hospital continues to average four weeks, which is more than twice the time required by internal fixation.

Good or excellent results have been reported in only 43% to 86% of cases. Complications are frequent and generally related to shortening, malalignment, and knee stiffness. The mean shortening reported in most series is more than 1 cm. Angulation of more than 10% in either the coronal or sagittal plane is common. Use of traction and cast braces in the treatment of femoral shaft fractures is becoming increasingly limited, especially in the patient with multiple injuries. This method is now limited to comminuted fractures of the distal third of the femur with minimal shortening on initial radiographs or to communities in which sophisticated fracture care is not available.

External Fixation External fixation of femoral shaft fractures continues to have limited application. The device is easily and quickly applied with low risk. The method allows early mobilization but often does not allow adequate knee motion. Late problems with this method include knee stiffness, pin-tract infection, delayed union, and malalignment. If significant pin-tract infection occurs, it may preclude surgical intervention with other methods. These problems make this technique less attractive.

With external fixation, 50% of patients lose knee motion. The fixator should be applied on the lateral aspect of the femur. Care should be taken not to impale the vastus lateralis or other quadriceps musculature, but to place pins beneath the muscle. Use of the Wagner apparatus, which is adjustable in the longitudinal plane, has been described by several authors. Its drawback is that pin clusters are placed far from the fracture site, not allowing adequate control of alignment in the frontal plane. A unilateral half-pin frame with stacked bars placed laterally is more stable but is not adjustable (Fig. 2). With either device, the overall alignment of the femur should be good before application of the frame.

Recent studies on the use of external fixation in complex femoral fractures (open fractures, comminuted fractures, shortening in traction, and spinal cord injury) have reported satisfactory outcomes in most cases. In some of these instances, locked intramedullary nailing is clearly more advantageous.

The ideal application for an external fixator is the severely contaminated Gustilo grade III open fracture when simultaneous debridement is performed. In areas where locked nails are unavailable, an external fixator may be indicated in complex fractures. Once an external fixator has been used, the surgeon must be cautious when contemplating future internal fixation because of contaminated pin sites.

Compression Plates The use of compression plates for femoral shaft fractures can fulfill the initial goals of early mobilization and functional range of motion. Stable anatomic reduction is provided early with maintenance of normal axial and length alignment. A single broad compression plate should be applied to the lateral aspect of the femur with a cancellous bone graft routinely applied along the medial aspect of the femur. Two plates cause excessive stress-shielding and require extensive dissection. Devices that apply intraoperative distraction can be helpful when a plate is applied. A broad plate bridging comminuted fractures, with stable fixation provided by screws that engage eight cortices both proximally and distally with minimal dissection, may achieve results superior to those of an "anatomic" reduction that requires more extensive dissection.

The liberal use of bone grafts should be encouraged when compression plates are applied.

Compression plates have many disadvantages. The infection rate is high. The incidence of late complications (such as plate failure, refracture at the end of the plate, refracture after plate removal, screw failure, nonunion, and delayed union) makes the method less than ideal. Most complications indicate that the method is not mechanically sound and requires excessive surgical dissection. Use of compression plates should be restricted to intra-articular fractures that extend into the knee joint and require anatomic reduction for congruity and stable fixation so that knee motion can begin. They may be used occasionally in femoral shaft fractures associated with complex proximal fractures that take precedence over the shaft fracture or in patients undergoing vascular repair associated with a distal-third femoral fracture.

Compression plates may have a role in the treatment of ipsilateral femoral shaft and neck fractures or in the patient with a concomitant femoral shaft fracture and arterial injury requiring repair.

Intramedullary Nails

Intramedullary nailing has become the treatment of choice for most femoral shaft fractures. The best results have been reported with the closed technique. However, similar results can be achieved with an open technique if the incision is used primarily to obtain reduction and minimal soft-tissue dissection is performed. The technique of nailing is otherwise similar for closed and open procedures. Reaming of the femoral canal allows the placement of a stiffer nail of larger diameter. This then expands the indications of the technique to complex fracture patterns by allowing the use of locked intramedullary nails that have proximal and distal holes for cross-bolts (Fig. 3).

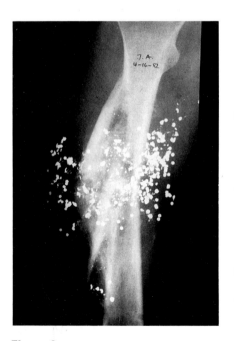
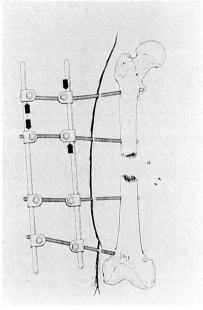
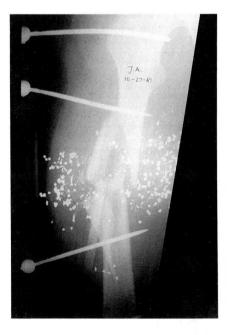

Figure 2
Stacked external fixation used for management of comminuted, open femoral fracture caused by a close-range shotgun blast.

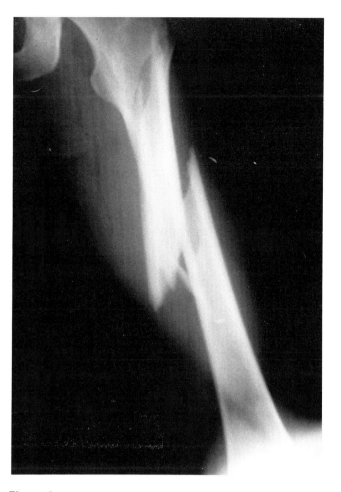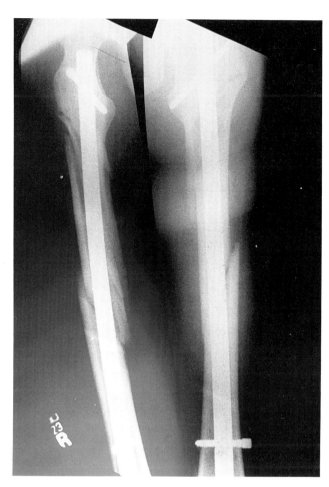

Figure 3
Locked intramedullary nail for management of comminuted femoral shaft fracture.

The use of intramedullary nails in the unreamed femur is advocated by some authors. The technique uses either a single nail of smaller diameter or multiple round nails of even smaller diameter. The use of nails in the unreamed femur should be reserved for simple fracture patterns (transverse or short oblique) that occur in the midshaft area. When these nails are used for proximal, distal, or more comminuted fractures, the results are inconsistent and unsatisfactory.

Reaming of the intramedullary canal destroys the endosteal blood supply to the bone, but this has been shown to be reestablished by six to eight weeks. Reaming does not increase the incidence of fat emboli in the fractured femur after stable intramedullary nailing. Abundant periosteal callus formation occurs at the periphery of the fracture site where cortical bone is well perfused. This brings further stability to the fracture site, and further revascularization of any devitalized bone then occurs.

Reamed, Locked Intramedullary Nails A marked expansion in the use of reamed, locked intramedullary nails has occurred in the past five years. These nails require reaming to allow placement of a nail with a relatively large diameter and holes for cross-fixation both proximal and distal to the fracture, usually with bolts but occasionally with blades.

They stabilize almost all fractures of the shaft of the femur, with the exception of those that extend into the joint proximally or distally. This form of fixation allows early mobilization. The infection rate is low and the union rate is high when the technique is performed with the closed method. They stabilize the complex shaft fracture by locking the intramedullary nail to the proximal and distal fragments. These nails allow better control of length and rotation than unlocked nails and are quite stable biomechanically. The disadvantage of the technique is the fact that a large amount of special equipment is required, such as an image intensifier, a fracture table, and a large inventory of implants. The use of these complex locked nails also requires a significant amount of experience, a second assistant, and experience with radiography in the operating room. This form of treatment is essentially the treatment of choice for all femoral shaft fractures in the United States today.

Because of the intramedullary nail, the indications for open reduction and cerclage wires in closed, comminuted shaft fractures are limited. One exception might be proximal or distal spiral fractures originating in the metaphysis and extending into the diaphysis.

Biomechanics There is no need for straight, solid intramedullary nails. These nails are placed without reaming, are weak, and tend to suffer fatigue failure with bending or breakage of the implant. Larger-diameter, hollow-section intramedullary nails require reaming of the intramedullary canal for insertion because the intramedullary canal is neither straight nor smooth. Reaming uniformly increases the diameter of the intramedullary canal and allows the insertion of this large nail. Reamed nails all use the original Küntscher design of a cloverleaf cross section with an open longitudinal slot that can be placed either anteriorly or posteriorly. When the slot is placed posteriorly, the nail has a high degree of bending stiffness but little flexibility. When placed anteriorly, the nail has less bending strength but more flexibility.

Recent investigators have made major changes in the design of intramedullary nails by removing the longitudinal slot. This leaves a closed cross section that is cannulated throughout the length of the nail. This markedly increases the torsional stiffness of these nails and, to a lesser degree, increases the bending strength of these nails as well. By doing this, the overall strength of the nail is increased, thereby creating the possibility of cross-locking. However, closing this cross section also increases the stiffness of the nail, thereby increasing the potential for additional comminution during insertion. Therefore, these nails must be overreamed by 1 to 2 mm. Closing the cross section of the nail also allows variation of the wall thickness. This aids in the control of the mechanical properties of the intramedullary nail. This design may make unreamed, locked nails a more attractive alternative in the future.

Other new designs have affected the biomechanics of these nails. Almost all intramedullary nails have an anterior bow. The radius of curvature varies from manufacturer to manufacturer. This anterior bow allows the nail to fit more anatomically within the femur when fully inserted, but does require some increased force that actually straightens the nail during insertion. A relatively stiff nail with a large radius of curvature can create a large hoop stress at the fracture site during insertion if the starting point is not carefully selected. An anterior starting point increases hoop stress at the fracture site and causes comminution of the fracture when the nail is inserted (Fig. 4). The stiffer the nail and the larger the radius of curvature, the more attention that must be paid to selection of the appropriate starting hole. The cross section of the nail, at least in the proximal 5 cm, has been closed routinely by several manufacturers to allow the attachment of a proximal targeting device by threading it directly onto the nail. This can create a stress concentrater that may cause a fatigue fracture of the nail at the proximal end even after the fracture has healed. Although many nails now have this type of design, current manufacturing techniques allow all intramedullary nails to be manufactured by the gundrill method. This means that the nails are formed from solid bar stock and the hollow portion of the nail is created by drilling out the internal diameter, similar to manufacture of a gun barrel. This improves the fatigue properties of the nail and places no welds in the nail where fatigue fractures can occur. Fatigue fracture of these intramedullary nails can also occur at the more distal screw holes. This is true with slotted nails when the fracture site is within 3 to 5 cm of the most proximal of the distal screw holes. This can be avoided by increasing the diameter of the nail to 13 or 14 mm and by preventing full weight-bearing until solid fracture union is achieved.

In the field of intramedullary nailing of femoral shaft fractures, the most recent development has been the elimination of slotted intramedullary nails. This revolutionary design change allows the manufacturer to decrease the diameter of the nails while maintaining enough strength to allow cross-fixation and cannulation. This is done, however, at the expense of flexibility but does not appear to decrease the rate of fracture healing.

Preoperative Management All femoral fractures should be treated at the earliest possible time. Even isolated femoral shaft fractures should be stabilized in the initial 24 hours if at all possible. If treatment is delayed, skeletal traction should be applied through either a proximal tibial or distal femoral traction pin. Femoral length should be kept as close as possible to normal in the preoperative period to allow ease of closed reduction and intramedullary nailing. Appropriate length determination can be made by a lateral radiograph performed with the patient in traction. Preoperative radiographs of the fractured femur should include the entire femur on both the anteroposterior and lateral views. An anteroposterior view of the pelvis must be obtained to rule out abnormalities of the hip or pelvis. The approximate diameter of the intramedullary nail needed can be determined by measuring the intramedullary canal on the lateral radiographs. Excessive comminution of the femoral shaft may make appropriate length determination difficult. The correct length of nail can be determined from a radiograph of the intact normal femur. The length of the nail is selected by measuring from the tip of the greater trochanter to the proximal pole of the patella or to the line up the posterior condyles on the anteroposterior radiograph. Magnification must be taken into account.

In patients with multiple injuries, femoral shaft fractures must be stabilized in the initial 24 hours. This allows mobilization of the patient and significantly reduces the incidence of pulmonary complications. All patients with closed femoral head injuries in addition to femoral shaft fractures require internal fixation and closed intramedullary nailing. A comatose patient with a femoral fracture

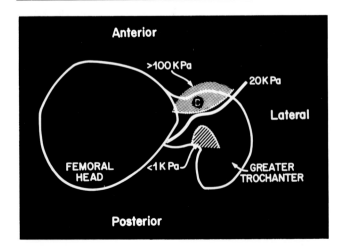

Figure 4
Anterior starting point that leads to increased hoop stress at the fracture site and comminution of the fracture with insertion of the nail.

should be treated with the expectation that complete neurologic recovery will occur. All patients over the age of 12 years are treated as adults when a femoral fracture occurs. Children under 10 years of age are still best managed with initial skeletal traction followed by spica cast application. Patients between the ages of 10 and 12 years require treatment based on size, concomitant injuries, and fracture pattern.

Surgical Technique Surgery is generally performed on a fracture table with the use of image intensification. The patient may be placed in either the supine position or the lateral position for placement of a nail. The supine position is a more physiologic position that is easier on patients with multiple injuries and should always be used for patients with significant pulmonary or spinal injuries. Fracture reduction and control of rotation is generally easier when the supine position is used. Unfortunately, the correct starting hole is sometimes difficult to define with the supine position because access to the greater trochanter is more difficult, particularly in the obese patient. The lateral position allows easier access to the tip of the greater trochanter for definition of the correct starting point. Generally, fracture reduction is more difficult, as is the definition of correct rotational alignment. The lateral position is best for isolated femoral shaft fractures and reconstructive surgery on the femur using intramedullary nails or saws.

Prophylactic intravenous antimicrobial therapy should always be used when large foreign-body implants are used. This is true for closed intramedullary nailing of a femoral shaft. Antibiotics should be begun perioperatively and continued for 24 to 48 hours postoperatively.

Locked intramedullary nails generally require placement of both proximal and distal bolts unless the fractures are stable enough to require neither proximal nor distal bolts. Fracture patterns that are stable (transverse, short oblique, or grade 0 and 1) can be treated with a simple nail with no cross-fixation or by a dynamic locked nail. For any degree of comminution or in proximal and distal fractures, nails should be placed in the static locked mode, which allows greater control of both length and rotation. Recent studies have shown that the criteria for dynamic intramedullary fixation (the placement of either proximal or distal bolts but not both) should be precise and exact. Dynamic intramedullary femoral stabilization should be performed only in transverse or short oblique fractures of the femoral isthmus with type 1 or type 2 comminution. Any increase in comminution at the site of the fracture is an indication for static locking (both proximal and distal bolts) of the nail. Essentially the surgeon should be compelled to find reasons not to perform static locking for a femoral shaft fracture. When dynamic locking nailing is performed, postoperative radiographs of the entire femur should be obtained before termination of anesthesia or removal of the skeletal traction. Any additional comminution that has occurred during the surgical procedure should lead the surgeon to apply static locking bolts (Fig. 5).

Placement of the proximal locking bolt is generally performed through a proximal targeting device attached directly to the nail. This aiming device works well for most nails and one or two proximal locking bolts can usually be placed without significant difficulty. Final placement of the bolt should be assessed in two planes to ensure that the bolt is located in its correct position through the nail. Distal

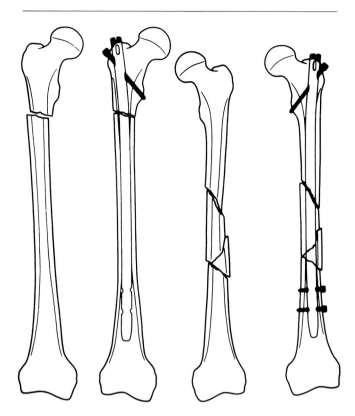

Figure 5
Static and dynamic locking of an intramedullary nail.

bolt placement is more difficult. All intramedullary locked nail systems have distal targeting devices that work reasonably well. Some of these devices are attached to the proximal end of the nail, others are hand-held, and others can be attached directly to an image intensifier. In general, all of these targeting devices can work. However, because of the added surgical time and the extra problems that targeting devices bring to the surgical procedure, most orthopaedic surgeons use a free-hand method of placement of distal bolts because it is simpler and less time-consuming. All methods of distal bolts placement require that the image intensifier project a perfectly round hole before the procedure begins. The image intensifier should be able to rotate through a 90-degree arc before the procedure begins. For free-hand targeting of the distal hole, a sharp awl or Steinmann pin is placed on the cortex of the bone directly in the center of the hole projected on the image-intensifier screen. An indentation or hole is made in the near cortex with the awl or pin after the awl is placed in a direct line with the X-ray beam (with the beam turned off). After this indentation or proximal hole is completed, a drill bit is then placed into the indentation or the hole and drilled through the nail and the far cortex, with the drill bit kept in a direct line with the image-intensifier beam. The drill is removed from the bit and the X-ray beam is used to verify placement. A depth gauge is used to determine the correct size of the bolt and a bolt is then placed across the femur.

Postoperative Management Patients with femoral shaft fractures require physical therapy if lower-extremity function is to be regained. The time spent in the hospital can be decreased by a continuous passive motion machine that restores knee motion as soon as possible. Quadriceps-strengthening exercises are begun on the first postoperative day. The goal is the ability to perform at least one unassisted straight leg raise before discharge. Electrical stimulation can help the patient to perform a quadriceps contraction. The patient is discharged from the hospital when adequate control of the lower extremity is obtained and crutches or a walker can be used safely. Generally, static locked nails are protected from full weightbearing for six to eight weeks. If dynamic locked nails or intramedullary nails placed in stable fractures are used, full weightbearing ambulation can be permitted immediately.

The maintenance of a full arc of motion of 90 to 100 degrees can prevent excessive callus formation from binding the quadriceps mechanism and limiting the range of motion of the knee. Knee manipulation for loss of knee motion or binding of the quadriceps mechanism is not recommended. These patients should be given physical therapy to restore motion gradually over several months. If progress cannot be obtained, an open quadricepsplasty and knee manipulation should be performed with the patient under general anesthesia.

Results Femoral shaft fractures treated by intramedullary nailing should be expected to heal within 16 to 20 weeks regardless of the amount of comminution. Expected mean range of motion of the knee is 0 to 125 to 135 degrees. Generally, 90% of patients will obtain a full range of motion. Seventy-eight percent of patients return to work within six months, and 96% return to work within 12 months. Eighty-eight percent of patients have no subjective pain, and 91% are able to walk normally. Two thirds of patients can be expected to return to normal daily activities and previous sports activities.

Complications After closed intramedullary nailing, including locked nails, infection rates are reported to be 0.5% to 1.5%. The infection rate after intramedullary nailing of open femoral shaft fractures following irrigation and debridement is 0% to 4%. This is true whether the intramedullary nailing is performed seven to ten days after initial irrigation and debridement or whether the intramedullary nailing is performed immediately after irrigation and debridement.

Treatment of an acutely infected intramedullary nail includes irrigation and debridement at the fracture site. The insertion site for the nail should be opened and a guide rod should be placed down the intramedullary canal. The nail should then be removed and the intramedullary canal thoroughly irrigated and debrided. This may include over-reaming of the intramedullary canal to remove infected granulation tissue around the nail. It may be necessary to open a hole in the distal medial aspect of the femur to allow thorough irrigation of the canal. If the intramedullary nail cannot be expected to reduce and stabilize the fracture adequately, it should be replaced. A slightly larger nail may be necessary to compensate for the extra reaming. After fracture union, which can be expected despite the infection, the intramedullary nail may need removal. If persistent drainage occurs after union, debridement, including permanent removal of the nail, should be done. This treatment is adequate for most infected intramedullary nails and generally results in a healed femoral shaft fracture

without residual infection. An intramedullary nail seldom requires complete removal before fracture union.

Delayed union or nonunion after intramedullary nailing is infrequent. This has been reported in 0% to 2% of cases. Nonunion is treated by removal of the intramedullary nail, reaming of the intramedullary canal, and replacement with a larger nail (approximately 2 mm larger than the original). Delayed union has been reported in 1% to 2% of cases. Recent studies have not shown a higher incidence of nonunion or delayed union. Dynamic nailing is not necessary unless there is clear radiographic evidence of nonunion at four to six months.

If nonunion persists, the intramedullary nail may fail. The intramedullary nail can break at a proximal weld site or at the most proximal distal bolt hole. Occasionally, an intramedullary nail bends or breaks at the fracture site. This is relatively rare. Removal of broken screws and nails can be difficult but can be accomplished with hooks that reach down to catch the end of the nail and allow it to be retrieved through the intramedullary canal. Isolated broken tops of nails or screws are not routinely removed when the hardware is buried well within the bone unless this is associated with a significant infection.

Malunion is the most frequent complication of intramedullary nailing. With the introduction of locked intramedullary nailing, the incidences of malrotation and shortening decreased markedly. When any type of shortening or malrotation can be anticipated, a static locked nail is always used. If a dynamic locked nail is used and shortening or malrotation is evident in the immediate postoperative period (one to two weeks), the patient should be returned to the operating room for realignment with skeletal traction and placement of static locking bolts. Recent studies have demonstrated that, in most femoral shaft fractures, static locking bolts provide better overall control of the fracture and guarantee normal alignment and fracture union.

Supracondylar Fractures of the Femur

Fractures that occur in the distal third of the femur and involve the distal metaphysis or junction of the distal diaphysis and metaphysis are commonly referred to as supracondylar fractures. These often occur in association with intra-articular extensions of the fracture line that may be more or less displaced depending on the level of energy that created the fracture. These fractures are most often the result of high-energy vehicular trauma in the younger patient, and the result of low-energy injuries in the elderly, most often from a fall. Because of the intra-articular extension of the fracture and the difficulty of immobilizing it, knee stiffness is common, as is degenerative osteoarthritis at the knee.

Classification

Supracondylar fractures can be classified as intra-articular or extra-articular and as involving either one or two condyles. The ASIF classification system divides fractures according to whether they are extra-articular (type A), unicondylar (type B), or bicondylar (type C) (Fig. 6).

Functional Bracing

Hinged casts and functional bracing have been used in nondisplaced extra-articular supracondylar fractures, generally in elderly patients in whom internal fixation with plates or screws can result in significant complications because of poor fixation in osteopenic bone. However, the technique has also been used in young patients with comminuted extra-articular fractures that have minimal malalignment problems with shortening or angulation. This method follows an initial period of skeletal traction with a distal femoral pin to allow for better control. Traction is used for at least three to four weeks and can be extended to six weeks if necessary. Functional bracing is then applied with either a hinged cast brace or a functional brace. This treatment method is not suited for most comminuted and intra-articular supracondylar fractures. Better results have been reported with internal fixation techniques.

Flexible Intramedullary Devices

Flexible intramedullary devices are indicated primarily for elderly patients and patients with noncomminuted distal femoral shaft fractures with articular injuries. Good axial alignment of the fracture can be obtained with these devices in both the anteroposterior and the mediolateral planes. Early mobilization of the patient is possible but anatomic fracture reduction and rigid stabilization should not be expected. If the fracture is at all comminuted, shortening usually occurs with this method. The ideal patient is elderly and has an extra-articular supracondylar fracture that is transverse without evidence of comminution. Devices available include Rush rods, Ender nails, and the Zickel supracondylar device. Cross-screws in the Zickel supracondylar device allow reduction and fixation of an intra-articular extension of the fracture (Fig. 7). These cross-bolts or cross-screws also prevent backing out of the nail and the impaction that can be expected with weightbearing.

These devices can be inserted without opening the fracture site by means of image intensification. The two intramedullary devices must cross the fracture simultaneously. If Ender nails or Rush rods are used, a functional fracture brace can be added for additional stability. An additional fracture brace is generally not necessary with the use of the Zickel supracondylar device. The patient can be mobilized soon after fixation, although weightbearing ambulation is avoided until early fracture union has occurred. Deep infections occur infrequently and nonunion is rare. Good or excellent results should be expected in approximately 70% of patients.

Patients with distal-third femoral fractures in whom major vascular injuries required a large medial approach for repair are good candidates for fixation with a Zickel supracondylar device. Fracture reduction can be obtained through the open wound, and a medial starting position is generally easily achieved through the exposed medial femoral condyle. The only extra incision necessary is a small 1-inch incision over the lateral femoral condyle for insertion of the lateral intramedullary device. This method is adequate for stabilization of simple transverse or short oblique fractures without extensive comminution. Fixation is adequate for early knee mobilization, and tends not to complicate fracture fixation when the additional complexity of the vascular injury and repair is present.

Angle Blade Plate

The angle blade plate or condylar blade plate generally provides the most rigid stabilization of comminuted, intra-

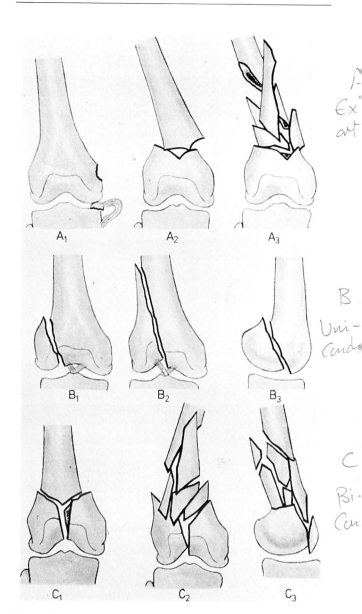

Figure 6
AO/ASIF classification of supracondylar fractures.

articular supracondylar fractures in young adults. This device originated in Europe, and extensive experience with the device is available. The device is generally used in intra-articular fractures with additional lag screws placed to fix the intra-articular or T-condylar extension. It requires an extensive surgical incision. The original "Mercedes incision" has been associated with a high incidence of wound breakdown, and the use of a universal longitudinal midline incision over the knee is currently recommended. If this is not used, a separate lateral incision with an additional medial incision may be necessary. The initial surgical step is open reduction of the displaced condylar fractures and fixation with lag screws. Lag screws are placed so that they do not interfere with subsequent application of the plate.

After internal fixation of the intra-articular fracture extension, the blade plate is applied. Correct placement of

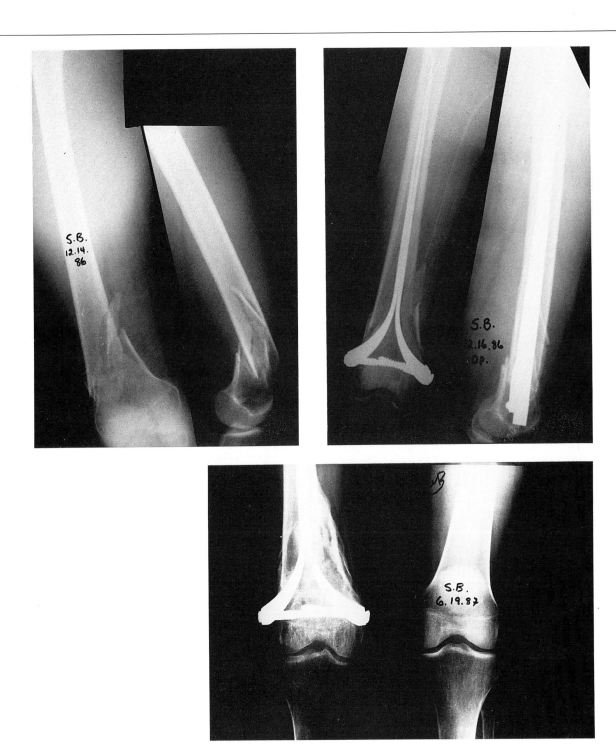

Figure 7
Zickel supracondylar device in elderly patient with bilateral distal femoral fractures. Note significant bilateral shortening.

the blade plate is difficult and requires alignment in all three planes. When the blade plate is correctly applied, good to excellent results can be expected in 75% of patients. Complications are usually technical and result from inadequate reduction of the articular surfaces, inaccurate positioning of the blade plate, and failure to apply an additional cancellous bone graft. Long-term complications include nonunions, which generally result in failure of the implant, knee joint stiffness, and degenerative osteoarthritis. Infection is uncommon, but may result in the loss of function in the knee joint.

Condylar Compression Screw
A condylar compression screw applied like an angle blade plate is commonly used in the United States. The indi-

cations for using the compression screw are similar to those for the blade plate, but the condylar compression screw is easier to apply and can be placed over a guide wire. The condylar compression screw needs accurate placement in only two of three planes. The device itself can allow for compression and stabilization across the intercondylar fracture but the addition of interfragmentary compression lag screws outside the plate is recommended. Rotation of the screw can be adjusted, allowing easier application of the plate to the femoral shaft. The disadvantage of the technique is that stabilization of the distal fragment is less rigid than that of the angle blade plate. Insertion of the large compression screw requires removal of a large amount of metaphyseal bone, which can never be replaced. If the device fails, the loss of metaphyseal bone makes reconstruction difficult. Satisfactory results have been reported in 70% of cases when the device is applied correctly.

Condylar Buttress Plate

The condylar buttress plate is designed to fix intra-articular fractures of the femur that have extensive comminution and may also involve either condyle in the anteroposterior plane. This device is generally used for the most difficult and most comminuted of distal intra-articular comminuted fractures. The condylar buttress plate is easy to apply and uses multiple lag screws across the distal intra-articular fracture component. The device itself is not as mechanically rigid as the angle blade plate or condylar compression screw. Anteroposterior lag screws may be needed to fix the fracture of the medial or lateral condyle in the frontal plane. The device must be aligned longitudinally to prevent fixation of the fracture in varus or valgus alignment. Because of the decreased strength of the device, weightbearing ambulation on an unhealed fracture results in a varus deformity because of bending of the side plate, usually at the screw-plate junction. Therefore, patients with this device should have more protection of the limb in the postoperative period, including a functional fracture brace. Early, gentle range of motion is allowed. The patient should avoid weightbearing ambulation until the fracture hais healed. All of these laterally placed plate-type devices require a bone graft at the junction of the diaphyseal and metaphyseal fracture lines. Occasionally, when comminution is severe, a medial T buttress plate is required. It is inserted through a medial approach with minimal soft-tissue stripping.

Controversies

Management of Open Fractures

Open fractures of the femoral shaft have been traditionally managed by debridement followed by traction, external fixation, or delayed internal fixation. Recent studies have noted a high union rate and low incidence of infection with immediate nailing after thorough fracture wound debridement. Although the 1% to 2% rate of infection after immediate nailings of grades I, II, and IIIA fractures is equivalent to that reported for delayed nailing, there has been a higher incidence of infection (as much as 10%) for grade IIIB and grade IIIC injuries. If complete surgical debridement of a lesser-grade fracture wound can be accomplished, immediate nailing appears to be an especially attractive alternative in patients with multiple injuries. For grossly contaminated wounds or wounds associated with extensive soft-tissue stripping of long segments of the femoral diaphysis, alternative stabilization techniques such as external fixation are preferred. Future clinical work in this field should help clarify the precise indications and contraindications for immediate intramedullary nailing of open fractures.

Indications for Static Locking and Dynamization

Initial speculation that static locking of intramedullary nails would predispose to stress-shielding and delayed union of fractures has not proven to be valid. Large North American series have confirmed that static locking of comminuted fractures of the femoral shaft does not retard either fracture healing or bone remodeling. Routine static locking of fractures, therefore, is indicated in any fracture pattern that may lead to postoperative shortening or malrotation if an unlocked nail is used. Dynamization of a statically locked nail by removal of either the proximal or distal bolts is unnecessary except in cases in which there is radiographic evidence of delayed healing three to six months after nailing.

Technique of Distal Locking

Four techniques for distal targeting have been tested during the last ten years in the United States. The nail-mounted targeting devices and C-arm-mounted targeting devices have been largely abandoned because of imprecise techniques. Deformation of the nail as it is driven down the femoral canal has frustrated attempts to use a targeting device attached to the proximal end of the nail. A third technique using hand-held targeting devices is still widely used but requires a delicate touch and involves a risk of prolonged exposure of the surgeon's hand to radiation. A free-hand technique in which an incision is made down to the lateral cortex of the distal femur at the site of the locking screws has largely supplemented the other targeting methods. With good radiographic assistance and proper use of instrumentation, predictable, accurate placement of the distal locking screws can be achieved.

Annotated Bibliography

Keywords

Compression plate; Compression screw; External fixation; Femoral neck fracture; Femoral shaft fracture; Hip fracture; Intramedullary nails; Polytrauma; Supracondylar fracture; Tibial shaft fracture; Vascular injury

Femoral Shaft Fractures

General Considerations

Garland DE, Rieser TV, Singer DI: Treatment of femoral shaft fractures associated with acute spinal cord injuries. *Clin Orthop* 1985;197:191–195.

Surgical stabilization of the femur within six weeks of injury produced the most favorable outcome with the least number of orthopaedic and other complications in patients with both complete and incomplete cord lesions.

Kessler SB, Hallfeldt KK, Perren SM, et al: The effects of reaming and intramedullary nailing on fracture healing. *Clin Orthop* 1986;212:18–25.

The process of reaming causes circulatory disturbances in the inner two thirds of the diaphyseal cortex. However, this does not impede the formation of external callus. The parts of bone that have sustained vascular damage by trauma or surgery are revascularized. Most patients are able to bear weight a few days after surgery.

ten Duis HJ, Nijsten MW, Klasen HJ, et al: Fat embolism in patients with an isolated fracture of the femoral shaft. *J Trauma* 1988;28:383–390.

Two groups were distinguished, those with open or closed fractures treated surgically within 24 hours of the accident (decompression group) and those with closed fractures treated conservatively for ten days (nondecompressed group). Clinical fat embolism occurred only in patients in the nondecompressed group (3.5%). Although the pathophysiologic mechanism of the onset of fat embolism remains unclear, initial temperature increases in combination with "typical" fracture localization and fracture type appear to have a predictive value.

Patients With Multiple Injuries

Bone LB, Johnson KD, Weigelt J, et al: Early versus delayed stabilization of femoral fractures: A prospective randomized study. *J Bone Joint Surg* 1989;71A:336–340.

A total of 178 acute femoral fractures in adults were randomly assigned to early or delayed fracture stabilization. When patients with multiple injuries had delayed fracture stabilization, the incidence of pulmonary complications (adult respiratory distress syndrome, fat embolism, and pneumonia) was higher, the hospital stay was longer, and the number of days in the intensive care unit was increased. The cost of hospital care showed a statistically significant increase for all patients with delayed fracture treatment compared with those with early fracture stabilization.

Johnson KD, Cadambi A, Seibert GB: Incidence of adult respiratory distress syndrome in patients with multiple musculoskeletal injuries: Effect of early operative stabilization of fractures. *J Trauma* 1985;25:375–384.

A significant increase in the incidence of adult respiratory distress syndrome was associated with delayed surgical stabilization of major fractures in patients with multiple orthopaedic injuries. This was particularly true for more severely injured patients (Injury Severity Score, > 40). This score is of prognostic value in predicting the incidence of adult respiratory distress syndrome, particularly when extremity and neurologic injuries are evaluated in the emergency room.

Seibel R, LaDuca J, Hassett JM, et al: Blunt multiple trauma (ISS 36), femur traction, and the pulmonary failure-septic state. *Ann Surg* 1985;202:283–295.

Pulmonary failure sepsis can be defined as an alveolar vs arterial difference in oxygen tension of more than 100 mm Hg, plus fever and leukocytosis. Thirty days of femoral traction significantly increased the duration of the sepsis compared with immediate fracture stabilization. Femoral shaft traction should be avoided in patients with blunt, multiple trauma because it greatly increases the cost of care and the risk of multiple-system organ failure.

Talucci RC, Manning J, Lampard S, et al: Early intra-

medullary nailing of femoral shaft fractures: A cause of fat embolism syndrome. *Am J Surg* 1983;146:107–111.

No cases of fat embolism syndrome were seen after immediate (less than 24 hours) intramedullary nailing of femoral shaft fractures. In contrast, five cases of fat embolism were found in patients treated in the traditional manner with initial balanced skeletal traction and delayed intramedullary nailing.

Vascular Injury

Barr H, Santer GJ, Stevenson IM: Occult femoral artery injury in relation to fracture of the femoral shaft. *J Cardiovasc Surg* 1987;28:193–195.

The femoral artery is injured in 2% of patients with fracture of the femoral shaft. Thirty patients who had suffered fracture of the femoral shaft six to 20 months before examination underwent hemodynamic assessment with Doppler ankle-arm pressure indices to determine the incidence of undetected femoral artery injury. Six patients exhibited hemodynamically significant abnormalities, all in the previously injured limbs.

Classification of Injuries

Milgrom C, Giladi M, Stein M, et al: Stress fractures in military recruits: A prospective study showing an unusually high incidence. *J Bone Joint Surg* 1985;67B:732–735.

A prospective study of 295 Israeli military recruits showed a 31% incidence of stress fractures. Eighty percent occurred in the tibial or femoral shafts. Sixty-nine percent of the femoral stress fractures were asymptomatic. Symptomatic stress fractures need treatment.

Winquist RA, Hansen ST Jr, Clawson DK: Closed intramedullary nailing of femoral fractures: A report of five hundred and twenty cases. *J Bone Joint Surg* 1984;66A:529–539.

A large series of femoral fractures was studied. A classification was developed for comminuted fractures. The union rate was 99% with a 0.9% infection rate. Shortening and malrotation were the most common complications.

Open Fractures

Chapman MW: The role of intramedullary fixation in open fractures. *Clin Orthop* 1986;212:26–34.

The author studied a consecutive series of 60 open fractures of the femur over a six-year period. These fractures were treated with immediate debridement followed by delayed reamed nailing ten to 14 days after injury. There was one infection. Acute reamed nailing in types I and II open fractures is justified when salvage of life or limb is a consideration and when other injuries make stabilization of the femur necessary.

Lhowe DW, Hansen ST: Immediate nailing of open fractures of the femoral shaft. *J Bone Joint Surg* 1988;70A:812–820.

Debridement of the wound and immediate reamed nailing were performed in 67 patients with open fractures of the femoral diaphysis from 1980 to 1985. There were 15 grade I, 19 grade II, and eight grade III soft-tissue injuries. Perioperative complications included loss of fixation in four patients, infection in two patients, and wound seroma in two patients. Other complications were routine for intramedullary nailing during that period. The authors concluded that immediate reamed nailing of open fractures of the femur was not associated with an increased rate of infection in their series.

Ipsilateral Fractures

Barquet A, Fernandez A, Leon H: Simultaneous ipsilateral trochanteric and femoral shaft fracture. *Acta Orthop Scand* 1985;56:36–39.

Delay in diagnosis of the hip fracture occurred in 15% of cases. Osteosynthesis of both fractures is recommended.

Friedman RJ, Wyman ET Jr: Ipsilateral hip and femoral shaft fractures. *Clin Orthop* 1986;208:188–194.

All fractures resulted from high-force impact (motor-vehicle accidents and falls); 25% were open. The many associated injuries required multiple operations. Delay in diagnosis occurred in three of 24 patients. Patients treated by fixation of one or both fractures had a significantly shorter hospital stay than those treated by traction alone. Extracapsular fractures had a high incidence (43%) of associated knee injuries. Treating both fractures with internal fixation allows early mobilization and easier patient care with fewer complications and a shorter hospital stay.

Swiontkowski MF: Ipsilateral femoral shaft and hip fractures. *Orthop Clin North Am* 1987;18:73–84.

Ipsilateral injury occurs in 5% of all patients with femoral shaft fractures. Management of the femoral shaft fracture should not interfere with treatment of the femoral neck or hip fracture.

Methods of Treatment

Baird RA, Kreitenberg A, Eltorai I: External fixation of femoral shaft fractures in spinal cord injury patients. *Paraplegia* 1986;24:183–190.

In patients with acute spinal-cord injury, external fixation should be considered for the treatment of closed femoral shaft fractures with marked comminution, and for open femoral shaft fractures with significant contamination or soft-tissue loss. In long-term spinal cord injury, external fixation of a femoral shaft fracture may increase the patient's level of independence and mobility during fracture healing and may permit a more rapid return to the patient's prefracture functional level.

Breederveld RS, Patka P, van Mourik JC: Refractures of the femoral shaft. *Neth J Surg* 1985;37:114–116.

An analysis of refracture in 148 femoral shaft fractures showed that 13% occurred after plate fixation. Cancellous bone grafting should be carried out in all fractures of the medial cortex and those in which there is devascularization of bone fragments. A delayed cancellous bone graft (eight to 12 weeks after primary surgery) is advocated in some of these fractures.

Cheng JC, Tse PY, Chow YY: The place of the dynamic compression plate in femoral shaft fractures. *Injury* 1985;16:529–534.

Traumatic femoral shaft fractures treated by dynamic compression plate were evaluated. Complications were failure of the implant (6.3%), loosened screws (3%), refracture (3%), and nonunion (3%). Average time to union was 5.5 months. Results were good to excellent in 91% of cases.

Gottschalk FA, Graham AJ, Morein G: The management of severely comminuted fractures of the femoral shaft, using the external fixator. *Injury* 1985;16:377–381.

Closed, comminuted fractures of the femoral shaft were treated with the ASIF tubular external fixator or the Wagner apparatus. All fractures united within eight months in a good position without shortening and none required an additional operation. Use of the external fixator reduced time in the hospital and facilitated postoperative rehabilitation by allowing uncomplicated healing.

Heitemeyer U, Kemper F, Hierholzer G, et al: Severely comminuted femoral shaft fractures: Treatment by bridging-plate osteosynthesis. *Arch Orthop Trauma Surg* 1987;106:327–330.

Surgical stabilization by plate osteosynthesis in 71 severely comminuted femoral shaft fractures was performed in two groups. One group had anatomic reduction and the other had bridging-plate osteosynthesis without preparation of the fracture zone. Fracture healing occurred within 23 weeks of bridging-plate use and within 36 weeks of anatomic reduction. Bridging-plate osteosynthesis is recommended in severely comminuted femoral fractures in patients with multiple injuries.

Marsh CH, Regan MW: Late positional correction of uniting femoral fractures using the Wagner external fixator. *Injury* 1986;17:248–250.

Good fixation of segmental fractures of the femoral shaft was obtained as much as ten weeks after the injury with the Wagner external fixator. Distraction and lengthening of the early reparative callus was possible and the method is recommended for those patients in whom shortening and malalignment of the fracture persist as union proceeds.

O'Beirne J, O'Connell RJ, White JM, et al: Fractures of the femur treated by femoral plating using the anterolateral approach. *Injury* 1986;17:387–390.

Fifty-six fractures of the femur were plated via an anterolateral approach. The final results were graded as excellent to good in 66% of cases. Patients with open fractures or with other fractures in the same femur tended to have poor final results. The late complication rate was 18%, similar to that for the posterolateral approach to plating of the femoral shaft.

Terjesen T, Nordby A, Arnulf V: Bone atrophy after plate fixation: Computed tomography of femoral shaft fractures. *Acta Orthop Scand* 1985;56:416–418.

Twelve patients with previous femoral shaft fractures treated by rigid plate fixation were examined by computed tomography one to two days after plate removal. An average reduction in cortical density of 11% was found. No reduction in cortical thickness of the plate occurred. Proximal and distal to the set of the plate in the ipsilateral tibial shaft, there was a slight reduction in cortical density and thickness (an average of 2% to 3%).

Thompson F, O'Beirne J, Gallagher J, et al: Fractures of the femoral shaft treated by plating. *Injury* 1985;16:535–538.

Seventy-seven fractures of the femoral shaft treated by plates were reviewed 12 to 72 months after surgery. There was no case of deep infection. The most common complication was a fatigue fracture of the plate, which occurred in five cases. Primary bone grafting is essential if rigid internal fixation is not obtained. Plating is an excellent method of treating fractures of the femoral shaft in patients under the age of 60 years.

Webb LX, Gristina AG, Fowler HL: Unstable femoral shaft fractures: A comparison of interlocking nailing versus traction and casting methods. *J Orthop Trauma* 1988;1:10–12.

Sixty complex femoral fractures were treated, 30 with traction and casting and 30 with interlocking nailing. Failure occurred in 67% of the traction group and 3% of the nailing group. Interlocking nailing is the treatment of choice for managing unstable femoral shaft fractures.

Intramedullary Nails

Bray TJ: Indications for locked intramedullary nailing. *Techn Orthop* 1988;3:943.

Interlocked intramedullary nailing has expanded the indications for closed intramedullary fixation of femoral and tibial shaft fractures. The indications for closed femoral fractures include most closed Winquist types 3 and 4 fractures, acute fractures, long oblique fractures, and closed reconstructed defects or malrotations.

Brumback RJ, Handal JA, Poka A, et al: Radiographic analysis of the Brooker-Wills interlocking nail in the treatment of comminuted femoral fractures. *J Orthop Trauma* 1987;1:120–129.

Forty-three patients were treated with the Brooker-Wills bladed type of locked nail. Nail deformation occurred in nine patients (21%) and was seen only in nails with 13- or 14-mm diameters. The distal lock controlled rotation clinically but played only a minor role in preventing shortening.

Brumback RJ, Reilly JP, Poka A, et al: Intramedullary nailing of femoral shaft fractures: Part I. Decision-making errors with interlocking fixation. *J Bone Joint Surg* 1988;70A:1441–1452.

The criteria for dynamic intramedullary fixation should be precise and exact. Dynamic intramedullary femoral stabilization should be performed only for transverse or short oblique fractures of the femoral isthmus, with type I or type II comminution. Any increase in comminution at the site of the fracture noted during the procedure is an indication for static interlocking. The threshold for the use of static interlocking fixation of an apparently stable femoral fracture should be extremely low.

Brumback RJ, Uwagie-Ero S, Lakatos RP, et al: Intramedullary nailing of femoral shaft fractures: Part II. Fracture-healing with static interlocking fixation. *J Bone Joint Surg* 1988;70A:1453–1462.

Ninety-eight percent of 87 comminuted femoral fractures treated with static interlocking fixation were followed up. In two cases conversion from static to dynamic interlocking fixation was required because of inadequate fracture healing; both progressed to uneventful union. Static interlocking of intramedullary nails in femoral shaft fractures does not appreciably inhibit the process of healing of the fracture, and routine conversion to dynamic intramedullary fixation is not needed.

Bucholz RW, Ross SE, Lawrence KL: Fatigue fracture of the interlocking nail in the treatment of fractures of the distal part of the femoral shaft. *J Bone Joint Surg* 1987; 69A:1391–1399.

Fatigue fracture of an interlocking nail at the more proximal of the two distal screw holes was studied in seven patients. In all patients the fracture of the femur was 5 cm or less from the level of the fatigue fracture. Finite-element analysis revealed that the stress on the nail exceeded its fatigue-endurance limit with weightbearing, and that the femur had to regain 50% of its original stiffness through healing to accommodate weightbearing without the risk of fatigue failure of the nail. The risk of fatigue failure may be minimized by using nails that have a larger diameter and by avoiding early weightbearing.

Christie J, Court-Brown C, Kinninmonth AWG, et al: Intramedullary locking nails in the management of femoral shaft fractures. *J Bone Joint Surg* 1988;70B:206–210.

A total of 117 patients with 120 femoral shaft fractures were treated with intramedullary locking nails; there were 20 open fractures, 13 pathologic fractures, and two nonunions. No infections occurred. Rehabilitation and union rates were satisfactory. Comminution of the proximal femoral fracture occurred in six patients, and there were three femoral neck fractures. All healed without further complications.

Eriksson E, Wallin C: Immediate or delayed Küntscher-rodding of femoral shaft fractures. *Orthopedics* 1986;9: 201–204.

No significant differences in results were found between two groups of patients, but those operated on within 12 hours returned to work an average of two months earlier than those operated on ten days after injury. If proper treatment for shock is given and concomitant injuries with higher priority are treated first, early Küntscher rodding does not seem to impair the healing of femoral fractures.

Franklin JL, Winquist RA, Benirschke SK, et al: Broken intramedullary nails. *J Bone Joint Surg* 1988;70A:1463–1471.

Sixty broken intramedullary nails in 56 patients were evaluated. There was a major correlation between the types and diameters of the nails and the incidence of breakage. Locking nails with distal interlocking holes and an anteriorly placed slot may leave too little metal in the anterior aspect of the nail, predisposing them to fatigue fracture. Proximal welds in the nail predispose nails to breakage. The design of the nail is an important factor. Nail design, technical errors in insertion, improper choice of starting point, underreaming the canal, and defects in fabrication can contribute to nail breakage. Recommendations for removal of broken nails are provided.

Green SA, Larson MJ, Moore TJ: Chronic sepsis following intramedullary nailing of femoral fractures. *J Trauma* 1987;27:52–57.

Chronic drainage after intramedullary nailing of a femoral shaft fracture was reviewed in 12 patients. All but one had been managed initially with the open nailing technique. Six patients were treated with the nail in place, and six patients were treated with nail removal, debridement, and external fixation of bone grafting. There was one persistent nonunion in each group. Drainage did not cease in either group until the nail and all sequestra had been removed.

Johnson KD, Greenberg M: Comminuted femoral shaft fractures. *Orthop Clin North Am* 1987;18:133–147.

Surgical intervention using locked intramedullary nails can lead to a consistently excellent outcome when the performance of the procedure is technically correct. The surgical procedure can eliminate a difficult management problem in patients with multiple injuries.

Johnson KD, Tencer AF, Blumenthal S, et al: Biomechanical performance of locked intramedullary nail systems in comminuted femoral shaft fractures. *Clin Orthop* 1986;206:151–161.

The biomechanical properties of commercially available locked nail systems designed for use in comminuted femoral shaft fractures were compared. The interlocking nail systems tested were comparable to each other and superior to Ender nails in bending and torsion. The distally bolted locked nails resisted significantly higher loads than either the distally bladed locked nail or Ender nails when tested to failure by axial loading.

Johnson KD, Tencer AF, Sherman MC: Biomechanical fractures affecting fracture stability and femoral bursting in closed intramedullary nailing of femoral fractures with illustrative case presentations. *J Orthop Trauma* 1987;1:1–11.

Mechanical variables affecting intramedullary nailing of femoral shaft fractures include insertion of the nail, stability provided by the implant, maximum load capacity, and modes of failure. The force necessary to insert an intramedullary nail into a reamed femur depends on the shape, length, and diameter of the intramedullary canal, the curvature of the nail, and the nail's stiffness and bending. Excessive insertion forces can cause the femur to burst. Anterior placement of a starting hole, combined with the use of the stiff nail, increases the likelihood of the femur bursting during insertion of the nail.

Klemm KW, Börner M: Interlocking nailing of complex fractures of the femur and tibia. *Clin Orthop* 1986;212:89–100.

Overall, 97% of femoral fractures and 94% of tibial fractures had an excellent or good result by clinical and radiographic criteria. Delayed union or nonunion requiring bone graft occurred in 2% of femoral fractures and 0.7% of tibial fractures. Deep infection developed in 2.4% of femoral fractures and 2.2% of tibial fractures. Rates of nonunion and infection were low and there was little risk of refracture after implant removal.

Leighton RK, Waddell JP, Kellam JF, et al: Open versus closed intramedullary nailing of femoral shaft fractures. *J Trauma* 1986;26:923–926.

The decision to use this specific type of internal fixation for femoral shaft fractures should be based on the fracture pattern, the surgeon's experience, and the equipment available. Opening the fracture site did not statistically increase the risk of complication in this series.

Mollica Q, Gangitano R, Longo G: Elastic intramedullary nailing in shaft fractures of the femur and tibia. *Orthopedics* 1986;9:1065–1077.

The authors propose using Ender nails as an alternative in the surgical management of shaft fractures of the femur. This technique achieves dynamic stabilization controlled by the elasticity of the nails, muscle tone, and weightbearing. Stabilization allows slight interfragmentary movement and produces the formation of periosteal bone callus.

Pankovich AM: Flexible intramedullary nailing of long bones: Part E. Flexible intramedullary nailing of femoral shaft fractures, in Griffin PP (ed): American Academy of Orthopaedic Surgeons *Instructional Course Lectures, XXXVI.* Park Ridge, Illinois, American Academy of Orthopaedic Surgeons, 1987, pp 324–338.

Simple flexible intramedullary nailing is a suitable method of fixation for femoral shaft fractures with stable configurations. Adjunctive measures must be used in the fixation of unstable fractures.

Patzakis MJ, Wilkins J, Wiss DA: Infection following intramedullary nailing of long bones: Diagnosis and management. *Clin Orthop* 1986;212:182–191.

Thirty patients with infected long-bone fractures after intramedullary nailing are described. After adequate surgical drainage and debridement with appropriate antibiotic coverage, union of the fracture is of great importance in controlling such infections.

Tencer AF, Johnson KD, Sherman MC: Biomechanical considerations in intramedullary nailing of femoral shaft fractures. *Techn Orthop* 1988;3:1–5.

A femur that has been stabilized with a slotted, interlocking intramedullary nail is about 2% as stiff as an intact femur in torsion, whereas a femur stabilized with a solid sectional locking nail is about 50% as stiff. In bending, the nails are about 80% as stiff as an average intact femur. Femur-locked nail constructs can support 300% to 400% of body weight in axial loading. The stiffness is unaffected by lack of bone contact at the fracture site.

Thoresen BO, Alho A, Ekeland A, et al: Interlocking intramedullary nailing in femoral shaft fractures: A report of forty-eight cases. *J Bone Joint Surg* 1985;67A:1313–1320.

Radiographic consolidation was seen in all fractures at a median of 16 weeks. Since there is a risk of rotational and longitudinal instability with a dynamic method of interlocking nails, the authors recommend that the static method be used whenever there is doubt about the stability of the fracture. No delay in bone healing was observed when the static method was used.

Tscherne H, Haas N, Krettek C: Intramedullary nailing combined with cerclage wiring in the treatment of fractures of the femoral shaft. *Clin Orthop* 1986;212:62–67.

Complications requiring surgical reintervention developed in 11 patients (6.6%). Intramedullary nailing and cerclage wiring significantly expand the indications for intramedullary fixation of fractures of the femoral shaft.

White GM, Healy WL, Brumback RJ, et al: The treatment of fractures of the femoral shaft with the Brooker-Wills distal locking intramedullary nail. *J Bone Joint Surg* 1986;68A:865–876.

There were intraoperative technical problems in 11 patients (12%) and postoperative complications in 18 patients (19.6%), including 14 patients (15%) with pulmonary emboli, infection, or heterotopic bone at the site of the insertion of the nail. Five patients (5%) had postoperative complications directly related to the proximal and distal fixation of the nail. The Brooker-Wills distal locking intramedullary nail proved to be an effective device for the stabilization of fractures of the femoral shaft.

Wiss DA, Fleming CH, Matta JM, et al: Comminuted and rotationally unstable fractures of the femur treated with an interlocking nail. *Clin Orthop* 1986;212:35–47.

Of the 112 nailings, 82 were static and 30 dynamic. Clinical and radiographic fracture union occurred in 98% of cases; there were two nonunions. There were no instances of deep wound infection or osteomyelitis. Immediate stabilization of the fracture allows immediate mobilization of the patient, early rehabilitation of the limb, and a shorter hospital stay.

Zuckerman JD, Veith RG, Johnson KD, et al: Treatment of unstable femoral shaft fractures with closed interlocking intramedullary nailing. *J Orthop Trauma* 1987;1:209–218.

Closed interlocking nailing is a safe, effective technique that provides stable fixation in most unstable femoral shaft fractures.

Supracondylar Fractures of the Femur

Johnson KD, Hicken G: Distal femoral fractures. *Orthop Clin North Am* 1987;18:115–132.

Surgical treatment of distal femoral fractures is recommended because of improved results. The implant is chosen on the basis of the nature of the fracture, soft-tissue status, surgical experience, and the patient's condition.

Siliski JM, Mahring M, Hofer HP: Supracondylar-intercondylar fractures of the femur: Treatment by internal fixation. *J Bone Joint Surg* 1989;71A:95–104.

Fifty-two fractures treated by a standard technique (angle blade plate and bone graft) were evaluated. Age did not influence results. Results were good to excellent in 75%. Infection accounted for three of four poor results; all were in patients with open fractures.

Zickel RE, Hobeika P, Robbins DS: Zickel supracondylar nails for fractures of the distal end of the femur. *Clin Orthop* 1986;212:79–88.

Results of 82 fractures of the distal end of the femur treated with a Zickel supracondylar device were reported. A high rate of union (98%) was achieved in the fracture group. Closed nailing is the procedure of choice because of decreased postoperative morbidity and increased knee motion. The device seems particularly helpful in elderly individuals.

41

Pelvis, Hip, and Femur: Reconstruction

Orthopaedic Knowledge Update I summarized the literature spanning late 1979 to mid-1982. Biomechanical studies of total hip replacements had defined optimal stem size, shape, and material properties although the controversy over relative stem stiffness remained unresolved. The value of anatomic positioning and metal backing of the acetabular component was strongly suggested. Improvement in surgical techniques, including grafting for osseous deficiencies, meticulous preparation of the bony bed, canal plugging, and cement pressurization, were discussed. Ten-year follow-up studies revealed revision rates from 1.3% to 20%. It appeared that acetabular loosening would be a more significant long-term problem than femoral loosening.

Success rates of 80% to 90% after two-stage reimplantation for infection were reported and the value of ultraclean air in the prevention of infection was recognized in various studies. Prophylaxis against thromboembolic disease in the form of aspirin, low-dose heparin, coumadin, and cyclical compression was studied, but the ideal protocol remained unresolved.

Revision total hip arthroplasty had become a subject unto itelf and initial reports of 14% failure rates at 3.5 years emphasized the importance of a durable result of primary total hip replacement. The enthusiasm with which surface replacement had been embraced during the mid-1970s was dampened by reports of failure rates as high as 34% after two years. Cementless total hip replacements had made their debut, but two-year results were not available.

Orthopaedic Knowledge Update 2 dealt with the literature through mid-1986. Serious concern over loosening in young patients (57% in one widely quoted study) and after ten- to 15-year follow-ups (5% to 20%) was being voiced, although it was realized that these studies represented early techniques and prosthetic designs. It was hoped that improved designs and techniques would lead to more durable results. Short-term studies suggested the value of metal backing on the acetabular side and optimizing cement technique. Mechanical studies on cement revealed improved strength after centrifugation and vacuum-mixing. It seemed that the problem of stem fracture might have been solved and infection rates were further decreased by adding total-body exhaust systems to ultraclean air and prophylactic antibiotics. The most effective prophylactic regimen against thromboembolic disease remained elusive. The feasibility and effectiveness of autologous blood donation were reported.

Longer-term follow-up of cemented revision arthroplasty revealed a 29% failure rate at 8.1 years. Such high failure rates after revision, and some reports of high failure rates after primary total hip replacement in young patients, led to great enthusiasm for fixation without cement. Press-fit, macrointerlock, and microinterlock (porous-ingrowth) devices were discussed. Poorly controlled studies from Europe suggested good early results with macrointerlock devices but disclosed problems with revision and bone loss. The major interest in the United States, however, was in porous-ingrowth devices. Experimental work identified the optimum pore size and revealed the occurrence of bone ingrowth into porous metals in canine models. Metallurgic problems were noted in that the addition of the porous surfaces significantly weakened the substrate. Follow-up studies were limited to one year and suggested an increased incidence of thigh pain in comparison with cemented devices.

The diagnosis of osteonecrosis was improved with the advent of magnetic resonance imaging. Early treatment with core decompression was supported by uncontrolled studies, but other studies failed to support these optimistic reports.

Total Hip Replacement With Implants

Biomechanics

Force data have been obtained from a telemeterized cemented total hip replacement. At one month postoperatively, joint-contact force equaled body weight during double-limb stance and measured 2.1 times body weight during ipsilateral single-limb stance, 2.6 to 2.8 times body weight during the stance phase of gait, and 2.6 times body weight during stair-climbing. Out-of-plane orientation of the resultant forces to the prosthesis was substantially increased during stair-climbing and straight leg raising. These measured forces were less than those that had been predicted previously by mathematical models.

Normalization of stress transfer from the pelvis through the prosthesis into the femur has been a goal of many stem designs. Theoretic and experimental studies before and after stem insertion have demonstrated that stresses and strains are closer to normal for uncemented than for cemented stems. The values are affected by relative tightness of fit in the proximal and distal regions and by the presence or absence of a collar. The average proximomedial bone strains for intact femur, press-fit, loose press-fit with collar, and proximally cemented (to simulate ingrowth) designs were 100%, 65%, 101%, and 54%, respectively, in one study. Collar "calcar" contact in another study of cemented stems increased proximal strains to 40% of normal.

Another school of thought suggests that cemented stems should be large with a high modulus of elasticity in order to protect the bone-cement interface from stresses that may result in loosening. One seven-year follow-up study of such a stem revealed a femoral loosening rate of only 2.3%, lending support to the hypothesis. The trade-off of calcar reabsorption as a result of stress-shielding was not a significant problem.

Debris resulting from damage to the surface of polyethylene components of total joint replacements has previously been shown to contribute to long-term problems such as loosening and infection. Surface damage is associated with fatigue processes caused by stresses arising from contact between the metal and polyethylene. Finite-element and elasticity models found much lower stresses in the acetabular component of a 28-mm hip replacement than in a 22-mm hip replacement. Stresses in polyethylene reinforced with carbon fiber were also higher by as much as 40%.

Imaging

The grid radiograph, a simple technique for consistent high-resolution visualization of the hip, allows reproducible positioning of the hip and the X-ray beam. Small changes in component position can be better detected with this method than with conventional radiographs. When used in conjunction with high-contrast radiographs and films, alterations at the bone-cement interface are more reliable indicators of true change at the interface.

Technetium bone scans of asymptomatic total hip replacements over time reveal that at six months activity surrounding the lesser trochanter and femoral stem becomes insignificant. By two years the activity about the greater trochanter, acetabular component, and femoral stem tip returns to normal. However, approximately 10% of asymptomatic hips showed some activity in one or more of these areas.

Technetium bone scans in total hip replacements in which heterotopic ossification was present showed persistently increased para-articular uptake for six months to as long as 15 years postoperatively in one study, clearly long after "maturity" of the heterotopic bone had been reached on plain radiographs. The authors suggested that radiophosphate imaging is not a reliable means of assessing maturation of heterotopic bone associated with hip arthroplasty.

Technetium radionuclide imaging of porous surface replacements demonstrated a predictable pattern in asymptomatic patients. An early increase in uptake is followed by a gradual decrease by one or two years postoperatively. Thus, the uptake remains increased for somewhat longer than that of stable cemented components. This is thought to result from persistent bone remodeling.

Preoperative computed tomographic scanning for both primary and revision total hip replacement has been found to be useful in defining acetabular wall defects in cases in which none were suspected after conventional radiographs. Preoperatively, the need for bone grafting can be determined more accurately. Additionally, acetabular component version can be easily evaluated in cases of recurrent dislocations.

Computed tomographic scanning has also been used to evaluate the femoral component in surface replacement hip arthroplasty. Image reconstruction using a high-frequency filter permits visualization of the bone-cement interface of the femoral shell. This provides an important tool in the evaluation of the painful surface replacement.

Surgical Approaches

A comparison of the anterolateral (Watson-Jones) and posterolateral (Gibson) approaches to the hip for total hip arthroplasty showed no significant differences in operating time, implant orientation, or complications in 74 consecutive patients.

Several new approaches have been described. An extensile approach based on an intact musculo-osseous-muscular sleeve constituted of the gluteus medius, greater trochanter, and vastus lateralis allows physiologic reconstruction of the hip's soft-tissue envelope. This approach is thought to be useful in revision surgery and in primary cases in which leg length must be adjusted.

A triradiate exposure of the hip was developed to allow complete anterior and posterior capsular visualization in revision and difficult primary cases. The greater trochanter routinely undergoes osteotomy as a component of the procedure.

Exposure of the hip by osteotomy of the anterior portion of the greater trochanter has been described. This maintains the continuity of the tendinous junction between the gluteus medius and the vastus lateralis, preserves the gluteus minimus insertion, retains good abductor function, and eliminates the problem of postoperative proximal migration of the greater trochanter.

Cemented Total Hip Replacements

Socioeconomic Factors

The cost-effectiveness of total hip and total knee arthroplasty in osteoarthritis was studied prospectively in a group of patients whose mean age was 66.4 years. On a purely economic basis, total joint arthroplasty could not be justified. Further, cost-effectiveness was judged greater for patients with poorer initial health status. Although this creates an argument for giving funding priority for total joint replacements to patients in poorer health, it is at odds with usual clinical decision-making, in which sicker patients are considered to be poor surgical risks.

Another study examined occupation after total hip replacement for osteoarthritis. Sixty-eight percent of patients younger than 60 years of age returned to work within two years. Long preoperative sick leave increased the likelihood of both long postoperative sick leave and retirement. The retirement rate was also greater in patients with physically demanding occupations. Age, sex, and bilaterality had no effect on postoperative sick leave or retirement.

Total hip replacement in the octogenarian carries acceptable risks in carefully selected patients. An 8% risk of major complications and a 2% mortality was found in one study of 100 consecutive cases.

Driving reactions in patients after total hip replacement were found to return toward normal by the eighth postoperative week in most patients. There were significant differences between patients with left and right hip replacements, and in a minority of patients with right total hip replacements recovery of reaction speed required a longer period of rehabilitation.

Long-Term Follow-up Studies

A 15-year follow-up study of 100 Charnley total hip arthroplasties revealed that 91% of the prostheses were intact at 15 years (Table 1). During that same period there was a 50% mortality in patients whose average age at surgery was 60 years. Of the patients who were available for evaluation at 15 years, 87.5% had good or excellent results. One socket and three femoral components were revised for

Table 1. Long-term follow-up studies of cemented total hip replacements

Site of Study	No. of Hips	Follow-up (yrs)	Revision Rate (%)	Radiographic Failure Rate (%)
New York	100	15	9	13
Exeter	426	11 to 16	11	65
California	700	14	17	54
California	479	11	8	21 F; 45 A*
New York	122	11	12	25
Eugene	156	12	15	20
San Francisco	100	15 to 17	16	20
Sweden	325	10 to 14	14	50
Wrightington	116	15 to 21	"Very low"	52
Wrightington†	49	10 to 15	18	26
South Africa	98	12	15	12

*F, femoral; A, acetabular.
†Patients less than 30 years old.

loosening. Seven percent of the remaining femoral components and 6% of the remaining acetabular components were radiographically loose.

An 11- to 16-year follow-up study of the Exeter total hip replacement revealed a 2% revision rate for loose stems and a 4% revision rate for loose sockets. Five percent of the stems fractured. Sixty-five percent of these collarless, polished, smooth, tapered stems subsided 1 to 10 mm, although this was rarely associated with significant pain.

A study of almost 700 cemented prostheses implanted before 1978 showed that 17% of all primary replacements required revision by 14 years postoperatively. When only patients under 40 years of age at the time of surgery were considered, the revision rate increased to 51%.

Another study compared the cobalt-chromium Charnley stem with both the curved and straight titanium STH stems. The 11-year survival rates for the Charnley and curved titanium prostheses were 91.5% and 92.7%, respectively; that for the straight titanium stem was 96.4%, a statistically significant difference. More generally, the titanium stem produced less calcar resorption and distal cortical hypertrophy but there was a statistically significant increase in radiolucencies at the bone-cement interface. The straight titanium stem performed better radiographically than the curved titanium stem on both the femoral and acetabular sides of the arthroplasty.

An average 11-year follow-up study of bilateral hip replacements found a 6.2% revision rate for aseptic loosening. Another 6.2% required revision for other causes. Radiographic loosening occurred in 7.8% of femoral components and 17.5% of acetabular components. Survivorship analysis predicted survival rates at 15 years of 87% for Charnley hips, 82% for T28 hips, and 78% for Charnley-Muller hips.

A well-controlled series of 156 total hip replacements followed up for an average of 12 years by a single surgeon revealed a revision rate for aseptic loosening of 8%. There was a 7% incidence of stem fracture and only one infection (delayed, secondary). In a group of patients under the age of 50 years followed up for ten to 15 years by the same surgeon, the revision rate for aseptic loosening was 19.6%.

A 15- to 17-year follow-up of 100 Charnley total hip replacements found a 16% revision rate (6% because of a fractured component and 7% for aseptic loosening). An additional 20% revealed radiographic loosening, with stems and sockets each accounting for one half of cases.

The authors thought that the clinical results paralleled the radiographic results.

A study of 325 consecutive Charnley total hip replacements followed up for ten to 14 years revealed a revision rate because of mechanical failure of 14%. Radiographic evidence of socket loosening was present in 11% and of stem loosening in 39%.

In another 15- to 21-year follow-up study, 23% of sockets were found to have migrated and 29% of stems were found to have subsided. There was a "very low" incidence of revisions for loosening of the components.

The results of 49 Charnley replacements performed in patients 30 years or younger followed up for ten to 15 years revealed failure of 14% of sockets and 4% of stems as a result of loosening. Most of these cases involved built-in restraints against overactivity.

A 12-year follow-up of 98 Charnley total hip replacements revealed a 15% revision rate for mechanical failure (mostly stem fracture) and a 12% overall loosening rate (both clinical and radiographic).

A series of 101 total hip replacements in active patients who were less than 55 years old was subjected to survivorship analysis. A success rate of 88% at ten-year follow-up was found.

A ten-year follow-up study of metal-backed acetabular components revealed a 12.5% revision rate for loosening and an additional 21% incidence of migration or impending radiographic failure.

Other ten-year follow-up studies have reported revision rates of 3% and 9%, with radiographic loosening rates of 34% and 29%, respectively. It can be concluded from these data that cemented total hip replacements perform well in the long-term, with revision rates for aseptic loosening generally under 10% at ten to 15 years of follow-up. The concern remains, however, that the radiographic evidence of loss of fixation in 20% to 50% in many of these studies may lead to higher numbers of clinical failures in the future.

Component Fracture

Sporadic reports of both femoral and acetabular component fracture continue to occur, but this problem has been minimized by improvements in design, metallurgy, and surgical technique.

An analysis of revision total hip replacement for fracture of the femoral component has been reported. The causes of failure were multifactorial and included patient size (large), sex (male), contralateral hip disease or replacement (present), component position (varus), and cement technique (too little cement, too much cancellous bone in the femoral neck region). Cantilever bending failure with proximal loosening and distal fixation was the predominant mechanism of failure. The long-term results of cemented revision for fracture of the femoral component are superior to the results of cemented revision for other modes of mechanical failures (P < .009).

Wear

Wear of the polyethylene acetabular components has received considerable attention but has usually been dismissed as an insignificant clinical problem. Although low mean radiographic wear rates of about 0.1 mm per year have been reported, individual components may erode at three to four times the average rate. These may be subject to failure through fracture of the component. Osteolysis and granulomatous destruction resulting from the release of large quantities of polyethylene debris are also concerns.

External wear of polyethylene cups in direct contact with bone (poor cement technique) has been reported. The authors suggested that this might be the mechanism for the generation of polyethylene wear debris at the bone-cement interface rather than the migration of particles from the metal-polyethylene articulation.

Wear of cemented cobalt-chromium stems produces higher levels of metal ions in urine and plasma than occurs in control subjects. However, the levels of cobalt and chromium were considerably lower than in occupationally exposed groups and do not appear to represent a toxic hazard for patients.

Failed cemented titanium stems with titanium bearing surfaces produce intense histiocytic and plasma cell reactions in pseudocapsular tissue. Titanium as a bearing surface may in some cases produce wear debris that contributes to loosening and infection. Once a titanium stem becomes slightly loose, a self-perpetuating cycle leading to gross loosening may be established.

Interface

Biopsy specimens from stable bone-cement interfaces in 13 patients revealed a spectrum of tissue reactions, ranging from direct bone-cement contact to a fibrous membrane as much as 1.5 mm thick. Any bone necrosis incurred at the primary operation had been largely resorbed and replaced by viable bone. Acetabular membranes were thicker than femoral membranes; both consisted primarily of dense fibrous tissue. However, toward the cement surface there were an increasing number of macrophages and foreign-body giant cells. These cell types are found even in the absence of wear debris. Since they are capable of bone resorption, their presence must give cause for concern. By contrast, macrophages are rarely seen in the membranes juxtaposed to uncemented devices. This has led some to use the term "cement disease," implying that the biomaterial properties of the cement used for fixation may also lead to a pathologic state that promotes loosening.

Membranes from cases in which cemented devices failed reveal histiocytosis, fibrosis, and necrosis. Other features include particles of cement and polyethylene debris. Failure is characterized by bone and cement microfracture. The process of loosening is characterized by the recruit-

ment of histiocytes into the interface and the subsequent resorption of bone around the prosthesis. The degree to which this occurs may depend on the rate of cement failure, particle size, and the immunologic predisposition of the host.

Others have noted the formation of a synovium-like membrane at the bone-cement interface. It contains high levels of prostaglandin E_2 and demonstrates enhanced bone-resorbing activity in tissue culture. These features suggest an active role in the bone lysis that may occur in association with loosening.

Total Hip Replacement for Special Problems

Acetabular Dysplasia Reports of total hip replacement in patients with acetabular dysplasia have noted success with various techniques, including the use of a mini-offset bore acetabular component, placement of the cup in the neoacetabulum with or without bone grafting for coverage, grafting laterally to cover the socket repositioned to the true acetabulum, and proximal release of the hip abductors combined with excision of the upper third of the ilium to allow adequate distal abductor repair and to provide a bone graft for reconstructing the true acetabulum. The most provocative report is an 8.5-year follow-up of reconstructions at the true acetabulum using large masses of cement instead of bone grafting, as had traditionally been recommended. In this study, no revisions for loosening were required in 66 hip replacements and only 9% showed radiographic evidence of loosening (Fig. 1).

Protrusio Acetabuli Reconstruction for protrusion defects of the acetabulum using morselized autogenous grafts and metallic reinforcement gave good results in 28 hips followed up for an average of three years. In all cases the graft was thought to have consolidated.

Sickle Cell Disease Eleven patients who had a form of sickle cell hemoglobinopathy underwent total hip arthroplasty for osteonecrosis of the femoral head. Four patients required revision and three more underwent resection arthroplasty. There were four serious postoperative infections. Another similar study projected a 50% failure rate at 5.4 years.

Tuberculosis Two studies reviewed the results of total hip replacement for tuberculous coxarthrosis. Results were generally good to excellent. Reactivation of disease occurred in 25% in one report and 14% in the other. Recurrences were controllable by chemotherapy in the second study but not in the first. The incidence of recurrence of infection is much higher in patients who have had inactive disease for less than ten years.

Paget's Disease Eighty patients with Paget's disease who had total hip replacements were followed up for ten years. The incidence of aseptic loosening requiring revision was 15%; radiographic evidence of loosening was present in 30% of the femoral components and 14% of the acetabular components. Compared with the overall experience with hip replacement at the same institution, these numbers represented an increased failure rate of only slight statistical significance.

Osteonecrosis A five- to ten-year (average, 7.6 years) fol-

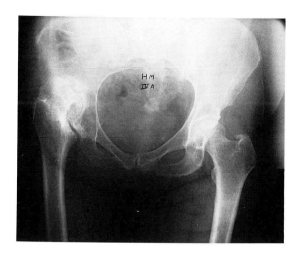 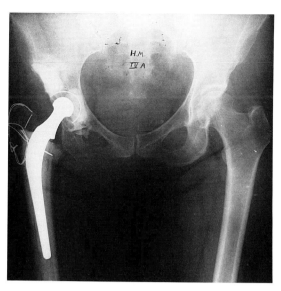

Figure 1

Left, Congenital dysplasia with secondary osteoarthritis, right hip. **Right**, Eight-year follow-up. Cement rather than bone grafting was used for lateral support of the acetabular component.

low-up study of 28 total hip arthroplasties for osteonecrosis of the femoral head revealed an overall failure rate of 37% (acetabular loosening in five cases, femoral loosening in one, femoral stem fracture in three, and late perioprosthetic infections in two). Patients with so-called idiopathic osteonecrosis, in whom no associated factors such as alcohol or corticosteroids could be identified, fared much better than the group as a whole, with a failure rate of 11%.

Lupus Erythematosus Hip replacement (total and bipolar) in 43 patients with systemic lupus erythematosus provided good to excellent results for most patients, but there was a high incidence of delayed wound healing (15%) and wound infection (10%).

Jehovah's Witnesses One hundred Jehovah's Witnesses underwent total hip replacement without transfusion. Hypotensive anesthesia was used in 89 of these patients and resulted in an intraoperative blood loss 30% to 43% less than that in normotensive controls. There were no deaths and only one complication that might have been related to hypotensive anesthesia, a case of acute renal tubular necrosis that resolved within one week.

Arthrodesis and Ankylosis Eighty total hip arthroplasties for spontaneous or surgical ankylosis of the hip were followed up for an average of 10.4 years. Failure occurred in 33% of those hips that had been surgically fused and in only 5% of those that had ankylosed spontaneously. Failure was also more common in patients who were 50 years old or younger at the time of the arthroplasty.

Juvenile Rheumatoid Arthritis Total hip replacement in juvenile rheumatoid arthritis gives good to excellent results in most cases. One study of 62 hips followed up for six years found only one revision for aseptic loosening although progressive radiolucencies or migration were noted in 26% of the acetabular and 8% of the femoral compo-

nents. Another study of 75 hips followed up for 5.4 years found one revision for a loosened femoral component and only two cases of radiographic loosening.

Cerebral Palsy Fifteen patients with cerebral palsy underwent total hip replacement because of pain. Thirteen patients were pain-free and functioning at a level consistent with their overall involvement after 67 years. Two patients had recurrent dislocations and underwent revisions. One patient had progressive femoral loosening radiographically but only mild pain.

Obesity A comparative study of total hip replacements in obese and nonobese patients revealed no increased risks of surgical complications or prosthetic loosening with obesity.

Infection

The use of ultraviolet light in the operating room was assessed bacteriologically in an open randomized study of 30 total hip replacements. The number of colony-forming units was found to be significantly reduced. Combining ultraviolet light with zonal ventilation and high air-exchange rates achieved "ultraclean air." The use of ultraviolet light in conventionally ventilated operating rooms, while decreasing bacterial count, does not achieve ultraclean air.

Recent randomized studies have confirmed that a considerable reduction in the infection rate can be obtained by operating in ultraclean air but that similarly low rates can be achieved with normal ventilation when prophylactic antibiotics are given. In addition, the two methods are effective independently; when they are used together, sepsis rates in the joint after total hip arthroplasty can be reduced to a few per thousand.

Surgical infections from total hip replacements at two community hospitals were reduced from 16% to 3% over a two-year period by operating-room surveillance. Intraoperative surveillance by an infection-control nurse at each hospital found too many persons in the operating room, excessive conversation, operating-room doors opened frequently, and inconsistent use of prophylactic antibiotics.

A study of the contamination of suction tips revealed a 35% rate of contamination by the time the femoral canal was prepared. The authors suggested that the rate of contamination was proportional to the length of time that the suction tip was in use. They recommended changing the suction tip at the time of preparation of the femoral canal.

The significance of surgical cultures in the development of deep infections in total hip arthroplasties performed for failures of previous operations was studied. Eleven percent of hips with positive cultures and 3% of hips with negative cultures subsequently developed infections. Failed total hip arthroplasties with positive cultures had a 40% rate of reinfection. Hips with a gram-negative growth at the time of reoperation had a higher infection rate than hips from which gram-positive organisms were cultured.

A retrospective review of 1,542 Charnley total hip replacements was done to compare the incidence of deep infection arising after plain and gentamicin-containing cement. There was no significant difference between the two groups in primary operations (1.72% vs 1.65%). However, in reoperations, the gentamicin-containing cement group had an infection rate of 0.81% compared with 3.46% for the plain cement group, a statistically significant improvement. All operations were performed in a clean-air enclosure using total-body exhaust suits.

Experimentally, in rabbits, antibiotic-impregnated cement significantly increased the size of the bacterial innoculum required to establish clinical infection.

The exact role of antibiotic-impregnated cement in total hip arthroplasty remains to be determined. Controversies exist over the best use of different antibiotics and cements. There is not sufficient evidence to support the use of antibiotic-impregnated cement for prophylaxis in primary total hip replacement. The most likely role for antibiotic-impregnated cement will be in the high-risk patient (multiple previous surgical procedures or impaired host defense) and in the treatment of established infections.

Failure to achieve adequate soft-tissue coverage after resection arthroplasty can be addressed by the use of a vastus lateralis flap. The vastus lateralis is dissected in a distal-to-proximal direction and is based on the vascular leash from the descending branch of the lateral femoral circumflex artery emerging from beneath the rectus femoris proximally. The distal portion of the vastus lateralis is secured to the acetabular area and the bulk of the muscle can then be rolled into the wound. Primary closure with or without skin grafting over drains completes the procedure.

Thromboembolic Disease

In a survey to assess current practices in regard to prophylaxis for thromboembolic disease, 84% of the surgeons used some form of pharmacologic or physical prophylaxis. Warfarin had been tried and abandoned by 50% because of bleeding complications. Aspirin was most widely used. More than 25% stated that at least one patient had died from a pulmonary embolus during the last five years.

There is experimental evidence that low-molecular-weight fractions of heparin are as effective as the standard form as far as thromboembolic prophylaxis is concerned, but cause fewer bleeding complications. A double-blind, randomized study comparing low-molecular-weight heparin to placebo in 100 patients undergoing total hip replacement revealed a 12% rate of thrombosis in the heparin group and a 42% rate in the placebo group (P = .0007). The bleeding rate was 4% in each group.

In a randomized, double-blind, placebo-controlled multicenter trial, the efficacy and safety of dihydroergotamine mesylate-heparin sodium as a prophylactic agent for deep venous thrombosis were evaluated in 148 patients undergoing total hip replacement. The incidence of venographically proven deep venous thrombosis was 25% in the treatment group and 52% in the placebo group (P = .002). There was no significant difference in the incidence of adverse reactions.

Another study compared the use of aspirin to placebo and dihydroergotamine-heparin. Aspirin and dihydroergotamine-heparin were significantly better than placebo but there were no differences between the aspirin and the dihydroergotamine-heparin groups.

Low doses of warfarin and external pneumatic compression boots were found to be as effective as high-dose warfarin in the prevention of proximal deep venous thrombosis. No major bleeding complications occurred with either method.

A study from Scandinavia suggested that the incidences of deep venous thrombosis and pulmonary embolism are lower in patients given continuous lumbar epidural anesthesia than in others given general anesthesia. Physiologic mechanisms that might explain this include hyperkinetic blood flow in the major vessels of the lower limbs, inhibition of platelet aggregation, and stabilization of endothelial cells.

The Greenfield vena cava filter has been used in patients who develop bleeding complications from heparin, have a recurrent embolism despite adequate anticoagulation, or in whom anticoagulant therapy is contraindicated.

Impedence plethysmography has been reported to be a useful noninvasive screening procedure for the detection of potentially fatal proximal venous thrombosis after total hip replacement. One study found a specificity of 96% and a sensitivity of 86%.

Heterotopic Ossification

A prospective study evaluated the efficacy of treatment with 10 Gy of radiation in the prevention of heterotopic ossification after total hip arthroplasty in patients who were at high risk. A previous study had demonstrated the effectiveness of 20 Gy instituted within four days of surgery in the prevention of heterotopic ossification in high-risk patients. No difference was found between the efficacy of 10 Gy (delivered in 2-Gy doses over five to seven days starting on the first postoperative day) and that of 20 Gy in the prevention of heterotopic ossification in high-risk patients. The 10-Gy protocol is preferable because it reduced the long-term cumulative effects of the radiation and halved the duration of hospitalization for treatment by radiation.

Indomethacin has been shown in a randomized, double-blind study to be significantly effective (P < .0005) in preventing heterotopic ossification. Twenty-five milligrams three times daily was administered daily for six weeks. Another uncontrolled study supported the effectiveness of indomethacin, finding only a 4% incidence of heterotopic ossification (grade IIA, mild) in a series of 47 total hip replacements in high-risk patients.

Diphosphonates have been shown to be ineffective in the prevention of postoperative heterotopic ossification. They do not prevent the formation of the osteoid matrix and, once treatment is discontinued, the matrix calcifies.

Other Complications

Evaluation of sciatic nerve compromise by intraoperative somatosensory evoked potentials was accomplished in 50 patients during total hip arthroplasty. There were 12 instances of temporary nerve compromise in ten patients—three during acetabular preparation because of retraction, one because of reamer contact, six during femoral reaming because of positioning, and two during trial reduction because of inadequate shortening of the femoral neck.

The incidence of sciatic and peroneal nerve palsy after total hip replacement was found to be 1.1% in one study. Sciatic palsies were associated with greater lengthening (average, 4.4 cm) than peroneal palsies (average, 2.7 cm). Electromyographic data placed the level of the lesion in peroneal palsies at the fibular neck.

Femoral neuropathy has been reported after use of an acetabular pressurizing device that forced large masses of cement anteriorly.

Cervical myelopathy resulting in quadriplegia and death has been reported after hip replacement in patients with rheumatoid arthritis who had unrecognized rheumatoid cervical instability.

The occurrence of urinary retention in men after total hip replacement could not be correlated with urologic history or physical examination but it was significantly increased in patients whose peak urinary flow rate was less than 17 ml per second. Another study found a correlation between inability to pass urine into a bottle while supine and previous bladder-outflow problems. Straight catheterization in the recovery room did not decrease the incidence of urinary complications in one study. In another, placement of an indwelling catheter immediately preoperatively with removal on the first postoperative day decreased the need for long-term catheterization in patients undergoing total hip replacement.

Femoral shaft fractures have been successfully treated by revision to a long-stem prosthesis or an Ogden-type plate, which consists of Parham-like band fixation around the shaft and plate in the region of the stem and bicortical screw-plate fixation distal to the stem (Fig. 2).

Leg-length inequality in 55 patients was radiographically measured as 8.7 mm in unilateral and 11.6 mm in bilateral total hip replacements. The authors suggested this as a possible cause of unexplained pain or aseptic loosening.

Pressure sores have been reported in 4% of patients undergoing total hip replacement.

Miscellaneous Considerations

An average 7.1-year follow-up study of the computer-aided-design prosthesis (a large, stiff, valgus stem) revealed a 7% revision rate for loosening and a 42% incidence of calcar reabsorption measuring 3 mm or more. Radiographic analysis revealed thinning of the bone stock of the proximal femur compared with the contralateral unoperated on hip. Survivorship analysis predicted a 77% survival rate at nine years.

In a consecutive series of 804 cases of trochanteric oste-

otomy, reattachment with two independent vertical wires and one transverse wire produced union in 99% of cases.

Pseudobursae surrounding total hip replacements, diagnosed by arthrography, may cause pain. Infection must be excluded and is more often associated with communicating, irregular cavities than with smooth, noncommunicating cavities. Occasionally these bursae are related to recurrent dislocations. In the absence of infection, loosening, or dislocation, symptoms caused by such bursae respond to local injections of anesthetic agents in about one half of cases.

Activation of complement, as indicated by anaphylatoxin release, has been noted during cemented total hip replacements but not during cementless total hip replacements. This may account, at least in part, for the hypotension and altered oxygen uptake noted in some patients undergoing cemented total hip replacement.

Intraoperative blood loss has been found to be significantly less with lumbar epidural anesthesia than with general anesthesia. This is most probably related to the arterial and venous hypotension induced with epidural anesthesia.

Follow-up of range of motion in total hip replacement revealed no improvement in flexion and abduction after one year, but adduction and rotation continued to improve for as long as 7.5 years.

Results With Improved Techniques

Several five-year follow-up studies are now available on improved techniques, including plugging the canal, pulsatile lavage, the use of Simplex P cement, centrifugation or vacuum-mixing of the cement, use of a cement gun, pressurization, use of a large superalloy stem with a broad medial border, the use of a metal-backed component with polymethylmethacrylate studs on the back, and pressurization of the cement mass. These studies show far better results than similar studies of older techniques. Reports of no revisions and radiographic failures in less than 5% of cases have come from several centers. Thus, there are reasons to believe that cement in an appropriate environment will not necessarily fail with time.

Uncemented Total Hip Replacements

Results

Minimum two-year follow-up studies have been reported for the PCA cementless total hip replacement (Table 2). In one review of 50 hips, there was a 16% incidence of mild thigh pain and a 28% incidence of moderate to severe limp, the latter thought to be secondary to surgical technique (straight lateral approach) rather than to the prosthesis. A progressive radiodense line surrounding the prosthesis developed in 41% of the femoral components and 8% of the acetabular components. Progressive bead loosening occurred in 24% of the femoral components and 18% of the acetabular components. Component shift occurred in 2% of each component and there was a 4% incidence of femoral shaft fracture. No components were revised.

A second study evaluated 118 PCA hips from several centers. Thigh pain was present in only 4% and limp in only 5%. One femoral component was revised for loosening. A second is pending. In retrospect, it was thought that the stem was undersized. No radiolucencies were seen in 35% of the femoral components and none of the re-

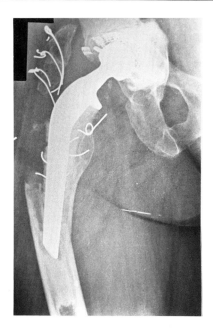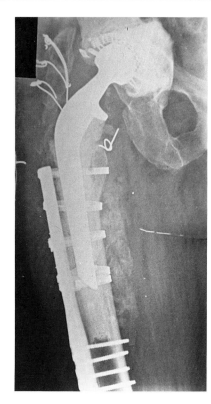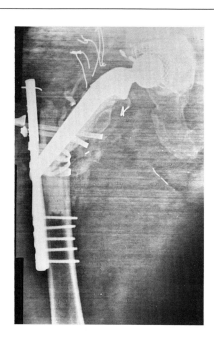

Figure 2

Left, Fractured femur surrounding cemented stem. **Center**, Repair using Ogden-type plate. **Right**, Eight weeks postoperatively, fixation has failed.

Table 2. Results of cementless total hip replacement

Site of Study	Prosthesis		Follow-up (yrs)	Comments
	Type	No.		
Washington, D.C.	PCA	50	>2	Pain, 16%; limp, 28%
Multicenter	PCA	118	>2	Pain, 4%; limp, 5%; failed, 6%
Arlington	AML	100	5	Pain, 14%; limp, 21%
Boston	HGP	—	1	Pain, 5%; limp, 9%
	Isoelastic	34	3.5	Revised, 32%

maining 65% had circumferential radiolucencies. No radiolucencies were seen in 48% of the acetabular components, again with none of the remainder having circumferential demarcation. Five femoral components have subsided. No acetabular components have migrated.

A five-year follow-up study of the AML prosthesis revealed a 14% incidence of pain (usually occasional and delayed in onset) and a 21% incidence of limp. Radiographic evaluation revealed probable bone ingrowth in 84%, fibrous ingrowth in 13%, and no ingrowth in 2%. There were no revisions. Pain and limp were significantly more common when bone ingrowth was not present. There was a 4% incidence of femoral shaft fracture.

A one-year follow-up study of the HGP prosthesis revealed moderate pain in 5% of cases and moderate or severe limp in 9%. Femoral shaft perforations or fractures occurred in 7%. There were no revisions.

A review of 34 RM isoelastic cementless total hip replacements revealed a femoral revision rate for loosening of 32%. Of the remaining cases, 69% had poor results because of pain and only 9% had good results after 3.5 years.

Problems

Loosening and fretting of sintered particles on porous-coated hip prostheses can cause excessive metal ion release. This results in reactive changes in surrounding tissue that may lead to bone loss, loosening, and infection. More serious is the possibility that increased levels of metallic debris may be carcinogenic. Reports of such bead loosening with both the AML and PCA prostheses are available. Pad separation from substrate in the HGP prosthesis has also been reported sporadically.

Proximal femoral stress-shielding has been seen with all three of the above cementless stems. With the proximally coated PCA and HGP prostheses, this has taken the form of calcar rounding, cancellization, and linear resorption in most cases. This is probably not clinically significant. With the more distally coated AML prosthesis, proximal bone-stock loss can be more extensive. In a review of 411 cases, "pronounced" bone resorption occurred in 18%, and this was thought to have potentially harmful clinical consequences such as pain, bone or stem fracture, and difficulty of revision. Stress-shielding was directly correlated with larger diameters and more extensively coated femoral components.

Disassociation of the polyethylene insert from the outer metal shell has been reported sporadically. Improvements in design should eliminate this complication.

Retrieval Data

Experimental studies in dogs have revealed that titanium fiber-mesh porous surfaces have greater amounts of bone ingrowth at six months than do beaded surfaces. Threaded cups are significantly looser than porous cups when retrieved at two and six months.

Retrieval data are somewhat difficult to interpret but, nonetheless, have been generally disappointing. The problems with these studies concern the multifactorial reasons for component removal and the multicenter sources of the retrieval specimens. In one study, one third of the retrieved implants had no bone ingrowth, one third had less than 2% ingrowth, and one third had 2% to 10% ingrowth. No implants had more than 10% ingrowth. These 28 hip implants were removed for a variety of reasons, including infection, dislocation, unexplained pain, and death. In another report of 36 components, the results were similar, and the authors observed that the reason for removal had no effect on the amount of ingrowth. One might suspect that those removed for pain would have less ingrowth than those removed for other reasons, but this was not the case. In another study of 226 retrieved porous-coated implants, 27% of the femoral components were at least partially ingrown by bone. This did not, however, preclude the presence of pain. Of the acetabular components, only 16% showed some bone ingrowth; none showed more than 50%.

Consideration has been given to hydroxyapatite coating of metal implants. In a canine total hip arthroplasty study, hydroxyapatite-coated stems had rigid fixation by bone growth up to the implant surface. Stems not coated with hydroxyapatite were surrounded by fibrous tissue and were easily extracted.

Investigation into porous polymeric coatings continues. Their low modulus allows a more uniform distribution of stress and the coating reduces metal ion release. Porous polytetrafluoroethylene-carbon fiber composite, porous polyethylene, and porous polysulfone are all under investigation. Poor clinical results have led to the discontinuation of one study using porous polyethylene. Clinical investigations of porous polysulfone are in progress. Their general use at the present time is not recommended.

Miscellaneous Considerations

A study of biologic ingrowth in 63 total hip replacements revealed a 6.3% incidence of intraoperative femoral fractures. There were five times more fractures during revisions than during primary operations. Treatment of the fractures consisted of cerclage wires or Parham bands and bone grafting in most cases. All fractures healed but 8% of stems required revision. Fractures were most frequent with the PCA stem (20%), intermediate with the osteonics (9%), and fewest with the HGP (6%) and Bias prostheses (4%).

These differences were probably related to the instrumentation used.

A study in femurs retrieved at autopsy into which collared and collarless uncemented devices had been implanted revealed distinct advantages for the collared device in terms of decreased subsidence and increased load to failure. Tightening of the collarless implant by subsidence could not be relied on to achieve fixation and may not be reliable in the clinical situation.

A technique of proximal femoral osteotomy to achieve correction of deformities combined with cementless total hip replacement has been described. Healing of the osteotomy is predictable and does not interfere with the clinical and radiographic impression of bone ingrowth.

Bone Grafting

Acetabulum

Of 21 patients who underwent allograft acetabular reconstruction, two had progressive bone-cement radiolucencies and one had a radiographic nonunion after 3.5 years. One allograft collapsed and required revision. Radiographic follow-up suggested incorporation in the other cases. Three-dimensional computed tomographic radioisotopic bone scans suggested revascularization and new bone formation. Femoral head allografting was believed to be a useful technique for the reconstruction of severely deficient acetabuli.

Of 47 femoral head autografts for severe congenital acetabular dysplasia (average follow-up, seven years), 10% failed because of either acetabular loosening or sepsis. Another 12% of sockets were definitely loose by radiographic criteria. Union of the graft appeared to be solid in all hips. Minor resorption occurred in 26 grafts, moderate resorption in eight, and major resorption in six.

Another study reviewed 29 frozen femoral head allografts followed up for two to seven (average, 3.9) years. Seventeen percent of the acetabular components had been revised or were definitely loose. All grafts appeared to be incorporated radiographically. Minor resorption had occurred in 11 hips, moderate resorption in three, and severe resorption in three. The technique was considered useful although the complication rate was somewhat high in this difficult group of patients.

At least one study suggested that significant numbers of allograft fail by seven years. Grafts that had functioned well at the five-year follow-up had failed by seven years, leading to failure of the arthroplasty and need for revision in 30% of cases. Careful studies are needed to evaluate the reliability of this potentially important observation.

A radiographic study of acetabular autografts concluded that union and revascularization occur uniformly but that standard radiographs are not reliable in the evaluation of graft reconstitution. By contrast, another study of 32 femoral head autografts revealed that although 30 grafts had united, 20 showed lateral resorption. In only three cases did the resorption involve the supporting portion of the autograft. These investigators believed that serial radiographs provided the best information about the integrity of acetabular roof reconstructions.

Several cautiously optimistic reports of small numbers of patients with massive allografts have appeared. Short-term success rates as high as 85% have been reported but infection and graft resorption are potential problems.

Femur

Allograft reconstructions of defects of the proximal portion of the femur in 28 patients were followed up for two to 15 years. Success was reported in 80% of the cases. Functional results were better when an allograft plus prosthesis rather than osteoarticular allograft was used.

In another study of failed total hip replacements revised with frozen proximal femoral allografts and cemented or uncemented femoral components, all grafts united by 16 to 30 months and no significant resorption was noted. Pain relief and functional improvement were significant. There were no infections.

An experimental study of cementless revision of cemented total hip replacement in dogs revealed enhanced ingrowth into a porous stem with both allografts and autografts. There was no significant difference between allografts and autografts.

Revision of Total Hip Replacements

Cemented Revisions

A series of 43 hips that underwent cemented revision of failed cemented total hip replacements and in which modern cementing techniques were used fared much better than expected. The revision rate in this group was only 2%. Thirteen percent were radiographically loose but clinical ratings for these hips were good or excellent. Dislocations occurred in 14%, trochanteric nonunions in 7%, and femoral shaft perforations in 19%. The reason for the improved results was thought to be a better technique.

Similarly, in a study of 68 acetabular reconstructions using an improved cement technique and metal reinforcement, no revisions were needed because of aseptic loosening. The infection rate was 3%. Radiographic loosening occurred in 3%. Allografts and autografts incorporated at equal rates. Again, the improved results were attributed to better techniques.

In one series of 45 patients, the rate of possible or probable radiographic loosening was very high, 45% on the acetabular side and 50% on the femoral side. The revision (or need for revision) rate was 7% after the second revision and 16% after the third revision. The prognosis in such cases is guarded. Cementless revision techniques or arthrodesis in younger patients may prove to be a better alternative in these difficult situations.

A comparison of function after revision surgery and function after primary surgery showed significantly improved walking performance, hip muscle strength, range of motion, forces applied to canes, and the amount of weight borne by the treated limb during quiet standing in both groups. The revision group, however, used more assistive devices, had more pain, walked more slowly, had less hip motion, and had more pronounced limps.

Uncemented Revisions

Results of revision of total hip replacements with newer cementless techniques are now appearing, although most reports are preliminary.

After an average follow-up of 1.7 years, a series of 61 cementless PCA revisions had a revision rate of 3% and radiographic failure rate of an additional 8%. Clinically, however, 90% were rated as good or excellent and 10% as fair or poor. The authors considered these results encour-

aging but noted that there are "definite candidates for cemented femoral components," especially elderly patients with first-time revisions.

In another series of 160 cementless AML revisions, followed up for an average of 4.4 years, 84% of the femoral components were graded as radiographically optimal (bone ingrowth), 12% as suboptimal (fibrous encapsulation), and 4% as failed. The acetabular results were poor, with 22.4% loose. This resulted primarily from the poor performance of the screw-in socket (42% loose) compared with those of the Anderson and the porous types (5% and 2.9% loose, respectively). Eight percent of the hips underwent revision because of symptomatic loosening (two stems and eight cups). Of patients in whom both components had an optimal radiographic appearance, 23% had pain and limped. Of patients in whom only the socket appeared optimal, 80% had painful limps; of those in whom only the stem appeared optimal, 55% had painful limps. The authors were optimistic about the predictability and durability of porous-coated acetabular components and distal fixation of porous-coated canal-filling stems in revisions.

In a series of 57 Bias stems, followed up for an average of 2.8 years, revision because of loosening was needed in 4%. An additional 12% were radiographically loose (subsided) but functioned well. Seventeen percent of the patients had some pain, 30% had moderate or severe limps, 27% used canes regularly, and only 60% could walk six blocks without limitation.

After an average follow-up of 17 months, no additional revisions were needed in a group of 60 patients who had undergone cementless revision with the HGP design. One patient required surgery because of unexplained pain. No cups had migrated but two were completely demarcated. One stem had subsided. Results were rated good or excellent in 71% of the patients, fair in 13%, and poor in 16%.

Surface Replacement

In one series of 584 hips followed up for one to ten years, the revision rate was 12.3%. In a three- to six-year follow-up study of Wagner surface replacements, a 26% failure rate was reported.

Several studies have compared surface replacements to total hip replacements. Functional hip improvement was thought to be equivalent. A survivorship analysis study of patients less than 40 years old showed similar patterns for both types of arthroplasty in low- and intermediate-risk groups. An advantage was found for conventional total hip replacement only in the highest-risk group (less than 30 years old, without rheumatoid arthritis or juvenile rheumatoid arthritis).

Thirty-four patients who underwent total hip replacement and surface replacement because of bilateral hip disease were followed up for five years. The revision rate for the total hips was 6% and that for the surface replacements was 26%. There was a statistically significant increased incidence of acetabular radiolucency on the surface replacement side.

Early results with a porous cementless surface replacement system have been encouraging. The bone of the femoral head in 25 surface replacement revisions for femoral-side failure was viable in 92% of cases. In the two cases in which the head was necrotic, the failure was secondary to a femoral neck fracture. Bone death is not an inevitable consequence of femoral head resurfacing with cement.

Bipolar Arthroplasty

The major role for this prosthesis is now in the treatment of displaced femoral neck fractures. However, this prosthesis has been used to revise femoral surface replacement failures in which the acetabular component remained well fixed. The metal outer bearing of the bipolar unit is thus articulated with the intact acetabular component of the surface replacement. Predictable short-term success has been reported in small series of patients.

Hip Reconstruction Without Implants

Biomechanics

Contact forces have been measured in vivo with a telemeterized femoral head replacement articulating with the acetabular cartilage. The data reveal very high (up to 18 MPa) local and nonuniform pressures, with abrupt spatial and temporal gradients. These correlate well with in vitro data and computerized simulations of joint mechanics. However, peak pressures are much higher than those measured in vitro. Because of these high peak pressures, rehabilitation protocols and design criteria for hemiarthroplasties and total hip replacements may need reevaluation.

An in vitro study measured intraosseous pressure in the femoral head in response to compressive loading of the joint. The juxta-articular cancellous bone of the femoral head becomes pressurized with compressive loading in vitro. In vivo, cyclic changes in intraosseous pressure may play a major role in the remodeling, perfusion, and load transmission of bone. In addition, load-induced pressure pulses may play a role in the development of atraumatic osteonecrosis.

Energy expenditure after arthrodesis of the hip has been measured. The average walking speed after hip arthrodesis was 84% of normal gait velocity. The mean oxygen consumption was 14.9 ml/kg of body weight per meter, which is 32% greater than normal. The oxygen cost, 0.223 ml/kg per meter, represented a gait efficiency of 53%. The physiologic energy expenditure after hip arthrodesis is greater than that reported after unilateral total hip arthroplasty for osteoarthritis.

Osteotomy

A computer-generated three-dimensional model has been developed to improve the results of osteotomy for hip dysplasia. The technique clearly establishes both deficiencies of osseous and cartilaginous coverage and congruence of pathologic hips and thus can be used to create a more precise definition and treatment of multiple congenital abnormalities.

A new periacetabular osteotomy in which cuts are made through the pubis and ischium at the acetabulum and innominate bone through the sciatic notch, all through a Smith-Peterson approach, has been described. The advantages include maintenance of the pelvic outlet, enhanced stability and vascularity of the acetabular fragment, and elimination of the significant pubic and ischial displacement seen with the Steele osteotomy. Complications in 75 patients included two intra-articular osteotomies, one femoral nerve palsy, one nonunion, and four cases of heterotopic ossification. The screws used for fixation of the acetabular fragment required removal in 13 patients.

Osteonecrosis

Mechanism of Disease

Clinical and experimental data accumulated during the last 20 years suggest a causal relationship between fat embolism and osteonecrosis. Evidence for fatty liver, coalescence of endogenous plasma lipoproteins, and/or disruption of depot or marrow fat, all resulting in continuous or intermittent fat embolism, is related to many different clinical conditions. These include hypercortisonism, Legg-Calvé-Perthes disease, Gaucher's disease, alcoholism, halogenated hydrocarbon poisoning, pregnancy, obesity, diabetes mellitus, dysbaric phenomena, hemoglobinopathies, pancreatitis, and injuries with unrelated antecedents. Intraosseous fat embolism appears to trigger a three-phase thrombotic process of focal intravascular coagulation that results in osteonecrosis.

An alternate hypothesis likens osteonecrosis to a compartment syndrome with increased intravenous pressures causing a venous outflow obstruction and secondary ischemia. Such increased pressures are observed in osteonecrosis and there is evidence that relief of pressure by core decompression also relieves pain.

In fact, however, the pathogenetic causes of osteonecrosis can be multifactorial and include arterial insufficiency (fractures, dislocations, slipped capital femoral epiphysis), venous occlusion (whether this ever occurs in isolation is questionable), intravascular sinusoidal occlusion (sickle cell disease, polycythemia, dysbaric ischemia, fat embolism), and extravascular sinusoidal occlusion (Gaucher's disease, corticosteroids, alcohol).

A study of 30 rabbits given high-dose steroids revealed no significant increases in intraosseous pressure or venous outflow resistance. The investigators suggested the possibility of a direct cytotoxic effect of steroids on osteocytes.

By contrast, another study demonstrated that clofibrate, a lipid-clearing agent, could increase femoral-head blood flow in rabbits treated with steroids. This suggests that the mechanism of steroid-induced osteonecrosis is ischemia caused by enlarged, space-occupying marrow fat cells and reversed by clofibrate.

Two cases of osteonecrosis of the acetabulum have been reported after radiation treatment.

Diagnosis

Bone scanning with technetium detects osteonecrosis of the femoral head before changes appear on conventional radiographs. The intensity of the increased isotope uptake does not correlate with the stage of the disease.

Magnetic resonance imaging has been shown to be very sensitive to early changes that occur within the marrow elements in osteonecrosis of the femoral head (Fig. 3). The marrow cavity in normal femoral heads emits a strong magnetic resonance signal because it contains large amounts of hydrogen-rich fat. In the early stages of osteonecrosis, magnetic resonance imaging detects changes arising from necrosis of marrow and ingrowth of vascularized mesenchymal tissue. These changes occur well before any alteration in trabecular architecture. Later, as the disease progresses, localized increases in bone density resulting from biologic and mechanical compaction further reduce the magnetic resonance signal.

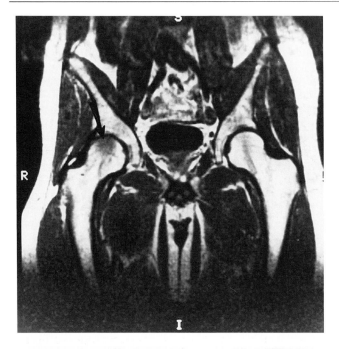

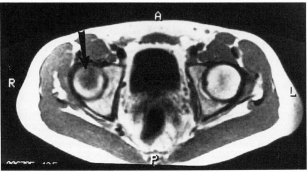

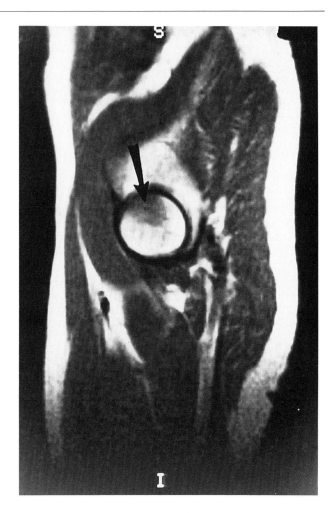

Figure 3

Osteonecrosis. **Top left**, Arrow points to dark avascular area in the right femoral head. **Bottom left**, Coronal view. **Right**, Sagittal view.

Magnetic resonance imaging may show abnormalities consistent with osteonecrosis in early cases in which technetium scans are still negative. Although magnetic resonance imaging is the most sensitive diagnostic technique and provides the earliest diagnosis, it is not useful for staging the disease.

Treatment

One retrospective review of 50 femoral heads found that only 6% stabilized with conservative management consisting of crutches and nonweightbearing. However, many of these heads had already reached stage III at the time treatment was begun. A prospective study of stage I and perhaps stage II lesions is necessary to define the natural history of osteonecrosis and to determine whether or not conservative management is effective.

Studies reviewing the results of core decompression have not supported previous work suggesting success rates of 80% to 90%. A 69% failure rate at 18 months with a 10% femoral fracture rate was noted in one group of 40 hips.

In a review of 21 core decompressions performed in Cincinnati, a 60% failure rate was also noted.

A five-year study of core decompression in 39 hips supported its use in Ficat stages 0, I, and IIA disease. Of hips with stage I disease, only 17% progressed; of those with stage IIA disease, 58% progressed. In contrast, 100% with stage IIB and 82% with stage III disease progressed.

A review of a series of patients who underwent core decompression and bone grafting with or without electrical stimulation via an implantable electrode showed no benefit from the electrode treatment.

Transtrochanteric rotational osteotomy was performed in 17 patients with stage III disease. Within three years, 56% of the patients required total hip arthroplasty. Failures were highest in patients with large necrotic fragments, degenerative joint disease, and steroid- or alcohol-related disease.

Cemented total hip replacement in 28 hips followed up for five to ten years (average, 7.6 years) had a failure rate of 37%. There is some hope that uncemented devices will improve on these results.

Miscellaneous Considerations

A 35-year follow-up study of hip arthrodeses revealed generally satisfactory results. Ipsilateral knee and back pain were present in 60% of patients, with onset at about 25 years postoperatively. Twenty-five percent had pain in the contralateral hip with onset about 20 years after the arthrodesis. Only one patient had severe pain. Seventy percent of patients were able to walk a mile and to sit for two hours. Six patients underwent total hip replacement because of back pain; all cases were successful.

Resection of the proximal end of the femur and interpositional arthroplasty were used in patients with cerebral palsy to enable them to sit. Ninety-seven percent of the patients had successful and durable results after two years.

Sepsis of the hip in nine paraplegic patients was treated successfully by resection of the head and neck of the femur, transposition of the vastus lateralis into the void, and external fixation across the resection for three to six weeks.

Controversies

Causes of Loosening in Cemented Total Hip Replacements

The cause of loosening of the cemented total hip replacement is disruption of the bone-cement or prosthesis-cement interface. The causes of these disruptions, however, remain somewhat controversial.

It is likely that the quality of the initial microinterlock is the major determinant of the long-term durability of the arthroplasty. Radiographic and clinical data examining modern cementing techniques support this.

Secondly, mechanical factors play a role. More flexible stems that highly stress the cement result in increased radiographic failures. Cups located superolaterally to the true acetabulum increase the joint reaction force and result in more failures, again because of excessive stresses at the level of the microinterlock. Diseased bone cannot support the normal stresses of a well-performed arthroplasty.

Finally, the biologic response to metal, plastic, and cement debris promotes osteolysis and progressive loosening. To what extent this is primary or secondary, or both in a cyclical fashion, is impossible to say.

Therefore, technical, mechanical, and biologic factors all cause loosening of cemented total hip replacement, probably in that order of importance. Is a cemented arthroplasty doomed to eventual failure? Probably not, unless biologic factors are of primary importance, a view not supported to date by the literature.

Cemented vs Uncemented Total Hip Replacements

The two methods of fixation should not be considered mutually exclusive. There may prove to be roles for both. The challenge lies in defining their indications.

At present, the comparison is somewhat unfair. There are ten- to 21-year follow-up data for cemented primary total hip replacements; many cases look good clinically and some look worrisome radiographically. Only two- to seven-year follow-up data are available for uncemented primary total hip replacement. Clinically, the outcomes can be considered inferior to those for cemented replacements, with more patients reporting pain or limp. Radiographically, the data are difficult to interpret, as many of the findings are of unknown significance.

Cementless total hip replacement is still in its early stages. On the basis of the long-term data for cemented replacements and the short-term data for uncemented replacements, the uncemented technique may be justifiable in young (less than 60 years old) patients, on the acetabular side, and in revision situations.

Autografts vs Allografts

Experimental work on the histology of incorporation and replacement of autografts and allografts supports an advantage for autografting. Revascularization and consolidation with new bone formation occur more rapidly than with allografting.

However, clinical studies using both large block autografts and allografts for replacement of major bone-stock deficiencies in total hip arthroplasty consistently fail to show any advantage of autografts over allografts.

Treatment of Osteonecrosis of the Femoral Head

When the cause and natural history of a disease remain obscure, a definitive treatment is unlikely to be obvious. Such is the case with osteonecrosis of the femoral head.

It has been shown that increased intraosseous pressures occur with osteonecrosis (a finding not unique to osteonecrosis since it occurs in osteoarthritis as well), that pain can be produced by increased pressures, and that core decompression can reduce pressures and relieve pain. It has not been shown that core decompression changes the natural course of the disease. Additionally, recent studies have not supported the predictable pain relief after core decompression that early studies suggested. Complication rates have been high in some series but suboptimal technique probably played a role in most of these instances.

Electrical stimulation should be viewed as experimental.

Annotated Bibliography

Keywords

Acetabular dysplasia; Ankylosis; Bipolar arthroplasty; Bone graft; Cerebral palsy; Heterotopic ossification; Infection; Juvenile rheumatoid arthritis; Lupus erythematosus; Obesity; Osteonecrosis; Osteotomy; Paget's disease; Protrusio acetabuli; Sickle cell disease; Total hip replacement; Tuberculosis

Total Hip Replacement With Implants

Biomechanics

Davy DT, Kotzar GM, Brown RH, et al: Telemetric force measurements across the hip after total arthroplasty. *J Bone Joint Surg* 1988;70A:45–50.

Force data obtained from a telemeterized total hip replacement revealed joint contact forces of 2.1 times body weight for ipsilateral single-limb stance and 2.6 to 2.8 times body weight during gait and stair-climbing.

Thomas BJ, Salvati EA, Small RD: The CAD hip arthroplasty: Five- to ten-year follow-up. *J Bone Joint Surg* 1986;68A:640–646.

A stem with a high modulus of elasticity used predominantly in young, active, heavy men had a low rate of mechanical failure.

Imaging

Amstutz HC, Ouzounian T, Grauer D, et al: The grid radiograph: A simple technique for consistent high-resolution visualization of the hip. *J Bone Joint Surg* 1986;68A:1052–1056.

This method allows the images of acetabular and femoral components to be superimposed over serial radiographs to detect subtle shifts in position.

Cemented Total Hip Replacements

Agins HJ, Alcock NW, Bansal M, et al: Metallic wear in failed titanium-alloy total hip replacements: A histological and quantitative analysis. *J Bone Joint Surg* 1988;70A:347–356.

Titanium surfaces can shed considerable amounts of wear debris into surrounding tissues, causing significant reactions when used as a bearing surface or when loosening occurs. This may contribute to infection and further loosening.

Ayers DC, Evarts CM, Parkinson JR: The prevention of heterotopic ossification in high-risk patients by low-dose radiation therapy after total hip arthroplasty. *J Bone Joint Surg* 1986;68A:1423–1430.

The authors found that 10 Gy delivered over five to seven postoperative days was as effective as 20 Gy.

Beisaw NE, Camerota AJ, Groth HE, et al: Dihydroergotamine/heparin in the prevention of deep-vein thrombosis after total hip replacement: A controlled, prospective, randomized multicenter trial. *J Bone Joint Surg* 1988;70A:2–10.

This combination is effective. The product is not currently commercially available in the United States.

Goldring SR, Jasty M, Roelke MS, et al: Formation of a synovial-like membrane at the bone-cement interface: Its role in bone resorption and implant loosening after total hip replacement. *Arthritis Rheum* 1986;29:836–842.

Histologic and histochemical evaluation of the interface membrane suggests its relationship to implant loosening.

Lidwell OM: Clean air at operation and subsequent sepsis in the joint. *Clin Orthop* 1986;211:91.

Recent randomized studies have confirmed that the sepsis rate can be considerably reduced by operating in ultraclean air but that a similarly low rate can be obtained with normal ventilation when prophylactic antibiotics are given. In addition, the two methods are effective independently and in combination. The sepsis rate in the joint after total arthroplasty was reduced to a few cases per 1,000.

McQueary FG, Johnston RC: Coxarthrosis after congeni-

tal dysplasia: Treatment by total hip arthroplasty without acetabular bone grafting. *J Bone Joint Surg* 1988; 70A:1140–1144.

The addition of a large, solid, superolateral bone graft above a cemented acetabular component does not decrease the likelihood of loosening and may increase it. At 8.5 years, no revisions were required in 66 total hip replacements when the acetabulum was restored to an anatomic position and the superolateral defect was filled with cement rather than bone graft.

Paiement G, Wessmyer G, Waltman AC, et al: Low-dose warfarin versus external pneumatic compression for prophylaxis against venous thromboembolism following total hip replacement. *J Arthop* 1987;2:23.

Both regimens were effective in preventing deep venous thrombosis, as were higher dosages of warfarin in earlier studies.

Poss R, Brick GW, Wright J, et al: The effects of modern cementing techniques in the longevity of total hip arthroplasty. *Orthop Clin North Am* 1988;19:591.

Modern prosthesis design and cementing techniques have dramatically improved femoral-component fixation.

Schmidt SA, Kjaersgaard-Andersen P, Pedersen NW, et al: The use of indomethacin to prevent the formation of heterotopic bone after total hip replacement: A randomized double-blind clinical trial. *J Bone Joint Surg* 1988; 7A:834–838.

Six weeks of postoperative treatment (25 mg three times a day) was highly effective in minimizing the formation of heterotopic ossification.

Schutzer SF, Harris WH: Deep-wound infection after total hip replacement under contemporary aseptic conditions. *J Bone Joint Surg* 1988;70A:724–727.

The incidence of early postoperative sepsis is low when prophylactic antibiotics, laminar air flow, and total-body exhaust suits are used in combination. Procedures involving major bone grafting increase the risk of infection.

Stone RG, Weeks LE, Hajdu M, et al: Evaluation of sciatic nerve compromise during total hip arthroplasty. *Clin Orthop* 1985;201:26–31.

Intraoperative monitoring of the nerve can detect temporary compromise and suggests those points during the procedure that place the nerve at risk.

Trippel SB: Current concepts review: Antibiotic-impregnated cement in total joint arthroplasty. *J Bone Joint Surg* 1986;68A:1297–1302.

The state of the art is discussed on the basis of the available literature.

Turpie AGG, Levine MN, Hirsch J, et al: A randomized controlled trial of a low-molecular-weight heparin (enoxaparin) to prevent deep-vein thrombosis in patients undergoing elective hip surgery. *N Engl J Med* 1986;315: 925–929.

This drug was shown to be safe and effective.

Wroblewski BM: 15–21-year results of the Charnley low-friction arthroplasty. *Clin Orthop* 1986;211:30–35.

Clinical results were good to excellent in 96.5% of patients. Radiographic loosening was present in 23% of sockets and 29% of stems. The revision rate was "very low."

Uncemented Total Hip Replacements

Callaghan JJ, Dysart SH, Savaory CG: The uncemented porous-coated anatomic total hip prosthesis: Two-year

results of a prospective consecutive series. *J Bone Joint Surg* 1988;70A:337–346.
  Clinical results were encouraging.

Collier JP, Mayor MB, Chae JC, et al: Macroscopic and microscopic evidence of prosthetic fixation with porous-coated materials. *Clin Orthop* 1988;235:173–180.
  The authors discuss the experimental and scientific bases of ingrowth.

Cook SD, Thomas KA, Hawddad RJ Jr: Histologic analysis of retrieved human porous-coated total joint components. *Clin Orthop* 1988;234:90–101.
  The amount of ingrowth bone in most of these retrieved components was alarmingly small.

Engh CA, Bobyn JD, Glassman AH: Porous-coated hip replacement: The factors governing bone ingrowth, stress shielding, and clinical results. *J Bone Joint Surg* 1987;69B:45–55.
  This is a comprehensive overview of experience with the AML prosthesis.

Glassman AH, Engh CA, Bobyn JD: Proximal femoral osteotomy as an adjunct in cementless revision total hip arthroplasty. *J Arthrop* 1987;2:47.
  The combination of proximal femoral osteotomy and cementless stem provides a good method of correcting deformity.

Hedley AK, Gruen TA, Borden LS, et al: Two-year follow-up of the PCA noncemented total hip replacement. *Hip* 1987;15:225–250.
  Good results are reported.

Bone Grafting

Gerber SD, Harris WH: Femoral head autografting to augment acetabular deficiency in patients requiring total hip replacement: A minimum five-year and average seven-year follow-up study. *J Bone Joint Surg* 1986;68A:1241–1248.
  The authors report favorable results.

Goldberg VM, Stevenson S: Natural history of autografts and allografts. *Clin Orthop* 1987;225:7–16.
  The histologic performance indicated that autografting is more advantageous than allografting.

Jasty M, Harris WH: Total hip reconstruction using frozen femoral head allografts in patients with acetabular bone loss. *Orthop Clin North Am* 1987;18:291–299.
  Results were favorable at an average follow-up of four years.

Jofe MH, Gebhardt MC, Tomford WW, et al: Reconstruction for defects of the proximal part of the femur using allograft arthroplasty. *J Bone Joint Surg* 1988;70A:507–516.
  Success was achieved in 70% to 80% of patients.

Hip Reconstruction Without Implants

Callaghan JJ, Brand RA, Pedersen DR: Hip arthrodesis: A long-term follow-up. *J Bone Joint Surg* 1985;67A:1328–1335.
  The authors report generally good long-term results.

Osteonecrosis

Camp JF, Colwell CW Jr: Core decompression of the femoral head for osteonecrosis. *J Bone Joint Surg* 1986;68A:1313–1319.
  Poor results and significant morbidity are reported.

Warner JJP, Philip JH, Brodsky GL, et al: Studies of nontraumatic osteonecrosis: The role of core decompression in the treatment of nontraumatic osteonecrosis of the femoral head. *Clin Orthop* 1987;225:104–127.
  Core decompression can be a useful procedure in certain situations.

42

Knee and Leg: Pediatric Aspects

Much of the recent literature regarding pediatric conditions about the knee and leg has dealt with traditional problems such as congenital deficiencies and pseudoarthroses. However, some worthwhile data have emerged with regard to osteochondritis dissecans and osteomyelitis. Certainly the treatment of leg-length irregularities with multiple-pin circular fixation frames is an exciting new innovation that will be a topic of interest for many years to come.

Congenital Abnormalities

Femoral Deficiency

Congenital deficiencies of the lower extremity that require orthopaedic management include femoral deficiency syndromes and deficiencies of the tibia, fibula, or foot. Knee ligaments (especially the cruciates) are often absent in these syndromes and may lead to unexpected disability. In mild femoral deficiency, simple limb equalization may suffice (femoral lengthening, contralateral epiphysiodesis), whereas more severe deficiencies may require knee fusion, fusion of the femoral remnant to the ilium, or Syme's amputation or the Van Ness rotationplasty. The potential for improved limb function with successful rotationplasty has led to a modest resurgence in the popularity of this procedure; however, function is better in patients who undergo Syme's amputation than in those who undergo rotationplasty.

Fibular Hemimelia

Fibular hemimelia often includes a deficient foot; in more complete forms, absence of the fibula makes foot and ankle reconstruction or stabilization difficult. In mild cases, the foot can be maintained by traditional methods used to equalize limb length. In severe cases, most investigators recommend a Syme's or Boyd-type amputation when the limb-length discrepancy at maturity is projected to be more than 12 to 15 cm. Excellent function has been documented in patients treated with Syme's amputation and a correctly fitting prosthesis.

In intermediate cases, in which the severity of limb-length discrepancy and ankle instability are difficult to predict accurately, the Gruca procedure, in which the distal tibia is split through the physis to provide medial and lateral support to the talus, has been recommended.

Tibial Hemimelia

Tibial hemimelia is less common than fibular hemimelia. Congenital diastasis of the tibia is part of the spectrum of this syndrome. In severe forms, the associated severe clubfoot deformity cannot be corrected because there is no tibia to aid in stabilizing the ankle. The Brown procedure, involving early transfer of the fibula to the proximal tibial remnant (or to the distal femur itself), has not been predictably successful. Instead, early disarticulation at the knee level and prosthesis use are recommended.

Angular Deformities of the Tibia

Infants may have tibial deformity (not physiologic genu varum) that requires accurate diagnosis and prognostication.

Tibial Bowing

Congenital posteromedial tibial bowing usually corrects spontaneously; however, in many patients a limb-length inequality develops that is great enough to require contralateral epiphysiodesis in adolescence. Parents should be advised of this possibility. Anteromedial bowing occurs in association with fibular hemimelia. Anterolateral bowing suggests congenital pseudarthrosis of the tibia, often associated with neurofibromatosis.

Congenital Pseudarthrosis of the Tibia

Often children with this condition initially have only a bowed tibia (prepseudarthrosis) but then progress to pseudarthrosis. After the diagnosis is made, a young child should be treated with a total-contact orthosis. Once complete pseudarthrosis develops, treatment is difficult and only partially successful.

Current traditional treatment methods include intramedullary rod fixation of both the tibia and the fibula, excision of the hamartomatous fibrous tissue, bone grafting, and possible placement of an electronic coil to stimulate bone formation. Clearly, long intramedullary rods provide more resistance to angular forces than do plates or dual-onlay bone grafts. The efficacy of electrical stimulation alone, or in conjunction with corrective surgery, remains uncertain.

A more aggressive approach includes a free vascularized fibular graft from the opposite normal limb. This method shows promise but has not yet achieved widespread use because follow-up has been short and complications, such as nonunion at the distal anastomosis site and fractures of the graft, have been common. Also parents are reluctant to have the opposite normal limb used as a donor site until the long-term efficacy of the procedure has been clarified.

Amputation and a prosthesis are advised after two or three failed surgical attempts to gain union. An amputation at the level of the ankle joint, rather than at the level of the pseudarthrosis, prevents bony overgrowth and frequent stump revision in the growing child.

Tibia Vara (Blount's Disease)

Most children have physiologic genu varum (bowlegs) early in life; this evolves naturally to genu valgum by the age of 3 to 4 years. There is a gradual return to neutral alignment by the age of 7 to 8 years. Parents must be advised of this natural sequence.

In a few cases of severe genu varum, spontaneous correction fails to occur, and progressive varus develops with a lateral thrust in stance phase. Asymmetric weightbearing leads to medial physeal injury, growth suppression, and further varus. This disorder, known as Blount's disease, must be recognized and treated in its early stages to prevent permanent physeal closure. Infantile tibia vara can be recognized when the child is 2 to 3 years old. Initial treatment can include progressive corrective bracing (long leg braces and pelvic band to control rotation—adjusted into further valgus every one to two months) worn while the child is weightbearing. Night bracing does not control pathologic forces and is ineffective. Brace treatment is difficult, and many parents and children are unable to cooperate. In such cases, surgical intervention with tibial-fibular osteotomy is required to avoid progression to irreversible growth plate arrest. Often the osteotomy is done too late or too little valgus is provided.

Adolescent Tibia Vara

Occasionally the pathophysiologic cycle of growth suppression-further varus-further growth suppression does not occur until the adolescent growth spurt. Adolescent Blount's disease is most common in overweight boys who maintain minor degrees of physiologic genu varum throughout childhood. Weight gain or increased activity leads to growth suppression of the medial tibial physis in the adolescent. Treatment consists of corrective osteotomy below the growth plate before a permanent bony bar forms.

Once a permanent bar has formed, treatment becomes more difficult. Although successful resection of the physeal bar in three children with infantile tibia vara has been reported, other investigators found this difficult to reproduce, further emphasizing the need for early corrective osteotomy to avoid permanent physeal closure in both infantile and adolescent tibia vara.

Genu Valgum

Physiologic Occasionally, the normal physiologic genu valgum seen in children 4 to 8 years old fails to correct and instead worsens. Teenagers with severe physiologic genu valgum appear awkward and in severe cases may be at risk for early lateral compartment arthritis. When the condition is recognized before growth ends, it can be corrected by stapling the medial distal femoral physis. Hemi-epiphysiodesis has been advocated to avoid the problem of staple removal.

Posttraumatic Transverse, unicortical fractures of the proximal tibial metaphysis often lead to asymmetric growth plate stimulation and progressive genu valgum. Many etiologic theories have been proposed, with most authors accepting asymmetric growth stimulation of the medial physis as a final common factor. One group reported gradual, spontaneous correction of the deformity one to three years after the fracture in five of six cases. Also, early attempts at corrective osteotomy in this condition commonly lead to recurrence of the deformity. In cases that fail to correct spontaneously, it is probably better to wait until the patient reaches adolescence and then perform medial tibial epiphysiodesis.

Abnormalities of the Knee

Knee pain is common in children and adolescents, particularly today when both sexes participate in vigorous sporting activities. Because hip disorders are common in the pediatric population and because knee complaints may be caused by referred pain, children who complain of knee pain should undergo a careful hip examination before the knee is inspected. Inappropriate knee arthroscopy in an adolescent with hip disease (for example, slipped capital femoral epiphysis) is, unfortunately, becoming increasingly common.

Radiographs should include a notch (tunnel) view to help identify osteochondritis dissecans. Unfortunately, the normal irregularity of ossification in the posterior area of the femoral condyles is sometimes misinterpreted as osteochondritis dissecans. True osteochondritis dissecans in children can range from a mild self-limiting disorder to severe involvement requiring arthroscopic assessment, surgical drilling, bone peg fixation, or excision of loose fragments. Most children under 12 years of age do well with conservative treatment; teenagers, however, have a greater risk for separation of the fragment.

Magnetic resonance imaging of the knee provides good detail in most osteochondritis dissecans lesions and may help to differentiate intact from separated lesions (Fig. 1). Unexpected lesions, such as congenital discoid meniscus, are also readily identified by magnetic resonance imaging (Fig. 2). The risk-cost-benefit ratio of arthroscopic vs magnetic resonance imaging evaluation of knee disorders in children remains unsettled.

Osgood-Schlatter disease, a probable overuse injury of the tibial tubercle apophysis, can usually be treated symptomatically. A knee sleeve provides relief in more chronic cases. In one study, five of 12 adolescents with tibial tuberosity fracture had had Osgood-Schlatter disease previously, suggesting that adolescents with active, symptomatic Osgood-Schlatter disease be restricted from jumping sports.

Joint Sepsis and Osteomyelitis

Joint Sepsis

Septic arthritis commonly affects the knee in infancy and childhood. The child often has an externally rotated hip and a flexed knee because this posture decreases intracapsular pressure. This is the same posture that a child with hip sepsis adopts and has led unwary physicians to mistakenly aspirate the hip joint in a child with early knee sepsis. As in all joint infections, suspected knee sepsis requires aspiration and fluid analysis. Confirmation of joint sepsis is an indication for intravenous antibiotics and aggressive joint decompression by open arthrotomy, arthroscopic drainage, or repeat needle aspiration. Traditional orthopaedic teaching advises open arthrotomy but there is convincing evidence that arthroscopic lavage and drainage of knee sepsis provide results equal to surgical drainage in children (Fig. 3).

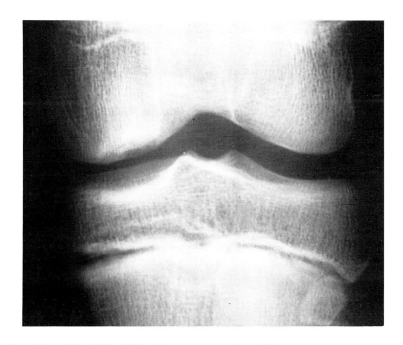

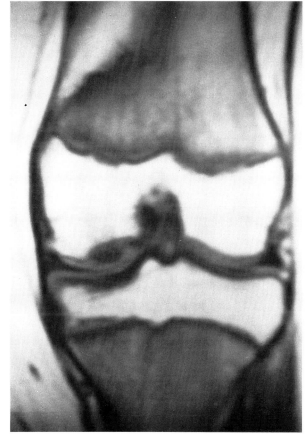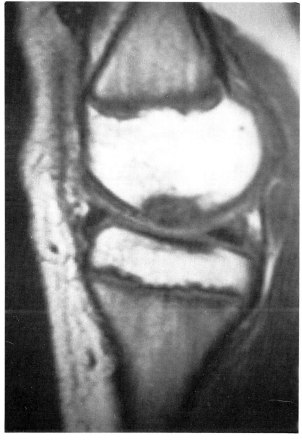

Figure 1

Osteochondritis dissecans lesion in the medial formal condyle of a 13-year-old boy is apparent on an anteroposterior radiograph (**top**) and anteroposterior (**bottom left**) and lateral (**bottom right**) magnetic resonance imaging views.

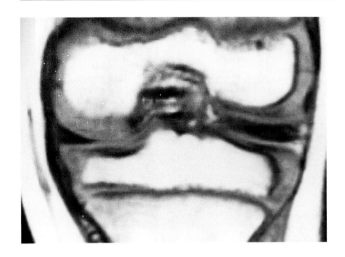

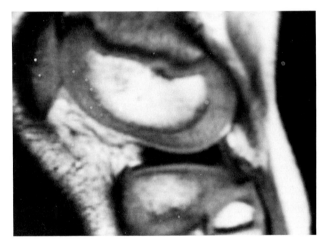

Figure 2

Anteroposterior (**top**) and lateral (**bottom**) magnetic resonance imaging views of the right knee of a 2-year-old child who had severe clicking in both knees. The widened lateral cartilage space is consistent with a congenital discoid meniscus. The same problem was noted in the left knee.

Lyme Arthritis

In assessing an inflamed joint in a child, orthopaedic surgeons must consider Lyme arthritis, a disorder caused by the tick-borne spirochete, *Borrelia burgdorferi*. Affected children have intermittent attacks of swelling in one or more large joints and may also have a characteristic skin rash (erythema chronicum migrans) that precedes the arthritis. Treatment includes tetracycline, penicillin, or erythromycin.

Osteomyelitis

Osteomyelitis commonly affects the distal femoral or proximal tibial metaphysis in children. Technetium bone scanning helps with early diagnosis; however, the scan is often falsely negative in neonates. Blood cultures are mandatory. Needle aspiration of both the subperiosteal space and the marrow cavity (thin metaphyseal cortex easily penetrated in children) provides material for Gram stain and culture studies (and occasionally produces pus). In an animal model, it was found that needle aspiration of a joint or bony cortex is unlikely to produce a false-positive bone scan.

Patients with osteomyelitis who have had symptoms for less than 72 hours, with no pus detected at aspiration, are treated with high-dose intravenous antibiotics. In cases in which diagnosis is delayed, particularly those with radiographic changes (a late finding), surgical decompression is required. When diagnosed and treated early in its course, joint sepsis or osteomyelitis requires only five to seven days of intravenous antibiotics if the organism is sensitive. Additional oral therapy is needed for three to six weeks. In more chronic cases requiring a lengthy course of intravenous drugs, a Hickman catheter can be placed and intravenous antibiotics administered at home. This method is highly successful in communities where home intravenous programs are functioning.

Children occasionally develop chronic multifocal osteomyelitis, a puzzling condition in which lytic lesions of bone are found at many sites, yet cultures are negative and biopsy specimens nonspecific. This rare inflammatory condition eventually resolves and neither antibiotics nor repeat surgical biopsy drainage is needed. This is a distinct entity, separate from subacute osteomyelitis.

Trauma

Physeal injuries about the knee are more common than ligamentous injuries. Stress views help to localize the injury. Significant ligamentous injuries can occur in the skeletally mature adolescent and should be treated like those in adults.

Salter-Harris type II injury to the distal femoral physis is relatively common. Even when anatomic reduction is achieved, there is at least a 30% chance of growth arrest. The usual treatment includes manipulative reduction, often supplemented by percutaneous K-wire fixation and cast immobilization. These injuries must be monitored radiographically for several years to determine outcome.

Fractures of the proximal tibial physis are rare but important injuries because they represent the childhood equivalent of knee dislocation with the associated risk for popliteal artery injury. Careful monitoring of vascular and compartment status is required.

Fractures of the tibial spine (intercondylar eminence) occasionally occur in adolescents. Hyperextension caused by a fall from a bicycle seems the most common pattern, producing fracture of the anterior spine. Anterior tibial spine fractures are graded according to displacement. Closed reduction with extension casting is advised for a minimally displaced fracture and open reduction for significant displacement. In one study of this injury, many patients continued to have anterior cruciate laxity and a mild loss of full extension, even when anatomic reduction had been achieved originally.

Fractures of the tibial tubercle can occur in adolescents; these usually require open reduction with K-wire and tension band fixation to avoid growth plate closure (Fig. 4).

Severe motor-vehicle accidents can produce a complete fracture of the femur and tibia ("floating knee") in childhood. Management is easier and the results better if at least one of the fractures is treated by open reduction and internal fixation.

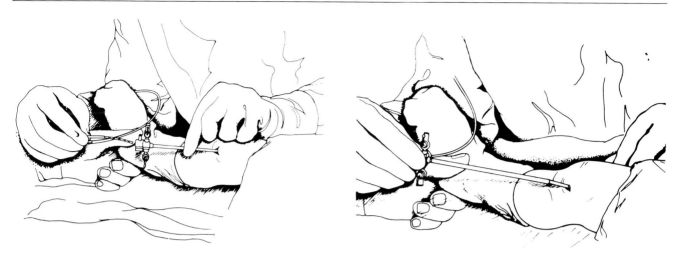

Figure 3

Arthroscopic lavage for septic arthritis of the knee in children. **Left**, A Hemovac drain is inserted through the arthroscope. **Right**, The arthroscope is then withdrawn, leaving the Hemovac in the joint. (Reproduced with permission from Skyhar MJ, Mubarak SJ: Arthroscopic treatment of septic knees in children. *J Pediatr Orthop* 1987;7:647–651.)

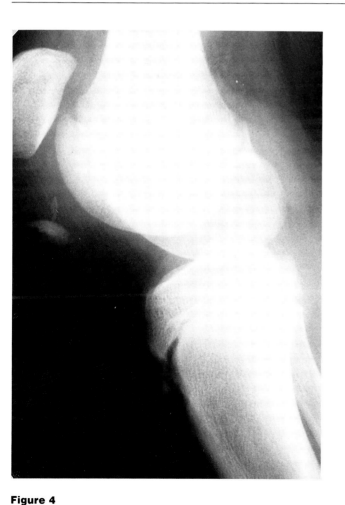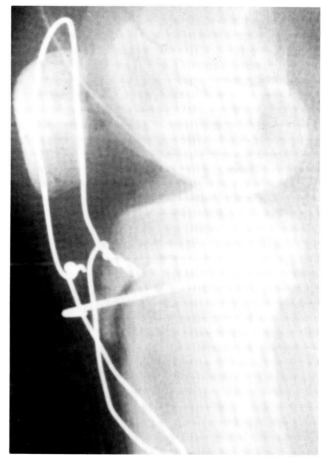

Figure 4

Lateral knee radiographs before (**left**) and after (**right**) surgical reduction in a 10-year-old child who jumped from a wall, resulting in a displaced tibial tubercle fracture.

Physeal Bridge Resection for Premature Closure of the Growth Plate

A diverse group of conditions can lead to growth plate closure. They have in common the fact that either by malposition of bony fragments or physeal cartilage death, bone forms across the growth plate. This, in turn, acts as a tether, leading to either partial or total cessation of growth or malalignment because of asymmetric growth.

Indications

At least two years or 2 cm of growth should remain for a patient to be considered for bridge resection. Less than 2 cm of discrepancy is generally well tolerated by patients. Accurate determination of the amount of growth remaining usually requires a bone-age film of the wrist.

Imaging

Accurate measurement of length and deformity of the involved bone can be accomplished by a variety of techniques. True scanograms have advantages is terms of accurate assessment of both length and alignment on one film.

Bridges larger than 50% are not amenable to resection. Plain radiographs are not sufficiently accurate to determine the extent of the bone bridge. Several alternative specialized radiographic techniques are available. Hypocycloidal tomography is the most accurate tomographic technique for estimating the amount of bridging bone.

Bone Scan Several techniques have been described for evaluation of the growth plate by bone scans. Apex views have provided useful information.

Computed Tomography Computed tomography using 1- and 2-mm cuts through the area in question with reformatting in 5-mm sagittal and coronal cuts gives clear images of the bridge. In many instances, these are superior to the visualization obtained by tomography, and allow a more accurate delineation of the epiphyseal bridge.

Magnetic Resonance Imaging To date, experience with magnetic resonance imaging is insufficient for its efficacy to be assessed.

Surgery

The goal is atraumatic resection of the physeal bridge and realignment of the extremity.

Bridge Resection In resecting the bridge, it is of paramount importance that the bar be removed without unnecessary damage to the residual viable growth plate. Hemostasis in the surgical field by means of a tourniquet is generally advisable. To remove the bridge as expeditiously yet as atraumatically as possible, sharp dental burrs and small sharp curettes to complete the removal are useful. Dental mirrors can be used to see into the recesses of the cavity.

The surgical exposure of the bridge depends somewhat on the nature of the bridge. Central bridges are best exposed through the metaphysis, either a metaphyseal window or the metaphyseal surface of an osteotomy if it is thought that realignment of the extremity is indicated at the time of the procedure. The metaphyseal exposure should be located well away from the perichondrial ring to prevent inadvertent damage to the growth plate by perichondrial ring disruption.

With a peripheral or a combined peripheral-central bridge, entry through the perichondrial ring is required. To prevent a recurrent peripheral bridge, the perichondrial ring should be resected rather than reflected and reapproximated.

In resecting the bridge, damage to the intact physis should be minimized. The growth plate should be identified through the physeal bridge and then exposed circumferentially, removing the bar in a centrifugal pattern. After the growth plate is identified around the circumference of the bar, it should be undercut on both the epiphyseal and metaphyseal surfaces to ensure intimate contact of the interposition material. Obviously, overzealous undercutting may lead to further physeal damage and be counterproductive.

The decision as to whether or not realignment osteotomy is required at the time of bridge resection must be made on a case-by-case basis. Generally, as much as 30 degrees of deformity can be tolerated if it is in the plane of motion of the adjacent joint, whereas deformity not in the plane of the joint probably requires realignment if it exceeds 10 to 15 degrees. Other factors that enter into the decision include the age of the child (remodeling of the deformity is probably more likely in younger children with successful bridge resections) and the type of interposition material used (if the interposition material must be removed at maturity, correction of the residual deformity, if necessary, could be carried then.)

Prevention of Recurrent Bridge Formation Prevention of recurrent bridge formation requires prevention of a hemotoma collection in the cavity. After the resection is completed, the tourniquet should be released and the cavity filled with thrombin-soaked Gelfoam or some other hemostatic material. After hemostasis has been obtained, this material should be removed before insertion of the interposition material.

To prevent recurrent bridge formation over the long-term, insertion of some inert interposition material is necessary. Currently three substances are in clinical use: fat, medical elastomer 328 (Silastic), and Cranioplast. Additionally, cartilage has been used experimentally by several investigatrs. Each has advantages and disadvantages (Table 1). Fat is readily available, but perhaps slightly less effective than Cranioplast or Silastic. It lends no inherent support to the bone but has been shown histologically to remain viable for long periods. Cranioplast and Silastic appear to be equally effective, with Cranioplast perhaps lending more intrinsic support and stability to the bone. Both substances require fixation to the epiphysis to prevent migration into the metaphysis, which has been associated with recurrent bridge formation. They both require removal at skeletal maturity. In laboratory studies, cartilage has been superior to fat.

Results

Follow-up to skeletal maturity is indicated because premature closure of the physis can occur after several years of "normal" growth. Trying to compare the clinical results of published reports of bridge resection is difficult. Nevertheless, certain trends are evident. Good results are more

Table 1. Comparison of interposition materials*†

Clinical Data	Materials			
	Fat	Silastic	Cranioplast	Cartilage
Availability	+++	Protocol	Protocol (?)	?
Efficacy	++, +++	+++	+++	++++
Stress raiser	++	++	+	++
Fixation required	No	Yes	Yes	No
Removal required	No	Yes	Yes	No

*Reproduced with permission from Burke SW: Principles of physeal bridge resection, in Barr JS Jr (ed): American Academy of Orthopaedic Surgeons *Instructional Course Lectures, XXXVIII.* Park Ridge, Illinois, American Academy of Orthopaedic Surgeons, 1989, pp 337–341.
†Materials are rated as excellent = ++++, good = +++, fair = ++, and lowest = +.

likely with a newly formed bridge, a bridge caused by trauma, a central bridge, a smaller bridge, and a bridge in a younger child.

Resection of partial epiphyseal bridges is effective both in terms of laboratory experimentation and clinical experience. Careful attention to detail in terms of remaining growth, delineation of extent of involvement, and careful surgical technique lead to predictable satisfactory results in most patients.

Limb-Length Inequality

Limb-length inequality can be congenital or acquired, with physeal fracture and delayed treatment of osteomyelitis common acquired causes. The orthopaedist's task is to monitor the limb-length discrepancy and to plan intervention for inequality that will be greater than 2 to 2.5 cm at maturity. Clinical measurements are adequate until the child is 5 or 6 years old. A 6-year-old child with a significant discrepancy should undergo yearly scanograms and wrist films to determine bone age.

Alternatively, microdose radiography and computed tomographic scanning techniques can be used to document limb-length inequality with accuracy.

Either the Green-Anderson tables or the Moseley straight-line graph can be used to chart growth and calculate the correct timing for epiphysiodesis. For discrepancies projected to be less than 5 or 6 cm at maturity, contralateral epiphysiodesis provides a simple, predictable way to correct the inequality. Several centers have begun performing percutaneous epiphysiodesis with a power burr guided by an image intensifier introduced via a minimal stab incision. The predictability and long-term efficacy of the method are unknown; thus, its application remains controversial, especially since the traditional Phemister method has few complications and results in excellent cosmesis, particularly if the two small incisions are closed with a subcuticular suture.

Limb Lengthening

For greater discrepancies, limb lengthening of either the femur or tibia can be performed, often in combination with contralateral epiphysiodesis. The many new methods of lengthening are still controversial.

Controversies

Managing Knee Sepsis

Traditionally, orthopaedic surgeons have opposed using antibiotics and knee aspiration alone for the treatment of joint sepsis. Both Herndon and associates and Wilson and Di Paola reviewed series of patients with septic arthritis and reported that joint aspiration and antibiotics provide satisfactory results for joints other than the hip. This controversial viewpoint is not widely accepted in North American orthopaedic centers. Also, the problem of repeat aspiration in the frightened child must be considered. The arthroscopic method described by Skyhar and Mubarak seems a logical compromise for knee sepsis.

Duration of Intravenous Antibiotic Treatment in Children

Few topics engender more controversy in pediatric orthopaedics than the duration of intravenous anibiotic treatment for joint sepsis or osteomyelitis. Opinions vary widely and physicians within a single institution often disagree completely as to when it is safe to switch to oral antibiotics. Commonly, the battle is between orthopaedic surgeons and infectious disease consultants. The important early work on this subject was performed at Southwestern Medical Center in Dallas, where Nelson and associates and Tetzlaff and associates demonstrated that a five-day course of intravenous antibiotics was adequate in early, uncomplicated cases of both joint sepsis and osteomyelitis when appropriate surgical drainage (for joint sepsis) and other supportive measures were used. After five days, if the organism has been identified and is sensitive, the patient's fever and erythrocyte sedimentation rate are declining, and the joint (or wound) appears benign, treatment can be switched to oral antibiotics. The parents must be trustworthy and adequate antibiotic levels must be confirmed.

Use of this regimen for the last eight years has produced only rare problems and few relapses or recurrences. The method probably works well because in large North American cities, with increasing numbers of well-trained pediatricians and orthopaedic surgeons, most cases of childhood joint sepsis and osteomyelitis are diagnosed early when intravenous antibiotics are maximally effective. Also, contemporary oral antibiotics have good bone and joint penetration.

It should be noted that many oral antibiotic suspensions (especially oxacillin and dicloxacillin) have an unpleasant metallic taste that most young children cannot tolerate. The oral cephalosporin elixirs taste much better. Orthopaedic surgeons might take the time to do an "antibiotic tasting" before deciding which oral suspension should be prescribed for a small child.

Percutaneous Epiphysiodesis

Encouraged by positive experience with knee arthroscopy, which permits surgery to be performed with almost invis-

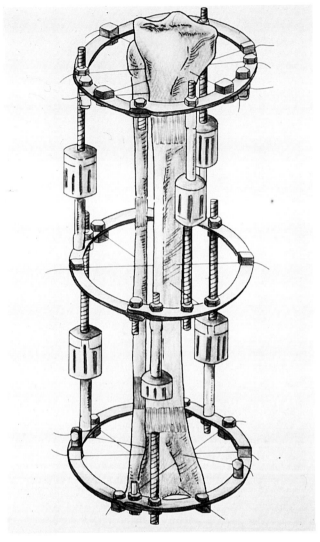

Figure 5

The Ilizarov apparatus that is applied to the tibia for leg lengthening. (Reproduced with permission from Paley D: Current techniques of limb lengthening. *J Pediatr Orthop* 1988;8:73–92.)

ible skin incisions, orthopaedic surgeons have begun to perform percutaneous epiphysiodesis when growth arrest is desired to equalize limb length. The procedure is performed under image-intensifier control, using a small power burr introduced through a tiny medial and lateral stab wound.

The procedure remains controversial because it is new and the results are as yet short-term. Long-term results are required because even open Phemister epiphysiodesis does not always succeed in closing the growth plate. Hemifailure (one side closes while the other does not) results in varus or valgus deformity. Thus, the percutaneous method must be carefully studied to confirm its predictability.

In addition, the surgeon's hands may be exposed to substantial irradiation since the procedure is performed under image-intensifier control.

Finally, many surgeons who prefer traditional Phemister

epiphysiodesis claim that their procedure can be performed through incisions of 2 cm or less.

Limb Lengthening

Many recently developed methods have provided controversy concerning the best method of lengthening a limb in a child (or adult). All methods for limb lengthening are complex and require extensive experience as well as intense attention to detail to achieve predictable results.

The Wagner technique of mid-diaphyseal lengthening has been the standard, allowing lengthening of as much as 15% of the original bone length (femur, 6 cm; tibia, 5 cm). This method requires a minimum of three operations (apparatus applied, fixation plate and bone grafting, and plate removal several years later) and relies on large Schanz pins that require great attention if skin problems and/or pintract infections are to be avoided.

Recently, newer methods have become popular. Physeal distraction (chondrodiastasis) requires long-term pin fixation very near a joint. This technique remains controversial and is not widely used in North America.

In contrast, the "callotasis" method described by De Bastiani and associates of gradual lengthening via a metaphyseal osteotomy, at a rate slow enough to allow callus formation in the distracted site, has quickly achieved wide acceptance. The advantages over Wagner's method are significant in that bone grafting, plate fixation, plate removal, and the complications of plate removal (late fracture) are avoided.

Ilizarov developed a limb-lengthening method that includes percutaneous metaphyseal corticotomy (cortex cut and medullary canal and medullary blood supply left intact) followed by gradual lengthening via thin proximal and distal K-wires attached to circumferential metal hoops (Fig. 5). The limb is slowly lengthened, allowing callus to form in the gap. Ilizarov and his colleagues claim a new understanding of the biology of lengthening, not only of bone but of soft tissues (especially nerves and vessels) as well.

The biologic principles of the callotasis performed by De Bastiani and associates and the Ilizarov methods are similar (slow lengthening, metaphyseal osteotomy, no plating required); however, the Ilizarov method has the advantage of using many very small K-wire transfixation pins, with fewer associated skin problems and infections. In addition, the complex circumferential hoop system allows simultaneous correction of rotational and angular deformities. In contrast, the callotasis method uses a typical external fixator with large Schanz-type pins (as in Wagner's method) that more readily become infected. The Ilizarov method has so far been used primarily in teaching centers because of its extreme complexity. It requires great technical prowess and long operating room times for correct application.

Both Russian and Italian investigators have applied their method to achondroplastic dwarfs, reporting a 30% increase in lower-limb length in some patients (De Bastiani and associates). The method remains controversial because lengthening of such magnitude carries an increased risk for morbidity (neurovascular, foot drop, joint dislocation) and these children still appear disproportionate unless the upper extremities are also lengthened. The psychological stress associated with this complicated, lengthy treatment is great. Despite these difficulties, many North American dwarfs have gone to Europe for limb lengthening. The few American centers that have begun this controversial treatment method are proceeding with great caution.

Annotated Bibliography

Keywords

Blount's disease; Congenital pseudarthrosis; Femoral deficiency; Fibula; Genu valgum; Genu varum; Hemimelia; Limb lengthening; Lyme arthritis; Osteochondritis dissecans; Osteomyelitis; Tibia vara

Congenital Abnormalities

Crawford AH Jr, Bagamery N: Osseous manifestations of neurofibromatosis in childhood. *J Pediatr Orthop* 1986;6:72–88.

This is a comprehensive review of neurofibromatosis that clearly analyzes current treatment and results of skeletal abnormalities associated with the condition.

Herring JA, Barnhill B, Gaffney C: Syme amputation: An evaluation of the physical and psychological function in young patients. *J Bone Joint Surg* 1986;68A:573–578.

Cybex testing, functional evaluation, and psychological testing demonstrated that, in a well-adjusted family, the athletic and psychological function of a child with Syme's amputation and a prosthesis closely approaches that of a nonhandicapped child of the same age.

Kalamchi A, Dawe RV: Congenital deficiency of the tibia. *J Bone Joint Surg* 1985;67B:581–584.

The authors provide a new classification that correlates well with treatment recommendations. Type I is total absence, type II is distal absence, and type III is distal absence with tibiofibular diastasis.

Loder RT, Herring JA: Fibular transfer for congenital absence of the tibia: A reassessment. *J Pediatr Orthop* 1987;7:8–13.

Early follow-up of six patients (nine knees) treated with the Baron procedure (fibula transfer) indicated fair results; however, at final follow-up (20 to 123 months), all had failed. The authors now advise knee disarticulation for severe tibial hemimelia.

Minami A, Ogino T, Sakuma T, et al: Free vascularized fibular grafts in the treatment of congenital pseudarthrosis of the tibia. *Microsurgery* 1987;8:111–116.

Three of five cases achieved union after a free vascularized fibular graft. Most cases developed fractures after union had been achieved. The authors conclude that several unresolved problems remain with this new method.

Paterson DC, Simonis RB: Electrical stimulation in the treatment of congenital pseudarthrosis of the tibia. *J Bone Joint Surg* 1985;67B:454–462.

The authors report early union in 20 of 27 cases in which classic surgery (excision of pathologic tissue, intramedullary fixation, bone grafting) was augmented by an implantable electrical stimulator. This report must be viewed critically because late recurrence is common in congenital pseudarthrosis.

Steel HH, Lin PS, Betz RR, et al: Iliofemoral fusion for proximal femoral focal deficiency. *J Bone Joint Surg* 1987;69A:837–843.

The authors advise fusion of the extremely shortened femoral stump to the ilium with the original knee, now at the level of triradiate cartilage, functioning as a hip. Patients who underwent Syme's amputation functioned better than those who underwent Van Ness rotationplasty (foot maintained and reversed to function as a "knee" in the prosthesis).

Thomas IH, Williams PF: The Gruca operation for congenital absence of the fibula. *J Bone Joint Surg* 1987; 69B:587–592.

The authors achieved satisfactory results in eight of nine patients with the Gruca method, in which the distal tibia is split vertically (through the physis) and the tilted talus placed in the newly created ankle. They recommend this foot-sparing method for all bilateral cases and for moderately involved unilateral cases when the surgeon or family is hesitant about Syme's amputation.

Angular Deformities of the Tibia

Beck CL, Burke SW, Roberts JM, et al: Physeal bridge resection in infantile Blount disease. *J Pediatr Orthop* 1987;7:161–163.

The authors describe three cases of infantile Blount's disease (Langenskiold VI with bony bar formed) corrected by bridge excision and placement of a fat graft. Their finding may have been somewhat optimistic because others have had difficulty reproducing these results.

Beskin JL, Burke SW, Johnston CE II, et al: Clinical basis for a mechanical etiology in adolescent Blount's disease. *Orthopedics* 1986;9:365–370.

This is a clear analysis, applying Heuter-Volkmann and Delpech's laws, explaining the growth abnormalities in adolescent tibia vara.

Loder RT, Johnston CE II: Infantile tibia vara. *J Pediatr Orthop* 1987;7:639–646.

Infantile Blount's disease is often rapidly progressive at an earlier age than expected. Also, brace treatment is often ineffective and early osteotomy is advised.

Robert M, Khouri N, Carlioz H, et al: Fractures of the proximal tibial metaphysis in children: Review of a series of 25 cases. *J Pediatr Orthop* 1987;7:444–449.

The authors noted recurrence of the deformity after attempted corrective osteotomy; therefore, they advise that time be allowed for spontaneous correction. The deformity, if still present, can be corrected by medial tibial epiphysiodesis in adolescence.

Zionts LE, MacEwen GD: Spontaneous improvement of post-traumatic tibia valga. *J Bone Joint Surg* 1986;68A: 680–687.

Valgus may worsen until one year after surgery but then spontaneously improves in most cases (six of seven in this series). Early corrective osteotomy should be avoided.

Abnormalities of the Knee

Eiskjaer S, Larsen ST: Arthroscopy of the knee in children. *Acta Orthop Scand* 1987;58:273–276.

The authors performed arthroscopy in 174 consecutive patients less than 18 years old and concluded that diagnostic arthroscopy is accurate in children's knee disorders.

Mesgarzadeh M, Sapega AA, Bonakdarpour A, et al: Osteochondritis dissecans: Analysis of mechanical stability with radiography, scintigraphy, and MR imaging. *Radiology* 1987;165:775–780.

The authors clearly demonstrate the value of magnetic resonance imaging in the evaluation of osteochondritis dissecans abnormalities of the knee.

Polakoff DR, Bucholz RW, Ogden A: Tension band wiring of displaced tibial tuberosity fractures in adolescents. *Clin Orthop* 1986;209:161–165.

In this report of 12 adolescent boys wih avulsion fractures of the tibial tubercle, the authors found that five had prior Osgood-Schlatter disease. They conclude that adolescents with active Osgood-Schlatter disease be restricted from jumping sports.

Joint Sepsis and Osteomyelitis

Canale ST, Harkness RM, Thomas PA, et al: Does aspiration of bones and joints affect results of later bone scanning? *J Pediatr Orthop* 1985;5:23–26.

This animal model demonstrated that needle aspiration of the hip joint never produces an iatrogenic false-positive scan. Similarly, metaphyseal drilling did not produce a positive scan when the scan was performed within two days of the drilling.

Culp RW, Eichenfield AH, Davidson RS, et al: Lyme arthritis in children: An orthopaedic perspective. *J Bone Joint Surg* 1987;69A:96–99.

In 43 children with clinical and serologic evidence of Lyme arthritis, arthritis was the presenting feature in more than one half the cases. Also, 50% of the children had initially been examined by orthopaedic surgeons, none of whom made the correct diagnosis.

Gamble JG, Rinsky LA: Chronic recurrent multifocal osteomyelitis: A distinct clinical entity. *J Pediatr Orthop* 1986;6:579–584.

In five cases of this puzzling chronic and recurrent condition, antibiotics and repeat biopsy of drainage were not helpful. The condition eventually resolves.

Herndon WA, Knauer S, Sullivan JA, et al: Management of septic arthritis in children. *J Pediatr Orthop* 1986;6:576–578.

In this report of treatment of joint sepsis in joints other than the hip in 45 children (49 joints), 34 joints were successfully treated by aspiration and antibiotics. The remainder required arthrotomy after failing to respond to nonsurgical treatment.

Skyhar MJ, Mubarak SJ: Arthroscopic treatment of septic knees in children. *J Pediatr Orthop* 1987;7:647–651.

The authors demonstrate that arthroscopic lavage with drainage provides results equal to those of open arthrotomy.

Wilson NI, Di Paola M: Acute septic arthritis in infancy and childhood: 10 years' experience. *J Bone Joint Surg* 1986;68B:584–587.

After reviewing 61 cases treated by joint aspiration and antibiotics, the authors believe that arthrotomy should be selective and nonmandatory. They still advise arthrotomy for the hip in younger children.

Trauma

Baxter MP, Wiley JJ: Fractures of the tibial spine in children: An evaluation of knee stability. *J Bone Joint Surg* 1988;70B:228–230.

In this review of 45 patients followed up for three to ten years after injury, the authors found some degree of anterior cruciate laxity and lack of full knee extension in many patients, even when anatomic reduction had been achieved.

Letts M, Vincent N, Gouw G: The "floating knee" in children. *J Bone Joint Surg* 1986;68B:442–446.

In this review of 15 patients with combined severe femoral and tibial fractures caused by motor-vehicle accidents, the authors found that open reduction and internal fixation of at least one of the fractures greatly facilitated treatment.

Limb-Length Inequality

Altongy JF, Harcke HT, Bowen JR: Measurement of leg length inequalities by Micro-Dose digital radiographs. *J Pediatr Orthop* 1987;7:311–316.

The authors describe a microdose digital scan that can be used to determine limb length accurately. The method requires 1% of the radiation dose used for conventional arthroroentgenograms.

Canale ST, Russell TA, Holcomb RL: Percutaneous epiphysiodesis: Experimental study and preliminary clinical results. *J Pediatr Orthop* 1986;6:150–156.

In this laboratory and clinical study (13 children) of percutaneous epiphysiodesis, the authors noted that their follow-up was short and that their patients must be followed up until growth plate closure to confirm efficacy and predictability.

De Bastiani G, Aldegheri R, Renzi-Brivio L, et al: Limb lengthening by callus distraction (callotasis). *J Pediatr Orthop* 1987;7:129–134.

The authors describe the currently widely accepted gradual distraction method via metaphyseal osteotomy. The authors report their results in 83 patients, 23 of whom had achondroplasia.

Huurman WW, Jacobsen FS, Anderson JC, et al: Limb-length discrepancy measured with computerized axial tomographic equipment. *J Bone Joint Surg* 1987;69A: 699–705.

The authors describe an accurate method of documenting limb length with less radiation exposure than is required for conventional scanograms.

Paley D: Current techniques of limb lengthening. *J Pediatr Orthop* 1988;8:73–92.

This comprehensive, completely referenced review describes theoretical and practical aspects of all current limb-lengthening methods.

Controversies

Managing Knee Sepsis

Herndon WA, Knauer S, Sullivan JA, et al: Management of septic arthritis in children. *J Pediatr Orthop* 1986;6:576–578.

Skyhar MJ, Mubarak SJ: Arthroscopic treatment of septic knees in children. *J Pediatr Orthop* 1987;7:647–651.

Wilson NI, Di Paola M: Acute septic arthritis in infancy and childhood: 10 years' experience. *J Bone Joint Surg* 1986;68B:584–587.

Duration of Intravenous Antibiotic Treatment in Children

Nelson JD, Bucholz RW, Kusmiesz H, et al: Benefits and risks of sequential parenteral-oral cephalosporin therapy for suppurative bone and joint infections. *J Pediatr Orthop* 1982;2:255–262.

Tetzlaff TR, Howard JB, McCracken GH Jr, et al: Antibiotic concentrations in pus and bone of children with osteomyelitis. *J Pediatr* 1978;92:135–140.

Tetzlaff TR, McCracken GH Jr, Thomas ML: Bioavailability of cephalexin in children: Relationship to drug formulations and meals. *J Pediatr* 1978;92:292–294.

Percutaneous Epiphysiodesis

Canale ST, Russell TA, Holcomb RL: Percutaneous

epiphysiodesis: Experimental study and preliminary clinical results. *J Pediatr Orthop* 1986;6:150–156.

Limb Lengthening

De Bastiani G, Aldegheri R, Renzi-Brivio L, et al: Limb lengthening by callus distraction (callotasis). *J Pediatr Orthop* 1987;7:129–134.

Paley D: Current techniques of limb lengthening. *J Pediatr Orthop* 1988;8:73–92.

43

Knee and Leg: Soft-Tissue Trauma

Advances in the management of knee injuries include improved diagnosis of soft-tissue injuries, a better understanding of the natural history of these injuries, and improved surgical techniques for achieving anatomic restoration of injured structures.

Diagnosis of Ligament Disruption

Disruption of a ligament alters the limits of joint motion. The motion resulting from a clinical test depends on the position of the limb at the initiation of the test, the force applied, the point of application of the force, and the point of detection of the displacement. For example, both the anterior cruciate ligament (ACL) and the posterior cruciate ligament (PCL) limit the total anteroposterior displacement of the tibia. PCL disruption results in greater posterior displacement of the tibia from its anatomic resting position; ACL disruption allows greater anterior displacement. To determine which structure or structures are disrupted, the clinician must be able to determine the neutral position.

The neutral position can be determined when the patient is lying supine with the knee flexed 90 degrees. The neutral position is the resting position of the tibia supported by the intact PCL. The resting position of the injured knee must be compared with that of the contralateral normal knee. If the PCL is disrupted, the tibia sags posteriorly. This sagging can be seen by looking at the distorted knee profile, palpated by feeling the posterior displacement of the tibia on the femoral condyle, and confirmed by noting that contraction of the quadriceps pulls the tibia anteriorly (Fig. 1). In the coronal plane, the neutral position for varus-valgus tests is the position in which the normal medial and lateral joint surfaces are in contact. The joint's axial-rotation neutral position has not been defined with precision. The rotational position of the tibia can be determined by reference to the tibial tubercle, the malleolar axis, and the foot, but the precise rotational position of the femur cannot be determined. Therefore, when axial-rotation tests are performed, the axis around which the joint is rotating is difficult to discern. For example, assume that there is an increased amount of tibial external rotation. This motion may be secondary to anterior subluxation of the medial tibial plateau (secondary to injuries to anteromedial structures), posterior subluxation of the lateral tibial plateau (secondary to injuries to the posterolateral structures), or both. The relative displacement of each of the tibial plateaus in relation to the femoral condyles can be evaluated manually or, more precisely, with lateral stress radiographs.

Table 1 summarizes the principal capsular and ligamentous structures around the knee, along with the alterations in motion limits that are most diagnostic of an isolated disruption. When a ligament is sectioned or disrupted, the limits of knee motion are determined by the remaining structures; these structures have been termed the secondary restraints. A ligament can be a primary restraint to one motion and a secondary restraint to another. For example, the medial collateral ligament (MCL) is the primary restraint to valgus angulation when the knee is in 30 degrees of flexion. Sectioning the MCL does not affect anterior displacement, which is controlled by the ACL. However, if the ACL is disrupted, the MCL is one of the structures that limit anterior displacement. If the MCL is then disrupted, anterior tibial displacement increases.

It is important to note that the amount of increased motion resulting from disruption of a single structure varies considerably from specimen to specimen and from patient to patient. For example, in the laboratory, 20-lb anterior-displacement tests with the KT-2000 revealed that sectioning the ACL increases motion 3 to 13 mm (Fig. 2). In another study, 20-lb anterior-displacement tests with the KT-1000 in 136 anesthetized patients with acute ACL disruption and no other apparent ligamentous disruptions demonstrated a right-left difference ranging from 0 to 12 mm (mean, 4.3 mm).

A thigh support to position the knees in 20 to 30 degrees of flexion is recommended to standardize the knee's flexion position for a varus-valgus stress test, an anterior-displacement test in early flexion, or an axial-rotation measurement (Fig. 3). Figure 4 shows the International Knee Documentation Committee's recommended techniques for performing a number of clinical tests. A manually detected right-left displacement difference or a perceived difference in end-point stiffness is indicative of ligament injury. On instrumented or stress radiographic measurements, a right-left difference of 3 mm or more is indicative of a ligament injury.

Ligament injury can be diagnosed with more than 90% accuracy by an experienced clinician using a manual examination, instrumented measurement, or stress radiographs. These examinations also provide the clinician with the abnormal motion measurements that are one factor guiding management decisions. Recently, magnetic resonance imaging has been used to diagnose ligament disruptions but this technique is seldom necessary.

The Natural History of Knee Ligament Injuries

Medial Collateral Ligament

An isolated MCL injury heals satisfactorily without surgical intervention. Treatment with a hinged cast or brace for three to six weeks may be indicated, depending on the amount of pathologic valgus motion, to prevent valgus angulation. Unless there is excessive valgus alignment that

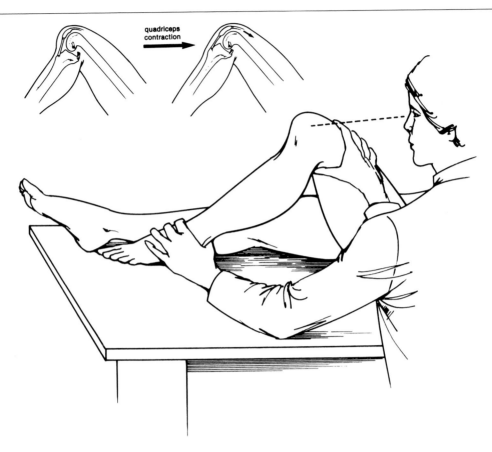

Figure 1

The 90-degree quadriceps active test. Keeping the eyes at the level of the subject's flexed knee, the examiner rests an elbow on the table and uses the ipsilateral hand to support the subject's thigh and to confirm that the thigh muscles are relaxed. The foot is stabilized by the examiner's other hand, and the subject is asked to slide the foot gently down the table. Anterior tibial displacement resulting from the quadriceps contraction indicates a PCL injury.

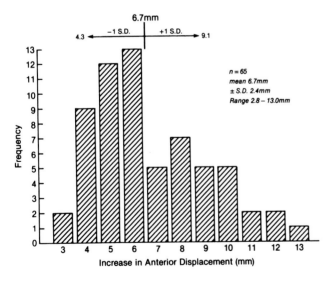

Figure 2

Increase in anterior tibial displacement after ACL sectioning in cadaveric specimens. The test instrument was the KT-2000.

Table 1. Primary clinical limits of motion tests

Test	Isolated Injuries*				
	ACL	PCL	MCL	LCL	PLC
Lachman	Yes	—	—	—	—
Pivot shift	Yes	—	—	—	—
Tibial posterior subluxation	—	Yes	—	—	—
Abduction (25 degrees)	—	—	Yes	—	—
Adduction (25 degrees)	—	—	—	Yes	—
Reverse pivot shift	—	—	—	—	Yes

would place a valgus stress on the knee, weightbearing can be permitted.

Lateral Ligamentous Complex

Disruption of the lateral ligamentous complex is usually associated with a cruciate ligament injury. The lateral injury may be associated with a posterolateral corner (arcuate complex and popliteus tendon) injury that is difficult to diagnose unless the patient is examined while under anesthesia. In a complete lateral complex injury, surgical exploration and repair are recommended.

Posterior Cruciate Ligament

The ratio of PCL injuries to ACL injuries in the general population is about one to ten. The injury is not usually

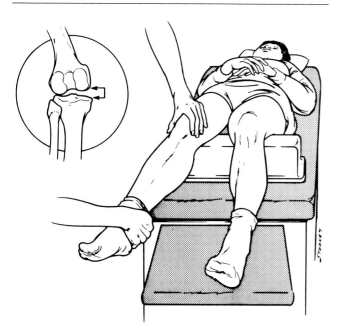

Figure 3
Patient supine with the thigh supported in 25 degrees of flexion.

associated with meniscal injuries, but may be associated with articular cartilage injury. Repairs of a midsubstance tear of the PCL have not been successful and reconstructions have been inconsistently successful. Many patients with an isolated PCL disruption are only modestly impaired and may return to sports activity. With the tibia displaced posteriorly, the posterior horns of the menisci are not loaded, which increases the load on the articular cartilage. As the tibia is pulled forward by the quadriceps from the posteriorly displaced position, there is increased shear stress on the hyaline cartilage. Both of these pathologic conditions probably contribute to the high incidence of degenerative arthritis of the patellofemoral articulation and the medial compartment of the knee observed in long-term PCL injury. If a PCL is avulsed with a bone fragment, surgical repair is recommended. In an isolated PCL injury, in the absence of a bone avulsion, the evidence is insufficient at this time to prove that surgical treatment is superior to nonsurgical treatment.

Anterior Cruciate Ligament

The most common disabling knee injury in athletes is ACL disruption. In the general population, 70% of ACL injuries are sustained during sports activities, specifically sports that involve jumping and cutting or those that use shoes with cleats or attach the foot to a ski. Most single-ligament ACL injuries do not involve contact with another player. The patient with an acute ACL injury also has a hemarthrosis. The patient with an acute traumatic hemarthrosis in the absence of a demonstrable fracture or patellar injury has a 70% chance of having an ACL injury. About 50% of patients with acute ACL disruption have an associated meniscus tear; however, many of these lesions are small tears that require neither excision nor repair. ACL disruption in children less than 12 years old is usually accompanied by avulsion of the tibial spine.

The natural course of the knee with an ACL injury varies.

Multiple-Ligament Injury

An evaluation of the knee with injuries to multiple ligaments includes a careful evaluation of the neurovascular

Tests of Motion Limits
International Knee Documentation Committee

| Force[1] | | | | Moment[1] | | | | Measurement Site[2] | Displacement Measured[3] | Knee Flexion Position | | |
Ant	Post	Med	Lat	IR	ER	Valgus	Varus			25°	90°
++								TT (1)	Anterior	_____	_____
++						+		MC (2)	Anterior	_____	_____
++					+			LC (3)	Anterior	_____	_____
	++							TT (1)	Posterior	_____	_____
	++					+		MC (2)	Posterior	_____	_____
	++				+			LC (3)	Posterior	_____	_____
										0°	25°
				−	−	++		MC (4)	Medial JSO[4]	_____	_____
				−	−		++	LC (5)	Lateral JSO[4]	_____	_____

[1] ++ = *primary force/moment*
+ = *secondary moment to maximize displacement*
− = *motion constrained*

no mark indicates motion unconstrained

[2] *Measurement site noted on knee figure*

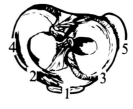

[3] *Millimeters of displacement (measured or estimated) from the anatomic supine resting position.*

[4] *Joint space opening referenced from joint surface contact position.*

Figure 4
Displacements are estimated or measured for each knee and the right-left difference calculated. TT, tibial tubercule; MC, medial compartment; LC, lateral compartment.

status of the limb. Anterior dislocation of the tibia in relation to the femur may cause traction injuries to the vessels; posterior dislocations may cause complete tears of these structures. The vascular injury may result in an intimal tear and/or an intraluminal thrombus with compromised circulation developing immediately or days after the injury. If there is a definite history of joint dislocation or if the patient has an injury to both cruciates and a collateral ligament and there is any suggestion of vascular compromise, an arteriogram is recommended. In the young active patient, the recommended management of the disrupted ligaments is surgical repair or reconstruction. When both cruciate ligaments are disrupted they are frequently avulsed with bone and can be repaired. Injuries to the posterolateral ligamentous complex, especially in association with a PCL injury, are especially disabling and should be repaired. A knee that has undergone surgical repair of multiple ligaments is at especially high risk for stiffness after surgery. To avoid this complication, surgical repairs should be as secure as possible so that an early postoperative passive motion program can be initiated.

Ligament Repair and Reconstruction

The goal of knee ligament surgery is to establish the normal limits of knee motion. After each damaged structure is repaired or reconstructed, the knee should be moved through 0 to 120 degrees of flexion to confirm that joint flexion and extension have not been restricted. Disruption of repaired or reconstructed structures when the knee is placed through a flexion arc reveals that the position and/or amount of tension is incorrect. Optimally, the strength of graft repairs and reconstructions allows gentle testing of the limits of knee motion at the conclusion of the surgical procedure as well as the institution of an early passive motion program.

The morbidity of ligament surgery is associated with the extent of surgical dissection required to expose injured structures, graft harvest, graft implantation, and restriction of limb function to protect the graft during the healing process. The surgical dissection should be minimized exposing only those ligamentous structures that will benefit significantly from surgical repair. Midsubstance repairs of injured ligaments have not been demonstrated to be of benefit. Healing of a midsubstance tear of the MCL is not improved by surgery. Reports on the results for cruciate ligaments with repaired midsubstance tears are mixed. A midsubstance repair without augmentation with a ligament graft has poor tensile strength and is at risk for disruption with an early motion program.

Ligament surgery, therefore, consists principally of repairing avulsed ligament structures and reconstructing midsubstance disruptions of the cruciate ligaments. Important technical aspects of surgery are graft selection and placement, prefixation tension, and soft-tissue fixation.

Graft Selection

Ligaments have been reconstructed with biologic tissues (autograft, xenograft, and allograft), synthetic materials, and combinations of these. Experience with material other than autograft tissue is limited and at this time should be considered experimental. The most frequently used autograft tissues are the semitendinosus tendon, a portion of the patellar tendon, and a portion of the distal iliotibial

tract. Factors to consider in selecting an autograft are the tissue's mechanical characteristics (strength and stiffness), potential for graft fixation, and the morbidity of tissue harvest and tissue loss. There is a considerable loss of tissue strength after graft implantation and, therefore, it is desirable to begin with a graft stronger than the tissue to be replaced. A graft with attached bone, such as the patellar tendon, provides greater strength at the fixation site. The morbidity of graft harvest must also be considered. The incidence of anterior knee pain, knee flexion contracture, and extensor weakness is greater one year after ACL surgery in cases in which more than one third of the patellar tendon was harvested than in cases in which a hamstring graft was harvested.

Graft Placement

Reconstruction of the cruciate ligaments consists of replacing a complex ligamentous structure with a cord of tissue or a prosthetic device. Within each of the cruciate ligaments there is a hypothetical neutral fiber that remains at almost constant length with passive knee motion. It is probably best to center the graft at the attachment sites of this hypothetical fiber to minimize length changes in the fibers anterior and posterior to the neutral fiber. The surgical technique for achieving this goal is to drill 2- to 4-mm pilot holes in the tibial and femoral attachment sites and then to measure the change in length between these attachment sites as the knee is passed through a range of motion (Fig. 5). If flexion of the joint increases the distance between attachment sites, then the course of the graft is anterior to the flexion axes. If the distance between attachment sites decreases with joint flexion, then the course of the graft is posterior to the flexion axes (Fig. 6). Optimum placement of the pilot holes results in 2- to 3-mm decrease in attachment site distance as the knee is flexed from 0 to 90 degrees.

Graft Tension

Most authors have stated the need to apply some tension on the graft at the time of fixation. Tension can be sustained for a time before fixation to precondition the graft. The relationship between the tension applied and joint stability depends on the length of the graft and the graft's stiffness. The precise relationship between the graft's tension at surgery and follow-up displacement measurements and knee function is unknown.

Graft Fixation

For a number of weeks after surgery, the weak links in the repaired or reconstructed ligament are probably the points of fixation. An autograft can resist 1,000 to 2,000 N of force whereas initial fixation resistance is 50 to 500 N. Strength at the attachment site decreases during the early stages of wound healing and then gradually increases until it exceeds graft strength. The surgeon should try to achieve maximum fixation strength, especially if the rehabilitation program includes an early motion program. Bone plugs with interference screws or heavy sutures passed through bone holes in the bone plug and then tied around a screw or through a button provide good fixation (Fig. 7). Soft tissue can be securely fixed to bone with a screw and spiked washer (Fig. 8) or with an interlocking heavy suture passed through the tissue and tied to a screw or button. Staple fixation of soft tissue is less secure.

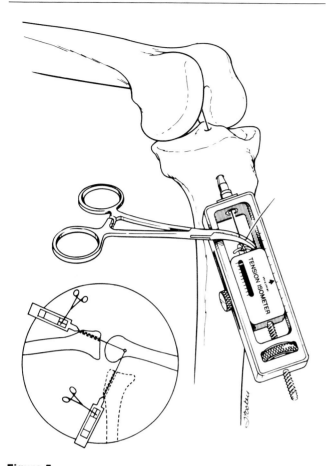

Figure 5

An isometer is used to measure the change in distance between the suture attachment sites from 0 to 90 degrees of flexion.

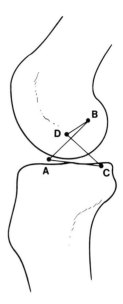

Figure 6

Kinematics of the knee in the sagittal plane can be modeled as a four-bar linkage assuming that a neutral fiber in each ligament remains isometric throughout flexion. AB represents the ACL "neutral fiber" and CD the PCL "neutral fiber." The instant center of flexion (flexion axis) is at the intersection of the two cruciate ligament links.

Graft Impingement

Bone tunnels should be oriented and fashioned to minimize impingement of the graft against bone. Entrances into bone tunnels should be chamfered. The anterior portal of the intercondylar notch may require enlargement to prevent graft impingement as the knee passes into extension. The normal ACL splays out as it inserts on the tibia. If a graft site is selected at the anterior attachment site of a normal ACL, the intercondylar notch will impinge superiorly on the graft as the knee goes into extension unless the notch is enlarged.

Arthroscopic Cruciate Ligament Surgery

Arthroscopic treatment of cruciate ligaments may decrease the surgical morbidity of certain procedures. For example, when a semitendinosus graft is used to reconstruct the ACL, it is less traumatic when the graft tunnels are prepared and the graft passed under arthroscopic observation than with an arthrotomy. In contrast, when a middle-third patellar tendon graft is used, there is little difference in joint morbidity between arthroscopic graft placement and operating through the patellar tendon defect. Further, direct visualization through the patellar tendon defect allows optimum evaluation of graft impingement on the apex of the intercondylar notch as the knee goes into extension.

Rehabilitation

The goal of the rehabilitation program is to reestablish full joint motion and muscle function quickly without disrupting repaired or reconstructed ligamentous structures. In developing a rehabilitation program, the surgeon must consider graft placement and strength and muscle-ligament interaction.

If grafts are placed so that the distance between attachment sites is constant throughout the flexion arc, passive motion places little strain on the graft. However, if the distance between graft attachment sites changes by more than 10% percent with joint motion, flexion or extension is limited or the graft will stretch or become disrupted. If the graft fails immediately after surgery, it will be at the attachment sites. As the attachment sites heal, the weak section of the graft is the revascularizing graft tissue, which takes months to remodel in animal models.

The pull of tendons crossing the knee joint can place an anterior or posterior displacing force on the joint; this is resisted by the cruciate ligaments. In early flexion, the pull of the patellar tendon results in an anterior vector, thus loading the ACL. Beyond 90 degrees of flexion, the pull is posterior and the PCL is loaded. The pull of the hamstrings is posterior when the knee is flexed beyond 15 degrees, thus loading the PCL. After ACL grafting, therefore, quadriceps exercises should be performed with the knee flexed beyond 45 degrees in the early postoperative period. After a PCL reconstruction, hamstring exercises should not be performed in the early postoperative period.

Knee Braces

Several types of knee orthosis are commercially available.

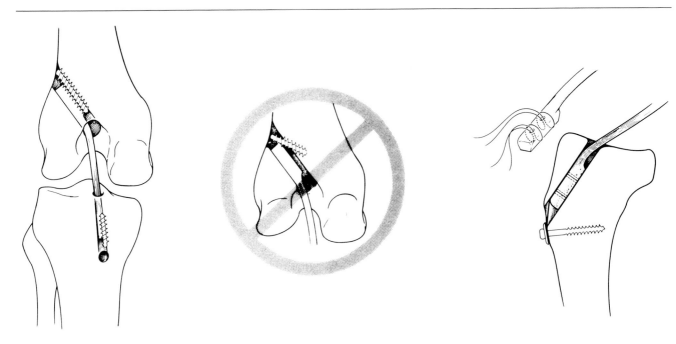

Figure 7
Patellar tendon graft fixation. **Left**, Interference screw technique. **Center**, Screw diverges, providing inferior fixation. **Right**, Suture fixation.

Prophylactic Braces

No knee brace has been shown to protect the normal knee against ACL injury. Several investigators have studied a single-sided hinge brace in an attempt to reduce the incidence of MCL injuries sustained in football. The routine use of prophylactic knee braces currently available has not reduced the number or severity of knee injuries. In some circumstances, such braces may even contribute to injury.

Functional Braces

Functional knee braces are used to limit functional instability. Functional braces have been recommended for patients with abnormal knee motion secondary to ligament disruptions and for patients who have undergone knee ligament surgery. The proposed mechanisms of action are a mechanical constraint of joint motion and improvement in joint position sense (proprioception). Many patients state they feel more secure in a functional knee brace. Instrumented measurement of anterior subluxation of patients with an ACL brace revealed a reduction of joint subluxation at low loads and less effect at moderate loads. It has not been demonstrated that the braces can control posterior joint subluxation or axial rotation. There is no evidence that functional knee braces decrease the incidence of knee injury.

The Meniscus

The fibrocartilaginous structures between the femur and tibia are composed of collagen and a proteoglycan. The collagen fibers are oriented in a circumferential manner that allows the meniscus to withstand tensile loading. This arrangement of collagen fibers allows the translation of vertical compressive load into circumferential or hoop stresses. The meniscus increases joint congruency, stabi-lizes the joint, and improves nutrition and lubrication of the articular cartilage. The menisci transmit between 50% and 70% of the load applied across the knee during axial loading.

The meniscus receives its nutrition from the joint fluid and from its peripheral vascular supply. The vascular supply depends on age. In a newborn, 50% of the periphery of the meniscus is vascularized but by the age of 40 to 60 years vascularization decreases to less than 20% of the total area of the meniscus. India ink injection studies have demonstrated that the peripheral 2 to 3 mm of meniscus does have a vascular supply. Recent measurements of meniscal blood flow with the laser Doppler indicate more vascularity than previously reported. As these investigations proceed in animal models, more confidence may be placed in a more aggressive approach to meniscal repair.

The presurgical diagnosis of meniscal tears is primarily by history and physical examination. A variety of noninvasive methods have been used to confirm the clinical impression of meniscal tear. These include computed tomography and magnetic resonance imaging, the newest noninvasive tool for evaluating the integrity of the menisci. Magnetic resonance imaging is more expensive than other imaging techniques and its accuracy is variable. One cadaver study showed that the results of magnetic resonance imaging are similar to those of conventional arthrography. In clinical studies, computed tomography and magnetic resonance imaging have similar accuracy rates. Magnetic resonance imaging may miss internal derangement such as articular cartilage defects and small loose bodies while overestimating meniscal lesions. Grading meniscal lesions according to the signal intensity improves accuracy and decreases false-positive findings. Grades I and II lesions are intrameniscal and are not usually treated surgically. These lesions are found on magnetic resonance imaging of nonsymptomatic knees; their incidence increases with age. Grade III meniscal lesions are those that penetrate the meniscal surface and can be confirmed visually at surgery. The results of magnetic resonance imaging depend on interpretation. Only if the clinician learns to interpret the findings by correlating the images with surgical findings will magnetic resonance imaging become a dependable tool for identifying patients who require surgical treatment. More experience and decreased costs are necessary before magnetic resonance imaging is used routinely to evaluate meniscal problems.

The meniscus has an important role in weightbearing and transmission of axial load and thus spares articular cartilage. Clinical and animal studies confirm the increased potential for osteoarthritis after meniscectomy. In patients with ACL instability, complete meniscectomy increases instability as well as symptoms. Every effort should be made to maintain the integrity of the menisci. Partial meniscectomy offers a rapid return to activity with minimal short-term morbidity, particularly for patients with bucket-handle or other large-fragment lesions. Patients with complex tears, associated instability, or arthritis may have more problems and have a more difficult postoperative course. The benefit of partial meniscectomy, whether it is done in an open fashion or arthroscopically, appears to be established. Failure of an arthroscopic partial meniscectomy cannot definitely be related to age, the number of previous operations, the duration of symptoms, range of motion, or the amount of degenerative change. Good and excellent results have been reported after a second arthroscopic procedure in cases of mechanical complaints or reinjury.

The success of meniscal repairs at or near the periphery is well established. The focus of investigation is currently on improvement of the healing response within the meniscus body. The techniques, which are all successful to varying degrees, include abrasion of the rim of the tear with a rasp, trephination of the rim, and, most recently, the use of fibrin clot as a scaffold and a chemotactic stimulus for healing. Results in animal models indicate that such additional stimulation may improve healing.

Factors that affect healing include the stability of the knee, coaptation of the edges of the tear, the size of the tear (less than 40 mm), the use of a mechanical or chemical stimulus, and the complexity of the tear. Studies have shown that 62% of repaired menisci heal, 17% heal incompletely, and 21% do not heal. However, 92% of the repaired menisci are clinically stable and 80% of patients return to active sports participation. There is general agreement that results are best in vertical longitudinal tears in the peripheral third of the meniscus. Arthroscopic techniques can be used safely as long as a soft-tissue dissection is done so that the needles can be visualized as they penetrate the posterior capsule.

Meniscal transplantation and meniscal regeneration are experimental techniques at the present time. These concepts have been applied in a limited, investigational setting in humans. The techniques of transplantation, substitution, or regeneration of the meniscus offer opportunities for the future.

Symptomatic Plica

A rare cause of internal derangement of the knee is symptomatic plica or shelf syndrome. About 2% of patients with internal derangement symptoms of the knee have symptomatic plica.

When the symptoms and abnormalities are primarily medial, symptomatic plica is called medial shelf syndrome. The normal synovial folds are suprapatellar, mediopatellar, or lateral patellar. Normal synovial folds become symptomatic because of an acute or repetitive-use injury that leads to inflammation, fibrosis, and impingement on the patella or femoral condyle. The symptoms are those of patellofemoral pain syndrome or internal derangement; they may respond to nonsteroidal anti-inflammatory drugs and quadriceps exercise.

When symptoms persist, the recommended treatment is complete excision. Mild to moderate recurrent pain can be expected because of scar formation in the capsule. The orthopaedist must rule out other potentially more serious problems and confirm this diagnosis by visualizing a fibrotic plica before attributing symptoms to it.

The Patella

Normal function of the patellofemoral joint depends on the interaction of at least four elements: alignment, stability, articular cartilage, and muscles. A formula relating each of these four to the others remains to be developed. It is useful to consider all new information as it relates to each of these four components. The terms malalignment, maltracking, instability, subluxation, dislocation, chondro-

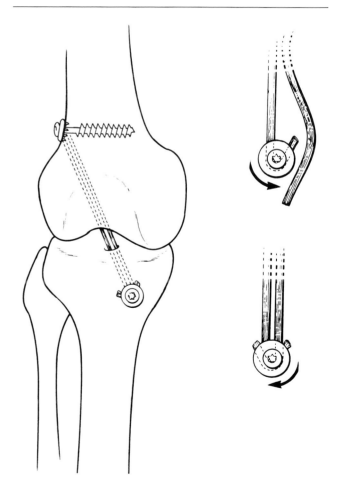

Figure 8
Free semitendinosus tendon fixed with screw and spiked washer.

malacia, and anterior knee pain must be used with precision.

Alignment

Alignment as applied to the patellofemoral joint indicates malposition of the patella on the femur and malposition of the axis of the limb with respect to the trunk and the ground-reaction forces. The presence of excessive femoral anteversion, excessive external tibial torsion, or increased varus or valgus abnormalities has a definite effect on the patellofemoral joint.

Alignment of the patella on the lower extremity should be viewed in three dimensions. The patella can translate along and rotate around three axes: the proximal-distal axis, the mediolateral axis, and the anteroposterior axis (Fig. 9). Rotation about the proximal-distal axis allows the patella to tilt medially or laterally. Rotation about the mediolateral axis allows the patella to flex or extend. Rotation about the anteroposterior axis allows the patella to spin (rotate) medially or laterally (clockwise or counterclockwise). Translation along the proximal-distal axis results in a high or low patella (alta or baja). Translation along the anteroposterior axis places the patella closer to or farther from the knee joint axis, thus increasing or decreasing joint reaction force.

As a result of flexion and extension of the knee, the patella follows a complex motion pattern or track down the femur. Bony constraints largely determine the tracking patterns. During tracking the patella flexes about 20 degrees more than knee flexion, tilts medially 2 to 8 degrees for the first 40 to 90 degrees of knee flexion, then tilts laterally as much as 15 degrees, rotates as much as 20 degrees medially, shifts medially as much as 4 mm, and then shifts laterally as much as 17 mm. This tracking pattern involves patellar flexion, shift, tilt, and spin (rotation). Anteroposterior rotation was found to be absent in 119 consecutive knees with chondropathy. Rotation of the tibia on the femur has been shown to be one of the greatest factors influencing patellar tracking. When the term "maltracking" is used, the variation from this normal pattern should be defined.

Both the congruence angle of Merchant, taken at 45 degrees of knee flexion, and the lateral patellofemoral angle of Laurin, taken at 20 degrees of knee flexion, have been used to demonstrate patellar subluxation radiographically. More recently, computed tomography with the knee in 0 degrees of flexion has been used to show tilt of the patella, which is assumed to represent symptomatic subluxation. Values for congruence angle and patellar tilt angles differ on a computed tomography scan taken at 0 degrees and on an axial view, and normal limits must be defined. Why patients whose radiographs show bilateral patellar subluxation can be symptomatic on only one side is still unknown.

Arthroscopists have evaluated patellofemoral alignment by noting the patella's position in the femoral trochlea. Some have stated that if the median ridge of the patella is seated in the femoral trochlea at 45 degrees of knee flexion, tracking is normal. Others have defined normal as centralization of the patella in the trochlea at 20 or 30 degrees or no overhang of the lateral facet over the lateral condyle. Tilt, flexion, and rotation have not been measured arthroscopically and, in light of the abnormal spin noted radiographically, arthroscopic evaluation of patellofemoral alignment may be incomplete.

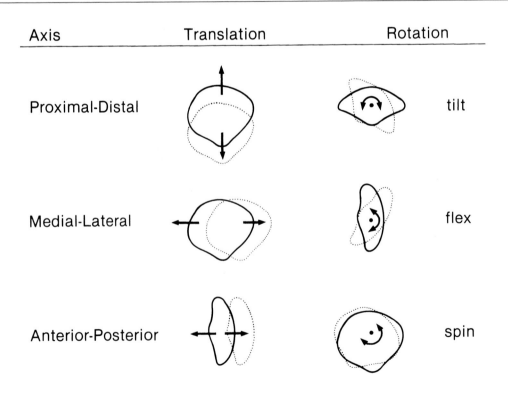

Axis	Translation	Rotation	
Proximal-Distal			tilt
Medial-Lateral			flex
Anterior-Posterior			spin

Figure 9
Patellar motion.

Stability

Stability of the patella on the femur is provided by a combination of bone and ligamentous restraints. The diagnosis of instability should depend on the demonstration of an abnormal displacement of the patella on the femur. The degree of displacement can be estimated clinically or measured with stress radiographs (Fig. 10). The diagnosis of subluxation or instability should not be based on such non-specific, subjective criteria as anterior pain swelling, giving way, difficulty on stairs, theater sign (an inability to sit comfortably for a few hours with the knee flexed), or apprehension with stress. These findings can strongly suggest a patellofemoral disturbance, but are not pathognomonic of patellar instability. A documented history of patellar dislocation is definitive evidence of instability. After nonsurgical treatment, the incidences of recurrent patellar dislocation and continuing patellofemoral symptoms are higher in patients with an anatomic predisposition to dis-

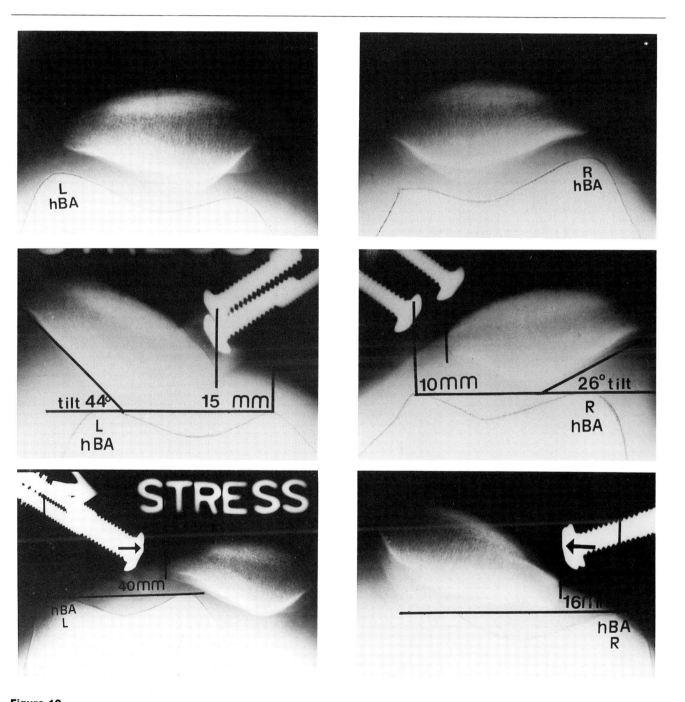

Figure 10

Top, Axial radiographs taken with the Merchant technique show a normal congruence angle and a normal patellofemoral angle. **Center**, Stress radiographs using a quantitative stress device show a 50% (5 mm) increase in lateral excursion of the symptomatic left knee. A difference in lateral tilt is also apparent. **Bottom**, Stress radiographs medially show a complete medial dislocation of the left patella after arthroscopic lateral release.

location than in patients without an anatomic predisposition (43% vs 20% for recurrence and 48% vs 25% for continuing symptoms, respectively). Nonsurgical treatment of recurrent dislocation of the patella has a better outcome than surgery for recurrent subluxation.

Articular Cartilage

Chondromalacia of the patella has been evaluated by electron microscopy and the findings shown to be compatible with injury resulting from mechanical overload. Initially, swelling of the superficial matrix is associated with breakdown of the collagen fiber network, especially in the superficial and transitional zones. Evidence of cellular hyperplasia and hypertrophy is present with only limited repair reaction. Both the thickness and the surface characteristics of the articular cartilage of the patella are readily apparent on computed tomographic scans (Fig. 11). Axial magnetic resonance imaging views also show the patellar articular cartilage but not to greater advantages than contrast-enhanced computed tomography.

A reduction in the surface area of the patella or an imposed load that is higher than normal increases articular cartilage pressure. In one instance, a reduction in the surface area of the patella of 35% was associated with articular degenerative change. The management of chondromalacia remains an enigma. Histologic analysis of patellas removed after shaving of chondromalacia cartilage failed to reveal any evidence of fibrocartilage healing, although one clinical study of arthroscopic shaving reported good or excellent results in 49% of cases. Chondromalacia patellae produced in rabbits by a lateral transfer of the tibial tubercle continued after the tubercle was repositioned six weeks later. Clinical studies have shown that surgery for chondromalacia fails when it does not lead to biomechanical improvement. In another study, realignment operations for anterior knee pain unrelated to instability all failed. As this condition appears to be multifactorial, no specific treatment can yet be recommended.

Other methods used to evaluate arthritis of the patellofemoral joint include bone scanning, interosseous pressure measurements, and thermography. Bone scans sometimes confirm the presence of an isolated unilateral area of uptake in the symptomatic patella, but one study suggested that their sensitivity, specificity, and predictive values are so low that their value is limited. Similarly, interosseous pressure measurements are not specific enough to be of value. Osteotomy of the patella in the coronal plane has been suggested because it reduces the interosseous pressure. Thermograms of osteoathritic or rheumatoid knees may show a diffuse increase in heat; in 28 of 30 athletes with anterior knee pain, there was a temperature increase along the medial border of the patella and radiating into the vastus medialis. Again, sensitivity, specificity, and predictive value remain to be defined.

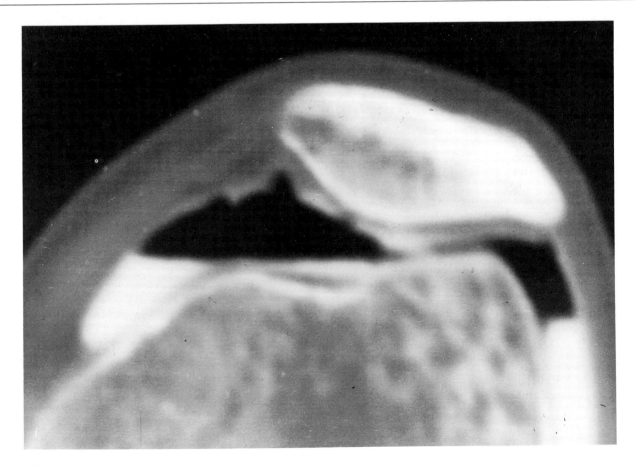

Figure 11

Contrast-enhanced image showing lateral subluxation of the patella and loss of articular cartilage.

Muscle

The knee does not function normally when there is a major deficiency in thigh or calf musculature and it has been assumed that synchronous contraction of the parts of the quadriceps contributes to preventing patellar subluxation. Electromyographic studies of patients with subluxating patellas have shown no evidence of an imbalance in the ratio of vastus medialis activity to vastus lateralis activity. In one study using axial radiographs, it was possible to view centralization of a subluxated patella by contraction of the quadriceps but in other studies using computed tomographic scans quadriceps contraction did not centralize the laterally subluxated patella. In one series, fewer than 23% of patients with either subluxating patellas or chondromalacia patellae improved after quadriceps exercise; in another series, however, symptoms improved in 40%. The value of a strong quadriceps in patellofemoral disorders may be nonspecific and its contribution to the actual stabilization of the unstable patella during activity should be reevaluated.

Treatment

Treatment is best based on an accurate diagnosis, but this is hampered by the difficulty of analyzing all the contributing factors. There is increasing agreement that modification or limitation of activity produces the most consistent improvement in symptoms. Strengthening exercises, stretching exercise of the quadriceps, hamstrings, iliotibial band, and gastrocsoleus muscles, anti-inflammatory medication, knee bracing, either parapatellar or infrapatellar, and foot orthoses have been tried with varying success. Two recent studies reported that patellar symptoms were decreased in 22% and 35% of patients who used braces.

Surgery has been directed at shaving or drilling the articular cartilage, tightening or loosening the medial or lateral retinaculum, advancing the quadriceps muscle, pes transfers, altering the Q angle by tubercle transfer medially, distally, or anteriorly, or a combination of these.

In selected patients, advancement of the tibial tubercle (Maquet or Bandi procedure) yields good results (varying in different reports from a high of 98% of cases to a low of 68%). Anterior displacement results in the contact surface on the patella moving proximally at the same time the contact surface on the femur moves slightly distally. Increasing the elevation makes the contact surface areas of both the patella and femur progressively smaller, decreasing joint reaction forces near knee extension but increasing joint reaction forces with greater knee flexion. An elevation of approximately 1 cm is recommended. Tibial tubercle elevation alters patellar tracking primarily through the great increase in rotational potential. This increases the Q angle on external rotation of the tibia and decreases it on internal rotation. These alterations lead to unpredictable contact areas and occasionally peak pressures that are higher than normal. Osteotomy of the patella, tibia, or femur has a beneficial effect in some cases. The correct approach depends on the contributing factors.

Running Injuries

Running is important in the lives of 20 million North Americans. In 1987 it was estimated that 2.8 million Americans entered at least one race a year and 73,000 finished marathons. The examiner must be familiar with the biomechanical aspects of running, "training errors," orthotic devices, and running footwear. "Overuse" injuries from training errors and/or biomechanical causes remain the bane of the runner's existence. Conservative treatment measures consist of rest, icing, stretching, nonsteroidal anti-inflammatory medications, orthotic devices, and a gradual return to running. Forty percent of the injuries involve the knee, 15% are classified as "shin splint syndrome," 15% are classified as Achilles tendinitis, and 10% involve subcalcaneal pain.

"Patellofemoral pain syndrome" is preferred to "chondromalacia" to describe the peripatellar or anterior knee pain frequently associated with malalignment problems. Chondromalacia is a pathologic term describing histologic evidence of articular damage. This is rare in running problems. Routine diagnostic arthroscopy is inappropriate. Iliotibial band friction syndrome is manifested as lateral knee pain, usually associated with a varus configuration of the tibia, and results from a rapid increase in running speed and distance, often on a banked surface. Symptoms usually occur laterally over the lateral femoral epicondyle, beginning late in the run and becoming severe the next day. Treatment involves stretching, local heat and/or ice, nonsteroidal anti-inflammatory medications, and local steroid injections. If the foot is hyperpronated, orthotic devices may be helpful. Surgery is rarely indicated.

Leg pain in runners must be accurately diagnosed. "Shin splint syndrome" (chronic medial tibial stress syndrome) refers to pain along the mid to distal areas of the medial tibia. Tibial stress fracture, tibial periostitis, and chronic posterior compartment syndrome are the most common causes. Periostitis and compartment syndrome can be differentiated on both physical examination and technetium bone scans. Tenderness on the medial edge of the bone indicates periostitis (periostalgia), whereas most posterior pain along the deep muscle belly indicates a compartment syndrome. A stress fracture shows up on the scan as a localized area of increased uptake, whereas periostitis shows up as "linear streaking" along the cortex. Conservative care (rest, ice, nonsteroidal medications, orthotic devices, taping, and stretching) usually resolves the problem. Compartment pressures are not increased in periostitis. Fasciotomy with cauterization of the periosteum can be beneficial in cases that repeatedly fail to respond to the usual measures.

Pressure-monitoring devices are helpful in diagnosing exertional compartment syndromes. Measurements are made with the patient at rest (normal, 0 to 4 mm Hg) and after running (treadmill, track, road) for a given period or until symptoms occur. A postexercise reading of 25 to 35 mm Hg is highly suspect and one of 40 mm Hg or more is diagnostic.

Achilles tendinitis or peritendinitis should be managed conservatively. Heel lifts and orthotic devices for a hyperpronated foot are helpful. Surgery in recalcitrant cases involves a J- or L-type incision so that both sides of the tendon, as well as the retrocalcaneal bursa, can be examined. In such cases the peritendon is usually hyperemic, thickened, and fibrotic as well as adherent to the underlying tendon. The posterior portion of periotendon is freed by sharp dissection and the tendon itself is inspected. Nodular, disrupted areas of mucoid and fibroid degeneration (tendinosis), if present, are removed, via longitudinal splitting incisions in the tendon. The tendon is then reapproximated in a side-by-side fashion. The athlete must understand preoperatively that a return to the previous level of running may not be possible.

Subcalcaneal pain constitutes about 80% to 90% of all foot pain in runners. It may be caused by plantar fasciitis, medial calcaneal neuritis, tuber calcanei pain, tarsal tunnel syndrome, stress fracture, or tarsal coalition. Careful history, physical examination, radiographs, bone scans, and electromyography should establish the correct diagnosis. Conservative management should be tried for at least one year before surgery is considered. It is essential that an accurate diagnosis be made before surgery is undertaken.

Running Shoes

The running-shoe industry has continued to improve its products. The training shoe provides motion control (stability), shock absorption (cushioning), and flexibility for ease of toe-off. The upper is made on a wooden or plastic last. In the modern training shoe, the configuration is either straight, slightly curved, or curved (7 degrees). If the nylon upper material is sewn on the wooden last, the shoe is termed slip-lasted; if it is placed on a piece of cardboard on the undersurface, the shoe is termed board-lasted (stable). In addition, a combination shoe consists of a board-lasted rearfoot and a slip-lasted forefoot. The mid-sole (including the heel wedge) is the area most important in cushioning the foot. Materials such as ethylene vinyl acetate of various densities, polyurethane, encapsulated air, encapsulated gel, and ethylene vinyl acetate with gel provide excellent shock absorption. The outer sole is of blown ruber, carbon rubber (heel plugs), and solid rubber.

Running shoes for the pronated foot should control excessive motion. The shoe should be board-lasted and straight-configured, have a stable heel counter, extra medial support, and a wider flare than shoes for the cavus foot. Because the cavus foot is more rigid, the shoe should be flexible; this usually requires slip-lasting of a curved configuration with an ethylene vinyl acetate mid-sole and a narrow flare at the heel.

Orthotic Devices

"Prescription" orthotic devices are of three major types: flexible, semirigid and rigid. Well-constructed soft or semirigid orthotic devices are most useful, especially for the runner with biomechanical abnormalities. A soft orthotic device can be made from precut material, molded, and cut to the runner's foot in the office. Both the semirigid and rigid types are made from a neutral plaster cast of the foot (subtalar joint in neutral position) and fabricated at an orthotic laboratory. A rigid device is rarely used for a runner.

Controversies

Instrumented Measurement of Anteroposterior Tibial Translation

The accuracy with which a cruciate ligament injury can be diagnosed by physical examination has ranged in different reports from less than 20% to more than 90%. In an effort to improve diagnostic accuracy and allow quantification of pathologic motion, instruments to measure joint motion have been developed. Instrumented measurement has been widely used in research centers to quantify joint motion before and after knee ligament surgery. The accuracy of testing depends on the skill of the person using the testing device. The tester must ensure that the patient is relaxed and that the instrument is properly positioned and stabilized on the limb if reproducible measurements are to be obtained. Some centers have reported that a cruciate ligament disruption can be diagnosed with an accuracy of more than 90%. Anteroposterior-displacement measurements have proven to be more reproducible than measures of axial rotation. Although it is believed that there is a correlation between the amount of pathologic joint motion and the probability of reinjury and degenerative arthritis, which measures of joint motion are most predictive of joint deterioration has yet to be determined.

Indications for ACL Surgery

The fate of the knee with an ACL injury depends on the degree of abnormal motion, the patient's age, and the activity. Sports that involve jumping or hard cutting place the patient at high risk for further injury. Sports that involve lateral motion without jumping or hard cutting are classified as moderate-risk sports. Running, bicycling, and swimming are examples of low-risk sports. The style of participation is also an important variable. Sports such as tennis can be low risk, moderate risk, or high risk depending on the way the patient plays. Age can affect participation (choice of sport, style, and hours played) and is also important because of changes in knee mechanics with aging.

There is general agreement that a knee with an ACL injury should be repaired or reconstructed if the following criteria are met: (1) closed growth plates and age less than 25 years; (2) moderately to severely abnormal motion (pivot shift grade, 2 to 3 on a 0 to 3 scale, and/or a right-left anterior-displacement difference of more than 5 mm); and (3) vigorous participation in high-risk sports. If the knee is not stabilized, there is a high likelihood of repeated injury, resulting in meniscus tears, progressive joint instability, and early degenerative arthritis. However, the indications for acute ACL surgery in patients with less abnormal motion, older or less active patients, and patients with open growth plates are more controversial. Data are not sufficient for firm recommendations to be made. When the ACL is disrupted and the meniscal tear can be repaired, ACL surgery in conjunction with the meniscus repair is recommended for patients participating in moderate-or high-risk sports.

Technique of ACL Surgery

An ACL reconstruction is usually more successful than an ACL repair. A well-fixed graft is immediately stronger than an ACL repair and is less likely to be disrupted by early joint mobilization. Some surgeons have advocated ACL repair in conjunction with a ligament reconstruction in hopes of maintaining the ligament's nerve supply as well as enhancing the graft's bulk and circulation. Others have confined the surgery to ACL reconstruction to minimize operating time and morbidity and to avoid compromising the graft's size or placement in an effort to preserve ruptured ACL tissue. There are no published data comparing outcomes with different graft sources in terms of joint stability or limb function. There appears to be a strong trend away from extra-articular procedures and toward intra-articular ACL procedures. In a recent review on the use of extra-articular procedures to augment intra-articular ACL reconstruction, extra-articular surgery did not enhance the results of an intra-articular patellar tendon or hamstring procedure.

Management of MCL Injury

There is firm laboratory and clinical evidence that an isolated MCL injury can be treated successfully without surgical repair. The management of the combined MCL-ACL injury is controversial. Many clinicians are more likely to manage a combined MCL-ACL injury surgically than an isolated ACL injury, although there are no data indicating that the combined injury produces a greater risk of impairment and repeated injury. When a combined injury is treated surgically, some surgeons repair or reconstruct both structures, whereas others repair only the ACL or only the MCL. An isolated MCL injury heals satisfactorily without surgical repair; therefore, reconstruction of the ACL alone seems reasonable. The success of this approach, however, is yet to be documented. Because ACL injuries do not heal and may result in significant joint impairment, surgical management of a combined MCL-ACL injury should include repair or reconstruction of or compensation for the ACL injury.

Lateral Release of the Extensor Mechanism

Lateral retinacular release has often been performed for lateral patellar subluxation and dislocation and anterior knee pain. Recent laboratory and clinical studies have questioned the benefit of lateral release and the number of cases of symptomatic medial patellar subluxation and dislocation after lateral release has increased. Studies in normal cadaveric knees before and after lateral release have revealed no change in tracking patterns. In some cases, actual increases in contact pressures have been noted, with what began as a uniform distribution of pressure becoming nonuniform with high peaks after release. Some recent clinical studies have questioned the benefit of lateral release. In one instance, the percentage of poor results increased from 24% to 70% after a follow-up of 4.6 years in a group of patients with patellar subluxation. In a second study, there was no difference between matched groups (one treated with lateral release and the other with physical therapy). Both groups had 60% fair or poor results. A third study reviewing the level of activity after lateral release noted that only 7% of patients had increased physical activity after lateral release, whereas 54% became less active, suggesting that any symptomatic improvement might be the result of reduced activity rather than the surgery. In a fourth review, 30 of 54 patients with continued pain after lateral release were shown to have medial subluxation of the patellas. The indications for lateral release surgery must be defined more precisely and the recovery course and results of surgery documented more objectively. It has been suggested the benefit of a lateral release might be best explained by denervation resulting from cutting the sensory nerves during the operation.

Annotated Bibliography

Keywords

Anterior cruciate ligament; Articular cartilage; Chondromalacia; Grafting; Knee brace; Medial collateral ligament; Meniscus; Patella; Plica; Posterior cruciate ligament; Sports medicine

General Considerations

Noyes FR, Grood ES, Torzilli PA: Current concepts review: The definitions of terms for motion and position of the knee and injuries of the ligaments. *J Bone Joint Surg* 1989;71A:465–472.
  The authors discuss and define position terms (position, dislocation, and subluxation), motion terms (motion, displacement, translation, rotation, range of motion, limits of motion, coupled motion, constrained motion, force, moment, laxity, and instability), and injury terms (sprain, rupture, and deficiency). Application of the terms to the clinical examination is discussed.

Diagnosis of Ligament Disruption

Daniel DM, Stone ML, Barnett P, et al: Use of the quadriceps active test to diagnose posterior cruciate-ligament disruption and measure posterior laxity of the knee. *J Bone Joint Surg* 1988;70A:386–391.
  With the knee joint in 90 degrees of flexion, contraction of the quadriceps resulted in an anterior translation of the tibia in 41 of 42 knees that had documented disruption of the PCL. Anterior translation did not occur in the contralateral normal knees of the same subjects, in the knees of 25 normal subjects, or in 25 knees with known unilateral ACL disruption.

Daniel DM, Stone ML, Sachs R, et al: Instrumented measurement of anterior knee laxity in patients with acute anterior cruciate ligament disruption. *Am J Sports Med* 1985;13:401–407.
  Anterior laxity measurements (KT-1000) were suggestive or diagnostic of pathologic anterior laxity in 50 of 53 patients with complete ACL tears. When examination with the patient under anesthesia included the maximum measurement obtained manually, the examination was diagnostic in all cases.

Sherman OH, Markolf KL, Ferkel RD: Measurements of anterior laxity in normal and anterior cruciate absent knees with two instrumented test devices. *Clin Orthop* 1987;215:156–161.
  A single examiner measured anteroposterior motion in 48 normal subjects and 19 patients with unilateral ACL disruption with two instrumented testing devices—the UCLA device and the KT-1000. The authors found that 95% of the normal subjects had a side-to-side difference of less than 2 mm with both devices. Both identified absent ACLs in 90% to 95% of cases outside the normal range.

The Natural History of Knee Ligament Injuries

Gollehon DL, Torzilli PA, Warren RF: The role of the posterolateral and cruciate ligaments in the stability of the human knee: A biomechanical study. *J Bone Joint Surg* 1987;69A:233–242.

At all angles of flexion the LCL and deep ligamentous complex functioned together as the principal structures preventing posterior translation. Sectioning the LCL and deep ligamentous complex alone resulted in a marked increase in external rotation of the tibia with posterior subluxation of the lateral tibial plateau. This was greatest at 30 degrees of flexion. When the PCL was sectioned after the LCL and deep ligamentous complex, the amount of external rotation at 90 degrees increased.

Grood ES, Stowers SF, Noyes FR: Limits of movement in the human knee: Effect of sectioning the posterior cruciate ligament and posterolateral structures. *J Bone Joint Surg* 1988;70A:88–97.

Removal of the PCL alone increased the limit of posterior tibial translation with no change in the limit of tibial rotation or varus and valgus angulation.

Hawkins RJ, Misamore GW, Merritt TR: Followup of the acute nonoperated isolated anterior cruciate ligament tear. *Am J Sports Med* 1986;14:205–210.

Forty patients who were examined within four weeks of acute ACL disruption and treated nonsurgically were reexamined an average of four years later. There were 31 males and nine females. The average age was 22 years (range, 15 to 43 years). Four patients were more than 30 years old and 17 were less than 22 years old. Giving way was a problem for 36 patients, but pain and swelling were not significant problems for most. Full return to unlimited athletic activities occurred in only four of the patients.

Kannus P, Järvinen M: Long-term prognosis of nonoperatively treated acute knee distortions having primary hemarthrosis without clinical instability. *Am J Sports Med* 1987;15:138–143.

A multidimensional follow-up analysis was done for 84 patients wihout clinical instability, fracture, or patellar luxation an average of eight years after an acute traumatic hemarthrosis. During the follow-up period, 67 patients (80%) had no surgery on the injured knee. Of the 72 patients (86%) who were asymptomatic, physical activity was at the preinjury level or better in 67 (93%). Ten of the 12 symptomatic patients had grades II to IV pathologic anterior knee laxity.

Parolie JM, Bergfeld JA: Long-term results of nonoperative treatment of isolated posterior cruciate ligament injuries in the athlete. *Am J Sports Med* 1986;14:35–38.

Twenty-five patients whose isolated PCL injuries were treated nonsurgically were examined 2.2 to 16 years after injury (mean, 6.2 years). At follow-up, 80% of the patients were satisfied with their knees and 84% had returned to their previous sport.

Satku K, Kumar VP, Ngoi SS: Anterior cruciate ligament injuries: To counsel or to operate? *J Bone Joint Surg* 1986;68B:458–461.

Untreated ACL injuries in 97 knees (87 patients) were reviewed after a mean interval of six years. After the initial recovery, 63% of the patients were able to return to their pre-injury sport; six years later, however, 27% could no longer perform at the same level. Radiologic deterioration was maximal in those who had undergone meniscectomy more than five years before review. Knees with intact menisci were often radiologically normal despite continuing instability.

Woo SL-Y, Inoue M, McGurk-Burleson E, et al: Treatment of the medial collateral ligament injury: II. Structure and function of canine knees in response to differing treatment regimens. *Am J Sports Med* 1987;15:22–29.

Thirty-two canine MCLs were surgically transected and treated using one of three regimens: (1) no repair or immobilization; (2) repair with three weeks of immobilization; and (3) repair with six weeks of immobilization. Results were best in group 1. The varus-valgus laxity of the knee joint and the structural properties of the ligament complex returned to values comparable to those for the contralateral control by 12 weeks. Recovery of the mechanical properties of the MCL substance was slower and not complete even at 48 weeks. Prolonged immobilization was shown to have deleterious effects on MCL healing.

Ligament Repair and Reconstruction

Bradley J, FitzPatrick D, Daniel D, et al: Orientation of the cruciate ligament in the sagittal plane: A method of predicting its length-change with flexion. *J Bone Joint Surg* 1988;70B:94–99.

The kinematics of the knee in the sagittal plane was studied with a four-bar linkage model.

Garrick JG, Requa RK: Prophylactic knee bracing. *Am J Sports Med* 1987;15:471–476.

The authors compared six studies to determine the effectiveness of prophylactic knee braces in preventing MCL injuries in football. They concluded that no consensus was possible because of conflicting results and problems with methodology. The role of prophylactic knee bracing, in their opinion, remains uncertain.

Gillquist J, Odensten M: Arthroscopic reconstruction of the anterior cruciate ligament. *Arthroscopy* 1988;4:5-9.

Arthroscopic reconstruction of the ACL was compared with reconstruction through a miniarthrotomy. Arthroscopic reconstruction offered no major advantage in terms of rehabilitation. The miniarthrotomy was preferred because it allowed better evaluation of graft impingement and execution of a notchplasty.

Kurosaka M, Yoshiya S, Andrish JT: A biomechanical comparison of different surgical techniques of graft fixation in anterior cruciate ligament reconstruction. *Am J Sports Med* 1987;15:225–229.

Using cadaveric material, the authors studied the holding power of staples, sutures in soft tissue, sutures through bone holes, and interface friction fixation of bone plug in a bone tunnel. With young bone, interface friction screw techniques provided the strongest fixation. Load-to-failure studies of all grafts revealed failure at the point of fixation, indicating that the mechanically weakest regions of the reconstructed graft are located at the fixation sites.

McFarland EG, Morrey BF, An KN, et al: The relationship of vascularity and water content to tensile strength in a patellar tendon replacement of the anterior cruciate in dogs. *Am J Sports Med* 1986;14:436–448.

Patellar tendon grafts implemented in dogs were studied at 37, 57, and 120 days after surgery. The graft strength decreased about 50% by 37 days and at 120 days was 40% of that of the control patellar tendon.

Paulos LE, Rosenberg TD, Drawbert J, et al: Infrapatellar contracture syndrome: An unrecognized cause of knee stiffness with patella entrapment and patella infera. *Am J Sports Med* 1987;15:331–341.

The infrapatellar contracture syndrome can occur as an exaggerated pathologic fibrous hyperplasia of the anterior soft tissues of the knee beyond that associated with normal healing. In 21 of the 28 patients in this series, the condition was secondary to knee ligament reconstruction. The signs include the restriction of knee extension and flexion associated with patellar entrapment.

Robertson DB, Daniel DM, Biden E: Soft tissue fixation to bone. *Am J Sports Med* 1986;14:398–403.

Cadaveric soft tissue was used to evaluate the holding power of sutures, staples, and screws with spiked washers or fixation plates. Loads at failure were greater with screws than with the other techniques. Sutures through bone holes in the patellar tendon graft had fixation failure loads similar to those for the screws.

Roth JH, Bray RC, Best TM, et al: Posterior cruciate ligament reconstruction by transfer of the medial gastrocnemius tendon. *Am J Sports Med* 1988;16:21–28.

Thirty-one patients undergoing gastrocnemius tendon transfer for symptomatic PCL instability were compared with a group of eight patients managed conservatively while awaiting surgery. The mean interval between surgery and follow-up was 53 months. Of the surgically treated patients, 69% were subjectively improved but 91% continued to have pain and continued to experience giving way. Medial gastrocnemius transfer did not significantly reduce anteroposterior translation.

The Meniscus

Arnoczky SP, Warren RF, Spivak JM: Meniscal repair using an exogenous fibrin clot: An experimental study in dogs. *J Bone Joint Surg* 1988;70A:1209–1217.

In these animal experiments, fibrin clot was used to stimulate the healing of surgically created meniscal tears in the canine meniscus. The authors believe that the clot provides a scaffold and chemotactic stimulus to healing.

Ghosh P, Taylor TKF: The knee joint meniscus: A fibrocartilage of some distinction. *Clin Orthop* 1987;224:52–63.

This article reviews the function of the meniscus and the way its anatomy provides for these functions. The authors also describe the effects of meniscectomy and the rationale for the preferred methods of treatment.

Hajek PC, Gylys-Morin VM, Baker LL, et al: The high signal intensity meniscus of the knee: Magnetic resonance evaluation and in vivo correlation. *Invest Radiol* 1987;22:883–890.

High signal intensity magnetic resonance imaging was used to evaluate the menisci of 40 cadavers and 14 patients. The conclusion was that magnetic resonance imaging remains inferior to conventional arthrography in the evaluation of meniscal abnormalities.

Jackson DW, Jennings LD, Maywood RM, et al: Magnetic resonance imaging of the knee. *Am J Sports Med* 1988;16:29–38.

The authors graded meniscal tears seen on magnetic resonance imaging on a scale of 1 to 3. The scale rates the change in signal-intensity characteristics. This grading system significantly improved the accuracy of prediction. For grade 3 tears the accuracy was 93.1% on the medial side and 96.6% on the lateral side. The authors emphasize the importance of recognizing the meaning of signal-intensity changes on magnetic resonance imaging scans.

Jakob RP, Stäubli HU, Zuber K, et al: The arthroscopic meniscal repair: Techniques and clinical experience. *Am J Sports Med* 1988;16:137–142.

The authors thought that vertical longitudinal tears were most suitable for repair and considered the use of a rasp to abrade the surfaces of the tear to be important. There was a 22% recurrence rate along the lines of the old tear.

Manco LG, Kavanaugh JH, Lozman J, et al: Diagnosis of meniscal tears using high-resolution computed tomography: Correlation with arthroscopy. *J Bone Joint Surg* 1987;69A:498–502.

High-resolution computed tomography used to evaluate 840 knees in 450 patients with meniscal abnormalities had an overall accuracy rate of 91%. However, the overall specificity was only 87%.

Mandelbaum BR, Finerman GAM, Reicher MA, et al: Magnetic resonance imaging as a tool for evaluation of traumatic knee injuries: Anatomical and pathoanatomical correlations. *Am J Sports Med* 1986;14:361–370.

Magnetic resonance imaging was performed on 105 patients with preoperative diagnoses of meniscal tears, ACL and/or PCL tears, tibial plateau fractures, and patellar and quadriceps injuries. Magnetic resonance imaging was 90% accurate for the medial meniscus, 91% accurate for the lateral meniscus, and 100% accurate for the ACL. The authors concluded that magnetic resonance imaging, in conjunction with clinical evaluation, can contribute to the decision-making process and assist in preoperative planning.

Morgan CD, Casscells SW: Arthroscopic meniscal repair: A safe approach to the posterior horns. *Arthroscopy* 1986;2:3–12.

The authors emphasize the anatomic conditions needed for a safe approach to peripheral meniscal tears. In 70 meniscal tears followed up for 18 months, the recurrence rate was 1.5%. There were two neurovascular complications but neither was permanent.

Scott GA, Jolly BL, Henning CE: Combined posterior incision and arthroscopic intra-articular repair of the meniscus: An examination of factors affecting healing. *J Bone Joint Surg* 1986;68A:847–861.

The results of meniscal repair in 167 patients were determined by postoperative arthroscopy or arthrography. Sixty-two percent of the menisci healed, 17% healed incompletely, and 21% did not heal. Ninety-two percent of the menisci were categorized as clinically stable and 80% of the patients returned to active sports.

Shoemaker SC, Markolf KL: The role of the meniscus in the anterior-posterior stability of the loaded anterior cruciate-deficient knee: Effects of partial versus total excision. *J Bone Joint Surg* 1986;68A:71–79.

In the ACL-deficient knee in which control of anterior tibial displacement has been compromised, the menisci helped the tibia maintain a balanced position on the femur. Therefore, the posterior horn of the medial meniscus in particular should be preserved whenever possible because of its effectiveness in resisting applied anterior tibial force.

Silva I Jr, Silver DM: Tears of the meniscus as revealed by magnetic resonance imaging. *J Bone Joint Surg* 1988;70A:199–202.

Forty-four patients were examined by magnetic resonance imaging and arthroscopy to detect tears of the meniscus. Magnetic resonance imaging had an accuracy rate of 45% for the 28 patients who had had no previous surgery and 49% in the 16 patients who had had previous operations. When false-negatives were eliminated, the accuracy rates were 65% and 55%, respectively.

Watanabe AT, Carter BC, Teitelbaum GP, et al: Common pitfalls in magnetic resonance imaging of the knee. *J Bone Joint Surg* 1989;71A:857–862.

Magnetic resonance imaging scans of 200 knees were studied retrospectively to determine the frequency with which normal ligamentous and tendinous structures mimic pathologic changes in the meniscus or elsewhere in the knee. The transverse geniculate ligament simulated an anterior horn of the lateral meniscus in 22% of cases. The bursa of the popliteus tendon simulated a tear of the posterior horn of the lateral meniscus in 27.5% of cases. The ligament of Humphrey was visualized in 33% of cases and the ligament of Wrisberg in 32.5% of cases. On sagittal images these structures can be mistaken for a loose body.

Symptomatic Plica

Bough BW, Regan BF: Medial and lateral synovial plicae of the knee: Pathological significance, diagnosis and treatment by arthroscopic surgery. *Ir Med J* 1985; 78:279–282.

This paper is a good review of the various kinds of plica and how they are manifested when symptomatic. The emphasis is on the similarity of symptomatic plica to internal derangement of the knee.

Muse GL, Grana WA, Hollingsworth S: Arthroscopic treatment of medial shelf syndrome. *Arthroscopy* 1985;1: 63–67.

Fifty-one knees (42 patients) were examined two years after arthroscopic treatment of the medial shaft syndrome. Although most patients had improved by one or more functional levels, there were only four satisfactory results. Some patients had mild persistent pain. Complete wide resection is needed to prevent recurrence of symptoms.

The Patella

Cash JD, Hughston JC: Treatment of acute patellar dislocation. *Am J Sports Med* 1988;16:244–249.

In this follow-up study of 103 knees, the patients were divided into those with and those without a predisposing anatomic factor. In the group with a predisposing factor, the recurrence rate was 36% (43% in those who had surgery, 0% in those who had open surgery, and 50% in those who had arthroscopic surgery) and the rating was excellent or good in 58%. In the group without an obvious predisposing anatomic factor, the recurrence rate was 15% and the rating was excellent or good in 79%. These findings indicate the importance of the predisposing anatomy. The Q angle was not as important as lateral mobility, a dysplastic vastus medialis oblique muscle, a high or lateral patella, or a history of dislocation or subluxation in the opposite knee.

Cerullo G, Puddu G, Conteduca F, et al: Evaluation of the results of extensor mechanism reconstruction. *Am J Sports Med* 1988;16:93–96.

A total of 116 patients were operated on for extensor mechanism malalignment associated with a dislocating, subluxating, or painful patella. The results were poor in those with stable patellas who were operated on for pain. In patients with dislocation, results were good in 100% of those who underwent proximal and distal reconstruction but satisfactory in only 75% of those with subluxation who underwent proximal reconstruction.

Inoue M, Shino K, Hirose H, et al: Subluxation of the patella: Computed tomography analysis of patellofemoral congruence. *J Bone Joint Surg* 1988;70A:1331–1337.

The sensitivity and specificity of computed tomographic scanning in the diagnosis of subluxation of the patella in extension greatly exceeded the sensitivity and specificity of diagnosis by routine radiography.

Kujala UM, Kvist M, Österman K, et al: Factors predisposing army conscripts to knee exertion injuries incurred in a physical therapy program. *Clin Orthop* 1986;210: 203–212.

The authors reviewed anatomic alignment factors in the lower extremity. The examination included a patellar stress device. They concluded that an increase in passive mobility of the patella, increased knee laxity, leg-length inequality, and increasing height were correlated with the development of exertional injuries of the knee during physical training.

Møller BN, Jurik AG, Tidemand-Dal C, et al: The quadriceps function in patellofemoral disorders: A radiographic and electromyographic study. *Arch Orthop Trauma Surg* 1987;106:195–198.

An exercise program increased strength but improved symptoms in only 15% of the patients with subluxation and 28% of those with chondromalacia. There was no change in the balance of the vastus medialis or vastus lateralis in either group.

Takai S, Sakakida K, Yamashita F, et al: Rotational alignment of the lower limb in osteoarthritis of the knee. *Int Orthop* 1985;9:209–215.

The authors measured the rotation of the lower extremities by computed tomographic scanning and correlated the findings with knee osteoarthritis. The patients were grouped into three categories: those with medial compartment disease, those with lateral compartment disease, and those with patellofemoral compartment disease. There was a significant relationship between increased internal femoral torsion and patellofemoral arthritis.

Running Injuries

Cox JS: Patellofemoral problems in runners. *Clin Sports Med* 1985;4:699–715.

Stress-related patellofemoral problems are common in runners, in whom the patellofemoral joint reaction force may reach 3.3 times body weight. The term "chondromalacia" is used to describe the anatomic and histologic characteristics of cartilage. The signs, symptoms, radiologic findings, and differential diagnosis are reviewed along with malalignment problems that can cause patellofemoral problems. Nonsurgical treatment consists of salicylates or other anti-inflammatory drugs, patellar stabilizing devices, orthotics, ice, heat, quadriceps exercises, stretching, and electrostimulation of the vastus medialis. Intra-articular steroids should not be used. Surgery should be contemplated only when all else fails. Diagnostic arthroscopy (for chondromalacia) with lavage can be combined with arthroscopic surgery on the patellar surface or with the treatment of malalignment problems by open surgery.

Detmer DE: Chronic shin splints: Classification and management of medial tibial stress syndrome. *Sports Med* 1986;3:436–446.

A clinical classification and treatment program for chronic medial tibial stress syndrome are discussed. The classification includes tibial stress fracture (type I), tibial periostitis (type II), and chronic distal deep posterior compartment syndrome (type III). Types II and III sometimes occur together. Surgery was performed on 41 patients with types II and III injuries who did not respond to a conservative program (rest, graded exercise, orthotics, ice). Those with type II or combined injuries underwent fasciotomy and periosteal cauterization; those with type III injuries underwent fasciotomy only. All surgery was done with the patient under local anesthesia. Complete cures were achieved in 78% of type II injuries, 57% of combined injuries, and 75% of type III injuries. Performance improved in 93%, 86%, and 100%, respectively.

Frederick EC: Biomechanical consequences of sports shoe design. *Exerc Sport Sci Rev* 1986;14:375–400.

The author emphasizes the methods used to characterize the mechanical properties of sports shoes and the observed effects of these properties on performance and on various sports injuries. This is an excellent review article on the biomechanical aspects of the foot and the shoe.

Lutter LD: Surgical decisions in athletes' subcalcaneal pain. *Am J Sports Med* 1986;14:481–485.

The author bases the decision for surgery on (1) correct diagnosis, (2) approximately 12 months of conservative treatment, (3) electromyography for diagnosis and appropriate nerve blocks, (4) thorough knowledge of anatomy, (5) the patient's understanding that surgery may not give a good enough result to allow a return to high-performance athletics, and (6) correct and appropriately directed surgery. The differential diagnosis includes plantar fasciitis, tarsal tunnel syndrome, tuber calcanei pain and medial calcaneal neuritis, calcaneal stress fracture, and tarsal coalitions. Of 182 patients with this diagnosis reviewed, four underwent surgery.

McBryde AM Jr: Stress fractures in runners. *Clin Sports Med* 1985;4:737–752.

This injury is a partial or complete fracture of bone resulting from its inability to withstand nonviolent stress applied in rhythmic, repeated, subthreshold manner. There are three types: (1) compression impact, (2) distraction with pulling of the periosteum (shin splint), and (3) muscle concentration. Runners who have a leg-length discrepancy, hyperpronation, or lower-extremity malalignment, or who use improper running shoes, who run on irregular or canted surfaces, or who are in poor physical condition are at risk for this injury. There is local pain and tenderness. Technetium bone scanning, tomography, xeroradiography, computed tomographic scanning, and magnetic resonance imaging can be used diagnostically. The author believes that general treatment involves cessation of running in some cases and keeping the level of running below the symptom threshold in other cases. The appropriateness of alternative training (swimming, biking, and so forth) depends on the site of fracture.

McKenzie DC, Clement DB, Taunton JE: Running shoes, orthotics, and injuries. *Sports Med* 1985;2:334–347.

In this extensive review article on the causes of running injuries, the authors report a 13-year increase in knee injuries from 18% to 50% of all injuries. Training errors accounted for 60% of the knee injuries. They emphasize footwear, biomechanical control, and a comprehensive rehabilitation program that considers other causative factors. They review the biomechanics of different foot types (such as hyperpronated or cavus feet).

Schepsis AA, Leach RE: Surgical management of Achilles tendinitis. *Am J Sports Med* 1987;15:308–315.

The authors present a retrospective study of 45 operations on 37 patients (24 for Achilles tendinitis and/or tenosynovitis, 14 for retrocalcaneal bursitis, and seven for both). Surgery was done after conservative measures (rest, ice, heel lifts, nonsteroidals, orthotics) failed. Average duration of symptoms was three years. In cases of Achilles tenosynovitis or tendinitis, the tendon sheath was excised except anteriorly and any fibrotic foci within the tendon were excised via a longitudinal incision and then reapproximated. In retrocalcaneal bursitis, the bursa and posterior superior angle of the os calcis were removed via a J-shaped incision. Overall results were excellent in 27 cases (60%), good in 12 cases (27%), fair in five cases (11%), and poor in one case (2%).

Controversies

Instrumented Measurement of Anteroposterior Tibial Translation

Daniel DM, Stone ML, Sachs R, et al: Instrumented measurement of anterior knee laxity in patients with acute anterior cruciate ligament disruption. *Am J Sports Med* 1985;13:401–407.

Hanley ST, Warren RF: Arthroscopic meniscectomy in the anterior cruciate ligament-deficient knee. *Arthroscopy* 1987;3:59–65.

Sherman OH, Markolf KL, Ferkel RD: Measurements of anterior laxity in normal and anterior cruciate absent knees with two instrumented test devices. *Clin Orthop* 1987;215:156–161.

Indications for ACL Surgery

Hawkins RJ, Misamore GW, Merritt TR: Followup of the acute nonoperated isolated anterior cruciate ligament tear. *Am J Sports Med* 1986;14:205–210.

Satku K, Kumar VP, Ngoi SS: Anterior cruciate ligament injuries: To counsel or to operate? *J Bone Joint Surg* 1986;68B:458–461.

Technique of ACL Surgery

Clancy WG Jr, Ray M, Zoltan DJ: Acute tears of the anterior cruciate ligament: Surgical versus conservative treatment. *J Bone Joint Surg* 1988;70A:1483–1488.

Odensten M, Hamberg P, Nordin M, et al: Surgical or conservative treatment of the acutely torn anterior cruciate ligament: A randomized study with short-term follow-up observations. *Clin Orthop* 1985;198:87–93.

Management of MCL Injury

Woo SL-Y, Inoue M, McGurk-Burleson E, et al: Treatment of the medial collateral ligament injury: II. Structure and function of canine knees in response to differing treatment regimens. *Am J Sports Med* 1987;15:22–29.

Lateral Release of the Extensor Mechanism

Hille E, Schulitz K-P, Henrichs C, et al: Pressure and contact-surface measurements within the femoropatellar joint and their variations following lateral release. *Arch Orthop Trauma Surg* 1985;104:275–282.

Huberti HH, Hayes WC: Contact pressures in chondromalacia patellae and the effects of capsular reconstructive procedures. *J Orthop Res* 1988;6:499–508.

Hughston JC, Deese M: Medial subluxation of the patella as a complication of lateral retinacular release. *Am J Sports Med* 1988;16:383–388.

Unneberg K, Reikeras O: The effect of lateral retinacular release in idiopathic chondromalacia patellae. *Arch Orthop Trauma Surg* 1988;107:226–227.

44
Knee and Leg: Bone Trauma

Although tibial fractures are common, opinions about their optimal treatment vary considerably. To the traditional goals of proper length, alignment, and joint congruity, optimal functional outcome and minimal loss of wages have been added. These demanding objectives have increased interest in the long-term results of surgical and nonsurgical approaches and led to the development of new implants, such as flexible, unreamed, and locked nails.

Fractures of the Tibial Plateau

The age of the patient largely determines the incidence, fracture patterns, and associated injuries in tibial plateau fractures. Most fractures occur in the fifth or sixth decades of life or later. In younger patients, tibial plateau fractures are often caused by vehicular accidents or falls from heights; in the elderly or those with osteopenic bone stock, minor missteps can shatter the proximal tibia. Sixty percent of these fractures involve the lateral plateau, 15% the medial plateau, and about 25% are bicondylar. The prevalence of lateral involvement results from the slight valgus alignment of the lower extremity and the fact that most deforming forces are directed from lateral to medial. Regardless of location or extent, these lesions can be classified as simple split, depression, or split-depression fractures.

Split fractures typically occur in young patients with strong bones of high rigidity. As many as 30% of simple split fractures, therefore, are accompanied by ruptures of the opposite collateral and/or cruciate ligaments. With advancing age, bone strength and stiffness decrease, split-compression fractures become more frequent, and the rate of associated ligamentous injury decreases. In the last decades of life, simple compression fractures without associated ligamentous injuries are most common.

In addition to partial or complete ligamentous ruptures, which occur in about 15% of all tibial plateau fractures, there is about a 5% to 15% incidence of meniscal lesions, generally in the form of peripheral tears. Neurologic lesions, vascular injuries, and compartment syndromes are rare. The latter may, however, develop after open reduction and internal fixation. Some other injury patterns around the knee carry a much higher incidence of ligamentous and neurovascular involvement. These fracture-dislocations, as they have been termed, may appear as minor avulsion fractures on initial radiographs, but are in fact much more serious injuries and require further investigations of associated injuries to ligaments, vessels, and nerves.

Assessment

Apart from assessing the patient's general status and associated injuries, the initial clinical evaluation of a patient with a tibial plateau fracture should focus on the location and extent of swelling, tenderness, and ecchymosis and the integrity of muscle compartments, nerves, and vessels. Radiographically, anteroposterior and lateral views in line with the tibial plateaus are basic. The extent and severity of the fractures can be clarified by tomographs in both planes and a computed tomographic scan extending from the knee joint to the most distal fracture line. These studies are of particular importance when internal fixation is considered. For medial and bicondylar fractures, which can easily heal in misalignment, anteroposterior views of the injured and uninjured knee on long films should be obtained for reference purposes. Preoperative stress films with the patient under anesthesia are helpful in identifying associated lesions of the collateral ligaments. If the ligamentous structures are intact, stress films in full extension indicate the degree of instability resulting from the fracture itself and thus can aid in the selection of conservative or surgical management.

Treatment

There are no clear criteria for selecting conservative management or surgical intervention. Since the introducton of more refined implants by the AO-ASIF group two decades ago, there has been an ongoing controversy about the merits of cast and traction vs open reduction and internal fixation. The opinions range from those who believe that most fractures can be treated nonsurgically to those who advocate open reduction and internal fixation for all lesions that are not anatomically aligned. Although the latter group has been more vocal, most long-term studies tend to support the former opinion. On balance, it appears that any patient who has intact collateral ligaments and less than 10 degrees of instability (roughly equivalent to 10 mm of vertical depression at the medial or lateral joint line) is a candidate for nonsurgical treatment, particularly if the patient is more than 50 years of age, has osteopenic bone, a sedentary profession, and mild to moderate recreational needs. Conversely, major ligamentous disruption, instability of more than 10 degrees with a fully extended knee, age of less than 50 years, firm bone stock, a profession that involves moderate to heavy physical demands, and the enjoyment of vigorous recreational activities are all factors suggesting that open reduction and internal fixation is preferable. However, open reduction of tibial plateau fractures can present formidable difficulties and may result in disastrous soft-tissue complications. Open reduction and internal fixation of tibial plateau fractures is a procedure that should only be undertaken once the patient is stable and all the ancillary studies have been incorporated into a careful surgical plan.

The knee joint is approached through a longitudinal parapatellar incision. Progressively more extensive exposure is possible through an osteotomy of Gerdy's tubercle, detachment of the anterior horn of one or both menisci, and elevation of the quadriceps mechanism through an osteotomy of the tibial tubercle. Once anatomic reduction and rigid internal fixation are obtained, the knee should be clinically and radiographically examined for collateral instability. A completely avulsed ligament should be repaired. Postoperatively, the limb is moved in a continuous passive motion machine. Later, active range-of-motion exercises and—if the fixation was suboptimal or the bone osteoporotic—a cast brace are added. Full weightbearing is rarely possible before eight to ten weeks.

An arthroscope-aided technique may minimize surgical exposure in some fractures. The joint surface is visualized arthroscopically. Through a cortical bone window, the joint surface can be elevated and supported with a bone graft. The fracture can then be stabilized with percutaneous screws.

For the rare tibial plateau fracture associated with a popliteal artery injury or extensive local soft-tissue destruction, temporary immobilization of the knee joint with an anterior external fixator reaching from the mid-femur to the mid-tibia may be indicated. After consolidation of the associated soft-tissue lesions, secondary internal fixation with plates and screws may follow.

Split Fractures Some simple split fractures can be reduced by applying a varus force in full extension with the patient under general anesthesia. If a reduction is achieved, the fracture can be stabilized with percutaneous screws or the leg can be held in a long leg cast for three to four weeks. The cast can then be replaced by a cast brace. If the horizontal gap between the two fragments cannot be closed, an incarcerated meniscus should be suspected. Some of these fractures can be managed arthroscopically with closed reduction and percutaneous screw fixation. In other cases, multiple screws and/or a lateral L-shaped buttress plate have been useful.

Depression Fractures These fractures typically occur in the elderly and in patients with osteoporotic bone. Stable fractures are often best managed in a cast brace. In younger patients, particularly when on the lateral view the whole plateau is involved, the articular surface should be elevated into an anatomic position. It can be held there by multiple Kirschner wires and a supporting corticocancellous bone graft. Buttressing with a plate or a cast brace prevents recurrence of the deformity in the early postoperative period.

Split-Depression Fractures The most complex of the lateral plateau fractures, these lesions may extend into the intercondylar area and can be associated with lesions of the medial collateral or anterior cruciate ligaments. In the elderly, they are best treated as simple depression fractures but most lesions in younger patients require open reduction and internal fixation. An extensile exposure that severs the anterior meniscal horns and elevates the tibial tubercle may be needed. A loose intercondylar eminence or detached anterior cruciate ligament should be stabilized with either a screw or heavy sutures through drill holes. Multiple K-wires, bone grafts, and buttress plates are often needed for proper stabilization. Nonrigid fixation and uncooperative patients must be protected with a cast brace postoperatively.

Fractures of the Medial Tibial Plateau Although the fracture patterns on the medial side are not unlike those observed laterally, most fractures of the medial tibial plateau have a worse prognosis. Restoration of the articular surface is not more difficult; nonetheless, slight varus alignment occurs often. This problem is seen with nonsurgical management and, unfortunately, is not uncommon after open reduction and internal fixation. Varus malalignments of as little as 5 degrees can lead to severe medial joint pain and posttraumatic arthritis that can only be relieved by a valgus osteotomy or total knee replacement. If these fractures are treated by open reduction and internal fixation, a slight valgus overreduction is advisable. Proper alignment can be ascertained only with long-cassette intraoperative anteroposterior radiographs compared with those of the normal side. As in other tibial plateau fractures, weightbearing should be delayed until complete fracture consolidation has occurred because secondary medial collapse is not unusual.

Bicondylar Fractures In younger patients, these fractures generally result from high-impact injuries and may be accompanied by a massive soft-tissue contusion or disruption. In the elderly and those with osteopenic bone, they often occur after minor mishaps. Lack of cooperation and osteopenia are good indications for distal tibial pin traction until early consolidation has occurred. Further immobilization is achieved with a long leg cast or a cast brace. With this approach, secondary remodeling of the joint surface often leads to a satisfactory result. Because proper bone stock and the clean environment have been preserved, total knee replacement or an osteotomy can be done safely at a later time. In younger patients restoration of the joint surface and fracture alignment are often possible only with open reduction and internal fixation. An extensile exposure is routine rather than an exception. Complications in the form of postoperative infection or soft-tissue necrosis are not unusual. Because postoperative malalignment is one of the principal causes of unsatisfactory late results, proper tibiofemoral alignment is critical.

Fractures of the Tibial Shaft

The tibia is the most commonly fractured long bone. In children, union is quite rapid and complications are rare. Healing delays and unsatisfactory results are more often seen in adults in whom infection, displacement, or an open soft-tissue wound and comminution are the principal variables that lead to delayed union or nonunion. Of tibial fractures treated in casts, about 6% heal with an angulation exceeding 10 degrees in the sagittal or frontal planes, 2% to 3% shorten more than 2 cm, and 25% of all patients lose about 25 degrees of knee or ankle motion. Although open fractures represent only 10% to 20% of all broken tibias, they have the highest rate of complications and nonunions. The widely held belief that tibial fractures involving the distal third and those associated with an intact fibula heal more slowly remains unsubstantiated. In fact, an intact fibula generally means a shorter healing time but an increased tendency for varus misalignment.

Closed Tibial Fractures

The treatment of most closed tibial fractures starts with the application of a long leg cast. After two to three weeks the long leg cast is often replaced by a snugly fitting short leg cast or a cast brace. With this approach, healing times average 20 weeks and the nonunion rate is between 2% and 5%. Malalignment occurs in 3% to 8% of cases and shortening of more than 1 cm occurs in as many as 10%. Because of associated injuries or unacceptable shortening and displacement in the cast, about 20% to 30% of all closed tibial fractures are presently treated with primary or secondary internal fixation. Plates seem best suited for the proximal and distal tibia. When they are used in tibial shaft fractures, however, the rate of major complications such as nonunions, implant failures, and infections is around 15% to 20%. Intramedullary nails appear to be safer. For stable fractures (Winquist types 1 or 2), multiple thin elastic nails or single stiff nails with and without reaming seem to be equally advantageous. Unstable fractures (such as Winquist types 3 or 4) are best managed with locking nails. Closed fractures associated with compromised soft tissues should be temporarily treated with a splint, traction, or an external fixator.

Open Tibial Shaft Fractures

Advanced age, displacement and comminution, the severity of the soft-tissue injury, the extent of bone loss, the disruption of a major artery, and the presence of a superficial or deep infection adversely affect the outcome of open tibial fractures. Open fractures are classified into three main groups and three subgroups according to the severity of the soft-tissue injury. Grade I fractures have a small skin perforation from inside out. Grade II lesions have a large opening with associated muscle laceration and skin contusions. Grade IIIA lesions are even more extensive, have larger soft-tissue flaps, and a considerable amount of crushed muscle. Grade IIIB indicates initial soft-tissue loss and extensive areas of denuded bone that make later flap coverage necessary. Grade IIIC fractures are associated with a disruption of a major vessel. Several investigators are presently developing criteria separating those grade IIIB and grade IIIC fractures best managed by extensive soft-tissue or microvascular reconstruction from those faring best with early amputation.

As in other open fractures, antibiotics, extensive and repeated debridement, early stabilization, the use of local or free muscle flaps, and bone grafts are all crucial to the successful management of severe open tibial fractures. The debridement must be radical, including all dead tissues and foreign material. Because continued soft-tissue swelling can cause additional muscle necrosis after the initial treatment, repeated debridements are needed at intervals of 36 to 48 hours until the wound is clean.

Antibiotic coverage should start when the patient arrives in the emergency room and should take into account the characteristics of the patient's injuries and the severity of the wound contamination. For most injuries a broad-spectrum cephalosporin should be supplemented by an aminoglycoside. Penicillin is added for farm-related injuries and major clostridial contamination. Antibiotics are discontinued within three days if the wound appears to be clean, or adjusted according to the results of earlier wound cultures.

Most wounds of grade IIIA or less can be closed eventually, on a delayed primary basis, using a split-thickness skin graft. All grade IIIB and many grade IIIC wounds, however, require flap coverage. For the proximal third of the leg, such coverage is best achieved with a gastrocnemius flap; a soleus flap is required for soft-tissue defects extending towards the mid-aspect of the tibia and a free flap is required for defects extending further distally in the leg. If the soleus or gastrocnemius muscles have been damaged by the injury, they are unsuitable for local coverage, and a free flap is then substituted.

There is good evidence that early fracture stabilization decreases additional local vascular damage, soft-tissue necrosis, and the propagation of infection. Because they make wound access difficult, casts are usually ill suited for this purpose. Although early internal fixation has led to good results at some institutions, most authors have discontinued plating of shaft lesions because of high infection and secondary complication rates. The place of early intramedullary nailing with either unreamed solid nails or thin elastic nails awaits further evaluation. There is also evidence that metal implants foster the formation of biofilms that may encapsulate bacteria, making them less accessible to systemic antibiotics. Although a number of methods may be suitable for stabilizing grade I and grade II injuries, there is general agreement that grade III lesions, particularly grades IIIB and IIIC, are best managed with external fixation.

The fixator chosen should have stiff connecting rods and stainless steel pins at least 4.5 to 5 mm in diameter. The pins should be inserted within the "safe corridor" to provide minimal obstruction to debridements and secondary procedures (Fig. 1). This means that, with few exceptions, one- or two-plane unilateral frames are safe. The rigidity of these frames is increased if the pins in each bony fragment are placed as far apart as possible and the longitudinal rods are close to the tibial shaft. Two-plane unilateral frames are needed only when there are long areas of comminution or segmental defects (Fig. 2).

With most half-frames, patient mobilization and early progressive weightbearing is safe. The predrilling of pin holes with sharp drill bits, the use of mechanically sound frames, patient education, and simple pin-care protocols have greatly reduced the rate of pin-tract infections and ring sequestra. However, the rate of nonunions in open tibial fractures treated with external fixation remains high unless denuded bone is covered with local or free muscle flaps early in the treatment and bony consolidation is facilitated by the placement of a cancellous bone graft. Mechanical methods that may reduce healing time and the rate of nonunion include transfer of the limb from an external fixator to a weightbearing cast as soon as the soft tissues have consolidated, reduction of axial frame resistance during early callus formation, gradual frame build-down, and the early introduction of load-sharing at the fracture site.

Tibial Shaft Nonunions

Uninfected Nonunions

Hypertrophic nonunions in which the fibula is intact are best managed with a partial fibulectomy (1 cm) and early weightbearing in a plaster cast. This approach carries little risk, has a success rate of 75% to 80%, and does not preclude more invasive measures later. Nonunions with mild to moderate malalignment can be treated with a bone graft and a cast or a reamed intramedullary nail, but major malalignments often need a local osteotomy, a bone graft, and a plate or nail for stabilization.

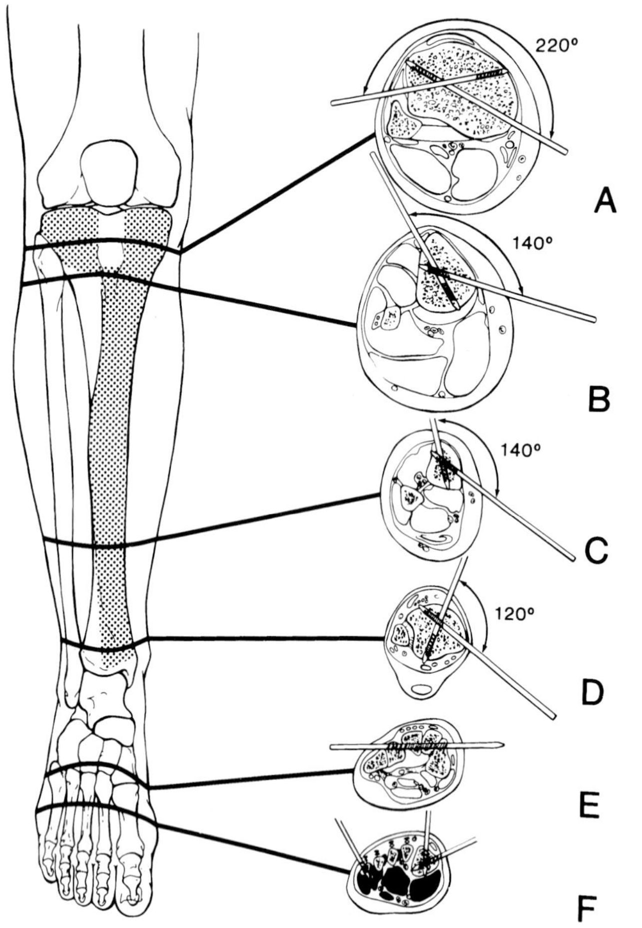

Figure 1

The "safe corridor" for pin insertion in the lower leg. At level A, proximal to the tibial tubercle, pins can be safely inserted within an arc of 220 degrees. At level B, just below the tibial tubercle, the safe arc deceases to 140 degrees. At C, in the distal third of the leg, the safe arc remains 140 degrees, but the anterior tibial vessels and deep peroneal nerves become vulnerable as they cross the lateral tibial cortex. At levels E and F, pins in the tarsal or metatarsal bones may be used to splint the ankle joint if neurologic or soft-tissue injuries prevent the application of an external support. The dotted area indicates where the tibia lies subcutaneously and pin insertion is safe. (Reproduced with permission from Behrens F, Searls K: External fixation of the tibia: Basic concepts and prospective evaluation. *J Bone Joint Surg* 1986;68B:246–254.)

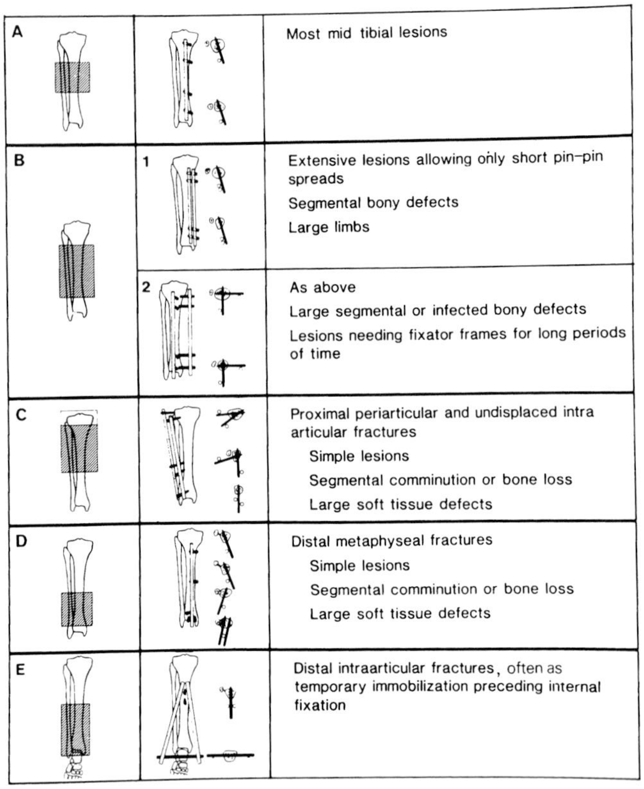

A		Most mid tibial lesions
B	1	Extensive lesions allowing only short pin–pin spreads Segmental bony defects Large limbs
	2	As above Large segmental or infected bony defects Lesions needing fixator frames for long periods of time
C		Proximal periarticular and undisplaced intra articular fractures Simple lesions Segmental comminution or bone loss Large soft tissue defects
D		Distal metaphyseal fractures Simple lesions Segmental comminution or bone loss Large soft tissue defects
E		Distal intraarticular fractures, often as temporary immobilization preceding internal fixation

Figure 2

Diagrams showing the recommended configuration of fixator frames for different bone and soft-tissue injuries. The location and extent of the lesion are indicated on the left, by the cross-hatched area. In the middle is the preferred frame with solid bars representing the pins. On the right are the specific indications for the use of the configuration. (Reproduced with permission from Behrens F, Searls K: External fixation of the tibia: Basic concepts and prospective evaluation. *J Bone Joint Surg* 1986;68B:246–254.)

Infected Nonunions

For infected nonunions of the tibia, particularly those associated with soft-tissue defects and segmental bone loss, amputation must be considered. Another option is wide local resection, stabilization with an external fixator, coverage with a local or free muscle flap, and application of a local bone graft or a free vascularized fibular graft. Although this approach has a 60% to 80% success rate, the time to union may exceed a year and the result may still be an atrophic limb with stiff joints. A new and exciting solution to these difficult problems is local bone transport by the Ilizarov technique. Traditionally carried out with a ring fixator, the procedure can be successfully completed with any properly engineered unilateral device.

Fractures of the Tibial Plafond

Fractures of the tibial plafond remain among the most challenging intra-articular lesions. In addition to malalignment of the distal tibia and comminution of the talar articular surface, most tibial plafond fractures are accompanied by local soft-tissue crushing or interruption of major neurovascular structures. If isolated, most closed fractures with compromised soft tissues can be held in Böhler's traction until the condition of the soft tissue improves and supplementary tomograms or computed tomographic scans have been obtained. If early mobilization is desirable, as in the patient with multiple injuries, an external fixator is superior. Surgical intervention generally follows a week or ten days after the original injury, when there is less risk of wound complications. Despite this cautious approach, difficulties in closing the incision are not uncommon; closure with a free flap is necessary in about 5% to 20% of surgically treated tibial plafond fractures.

Most open fractures are managed by immediate debridement and reduction and internal fixation. The wound is left open and secondary closure or a free flap should follow within three to five days. In lesions characterized by severe soft-tissue crushing and massive contamination, it may be wise to focus on wound debridement, foregoing open reduction and internal fixation and salvaging the extremity with a tibiotalar fusion. In this situation, the external fixator is the most suitable means of fracture stabilization.

Controversies

Surgical vs Nonsurgical Management of Split-Depression Fractures of the Tibial Plateau

The past decade has provided us with new diagnostic modalities (arthroscopy, computed tomography, magnetic resonance imaging), more extensive surgical approaches, and specialized implants.

These advances have made it easier to assess complex fractures of the tibial plateau, reduce them, and achieve exercise-stable internal fixation. Yet, the past decade has also shown that osteopenia, soft-tissue contusions, and lack of experience can lead to disastrous postoperative complications despite the best intentions. It has also been shown that nonsurgical management based on simple guidelines (stability in full extension) can often give surprisingly functional short- and long-term results.

It is likely that, in the future, advanced surgical techniques will be most appropriate and successful in the hands of those experienced in these techniques and employed in treating young patients who have solid bone stock and who have suffered devastating injuries in high-energy accidents. Similar injuries in the elderly may be better treated with nonsurgical approaches focusing on proper limb alignment and maintenance of adequate bone stock.

Treatment of Closed Tibial Fractures

Most closed tibial fractures can be managed with weight-bearing plaster casts or braces. Recently, internal fixation has gained favor, particularly for displaced and comminuted lesions that have higher rates of nonunion and malunion when treated in casts. If internal fixation is used, traditional locked and unlocked nails seem safest and most effective for fractures of the tibial shaft; unstable lesions of the proximal and distal metaphyseal areas are still best handled with plates. Indications for external fixation include severe soft-tissue crushing, impending compartment syndromes, and "bumper fractures" of the proximal tibia. Other indications are closed tibial shaft fractures with skin infections, burns, or dermatologic conditions.

Treatment of Open Tibial Fractures

The experience of the past five to ten years has shown that most grade III open fractures of the tibia can be safely managed with current methods of external fixation. Conversion from external fixation to intramedullary fixation of open tibial fractures should be performed cautiously. The length of time after injury during which such conversions can be done safely, without an unacceptable risk of infection from contaminated pin tract, is unknown. The minimum time that should be allowed for healing of pin tracts before conversion is also unknown. Nonetheless, fixator-related complications, the demands of constant patient supervision, and the need for secondary intervention to achieve bony union in about 20% to 30% of cases have rekindled interest in the use of intramedullary nails for grades I and II injuries. At present, it is unclear what type of nail—elastic, reamed, unreamed, or locked—is preferable. Casts and plates are currently out of favor because they appear to be less reliable and have a higher complication rate than other methods of bone stabilization.

Indications for Nonsurgical Management of Tibial Plafond Fractures

For minimally displaced, well-aligned tibial plafond fractures, a cast or brace followed by early range-of-motion exercises is safe and gives good results. Most comminuted plafond fractures do best with exact open reduction and rigid internal fixation. An exception is the extremely comminuted lesions that are occasionally seen in osteopenic bone and some high-energy accidents. Here, proper alignment of the fracture fragments with an external fixator, followed by early range-of-motion exercises, is safest. This approach allows adequate function in many cases and does not jeopardize the option of successful secondary tibiotalar fusion.

Annotated Bibliography

Keywords

Bicondylar fracture; Depression fracture; Fracture; Infection; Ligament injury; Split-depression fracture; Split fracture; Tibial plafond fracture; Tibial plateau; Tibial shaft fracture

Fractures of the Tibial Plateau

Dias JJ, Stirling AJ, Finlay DBL, et al: Computerised axial tomography for tibial plateau fractures. *J Bone Joint Surg* 1987;69B:84–88.
  Computed tomographic scans of tibial plateau fractures are helpful in classification, evaluation of comminution, and measuring displacement. Because the limb is kept in a single position throughout, the patient experiences less pain than with other assessment procedures.

Fernandez DL: Anterior approach to the knee with osteotomy of the tibial tubercle for bicondylar tibial fractures. *J Bone Joint Surg* 1988;70A:208–219.
  Elevation of the quadriceps mechanism through an osteotomy of the tibial tubercle results in better exposure and reduction and, therefore, a lower rate of complications. The author describes six bicondylar tibial plateau fractures and two fracture-dislocations with short-term follow-up.

Lansinger O, Bergman B, Körner L, et al: Tibial condylar fractures: A twenty-year follow-up. *J Bone Joint Surg* 1986;68A:13–19.

In this long-term follow-up of 120 tibial plateau fractures, fractures with less than 10 degrees of lateral and medial deviation in full extension were considered stable and treated nonsurgically. Unstable fractures and most bicondylar fractures were treated by open reduction and internal fixation. Ninety percent of the patients were rated as having a good result after 20 years. This means that they had occasional stabbing pain, were able to walk outdoors for at least an hour, and had a total range of motion of at least 90 degrees and less than 10 degrees of instability in full extension. The best results were seen in split fractures of the lateral condyle and depression fractures when the depression was confined either to the anterior or to the posterior part of the tibial plateau. For patients with stable fractures, the authors strongly recommend nonsurgical management.

Fractures of the Tibial Shaft

Blick SS, Brumback RJ, Poka A, et al: Compartment syndrome in open tibial fractures. *J Bone Joint Surg* 1986;68A:1348–1353.

A retrospective review of 198 acute open fractures showed associated compartment syndromes in 9.1%. Of these patients, 83% had sustained grade III injuries. All compartment syndromes were managed by four-compartment fasciotomies.

Bone LB, Johnson KD: Treatment of tibial fractures by reaming and intramedullary nailing. *J Bone Joint Surg* 1986;68A:877–887.

In this review of 100 acute tibial fractures and nonunions treated by intramedullary nailing, all but one united. Infection rates were 2.9% in closed or grade I fractures and 25% for grades II or III open fractures. Open surgical techniques were associated with a higher infection rate.

Böstman OM: Spiral fractures of the shaft of the tibia: Initial displacement and stability of reduction. *J Bone Joint Surg* 1986;68B:462–466.

In this analysis of 192 spiral fractures of the tibia, satisfactory closed reduction was possible in only 18% of the cases with initial anterior or posterior displacement of more than 50% of the width of the shaft. The author states that such fractures are best managed by open reduction and internal fixation or a few weeks of initial calcaneal traction.

Böstman O, Vainiopää S, Saikku K: Infra-isthmal longitudinal fractures of the tibial diaphysis: Results of treatment using closed intramedullary compression nailing. *J Trauma* 1984;24:964–969.

In this follow-up study of 103 long spiral fractures of the distal tibia, 71 fractures with slight or minimal displacement were treated in weightbearing long leg casts and 32 fractures with moderate displacement were treated with Kaessmann compression nails. Despite more severe initial displacement, fractures treated with intramedullary nailing had shorter healing times, fewer malunions (9% vs 27%), and lower rates of decreased ankle function.

Caudle RJ, Stern PJ: Severe open fractures of the tibia. *J Bone Joint Surg* 1987;69A:801–807.

In this review of 62 type III open fractures followed up for seven to 51 months, nonunions occured in 27% to 30%, infections in 10% to 59%, and secondary amputation in 0% to 78%. The best results were achieved in seven grade IIIA and in seven grade IIIB injuries treated by vigorous debridement and the early application of local flaps or free tissue transfers. Of nine grade IIIC injuries, seven ultimately required secondary amputation.

Gregory RT, Gould RJ, Peclet M, et al: The mangled extremity syndrome (M.E.S.): A severity grading system for multisystem injury of the extremity. *J Trauma* 1985; 25:1147–1150.

From this retrospective review of 17 patients, the authors believe that the need for amputation and success with functional limb salvage can be predicted.

Klemm KW, Börner M: Interlocking nailing of complex fractures of the femur and tibia. *Clin Orthop* 1986;212: 89–100.

In 401 unstable tibial fractures treated with interlocking nails, the average follow-up was 21 months. Delayed unions or nonunions occurred in 0.7% and deep infections in 2.2%; 94% had excellent or good clinical results.

Lange RH, Bach AW, Hansen ST, et al: Open tibial fractures with associated vascular injuries: Prognosis for limb salvage. *J Trauma* 1985;25:203–208.

In this retrospective analysis of 23 cases, unfavorable outcome was related to crush injuries, segmental tibial fractures, and revascularization delayed for more than six hours. Guidelines for primary amputation were developed but not prospectively evaluated.

Leffers D, Chandler RW: Tibial fractures associated with civilian gunshot injuries. *J Trauma* 1985;25:1059–1064.

Low-energy missiles caused simple fracture patterns, often with unicortical comminution. Medium- and high-energy missiles caused comminuted fractures, many grades II and III wounds, neurologic deficits, more infections, and prolonged times to union.

Mayer L, Werbie T, Schwab JP, et al: The use of Ender nails in fractures of the tibial shaft. *J Bone Joint Surg* 1985;67A:446–454.

A review of 51 severe tibial fractures treated with multiple intramedullary nails 4 to 4.5 mm in diameter found nonunions in 4%, shortening in 6%, angulation of more than 6 degrees in 4%, and infections after open fractures in 8%.

Nkele C, Aindow J, Grant L: Study of pressure of the normal anterior tibial compartment in different age groups using the slit-catheter method. *J Bone Joint Surg* 1988;70A:98–101.

In 30 volunteers the average resting pressure was +5.1 mm Hg (range, –2.01 to +17.5 mm Hg). Average peak pressure during foot exercise was 25.4 mm Hg (range, –3 to +81 mm Hg). Exercise-induced increase in pressures returned to normal within 3.4 minutes after the exercise was stopped. For reliable resting pressures to be obtained, the patient should be supine and the big toe should be pointing upward.

Smith MA, Jones EA, Strachan RK, et al: Prediction of fracture healing in the tibia by quantitative radionuclide imaging. *J Bone Joint Surg* 1987;69B:441–447.

Uptake of technetium was studied in 73 patients with fresh tibial fractures. Images obtained between one and four weeks after fracture were related to the incidence of nonunion six months later. A ratio of 1.3 between the uptake at the fracture site and normal bone adjacent to it predicted a nonnion with a sensitivity of about 70% and a specificity of about 90%.

Swartz WM, Mears DC: The role of free-tissue transfers in lower-extremity reconstruction. *Plast Reconstr Surg* 1985;76:364–373.

An analysis of 85 free flaps for clean and infected soft-tissue and bony defects found that the flaps were lost in 20%, persistent oseomyelitis occurred in 8%, and amputations were needed in 12%. Thus, indications for extensive procedures for grade IIIB injuries, with large segments of infected bone and absence of plantar sensation, are limited.

Tibial Shaft Nonunions

Galpin RD, Veith RG, Hansen ST: Treatment of failures after plating of tibial fractures. *J Bone Joint Surg* 1986;68A;1231–1236.

Eighteen patients with plated tibial fractures that failed to unite were treated with reamed open intramedullary nailing after plate and screws were removed. Fifteen of 16 fractures with sufficient follow-up healed. One patient needed a later bone graft.

Gordon L, Chiu EJ: Treatment of infected tibial nonunions and segmental defects of the tibia with staged microvascular muscle transplantation and bone-grafting. *J Bone Joint Surg* 1988;70A:377–386.

Of 14 infected tibial nonunions with or without segmental defects, all healed after debridement and local or free muscle flaps. Of the eight infected nonunions with segmental defects, three failed to unite or needed a below-knee amputation despite the use of bone graft or a free fibular graft.

Johnson EE, Marder RA: Open intramedullary nailing and bone-grafting for non-union of tibial diaphyseal fracture. *J Bone Joint Surg* 1987;69A:375–380.

Of 22 uninfected tibial nonunions treated with open reduction and intramedullary nailing augmented by local bone grafting, all went on to union with bridging callus at an average of 12.5 weeks.

Fractures of the Tibial Plafond

Ovadia DN, Beals RK: Fractures of the tibial plafond. *J Bone Joint Surg* 1986;68A:543–551.

This is a collective review of 145 fractures of the tibial plafond treated by many orthopaedic surgeons and followed up for an average of a 4.9 years. The clinical outcomes were directly related to the severity of comminution and ranged from 100% good results for minimally displaced fractures to 10% to 40% good results for severely comminuted wounds. Patients with simple fractures did equally well with nonsurgical treatment and internal fixation. In comminuted and displaced lesions, the end results were clearly superior when treatment was based on AO principles. Fractures with incomplete reduction or residual gaps in the articular surface also had poorer outcomes. Seven of 12 patients who were known alcoholics had poor results. About 20% of the patients with the most severe fractures needed an arthrodesis after an average of 2.5 years.

45

Knee and Leg: Reconstruction

Significant advances in the areas of synovectomy, debridement, realignment, and total knee arthroplasty have been documented in the recent literature. The results of current total knee arthroplasty with condylar prostheses are predictable if the procedure is correctly performed in appropriately selected patients. The results of total knee arthroplasty are equal to those of total hip arthroplasty. Complications at the present time are related primarily to wear, infection, and the extensor mechanism. Some of these complications are preventable by correct surgical technique. The results of salvage with revision arthroplasty are satisfactory at five years in approximately 70%. The results of revision vary, depending on the reason for failure and the type of previous implant.

Synovectomy

The techniques of synovectomy in the management of synovial proliferative disorders have expanded. Synovial proliferative disorders suitable for synovectomy include rheumatoid arthritis, pigmented villonodular synovitis, synovial chondromatosis, and hemophilic synovitis. The indications for synovectomy in rheumatoid arthritis are failure of medical management after a trial of six to eight months, persistent synovitis, and stage I or II arthropathy (little or no bone involvement) on radiographs. Once the disease has progressed with loss of the joint space, the results of synovectomy are unpredictable.

The long-term (14-year) results of open synovectomy in rheumatoid arthritis are satisfactory in 49%. Diminished pain and swelling can be anticipated after synovectomy, but motion is unchanged or decreased. In juvenile rheumatoid arthritis, 77% of patients have satisfactory pain relief at 7.5 years. A prospective study of medical management alone compared with open synovectomy in juvenile rheumatoid arthritis found better local disease control in the synovectomy group at two years. The greater the disease activity at the time of surgery, the greater the risk of subsequent deterioration of the result. Radiographic joint degeneration is not prevented by synovectomy. Similar degrees of joint-space narrowing were observed in patients with bilateral knee disease but unilateral synovectomy. The major problems with open synovectomy techniques are a prolonged recovery, stiffness, long hospitalization, and difficulty in regaining motion.

Arthroscopic synovectomy techniques have been developed to decrease morbidity. Outpatient surgery is possible. Recovery is more rapid after arthroscopic synovectomy and the complication rate is low. Arthroscopic synovectomy requires a knowledge of multiple-portal placement and use of a high-speed synovial resector. Results after two years were satisfactory in 80% of cases.

Alternative techniques include chemical and radiation synovectomy. Chemical synovectomy with alkylating agents or osmic acid is rarely used because of potential articular cartilage damage. Radiation synovectomy with gold or yttrium has provided satisfactory results in 58% of properly selected patients at three years. The best results are in patients with minimal radiographic abnormalities and low systemic disease activity. The disadvantages of these agents are their long half-life (two to three days) and some diffusion of the agents to the regional lymph nodes and liver. A three-day hospitalization has been required. Dysprosium 165, a new agent with a half-life of two hours, has been attached to ferric hydroxide macroaggregates. The short half-life and larger carrier size minimize diffusion of the agent from the knee. Hospitalization has been decreased to one day. Satisfactory results have been found in 66% of patients at two years. When repeat radiation synovectomy was required, results were good in 54%.

Synovectomy in hemophilia is indicated in the patient with recurrent hemarthrosis and subacute or chronic synovitis. The best results occur in patients with stages I to III arthropathy. Open synovectomy has consistently resulted in a decreased frequency of hemarthrosis. However, open synovectomy has resulted in loss of motion in as many as 85% of patients and has been associated with complications in as many as 50%. Arthroscopic synovectomy effectively decreases the incidence of recurrent hemarthrosis but has been associated with loss of motion in as many as 40% of knees. Neither open synovectomy nor arthroscopic synovectomy has been shown to prevent progression of arthropathy. Progression of arthropathy after synovectomy occurs in 20% to 60% of knees.

Arthroscope-guided intervention for limited degenerative gonarthrosis or for degenerative meniscal tears continues to be a useful tool. Attempts to alter the underlying process by osseous debridement to bleeding bone (abrasion arthroplasty) have not proven to be successful. There are no recent reports substantiating the use of this procedure, even for the localized defects for which it continues to be used. The debridement of synovial and meniscal tissue, however, continues to be perceived as an effective treatment in some instances. There is little objective documentation of its value but the clinical impression is that 50% to 60% of patients benefit from this procedure for several months to several years.

Osteotomy About the Knee

The role of osteotomy about the knee for unicompartmental tibiofemoral gonarthrosis has undergone refinements in recent years. Controversy still exists as to whether the osteotomy should be performed on the tibial or femoral side and which techniques of fixation are best.

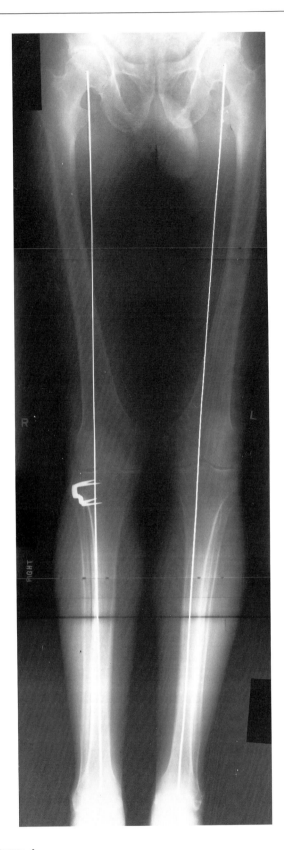

Figure 1

Full-length anteroposterior radiograph demonstrating the mechanical axis of the limb. Previous upper tibial osteotomy of the right knee has corrected the mechanical axis to the lateral compartment.

Biomechanics

Significant loads occur across the knee in the range of two to four times body weight with approximately 60% of the load passing through the medial compartment. In unicompartmental tibiofemoral arthritis, there is wearing away of the articular cartilage and some of the subchondral bone, further changing limb alignment. This redistribution of the load across the joint produces even further loading on damaged articular cartilage and thus perpetuates a vicious cycle.

Osteotomy attempts to resolve this problem by redistributing forces across the joint to a more normal level. This results in unloading of the damaged compartment with the potential for regeneration of reparative fibrocartilage. Unfortunately, static assessment of loads across the joint are inaccurate. Short standing radiographs of the knee are inadequate to assess overall limb alignment; full-length radiographs of the lower extremity are needed to determine the mechanical axis of the limb (Fig. 1). The objective of osteotomy should be to correct the mechanical axis into the opposite compartment to unload the diseased side. Such determinations are usually made on the basis of static loads on the affected limb. However, dynamic evaluation has shown that static analysis alone is inadequate to assess true forces across the joint and that most of the load may pass through the medial compartment even after a seemingly appropriate valgus realignment. Therefore, some surgeons are combining dynamic gait analysis, full-length radiographs, and computer programming to determine the optimum degree of correction to be achieved with the osteotomy. At the very least, a full-length radiograph of the lower extremity should be used and the desired correction should be based on correction of the mechanical axis of the limb. Whether the full-length radiograph is taken with the patient standing with equal weight on both legs or in a one-leg stance remains a controversial issue.

Patient Selection

In selecting a patient for osteotomy about the knee, the most important considerations in determining the site of osteotomy should be that adequate correction of the mechanical axis of the limb can be achieved and that the resulting orientation of the joint line is not oblique.

Valgus Osteotomy

Upper tibial valgus osteotomy for varus deformity is the most frequently performed osteotomy about the knee. In selecting a patient for upper tibial osteotomy, several factors should be considered. Favorable characteristics include unicompartmental tibiofemoral arthrosis, younger age (usually less than 60 years), optimal weight, vigorous occupation, satisfactory knee motion, and no severe angular deformity. The ideal patient must have an adequate range of motion with no more than a 10- or 15-degree flexion contracture and at least 80 to 90 degrees of knee flexion. Knee motion is unlikely to be improved after osteotomy. The patient's pain should be localized to the radiographically involved compartment. If there is a question concerning the isolated nature of the disease, a technetium bone scan may be helpful in further evaluation of the extent of the disease process. Varus deformity should be 15 degrees or less (tibiofemoral); otherwise it will be difficult to achieve adequate correction with a proximal tibial wedge osteotomy and the bone loss resulting from such a large wedge resection may lead to dynamic instability during gait. On physical examination, the patient who walks with a lateral thrust has evidence of dynamic instability and high medial compartment loading. This individual will not do as well after osteotomy as the individual who has a stable knee during gait.

Technique Osteotomy of the proximal tibia is performed proximal to the tibial tuberosity through cancellous bone, which heals rapidly. Either a wedge or a dome-shaped osteotomy can be performed. More distal dome or Wagner osteotomies may correct larger angular deformities. Anterior displacement of the distal fragment has been used to decrease patellofemoral contact pressures, but has the distinct disadvantage of making the contour of the anterior tibia abnormal, making subsequent total knee arthroplasty more difficult. Because patellofemoral tracking is altered by the change in limb alignment after osteotomy, there are few indications for combining anterior tibial displacement with the valgus osteotomy.

Fixation Although many different devices have been advocated for fixation of the osteotomy, more rigid fixation is used to allow early motion. Step staples have proven to be effective in providing stability adequate to allow early motion with the use of a brace or a cast brace. External fixation is used less frequently because of problems with pin sites. Plate fixation requires extensive dissection and is more difficult to remove if subsequent arthroplasty is required. Improved fixation allowing early motion may prove to be a valuable adjunct to osteotomy. Although the overall recovery time has been shortened, the final range of motion has not been shown to be significantly different from that after longer periods of immobilization. Contraindications to osteotomy include significant peripheral vascular disease, a flexion contracture of more than 15 to 20 degrees, flexion of less than 70 to 80 degrees, significant ligamentous instability, lateral subluxation of the tibia on the femur of more than 1 cm, and bone loss from the tibial plateau.

Results The results of upper tibial valgus osteotomy are difficult to interpret. Reported long-term series included patients who today would no longer be considered optimal candidates. Additional problems in interpreting long-term results are that the adequacy of the surgical technique and calculation of the optimal degree of correction were not appreciated at the time of the patient's initial procedure. Despite these limitations, satisfactory results as high as 60% at ten-year follow-up have been reported. There is a general tendency for the results to deteriorate with time as the degree of arthrosis progresses. The single most important factor in influencing the long-term results has been the adequacy of correction of the malalignment, with the best results occurring when the mechanical axis of the limb is overcorrected by 2 to 3 degrees beyond a neutral position. Significant overcorrection, as well as undercorrection, has been correlated with less satisfactory results. The age of the patient at the time of osteotomy has been thought not to influence the end result in some series, whereas in others older patients have had less satisfactory results than younger patients. A recent report specifically addressed the issue of osteotomy for secondary gonarthrosis from men-

iscectomy, for osteochondritis dissecans, and after trauma in patients less than 40 years old. After six years of follow-up, 75% had satisfactory results. Obese patients are less likely to have continued satisfactory results than patients closer to their ideal weight.

Complications Complications associated with osteotomy include infection, compartment syndromes, and peroneal nerve palsy, especially after dome osteotomy and the use of external fixation pins. Delayed union can often be attributed to poor apposition of the osteotomy site or inadequate fixation. Osteonecrosis and collapse of the tibial plateau may occur if the osteotomy is done too close to the joint. Fracture into the joint results from a technical error related to failure to use radiographic control at the time of the osteotomy or failure to complete the osteotomy through the tibia before closing the osteotomy.

Varus Osteotomy

The role of varus osteotomy in correcting valgus deformities about the knee has been more controversial than that of valgus osteotomy for varus deformity. The distal femur has an inherent valgus angulation that continues to exert a force across the joint. If a valgus deformity of more than 12 degrees is corrected by osteotomy through the proximal tibia, an oblique joint line results. With more than 10 degrees of medial tilting of the joint line, there is a tendency for subluxation of the joint and an unsatisfactory result. Therefore, in selecting a patient for a varus osteotomy for unicompartmental lateral disease, careful attention should be paid to the position of the joint line if the correction is performed at the proximal tibia. For varus osteotomy of the proximal tibia to be effective, the patient must have less than 12 degrees of valgus alignment of the knee and a satisfactory range of motion similar to that required for the valgus osteotomy. The optimal degree of correction is to 0 degrees of anatomic tibiofemoral alignment with the mechanical axis of the limb in the medial compartment. Proximal tibial varus osteotomy produced satisfactory pain relief in 77% of cases after an average nine-year follow-up in one study.

Varus osteotomy of the distal femur is needed in the individual with more than 12 degrees of valgus deformity. Initial attempts at varus osteotomy of the distal femur using staple fixation were subject to problems of prolonged cast immobilization. Results were satisfactory in only 41% of cases after a four-year follow-up. Current surgical techniques use plate fixation for the distal femur followed by early range of motion. This provides better results. Distal femoral varus osteotomy for valgus deformities of more than 12 to 15 degrees gave satisfactory results in 83% to 92% of cases after a four-year follow-up. Complications associated with the distal femoral varus osteotomy are similar to those associated with upper tibial valgus osteotomy. It is an exacting technique that must be performed with extreme care to achieve satisfactory results.

Arthroscopy

The role of arthroscopy in patients being treated by osteotomy about the knee remains controversial. The extent of arthritic involvement of the patellofemoral and contralateral compartment of the knee does not correlate well with the clinical results of osteotomy. The most important factor in the results appears to be the degree of overall correction of alignment. Arthroscopy has been useful in documenting fibrocartilaginous resurfacing of the unloaded portion of the joint by six years after osteotomy. Determining whether or not arthroscopic debridement procedures with removal of degenerative menisci, osteophytes, and loose bodies improves the results of osteotomy requires a randomized prospective study with long-term follow-up. At the present time, arthroscopy must be considered an investigative tool for the patient being treated by osteotomy rather than as an adjunctive treatment.

Effect of Osteotomy on Subsequent Arthroplasty

If osteotomy is used as a technique to delay total knee arthroplasty, it is important that the osteotomy does not compromise the subsequent arthroplasty. Technical problems identified at the time of total knee arthroplasty after upper tibial osteotomy include patella infera, the presence of tibial bone deficiencies, and posterior displacement of the proximal tibial fragment relative to the tibial shaft. Additional potential problems are related to malalignment from technical errors, nonunions, and fracture complications of osteotomy. The results of total knee arthroplasty after osteotomy have been satisfactory in 73% of 45 knees and 89% of 35 knees in different series. In most patients, it is possible to achieve a satisfactory result with total knee arthroplasty after osteotomy but the number of excellent results is lower and the procedure is technically more difficult. This may influence patient selection when osteotomy and total knee replacement are both appropriate options.

Arthroplasty

Hemiarthroplasty

The theoretic advantage of hemiarthroplasty over total knee arthroplasty is that it requires minimal bone resection. Indications for a hemiarthroplasty (for example, McKeever or MacIntosh procedures) are a young patient or obesity in a patient with disability from osteoarthritis, posttraumatic arthritis, or previous sepsis. Contraindications to hemiarthroplasty are previous sepsis, erosion or cystic change on the tibial or femoral surface, ankylosis, neuropathic arthropathy, angular deformity that is not passively correctable, or a poorly motivated patient. The results of hemiarthroplasty at eight to ten years are satisfactory in 70% with a 15% to 25% revision rate. The results of hemiarthroplasty are less predictable than those of total knee arthroplasty but revision of the hemiarthroplasty to total knee arthroplasty provides excellent results in most patients.

Unicompartmental Arthroplasty

Comparative studies of unicompartmental arthroplasty and osteotomy are difficult to perform. There are no randomized, prospective studies showing any advantage of unicompartmental replacement over osteotomy. The results depend on patient selection, optimal design of the prosthesis, and restoration of limb alignment and accurate soft-tissue balance.

Unicompartmental total knee arthroplasty has some potential advantages over tricompartmental total knee replacement. Unicompartmental knees tend to have a greater range of motion preoperatively and postoperatively and may feel more "normal" than those treated with tricompartmental replacement. It has been stated that unicompartmental arthroplasty preserves bone stock more than tricompartmental replacement because the contralateral compartment and patellofemoral joint are not treated.

Indications The indication for performing a unicompartmental arthroplasty is unicompartmental tibiofemoral disease, usually in the older patient who is sedentary. Preferably, patients should be at their ideal weight and should not have severe fixed deformities that require extensive soft-tissue releases for correction. The knee should have a reasonable range of motion, but unicompartmental arthroplasties are successful in patients with less than 90 degrees of flexion or flexion contractures of more than 15 degrees if these can be corrected at the time of arthroplasty by appropriate debridement. The rationale for unicompartmental arthroplasty is that articular cartilage that is visually normal is chemically, histologically, and metabolically normal. However, the mechanical characteristics of the articular cartilage have not been investigated in detail.

Contraindications Contraindications to unicompartmental arthroplasty include inflammatory arthritis in the young patient, high activity demands, obesity, a fixed deformity that requires extensive soft-tissue release for correction, dynamic instability as evidenced by a lateral thrust to the gait or tibial subluxation, and severe limitation of motion.

Results The overall results of unicompartmental arthroplasty with older, cemented designs were approximately 78% satisfactory at five years (Fig. 2). However, the reported results have ranged widely from as few as one third of the patients improved to as many as 95% with satisfactory outcomes. In one series, only 63% of the unicompartmental arthroplasties were satisfactory after a minimum follow-up of ten years. In studies of the St. George unicompartmental replacement, results after eight years of follow-up were satisfactory in 70%. The initial design of the Brigham unicompartmental replacement had a 10% failure rate at ten years. The revised Brigham unicompartmental replacement had 92% satisfactory results at five years. The revised design incorporates metal backing of the tibial compartment. Whether or not improved results will be obtained with newer designs and improved surgical techniques remains to be determined.

Complications The complications associated with unicompartmental arthroplasty are largely related to implant loosening (7.5%); the overall revision rate is 5%. The incidence of deep infection has been extremely small, in the range of 0.3%. Failure mechanisms in unicompartmental arthroplasty are primarily loosening, implant subsidence, tibial subluxation, patellar impingement by the femoral component, bony fracture of either the femoral or tibial condyles, breakage of the prosthesis, and degeneration of the opposite compartment. Almost all these complications and failure mechanisms can be related to errors in surgical technique or patient selection.

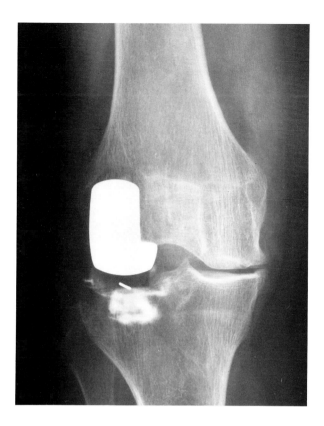 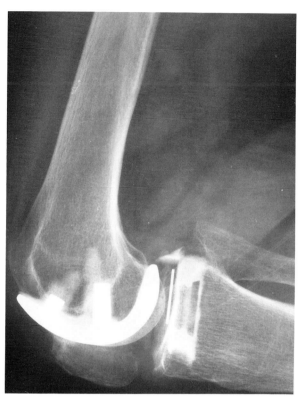

Figure 2

Anteroposterior (**left**) and lateral (**right**) radiographs of lateral unicompartmental geometric total knee replacement after ten years.

Surgical Considerations Overall tibiofemoral alignment is critical. It is important to correct the underlying varus or valgus deformity but overcorrection must be avoided or degeneration of the contralateral compartment will occur. Soft-tissue balancing must be achieved without the use of extensive soft-tissue releases. There should be excellent stability of the tibial components with no tendency toward lift-off through 120 degrees of flexion. The femoral component must be centered on the condyle, cover the weight-bearing surface, and reproduce the anteroposterior dimension of the femur. The femoral component should not impinge against the patella during motion. The tibial component must be congruent with the femoral component, cover the tibia, and replace lost bone. Most current designs incorporate metal backing.

Fixation Currently, unicompartmental arthroplasty uses cemented components. Cementless components have been developed and used investigationally. One design had a 25% failure rate within two years; results were satisfactory in 74%. In another study with a different implant design, the results were satisfactory in 94% after a follow-up of 3.8 years. Longer follow-up of the newer cementless replacements is needed to determine whether there is a role for these prostheses. The small surface area available for porous ingrowth may well be a limiting factor.

Total Knee Arthroplasty: Indications and Results

Indications

The indications for total knee arthroplasty are disabling knee pain and functional impairment from osteoarthritis, rheumatoid arthritis, posttraumatic arthritis, and other arthropathies. There should be clinical and radiographic involvement of two or more compartments of the knee. The patient should have failed a course of nonsurgical management and not be a candidate for less extensive procedures such as debridement or osteotomy. Contraindications to total knee arthroplasty are a nonfunctioning extensor mechanism, severe neuromuscular dysfunction preventing control of the knee, active sepsis, previous surgical arthrodesis, and neuropathic arthropathy.

Results

The results of total knee arthroplasty can be considered in relation to implant type, preoperative diagnosis, or survival analysis techniques. Survival analysis is a statistical technique that includes all patients entered into a study group regardless of the duration of follow-up. Survival analysis has been widely used in oncology studies and has been applied to total joint arthroplasty. A 50% implant survival at six to eight years has been reported for an early four-compartment Liverpool total knee replacement. The geometric prosthesis had a 69% survival rate at ten years. Implant survival has improved with newer surface replacement designs in both osteoarthritis and rheumatoid arthritis. Survival rates of 87% in osteoarthritis and 90% in rheumatoid arthritis at six years have been reported for tricompartmental total knee replacements. A 94% 11-year survival has been found for the total condylar prosthesis.

The ten-year results for the total condylar prostheses are now being reported. Satisfactory results have been reported in 70% to 90% of total condylar knees with an all-polyethylene tibial component. The variant of the total condylar prosthesis that spares the posterior cruciate ligament has provided 90% to 95% satisfactory results at five years. The posterior stabilized prosthesis has provided 94% to 96% satisfactory results at six to ten years. The similarity of results suggests that condylar total knee replacement provides highly predictable results for five to ten years in patients with osteoarthritis or rheumatoid arthritis.

Satisfactory results have been reported in 91% of knees with osteonecrosis and in 70% to 90% of those in hemophiliacs. For arrested septic arthritis, the results of total knee arthroplasty are satisfactory in 86% with a history of quiescent tuberculosis and 92% of those with nonmycobacterial septic arthritis. In the young patient less than 40 years old who has rheumatoid arthritis, a functional improvement and 86% good to excellent results can be anticipated at five years.

Bilateral total knee arthroplasty done at a single session provides satisfactory clinical results with a complication rate similar to those of staged and unilateral arthroplasties. Hospitalization and cost are lower in simultaneous arthroplasties than in staged arthroplasties.

Design of Total Knee Replacements

Total knee replacement designs have improved greatly from the initial hinged prostheses. Current implant designs are variations on the total condylar prosthesis concept. However, the multiplicity of designs suggests that no single design is optimal.

Two current areas of concern in implant design are implant fixation and polyethylene wear. Implant fixation and polyethylene wear are interrelated problems. Cemented tibial implant fixation has been improved by the use of a central stemmed component, metal backing of the tibial component, and multiple implant sizes to provide maximum coverage of the tibial plateau. Maximum coverage of the tibial plateau by the tibial implant is essential. Failure to achieve this results in a deleterious strain distribution. Metal backing of the component allows more uniform tibial loading of the knee when it is correctly aligned but allows increased tensile forces if the implant is asymmetrically loaded. Metal backing of the tibial component results in a decreased polyethylene thickness and increased polyethylene stresses. An intramedullary stem improves fixation by assisting in control of bending forces, but the stem length must be limited because stress-shielding of the tibial cortex occurs along the entire length of the tibial stem.

Polyethylene wear (Fig. 3) and polyethylene breakage (Fig. 4) are being recognized with increased frequency. Polyethylene wear damage occurs more frequently in heavy individuals, with malalignment of implants, and with long duration of implantation. High conformity of the tibiofem-

oral surface increases the contact area and decreases stresses on the polyethylene. Unfortunately, high conformity also alters ligament tension, alters knee kinematics, decreases motion, and increases bone-cement stresses that lead to loosening. Low conformity of the tibiofemoral surface increases polyethylene wear and results in edge loading of the components as well as instability. A foreign-body reaction to the wear debris may result in late implant loosening. An optimal compromise is partial conformity of the implant, but the ideal degree of conformity has not been determined. Other factors leading to polyethylene wear are a thin polyethylene component and carbon-fiber-reinforced polyethylene.

Wear cannot be eliminated because moving contact points result in cyclic stresses on the polyethylene. The maximum shear stresses on the polyethylene occur 2 mm below the surface, which predisposes to the formation of subsurface cracks. In total knee arthroplasty, the stresses on the polyethylene may exceed the yield point of the polyethylene, usually in knee flexion when the contact areas are minimal.

Surgical Technique in Total Knee Arthroplasty

Correct surgical technique is essential to achieve predictable and durable results in total knee arthroplasty. The goals are to achieve proper limb and component alignment, soft-tissue stability throughout the range of motion, and motion adequate for the activities of daily living. The surgical incision should incorporate previous incisions when possible. For the knee without previous surgical incisions, either a medial parapatellar or midline longitudinal incision with an anteromedial capsular incision suffices. Wound healing is similar with both. A curved medial incision has a higher incidence of delayed wound healing and poor oxygenation of the lateral skin flap.

Optimal position and alignment of the limb and the prosthesis are necessary for satisfactory results. Optimal limb alignment is present when the mechanical axis of the limb falls through the center of the joint or slightly toward the lateral compartment (Fig. 5). It is currently thought that the most accurate method of achieving the correct degree of femoral valgus is the use of an intramedullary alignment system combined with an extramedullary alignment system. A radiographic marker over the femoral head allows intraoperative determination of the mechanical axis of the limb. The position of the femoral and tibial components can be incorrect despite a correct mechanical axis. The correct coronal orientation of the tibial and femoral components is controversial.

If the tibia is cut at 90 degrees to its axis in the coronal plane, there may be a slight tilt of the joint line relative to the ground in the standing position. If a 90-degree tibial cut is selected, a 5- to 7-degree valgus cut on the distal femur usually provides a correct mechanical axis of the limb. If a 3-degree varus cut in the coronal plane is performed on the tibia, the joint line may be oriented parallel to the ground but requires a greater degree of valgus for the distal femoral cut. The increased valgus orientation of the femoral component may adversely affect patellar tracking. It is extremely difficult to achieve a 3-degree varus tibial cut. The usual surgical error involves too much varus. A varus tibial angulation of more than 3 degrees has

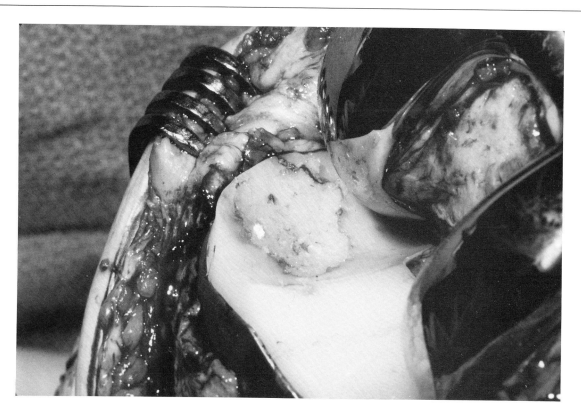

Figure 3

Wear of kinematic condylar polyethylene tibial component in vivo after two years.

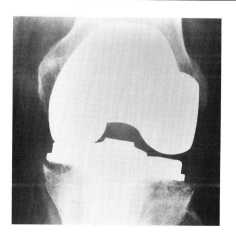

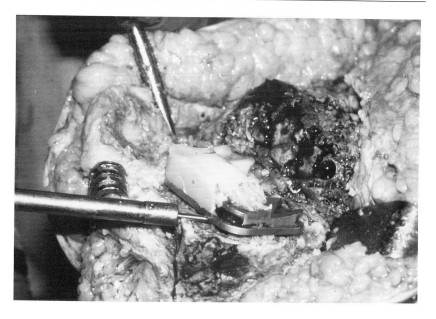

Figure 4

Left, Anteroposterior radiograph of polyethylene breakage after five years. **Right,** Intraoperative photograph of polyethylene breakage.

been associated with an increased incidence of tibial loosening in a wide variety of total knee designs.

In the sagittal plane, a slight posterior tilt of the tibial cut improves motion and prevents impingement against the femur in flexion. The degree of the posterior slope depends on the implant design. Tibial implant positioning should be centered on the plateau in the mediolateral direction and centered or slightly posterior in the antero-

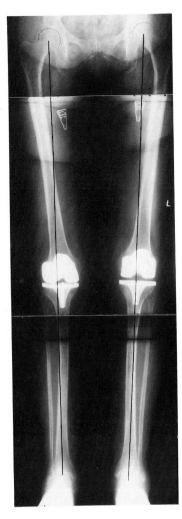

Figure 5

Correct mechanical axis of the limb after arthroplasty.

posterior plane. The implant should cover the tibial surface as completely as possible without overhanging the bone edges. The femoral component should reproduce the anteroposterior dimension of the femur. The femoral component should be in contact with the posterior femoral condyles or support will be inadequate in flexion, predisposing to femoral component loosening.

Soft-tissue releases are best performed in a staged manner. Soft-tissue balance must be present throughout a range of motion and depends on maintenance of the correct height of the joint line. Soft-tissue balance affects limb alignment and must be considered in its assessment. Correct soft-tissue balance is usually achieved by sequential release of tight structures from the concave side of the deformity. On rare occasions, advancement of soft tissues may be necessary.

Bone deficiencies are frequently present in long-standing varus or valgus deformities, previous upper tibial osteotomy, and revision surgery. Tibial bone strength is less in rheumatoid patients than in osteoarthritic patients. Tibial bone strength decreases with increased depth of resection. Therefore, resection of more than 5 to 8 mm of tibial bone is inadvisable as it compromises implant fixation. Bone

grafting has been used to fill large peripheral bone deficiencies with a 90% success rate (Fig. 6). Bone grafts are indicated for defects constituting 50% of the tibial plateau and when a cement column would exceed 5 mm in height. Small bone deficiencies can be managed by shifting of the prosthesis but this necessitates using a small tibial component and may alter joint loading. Screws and cement filling have been used successfully for bone defects of as much as 9 mm with a 26% incidence of radiolucent lines at three years. A custom-augmented prosthesis to fill the deficiency provides excellent loading across the defect without the uncertainty of bone graft incorporation.

Uncemented Total Knee Replacements

Uncemented fixation of total knee replacements was developed in an attempt to improve implant fixation. As experience has been gained with uncemented fixation, problems have been identified. Although femoral components have demonstrated secure fixation, patellar and tibial component fixation has been difficult to achieve in a predictable manner (Fig. 7). Problems with tibial implant subsidence have been reported with several different designs. Retrieval analysis of fibrous tissue has demonstrated limited tibial bone ingrowth. Perhaps the failure of tibial component ingrowth is related to micromotion between the implant and bone. Experimentally, movement of more than 150 μ results in ingrowth of only fibrous tissue.

Clinical comparisons of cemented vs uncemented implants have revealed a longer recovery time for the uncemented implants. The knee scores for the implants fixed without cement are lower than those for cemented implants. The frequency of reoperation is higher for uncemented than for cemented knees.

Complications of uncemented replacements include patellar loosening and polyethylene wear to the metal backing of the porous implant. Tibial-tray breakage has been reported with the implication that porous coating of the tray may have weakened the prosthesis. Cementless fixation should be used with caution in osteoporotic bone.

Loosening of the porous coating has been identified in 50% to 75% of patients. Loose beads are correlated with radiolucent lines at the bone-prosthesis interface (Fig. 8). Bead loosening has been more frequently observed adjacent to the tibial component. The loose beads probably represent micromotion of the implant.

The initial cementless implants have been modified in an attempt to improve tibial fixation. Screws, keels, and large stems have been added. No long-term data are yet available to confirm that these modifications have improved implant fixation. Therefore, some surgeons have elected to perform "hybrid" operations with cemented tibial and patellar components and cementless femoral components. Initial results with these hybrid knees have been similar to those with cemented prostheses.

Because porous-coated component fixation has led to bone ingrowth problems, other coatings such as hydroxyapatite are being studied in experimental animals. Direct bone bonding to hydroxyapatite-coated titanium transcortical plugs has been observed. Whether or not hydroxyapatite-coated tibial implants will have results similar to those of transcortical plugs requires further investigation.

A long-term concern with the porous-coated implants is

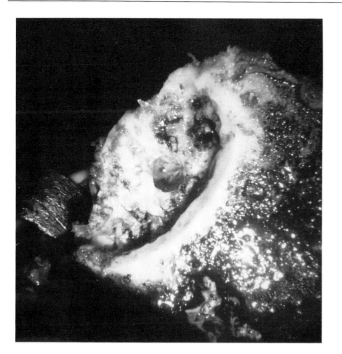

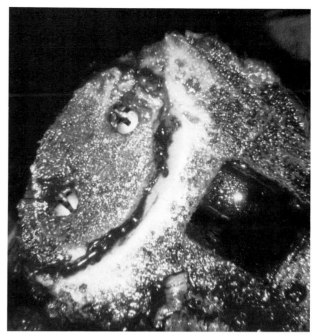

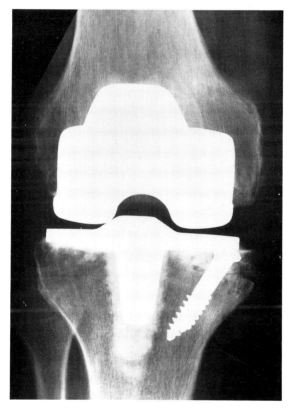

Figure 6
Top left, Intraoperative photographs of tibial bone deficiency. **Top right,** The bone graft used to treat it. **Bottom,** Postoperative radiograph.

metal corrosion. The surface area of the porous implant is substantially increased over that of a nonporous prothesis. The immunologic and oncologic consequences of high local metal ion concentrations in the soft tissues remains to be determined.

Patellar Resurfacing

The indications for patellar resurfacing during total knee arthroplasty remain controversial. Forces of one to four times body weight are transmitted across the patellofem-

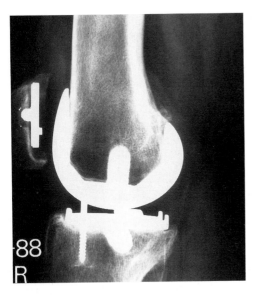

Figure 7
Lucent lines adjacent to patellar implant of PCA prosthesis.

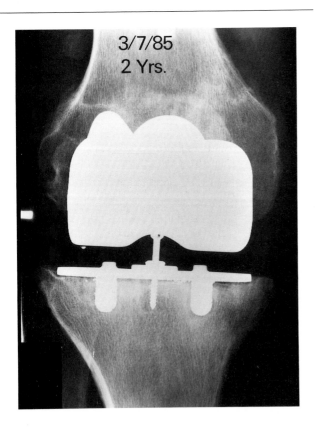

Figure 8
Loose beads and subsidence of tibial component of the PCA prosthesis.

oral joint. These forces are substantial for articular cartilage or for a polyethylene component articulating with the trochlear portion of the femoral component of a total knee replacement. Surface strains on the patella are maximal

between 45 and 90 degrees of flexion. Patellar resurfacing increases the stresses on the patella.

Older total knee prostheses produced patellofemoral pain in as many as 20% of resurfaced and 50% of hinged designs. With current condylar implants, patients with patellar resurfacing have less pain and better stair-climbing ability than patients without patellar resurfacing. Without patellar resurfacing, one third of patients with a total condylar prosthesis have difficulty ascending stairs. In osteoarthritic knees, patellar resurfacing may be optional, but all rheumatoid knees with adequate patellar bone stock should be resurfaced. Patellar tracking and congruency with the femoral component are probably the most important factors in deciding on patellar resurfacing. Patellar tilt or displacement adversely affects patellofemoral function. There has been poor correlation between the extent of chondromalacia at surgery and the clinical knee score after arthroplasty. A reoperation rate of 2.5% for patellar problems has been identified with or without patellar resurfacing.

Complications affecting the patellofemoral joint after total knee arthroplasty occur in as many as 10% of patients and include instability, fracture, wear, patellar ligament rupture, and soft-tissue impingement. Patellar subluxation or dislocation occurs in 0.4% to 0.8% of arthroplasties and may occur with or without patellar resurfacing. The instability may be caused by errors in surgical technique, quadriceps imbalance, trauma, or poor implant design. Internal rotation of either the femoral or the tibial component places the tibial tuberosity laterally, increasing the "Q" angle and leading to subluxation. Malrotation of an asymmetric, anatomic patellar design can result in instability caused by failure to articulate concentrically with the trochlear groove. Quadriceps imbalance most often results from failure to perform a lateral release during correction of a valgus knee. Other causes of quadriceps imbalance include vastus medialis weakness, vastus lateralis hypertrophy, and contracture of the iliotibial band. Postoperative trauma may tear the medial retinaculum or the repair may fail to heal. Older fixed-hinge implants had a high frequency of patellar instability, as did other early designs that provided a trochlear flange without a groove. Designs with unlimited rotation have had a high incidence of patellar instability because of the difficulty of achieving perfect soft-tissue balance at surgery.

Treatment of patellar instability after total knee arthroplasty must be directed at its cause. Malpositioned or malrotated components must be revised. Soft-tissue imbalance in the presence of correct implant position is best treated by proximal soft-tissue realignment procedures. Distal realignment techniques are best avoided because soft-tissue healing is unpredictable, with a high frequency of patellar ligament avulsion.

As much as possible of the original patellar thickness should be retained to optimize extensor mechanics and maintain patellar strength. Patellar fracture after total knee arthroplasty occurs with a frequency of less than 2%. Fractures occur more frequently in resurfaced patellas than in patellas without resurfacing (Fig. 9). The incidence of fracture is similar in osteoarthritic and rheumatoid patients. Factors predisposing to fracture include osteonecrosis, excess bone resection, a large central fixation lug, an excessively large femoral component, component malalignment, and trauma.

Whether treatment should be surgical or nonsurgical depends on the integrity of the extensor mechanism and the

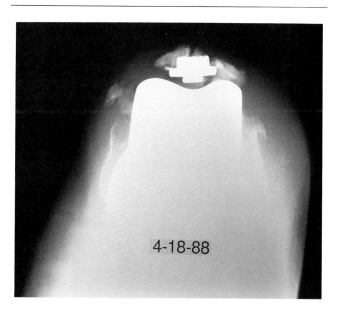

Figure 9

Patellar fracture after total knee arthroplasty with patellar resurfacing.

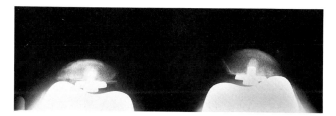
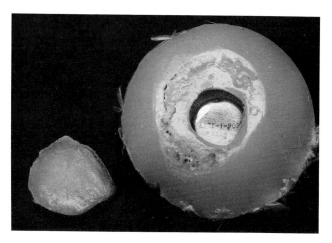

Figure 10

A Merchant radiograph (**top**) and photograph (**bottom**) of polyethylene wear exposing the metal backing of the patellar implant.

fixation of the implant. Nonsurgical treatment is used when the extensor mechanism is intact, the implant is secure, displacement is less than 2 cm, and there is no fracture comminution. Surgery should be selected in the absence of these factors.

Open reduction and internal fixation is a poor choice for these fractures. Open reduction and internal fixation has been associated with frequent problems of failure of fracture union, failure of wound healing, and deep infection. Partial patellectomy with repair of the extensor mechanism should be used for a single major fragment with a secure implant. Comminuted fractures with a loose implant are best managed by patellectomy. The results have been satisfactory in 96% of nonsurgically treated cases compared with 55% in surgically treated cases. Surgery has had complication rates as high as 42%. Complications include deep sepsis, implant loosening, and patellar ligament rupture.

Patellar implant loosening occurs in 0.5% of cases. Factors leading to loosening include deficient bone stock, asymmetric patellar bone resections, a small patellar fixation lug, and excessive loading by the patient's activities. Treatment by patellar implant revision depends on adequate bone stock but provides the best results. If patellar bone stock is deficient, patelloplasty or patellectomy should be selected.

Failure of metal-backed patellar components is occurring with increasing frequency (Fig. 10). All designs are potentially at risk, with failure being reported for at least seven different designs. Failure may occur by wearing through to the metal backing, fracture of the polyethylene that exposes the metal backing, or separation of the polyethylene from the metal backing. The metal backing of the patella then articulates with the femoral component, causing wear and a metallic synovitis. Symptoms include pain, swelling, and a metallic crepitation in the knee. The most important causative factor is malalignment of the patella with maltracking. Other associated factors are overweight, osteoarthritis, high activity level, and increased

thickness of the patellar component. Aspiration of the knee reveals metallic debris in long-standing cases. Arthroscopy is useful for early diagnosis of suspected polyethylene failure. Treatment consists of correction of the patellar tilt or malalignment, revision to an all-polyethylene patellar implant, and synovectomy. Revision of the femoral component is performed only if the wear is severe. The best results occur with early diagnosis before severe synovitis and foreign-body reaction develop.

Patellar tendon rupture occurs in less than 0.2% of knees. Patients with limited preoperative motion or those who are treated with a distal extensor mechanism realignment for patellar dislocation after arthroplasty are at high risk for this complication. The optimal treatment is reattachment of the tendon with augmentation as necessary to allow early motion. Problems with wound healing and secondary infection are frequent. These can be prevented by a turndown of the extensor mechanism when the ankylosed knee is exposed.

Revision Total Knee Arthroplasty

Failure of total knee arthroplasty requiring revision has largely been the result of prosthetic loosening, instability, or infection. Failure may result from poor patient selection, incorrect implant design, or improper surgical technique. The principles of revision arthroplasty are the same as those of primary arthroplasty but they are more difficult to achieve because of soft-tissue scarring and bone loss. Bone grafting or augmented femoral components compensate for femoral bone loss and allow restoration of the joint line. Long intramedullary stems help relieve stress in areas of bone deficiency and allow fixation in intact bone. Patellar bone loss may necessitate patelloplasty or patellectomy. The least constrained implant possible should be selected to minimize stresses on the bone-cement interface and subsequent loosening.

The results of total knee revision are not as good as those of primary surgery, being satisfactory in 70% to 80% of cases. Results are better for less constrained implants. Revision with a condylar-type prosthesis with minimal bone loss provides the best results. Conversely, revision of failed hinge implants to new rotating-hinge implants provides the least satisfactory results. Revisions with uncemented implants with long intramedullary stems have relieved pain in 77% to 91% of cases after short-term follow-up. Further follow-up is needed to assess the value of this technique.

Complications are more frequent after revision surgery than after primary surgery. An infection rate of 2% to 5% can be anticipated with resurfacing implants; infection rates are higher with larger implants such as rotating-hinge designs. Extensor mechanism problems of pain, patellar maltracking, and impingement between the patella and the tibial component are common because of the difficulty of restoring the joint line. Radiolucent lines are present in 20% to 80% of knees and reflect the difficulty of achieving cement penetration into sclerotic bone. Therefore, subsequent implant loosening can be anticipated more often than in primary arthroplasty.

Imaging After Total Knee Arthroplasty

Radiographic evaluation of total knee replacements is difficult to perform accurately because of their complex geometries. Therefore, the significance of radiolucent lines and assessment of loosening are difficult. A standard radiograph fails to reveal a 1-mm lucent line adjacent to an all-polyethylene tibial component if there is (1) flexion or rotation of the prosthesis of more than 5 degrees, (2) angulation of the roentgen beam of more than 6 degrees, or (3) offsetting of the beam of more than 2.5 cm. More than 4 degrees of flexion obscures a lucent line adjacent to a metal-backed component. Incomplete radiolucent lines of 1 mm or less do not correlate with clinical results but complete lucent lines of 2 mm correlate with poor clinical results. Radiolucent lines correlate with malalignment of the limb or implant. Lucent lines are frequent in areas of bone deficiency filled with cement. A shift of implant position on sequential radiographs is indicative of loosening. The histologic characterization of the radiolucent lines varies from inert fibrous tissue to active tissue with either giant cells or foam cell proliferation. With mechanical instability, with or without polyethylene and cement debris, the interface tissue is usually composed of inflammatory cells.

Bone scanning is used to evaluate loosening. In asymptomatic knees, increased activity on a diphosphonate scan can be expected for one year after surgery. Increased activity on the diphosphonate scan after one year is present in 89% of tibial and 63% of femoral components. Therefore, bone scans must be carefully interpreted in conjunction with the clinical examination and radiographs. The increased activity visualized on bone scans within a year of surgery reflect bone remodeling adjacent to the implant. Gallium or indium bone scans combined with technetium diphosphonate scans are helpful in differentiating infection from asymptomatic loosening. Quantitative computed tomography has revealed an expected loss of tibial bone of

1.6% per month after arthroplasty. This stabilizes by one year.

The stability of the implant and the bone-cement interface is important in the development of radiolucent lines. High-resolution roentgen stereophotogrammetric analysis has revealed micromotion of cemented implants with reversible displacement of the tibial component on loading of 0.2 to 1.0 mm. Reversible displacement was greatest for rotatory stresses. Migration was documented for all total condylar prostheses, with 70% stabilizing by one year. For the cementless Freeman-Samuelson prosthesis, migration ranging from 0.7 to 4.8 mm occurred, primarily in the first six weeks after implantation. Reversible displacement is larger with cementless implants than with cemented implants. Migration and reversible displacement occur within the fibrous tissue layer between either the cement and bone or the implant and bone.

Rehabilitation After Total Knee Arthroplasty

Function after total knee arthroplasty depends on correct surgical technique and postoperative rehabilitation. Knee motion affects the total knee score, stair-climbing ability, and walking ability. Significant improvement in knee flexion occurs between three months and one year, with some patients improving as long as three years after arthroplasty. A major determinant of the ultimate range of motion is the preoperative range of motion. Flexion contractures must be corrected soon after surgery. After hospital discharge, little improvement or progression in flexion contractures occurs. Implant design affects the ultimate motion achieved. Flattening of the posterior aspect of the tibial plateau allows increased knee flexion but may contribute to anteroposterior laxity.

Continuous passive motion is being used as an adjunct to physical therapy to rehabilitate the patient after total knee arthroplasty. Continuous passive motion allows the patient to achieve 90 degrees of knee flexion earlier than physical therapy alone. Hospitalization may be shortened. However, the ultimate range of motion after total knee arthroplasty is not influenced by use of continuous passive motion. Wound healing and thromboembolism are also uninfluenced by continuous passive motion.

The use of postoperative suction drainage has been controversial. No significant differences in wound healing or range of motion have been found in knees treated with and without suction drainage; blood loss, however, was increased with suction drainage. Early weightbearing after arthroplasty has no apparent adverse effect on cemented implant fixation. Activity levels must be considered in relation to soft-tissue healing.

Periprosthetic Fractures of the Femur After Total Knee Arthroplasty

Supracondylar fractures of the femur after total knee arthroplasty occur in 0.6% of primary and 1.6% of revision arthroplasties. The important factors are osteoporosis (40% of cases) and notching of the anterior femoral cortex (27% of cases). As many as 42% of patients with rheumatoid arthritis undergoing total knee arthroplasty who have surgical notching of the anterior femoral cortex sustain a fracture.

Treatment of the fracture depends on the adequacy of implant fixation and the quality of reduction that can be achieved. Nondisplaced fractures or fractures in which an anatomic reduction can be achieved and in which the implant is not loose can be managed nonsurgically with cast immobilization. Nonsurgical management has provided satisfactory results in 42% of cases. Open reduction and internal fixation is indicated for displaced fractures that cannot be adequately reduced by closed means and in which the prosthesis is not loose (Fig. 11). Open reduction and internal fixation provides satisfactory results in 64% of cases. For open reduction and internal fixation to be successful, the quality and size of the metaphyseal bone fragment must be adequate to achieve surgical fixation that allows early motion. If the implant is loose, revision of the arthroplasty is required. A long-stemmed condylar type femoral component to bridge the fracture site is preferable to resection of the metaphyseal fragment and use of a custom-hinged implant.

Vascular Complications After Total Knee Arthroplasty

Vascular complications after total knee arthroplasty are either arterial ischemia or venous thrombosis. Arterial injuries are infrequent, with an incidence of 0.3%. Preexisting arteriosclerotic disease or correction of preexisting flexion contractures predispose to this complication.

Venous thrombosis, pulmonary embolism, and fat embolism do occur after total knee arthroplasty. The clinically significant venous thrombosis or pulmonary embolism is rare, occurring in less than 2% of patients. Venographically documented deep venous thrombosis occurs in 50% to 70% of patients. The 32% incidence of deep venous thrombosis with cementless fixation was significantly less than the 49% incidence with cement fixation in one study. Asymptomatic pulmonary emboli have been found with ventilation perfusion lung scans in 17% of patients. Risk factors for venous thrombosis are difficult to identify. No single prophylactic regimen has proven satisfactory in the prevention of thrombosis. Continuous passive motion after arthroplasty has not been proven to be beneficial in prevention of venous thrombosis. Prophylaxis with warfarin has a 17% incidence of complications. In view of the low incidence of clinically symptomatic pulmonary emboli, the inability to identify high-risk patients, and the frequent complications with therapeutic anticoagulation regimens, the indications for thromboembolic prophylaxis are unclear.

The use of intramedullary instrumentation for total knee arthroplasty has improved the accuracy of surgical technique. Prostheses with long intramedullary stems are being used in revision surgery. Fat embolization is associated with total knee arthroplasty when large-stemmed implants are used. Lavage of the medullary canal and slow insertion of intramedullary devices should be performed to minimize this complication.

Infection After Total Knee Arthroplasty

Administration of systemic antibiotics at least five minutes before tourniquet inflation remains the current technique for prophylaxis against infection. The role of antibiotic-impregnated cement for prophylaxis against infection in routine total knee arthroplasty remains controversial because of possible allergies to the antibiotic and the development of antibiotic-resistant bacteria.

Infection after total knee arthroplasty remains a major cause of failure. The incidence of infection has been 1% to 2% in large series. The highest infection rate has been found with hinged prostheses, revision surgery, immunocompromised patients, previous septic arthritis, and previous surgery. Hematogenous spread of infection also causes failure.

Aspiration of the knee is useful when the culture is positive but a negative culture does not exclude infection. Hematologic studies and bone scanning are useful adjuncts but are insufficient by themselves. Gram-positive organisms constitute 50% to 70% of the infecting organisms but gram-negative organisms, anerobes, fungi, and mycobacteria also cause infections. Therefore, cultures should be done for all these organisms.

Treatment options include antibiotic suppression, debridement, resection arthroplasty, implantation of a new prosthesis, arthrodesis, and amputation. Antibiotic suppression is indicated only for patients unfit for surgical management. Antibiotics alone will not cure the infection. Surgical debridement with retention of the prosthesis is successful in 80% of acute infections but in only 10% of chronic infections.

Resection arthroplasty (implant removal without an attempt at arthrodesis) is indicated for the severely afflicted patient with polyarticular disease and limited ambulatory demands. Resection arthroplasty controls systemic infec-

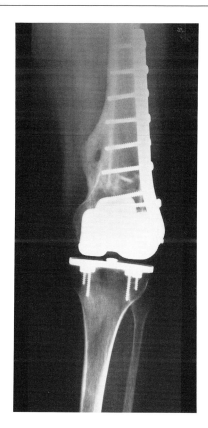

Figure 11

Miller-Galante total knee replacement after open reduction and internal fixation of femoral fracture with residual varus alignment.

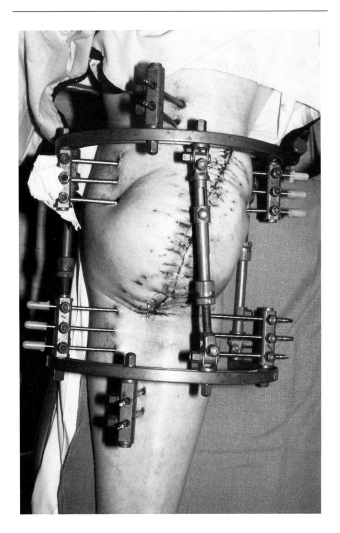

Figure 12
Biplanar external fixation for arthrodesis in acute infection.

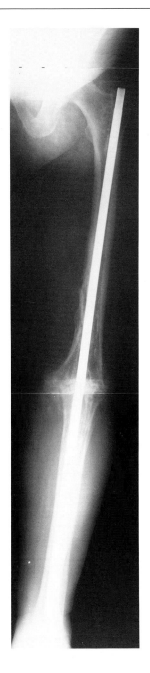

Figure 13
Inramedullary arthrodesis for quiescent infection after total knee arthroplasty.

tion but local wound drainage persists in 10% to 20% of cases. Subsequent arthrodesis is required in 21% of cases.

Reimplantation of a new prosthesis is best performed as a two-stage procedure with a delay of three to six weeks between procedures. Polymethylmethacrylate beads and a spacer containing antibiotics specific for the infecting organism are placed in the wound after debridement. Antibiotic-impregnated cement is used when the new prosthesis is implanted. A success rate of 80% can be anticipated with this approach.

The extent of bone loss is the single most important factor influencing the union rate after arthrodesis. Shortening after arthrodesis averages 3 cm. Biplanar external fixation in acute sepsis has a success rate of 68% (Fig. 12). Secondary attempts at arthrodesis have a 50% success rate. Intramedullary nail fixation is reserved for noninfected failures or as a secondary technique after infection has been resolved. The success rate of intramedullary arthrodesis is 90% (Fig. 13).

Ablative procedures are reserved for massive bone loss combined with persistent sepsis, persistent severe pain, or life-threatening infection. Amputation is necessary in less than 5% of patients with infection after arthroplasty.

Controversies

Patellar Resurfacing

Patellar resurfacing remains controversial. Most surgeons recommend resurfacing in inflammatory arthritis and a selective approach to patellar resurfacing in osteoarthritis. With higher ranges of motion obtained by improved surgical techniques and better prosthetic designs, more demands and larger forces are being placed on the patellofemoral joint. More attention given to lateral releases to improve patellar tracking has decreased patellar problems but resurfaced patellas continue to have loosening problems. Trochlear grooves on femoral components must be designed for both resurfaced and unresurfaced conditions. At the present time, metal-backed patellar implants of all designs are suspect because of problems with polyethylene wear exposing the metal backing.

Implant Fixation

Cemented vs uncemented fixation has continued to be a controversial issue. At the present time, cementless fixation of the femoral component appears to provide results similar to those obtained with a cemented component. The long-term advantages of cementless femoral fixation remain to be determined. Removal of cementless knee components does not necessarily protect bone stock any more than removal of cemented components and may actually result in increased bone loss during extraction. Cementless fixation of tibial components, regardless of design, has been a problem and, since most arthroplasties are done in an elderly population, cemented fixation of the tibia provides more predictable results. The promised of enhanced cementless fixation with various surface treatments and/ or screws requires further experimental investigation, both clinically and in the laboratory.

Retention vs Sacrifice of the Posterior Cruciate Ligament

Whether to retain or sacrifice the posterior cruciate ligament remains an unresolved issue. Both types of arthroplasty provide satisfactory results when correctly performed. Clinical studies to date show no long-term differences. Findings of gait studies imply higher interface forces associated with designs that sacrifice the posterior cruciate, and some functional activities are diminished. Whether these higher forces will contribute to increased loosening rates after longer-term follow-up is unknown. On the other hand, less conforming surfaces used in designs that spare the posterior cruciate increase wear of polyethylene surfaces. It is possible that direct wear of polyethylene surfaces and/or the biologic response to wear particles may lead to higher failure rates after longer-term follow-up. These unresolved questions will become even more important as total knee arthroplasty is extended to younger and more active patients.

Infection

Reimplantation and arthrodesis appear to be satisfactory modes of salvage for the infected total knee arthroplasty. Reimplanation should be selected when feasible over arthrodesis because it provides improved functional results. The optimal interval between removal and reimplantation is controversial. This decision depends on individual considerations such as the virulence of the organism, the status of the host tissue, and the immunocompetence of the patient.

Revision Total Knee Arthroplasty

Although the overall principles of revision knee arthroplasty are the same as those of primary arthroplasty, the handling of defects and poor quality of bone assumes great importance. Bone grafting techniques seem to work well and offer almost limitless adaptations for repairing defects. Long-term survival of both small and large grafts needs investigation. Modular prosthetic systems pose mechanical and design problems that seem to be minimal in the short run, but longer-term results are lacking. The results of custom designs also need scrutiny. Firmer guidelines about when each of these methods is most advantageous should be developed.

Annotated Bibliography

Keywords

Femoral fracture; Hemiarthroplasty; Infection; Ischemia; Osteotomy; Patellar resurfacing; Roentgenography; Synovectomy; Total knee replacement; Unicompartmental arthroplasty

Synovectomy

Ishikawa H, Ohno O, Hirohata K: Long-term results of synovectomy in rheumatoid patients. *J Bone Joint Surg* 1986;68A:198–205.
A 14-year study of synovectomy in 78 knees in 55 patients with rheumatoid arthritis revealed satisfactory results in 48%. There was no significant difference in radiographic degenerative joint disease between knees that had undergone surgery and those that had not. The best results were achieved in stage I disease.

Montane I, McCollough NC III, Lian EC: Synovectomy of the knee for hemophilic arthropathy. *J Bone Joint Surg* 1986;68A:210–216.
Synovectomy of the knee for hemophilic arthropathy had relieved pain in 66% at a seven-year follow-up. Of the 13 patients treated by synovectomy, 85% had a loss of motion. The overall complication rate was 46%.

Rydholm U, Elborgh R, Ranstam J, et al: Synovectomy of the knee in juvenile chronic arthritis: A retrospective, consecutive follow-up study. *J Bone Joint Surg* 1986; 68B:223–228.
Pain relief was satisfactory after 7.5 years in 77% of 60 synovectomies in 51 children with juvenile rheumatoid arthritis. Progression of radiographic joint damage correlated with older age or high activity level of disease.

Sledge CB, Zukerman JD, Shotkroff S, et al: Synovectomy of the rheumatoid knee using intra-articular injection of dyprosium-165-ferric hydroxide macroaggregates. *J Bone Joint Surg* 1987;69A:970–975.
Results were satisfactory in 66% of cases two years after radiation synovectomy using dysprosium 165. The best results occurred with early disease activity.

Osteotomy About the Knee

Coventry MB: Proximal tibial varus osteotomy for osteoarthritis of the lateral compartment of the knee. *J Bone Joint Surg* 1987;69A:32–38.

After 9.4 years of follow-up, pain was relieved in 77% of 24 knees treated by varus upper tibial osteotomy. This technique is recommended only if the valgus deformity is less than 12 degrees and if the tilt of the tibial articular surface will be less than 10 degrees after the osteotomy.

Coventry MB: Upper tibial osteotomy for osteoarthritis. *J Bone Joint Surg* 1985;67A:1136–1140.

The results of upper tibial valgus osteotomy were 62% satisfactory at ten years. Careful patient selection and consideration of dynamic loading are essential in achieving optimum results.

Holden DL, James DL, Larson RL, et al: Proximal tibial osteotomy in patients who are fifty years old or less: A long-term follow-up study. *J Bone Joint Surg* 1988;70A: 977–982.

Upper tibial valgus osteotomy in patients under the age of 41 years provided 70% satisfactory results at a ten-year follow-up. The most important factor influencing the result of the procedure was the overall level of disease activity. Deficiency of the anterior cruciate ligament did not prevent a satisfactory result.

Prodromos CC, Andriacchi TP, Galante JO: A relationship between gait and clinical changes following high tibial osteotomy. *J Bone Joint Surg* 1985;67A:1188–1194.

Correlation between the clinical results of osteotomy and preoperative gait analysis revealed that the best results were achieved when the preoperative adduction moment was low. The overall geometry of the joint and alignment did not directly correlate with dynamic loading that occurred during walking.

Staeheli JW, Cass JR, Morrey BF: Condylar total knee arthroplasty after failed proximal tibial osteotomy. *J Bone Joint Surg* 1987;69A:28–31.

Results were satisfactory in 89% of cases after condylar-type total knee arthroplasty in patients who had undergone a previous upper tibial osteotomy. The intraoperative and postoperative complication rates were no higher than those of primary total knee arthroplasty.

Arthroplasty

Hemiarthrolasty

Scott RD, Joyce MJ, Ewald FC, et al: McKeever metallic hemiarthroplasty of the knee in unicompartmental degenerative arthritis: Long-term clinical follow-up and current indications. *J Bone Joint Surg* 1985;67A:203–207.

Results were satisfactory at an eight-year follow-up in 70% of 44 knees treated by McKeever hemiarthroplasty. The revision rate was 14%. It was thought that obese and young patients were candidates for this procedure.

Swanson AB, Swanson GdeG, Powers T, et al: Unicompartmental and bicompartmental arthroplasty of the knee with a finned metal tibial-plateau implant. *J Bone Joint Surg* 1985;67A:1175–1182.

Results were satisfactory five years after hemiarthroplasty in 94% of 32 knees. One patient required revision of the hemiarthroplasty because of progression of pain during this time.

Wordsworth BP, Shakespeare DT, Mowat AG: MacIntosh arthroplasty for the rheumatoid knee: A 10-year follow-up. *Ann Rheum Dis* 1985;44:738–741.

Results of the MacIntosh hemiarthroplasty in rheumatoid patients were satisfactory in 71% at ten years. The procedure was thought to be contraindicated in patients with large angular deformities or pronounced articular cartilage damage.

Unicompartmental Arthroplasty

Larsson S-E, Larsson S, Lundkvist S: Unicompartmental knee arthroplasty: A prospective consecutive series followed for six to 11 years. *Clin Orthop* 1988;232:174–181.

A prospective study of 102 unicompartmental St. George prostheses followed up for eight years revealed a 4% loosening rate, 11% subsidence, and 4% degeneration of the contralateral compartment. Satisfactory overall clinical results were achieved in 78%.

Marmor L: Unicompartmental arthroplasty of the knee with a minimum ten-year follow-up perod. *Clin Orthop* 1988;228:171–177.

Of 81 unicompartmental total knee arthroplasties with an 11-year follow-up, 47% had satisfactory results, 27% had unsatisfactory results, and 26% failed. The failure was correlated with too severe initial disease, component malpositioning, or use of a component that was too thin.

Total Knee Arthroplasty: Indications and Results

Bryan RS: Total knee arthroplasty revisited: One surgeon's 14 years of experience, in Rand JA, Dorr LD (eds): *Total Arthroplasty of the Knee: Proceedings of the Knee Society 1985–1986*. Rockville, Maryland, Aspen Publishers, 1987, pp 83–106.

Actuarial survival analysis techniques showed that failures were exremely rare after condylar knee implants. Results were much better for condylar knees than for earlier total knee replacement designs or cemented total hip replacement designs.

Goldberg VM, Figgie MP, Figgie HE III, et al: Use of a total condylar knee prosthesis for treatment of osteoarthritis and rheumatoid arthritis: Long-term results. *J Bone Joint Surg* 1988;70A;802–811.

Of 109 total condylar knees followed up for nine years, 74% had good to excellent results. The infection rate was 0.6%. Better clinical results were achieved with patellar resurfacing than without patellar resurfacing.

Insall JN, Kelly M: The total condylar prosthesis. *Clin Orthop* 1986;205:43–48.

A ten-year evaluation of 40 total condylar knee replacements found satisfactory results in 88%. Failures were correlated with technical errors or improper patient selection. Lucent lines were present in one third of the patients at ten years.

Morrey BF, Adams RA, Ilstrup DM, et al: Complications and mortality associated with bilateral or unilateral total knee arthroplasty. *J Bone Joint Surg* 1987;69A: 484–488.

A comparative review of 1,000 total knee arthroplasties showed a 9% incidence of complications with simultaneous bilateral arthroplasty, 7% with bilateral procedures done at different times during the same hospitalization, and 12% with bilateral procedures done during separate hospitalizations. Because the morbidity and mortality associated with simultaneous bilateral total knee arthroplasty were about the same as those associated with arthroplasty performed at different times, cost analysis favors simultaneous bilateral arthroplasty when bilateral surgery is indicated.

Ranawat CS, Boachie-Adjei O: Survivorship analysis and results of total condylar knee arthroplasty: Eight- to 11-year follow-up period. *Clin Orthop* 1988;226:6–13.

A survivorship analysis of 112 total condylar knees after follow-ups of as long as 11 years showed 89% of the replacements to be functioning. Actual results at follow-up were clinically satisfactory in 9%. Radiolucent lines were observed in 60%. Increased body weight correlated with radiolucent lines.

Scott WN, Rubinstein M, Scuderi G: Results after knee

replacement with a posterior cruciate-substituting prosthesis. *J Bone Joint Surg* 1988;70A:11633-1173.

Of 119 knees treated with a posterior stabilized prosthesis, 83% had good or excellent results after two to eight years. Radiolucent lines were seen in 76% but did not correlate with the clinical result. The overall range of motion was 107 degrees.

Stuart MJ, Rand JA: Total knee arthroplasty in young adults who have rheumatoid arthritis. *J Bone Joint Surg* 1988;70A:84-87.

After an average follow-up of five years, good or excellent results were achieved in 86% of 44 condylar replacements in patients with rheumatoid arthritis who were less than 40 years old. Only 18% had radiographic lucent lines. No failures were caused by implant loosening.

Design of Total Knee Replacements

Bartel DL, Bicknell VL, Wright TM: The effect of conformity, thickness, and material on stresses in ultra-high molecular weight components for total joint replacement. *J Bone Joint Surg* 1986;68A:1041-1051.

Stresses associated with surface damage to the polyethylene in total knee replacements are higher than those in total hip replacements. Contact stresses are a function of the thickness of the polyethylene insert and are high for thicknesses of less than 8 to 10 mm. A combination of high stresses and a moving contact area predispose to wear of the polyethylene of the tibial components. Contact stresses can be reduced by making the tibiofemoral articulation more conforming in the mediolateral direction.

Bourne RB, Finlay JB: The influence of tibial component intramedullary stems and implant-cortex contact on the strain distribution of the proximal tibia following total knee arthroplasty: An in vitro study. *Clin Orthop* 1986;208:95-99.

Contact between the tibial component and the peripheral cortical rim decreases strain values in the proximal tibia. Therefore, implant coverage of the proximal tibia should be maximized. Intramedullary stems stress-shield along the entire length of the tibial stem. Therefore, they should be no longer than necessary to achieve fixation to prevent problems of long-term stress-shielding.

Walker PS, Reilly D, Soudry M, et al: Femorotibial contact location in condylar replacement knee implants, in Dorr LD (ed): *The Knee: Papers of the First Scientific Meeting of The Knee Society.* Baltimore, University Park Press, 1985, pp 95-108.

Retention of the posterior cruciate ligament in total knee arthroplasty results in a more central contact area as well as higher contact stresses on the tibial polyethylene. Implant design should include semiconformity between the femoral and tibial surfaces to prevent excessive wear on the surface or increased stresses at the bone-cement interface.

Wright TM, Bartel DL: The problem of surface damage in polyethylene total knee components. *Clin Orthop* 1986;205:67-74.

A review of retrieved tibial components showed a correlation of damage with the weight of the patient as well as with the time of implantation. Three variables were found to influence the degree of wear: (1) conformity of the articular surface, (2) the elastic modulus of the polyethylene, and (3) the thickness of the polyethylene.

Surgical Technique in Total Knee Arthroplasty

Dorr LD, Boiardo RA: Technical considerations in total knee arthroplasty. *Clin Orthop* 1986;205:5-11.

The technique used in total knee arthroplasty is critical.

There is an increased frequency of lucent lines after total knee arthroplasty with bone resection more than 5 mm from the tibia. Varus placement of the tibial component should be avoided. The anteroposterior height of the femur should be maintained. The deformity should be corrected by soft-tissue balancing rather than by excessive bone resection.

Dorr LD, Ranawat CS, Sculco TA, et al: Bone graft for tibial defects in total knee arthroplasty. *Clin Orthop* 1986;205:153-165.

Twenty-two of 24 bone grafts for bone deficiencies at total knee arthroplasty were satisfactory. Two failures occurred: one because of varus alignment of the limb and the other because no vascular bed was prepared for the bone graft. Bone grafting is indicated for bone deficiencies of more than 5 mm after completion of the bone cuts.

Figgie HE III, Goldberg VM, Heiple KG, et al: The influence of tibial-patellofemoral location on function of the knee in patients with the posterior stabilized condylar knee prosthesis. *J Bone Joint Surg* 1986;68A:1035-1040.

When a posterior stabilized total knee replacement design was used, the best clinical results occurred when the joint line height was restored to within 8 mm of the preoperative position. The frequency of patellofemoral problems increased and motion decreased in knees in which the joint line was malpositioned.

Uncemented Total Knee Replacements

Haddad RJ Jr, Cook SD, Thomas KA: Biological fixation of porous-coated implants. *J Bone Joint Surg* 1987;69A:1459-1466.

Fixation of most porous total knee implants has been by fibrous tissue, especially on the tibial component. The most consistent site of bone ingrowth has been adjacent to fixation pegs in both the femoral and the tibial components.

Hungerford DJ, Krackow KA, Kenna RV: Two and five year experience with a cementless porous coated total knee prosthesis, in Rand JA, Dorr LD (eds): *Total Arthroplasty of the Knee.* Rockville, Maryland, Aspen Publishers, 1987, pp 215-235.

After two to five years of follow-up, the PCA prosthesis without cement provided good or excellent results in 95% of 63 patients with osteoarthritis and in 92% of 25 patients with rheumatoid arthritis. Problems with patellar implant fixation were noted with the early patellar implant design. Loose beads were seen adjacent to 20% of the femoral components and 60% of the tibial components.

Rorabeck CH, Bourne RB, Nott L: The cemented Kinematic-II and the non-cemented porous-coated anatomic prosthesis for total knee replacement: A prospective evaluation. *J Bone Joint Surg* 1988;70A:483-490.

A comparison of cemented kinematic condylar and uncemented PCA total knee replacements at 24 months showed higher knee scores for the cemented implant. Improved motion was also observed in the knees that had a cemented replacement. The reoperation rate for the cemented replacement was 4% compared with 12% for the uncemented replacement.

Rosenqvist R, Bylander B, Knutson K, et al: Loosening of the porous coating of bicompartmental prostheses in patients with rheumatoid arthritis. *J Bone Joint Surg* 1986;68A:538-542.

Thirty-four cementless PCA knees were followed up for 17 months. More than one half showed radiographic evidence of loose beads from the porous coating. In 14 knees, the beads had loosened by three months postoperatively, suggesting micromotion of the implants.

Patellar Resurfacing

Bayley JC, Scott RD, Ewald FC, et al: Failure of the metal-backed patellar component after total knee replacement. *J Bone Joint Surg* 1988;70A:668–674.

A comined multicenter experience with metal-backed patellar components in 25 total knee replacements showed that the factors contributing to failure were obesity and osteoarthritis. Failure occurred from wear, fracture, or dissociation of the polyethylene relative to the metal backing. Seven different implants failed at the patella, suggesting that this is a generic problem.

Brick GW, Scott RD: The patellofemoral component of total knee arthroplasty. *Clin Orthop* 1988;231:163–178.

Of 2,887 primary total knee replacements, 1.5% had complications related to the patellofemoral joint; the revision rate was 1.3%. Subluxation occurred in 0.8%, fractures in 0.3%, and patellar loosening in 0.6%.

Grace JN, Sim FH: Fracture of the patella after total knee arthroplasty. *Clin Orthop* 1988;230:168–175.

Fracture of the patella after total knee arthroplasty occurred with increased frequency in those with patellar resurfacing and after revision arthroplasty. Complications occurred in 42% of the knees after treatment for this problem.

Merkow RL, Soudry M, Insall JN: Patellar dislocation following total knee replacement. *J Bone Joint Surg* 1985;67A:1321–1327.

Patellar instability after total knee arthroplasty correlated with preoperative valgus deformity, trauma, incorrect tracking after replacement, and malrotation of the tibial component. In the absence of component malposition, proximal realignment provided satisfactory clinical results.

Soudry M, Mestriner LA, Binazzi R, et al: Total knee arthroplasty without patellar resurfacing. *Clin Orthop* 1986;205:166–170.

A comparison of total condylar knees with and without patellar resurfacing found better stair-climbing ability in those patients with patellar resurfacing. There was little functional differences between the two groups in terms of pain relief or knee scores.

Revision Total Knee Arthroplasty

Goldberg VM, Figgie MP, Figgie HE III, et al: The results of revision total knee arthroplasty. *Clin Orthop* 1988;226:86–92.

Of 65 total knee arthroplasties revised because of mechanical failure, only 46% had good or excellent results at five years. The most improvement occurred in those knees in which a posterior stabilized or total condylar replacement was used for the revision. The best results were achieved in those knees in which component positioning and alignment were restored toward normal. The overall infection rate was 4.5%.

Insall JN: Revision of total knee replacement, in Anderson LD (ed): American Academy of Orthopaedic Surgeons *Instructional Course Lectures, XXXV*. St. Louis, CV Mosby, 1986, pp 290–296.

Of 72 revision total knee arthroplasties, 89% had satisfactory results after two to five years. A constrained prosthesis is seldom required. The addition of stems to the implant is useful for fixation in deficient bone.

Rand JA, Bryan RS: Results of revision total knee arthroplasties using condylar prostheses: A review of fifty knees. *J Bone Joint Surg* 1988;70A:738–745.

After five years of follow-up, satisfactory results were achieved in 76% of 50 revisions using a condylar prosthesis.

There were no deep infections and lucent lines were present in only 17%.

Rand JA, Peterson LFA, Bryan RS, et al: Revision total knee arthroplasty, in Anderson LD (ed): American Academy of Orthopaedic Surgeons *Instructional Course Lectures, XXXV*. St. Louis, CV Mosby, 1986, pp 305–318.

A review of 427 revision total knee arthroplasty procedures with a variety of implants over a ten-year period showed the condylar-type devices had the best implant survival. The five-year probability of prosthetic function was 75% after a single revision and 62% for knees undergoing two revision procedures. Prosthetic survival was better for less constrained than for more constrained implants.

Imaging After Total Knee Arthroplasty

Ecker ML, Lotke PA, Windsor RE, et al: Long-term results after total condylar knee arthroplasty: Significance of radiolucent lines. *Clin Orthop* 1987;216:151–158.

In a clinical study of 123 total condylar prostheses, radiolucent lines were identified in 65% at five years. There was no correlation between radiolucent lines and clinical results. With metal-backed tibial components, more than 4 degrees of flexion or angulation between the radiographic beam and the component obliterates a 1-mm radiolucent line. With a polyethylene tibial component, more than 5 degrees of rotation, 6 degrees of angulation, or 2.5 cm of off-setting obliterates a radiolucent line.

Ryd L: Micromotion in knee arthroplasty: A roentgen stereophotogrammetric analysis of tibial component fixation. *Acta Orthop Scand* 1986;220(suppl):1–80.

Roentgen stereophotogrammetric analysis showed that cemented tibial components have micromotion on loading and/or reversible displacement. Metal support for the polyethylene did not decrease micromotion. Limb alignment, position of the prosthesis, and cortical bone support did not correlate with micromotion.

Ryd L, Albrektson BEJ, Herberts P, et al: Micromotion of noncemented Freeman-Samuelson knee prostheses in gonarthrosis: A roentgen-stereophotogrammetric analysis of eight successful cases. *Clin Orthop* 1988;229:205–212.

Analysis of cementless Freeman-Samuelson components showed component displacement ranging from 5 to 8 mm in all cases. In all cases, some migration had occurred two years after implantation.

Rehabilitation After Total Knee Arthroplasty

Romness DW, Rand JA: The role of continuous passive motion following total knee arthroplasty. *Clin Orthop* 1988;226:34–37.

A comparison of patients undergoing total knee arthroplasty with and without continuous passive motion was performed. The patients with continuous passive motion achieved 90 degrees of knee flexion earlier than the control group but at three months and one year there was no significant difference in motion between the two groups. There was no significant difference in the duration of hospitalization or blood loss between the two groups.

Schurman DJ, Parker JN, Ornstein D: Total condylar knee replacement: A study of factors influencing range of motion as late as two years after arthroplasty. *J Bone Joint Surg* 1985;67A:1006–1014.

Motion progressively improved for as long as one year after total knee arthroplasty. A flexion contracture was less likely to improve with time than knee flexion.

Periprosthetic Femoral Fractures After Total Knee Arthroplasty

Aaron RK, Scott R: Supracondylar fracture of the femur after total knee arthroplasty. *Clin Orthop* 1987;219:136–139.

Notching of the anterior femoral cortex as well as osteoporosis contributed to supracondylar fracture of the femur after total knee arthroplasty. Of 12 knees with significant anterior femoral cortical notching, 42% sustained supracondylar fractures.

Culp RW, Schmidt RG, Hanks G, et al: Supracondylar fracture of the femur following prosthetic knee arthroplasty. *Clin Orthop* 1987;222:212–222.

A review of 61 supracondylar fractures of the femur, half of which were treated surgically and half nonsurgically, found better clinical results with surgery. Notching of the anterior femoral cortex as well as neurologic disorders predisposed to supracondylar fracture.

Vascular Complications After Total Knee Arthroplasty

Arterial

Rush JH, Vidovich JD, Johnson MA: Arterial complications of total knee replacement: The Australian experience. *J Bone Joint Surg* 1987;69B:400–402.

Of a combined series of 12 arterial injuries associated with total knee arthroplasty, seven involved femoral and popliteal artery thrombosis and five involved direct trauma to the major vessels. Peripheral vascular disease should be carefully evaluated before total knee arthroplasty is performed.

Venous

Lynch AF, Bourne RB, Rorabeck CH, et al: Deep-vein thrombosis and continuous passive motion after total knee arthroplasty. *J Bone Joint Surg* 1988;70A:11–14.

A 40% incidence of deep venous thrombosis in the calf was associated with total knee arthroplasty. Continuous passive motion had no effect on the incidence of thrombosis. The thrombosis extended into the popliteal vessels in 5%. Deep venous thrombosis was more frequent in patients in whom the prosthesis was fixed with cement.

Sutherland CJ, Schurman JR: Complications associated with warfarin prophylaxis in total knee arthroplasty. *Clin Orthop* 1987;219:158–162.

A 17% incidence of complications was identified after warfarin prophylaxis was used in the prevention of deep venous thrombosis after total knee arthroplasty. Warfarin prophylaxis should be used only in highly selected patients.

Infection After Total Knee Arthroplasty

Bannister GC, Auchincloss JM, Johnson DP, et al: The timing of tourniquet application in relation to prophylactic antibiotic administration. *J Bone Joint Surg* 1988;70B:322–324.

Antibiotic levels in bone and fat were measured in patients undergoing total knee arthroplasty. At least five minutes is required after intravenous administration of antibiotics before tourniquet application so that the antibiotic can reach satisfactory levels.

Falahee MH, Matthews LS, Kaufer H: Resection arthroplasty as a salvage procedure for a knee with infection after a total arthroplasty. *J Bone Joint Surg* 1987;69A:1013–1021.

Implant removal without arthrodesis as a salvage procedure for the failed total knee arthroplasty provides the best results in severely afflicted rheumatoid patients with limited ambulatory demands. Resection arthroplasty provides inadequate stability for ambulation and inconsistent pain relief in most patients with osteoarthritis and single-joint disease. Only five of 24 patients who were ambulatory before surgery had a mobile joint that was stable enough for walking without support after resection arthroplasty.

Grogan TJ, Dorey F, Rollins J, et al: Deep sepsis following total knee arthroplasty: Ten-year experience at the University of California at Los Angeles Medical Center. *J Bone Joint Surg* 1986;68A:226–234.

Of 13 knees with infection after total knee arthroplasty, only four could be salvaged without implant removal. Debridement was most effective when the sepsis was treated within one week.

Petty W, Spanier S, Shuster JJ: Prevention of infection after total joint replacement: Experiments with a canine model. *J Bone Joint Surg* 1988;70A:536–539.

An in vivo canine experiment comparing antibiotic irrigation with systemic antibiotics and antibiotic-impregnated cement found a statistically significant reduction in the rate of infection with antibiotic-impregnated bone cement. The antibiotic cement proved superior for prevention of infection.

Rand JA, Bryan RS, Chao EY: Failed total knee arthroplasty treated by arthrodesis of the knee using the Ace-Fischer apparatus. *J Bone Joint Surg* 1987;69A:39–45.

A 68% success rate was achieved with biplanar external fixation in 28 patients. A 36% complication rate was encountered. Bone loss was the single most important factor influencing failure of the arthrodesis. Bone grafting is recommended to offset the effect of bone deficiencies at the time of arthrodesis.

Salvati EA, Callaghan JJ, Brause BD, et al: Reimplantation in infection: Elution of gentamicin from cement and beads. *Clin Orthop* 1986;207:83–93.

An in vivo study of gentamicin release from cement showed levels 17 times higher with cement beads and seven times higher with antibiotic-impregnated cement than could be achieved with systemic intravenous antibiotics. Although tissue levels were significantly higher with antibiotic-impregnated cement, serum and urine levels were considerably lower than those after intravenous administration. No toxic effects of the antibiotic-impregnated cement were identified.

46
Ankle and Foot: Pediatric Aspects

Topics of pediatric interest include congenital conditions such as clubfoot, tarsal coalition, metatarsus adductus, flatfoot, and congenital vertical talus, neuromuscular disorders such as cerebral palsy and myelomeningocele, and occurrences such as infection and trauma that affect the ankle and foot.

Clubfoot

Idiopathic clubfoot is a relatively common (one in 1,000 births) congenital defect consisting of rigid equinovarus hindfoot with an adducted supinated forefoot. Although the pathologic anatomy and causes of this deformity have been studied and debated for years, no definite conclusions have been reached. Inheritance is multifactorial and boys are affected twice as often as girls.

Cause

Clubfoot can occur as part of a syndrome, as in diastrophic dwarfism or the Freeman-Sheldon syndrome. Arthrogryposis, amniotic band syndrome, and myelomeningocele are highly associated with clubfoot.

The cause of idiopathic clubfoot remains elusive. Abnormalities in the vasculature, muscle, ligaments, and bone have been reported. The recent demonstration of abnormal arterial supply in 15 embryos with clubfoot suggested a possible primary vascular cause. Other investigators have reported primary abnormalities in the ossification and growth of the talus, suggesting a "germ-plasma defect in the cartilaginous anlage." Fiber type disproportion and ultrastructural abnormalities have been found in clubfoot muscle, suggesting a neurogenic origin to some. However, these findings may be secondary because electromyographic and nerve conduction studies have shown no neuropathic or myopathic alterations that might account for the development of a clubfoot. Abnormal tendon insertions and the absence of an anterior muscle compartment have been proposed as causes but are not commonly found. Another proposed cause is retracting fibrosis, which has recently been described as thick, shortened ligaments on the posterior and medial aspects of the ankle joint containing myofibroblasts like those seen in Dupuytren's contracture.

An attempt to define the abnormal anatomy by means of three-dimensional computer modeling of a single neonatal clubfoot found that the body of the talus was externally rotated 14 degrees in the ankle mortise with 45 degrees of internal rotation of the neck and head of the talus. In a normal foot, the body is internally rotated 5 degrees and the neck internally rotated 25 degrees. The calcaneus is externally rotated 5 degrees in a normal foot but internally rotated 22 degrees in the clubfoot. Others have emphasized the abnormal internal rotation of the calcaneus

so that the posterolateral aspect of this bone rotates toward the fibula (Fig. 1).

Treatment

Cast Correction Initial cast correction of a clubfoot requires that the adduction deformity of the forefoot be corrected first with firm pressure over the medial forefoot and counterpressure over the calcaneocuboid joint. The equinus and varus deformities of the hindfoot are then corrected. The correction should be confirmed radiologically. The longitudinal axis of the talus and calcaneus should diverge on the lateral view; on the anteroposterior view, the first ray should be aligned with the long axis of the talus and fifth ray should be aligned with the long axis of the calcaneus.

Surgery Specific surgical therapy for clubfoot remains controversial. Not all clubfeet require the same procedure. Some investigators ascribe the abnormality to the subtalar joint, whereas others believe that the position of the talus in the ankle joint is critical and that the subtalar joint requires no treatment. Most—but not all—authors recognize that talonavicular subluxation is a major component. One investigator found a laterally rotated talus to be the norm, whereas another found no talonavicular subluxation and attributed the deformity to an accentuation of full inversion.

It is generally recommended that surgery should be done when the child is 4 to 8 months old, although a few individuals prefer to do it sooner. The age of 4 to 8 months seems appropriate for a surgical release because the child will be ready to begin walking after the period of immo-

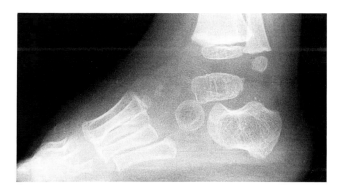

Figure 1

This 2-year-old patient underwent a clubfoot repair 18 months before this radiograph was taken. Notice that there is an anteroposterior view of the ankle and a lateral view of the foot. It is this problem of malrotation that has led to greater emphasis on the posterolateral corner and circumferential subtalar release in clubfoot.

bilization, and generally begins standing in the postoperative cast. The surgical procedure can be performed either via a Cincinnati incision or a straight medial incision with a short lateral incision if necessary. The procedure should, in general, be a posteromedial release with special attention paid to the posterolateral corner of the ankle. There may be limited situations in which a posterior release or a posterolateral release is all that is necessary. The procedure should always include isolation of the neurovascular bundle with release of the abductor hallucis muscle. The Achilles tendon is lengthened in a Z-fashion. The posterior tibial tendon is lengthened in a Z-fashion with preservation of the pulley or tendon sheath when possible. The flexor digitorum communis and the flexor hallucis longus may require lengthening. The posterior ligamentous structures released always include the tibiotalar joint, the talofibular and talocalcaneal ligaments, and a portion of the subtalar joint.

The medial and lateral extent of the subtalar release depends on the degree of deformity present. Many believe that a full lateral and sometimes circumferential release of the subtalar joint is of value in correcting the rotational deformity of the calcaneus. In feet with severe deformity,

satisfactory correction requires releases of the calcaneocuboid joint and the lateral talonavicular joint. A medial, dorsal, and plantar release of the talonavicular joint is done as part of the medial release in all feet. Most foot procedures keep the talocalcaneal or interosseous ligament intact; however, Simons' complete subtalar release sacrifices this ligament to obtain full correction. Kirschner-wire stabilization of the talonavicular joint is recommended to maintain alignment of the foot. At times, a talocalcaneal wire is used as well. At the conclusion of the procedure, radiographic documentation of alignment of the first ray with the talus on anteroposterior and lateral views, as well as alignment of the fifth ray with the calcaneus, is obtained. The patient may be placed in a splint initially with conversion to a cast after the initial swelling is decreased. A cast-brace apparatus has been recommended to preserve motion and increase tendon function, but most surgeons still favor immobilization for two to four months after a clubfoot release.

If the anterior compartment muscles are absent or if the anterior tibial or peroneal muscles are weak, a prolonged period of splinting with an ankle-foot orthosis is required to prevent recurrence.

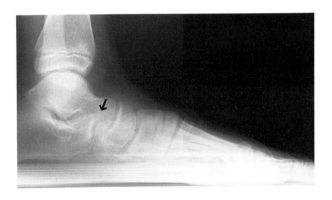

Figure 2
Anteater's nose.

Tarsal Coalition

Tarsal coalition is a condition in which the tarsal bones have fused. The most plausible cause is a congenital failure of segmentation in the cartilaginous anlage. Progressive ossification of the "bar" occurs with age. Patients experience symptoms in late childhood and adolescence, possibly because of a stress fracture in the coalition. Bone scans of coalitions frequently show increased uptake.

Foot and ankle pain is the common initial symptom. Pain may be localized to the area of the coalition or more diffuse over the midfoot and hindfoot. The pain is activity-related and responds poorly to anti-inflammatory drugs. A rigid flatfoot or peroneal spastic flatfoot is often associated with this structural abnormality. Although tarsal coalition may be the most common cause of peroneal spastic flatfoot, a differential diagnosis of the latter must include juvenile rheumatoid arthritis, osteoid osteoma, trauma, infection, neoplasm, and idiopathic causes. Recurrent ankle sprains can also be associated with tarsal coalitions.

The most common tarsal coalition is the calcaneonavicular fusion, in which the inheritance pattern is autosomal dominant. The second common coalition is fusion of the talocalcaneal middle facet. Radiologically, the calcaneonavicular coalition is best seen on an oblique plain radiograph of the foot. On a lateral plain radiograph, it can be seen as an extension of the calcaneal beak, resembling an "anteater's nose" (Fig. 2); on an anteroposterior view of the foot, it may be totally invisible. A sclerotic, angulated (more than 30 degrees), or absent middle facet joint demonstrates a talocalcaneal coalition. Computed tomography is now considered to be the best imaging technique for a talocalcaneal coalition (Fig. 3) and has largely replaced the conventional Harris view. The coalition can be seen on a coronal view through the middle facet. Magnetic resonance imaging may offer greater accuracy in the future, particularly for the diagnosis of cartilaginous and fibrous coalitions, but at present there are no reports comparing this technique with existing imaging techniques.

An asymptomatic tarsal coalition requires no treatment.

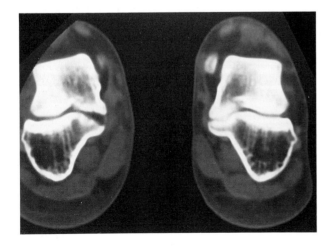

Figure 3
Talocalcaneal coalitions are seen best on a computed tomographic scan. The coalition on the left side was previously excised.

Symptomatic lesions should be treated with a trial of immobilization. The painful coalition without peroneal spasm or rigidity often becomes asymptomatic with immobilization, and may remain so with a simple arch support. A rigid peroneal spastic flatfoot associated with a tarsal coalition may also resolve with immobilization and this should be attempted before surgical intervention.

Surgical treatment of a calcaneonavicular coalition is excision. This generally has excellent results. Athletes are able to return to sports in most cases. Success requires that sufficient bone be resected through a sinus tarsae approach so that refusion does not occur. The excision site is prevented from reuniting by the use of an interposition material, either fat or short extensor muscles of the foot pulled through the bony gap. Talar beaking has previously been thought to represent a contraindication to excision, but it has been shown that this is not necessarily so. If degenerative arthritis is present within the tarsal joint, simple excision of the coalition is not indicated and a triple arthrodesis should be performed.

In the past, talocalcaneal coalition of the middle facet was treated primarily by triple arthrodesis when the symptoms did not resolve with immobilization. In the last five years there have been many reports that excision successfully relieved pain and restored function. To be resectable, the coalition should occupy less than 50% of the middle facet on computed tomography. The bed of the resected coalition is packed with fat to prevent reformation of the bony fusion. If support for the subtalar joint is insufficient after surgical excision, a triple arthrodesis should be performed. If the peroneal spasm and marked pronation deformity are not relieved postoperatively, triple arthrodesis is indicated. Talocalcaneal coalition excision is usually successful if normal hindfoot motion can be restored to the foot and pain relieved.

Another procedure that may have a significant role in the management of talocalcaneal coalition is subtalar arthrodesis. Satisfactory midfoot mechanics has been demonstrated after subtalar arthrodeses for hindfoot coalition. If the pain results from a stress fracture through the coalition, restoring integrity by fusion seems logical. An alternative in the foot with significant valgus malalignment of the hindfoot is the calcaneal osteotomy. As yet data are insufficient for either of these procedures to be recommended without reservation.

Cerebral Palsy

Foot deformity is often seen in patients with cerebral palsy. Chronic muscle imbalance produces an evolving pattern of deformity despite the static cerebral lesion. Management of the flexible mild deformity of childhood may prevent fixed bony deformity from occurring in adolescence and adulthood. Common deformity patterns are the equinovalgus foot that often occurs in spastic diplegia and the equinovarus foot that frequently occurs in spastic hemiplegia. The child with spastic quadriplegia or total-body involvement has a diffuse cerebral involvement with less predictable patterns of foot deformity. Treatment includes maintaining flexibility with physical therapy, bracing to prevent deformity and improve function, and surgery in selected cases. Surgery should be done to free a child from braces, to make bracing possible in cases in which it was impossible, or to correct an existing deformity and prevent

a worsening problem. Specific surgical procedures remain controversial. The soft-tissue surgical options include muscle lengthening, split transfers, and total tendon transfers. The surgeon must assess the flexibility of the foot while remembering that the rigid underlying deformities must be corrected before muscle-balancing procedures are undertaken.

A flexible equinus deformity can be managed by a brace. Heel-cord lengthening in general is reserved for the patient with equinus deformity secondary to myostatic contracture. Optimal time for lengthening is when the child is about 4 years old. The presence of an anterior tibial muscle under voluntary control correlates positively with postoperative brace-free status. The anterior tibial muscle can be strengthened as part of a standard postoperative physical therapy regimen. Equinus deformity in patients with movement disorders should be treated very cautiously because surgical treatment gives unpredictable results.

Varus deformity can accompany the equinus posturing of the foot, particularly in hemiplegia. This generally results from the overpull of the posterior tibial tendon but the anterior tibial tendon can also be implicated in the development of a varus foot. Management of this disorder in its flexible state includes the following possible tendon procedures: (1) Split posterior tibial tendon transfer (one half of the tibialis posterior to the peroneus brevis); this is ideal for the patient with an active anterior tibial muscle and a dynamic flexible varus deformity with posterior tibial spasticity. (2) Anterior transfer of the posterior tibial tendon through the interosseous membrane; the ideal patient for this procedure has a nonfunctioning anterior tibial muscle with a tibialis posterior muscle active during swing phase and minimal tightness in the gastrocnemius-soleus complex so that heel-cord lengthening is not required. (3) Split anterior tibial tendon transfer (transfer of one half of the anterior tibial tendon to the cuboid); an ideal patient for this procedure has a varus hindfoot and a supinated forefoot with weightbearing over the lateral aspect of the foot. This procedure is often accompanied by a lengthening of the posterior tibial and Achilles tendons.

Each of the tendon transfers for correcting a varus foot carries with it specific problems. The major limitation of the split posterior tibial tendon transfer is that it provides absolutely no foot dorsiflexion; it is, however, a safe, predictable transfer. The transfer of the posterior tibial tendon through the interosseous membrane carries a significant risk of a calcaneovalgus foot, particularly if the heel cord is lengthened simultaneously. A tonically firing posterior tibial muscle and a tight heel cord are contraindications to this procedure. Finally, the split anterior tibial tendon transfer is a safe procedure. If there is a rigid varus deformity, the varus must be corrected before the tendon transfer. This can be accomplished either by calcaneal osteotomy or by triple arthrodesis, depending on the age of the child and degree of deformity.

Valgus deformities can be caused by overpull of the peroneal muscles or underpull of the posterior tibial muscle. Once the valgus deformity is present, the force of the triceps surae, as well as gravity, tends to accentuate the deformity. Bracing with a UCB or ankle-foot orthosis may be effective in mild cases. Peroneus brevis lengthening combined with bracing has been beneficial in mild flexible cases in which the peroneal muscles overpulled. Realignment procedures to correct the valgus deformity in cerebral palsy include the calcaneal slide osteotomy in which the tuberosity of the calcaneus can be placed in proper alignment with respect to the subtalar and ankle joints; this may restore the proper axis of weightbearing. This is often combined with heel-cord lengthening and postoperative bracing. The Grice subtalar arthrodesis is problematic in the management of the valgus foot deformity in the young child because of both nonunion and malunion. It may, however, have a role in a child with severe involvement who has a severe valgus deformity. Another transfer used to correct the valgus deformity in cerebral palsy is the peroneus brevis to posterior tibial tranfer.

Forefoot deformities in cerebral palsy include cavus, metatarsus adductus, bunions, hallux valgus, and toe-flexion deformities. The flexible deformities can be treated by soft-tissue procedures and tendon lengthenings, but results are mixed. Arthrodesis and osteotomy are always required when fixed deformity is present and should always be accompanied by tendon-balancing procedures.

Hallux Valgus

Hallux valgus is a common problem in which a congenital predisposition can be aggravated by footwear, producing a painful foot deformity. Metatarsus primus varus may or may not accompany this deformity. Pain is the usual indication for therapeutic intervention. Therefore, the initial evaluation should concentrate on the cause of foot pain in the child. Possible causes include an osseous or soft-tissue lesion about the first metatarsal or metatarsophalangeal joint, infection, arthritis, and finally the bunion itself. In children, a pronated foot with loss of the longitudinal arch is often associated with hallux valgus. Treatment of the associated flatfoot with an arch support may resolve the foot pain in many children.

Surgical correction in adolescence has a high recurrence rate when compared with the accepted results in adults. The rate of recurrence is higher in the presence of a flatfoot deformity (56%). Although many procedures have been described for correction of hallux valgus, they can be divided into the proximal metatarsal osteotomies and the distal metatarsal osteotomies. There are no series comparing these procedures in a controlled fashion. From recent reports, the distal metatarsal osteotomy may have better overall results than the proximal osteotomy in adolescents.

Infection

After puncture wounds of the foot, there is a small risk of deep infection. In general, initial management should include debridement and irrigation of the puncture wound. The efficacy of antibiotic therapy as part of initial management is controversial but antibiotics are commonly administered. Deep *Pseudomonas* infections become evident an average of about nine days after injury. A cartilaginous surface is always involved in a *Pseudomonas* infection. Appropriate therapy requires that the involved joint be drained surgically and aminoglycoside antibiotics administered intravenously for ten to 14 days. Such short-term intravenous antibiotics require aggressive surgical drainage and debridement. The oral anti-*Pseudomonas* drug, ciprofloxacin, is not approved for treatment in children. Deep *Pseudomonas* infections are more common than deep staphylococcal infections after puncture wounds.

Hematogenous osteomyelitis commonly affects the calcaneous and should be considered in the differential diagnosis of heel pain in children. Signs of an acute febrile illness and localized bone pain are absent in 30% of all cases of hematogenous osteomyelitis at children's hospitals. *Staphylococcus* is the most common organism.

Metatarsus Adductus

Metatarsus adductus and skewfoot are the most common foot deformities in children. In general, spontaneous resolution of the deformity occurs in 85% to 90% of cases. Unfortunately, this leaves 10% to 15% of all patients with a significant residual defect if no treatment is recommended. The problem is most frequently identified by parents and pediatricians at the child's birth, and orthopaedic consultation sought. The foot deformity is differentiated from a clubfoot on the basis of absence of an equinovarus posture to the hindfoot with full dorsiflexion present.

The generally accepted criteria for treatment are (1) an abnormal-appearing foot with a deep medial crease and (2) enough rigidity that digital pressure fails to overcorrect the foot. Rigidity is an unreliable predictor of spontaneous resolution. The correction of the foot should be begun within the first eight months of life to be most effective.

Metatarsus adductus has been divided into four types on the basis of the relative alignment of the forefoot, midfoot, and hindfoot (Fig. 4). These types are (1) simple metatarsus adductus, (2) complex metatarsus adductus with lateral shift of the midfoot, (3) skewfoot in which metatarsus adductus is accompanied by a valgus hindfoot, and (4) complex skewfoot in which metatarsus adductus and valgus hindfoot are accompanied by a lateral shift of the midfoot. The types vary in the ease with which they can be corrected. Simple metatarsus adductus corrects either spontaneously or with casting within three weeks. The more complex forms of forefoot and midfoot deformities usually require more than seven weeks of casting to obtain correction.

In general, forefoot deformities should initially be treated with exercise. Residual or noncorrecting cases can be selected for corrective short leg casting within the first three months of life so that full correction is achieved before the child is 1 year old. A Denis Browne bar has been used by some to treat metatarsus adductus, especially when accompanied by internal tibial torsion, but this may result in an increased incidence of flatfoot. Surgical management of metatarsus adductus is rarely necessary, but is indicated if conservative management fails.

Risk factors for failure of conservative management in the young child include a deep medial crease and a short, broad first metatarsal.

Surgical correction can be achieved through metatarsal osteotomies. In the young child, one less than 3 years old, soft-tissue release may be useful, but metatarsal osteotomies appear to give better correction of the deformity, have better remodeling potential, and produce less rigidity in the foot postoperatively. In one series, unsatisfactory tarsal-metatarsal capsulotomies (Heyman-Herndon releases) produced unsatisfactory results in 50% of cases (Fig. 5).

Flatfoot

Flatfoot is a common finding in children but it is seldom a problem. Observation is the recommended management

NORMAL   ABNORMAL

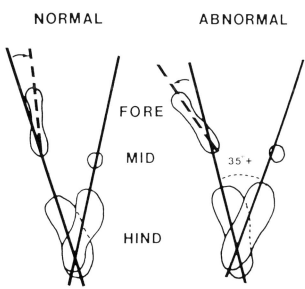

Figure 4

Metatarsus adductus ranges from simple metatarsus adductus, complex metatarsus adductus with lateral shift to the midfoot, skewfoot with a valgus hindfoot, to complex skewfoot with a lateral shift of the midfoot combined with a valgus hindfoot. The more severe the deformity, the longer casting is required. (Reproduced with permission from Berg EE: A reappraisal of metatarsus adductus and skew foot. *J Bone Joint Surg* 1986;68A:1185–1196.)

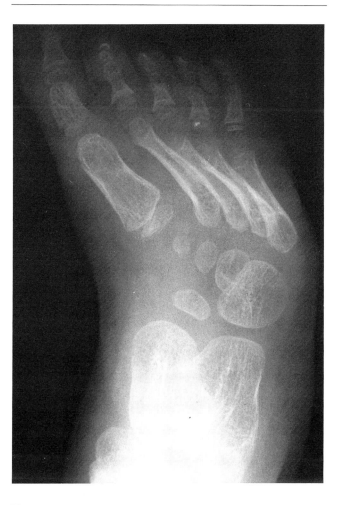

Figure 5

This child had metatarsal-tarsal capsulotomies for severe forefoot adduction. Recurrent deformity with dorsal prominence of the midfoot produced an unsatisfactory result. Metatarsal osteotomy is preferable for correcting severe deformity of metatarsus adductus.

of flexible flatfoot within the normal range. A normal longitudinal arch steadily develops during childhood. There is no evidence to suggest that treatment of a flexible flatfoot influences its eventual appearance.

Indications for treatment of a flexible flatfoot are (1) foot and leg pain, (2) excessive wear on shoes, (3) progressive deformity, (4) a family history of symptomatic flatfoot, and (5) presence of neurologic disease with muscle imbalance. Milder cases can be managed with a simple arch support or navicular "cookie," but these fail to control the hindfoot valgus. A custom-molded arch support may be required. Surgical choices include the calcaneal slide osteotomy and the Miller procedure with bone grafting of the navicular-cuneiform joint and advancement of the posterior tibial tendon. Although the Grice subtalar arthrodesis is not recommended for flexible flatfoot in childhood, it may have a role in neuropathic flatfoot. Surgical management is rarely indicated.

Congenital Vertical Talus

Congenital vertical talus is a foot deformity in which there is an irreducible dorsal dislocation of the navicular on the talus. Associated deformities of the foot include subluxation of the calcaneocuboid joint, a tight heel cord, tight anterior and lateral compartment muscles, and perhaps a tight posterior capsule. Congenital vertical talus should be suspected if a rigid flatfoot is discovered in a newborn child. The differential diagnosis includes a positional calcaneovalgus foot, an oblique talus, and perhaps a rigid valgus foot associated with fibular hemimelia. A plantar-flexion radiograph is used to diagnose the congenital vertical talus in which the talonavicular joint does not realign on forced plantar flexion (Fig. 6). In the child less than 3

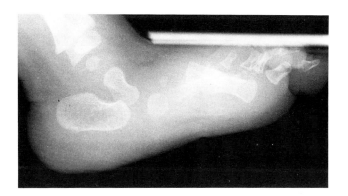

Figure 6

The diagnosis of congenital vertical talus is confirmed by the failure of reduction of the talonavicular joint on a forced plantar-flexion view. The navicular is not ossified in infancy. The failure of the cuboid and first metatarsal to align properly with the long axis of the talus is accepted as evidence of fixed dislocation of the talonavicular joint.

or 4 years of age, the navicular is not ossified so that the radiologic assessment is based on the presumed position of the navicular, using the cuboid and first metatarsal as markers.

Congenital vertical talus can be an isolated congenital abnormality or can be associated with a chromosomal abnormality, myelomeningocele, arthrogryposis, or malformation syndrome. A search for associated abnormalities should be part of the initial physical examination. There is an increased incidence in family members. Initial management generally includes corrective casting to stretch soft tissues, although this is rarely successful in managing the skeletal deformity. Cast correction is accomplished by using a long leg cast with the knee flexed 90 degrees and the foot in a position of maximum plantar flexion and inversion. Casting is continued for approximately three months or until the correction is achieved. Surgical therapy is delayed for four to eight months to allow the foot to grow, making the surgical procedure easier. Surgical correction should be performed before the child begins weightbearing.

The deformity should be corrected by releasing the talonavicular joint in all cases, and the calcaneocuboid joint in most cases. The heel cord is nearly always lengthened, as is the posterior tibial tendon. The anterior tibial tendon toe extensors and peroneals are lengthened in some cases. Posterior capsulotomy is sometimes, but not always, required. Some have recommended early Grice subtalar arthrodesis but most physicians use this fusion only in the older child or the child with recurrent foot deformity. In one series, the best results were achieved when the Grice subtalar arthrodesis was performed at the time of the initial surgery or at least within two to four years thereafter. K-wire fixation is accepted by all. Casting in a nonweight-bearing long leg cast with the foot in the corrected position is carried out for at least two months after surgery. When the child begins to walk, a UCB insert protects the foot and the repair, preventing return to a valgus hindfoot and abducted forefoot. These methods of initial treatment generally yield 60% to 70% good and excellent results.

In the older child (2.5 years to 6 years of age), a Grice subtalar arthrodesis is generally required to maintain the correction. Otherwise, the surgical procedure to release the deformity and provide reduction of the navicular on the talus is the same.

The degree of bony alteration or adaptation to this abnormal position is greater in the older child and restoration of normal alignment may be impossible. In children more than 6 years old, it may be simpler to prevent pain and protect the skin with appropriate footwear until the child is old enough to undergo a triple arthrodesis.

Myelomeningocele

Foot deformity is present at birth in 50% of patients with myelomeningocele. Included in the array are equinus, equinovarus, calcaneal, valgus, cavus, and vertical talus deformities. The deformities occur secondary to muscle imbalance, either from weakness or spasticity. Lack of sensation is a major problem, as its consequence is ulceration over areas of increased load-bearing. Rigid deformity leads to areas of increased pressure and may predispose to skin breakdown in an insensate foot. Bracing with a total-contact ankle-foot orthosis provides the key to stabiliza-

tion. The goal in caring for the foot in a child with myelomeningocele is a flexible plantigrade foot with intact skin, that is, a foot that can be braced.

In isolated equinus deformity, heel-cord lengthening may suffice, but in equinovarus deformity (neurogenic clubfoot) extensive posterior and medial releases are required. Division rather than lengthening of the tibialis posterior, tibialis anterior, and Achilles tendons has been recommended to avoid recurring deformity. In the rigid equinus foot with recurrent deformity not correctable by releases alone, procedures such as talectomy and talar decancellation have been recommended.

Triple arthrodesis should be reserved for a severe deformity in a patient with protective sensation in the foot. In the absence of sensation, producing a rigid foot by arthrodesis may lead to skin ulceration.

In the calcaneal deformity, ankle and subtalar valgus are common. The ankle valgus is generally associated with a short fibula. The valgus ankle can be corrected either by tibial osteotomy or by a partial Achilles tendon tenodesis to the fibula. The latter procedure is indicated if there is less than 10 mm of fibular shortening relative to the tibia. It is thought that weakness of the muscles attached to the fibula leads to too little stimulation for normal growth to occur. The validity of this unusual transfer has been demonstrated. Plantar-flexion power can be provided to the foot by transfer of an anterior tibial tendon through the interosseous membrane to the calcaneus. Unbalanced transfers, however, can lead to eventual deformity and certainly do not obviate the need for bracing.

Except for patients with low-level myelomeningocele, ankle-foot orthoses are required. These should control the alignment of the foot and protect it from ulceration.

Cavus Foot

The cavus foot is defined as one with an elevated longitudinal arch. Varus or calcaneal malalignment of the hindfoot is accompanied by midfoot and forefoot equinus and supination. Cock-up toes and soft-tissue contracture of the plantar fascia are uniformly present. The fat pads migrate from under the metatarsal heads and painful calluses are formed.

An imbalance between intrinsic and extrinsic muscles or between flexors and extensors is said to lead to this deformity. The exact muscle imbalance and resulting deformity are quite variable.

The cavus foot is common in neuromuscular diseases such as Charcot-Marie-Tooth disease and Friedreich's ataxia. It exists as a residual deformity in a partially treated or recurrent clubfoot. The idiopathic cavus foot is rare but, when it does occur, is usually bilateral. A tethered spinal cord or diastematomyelia may produce this foot deformity. Finally, it occurs as a posttraumatic problem either from a compartment syndrome or tendon lacerations. The differential dignosis and cause must be considered first, before correction can be undertaken.

Patients complain of foot pain under the metatarsal heads and over the lateral border of the foot or sinus tarsae. There is generally callus formation under the metatarsal heads and over the lateral border of the foot. Recurrent ankle sprains occur in some cases and excessive and ab-

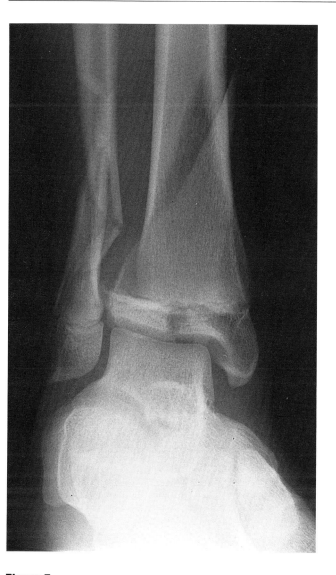
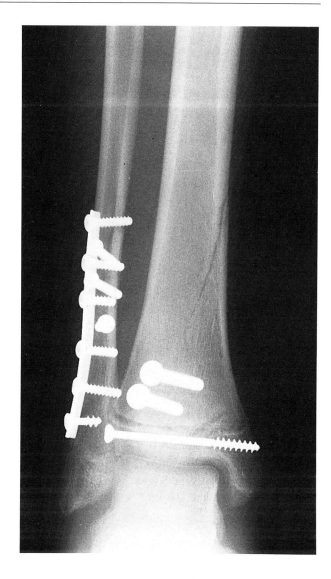

Figure 7

Triplane fracture. **Left**, A triplane fracture requires open reduction and internal fixation when significant displacement is present. Persistent displacement of 2 mm or more of the articular fragments has resulted in unacceptable long-term results. **Right**, A postoperative radiograph of open reduction and internal fixation of a triplane fracture. Both anterior and posterior approaches are required to obtain a satisfactory reduction and fixation.

normal wear on shoes is common. Radiographic documentation of the cavus foot deformity consists of a line between the talus and the first metatarsal. The apex is dorsal and the forefoot is relatively plantar-flexed in comparison with the hindfoot.

Flexibility should be assessed with the Block test, in which a lift is placed under the lateral border of the forefoot and hindfoot, forcing the hindfoot into valgus and the forefoot into a relatively pronated position while relieving pressure under the first metatarsal head. A full motor and sensory examination must be performed in all cases. The exact muscle imbalance should be isolated, the sensory deficit documented, and the degree of rigidity determined before treatment.

Treatment is directed at the muscle imbalance and the bony deformity within the foot by a combination of release and arthrodesis, depending on the underlying cause and

rigidity of the deformity. The imbalance is corrected by tendon transfer or tendon lengthening. In the adolescent, isolated soft-tissue releases to correct the cavus foot may be successful. The specific releases generally involve the plantar fascia with radical stripping of the intrinsic flexor muscles of the foot. Corrective casting is generally required postoperatively.

As the deformity becomes more rigid with the child's increasing age, bony procedures become necessary. Correction of the high-arched deformity necessitates plantar fascial release with intrinsic flexor release as well as osteotomies. Options include metatarsal osteotomies, midfoot wedge osteotomies, calcaneal opening or closing wedge osteotomies, and triple arthrodesis. Depending on the site and degree of deformity, each of these operations has a specific role. Recently, the Akron midfoot dome osteotomy has been advocated to correct this deformity. Certainly, midfoot osteotomies are a standard treatment and the midfoot dome offers a significant advantage in some cases. Finally, clawtoe deformities are approached after the main deformity of the foot is corrected. If, however, the flexion-extension couple is tight enough to prohibit satisfactory correction of the cavus foot independent of the toe deformity, toe deformities can be corrected simultaneously. However, this is not usually the case.

Trauma

Ankle fractures in children are frequently minimally displaced and require no or minimal reduction and simple cast immobilization. However, displaced intra-articular fractures and displaced physeal fractures deserve special attention. The Salter type II distal tibial fracture frequently proceeds to growth arrest because there is often an element of crush injury (Salter type V) associated with the initial injury. Gentle closed reduction to an anatomic position and sometimes internal fixation appear to be the best way to lessen the chance of growth disturbance. Computed tomography has helped to document the anatomy of complex distal tibial fractures, particularly triplane fractures. With computed tomography, a third fragment (epiphyseal) is often found.

Anatomic reduction by either closed or open means is mandatory in the treatment of triplane fractures (Fig. 7) because long-term follow-up studies have documented progressive joint deterioration in those that are poorly reduced. Open reduction should be done with a combined anterior and posterior approach to facilitate fixation. Just as computed tomography has outlined the anatomy of triplane fracture, it identifies fragments of bone or cartilage within joints in displaced intra-articular fractures. Such fragments must be reduced or excised to prevent future joint deterioration.

Controversies

Surgical Management of Clubfoot

Some of the most controversial aspects of pediatric foot surgery involve the management of clubfoot. Among the major controversies in this area are the following:

Age at Surgery Opinions as to the best age range from several days to 1 year. Most orthopaedic surgeons consider an age of 4 to 8 months optimal, but differences abound.

Incision of Choice The two incisions primarily used for clubfoot surgery are the Cincinnati incision and the medial incision along with a small lateral incision. Members of the Pediatric Orthopaedic Society of North America were divided on the use of these approaches at last polling. Any approach to the clubfoot must give access to the posterolateral corner for release of the peroneal tendon sheath and calcaneofibular ligament.

Extent of Subtalar Release The extent of this release should be based on the degree of deformity. Nonetheless, some surgeons do a total release in all cases whereas others do not open the subtalar joint at all. Most release the subtalar joint to some extent, generally leaving the interosseous ligament intact, to prevent valgus deformity. The exact extent of the subtalar release cannot be decided on the basis of published reports.

Postoperative Immobilization Since a report appeared concerning the use of an ankle cast brace in the postoperative period, the role of postoperative rigid immobilization has been questioned. Others have tried to use the cast brace without a documented increase in motion. Given that recurrent or residual deformity appears to be a much more significant problem than stiffness in most feet, early postoperative motion has not met with great acceptance.

Annotated Bibliography

Keywords

Cavus foot; Cerebral palsy; Clubfoot; Congenital vertical talus; Flatfoot; Hallux Valgus; Infection; Metatarsus adductus; Myelomeningocele; Tarsal coalition; Tendon transfer

Clubfoot

Cowell HR: The management of club foot, editorial. *J Bone Joint Surg* 1985;67A:991–992.
   This editorial further stresses the need for recognition of the varied causes and degrees of deformity in clubfoot when choosing the appropriate procedure. It places into perspective the various surgical procedures that have been recommended.

Herzenberg JE, Carroll NC, Christofersen MR: Clubfoot analysis with three-dimensional computer modeling. *J Pediatr Orthop* 1988;3:257–262.
   A three-dimensional model for clubfoot is analyzed. The external rotation of the body of the talus and relative internal rotation of the calcaneus in the clubfoot are nicely described and documented. The need for correction of the rotational deformity through the subtalar joint in clubfoot deformity is apparent from this analysis.

Simons GW: Complete subtalar release in club feet: Part I. A preliminary report. Part II. Comparison with less extensive procedures. *J Bone Joint Surg* 1985;67A:1044–1065.
   These articles outline the rationale and procedure for complete subtalar release in clubfoot deformity. The results of the complete subtalar release were superior to those of less extensive procedures. The disadvantage encountered was overcorrection. The advantage was superior alignment between foot and leg. The question remains as to when a complete subtalar release is necessary.

Tarsal Coalition

Herzenberg JE, Goldner JL, Martinez S, et al: Computerized tomography of talocalcaneal tarsal coalition: A clinical and anatomic study. *Foot Ankle* 1986;6:273–288.

This shows the value of computed tomographic scanning in the diagnosis of talocalcaneal coalition.

Mann RA, Baumgarten M: Subtalar fusion for isolated subtalar disorders: A preliminary report. *Clin Orthop* 1988;226:260–265.

Talocalcaneal subtalar arthrodesis preserves 50% of transverse tarsal motion. Functional pain ratings for patients with fusions for talocalcaneal bars were uniformly good or excellent in this series.

Morgan RC Jr, Crawford AH: Surgical management of tarsal coalition in adolescent athletes. *Foot Ankle* 1986;7:183–193.

Most patients are able to return to athletics after resection of tarsal coalition, either calcaneonavicular or talocalcaneal.

Olney BW, Asher MA: Excision of symptomatic coalition of the middle facet of the talocalcaneal joint. *J Bone Joint Surg* 1987;69A:539–544.

In this series of ten excisions of coalitions and fat graft, there were five excellent results, three good results, one fair result, and one poor result. Talar beaking was not thought to be a contraindication to this surgery. Incomplete excision was the cause of the one failure.

Scranton PE Jr: Treatment of symptomatic talocalcaneal coalition. *J Bone Joint Surg* 1987;69A:533–539.

Indications for resection of the talocalcaneal coalition are failure of nonsurgical treatment, involvement of less than 50% of the joint, and absence of degenerative changes in the talonavicular joint.

Cerebral Palsy

Hoffer M, Barakat G, Koffman M: 10-year follow-up of split anterior tibial tendon transfer in cerebral palsied patients with spastic equinovarus deformity. *J Pediatr Orthop* 1985;5:432–434.

This is an exceedingly successful procedure in resolving equinovarus deformity in cerebral palsy. It requires that the anterior tibial tendon be active and is often combined with heel-cord lengthening and posterior tibial tendon lengthening to correct the deformity.

Kling TF Jr, Kaufer H, Hensinger RN: Split posterior tibial-tendon transfers in children with cerebral spastic paralysis and equinovarus deformity. *J Bone Joint Surg* 1985;67A:186–194.

This procedure is designed to correct heel valgus. It does not affect dorsiflexion. It proved to be a safe, reliable procedure to eliminate hindfoot varus with no incidence of calcaneal valgus deformity postoperatively.

McCall RE, Lillich JS, Harris JR, et al: The Grice extra-articular subtalar arthrodesis: A clinical review. *J Pediatr Orthop* 1985;5:442–445.

There were 46% unsatisfactory results because of graft failure and clinical deformity. The procedure has a role in polio and cerebral palsy but not in myelodysplasia or flexible flatfoot.

Root L, Miller SR, Kirz P: Posterior tibial-tendon transfer in patients with cerebral palsy. *J Bone Joint Surg* 1987;69A:1133–1139.

Posterior tibial tendon transfer to the dorsum of the foot through the interosseous membrane was reported in 57 patients. Good or excellent results occurred in 27 of 30 hemiplegic patients but in only two of 11 quadriplegic patients. The incidence of calcaneal valgus deformity was remarkably low, attesting to the accuracy of patient selection. Exact criteria for patient selection are difficult to discern from this article.

Scott SM, James PC, Stephens PM: Grice subtalar arthrodesis followed to skeletal maturity. *J Pediatr Orthop* 1988;8:176–183.

Sixty-two feet (45 patients) were followed up to maturity with failure in 32% and poor results in 61%. A subtalar arthrodesis cannot compensate for ankle valgus and does not substitute for muscle-balancing procedures.

Winters TF Jr, Gage JR, Hicks R: Gait patterns in spastic hemiplegia in children and young adults. *J Bone Joint Surg* 1987;69A:437–441.

Four patterns of gait were defined in 46 patients with hemiplegia. A group was characterized in whom a plantar-flexion deformity in swing phase was followed by an initial contact of the toe with dorsiflexion through midstance. Heel-cord lengthening did not resolve the problem, because it resulted from deficiency of the anterior tibial tendon muscle. Such a patient should be braced; heel-cord lengthening is contraindicated. Ankle, knee, and hip problems related to hemiplegic gait are defined.

Infection

Jacobs RF, Adelman L, Sack CM, et al: Management of *Pseudomonas* osteochondritis complicating puncture wounds of the foot. *Pediatrics* 1982;69:432–435.

A short course (ten to 14 days) of aminoglycoside antibiotics combined with aggressive surgical debridement is satisfactory treatment for *Pseudomonas* osteochondritis. A cartilaginous surface is uniformly involved in *Pseudomonas* infections after a puncture wound of the foot.

Metatarsus Adductus

Berg EE: A reappraisal of metatarsus adductus and skewfoot. *J Bone Joint Surg* 1986;68A:1185–1196.

This paper defines four types of metatarsus adductus as simple and complex metatarsus and simple and complex skewfoot. The feet requiring treatment were uniformly corrected with casting, but the more complex deformities required more casting. Forty-three percent of simple metatarsus adductus required no treatment, whereas only 24% of the more complex deformities resolved spontaneously.

Peterson HA: Skewfoot (forefoot adduction with heel valgus). *J Pediatr Orthop* 1986;6:24–30.

Skewfoot represents a malalignment of the tarsal metatarsal bones, characterized by forefoot adduction, heel valgus, and translation of the midfoot. If surgery is required to correct this deformity, realignment of the tarsal bones and metatarsals should be supplemented by hindfoot realignment. Corrective casting of this condition in infancy should always include lateral pressure over the head of the talus to prevent exacerbation of the valgus hindfoot deformity at the time of forefoot correction.

Staheli LT, Chew DE, Corbett M: The longitudinal arch: A survey of eight hundred and eighty-two feet in normal children and adults. *J Bone Joint Surg* 1987;69A:426–428.

This paper documents the range of normal development of the longitudinal arch and the physiologic presence of flatfoot in early childhood.

Stark JG, Johansson JE, Winter RB: The Heyman-Herndon tarsometatarsal capsulotomy for metatarsus adductus: Results in 48 feet. *J Pediatr Orthop* 1987;7: 305–310.

The authors report 48 feet with 41% failures and 50% painful dorsal midfoot prominence. Sixty-eight percent of the patients with this procedure were difficult to fit with shoes.

Congenital Vertical Talus

DeRosa GP, Ahlfeld SK: Congenital vertical talus: The Riley experience. *Foot Ankle* 1984;5:118–124.

Treatment of ten feet with congenital vertical talus with soft-tissue release alone resulted in three excellent, three good, and four fair outcomes. No patient required subtalar arthrodesis.

Oppenheim W, Smith C, Christie W: Congenital vertical talus. *Foot Ankle* 1985;5:198–204.

Treatment of congenital vertical talus with soft-tissue release was most effective when it was combined with a subtalar arthrodesis within two to four years after the initial surgery.

Seimon LP: Surgical correction of congenital vertical talus under the age of 2 years. *J Pediatr Orthop* 1987;7: 405–411.

Seven patients (ten feet) with congenital vertical talus were followed up for five years. A single-stage soft-tissue release resulted in satisfactory outcomes in all patients. There were seven excellent and three good results. The surgical procedure was primarily a dorsal midfoot release with a posterior capsulotomy only done in one patient. No bony procedure was done. The author thought that there is no indication for two-stage surgery for a congenital vertical talus.

Walker AP, Ghali NN, Silk FF: Congenital vertical talus: The results of staged operative reduction. *J Bone Joint Surg* 1985;67B:117–121.

This article documents a satisfactory outcome in 12 of 15 feet after a two-stage release. Eight months of immobilization in plaster with foot plantar flexion was used between the anterolateral and posterior release.

Myelomeningocele

Carroll NC: Assessment and management of the lower extremity in myelodysplasia. *Orthop Clin North Am* 1987;18:709–724.

Foot deformity in myelodysplasia is very common. It is managed by soft-tissue releases and bracing, maintaining a flex-

ible plantigrade foot with stable skin. Such surgery is only an incidental event in the rehabilitation program of a child with myelodysplasia.

Dias LS: Valgus deformity of the ankle joint: Pathogenesis of fibular shortening. *J Pediatr Orthop* 1985;5:176–180.

Abnormal shortening of the fibula commonly leads to valgus deformity of the ankle joint in paralytic disease. The author studied 120 patients with myelomeningocele. The average shortening was 7.5 mm; shortening rarely exceeded 1 mm in children less than 8 years old. In children more than 8 years old, the average amount of shortening was 14 mm. The degree of fibular shortening was thought to be related to the weakness of the soleus muscle. The most common cause of fibular shortening was paralysis of calf muscles. Other causes include growth disorders and cerebral palsy.

Stevens PM, Toomey E: Fibular-Achilles tenodesis for paralytic ankle valgus. *J Pediatr Orthop* 1988;8:169–175.

Talar tilt was reduced (mean correction, 9 degrees; range, 4 to 21 degrees) and fibular length increased in 81.2% of feet. Some correction of hindfoot valgus was achieved.

Cavus Foot

Wilcox PG, Weiner DS: The Akron midtarsal dome osteotomy in the treatment of rigid pes cavus: A preliminary review. *J Pediatr Orthop* 1985;5:333–338.

The authors report 94% satisfactory results in patients more than 8 years old after this midfoot osteotomy. The underlying diagnosis in the majority of their patients was cerebral palsy or clubfoot.

Trauma

Ertl JP, Barrack RL, Alexander AH, et al: Triplane fracture of the distal tibial epiphysis: Long-term follow-up. *J Bone Joint Surg* 1988;70A:967–976.

Eight of 15 patients with confirmed triplane fractures were asymptomatic three months to 13 years later. Residual displacement of more than 2 mm led to unsatisfactory results. Computed tomographic scanning is an effective way of determining the exact anatomy of this difficult fracture. Satisfactory open reduction required a combined anterior and posterior procedure.

47

Ankle and Foot: Trauma

The goal of surgical intervention in the ankle and foot is to improve functional outcome and to provide early rehabilitation. Improvements in biomechanical investigational techniques have added to knowledge of the mechanics of the foot and led to a better understanding of these injuries. Internal fixation techniques found to be useful in other anatomic areas have been adapted for use in the foot.

Soft-Tissue Injuries

Tendon Injuries

A recent review provided support for aggressive surgical treatment of major tendon lacerations in the foot. Although often complicated by adhesions, primary repair of the tibialis anterior, tibialis posterior, and peroneal tendons is indicated, particularly in children. In the growing foot, the muscular imbalance that arises from major tendon disruption, if not repaired, can lead to progressive deformation of the foot. Surgical exploration and debridement allow further definition of the injured structures, as well as ensuring adequate removal of foreign bodies and contamination. Primary tendon repair should be undertaken at the time of wound exploration, although primary wound closure may not be possible because of contamination.

Lacerations of the flexor digitorum longus tendon in the plantar part of the foot produce minimal disability. In light of its complex interrelationship with plantar nerves and vessels, extensive exploration to bring about primary repair of this tendon is probably not justified. Similarly, laceration of the flexor hallucis longus is associated with minimal disability. Nonsurgical treatment or tenodesis of the flexor digitorum longus is satisfactory when primary repair cannot be performed.

Heel-Cord Rupture

Rupture of the Achilles tendon commonly occurs during forced dorsiflexion against a contracted heel cord. Often the patient notes a "pop," followed by difficulty in walking. There may be minimal discomfort. The diagnosis is made by careful examination. With the patient kneeling on a chair or examination table, and the foot hanging free, the calf is squeezed in its area of maximal girth. Lack of plantar function in the foot indicates a ruptured Achilles tendon. The extent of injury varies from complete disruption with a large gap to shredding of the tendon with considerable interdigitation of the tendon ends. The difficulty of documenting displacement makes treatment comparisons unreliable.

The choice of surgical or nonsurgical treatment depends on the activity requirements of the patient, the status of the blood supply, and the experience of the treating physician. Both treatments are effective. Sedentary patients or those with poor soft tissues or circulatory disorders can be treated in an equinus walking cast for eight weeks. A heel lift is then used for one to two months to diminish forces across the healing tendon. Although the use of a long leg bent-knee cast may reduce the number of cases with marked shortening, the quadriceps atrophy and knee stiffness that accompany this treatment may require considerable rehabilitation. Nonsurgical treatment leads to decreased strength in the gastrocsoleus complex because the tendon heals in a lengthened position. However, this has little functional significance. Larger differences in strength can be measured by objective techniques such as the Cybex, particularly in eccentric loading, in which patients treated nonsurgically are much weaker.

Surgical treatment is generally recommended for an active person who wishes optimal functional return. A posteromedial incision is recommended. Midline incisions are associated with skin slough and adhesions, and posterolateral incisions can be associated with sural nerve injury. A posteromedial incision also allows access to the plantaris tendon, which may be used to augment the repair. A modified Bunnell-type repair is advocated, augmented with peripheral absorbable suture. The tendon sheath and the subcutaneous tissue should be closed separately, in layers if possible. Except for unusual circumstances in which primary anastomosis of the divided segments cannot be obtained easily, a short leg equinus cast is adequate postoperative immobilization. Late repairs should be supplemented with plantaris tendon, fascia lata, or a strip of fascia turned down from the proximal gastrocsoleus complex. An infection rate of 1%, a rerupture rate of 2% to 7%, and a wound necrosis rate of 5% have been known to follow surgical treatment. Reported rerupture rates after nonsurgical treatment have ranged from 8% to 35% but are generally thought to be about 15%.

Rupture of the posterior tibial tendon may be associated with acute injury to the foot and ankle. More often it is an attritional disorder.

Tendon Dislocation

Dislocation of the peroneal tendons is the most common type of tendon dislocation about the ankle. The injury usually occurs during a twisting dorsiflexion movement of the ankle. The diagnosis is frequently missed initially. If the dislocation is recognized easily and is easily reduced and stable, treatment with a short leg cast for eight weeks is usually sufficient. Many surgical techniques have been described for recurrent dislocation. They involve re-creation of the peroneal tunnel with bone, periosteum, or local ligament or redirection deep to the calcaneofibular ligament. In some cases a lesion is present similar to that described by Bankart in recurrent dislocation of the shoulder. The retinaculum remains in continuity with the periosteum. Both are stripped from the bone, forming a redundant pouch with nothing to hold the posterior position of the tendons. Repair is by incising the peroneal retinaculum and attaching it to the posterolateral border of the fibula.

Ligamentous Injuries

Ligamentous injuries to the lateral aspect of the ankle are the most common ligamentous injuries in the body. Injury to the anterior talofibular ligament is most common. The calcaneofibular ligament may be torn during more severe injuries. These structures resist anterior drawer and talar tilt, respectively. The posterior talofibular ligament is rarely disrupted. The diagnosis of ligamentous injury is made on the basis of local tenderness supplemented by clinical examination and stress radiography. Early treatment consists of icing and a leg compression dressing followed by early functional bracing or taping. An occasional patient with a very severe injury may benefit from ten days to three weeks in a short leg cast. This is followed by exercises against resistance and work on a balance board to reestablish strength and proprioception.

Primary repair of lateral ligamentous injuries is rarely indicated. Both immediate repair and delayed reconstruction produce satisfactory outcomes. More than 85% of patients do not require surgical treatment and early repair has been shown to have no better results than delayed repair. Immediate surgical repair has been advocated for the elite athlete for whom the 15% to 20% chance of unsuccessful outcome of nonsurgical treatment is unacceptable and who may need the slightly improved objective result expected from surgery. However, this aggressive approach has not been justified in a scientific way. When reconstruction is required, many treatment options are available. The goal of treatment is to restore the stability provided by the anterior talofibular and calcaneofibular ligaments. Split peroneus brevis is usually used. A variety of techniques can provide a satisfactory outcome. Objective testing has failed to show a significant deficit in eversion strength in patients in whom the peroneus tendon was transferred, leading some investigators to suggest that the remaining peroneus tendon hypertrophies. A recently described reconstruction technique uses the plantaris tendon to re-create the calcaneofibular and anterior talofibular ligaments in an anatomic way. The plantaris is freed proximally and its attachment to the calcaneus is kept intact. It is then drilled through the calcaneus to the origin of the calcaneofibular ligament. It is then passed deep to the peroneal tendons, through the fibula, and into a tunnel on the talus. Next, it is doubled back through the fibula and secured to itself as it leaves the osteoperiosteal tunnel through the calcaneus. This technique places the reconstruction in the most nearly anatomic position, and spares the peroneal tendon. Whether the extra dissection is justified requires further study.

It is important, although difficult, to differentiate ankle instability from subtalar instability. For primary ankle instability, procedures that do not restrict subtalar motion are preferred. Subtalar instability should be suspected when the initial area of tenderness is distal and lateral to the ankle joint in the area of the sinus tarsi. The diagnosis of subtalar instability is made by stress Broden's views (45-degree internal rotation of the foot with the beam tilted 20 degrees caudad, while the heel is stressed into varus).

The joint capsule, interosseus ligaments, bifurcate ligament, and calcaneofibular ligament are the stabilizers of the subtalar joint. Should the subtalar joint prove to be unstable, a combined ankle ligament and subtalar repair may be required.

Distal tibiofibular syndesmosis rupture can occur as an isolated injury. The tibiofibular space in the normal ankle is rarely more than 4 mm. A 5-mm separation or a clear space between the tibia and fibula in a skeletally mature individual is evidence of a diastasis that may require screw fixation until the ligament heals.

Injuries of the distal tibiofibular syndesmosis can also accompany a more proximal fibular fracture. The goal of treatment is to restore the fibula and mortise to the reduced position. Reduction of the fibula includes restoration of length as well as rotation. If closed reduction can be performed, a screw inserted approximately 1 cm above the distal tibiofibular joint is used to maintain the reduction until the ligament heals. When closed reduction cannot be obtained, open reduction is required. Significant controversy surrounds the technique as well as the timing and necessity of screw removal. During normal motion of the ankle joint, some rotatory motion occurs in the tibiofibular articulation. Therefore, when walking is instituted with the screw between the tibia and fibula, stress fracture of the hardware can occur and the medial portion, which is embedded in the tibia, can be difficult to remove. This hardware failure can be avoided or diminished by using a shorter screw that does not engage the medial cortex of the tibia. It should be stressed that the screw should not be inserted in a lag fashion, which would distort the anatomy of the mortise, but rather that reduction should be performed first and the screw inserted to maintain the reduced position.

Compartment Syndrome

Compartment syndromes do occur in the foot and can be isolated to one or several compartments. As in compartment syndromes elsewhere, a high index of suspicion is the best diagnostic tool. Severe pain accompanied by an increase in intracompartmental pressure indicates the need for decompression. The foot contains at least four fascial compartments: the medial compartment containing the abductor hallucis and flexor hallucis brevis; the lateral compartment containing the abductor digiti and flexor digiti minimi; the interosseus compartment containing the interossei and the arterial arch and digital nerves; and the central compartment containing the long flexor tendons, the adductor hallucis, the flexor brevis, and the quadratus plantae. The geographic and functional separation of the compartments is not nearly as well defined in the foot as in the leg. As in the hand, direct compartmental pressure measurements may not be reliable. The compartments are small and muscle mass is meager. Pain experienced with passive motion can be difficult to distinguish from the pain of local trauma. Perhaps the most reliable sign is a palpably tense foot combined with pain out of proportion to the injury. The compartments can be released through a combination of dorsal and medial incisions combined with stabilization of bony injuries. Clawing of the toes is a common sequela of compartmental syndrome even with appropriate treatment.

Fractures and Fracture-Dislocations

Dislocation

Dislocation of the ankle without fracture is an uncommon injury. The mechanism of injury appears to be forced inversion of and axial load on the maximally plantar-flexed foot. It is most often posteromedial, occurs in young people, and generalized ligamentous laxity seems to be a predisposing condition. When the injury is closed, closed reduction and casting for six weeks leads to a satisfactory result. When open, debridement, reduction, and primary repair of the lateral ligaments are indicated. Syndesmosis rupture is uncommon but must be considered.

Fractures of the Ankle

Treatment of fractures of the ankle requires an understanding of the commonly used classification systems. Two such classification systems are currently in use (Fig. 1). The first was described by Lauge-Hansen in 1942 and later modified to include ligamentous injuries. His system evolved from cadaver experiments in which the foot was fixed and force was applied in different directions. Each of the four classes in Lauge-Hansen's system contain two descriptive anatomic words—the first describes the position of the foot at the time of injury and the second describes the direction of the deforming force. The strength of this system is its helpfulness in closed reduction. The position and direction of force are reversed to bring about reduction.

In 1949 Danis described an anatomic classification for surgical treatment. His system was then modified by Weber and is now commonly known as the AO classification. In the AO system injuries are divided into classes A, B, and C according to the relationship of the fibular fracture to the syndesmosis and interosseous ligaments. In this system, class A fractures are distal to both the interosseus ligament and the syndesmosis. Class B fractures involve part or all of the syndesmosis and are considered to have an unstable syndesmosis 50% of the time. Class C fractures are all unstable and the injury includes syndesmotic, ligamentous, and, at times, interosseous membrane disruption.

Both systems permit comparisons between different types of injuries. Lauge-Hansen's system has been criticized for being too comprehensive and difficult to use in clinical practice. The AO system, although much easier to use, leaves out important information.

Both classification systems recognize the importance of the lateral malleolus. Lateral malleolar reduction and stability are the key to successful treatment of ankle fractures. The fibular malleolus is responsible for maintenance of the talus within the ankle mortise. Lateral displacement of the talus of as little as 1 to 2 mm can reduce the contact surface of the tibiotalar joint by more than 40%. Radiographic attempts to confirm reduction of the mortise should be done with the ankle in the neutral position. When allowed to plantar flex, the talus becomes less stable within the mortise and may give a false impression of talar tilt.

In addition to the restoration of bony anatomy of the lateral malleolus and the weightbearing surface, the integ-

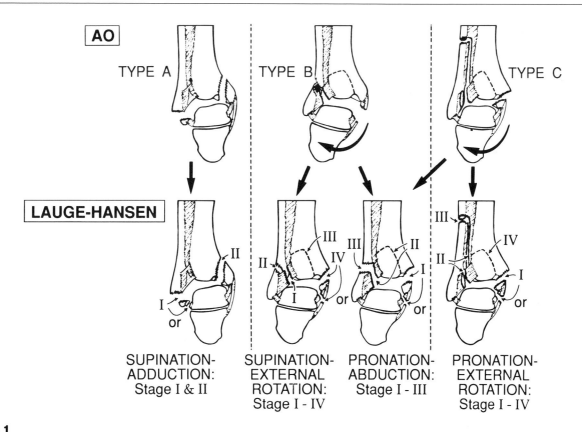

Figure 1

The AO (Danis-Weber) and Lauge-Hansen classification systems. Note that the AO system includes injuries of different Lauge-Hansen types in one category.

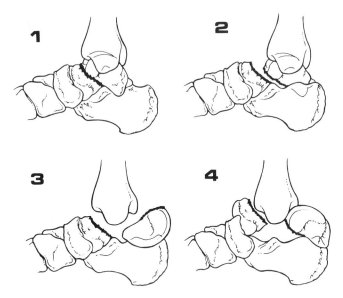

Figure 2

Vertical fractures of the talar neck were classified by Hawkins on the basis of displacement. Type 1 includes nondisplaced fractures. Type 2 includes injuries in which the talar neck is displaced and the subtalar joint is subluxated. Type 3 includes injuries in which both the subtalar joint and the ankle joint are subluxated. The body of the talus is frequently inverted and posterior to the tibia. Type 4, which was added later by Canale, includes displacement of the talonavicular joint. The types are correlated with an increasing likelihood of osteonecrosis.

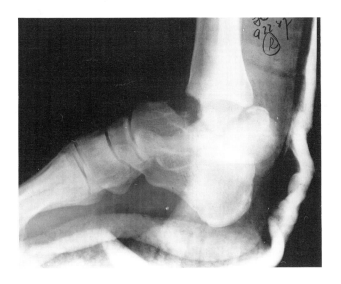

Figure 3

A lateral view of a Hawkins type 3 talar neck injury. The talar dome is extruded posteromedially and the medial malleolus is fractured.

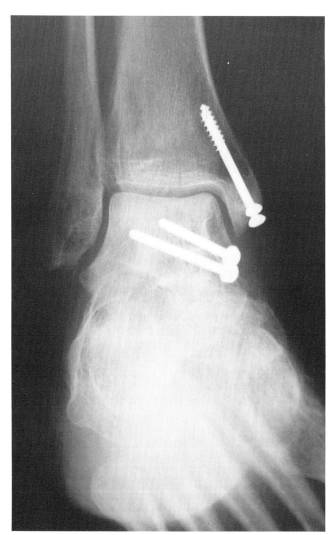

Figure 4

Same patient shown in Figure 3. Mortise view three months after surgery shows union of the fractures but dense sclerosis of the talus. The medial part of the dome shows evidence of revascularization.

rity of the syndesmotic ligament should be assessed. In injuries in which the fibular malleolus is fractured above the level of the plafond, the integrity of the syndesmotic ligament should be assessed at the time the fracture is surgically repaired. This can be done by grasping the repaired fibula with a reduction clamp and attempting to dislocate it from its tibial articulation. If found to be unstable, the distal tibiofibular joint should be reduced and fixed with a cortical screw inserted just proximal to the tibiofibular joint.

In deciding whether to treat displaced ankle fractures by closed or open means, the importance of the reduction of the lateral malleolus must again be emphasized. The fibula is the most important factor in determining the reduction of the talus within the mortise. If anatomic reduction is obtained by closed means, treatment in a long leg cast has long-term results similar to those of open reduction. If anatomic reduction of the mortise cannot be obtained by closed means, open reduction and internal fixation is required.

When surgical treatment is chosen, fixation should be selected to fit the fracture pattern. Most simple fracture patterns of the medial malleolus can be satisfactorily repaired with two 4-mm cancellous screws directed proximally from the tip of the malleolus. Because of the importance of fibular length and rotation, the fibula is best treated with a plate positioned to resist the deforming force. Skin problems and hardware morbidity are uncommon. The lateral plate advocated by the AO group is widely accepted, but the antiglide plate has some advantages for oblique fractures of the fibula. "Antiglide" refers to a technique rather than a specific plate. In the antiglide technique, a plate is fixed to bone in such a way that the distal fragment of an oblique fracture is blocked from gliding along the fracture when a load is applied. The plate is placed at the apex of the fracture, which wedges the distal fragment between the plate and the proximal fragment. When a deforming force is directed across the fracture line, it is converted to a compressive force. For AO class B fractures, the plate is positioned at the posterior or posterolateral fibula. This construct is significantly stiffer, absorbs more energy before failure, and does not require as much dissection as a laterally placed plate.

Restoration of fibular length in fractures with marked comminution (pronation-abduction, AO class C) is challenging. If the talus can be reduced into the mortise by first repairing the medial malleolus, the fibular facet of the talus can be used as a guide to the length. A plate is then applied to maintain the position of the fibula.

When deltoid disruption accompanies ankle injury, repair is unnecessary. If medial reduction is blocked by entrapped soft tissue, the medial side of the ankle joint should be inspected and entrapped portions of the deltoid ligament, or other tissues, removed. Under these circumstances the treating physician must rule out entrapped tibial tendon and nerve.

Fractures of the Talus

Two issues guide the treatment of talus fractures. A complex geometric relationship exists among the three articular surfaces of the talus—the ankle, subtalar, and talonavicular surfaces. Displaced vertical fractures through the substance of the talus, including the talar neck, disrupt this complex relationship and impair motion in the ankle, hindfoot, and midfoot. Secondly, the talus has no muscular insertions and is covered by articular cartilage on approximately 60% of its surface. As a result, areas of blood inflow are limited and injuries present a serious threat to its blood supply. The first issue dictates that absolute anatomic reduction must be restored and maintained until healing. The second mandates that reduction be performed with minimal dissection around the blood supply. The conflicting needs of reduction and exposure contribute to the considerable morbidity associated with this injury.

Three types of talar neck fractures have been described on the basis of increasing fracture displacement, progressive disruption of the blood supply, and an increasing incidence of osteonecrosis. Hawkins type 1 injuries include undisplaced vertical fractures of the talar neck and are not expected to be complicated by osteonecrosis. Type 2 injuries include fractures that are displaced and involve subluxation of the subtalar joint. In type 3 injuries, both the ankle and the subtalar joint are subluxated or dislocated. A fourth classification, added later, in which the talar head is also dislocated, includes complete disruption of the entire blood supply (Fig. 2).

Nondisplaced fractures of the talar neck and body can be treated in a nonweightbearing below-knee cast until healing occurs. The surgeon must be sure that the fracture

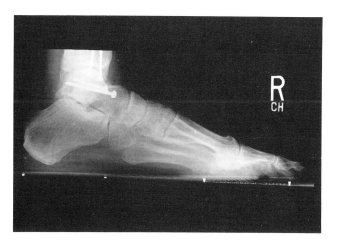

Figure 5

Same patient shown in Figures 3 and 4. Standing lateral view taken one year after the injury. The patient is symptom-free but the talus has not yet revascularized.

is truly nondisplaced. Even a small amount of displacement suggests that what is really an unstable fracture has returned to an almost reduced position after removal of the deforming force. The presence of any displacement represents a disruption of the complex geometric relationships of the subtalar transverse tarsal and ankle joints.

Displaced fractures should be treated by open reduction and internal fixation (Figs. 3 to 5). Laboratory studies indicate that screws resist displacement better than Kirschner wires and the intrinsic muscle forces generated across the ankle. K-wires provide fixation inadequate to resist muscle forces across the ankle joint and must be supplemented with a well-molded cast until healing. The approach to internal fixation varies with fracture type. Two medial screws, a medial and lateral crossed-screw configuration, and posterior-to-anterior lag screw fixation have all been advocated. Before surgery is undertaken, the anatomy of the blood supply must be understood. The fixation pattern that least threatens the remaining blood supply of the individual injury should be chosen. In general, displaced vertical fractures are reliably reduced through an anterolateral or anteromedial approach and fixed with lag screws. The anteromedial approach, between the anterior and posterior tibial tendons, is safe but provides limited visualization. The anterolateral approach risks injury to the superficial peroneal nerve. However, in most cases little dissection beyond the skin is required. The soft tissues are often stripped off the neck and anterior body and the fracture line easily visualized. A screw can be inserted at the root of the inferior extensor retinaculum through the talar neck.

For comminuted fractures, most often Hawkins type 2, a combined anteromedial and anterolateral approach is used and a bone graft is used primarily. A 6.5-mm screw inserted in a posterior-to-superior direction has undergone limited clinical testing. This technique may be most useful in the treatment of nondisplaced fractures that cannot be adequately immobilized in plaster.

Each of the articular surfaces can be disrupted by intra-articular fractures as well. Fractures not involving the neck include lateral and posterior process fractures. These injuries involve the subtalar joint. Plain radiographs gener-

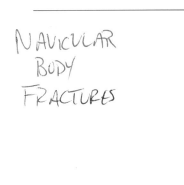

NAVICULAR
BODY
FRACTURES

Type I

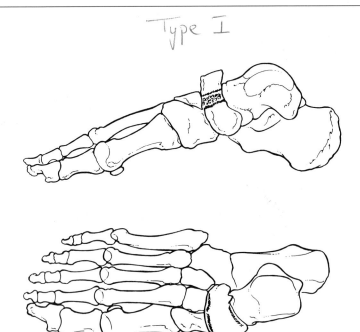

Type II

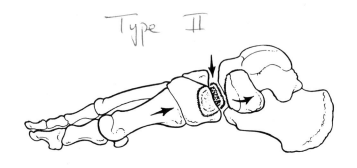

Type III

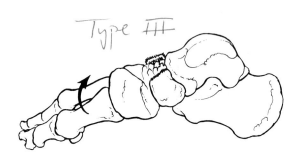

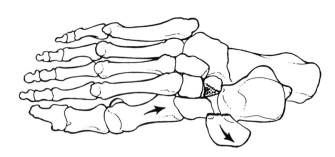

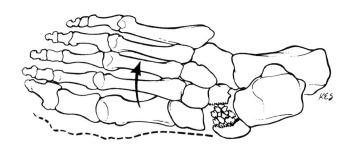

KES

Figure 6

Navicular body fractures. **Top**, Type 1. The fracture line is in the coronal plane of the foot. Less than 50% of the body is displaced, and displacement is primarily dorsal. Little deformity is visible on the dorsoplantar view. **Bottom left**, Type 2. This is the most common type. A large part of the body of the navicular is displaced dorsomedially. The smaller lateral fragment is often comminuted. The medial border of the foot is shortened. **Bottom right**, Type 3. There is substantial comminution. The naviculocuneiform joint is disrupted. The forefoot is laterally displaced.

ally underestimate the involvement of the articular surface and the diagnosis is commonly missed. Computed tomography or hindfoot rotation (Broden's) views, can be used to confirm the diagnosis. Anatomic reduction and sufficient stability to allow early motion are the goals of treatment. Fractures with less than 2 mm of displacement can be treated in a below-knee cast. Single large displaced fragments should be treated by open reduction and internal fixation with a small fragment screw. Comminuted fractures should be debrided to prevent late posttraumatic arthritis by intra-articular fragments.

Fractures of the Tarsal Navicular

Navicular fractures have been divided into four types: those involving the tuberosity, chip or avulsion fractures from the dorsal surface, displaced fractures of the body, and stress fractures. Tuberosity fractures, when nondisplaced, can be treated nonsurgically in a short leg cast. When displaced, or when the posterior tibial tendon has avulsed, fixation with a 3.5-mm or 4-mm lag screw and a soft-tissue washer may bring about a satisfactory result. Avulsion fractures should provoke suspicion of an undetected fracture on the lateral side of the foot. Oblique films of the midfoot may help to rule out anterior process fractures of the calcaneus, disruption of the calcaneocuboid joint, or a compression fracture of the cuboid. Undisplaced isolated ligamentous avulsion is treated with a short leg cast for six weeks.

Displaced fractures of the navicular body involve the talonavicular and navicular cuneiform articulations. They are usually the result of high-energy injuries and occur in three radiographic patterns (Fig. 6) that indicate an increasing risk of morbidity, including osteonecrosis and posttraumatic arthritis. Successful reduction of more than 60% of the articular surface on both the anteroposterior and lateral views gives a satisfactory result in more than 70% of cases. Treatment of these injuries is open reduction and internal fixation with screws supplemented with K-wires when necessary. For severely comminuted injuries, external fixation may be required. External fixation is provided for six to eight weeks and then mobilization is begun. A type 2 fracture with a large medial fragment and a small comminuted lateral fragment can be secured by a screw passing through the navicular into the cuneiform or cuboid.

Cuboid Fractures

Injuries of the cuboid are most often minimally displaced avulsion fractures that can be treated with simple cast immobilization. In contrast, an indirect "nutcracker" fracture can be caused by compression of the cuboid between the calcaneus and the metatarsals. With compression, the lateral column of the foot is shortened, placing the forefoot into an abducted position. This injury requires open reduction and bone grafting to maintain length and reduce the intra-articular component.

Fractures and Dislocations of the Tarsometatarsal (Lisfranc) Joint

Injuries to the transmetatarsal joint are diagnosed on the basis of a swollen foot with a history consistent with an axially loaded, plantar-flexed foot or a hyperpronation or supination injury. Anteroposterior lateral and oblique

radiographs are confirmatory. The medial border of the second metatarsal should align with the medial border of the intermediate cuneiform; if any question remains, stress radiography should be performed with the patient given analgesia or anesthesia. The goals of treatment are anatomic reduction and early motion. This is achieved by percutaneous pinning or open reduction and pinning supplemented with a cast. Recent data indicate an excellent success rate with open reduction and fixation with screws (Fig. 7). Results were poor in patients with articular comminution. Whether treatment is surgical or nonsurgical, symptoms can continue to improve for more than a year. Cases that fail to improve can be salvaged by arthrodesis.

Calcaneal Fractures

The calcaneus is the largest bone in the foot. The posterior third is extra-articular, and serves as the attachment site of the Achilles tendon. The middle third contains the posterior facet, which is supported by a structural thickening of cortical bone known as the thalamus. Because of this thickening, this is a relatively reliable area of the fractured bone to use for reduction and fixation.

Fractures of the calcaneus commonly result from a fall and almost always involve an axial load. The calcaneus is driven upward against the talus, often creating a fracture line through the sinus tarsi posterior to the interosseus ligament. This fracture is quite consistent and has been called the "separation fracture" or primary fracture line. The primary fracture line extends from anterolateral to posteromedial. It divides the tuberosity and lateral wall, along with a variable part of the posterior facet, from the sustentaculum with the middle and anterior facets. The sustentacular fragment remains in its normal position. Because the tuberosity is the site of first impact, the lateral fragment is displaced laterally; this is accompanied by some rotation of the tuberosity. As the impact continues, the tuberosity is driven upward, causing a relative downward rotation of the anterior portion of the posterior facet. If this force continues, the posterior facet may be driven through the interior cortex. Many secondary fracture lines occur. The number and locations of these lines are determined by the direction and force of impact as well as the position of the foot. Fracture lines can be vertical, horizontal, or oblique and can involve substantial compression of cancellous bone. Patterns of injury have been difficult to delineate. Several fracture classifications have been described, but none has been widely accepted. The fracture patterns are generally described in terms of the relationship of thalamic and sustentacular fragments to one another and to the fracture lines.

Minimum roentgenographic evaluation includes dorsoplantar, lateral, axial, and oblique views. The lateral view is the most helpful in assessment of the thalamic depression (position of the posterior facet). The dorsoplantar view shows displacement of the calcaneocuboid joint and the axial view demonstrates the direction of the primary fracture line as well as giving information about the relationship between the posterior facet and the sustentacular fragment. The axial view also demonstrates varus displacement and fibular abutment, and may give information about the subtalar joint when displacement is not too severe. The oblique view demonstrates the degree of comminution of the anterior process of the calcaneus and hidden injuries of the midfoot. If surgical treatment is

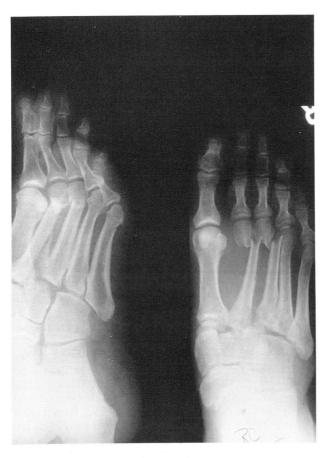
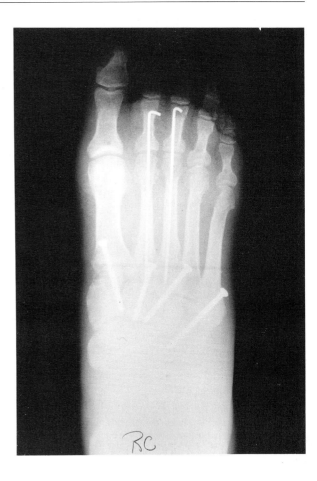

Figure 7

Fracture-dislocation of the tarsometatarsal (Lisfranc) joint. **Left,** Anteroposterior and oblique views of homolateral fracture-dislocation of the Lisfranc joint and metatarsal fractures. The second metatarsal base does not line up with the middle cuneiform and the first metatarsal is laterally displaced. **Right,** Postoperative anteroposterior view shows reduction and fixation with screws. The second metatarsal is reduced to the middle cuneiform but the first metatarsal is incompletely reduced.

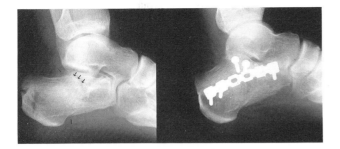

Figure 8

Lateral views of a joint depression injury. **Left,** Preoperative film. The arrows point to the major part of the posterior facet. It is depressed, causing a reversal of Böhler's angle. The calcaneus is shortened through the primary fracture line. **Right,** Postoperative film. There are two lag screws in the subchondral position (thalamus) beneath the posterior facet, and a laterally applied plate. The posterior facet is reduced and Böhler's angle is equal to that in the other foot.

contemplated, further information must be gathered. Computed tomography provides better information regarding displacement, comminution, and sagittal reconstruction than radiographs without the problems of positioning and patient discomfort and with less radiation than multiple Broden's views. It should be performed in two planes—in the plane of the plantar surface and perpendicular to the articular surface of the posterior facet. This allows evaluation of the shortening of the long axis, the displacement of the lateral wall, the position of the primary fracture line, comminution of the posterior facet, posterior facet depression, the size of the sustentacular fragment, and displacement in the calcaneocuboid joint.

Fractures of the calcaneus are serious injuries that require a prolonged recovery period. The general goal of treatment is pain-free function compatible with activities of daily living. It has not been established in an objective way that surgical treatment is superior to nonsurgical treatment. There are advocates of early motion without reduction, manipulative reduction, and open reduction through a medial or lateral approach. The goals of surgical treatment are restoration of the geometric relationships of the talocalcaneal and calcaneocuboid joints, reduction of the intra-articular surface, reduction of the tuberosity fragment, which restores the height of the foot, and reduction of the lateral wall to prevent lateral impingement. These factors have been associated with unsatisfactory results in nonsurgical treatment, and with difficulties in salvage.

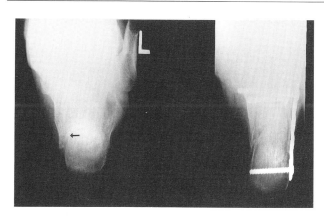

Figure 9

Axial views of the fracture shown in Figure 8. **Left,** Preoperative film. Shortening and lateral translation of the tuberosity are apparent. The arrow points to the medial wall of the calcaneus in its impacted position. The lateral wall is buckled outward under the fibula. **Right,** Postoperative film. Indirect reduction of the tuberosity with a traction pin has corrected the varus and lateral translation. Direct reduction of the posterior facet was achieved through a lateral approach, and a lateral plate was applied to maintain the reduced position. The lateral wall and trabecular pattern are now straight. Reduction through a medial approach would have been difficult because of the comminution of the medial wall.

These goals must be accomplished without the prolonged immobilization that leads to stiffness. Significant controversy exists as to the most effective means of achieving these goals. There is no universally accepted classification that allows meaningful comparisons of treatment or prognosis because early classification systems were outlined before the advent of computed tomography clarified complex intra-articular fragments.

A lateral incision plantar and dorsal to the peroneal tendons allows an extensive exposure of the lateral wall, posterior facet, and calcaneocuboid joint as well as sufficient exposure for rigid fixation. Fixation is provided by thalamic screws and a lateral plate. This approach has been very successful. However, the extensive flap created carries with it the potential for significant soft-tissue morbidity.

Retrospective studies have shown that the most important criteria for long-term satisfactory results are reduction of the joint, elevation of the posterior facet, reduction of the lateral wall, and early motion. Unless there is only a primary fracture line and little or no comminution, few of these goals can be accomplished through the medial approach. The lateral approach allows direct reduction of the posterior facet, lateral wall, and calcaneocuboid joint. When the lateral approach is used, care must be taken to avoid varus fixation. Prominence of the hardware under the peroneal tendons has not been a problem. A combined approach using the medial approach to restore the height of the tuberosity and a lateral approach to reduce and fix the joint surfaces and lateral wall is under evaluation.

After reduction, the fixation used should allow motion to be instituted within two weeks. A staple or an H-plate used on the medial side does not provide rigid fixation. A low-profile reconstruction plate and lag screws placed beneath the subchondral bone of the posterior facet are used on the lateral side. Lag screws in a subchondral position (the thalamus) generally provide stable fixation. Smooth

pins provide minimal stability and, when used across the joint, delay mobilization (Figs. 8 and 9).

The issue of whether to bone graft is equally unresolved; although the defect may eventually fill with bone, the critical issue is early motion and stability with institution of weightbearing. In general, if there is a bony defect after reduction large enough to delay healing or a structural defect, a bone graft should be used.

Controversies

Fixation of Syndesmosis Injuries

The anterior and posterior tibiofibular and interossei ligaments support the distal tibiofibular articulation. Disruption occurs as an isolated injury and as an accompaniment to fibular fracture. The goal of treatment is to restore the ankle mortise and to maintain its position until healing of the ligaments has taken place. There are many techniques of fixation, each with ardent advocates. Screw fixation using 3.5- or 4.5-mm screws is recommended. Whether to use one or two screws, to engage three or four cortices, to allow early weightbearing or to perform early screw removal has been debated.

Syndesmosis screws are subjected to significant bending stresses if walking is allowed. If weightbearing begins within six weeks after injury, there is a chance of fatigue failure of the screw. If the tricortical technique is used, the screw can be left in place for 12 to 16 weeks. Because the syndesmotic ligament is unlikely to heal in six weeks, the risk of early removal seems to overshadow the risk of screw fracture. This 4.5-mm screw is less likely to fail than the 3.5-mm screw, but the fibula has been known to fracture through the larger screw hole necessary for the 4.5-mm screw.

Successful treatment with little morbidity can be expected with the following approach. First, reduce the length and rotation of the fibula. Hold the position with a large reduction clamp. Place a 3.5- or 4.5-mm cortical screw through the fibula and into the tibia but do not engage the medial cortex of the tibia. Allow weightbearing with the screw in place six weeks postoperatively and remove the screw no sooner than eight weeks. Do not use a lag screw or a cortical screw placed in a lag or a compression fashion.

Calcaneal Fractures

Almost every aspect of fractures of the os calcis is controversial. There is no universally accepted classification of calcaneal fractures. There are advocates of surgical and of nonsurgical treatment and of medial and of lateral surgical approaches; there are arguments both for and against bone grafting. Nonsurgical treatment in some cases has unsatisfactory results that are inconsistent with the patient's expectations. Deformity, stiffness, and prolonged absence from the workplace are common. Surgical treatment carries a significant incidence of soft-tissue problems, infection, and nerve injury, but offers an opportunity to restore the anatomy and perhaps the function of the hindfoot. No prospective data on the relative merits of nonsurgical and surgical treatment are available to help define the proper treatment for a given fracture pattern and patient.

Stabilization of Posterior Malleolar Fractures

Fractures of the posterior aspect of the tibia associated with fractures of the medial and lateral malleolus (trimalleolar fractures) have traditionally been classified according to the percentage of articular surface on the fragment. Fractures that involve more than one quarter to one third of the articular surface are routinely reduced and internally fixed after stabilization of the medial and lateral malleolus.

Recent studies suggest that most posterior malleolar fragments reduce to within 1 to 2 mm of their anatomic position with anatomic reduction of the lateral malleolus. Long-term follow-up of patients treated nonsurgically suggests that routine stabilization of such posterior malleolar fragments, even in the presence of significant articular involvement, is unwarranted.

Annotated Bibliography

Keywords

Achilles tendon; Ankle fracture; Calcaneus; Compartment syndrome; Cuboid; Ligament injury; Lisfranc joint; Navicular; Talus; Tendon injury

Soft-Tissue Injuries

Anderson ME: Reconstruction of the lateral ligaments of the ankle using the plantaris tendon. *J Bone Joint Surg* 1985;67A:930–934.

In a small number of patients, the author used the plantaris tendon to reconstruct the calcaneofibular and anterior talofibular ligaments. The attachment of the plantaris to the heel cord is maintained while the proximal end of the plantaris is used to reconstruct the ligaments. The advantage of this technique is that it is the most nearly anatomic lateral ligament repair available and preserves the function of the peroneal musculature.

Barnes MJ, Hardy AE: Delayed reconstruction of the calcaneal tendon. *J Bone Joint Surg* 1986;68B:121–124.

The authors reviewed a small number of patients with late diagnoses of rupture of the calcaneal tendon. The 11 surgically treated patients compared favorably in isometric and isokinetic testing with two patients who declined surgery. There was no rerupture in the surgically treated group.

Boutti PM, Bell GR: Compartment syndrome of the foot: A case report. *J Bone Joint Surg* 1986;68A:1449–1451.

A case report of compartment syndrome in the foot with a review of the relevant anatomy and physiology.

Cass JR, Morrey BF, Katoh Y, et al: Ankle instability: Comparison of primary repair and delayed reconstruction after long-term follow-up study. *Clin Orthop* 1985;198:110–117.

No difference was found in objective and subjective outcomes between 25 ankle ligament reconstructions done acutely and 40 done as reconstructive procedures. Acute repairs were done by a ligament-to-bone repair and delayed repairs were done by the Evans/Watson-Jones or Chrisman-Snook technique. The authors advocate primary repair only for the high-performance athlete who may not be able to accept the 20% uncertainty of nonsurgical treatment.

Colville MR, Colville JM, Manoli A II: Posteromedial dislocation of the ankle without fracture. *J Bone Joint Surg* 1987;69A:706–711.

Six of eight patients followed up for two to eight years had no functional impairment and no symptoms. The injuries occurred in young people, often during athletic activities. Generalized ligamentous laxity was common. The mechanism of injury appeared to be forced inversion of the foot and axial loading of the foot in a plantar-flexed position. No injuries of the distal tibiofibular ligaments or syndesmosis occurred.

Das de S, Balasubramaniam P: A repair operation for recurrent dislocation of peroneal tendons. *J Bone Joint Surg* 1985;67B:585–587.

The authors describe the pathologic anatomy of recurrent peroneal tendon disruption as the formation of a false pouch by the retinaculum and periosteum pulling off the fibula to form a continuous pouch from posterior to anterior around the lateral aspect of the fibula. They liken this lesion to a Bankart lesion in the shoulder and describe an analogous repair.

Floyd DW, Heckman JD, Rockwood CA Jr: Tendon lacerations in the foot. *Foot Ankle* 1983;4:8–14.

This study indicates that good functional results can be achieved by aggressive surgical treatment of tendon lacerations. The authors advocate primary repair of the flexor hallucis longus, extensor hallucis longus, tibialis anterior, tibialis posterior, and peroneal tendons. Failure to repair these tendons often led to muscular imbalance and late deformity in skeletally immature patients.

Kellam JF, Hunter GA, McElwain JP: Review of the operative treatment of Achilles tendon rupture. *Clin Orthop* 1985;201:80–83.

Long-term review showed an incidence of rerupture of 3%; skin problems developed in 13% of 68 patients. The authors recommend nonsurgical treatment for unathletic patients more than 50 years old because of potentially serious problems with wound healing.

Larsen E: Experimental instability of the ankle: A radiographic investigation. *Clin Orthop* 1985;204:193–200.

In cadaver dissections, the author identified 10 degrees of plantar flexion as the position in which to best test the anterior drawer sign. The anterior talofibular ligament was found to be the most significant restraint against the anterior drawer. The authors recommend 10 degrees of plantar flexion and 25 degrees of inward rotation of the leg during radiographic examination of ankle instability.

Linsdjo U: Classification of ankle fractures: The Lauge-Hansen or AO system? *Clin Orthop* 1985;199:12–16.

The author discusses the history, strengths, and weaknesses of each of the two predominant classification systems now used. The former has the advantages of being more comprehensive and giving more information about mechanism and soft-tissue injury. The latter is easier to use and provides adequate information for planning surgical repair.

Myerson MS: Experimental decompression of fascial compartments of the foot. *Foot Ankle* 1987;8:308–314.

A laboratory study was performed involving decompression of the foot in simulated compartment syndrome. The dorsal approach was simpler but the medial approach allowed more rapid decompression and better access to plantar compartments.

Nada A: Rupture of the calcaneal tendon: Treatment by external fixation. *J Bone Joint Surg* 1985;67B:449–453.

Thirty-three patients were treated with an external fixation technique. Ninety percent had excellent to good results. Fair and poor results occurred in three patients—two with sural nerve injury and one with Sudeck's atrophy.

Sclafani SJ: Ligamentous injury of the lower tibiofibular syndesmosis: Radiographic evidence. *Radiology* 1985; 156:21–27.

Intact ankle specimens have a roentgenographic clear space of 4 mm or less at the distal tibiofibular joint. A space of 5 mm or more between the disal tibia and fibula indicates disruption of the syndesmosis.

van Rappard JH, Reinders JF, Mahabier C, et al: Operative treatment of persistent lateral instability of the ankle: Is it worse to sprain the ankle than to break it? *Neth J Surg* 1987;39:65–67.

Sixteen hundred lateral ligamentous injuries were treated nonsurgically with plaster and bandages. Thirty-five (21.1%) required surgical treatment because of persistent instability. Most patients with ligamentous ankle injuries do not require surgery.

Fractures and Fracture-Dislocations

Arntz CT, Veith RG, Hansen ST Jr: Fractures and fracture-dislocations of the tarsometatarsal joint. *J Bone Joint Surg* 1988;70A:173–181.

Forty-one injuries in 40 adults were treated by open reduction and internal fixation with AO screws. The authors correlated good results with anatomic reduction. Less than anatomic reduction in grade II or grade III open injuries was correlated with poor results.

Bauer M, Bergstrom B, Hemborg A, et al: Malleolar fractures: Nonoperative versus operative treatment. A controlled study. *Clin Orthop* 1985;199:17–27.

A prospective, randomized study carried out over seven years found that fractures treated with surgery had a more favorable outcome initially. However, at long-term follow-up little differences existed between the two forms of treatment.

Howie CR, Hooper G, Hughes SP: Occult midtarsal subluxation. *Clin Orthop* 1986;209:206–209.

Fifty percent of patients with navicular tuberosity avulsion were found to have a hidden injury at the calcaneocuboid joint. The diagnosis was initially missed in five of seven cases. All had prolonged symptoms, and degenerative changes developed in the calcaneocuboid joint.

Limbird RS, Aaron RK: Laterally comminuted fracture-dislocation of the ankle. *J Bone Joint Surg* 1987;69A: 881–885.

Although the lateral malleolus is the key to reduction of ankle fractures, severe comminution can make accurate reduction difficult. If the medial malleolus is reduced first in these injuries, the position of the talus in the mortise can be used as a guide to reduction of the fibula.

Mayo KA: Fractures of the talus: Principles of management and techniques of treatment. *Techn Orthop* 1987;2: 42–54.

The author reviews the anatomy, blood supply, classification, radiographic assessment, and treatment of talus fractures. A combined medial and dorsolateral approach is suggested to ensure anatomic reduction of talar neck fractures. Rigid internal fixation is recommended.

Sangeorzan BJ, Benirschke SK, Mosca V, et al: Displaced intra-articular fractures of the tarsal navicular. Presented at the meeting of the Orthopaedic Trauma Association, Dallas, October 1988.

Twenty-two patients with tarsal navicular fractures were reviewed in a retrospective fashion. Three radiographic patterns emerged and correlated well with long-term prognosis. The authors recommend an attempt to restore the talonavicular joint.

Schaffer JJ, Manoli A II: The antiglide plate for distal fibular fixation: A biomechanical comparison with fixation with a lateral plate. *J Bone Joint Surg* 1987;69A: 596–604.

The authors tested posterior vs lateral plating of distal oblique fibular fractures and found that the posterior antiglide plate was more stiff, absorbed greater torque, and failed at higher loads than the laterally placed plate. The authors recommended the antiglide plate for treating short, oblique fractures of the distal fibula.

Sondenaa K, Hoigaard U, Smith D, et al: Immobilization of operated ankle fractures. *Acta Orthop Scand* 1986;57:59–61.

Forty-three patients with stable internal fixation of ankle fractures were randomly assigned to cast or early mobilization groups. The two groups were followed up for a year. There were no significant differences in long-term outcome.

Stephenson JR: Treatment of displaced intra-articular fractures of the calcaneus using medial and lateral approaches, internal fixation, and early motion. *J Bone Joint Surg* 1987;69A:115–130.

The author reviews his treatment technique and results in 22 patients. A lateral approach supplemented at times by a medial approach, with internal fixation and early motion, was used. Twenty-one of 22 patients returned to work within six months.

Swanson T, Bray T: Talar neck fractures: A mechanical and histomorphometric study of fixation. Presented at the meeting of the Orthopaedic Trauma Association, Dallas, October 1988.

The authors tested a number of screw configurations as well as K-wire stabilization of laboratory-produced talar neck fractures. K-wires provide fixation strength inadequate to resist intrinsic muscle forces across the ankle joint. Fixation into the lateral head and inferolateral body provided the best bone quality for fixation. Posterior-to-anterior fixation with a 6.5-mm cancellous screw provided the strongest fixation.

Wuelker N, Zwipp H, Tscherne H: The operative treatment of intra-articular calcaneus fractures. Presented at the 55th Annual Meeting of the American Academy of Orthopaedic Surgeons, Atlanta, Feb 4, 1988.

Thirty-seven patients were treated by a combined medial and lateral approach and evaluated at an average of three years. A medial approach was used to elevate the subtalar joint. The intra-articular anatomy was restored through a lateral approach about the peroneal tendons. The lateral incision was also used for bone grafting. The reduction was stabilized with subarticular lag screws from the lateral side and a medial H plate; early motion was then instituted.

Controversies

Fixation of Syndesmosis Injuries

Finsen V, Saetermo R, Kibsgaard L, et al: Early postoperative weight-bearing and muscle activity in patients who have a fracture of the ankle. *J Bone Joint Surg* 1989;71A:23–27.

Stabilization of Posterior Malleolar Fractures

Harper MC, Hardin G: Posterior malleolar fractures of the ankle associated with external rotation-abduction injuries: Results with and without internal fixation. *J Bone Joint Surg* 1988;70A:1348–1356.

48
Ankle and Foot: Reconstruction

The adult foot and ankle are afflicted with many abnormalities that are painful and frequently disabling. The biomechanics and the anatomy of the foot and ankle are complex. Thus, the many disorders may be difficult to diagnose and treat.

Regional Anesthesia

Regional anesthesia is now increasingly used for operations involving the foot, particularly the forefoot. Since many of these procedures are done on an outpatient basis, this type of anesthesia appears to be effective while containing costs. The landmarks for the various nerves that cross the ankle and innervate the foot are usually fixed and easily identified. Frequently a 1:1 mixture of lidocaine and bupivacaine is used. The amount of local anesthetic is usually limited to 30 ml of a 1:1 mixture of 1% lidocaine and 0.25% bupivacaine on a single extremity. In bilateral procedures, 20 ml of this solution (40 ml total) has not caused any difficulties. It is a distinct advantage to have an anesthesiologist assist in performing the blocks. Also, the use of intravenous medications to relax the patient is often helpful. At times, nerve stimulators can help in identifying the nerves, particularly in patients who have had previous operations.

Hallux Valgus

Hallux valgus is still a difficult problem. For the most part, the patients are women and a great part of the problem is the pain and discomfort produced by wearing fashionable shoes. Unfortunately, many working women are required to dress in a certain style or fashion. Thus, it is reasonable to consider treatment that will alleviate the discomfort and allow patients to return to some sort of desirable shoe wear.

Many bunion operations have been described over the years. These basically consist of soft-tissue releases around the metatarsophalangeal joint and may be associated with either a proximal osteotomy of the hallux metatarsal or a distal osteotomy. The important blood supply to the first metatarsal head and metatarsophalangeal joint has been investigated and must be remembered whenever an extensive soft-tissue release or an osteotomy, particularly a distal osteotomy, is being considered in planning a hallux valgus correction.

The blood supply to the hallux metatarsophalangeal joint is both extraosseous and intraosseous. The extraosseous supply enters the bone primarily on the dorsolateral side. The main arteries are the first dorsal metatarsal artery and the first plantar metatarsal artery. These give off branches to the lateral capsule, which then course into the metatarsal head. These arteries run longitudinally along the metatarsal and eventually give off capsular branches.

Thus, any stripping of the dorsal and lateral part of the distal metatarsal may cause significant disruption of this extraosseous blood supply. The intraosseous blood supply consists of a diffuse network of fine periosteal arteries that surround the diaphysis of the metatarsal. A single nutrient artery perforates the first metatarsal at the lateral aspect of the shaft distally. Further, a system of metaphyseal and capital arteries also appears to constitute a major source of blood supply to the metatarsal head.

Assessment

A careful assessment of the patient by means of physical examination and radiography is essential in planning any type of hallux valgus correction. Preoperative evaluation of the bunion deformity is needed to plan the operation. This evaluation is based on the bunion deformity and the relationship of the foot to the leg and the rest of the body. Additionally, the patient's general condition, age, and expectations with regard to foot wear and level of activity postoperatively must be evaluated. Surgical procedures can be classified as distal soft-tissue realignments, metatarsal osteotomies, miscellaneous operations, and arthroplastic procedures. A combination of procedures is often required. Consistent weightbearing radiographs are essential. These should determine (1) the relative lengths of the first and second metatarsals, (2) the shape of the first metatarsal head (rounded and generally more unstable or more flat, and thus more stable), and (3) the shape of the metatarsal cuneiform joint (oblique and thus more resistant to realignment or transverse, making lateral displacement of the metatarsal head easier). The lateral weightbearing radiograph is important for determining the relationship between the forefoot and the hindfoot. A line drawn through the first metatarsal should pass directly through the midportion of the talus. If the line through the talus points below one drawn through the metatarsal, then a flatfoot deformity is present.

Treatment

In general, the most commonly performed distal soft-tissue realignment procedure is based on the original McBride procedure. This is used for mild to moderate deformities. The modification is based on retaining the lateral sesamoid. The most popular distal osteotomy is the chevron, which is used for mild to moderate deformities in the young or the middle-aged adult with tarsus primus varus. It is not recommended for patients more than 50 years old. Although this osteotomy produces a small degree of shortening of the first metatarsal, this shortening has not led to subsequent transfer metatarsalgia. When the first metatarsal is longer and the deformity is mild in a younger patient, this is an excellent operation. Opening and closing wedge osteotomies have limited applications because the former requires bone grafting and may tighten the soft tissues, and the latter causes a definite shortening of the first metatarsal. The concentric or curved type of osteotomy has gained considerable popularity (Figs. 1 and 2). The surgeon must be careful not to allow any dorsiflexion of the first metatarsal head when performing these osteotomies or a transfer metatarsalgia will result. These osteotomies require internal fixation.

Combinations of procedures are common. For example, the distal soft-tissue realignment of the modified McBride procedure is frequently combined with a curved proximal first metatarsal osteotomy. Additionally, a closing wedge osteotomy through the base of the proximal phalanx, the Akin procedure, is used to correct the deformity further. This osteotomy is also useful in correcting hallux valgus interphalangeus. However, the Akin procedure alone has been reported to be unsatisfactory for the correction of hallux valgus deformities.

By using radiographs to plan hallux valgus correction (measuring the length of the first metatarsal and the width of the osteotomy site), the surgeon can project the amount of correction of a distal metatarsal osteotomy. These measurements also provide the limits of angular corrections for which such osteotomies can be used. An intermetatarsal angle of more than 20 to 30 degrees cannot be corrected by a distal lateral displacement osteotomy and requires a corrective osteotomy performed more proximally, preferably at the base. A comparison of the effectiveness of five different osteotomies of the first metatarsal to correct hallux valgus deformities showed that satisfactory results were obtained with a biplanar osteotomy of the metatarsal neck, if the lateral displacement was between 4.5 to 5.5 mm. This

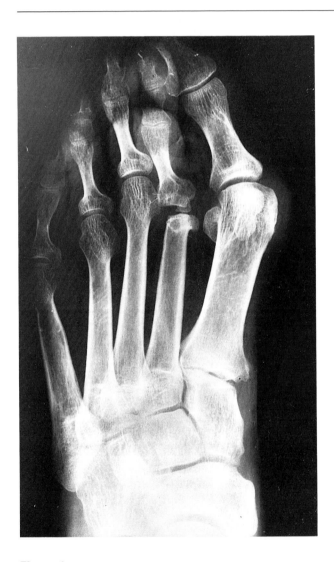
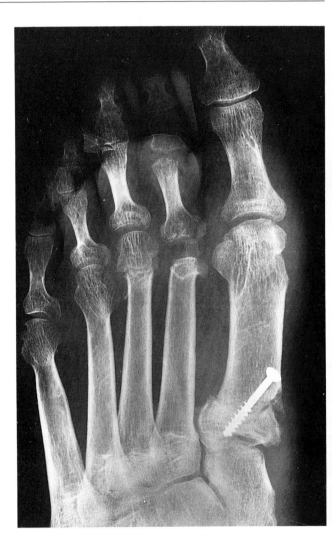

Figure 1

A 57-year-old man had symptomatic hallux valgus. His second metatarsal head had been removed several years earlier because of osteomyelitis. **Left,** The primary complaint was pain on the medial side of the bunion deformity and moderate pain on the dorsum of the proximal interphalangeal joint of the second toe. **Right,** Radiograph taken after a concentric osteotomy of the hallux metatarsal. The osteotomy, originally described with the convexity of the curve pointing proximally, has been reversed so that the curve points distally. The osteotomy was solidly fixed with a 4-mm cancellous screw. A small amount of the head of the proximal phalanx of the second toe was removed during soft-tissue repair of the hammertoe. Alignment was excellent and the symptoms were relieved.

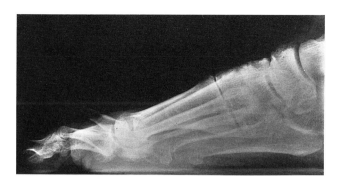

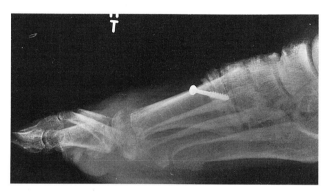

Figure 2

Same patient shown in Figure 1. **Top,** Preoperative lateral radiograph. **Bottom,** Postoperative lateral radiograph showing placement of the screw. The metatarsal head has not drifted dorsally.

gives consistently good results in metatarsus primus varus of as much as 13 degrees. In patients with metatarsus primus varus of more than 13 degrees, a basilar concentric osteotomy, to which a closing wedge is added, has been advocated. This seems to give more consistently satisfactory results and greater corrections than other osteotomies. Intraoperative and nonweightbearing postoperative radiographs are often misleading and give a false impression of full correction when no correction has actually occurred. Radiographs taken in a nonweightbearing fashion with even slight supination of the foot often give misleading measurements of correction of the metatarsus primus varus. The key to proper corrective surgery is rigid internal fixation and intraoperative measurements of the amount of correction in both the transverse and the horizontal planes.

Probably one of the most important factors in predicting the overall results of hallux valgus surgery is the laxity of a patient's joints. There is a statistically significant correlation between patients with symptomatic hallux valgus and generalized hypermobility of the joints. Hypermobility was measured by hyperextension at the metacarpophalangeal joint, passive opposition of the thumb to the flexor surface of the forearm, and hyperextension of the elbow and knee beyond 10 degrees. Such patients might be better treated with osteotomies, because their hypermobile soft tissues could conceivably result in recurrent deformity.

One of the major concerns regarding distal osteotomy of the first metatarsal is the potential for developing osteonecrosis of the metatarsal head. In a review of 60 feet

in 41 patients who underwent distal chevron osteotomy, postoperative radiographs showed some evidence of osteonecrosis in 20% (Fig. 3). Moreover, when the osteotomy was combined with a lateral adductor release, osteonecrosis was noted in 40%. Unfortunately, these investigators did not describe the surgical approach used and the operations were apparently done by many different surgeons. The presence of osteonecrosis did not correlate with the final results. Further, the osteonecrosis seen radiographically did not progress in all patients. Several patients apparently underwent internal fixation of the osteotomy and this might have contributed to the incidence of osteonecrosis.

Reasons for failure included preexisting osteoarthritis of the joint, injury to the dorsal proper digital nerve, and osteonecrosis. Metatarsophalangeal joint motion was decreased by only 17 degrees unless there was some evidence of osteonecrosis, when it was decreased by 28 degrees. However, the arc of motion was most acceptable at 61 degrees. As would be expected, there was no significant correction of the angle between the first and second metatarsals. There was a correlation between the amount of motion and final result. There were no transfer lesions and no shortening of the first metatarsal. However, patients with advanced abnormalities, such as those with angles between the first and second metatarsals of more than 15 degrees, had a higher incidence of surgical failure. Thus, of patients with a preoperative intermetatarsal angle of more than 12 degrees, only 74% achieved a satisfactory result compared with 94% of those with an intermetatarsal angle of less than 12 degrees. The patient's age did not

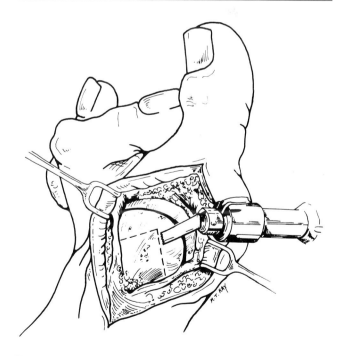

Figure 3

The chevron osteotomy is currently the most popular osteotomy for correcting hallux valgus with moderate deformity. The osteotomy is done within the head and neck of the hallux metatarsal at an angle of approximately 60 degrees. The distal fragment containing the head is then displaced laterally.

affect the final result. Finally, it is interesting to note that the average length of hospitalization was 5.6 days for the unilateral group and 6.9 days for those undergoing bilateral operations.

In another series of patients who underwent chevron osteotomy for bunion correction, 12.9% were satisfied with minor reservations and 8% were dissatisfied. Only those patients with some problem underwent postoperative radiographic analysis. Satisfaction was influenced in part by the age of the patient at the time of the operation. Twenty-five percent of patients in the sixth decade of life were somewhat dissatisfied with the procedure. Also, of patients with a preoperative metatarsophalangeal angle of 40 degrees or more, only 52% were completely satisfied; of those with a preoperative intermetatarsal angle of more than 15 degrees, only 68.9% were satisfied. Thus, older patients, those with more severe hallux valgus, and those with a wider angle between the first and second metatarsals may not be suited for this type of bunion correction. In those patients who underwent postoperative radiography, there was no evidence of osteonecrosis. Thus, if osteonecrosis was present, it was probably asymptomatic or the follow-up was too short for degenerative joint disease to have developed.

Despite published reports citing the disadvantages of excisional arthroplasty of the hallux metatarsophalangeal joint, one series had a success rate of 77%. This group of women (75 feet) had an average age of 66 years and an average follow-up of 31 months. Cock-up deformities of the hallux occurred but did not influence the overall results. There were no cases of transfer metatarsalgia. These were older patients who had very low activity levels and the operation was not recommended for young, active patients. This report probably represents a highly selected group of patients, because this type of resectional arthroplasty has been associated with a significantly high incidence of postoperative transfer metatarsalgia along with cock-up deformity of the toe and recurrence of the hallux valgus.

Salvage

Arthrodesis of the hallux metatarsophalangeal joint is a dependable salvage procedure for painful disorders affecting this joint. In one experimental study the arthrodesis site was maintained most effectively when 40-mm cancellous screws were used and when the adjacent bony surfaces were cut flat. Rigid fixation will fail if the screw head fractures the bony flange of the proximal phalanx.

Compression arthrodesis of the hallux metatarsophalangeal joint has been reported. These investigators used two 27-mm screws and fused all 20 toes. Others have used two 37-mm double-ended threaded Steinmann pins across the metatarsophalangeal joint to obtain fusion. These patients had undergone Keller arthroplasties that had failed and the proximal phalanx was quite short.

Salvage of a painful hallux metatarsophalangeal joint can also be accomplished with the use of a double-stemmed silicone implant. The majority of these implants are used in patients with reduced activity levels and generalized foot abnormalities like those seen in rheumatoid arthritis. Currently, such implants are inserted with the use of titanium grommets. These grommets protect the stem as it joins the hinge part of the implant. A silicone implant should be used only in a joint being considered for either arthrodesis

or excisional arthroplasty. It is never appropriate to use such implants in a joint that could be realigned via either soft-tissue releases or osteotomy. Unfortunately, the inappropriate use of these implants has led to complications. Among these is synovitis within the metatarsophalangeal joint when particulate silicone is produced. Injury to the implant from overuse or improper placement may lead to its deterioration and particulate materials. One such case has been reported with the use of a double-stemmed silicone implant. In addition to the synovitis, which was minimal, the patient exhibited granulomatous inguinal lymphadenopathy. This complication occurred because the implant was placed in a patient who should not have received one.

Hallux Rigidus

Conservative care is sometimes successful and consists of methods to reduce motion across the joint. This can be accomplished with an orthotic support placed just behind the joint; a rocker-bottom sole can also be helpful, along with mild analgesics or nonsteroidal anti-inflammatory drugs. Cheilectomy is the procedure of choice. All osteophytes, as well as the dorsal-most quarter to third of the metatarsal head must be removed. Because about one half of the motion will be lost postoperatively, it is important to gain as much motion as possible at the cheilectomy. Complete relief of pain was obtained in 22 of 31 joints in one series. There were only three failures. Motion also improved in 23 of the joints (average postoperative arc, 48 degrees).

In another series of 58 patients treated with cheilectomy, results were unsatisfactory in 27.6%. The final result appeared to correlate directly with the degree of preoperative joint abnormality. These investigators advised cheilectomy only in patients with mild degrees of hallux rigidus. In those with advanced abnormalities, they recommended arthrodesis.

Disorders of the Lateral Toes and Metatarsophalangeal Joints

Lateral toe joint disorders are all common problems and can be the source of severe pain and disability. Hammertoes, mallet toes, and clawtoes are common deformities that may require surgical correction.

Hammertoe

A hammertoe is a contracture of the proximal interphalangeal joint and is frequently associated with either some contracture or even dorsal subluxation of the metatarsophalangeal joint. It is usually an acquired deformity. Although the hammertoe deformity is usually fixed, that is, it cannot be passively corrected, in its early stages it may be flexible (passively correctable). Conservative treatment should be attempted. This usually requires a change in heel height and obtaining a shoe with an adequate toe box.

Surgical correction of a rigid hammertoe deformity usually requires removal of the head of the proximal phalanx and a dermadesis of the dorsal skin. It is important to be certain that the metatarsophalangeal joint is not left dorsally subluxated. A Kirschner wire may be necessary to maintain the corrected position. An arthrodesis of the imal interphalangeal joint is also possible. In either case, a flexor tenotomy can also be performed.

A flexible hammertoe deformity can be passively correctable. If surgical treatment is required, a flexor tendon transfer as described by Girdlestone can be performed, although it is a moderately difficult procedure. This transfer consists of releasing the flexor tendon distally through a transverse incision made on the plantar surface of the metatarsophalangeal joint. The tendon is thus released distally from its insertion and can then be split longitudinally through its normal median raphe. Each limb of the tendon is then passed dorsally around the most proximal portion of the proximal phalanx to the dorsum of the metatarsophalangeal joint. With the ankle in neutral position, the tendon is then sutured to itself. A K-wire may be required to stabilize the toe, and it may be necessary to remove a small portion of the proximal phalanx if a residual flexion deformity exists. It is essential that the neurovascular structures not be disrupted in this transfer.

In any of these procedures on the toe, subluxation or dislocation of the metatarsophalangeal joint must also be corrected. The joint should be approached through a dorsal curved incision or a Z-type incision so that subsequent contracture by the scar is not a factor. The extensor tendon is lengthened. Hypertrophic synovium should be excised. The dorsal capsule and collateral ligaments are usually released. It may also be necessary to stabilize the joint for a few weeks with a K-wire. K-wires are usually removed at about three weeks after surgery. The adjacent toes should then be taped together for about six weeks.

Mallet Toe

A mallet toe is a flexion contracture of the distal interphalangeal joint. This leads to pain at the tip of the toe. Surgical treatment consists of excision of the head of the middle phalanx and release of the long flexor tendon. The distal interphalangeal joint is stabilized by a K-wire and a dorsal dermadesis may be added.

Clawtoe

Clawtoe deformities usually involve several toes and may be associated with some type of neurologic abnormality. Nonsurgical treatment should be attempted because there is usually involvement of the entire foot with a cavus deformity usually present. Therefore, a shoe with a deep and wide toe box should be prescribed. Surgical correction usually involves several toes. Sufficient bone must be removed from the proximal phalanx to gain correction of these advanced deformities. This may require excising most of the proximal phalanx. Syndactylism of adjacent operated-on toes can also be used.

Second Metatarsophalangeal Joint

Subluxation One of the more important new developments in the diagnosis and treatment of forefoot disorders is recognition of subluxating toe at the metatarsophalangeal joint. This is usually associated with either a stretching of the plantar capsule (volar plate) or its actual rupture. The patient's foot may appear to be normal. Thus, the condition must be suspected on the basis of pain in the affected area (usually the second toe and the second metatarsophalangeal joint). The patients are usually active individuals. The instability at the joint probably evokes a sec-

ondary synovitis, and, if the volar plate is absent, it may cause tenosynovitis about the flexor tendon, which is directly underneath. This abnormality may also be associated with hallux valgus and a long second metatarsal. Physical examination can show some mild swelling of the joint and instability. The Thompson-Hamilton sign is an instability of the second metatarsophalangeal joint. The foot is stabilized and the proximal phalanx is grasped firmly and an attempt made to subluxate the base of the proximal phalanx dorsally. This should be done carefully because the area may be tender. The subluxation is usually palpable and reproduces the patient's discomfort.

Early treatment consists of stabilizing the toe either by modifying the patient's shoes or by using some type of pad that limits the amount of dorsiflexion of the proximal phalanx. This can be something like a toe retainer that places a plantar-directed force on the proximal phalanx. A rocker-bottom sole is frequently helpful, as is adding a full shank to the shoe. At this time, there is no procedure to repair the plantar capsule; if conservative care is not adequate, surgical stabilization is necessary. This is usually an exploration of the metatarsophalangeal joint, with a synovectomy if necessary, and transfer of the flexor to the extensor tendon. If the joint cannot be completely reduced, then removing a wafer of articular cartilage from the second metatarsal head (the DuVries procedure) is also helpful.

Nonspecific Synovitis Nonspecific synovitis of the second metatarsophalangeal joint can also develop. It is important to evaluate all patients with forefoot pain for this entity. There is usually no history of trauma. In one series, all patients had evidence of joint instability. The synovial hypertrophy was also thought to be the cause of neuritic symptoms, leading to resection of the interdigital nerve in three of seven patients. Conservative treatment was used in all cases; in only one did the synovitis subside. Six of the seven patients required synovectomy of this joint. It is important to treat this condition aggressively, before the joint becomes arthritic or dislocates.

Dislocation Dislocation of the second metatarsophalangeal joint makes conservative care difficult unless a shoe with an adequate toe box acceptable to the patient can be found. Surgical treatment is usually indicated and the course may be complicated if a hallux valgus deformity is present. In this case, the hallux valgus deformity should be corrected even if it is relatively asymptomatic. Correction of the hallux valgus creates adequate space for relocation of the second toe. The surgical approach to the second toe requires an extensor tenotomy, dorsal capsulotomy, and release of the collateral ligaments. In most cases, a fixed hammertoe is present, and should be surgically corrected as well. It is essential that the toe remain in the corrected position before it is stabilized with wires or other devices. K-wire fixation may be necessary to keep the corrected position, but should not be used to gain correction. The K-wire should only remain in place for a few weeks until soft-tissue healing has occurred.

Crossover Deformity A crossover deformity of the second toe is common and can be challenging to correct. A medially deviated second toe can occur either as an isolated phenomenon or in association with hallux valgus. This deformity has been attributed to deterioration of the lateral collateral ligament of the second metatarsophalangeal joint as well as the joint capsule. In a severe deformity, the second toe can also deviate dorsally and rest over the hallux. Radiographic evaluation of such patients usually shows a noncongruent second metatarsophalangeal joint articulation. Most patients also have excessively long second metatarsals in relation to the first and third metatarsals.

For a mild deformity, which is passively correctable, conservative care can be used, taping the second toe to the third toe. Although this may not correct the deformity, it may arrest its progression. Mild deformities needing surgical treatment require an extensor tenotomy or lengthening and a metatarsophalangeal joint capsulotomy. It may also be necessary to reef the lateral joint capsule. Usually, the joint is stabilized with a K-wire, which is removed after four weeks. Taping is then continued for an additional six weeks.

In a moderate deformity, there is usually hyperextension of the proximal phalanx or a flexible hammertoe. In such cases a flexor tendon transfer is added to the procedure. The lateral limb of the transferred flexor tendon is sutured under increased tension to help realign the medially deviated second toe. Although a K-wire can be used, it must not be relied on to obtain correction, but rather to hold the correction obtained by the soft-tissue procedure.

In severe subluxation, there is usually a fixed hammertoe deformity. Such cases usually require a metatarsophalangeal joint arthroplasty with removal of between 3 and 4 mm of the distal metatarsal articular surface. A DuVries hammertoe repair is also carried out to correct the fixed hammertoe deformity. The entire phalanx is stabilized by an intramedullary K-wire, removed after four weeks. Taping of the second toe to the third toe then continues for an additional four to six weeks. Such severe cases usually result in some stiffness of the toe, but correction of the deformity is usually maintained. Of 15 toes (11 patients), all of which underwent joint capsulotomy and extensor tenotomy or extensor lengthening with K-wire insertion to hold the repair, 73% also had a flexor tendon transfer and 33% had a metatarsophalangeal joint arthroplasty. A bony hammertoe repair was done in 55%. Of these, 90% were fully satisfactory at an average follow-up of 42 months.

Infraction This involves the second metatarsal head, and has an unknown cause, although trauma has been implicated by many authors. It occurs most often in the second and third metatarsal heads because these are the least mobile; they may be more frequently subjected to traumatic conditions. In the early stages, stages I and II, the pain on weightbearing may be caused by the infraction of the metatarsal head and an effusion within the joint. This can be treated by protected weightbearing using crutches or a weightbearing orthotic device. No studies are available to indicate the effectiveness of this conservative care.

In the early stages with radiographic changes, a dorsal cancellous bone graft has been inserted to restore the contour of the metatarsal head. Transfixion of the metatarsal head with a K-wire and a below-knee walking cast for six weeks have been advocated. In the later stages, stages III to V, symptoms result from metatarsalgia caused by an expanded metatarsal head or pain, producing the secondary osteoarthritis of the joint. Management of these later stages should be directed toward the cause of symptoms. If there is no pain on moving the joint and the symptoms

are caused by metatarsalgia, an osteotomy of the metatarsal may be indicated. If pain comes from motion of the arthritic joint, a replacement silicone arthroplasty is recommended. A debridement of the joint may be considered in a younger, more active patient.

Rheumatoid Arthritis

Patients with rheumatoid arthritis often have painful foot deformities. These usually involve the forefoot, with dislocated metatarsophalangeal joints, lateral drift of the toes, and toe deformities such as fixed hammertoes. Additionally, patients frequently have hindfoot disorders involving either the talonavicular joint alone or, more commonly, all three hindfoot joints. It is essential to evaluate the hindfoot in any rheumatoid patient. These patients may also have a ruptured posterior tibial tendon, but the synovial disease usually destroys the joints and leaves the hindfoot with a fixed valgus deformity. Patients with significant hindfoot deformity and pain usually complain of pain in the "ankle." Thus, it is essential to distinguish between ankle involvement and hindfoot involvement. If the patient has significant deformity in the hindfoot and the forefoot, it is important to decide which area should be corrected first. Should a forefoot deformity be corrected and the hindfoot deformity neglected, lateral drift of the toes may recur because of overall deformity of the foot.

The most common operation used to correct the rheumatoid forefoot is some type of an excisional arthroplasty. Although excisional arthroplasty of the lateral four metatarsophalangeal joints is frequently satisfactory, it is probably wise to stabilize the hallux metatarsophalangeal joint either with a double-stemmed silicone implant arthroplasty or with an arthrodesis. The medial side of the foot is the most stable; if the hallux is not stabilized and then begins to drift laterally, lateral drift of the lateral toes may recur. After excisional arthroplasty of the rheumatoid forefoot, significant changes in plantar forefoot pressures occur.

In a study of patients who underwent resectional arthroplasty and dynamic and static foot pressure studies, rheumatoid patients showed a loss of the rocking motion of the foot during gait. Heel strike and toe-off were often reduced or absent. Toe function was almost invariably absent as well. Postoperatively, pain relief was noted in 92% of feet at rest and in 73% of feet on walking. Sixty percent were more mobile after the operation, with only two patients claiming less mobility. Pressure studies showed a reduction of pressure under the central metatarsals, but this was shifted to the first and fifth metatarsals. These results indicate the need to emphasize adequate excision of the lateral metatarsals. Many of the high pressures under the first metatarsal were reduced to normal, but some never reached normal. In several feet, a new high-pressure area was created under the first metatarsal. There was a significant difference between the dynamic and static measurements relative to the site of maximum pressure. Postoperatively, maximum pressure was shifted to the first or the fifth metatarsal during standing, whereas it was confined to the first metatarsal during the dynamic studies. Thus, it may be important to stabilize the hallux metatarsophalangeal joint either with a double-stem silicone implant or a fusion.

In a retrospective study of 26 patients with rheumatoid arthritis who had 45 forefoot operations, the type of drug treatment the patient received and the duration of the disease at the time of surgery were used to establish a disease-severity index. The investigators arbitrarily assigned patients a low grade if they were taking drugs such as aspirin or nonsteroidal anti-inflammatory medications and a high grade if they were taking drugs such as cyclophosphamide. Added to this was the duration of disease. Those who had had the disease for less than five years were graded I and those who had had it for 15 years or more were graded IV. These two grading systems were then combined.

Unfortunately, the surgical procedures were quite varied and were done by eight different surgeons. Some of the procedures also involved a hindfoot fusion. Overall, the forefoot surgery seemed to be beneficial in patients with rheumatoid arthritis, although the procedures did not give long-lasting results as the rheumatoid disease progressed. The procedures did not improve gait or function, and in fact may have caused some deterioration in push-off. Most of these operations were excisional arthroplasties. Although they had no significant evidence, these investigators believed that fusion of the first metatarsophalangeal joint gave better results than resection of that joint and that stability of the first ray should be a primary goal for forefoot operations. A few silicone implants were used, but they were of the single-stem design and thus did not provide significant stability.

This study showed the difficulty of trying to classify rheumatoid patients. Such patients now receive a wide variety of medications depending on the aggressiveness of their medical care. For example, in some patients with long-duration rheumatoid arthritis, the disease can be well controlled with drugs such as aspirin whereas other patients with short-duration disease require more potent medications.

In a review of 21 patients (35 feet) who underwent excision of the metatarsal heads, mostly through a dorsal transverse incision with a mean follow-up of 29 months, K-wire fixation was used in only five feet. On the basis of a grading system that included the amount of walking, use of a walking aid, the type of shoes, the cosmesis of the foot, and the amount of pain relief, 16 feet (46%) had excellent results, 12 feet (34%) had good results, six feet (17%) had fair results, and one foot (3%) had a poor result. Postoperative radiographic examination revealed impingement of the metatarsal stump on the base of the proximal phalanx in 67%, but this was not correlated with the overall result. Recurrence of deformity with lateral toe deviation was found in 23%, and new bone formation on the resection metatarsal stump in 18%, but this showed no correlation with clinical success. None of the feet required revision surgery, two had a slight delay in wound healing, one developed a superficial wound infection, and there was no deep wound sepsis. Sixty-six percent of the patients wore shoes without support. Special shoes, pads, or bars were not routinely prescribed.

Hindfoot and Tendons

Radiographic evaluation of hindfoot abnormalities can be difficult and the advent of computed tomography has greatly aided in the diagnosis of such conditions as tarsal coalitions. Computed tomography is superior to plain radiographs for demonstrating coalitions of the cartilaginous type. Studies on fresh cadaveric feet comparing computed tomography, plain tomography, and plain radiographs showed that individualization of the subtalar facet joint was far superior with computed tomography. Thus, whenever hindfoot disorders are suspected, plain radiographs are usually helpful in at least screening the hindfoot, but computed tomography is the best method for detecting and interpreting the degree of abnormality.

Tendon Rupture

The diagnosis of posterior tibial tendon rupture can usually be made from the history and physical examination. In one study, patients with tendon avulsion at the insertion were treated by reinsertion of the tendon, those with midsubstance rupture had a flexor digitorum tendon transfer, and those with tenosynovitis had only a synovectomy. At times the diagnosis may be in doubt and ultrasonography has been used to detect posterior tibial tendon rupture. However, magnetic resonance imaging has also been reported to show tendon rupture and may be more reliable than tenography. Because the diagnosis is so clearly made on a clinical basis, the use of magnetic resonance imaging can only be justified if some other abnormality, such as a tumor, is suspected.

Many different operations have been described to reconstruct the lateral ligaments of the ankle and hindfoot. Long-term evaluation of these patients, most of whom are quite young, is essential. In a review of 42 consecutive patients who underwent the Evans procedure for chronic lateral instability of the ankle, only 21 patients had satisfactory long-term functional results and 12 patients with satisfactory early results showed deterioration after three to six years of follow-up. This operation seemed to control talar tilt more successfully than anterior subluxation of the talus. The Evans procedure uses the peroneus brevis tendon, which is passed through a tunnel in the lateral malleolus from anterior to posterior and then reattached under tension to the proximal portion of the tendon with the foot held in slight eversion. A positive anterior drawer sign was detected in 23 patients; of these, 19 had unsatisfactory results (four fair and 15 poor). In contrast, at about one year after operation, most patients had a negative anterior drawer sign. Thirteen patients required a second operation, five for repeat ligament reconstruction after two to six years. Thus, Evans tenodesis reduced subtalar movement at least in plantar flexion, but offered less control of anterior talar subluxation.

Rheumatoid Arthritis

Stabilization of the adult hindfoot (triple arthrodesis) is frequently indicated in patients with rheumatoid arthritis after a hindfoot fracture involving the subtalar joint and in some patients with rupture of the posterior tibial tendon. Some type of bone grafting is apparently important in gaining stability in these joints. It should also be remembered that any significant varus or valgus deformity should be corrected before the hindfoot joints are stabilized. Thus, a triple arthrodesis performed in adult patients should first correct the deformity, usually by soft-tissue release, and then stabilize the joints, usually by placing bone grafts at least in the subtalar joint and securing all three joints with some type of internal fixation. In a triple arthrodesis technique for patients with either a valgus deformity or no deformity, a K-wire is inserted through the sole of the foot from the calcaneus to the talus. This is done before cutting the lateral trough across the hindfoot joints and inserting a tibial graft.

Patients with rheumatoid arthritis who have isolated destruction of the talonavicular joint may benefit from talonavicular arthrodesis. It is essential that the hindfoot be correctable to neutral inversion-eversion when this procedure is done.

Midfoot Arthrodesis

After fracture-dislocation at Lisfranc's joint, degenerative arthritis can develop. Stabilization of these joints may be necessary in patients who have significant pain. A dowel-graft arthrodesis technique appears to be a satisfactory method of obtaining fusion. The surgical technique consists of removing a bone plug 7.5 mm in diameter from between the affected joints. The plug is discarded and solid 7.5-mm plugs of bone graft are removed from the iliac crest through a percutaneous approach, placed into the trephined defects of the tarsometatarsal joints, and then fixed with crossed wires. Of 13 patients followed up for a mean of 37 months, only two were dissatisfied with their pain relief. Complications included three nonunions and one postsurgical reflex sympathetic dystrophy syndrome. The mean interval to arthrodesis from the time of injury was 72 months. The mean total duration of cast immobilization was 11 weeks until radiographic evidence of union was seen.

This can be a difficult condition to treat and patients should be cautioned that they will be improved, but not returned to normal. At follow-up one patient had severe pain, nine had mild pain, and three were essentially pain-free. Eleven of the 13 patients said that they would undergo the procedure again. Good or excellent results were achieved in 70%; 15% had fair results and 15% had poor results. The more common articulations fused were at the base of the second and third metatarsals. The procedure made no attempt to correct any incongruity or deformity at the tarsometatarsal joints. Thus, the joints were fused in situ. Most patients had mild to moderate deformity and there was no correlation between the amount of hindfoot-forefoot deformity and the overall results.

Painful Afflictions of the Foot and Ankle

Chronic pain involving any part of the foot can pose a difficult diagnostic problem. Conservative care should be the rule while proper investigations are being carried out to determine, if possible, the specific cause of the pain.

Heel Pain

Patients with heel pain can be especially difficult to evaluate. Usually radiographic studies show little besides the presence of a heel spur. Technetium bone scans of 45 patients with painful heel syndrome who had no evidence of associated inflammatory arthritis showed increased uptake of the radioisotope at the calcaneum in 59.6%. These patients tended to have more severe heel pain and responded more frequently to local corticosteroid injections. A plantar spur was identified in 7%, but 63% of patients with contralateral foot radiographs and no pain also showed a spur. No evidence of stress fracture was seen. Thus, radioisotope bone scanning seems to have only a limited application in managing patients with a painful heel. However, it did appear that patients with positive scans responded better to corticosteroid injections than those with negative scans. Radioisotope bone scanning was most useful as a screening test when radiographs were normal in patients with unexplained foot pain. The scans permitted an earlier diagnosis of stress fractures, fractures of the sesamoids, and subtalar arthritis in patients with persistent foot pain after injury. Scans also helped to diagnose patients with reflex sympathetic dystrophy.

Tarsal Tunnel Syndrome

Although many reports of tarsal tunnel syndrome have appeared in the literature, this condition is still difficult to diagnose because of the variety of symptoms. Some investigators believe that the failure of conservative treatment such as injections of corticosteroids may be the result of a delay in making the diagnosis. A tight laciniate ligament, varices, exostosis, and adhesions may be causative factors.

Neuroma

The diagnosis of a painful "Morton's neuroma" is all too frequently made in the general population. Not all patients who undergo excision of an interdigital "neuroma" are cured. In a review of 34 patients (37 feet) who underwent reoperation for pain that persisted after excision of a neuroma, elements of either a primary interdigital neuroma or a neuroma in association with an amputation stump were uncovered in 67%. These patients probably had an incomplete initial nerve exision. Twenty-two patients (67%) had complete relief or marked improvement after the revision operation. Three (9%) had some improvement but had persistent pain and eight (24%) had no improvement or worse pain after the revision surgery. When there is no firm diagnosis, conservative care with a molded insole and a wide cushioned-sole shoe should be used, particularly if a revision procedure done through a plantar approach has failed.

Thirty patients (39 recurrent interdigital neuromas) were evaluated to determine whether a repeat operation would be successful and whether a dorsal approach through the previous scar or a transverse plantar approach proximal to the metatarsal heads would make any difference. Overall, significant improvement was reported in more than 80% of the patients; however, fewer than 50% gained complete pain relief and 58% experienced persistent discomfort in certain types of shoes. The plantar approach offers a simplified and less traumatic exposure of the nerve in a more proximal location. There were no healing problems. Thus, patients who are operated on for a so-called interdigital neuroma experience significant problems. Patients should be completely assessed before being offered this type of surgery because there are significant numbers of failures. Once the operation has failed, it is very difficult to make these patients completely pain-free and fully satisfied.

Controversies

Implant Arthroplasty

Considerable discussion continues as to whether there is a role for implant arthroplasty of the metatarsophalangeal joint at all, as satisfactory results of surgery, even salvage surgery, have been reported without the use of implants. There are signs that results of implant operations deteriorate clinically and radiologically with time. The resolution of this question awaits better implant designs with careful follow-up studies.

Bone Grafting in Triple Arthrodesis

Another current topic of discussion is whether bone grafting is routinely required in triple arthrodesis. Although few would argue with the use of a bone graft in a patient with rheumatoid arthritis who has a valgus deformity and significant bone loss, in many instances the arthrodesis can be accomplished without a tibial graft.

Second Metatarsophalangeal Joint Dislocation

The dislocated second metatarsophalangeal joint is an interesting topic, and there is some disagreement regarding the appropriate treatment. When the metatarsophalangeal subluxation is associated with rigid hammertoe deformity, many would consider distal hemiphalangectomy followed by soft-tissue releases at the metatarsophalangeal level such as extensor tenotomies and division of the dorsal capsule and collateral ligaments. If this is not adequate, then decompressing the joint by removal of a portion of the joint is necessary. This may include the distal-most portion of the metatarsal condyles or the base of the proximal phalanx. This area is controversial because some believe that simply removing the base of the phalanx addresses the subluxation problem, whereas others argue that the instability that this creates affects the stability of the joint and that syndactylization is usually required.

Revision of Neuroma Excision

The technique of revision surgery for failed plantar interdigital neuroma excision is the source of some discussion. There are some who remain strong advocates of revision surgery performed through the traditional dorsal incision, whereas more recently others have advocated plantar exposure.

Annotated Bibliography

Keywords

Anesthesia; Arthritis; Arthrodesis; Bunion; Clawtoe; Hallux rigidus; Hallux valgus; Hammertoe; Mallet toe; Metatarsophalangeal joint; Neuroma; Rheumatoid arthritis; Synovitis; Tarsal tunnel syndrome; Tendon rupture

Foot and Ankle Reconstruction

Alexander IJ, Johnson KA, Berquist TH: Magnetic resonance imaging in the diagnosis of disruption of the posterior tibial tendon. *Foot Ankle* 1987;8:144–147.
  Report of a single patient in whom magnetic resonance imaging demonstrated a complete disruption of the posterior tibial tendon in the absence of the commonly associated clinical findings.

Beskin JL, Baxter DE: Regional anesthesia for ambulatory foot and ankle surgery. *Orthopedics* 1987;10:109–111.
  Thirty patients with 39 recurrent neuromas were evaluated. Significant improvement occurred in more than 80% of the patients. However, less than 50% gained complete relief and 58% experienced discomfort in certain shoes. The plantar approach offered a simplified, less traumatic exposure of the nerve in a more proximal location. There were no healing problems.

Betts RP, Stockley I, Getty CJM, et al: Foot pressure studies in the assessment of forefoot arthroplasty in the rheumatoid foot. *Foot Ankle* 1988;8:315–326.
  Pressure studies showed significant changes after resection of the metatarsal heads in rheumatoid arthritis. Thus, there will be changes in forefoot pressure in rheumatoid patients after excisional arthroplasty.

Bordelon RL: Evaluation and operative procedures for hallux valgus deformity. *Orthopedics* 1987;10:38–44.
  The author describes a variety of surgical procedures available for the adolescent and adult patient with hallux valgus.

Carl A, Ross S, Evanski P, et al: Hypermobility in hallux valgus. *Foot Ankle* 1988;8:264–270.
  A statistically significant correlation was found between patients with symptomatic hallux valgus and patients having a mild generalized hypermobility of their joints. Ligamentous laxity seems to support the need for bony correction in such patients.

Citron N, Neil M: Dorsal wedge osteotomy of the proximal phalanx for hallux rigidus: Long-term results. *J Bone Joint Surg* 1987;69B:835–837.
  A dorsal wedge osteotomy of the proximal phalanx in the treatment of hallux rigidus produced some evidence of improvement. This osteotomy tends to improve postoperative extension.

Coughlin MJ: Crossover second toe deformity. *Foot Ankle* 1987;8:29–39.
  The crossover second toe deformity occurs when the lateral collateral ligament and joint capsule of the second metatarsophalangeal joint deteriorate. Most toes deviate in a medial direction and later deviate dorsally and cross up over the dorsum of the great toe. Satisfactory results were reported in 90% of cases.

Coughlin MJ: Lesser toe deformities. *Orthopedics* 1987;10:63–75.
  A scheme of classification and treatment of the various deformities of the lateral toes is given.

Coughlin MJ, Mann RA: Arthrodesis of the first metatarsophalangeal joint as salvage for the failed Keller procedure. *J Bone Joint Surg* 1987;69A:68–75.
  The authors report the success rate after arthrodesis of the first metatarsophalangeal joint as a salvage procedure for failed

Keller procedures. Arthrodesis tended to stabilize the first ray and was considered an excellent procedure.

Downey DT, Simkin PA, Marc LA, et al: Tibialis posterior tendon rupture: A cause of rheumatoid flat foot. *Arthritis Rheum* 1988;31:441–446.

Two patients with rheumatoid arthritis developed flatfoot deformities secondary to surgically confirmed rupture of the posterior tibial tendon.

el-Batouty MM, Aly EM, el-Lakkany MR, et al: Triple arthrodesis for paralytic valgus: A modified technique. *J Bone Joint Surg* 1988;70B:493.

The authors report a modification of a slot graft technique for triple arthrodesis. A slot cut through a lateral approach includes all three joints.

Funk DA, Cass JR, Johnson KA: Acquired adult flat foot secondary to posterior tibial tendon pathology. *J Bone Joint Surg* 1986;68A:95–102.

The authors report their success rate with flexor digitorum longus transfer for patients with ruptured posterior tibial tendon. The surgical procedure is described in detail.

Gainor BJ, Epstein RG, Henstorf JE, et al: Metatarsal head resection for rheumatoid deformities of the forefoot. *Clin Orthop* 1988;230:207–213.

The authors describe their results after metatarsal head resection for painful rheumatoid forefoot deformities. Results were excellent or good in 80% and poor in only 3%. No improvement was noted in patients whose toes were fixed temporarily with a smooth wire.

Goldberg I, Bahar A, Yosipovitch Z: Late results after correction of hallux valgus deformity by basilar phalangeal osteotomy. *J Bone Joint Surg* 1987;69A:64–67.

Results were poor in a long-term follow-up study. This operation does not correct the biomechanical abnormalities of hallux valgus.

Hasselo LG, Willkens RF, Toomey HE, et al: Forefoot surgery in rheumatoid arthritis: Subjective assessment of outcome. *Foot Ankle* 1987;8:148–151.

The initially high success rate in rheumatoid patients after resection of the metatarsophalangeal joints deteriorated.

Hattrup SJ, Johnson KA: Chevron osteotomy: Analysis of factors in patients' dissatisfaction. *Foot Ankle* 1985;5:327–332.

Chevron osteotomies with which the patients were dissatisfied failed to achieve correction of the deformity and included technical errors.

Hattrup SJ, Johnson KA: Subjective results of hallux rigidus following treatment with cheilectomy. *Clin Orthop* 1988;226:182–191.

Fifty-eight patients who were treated with cheilectomy were reviewed. Preoperative grading was established and correlated with the final result. Results were unsatisfactory in 27.6% of the cases.

Helal B, Gibb P: Freiberg's disease: A suggested pattern of management. *Foot Ankle* 1987;8:94–102.

This article establishes a grading system for Freiberg's disease as well as a method of treatment.

Herzenberg JE, Goldner JL, Martinez S, et al: Computerized tomography of talocalcaneal tarsal coalition: A clinical and anatomic study. *Foot Ankle* 1986;6:273–288.

This paper describes the advantages of computed tomography in talocalcaneal tarsal coalition.

Jahss MH, Troy AL, Kummer F: Roentgenographic and mathematical analysis of first metatarsal osteotomies for metatarsus primus varus: A comparative study. *Foot Ankle* 1985;5:280–321.

Five different first metatarsal osteotomies were evaluated radiographically for the treatment of hallux valgus. Surgical techniques and failures are discussed. The chevron osteotomy gave the least correction and did not permit plantar displacement of the head. A modification of the basilar concentric osteotomy is described.

Johnson JE, Johnson KA: Dowel arthrodesis for degenerative arthritis of the tarsometatarsal (Lisfranc) joints. *Foot Ankle* 1986;6:243–253.

A dowel-graft arthrodesis technique using iliac crest graft was used in patients with degenerative arthritis after Lisfranc fracture. Only two patients were dissatisfied.

Johnson JE, Johnson KA, Unni KK: Persistent pain after excision of an interdigital neuroma: Results of reoperation. *J Bone Joint Surg* 1988;70A:651–657.

The authors used a longitudinal and plantar incision as well as a dorsal web-space incision for reoperation in patients in whom treatment of interdigital neuromas had failed. The plantar incision was satisfactory in all but one patient and did not lead to a painful scar. Of the patients, 24% had no improvement or had worse pain; thus, reexploration may be hazardous.

Karlsson J, Bergsten T, Lansinger O, et al: Lateral instability of the ankle treated by the Evans procedure. *J Bone Joint Surg* 1988;70B:476–480.

In a long-term (average follow-up, 14 years) review of the Evan's operation for chronic lateral ankle instability, only 50% had satisfactory results.

Love TR, Whynot AS, Farine I, et al: Keller arthroplasty: A prospective review. *Foot Ankle* 1988;8:46–54.

In this review of 75 feet after a Keller arthroplasty, overall patient satisfaction was 77%.

Mann RA: Treatment of the bunion deformity. *Orthopedics* 1987;10:49–55.

The authors describe the basilar concentric osteotomy and the modified McBride technique for the correction of hallux valgus.

Mann RA, Clanton TO: Hallux rigidus: Treatment by cheilectomy. *J Bone Joint Surg* 1988;70A:400–406.

Of 25 patients with hallux rigidus who underwent cheilectomy, all but three had relief of pain. Cheilectomy is preferred as the best primary treatment for hallux rigidus.

Mann RA, Mizel MS: Monarticular nontraumatic synovitis of the metatarsophalangeal joint: A new diagnosis? *Foot Ankle* 1985;6:18–21.

Of seven patients with synovitis of the second metatarsophalangeal joint, six underwent synovectomy.

Maurice HD, Newman JH, Watt I: Bone scanning of the foot for unexplained pain. *J Bone Joint Surg* 1987;69B:448–452.

A bone scan can provide clues to the cause of foot pain that cannot be uncovered by routine radiographs and physical examination.

Meier PJ, Kenzora JE: The risks and benefits of distal first metatarsal osteotomies. *Foot Ankle* 1985;6:7–17.

Chevron and Mitchell osteotomies of the first metatarsal were used in the treatment of hallux valgus. Osteonecrosis was reported after the chevron osteotomy in 20%, but many of these patients had a lateral adductor release as well as the osteotomy. This emphasizes the anatomy of the blood supply to the first metatarsal head and how it can be disrupted by various surgical procedures.

Ricciaradi-Pollini PT, Moneta MR, Falez F: The tarsal

tunnel syndrome: A report of eight cases. *Foot Ankle* 1985;6:146–149.

Tarsal tunnel syndrome is probably an unusual condition and may be difficult to diagnose.

Sarrafian SK: A method of predicting the degree of functional correction of the metatarsus primus varus with a distal lateral displacement osteotomy in hallux valgus. *Foot Ankle* 1985;5:322–326.

The author describes a simple method of calculating preoperatively the maximum correction that can be obtained with an osteotomy in the treatment of hallux valgus.

Sartoris DJ, Resnick D: Pictorial review: Cross-sectional imaging of the foot and ankle. *Foot Ankle* 1987;8:59–80.

A number of examples show the use of computed tomography and magnetic resonance imaging in the diagnosis of foot abnormalities.

Shereff MJ, Yang QM, Kummer FJ: Extraosseous and intraosseous arterial supply to the first metatarsal and metatarsophalangeal joint. *Foot Ankle* 1987;8:81–93.

This was a cadaver study of the blood supply, both intraosseous and extraosseous, to the hallux metatarsal head.

Shiel WC Jr, Jason M: Granulomatous inguinal lymphadenopathy after bilateral metatarsophalangeal joint silicone arthroplasty. *Foot Ankle* 1986;6:216–218.

A patient developed bilateral inguinal granulomatous adenop-athy secondary to silicone implants that had been placed in the hallux metatarsophalangeal joint.

Sykes A, Hughes AW: A biomechanical study using cadaveric toes to test the stability of fixation techniques employed in arthrodesis of the first metatarsophalangeal joint. *Foot Ankle* 1986;7:18–25.

The authors describe the stability of various fixation techniques and bone preparation in order to stabilize the first metatarsophalangeal joint.

Thompson FM, Hamilton WG: Problems of the second metatarsophalangeal joint. *Orthopedics* 1987;19:83–89.

An important description of subluxation at the second metatarsophalangeal joint as well as other abnormalities involving this important joint.

Turan I, Lindgren U: Compression-screw arthrodesis of the first metatarsophalangeal joint of the foot. *Clin Orthop* 1987;221:292–295.

The technique of using screws in arthrodesis of the first metatarsophalangeal joint.

Williams PL, Smibert JG, Cox R, et al: Imaging study of the painful heel syndrome. *Foot Ankle* 1987;7:345–349.

Technetium bone scans were used in 52 patients with painful heels. Uptake over the calcaneus was increased in 59.6%. These patients responded more frequently to local hydrocortisone injections.

Index